CURRENT PERSPECTIVES ON

The Fetus as a Patient

Edited by

Frank A. Chervenak

The New York Hospital – Cornell Medical Center, New York, USA

and

Asim Kurjak

Ultrasonic Institute, University of Zagreb, Croatia

Published on behalf of
The International Society of
The Fetus as a Patient

The Parthenon Publishing Group

International Publishers in Medicine, Science & Technology

NEW YORK   LONDON

Library of Congress Cataloging-in-Publication Data
Current perspectives on the fetus as a patient, edited by
  Frank A. Chervenak and Asim Kurjak
      p.   c.m.
    Includes bibliographical references and index
    ISBN 1-85070-742-1
    1. Fetus—Diseases.   2. Fetus—Abnormalities.
3. Prenatal diagnosis.   4. Pregnancy—Complications.
I. Chervenak, Frank A.   II. Kurjak, Asim
    [DNLM: 1. Fetal Diseases—ultrasonography.
2. Ultrasonography, Prenatal.   3. Fetal
Diseases—therapy.   WQ 209 N532 1996]
RG626.N49   1996
618.3′2—dc20
DNLM/DLC
for Library of Congress   96-17371
                                           CIP

British Library Cataloguing in Publication Data
Current perspectives on the fetus as a patient
  1.Perinatology 2.Fetus
  I.Chervenak, Frank A. II.Kurjak, Asim
  618.3′2
  ISBN 1-85070-742-1

Published in North America by
The Parthenon Publishing Group Inc.
One Blue Hill Plaza
PO Box 1564, Pearl River
New York 10965, USA

Published in the UK and Europe by
The Parthenon Publishing Group Ltd
Casterton Hall, Carnforth
Lancs. LA6 2LA, UK

Copyright © 1996 The Parthenon Publishing
  Group Limited

First published 1996

Typesetting by AMA Graphics Ltd., Preston, UK
Printed and bound by Butler and Tanner, Frome, UK

Contents

List of principal contributors ix

Preface xiii

Color plates xv

1 An essential clinical ethical concept 1
  F. A. Chervenak, L. B. McCullough and A. Kurjak

Section 1   New dimensions in fetal imaging

2 Safety of obstetric ultrasound 13
  G. Kossoff and S. B. Barnett

3 Ultrasonic and Doppler studies of the human yolk sac 21
  A. Kurjak, S. Kupesic, M. Kos, V. Latin and M. Kos

4 Doppler studies of subchorionic hematomas in early pregnancy 33
  S. Kupesic, A. Kurjak and F. A. Chervenak

5 Color Doppler in prenatal diagnosis 39
  J. M. Carrera, R. Devesa, M. Torrents, C. Mortera, C. Comas and A. Muñoz

6 Current perspective on the evaluation of suspected intrauterine growth retardation 49
  W. J. Ott

7 Three-dimensional ultrasound in the evaluation of fetal anatomy and fetal malformations 75
  E. Merz

8 Tissue echogenicity 89
  M. Smith-Levitin, I. Blickstein and E. Gurewitsch

9 Fetal radiology 103
  B. R. Elejalde, M.-M. de Elejalde, R. R. Lebel, J. M. Acuna, J. Gomez and R. A. Elejalde

Section 2   Advances in prenatal screening and diagnosis

10 Molecular genetics in fetal medicine 119
  B. R. Elejalde and M. M. de Elejalde

11 Fetal echocardiography in the late first trimester of pregnancy 137
  I. A. L. Groenenberg, J. M. G. van Vugt and H. P. van Geijn

v

12   Fetal heart screening: a diagnostic challenge   147
      E. Tegnander and S. H. Eik-Nes

13   New dimensions in fetal neuroscanning   159
      A. Monteagudo and I. E. Timor-Tritsch

14   Congenital cerebral infections   185
      G. Nigro and E. V. Cosmi

15   Routine obstetric ultrasound examination: a clinical and ethical evaluation   203
      D. W. Skupski, F. A. Chervenak and L. B. McCullough

16   Malformations and karyotype   213
      G. D'Ottavio, M. A. Rustico, V. Pecile, A. Maieron, G. Conoscenti, R. Natale and
      G. P. Mandruzzato

17   Nuchal translucency screening for chromosomal abnormalities in the first trimester   229
      N. J. Sebire, R. J. M. Snijders, A. Kalogeropoulos, N. Psara and K. H. Nicolaides

18   The role of second-trimester ultrasound examination in the detection of fetal   243
      aneuploidy
      A. M. Vintzileos, J. C. Smulian and D. L. Day-Salvatore

Section 3   Challenges in fetal therapy

19   Fetal surgery   257
      K. J. VanderWall and M. R. Harrison

20   Endoscopic laser coagulation in the management of severe twin–twin transfusion   271
      syndrome
      N. J. Sebire, J. Hyett, Y. Ville and K. H. Nicolaides

21   Prenatal diagnosis and management of fetal tumors   281
      V. D'Addario and V. De Salvia

22   Fetal cardiac intervention in congenital heart disease   297
      T. Kohl

23   Thoracoamniotic shunting for fetal pleural effusions   317
      N. J. Sebire and K. H. Nicolaides

24   Techniques for pediatric and fetal surgery   327
      Z. Szabo, A. Cuschieri and G. Berci

Section 4   Assessment of the fetal condition

25   The embryo as a patient: early pregnancy loss   345
      J. C. Birnholz and F. B. Kent

26   New advances in understanding fetal hypoxia   359
     A. Salihagic, A. Fignon, A. Locatelli, J. Lansac and Ph. Arbeille

27   Improved fetal outcome by fetal monitoring: 17 years' experience in Yohka Hospital   379
     K. Maeda and T. Tsuzaki

28   Systematic antenatal functional evaluation   385
     B. Arabin, D. Oepkes and J. van Eyck

29   Monitoring fetal hypoxemia: Doppler flow measurement and computerized   393
     cardiotocography
     G. P. Mandruzzato, Y. J. Meir and L. Fischer Tamaro

30   Uterine Doppler waveform: prediction and management of pregnancy complications   405
     B. Haddad and S. Uzan

31   Actocardiographic assessment of the fetus   415
     K. Maeda

32   Systematic antenatal functional evaluation in pregnancies at risk of progressive fetal   423
     anemia
     D. Oepkes, H. Kanhai and B. Arabin

33   Abruptio placentae: from early pregnancy to term   433
     R. N. Laurini

34   Systematic antenatal functional evaluation in pregnancies at risk of progressive   445
     abruptio placentae
     B. Arabin, R. Aardenburg and J. van Eyck

35   What is fetal distress?   455
     D. W. Skupski

Section 5   Clinical perinatology
36   Calcium supplementation in the prevention of pregnancy-induced hypertensive   471
     diseases
     B. Haddad and S. Uzan

37   Preterm prelabor amniorrhexis   477
     N. J. Sebire, S. G. Carroll and K. H. Nicolaides

38   Clinical implications of automated blood pressure monitoring in pregnancy   497
     J. Rigó Jr and Z. Papp

39   Twinning and twins   507
     I. Blickstein and M. Smith-Levitin

40   Management of intrauterine growth retardation   527
     G. C. Di Renzo and G. Luzi

41 The diabetic fetus   539
    Y. Ezra and J. G. Schenker

42 Biochemical markers of preterm delivery   555
    S. R. Inglis

43 Early onset pre-eclampsia and HELLP syndrome   563
    J. van Eyck, W. P. F. Fetter and B. Arabin

44 Post-term pregnancy: fetal considerations   571
    H. N. Winn

45 Congenital toxoplasmosis: old and new perspectives   581
    E. Schiff and S. Mashiach

46 Fetal and neonatal aspects of myasthenia gravis   589
    V. Váradi

47 Surfactant therapy for neonatal respiratory distress syndrome   603
    T. Fujiwara

Index   617

List of principal contributors

B. Arabin
Sophia Ziekenhuis
8025 AB Zwolle
The Netherlands

Ph. Arbeille
Department of Nuclear Medicine and
    Ultrasound
Chu Trousseau
Tours 37044
France

J. C. Birnholz
12 Oak Brook Center
Oak Brook
IL 60524
USA

J. M. Carrera
Department of Obstetrics and Gynecology
Division of Maternal–Fetal Medicine
Instituto Universitario Dexeus
Passeig Bonanova 67
Sotano 2
08017 Barcelona
Spain

F. A. Chervenak
The New York Hospital–Cornell Medical
    Center
Department of Obstetrics and Gynecology
525 East 68th Street – M713
New York
NY 10025
USA

V. D'Addario
Department of Obstetrics and Gynecology
University of Bari
Piazza G. Cesare
70124 Bari
Italy

G. D'Ottavio
Department of Obstetrics and Gynecology
Istituto 'Burlo Garofolo'
Via del'Istria, 65/1
34100 Trieste
Italy

G. C. Di Renzo
Institute of Obstetrics and Gynecology
University of Perugia
Policlinico Monteluce
Via A Brunamonti
06122 Perugia
Italy

S. H. Eik-Nes
National Center for Fetal Medicine
Department of Gynecology and Obstetrics
Trondheim University Hospital
N-7006 Trondheim
Norway

B. R. Elejalde
Medical Genetics Institute, S. C.
4555 West Schroeder Drive, Suite 180
Milwaukee
WI 53223-1470
USA

T. Fujiwara
Department of Pediatrics
Iwate Medical University
Uchihmaru 19-1
Morioka 020
Japan

I. A. L. Groenenberg
Academisch Ziekenhuis Vrije Universiteit
Department of Obstetrics and Gynecology
PO Box 7057
1007 MB Amsterdam
The Netherlands

B. Haddad
Department of Obstetrics and Gynecology
C. H. I. Créteil
40 avenue de Verdun
94010 Créteil Cedex
France

S. R. Inglis
Department of Obstetrics and Gynecology
The New York Hospital–Cornell Medical Center
525 East 68th Street, Room J-130
New York
NY 10021
USA

T. Kohl
Division of Pediatric Cardiothoracic Surgery
505 Parnassus Avenue-Box 0118
San Francisco
CA 94143-0118
USA

G. Kossoff
Ultrasonics Laboratory
Division of Radiophysics
CSIRO
126 Greville Street
Chatswood NSW 2067
Sydney
Australia

S. Kupesic
Ultrasonic Unit
Department of Obstetrics and Gynecology
University of Zagreb
Sveti Duh Hospital
Sveti Duh 64
41100 Zagreb
Croatia

A. Kurjak
Department of Obstetrics and Gynecology
Medical School University of Zagreb
Sveti Duh Hospital
Sveti Duh 64
41000 Zagreb
Croatia

R. N. Laurini
Division of Developmental and Pediatric
    Pathology
Institute of Pathology
Rue de Bugnon 25
1011 Lausanne
Switzerland

K. Maeda
Department of Obstetrics and Gynecology
Seirei Hamamatsu Hospital
Sumiyoshi 2-12-12
Hamamatsu 430
Japan

G. P. Mandruzzato
Department of Obstetrics and Gynecology
Istituto 'Burlo Garofolo'
Via del'Istria 65/1
34100 Trieste
Italy

S. Mashiach
The Department of Obstetrics and Gynecology
Sheba Medical Center
Tel-Aviv University
Tel-Hashomer 52621
Israel

E. Merz
Department of Obstetrics and Gynecology
Center for Ultrasound Diagnosis and Fetal
    Therapy
Johannes Gutenberg-University
Langenbeckstrasse 1
D-55101 Mainz
Germany

A. Monteagudo
Columbia Presbyterian Medical Center
Department of Obstetrics and Gynecology
Division of OB/GYN Ultrasound
622 West 168th Street
New York
NY 10032
USA

G. Nigro
II Institute of Obstetrics and Gynecology and
   Pediatric Institute of 'La Sapienza'
   University
Viale Regina Elena 324
00161 Rome
Italy

D. Oepkes
Department of Obstetrics
University Hospital Leiden
PO Box 9600
2300RC Leiden
The Netherlands

W. J. Ott
Division of Maternal and Fetal Medicine
Department of Obstetrics and Gynecology
St. John's Mercy Medical Center
St. Louis
MO 63141
USA

J. Rigó
1 Department of Obstetrics and Gynecology
Semmelweis University Medical School
Baross Utca. 27
Budapest
Hungary H-1088

J. G. Schenker
Department of Obstetrics and Gynecology
Hadassah Medical Center
PO Box 12000
The Hebrew University
91120 Jerusalem
Israel

N. J. Sebire
Harris Birthright Research Centre for Fetal
   Medicine
King's College Hospital School of Medicine
Denmark Hill
London SE5 8RX
UK

D. W. Skupski
Department of Obstetrics and Gynecology
The New York Hospital–Cornell Medical
   Center
525 East 68th Street, Room J130
New York
NY 10021
USA

M. Smith-Levitin
Department of Obstetrics and Gynecology
The New York Hospital–Cornell Medical
   Center
525 East 68th Street, Room J130
New York
NY 10021
USA

Z. Szabo
University of California
Department of Pediatric Surgery
513 Parnassus Avenue, Room HW1601
San Francisco
CA 94143
USA

J. van Eyck
Sophia Ziekenhuis
8025 AB Zwolle
The Netherlands

K. J. VanderWall
The Fetal Treatment Center
University of California at San Francisco
513 Parnassus Avenue, Room 1601 HSW
San Francisco
CA 94143-0570
USA

V. Váradi
Department of Neonatology
St. Margaret Hospital
Bécsi u. 132.
H-1032 Budapest
Hungary

A. M. Vintzileos
Department of Obstetrics, Gynecology and
    Reproductive Sciences
Robert Wood Johnson Medical School/St.
    Peter's Medical Center
254 Eastern Avenue, MOB 4th Floor
New Brunswick
NJ 08903
USA

H. N. Winn
St. Louis University Health Sciences Center
Center for Fetal Diagnosis and Management
6420 Clayton Road
St. Louis
MO 63117
USA

Preface

The International Society of the Fetus As a Patient is an interdisciplinary group of physicians dedicated to improving all aspects of fetal diagnosis and therapy. This book bears testament to the excellent work produced by the Society's Board of Directors and invited speakers.

As ethics is essential to the appreciation of the fetus as a patient in a clinical context, the opening chapter presents a clinical ethical framework. Section 1 presents new dimensions in fetal imaging, emphasizing Doppler ultrasound, three-dimensional ultrasound, tissue echogenicity, and fetal radiology. The science of molecular genetics and screening for fetal anomalies is rapidly evolving, as demonstrated in Section 2. Section 3 presents the latest available information about the newest frontier for the fetus as a patient: fetal surgery. The assessment of the fetal condition has long challenged the obstetric profession and Section 4 provides a broad-based overview of the various modalities available. Section 5 presents up-to-date perspectives on the clinical management of especially controversial clinical areas in perinatology, both before and after birth.

We thank the Board of Directors and the invited speakers of The International Society of the Fetus As a Patient, who have worked so hard to improve fetal diagnosis and therapy, for making the effort to put together their special expertise. This collaboration by the world's leading authorities has resulted in *Current Perspectives on the Fetus As a Patient.*

Frank A. Chervenak
Asim Kurjak

Color plates

Color plate 1 Transvaginal scan, demonstrating a 7–8 weeks' gestational sac. Note the normal morphology of the yolk sac and vitelline duct. Vascular signals were obtained from the umbilical cord and living embryo

Color plate 2 Subtle pulsed Doppler signals (right) were obtained from the vitelline duct

Color plate 3 The same case as in Color plate 2. Pulsed Doppler signals derived from the umbilical cord are characterized by low velocity and absence of diastolic flow. Angle-independent indices such as the pulsatility index demonstrate different values for vitelline artery and umbilical artery in the same cohort of patients analyzed

Color plate 4 The yolk sac and vitelline duct vascularity. Color signals were displayed from the vitelline duct

Color plate 5 The absence of end-diastolic blood flow is a normal physiological finding at this gestational age (9–10 weeks' gestation)

Color plate 6 Pulsed Doppler signals obtained from the wall of the yolk sac demonstrate low velocity and absence of diastole

Color plate 7 Transvaginal color Doppler scan of the embryonic head and yolk sac at 10 weeks' gestation. Pulsed Doppler signals obtained from the yolk sac display no end-diastolic component of blood flow

Color plate 8 Pulsed Doppler signals derived from the yolk sac in a patient with missed abortion. Note the larger diameter (7 mm) of the yolk sac and irregular blood flow signals at its periphery

Color plate 9 Transvaginal scan of a gestation lasting 6 weeks, complicated by bleeding. The pulsed Doppler waveform analysis indicates permanent diastolic flow and moderate impedance to blood flow (resistance index 0.55). A few days after the examination was completed, spontaneous abortion occurred

Color plate 10 Venous blood flow signals obtained from the yolk sac at 10 weeks' gestation in a patient with missed abortion

Color plate 11 Transvaginal scan of a gestation that lasted 6–7 weeks and was complicated by a retrochorionic hematoma (left). Uterine perfusion (spiral artery blood flow) is displayed simultaneously

Color plate 12 Transvaginal scan, demonstrating a gestational sac. Note the color-coded area that represents the spiral arteries (left). The pulsed Doppler analysis shows a high-velocity and low-impedance signal (RI = 0.38) (right)

Color plate 13 Large-volume hematoma is demonstrated in the fundal corporeal region. Note the uterine blood flow signals on the side of the hematoma

Color plate 14 The same patient as in Color plate 13. High impedance to blood flow (RI = 0.87) was obtained from the spiral arteries

Color plate 15 Large-volume hematoma in the supracervical region. Uterine perfusion is displayed on the periphery of a gestational sac

Color plate 16 The same patient as in Color plate 15. Blood flow signals extracted from spiral arteries show absence of diastolic flow (RI = 1.0). Demonstrated changes are the secondary effects of perigestational hemorrhage

Color plate 17 Transvaginal scan, demonstrating a gestational sac (8–9 weeks' gestation) with live embryo. In close proximity, a well-defined oval fluid collection surrounded by an echogenic ring is visible. This is a typical appearance of a blighted twin (right). The thick wall separating the gestational sacs suggests a dichorionic gestation

Color plate 18 The bladder is always surrounded by the two fetal hypogastric arteries. Doppler color permits differentiation of the urinary bladder from other cystic images

Color plate 19 Aneurysm of the vein of Galen. Doppler color permits a differential diagnosis from an arachnoid cyst

Color plate 20 Isolated unilateral cleft lip and palate. (a) Axial scan through maxilla showing a cleft lip and an incomplete formation of the maxillary ridge indicating cleft palate; (b) same scan using color-coded Doppler. An amniotic fluid flow is demonstrated through the cleft lip/palate to the mouth

Color plate 21 Color Doppler imaging of the ventricles during diastole at 11 weeks and 4 days of gestation. Equal color flow into both ventricles is seen

Color plate 22 Real-time image of the fetal heart, with the function of color flow imaging superimposed, showing the right ventricular outflow tract at 13 weeks and 4 days. The main pulmonary artery and ductus arteriosus is outlined in color

Color plate 23 Color Doppler imaging in a case of single ventricle at 13 weeks' gestation. Forward flow on color Doppler is seen into one ventricle

Color plate 24 Color Doppler imaging of the right ventricular outflow tract in a fetus with transposition of the great arteries (15 weeks). The aorta is seen rising from the anterior right ventricle. the aortic arch is outlined in color

Color plate 25 Median image captures the color flow image of the vessels in the median plane. Internal carotid artery, 1; anterior cerebral artery, 2; pericallosal artery, 3; precuneal artery, 4; callosomarginal artery, 5

Color plate 26 Fetal aortic valve stenosis resulting in cardiac failure at 26 weeks of gestation. (a) The left ventricle is thin walled and extremely dilated; (b) Doppler color flow imaging shows mitral and tricuspid regurgitation; (c) pulsed Doppler interrogation of the mitral valvar regurgitation shows a low-velocity signal with slow upstroke indicating loss of contractile ventricular function. Further signs of cardiac failure are (d) retrograde flow with atrial contraction in the ductus venosus and (e) umbilical venous pulsations. Because of the advanced disease stage with severe left ventricular dysfunction and dilatation, this fetus may not receive any further benefit from prenatal cardiac intervention. LA, left atrium; RA, right atrium; LV, left ventricle; RV, right ventricle. (Courtesy of N. H. Silverman)

Color plate 27 Fetal aortic valve stenosis with hypoplastic left ventricle (LV) at 25 weeks of gestation. (a) The right ventricle forms the apex of the heart. The bright interior surface of the heart indicates the presence of endocardial fibroelastosis; (b) Doppler color flow imaging with high scale settings shows no apparent diastolic filling of the left ventricle and (c) tricuspid and mitral regurgitation (arrows); (d) pulsed Doppler interrogation of the mitral regurgitation shows a high-velocity signal with quick upstroke indicating that the obstructed ventricle still generates pressure; (e) shows the thickened and dysplastic aortic valve with a good-sized ascending aorta. Doppler color flow imaging shows antegrade flow across the stenotic valve (f) as well as flow disturbance (arrow) in the ascending aorta. Pulsed Doppler interrogation across the aortic valve (g) demonstrates near normal flow velocity but is generally not sensitive enough to provide information about the severity of the stenosis. Because of left ventricular growth failure, development of endocardial fibroelastosis in concert with sufficient systolic ventricular function and the long remainder of pregnancy, this fetus may benefit from balloon valvuloplasty. RA, right atrium; LA, left atrium; RV, right ventricle. (Courtesy of N. H. Silverman)

Color plate 28 Fetal pulmonary atresia with intact septum at 31 weeks of gestation. (a) The right ventricle is mildly hypoplastic and demonstrates decreased tricuspid valve growth. Increased trabeculation is visible at its apex; (b) the imperforate valve plate can be recognized with no evidence of subvalvar narrowing; (c) Doppler color flow imaging using high scale settings shows no apparent diastolic filling of the right ventricle and (d) retrograde filling of the pulmonary trunk via the ductus arteriosus. RA, right atrium; LA, left atrium; RV, right ventricle; LV, left ventricle; MPA, main pulmonary arteries. (Courtesy of N. H. Silverman)

Color plate 29 Ultrasound-guided balloon valvuloplasty of a severely stenotic aortic valve at 26 weeks of gestation. (a) Doppler color flow imaging displays the narrow jet of forward flow across the thickened dysplastic aortic valve into the ascending aorta (AAo) (b) as well as left to right atrial shunting; (c) the needle can be recognized in the left ventricle (LV) coaxial to the left ventricular outflow tract; (d) the guide wire (GW) has been advanced across the stenotic valve and can be seen in the proximal ascending aorta. Subsequently, the balloon catheter was introduced and successful valvuloplasty of the aortic valve was performed; (e) shows the broad jet across the aortic valve into the ascending aorta after the procedure. RV, right ventricle; LV, left ventricle; LA, left atrium; RA, right atrium. (Courtesy of R. Chaoui)

Color plate 30 Triptych of views between 8 and 11 weeks' gestational age. Energy Doppler maps the central circulation in the middle image. First-trimester views are the patient's introduction to the reality of pregnancy. The examination is an emotionally charged experience, especially as the human form and features are perceived

Color plate 31 A gallery of peak velocity Energy Doppler imaged saggital-plane images in the early to mid-first trimester. Image (c) is the same embryo shown 2 weeks earlier in Figure 3(b) in Chapter 25. The aorta is resolved before the start of the 7th week

Color plate 32 The flow void of the relatively thick septum facilitates Doppler imaging of separate ventricles before the end of the first trimester. Thoracic diameter is about 8 mm in this case

Color plate 33 Cardiac extrophy accounts for the upper body contor bulge. Arrhythmia and demise occurred 3 weeks after this examination

Color plate 34 Absent end-diastolic flow in the umbilical artery

Color plate 35 Reverse flow in the umbilical artery

Color plate 36 Fetal hemodynamic changes in severe intrauterine growth retardation at 28 weeks of gestation (left) and after 1 week (right) in the umbilical artery. The progression from absent to reversed end-diastolic flow can be seen

Color plate 37 Fetal hemodynamic changes in severe intrauterine growth retardation at 28 weeks of gestation (left) and after 1 week (right) in the ductus venosus. The high pulsatility can be seen

Color plate 38 Fetal hemodynamic changes in severe intrauterine growth retardation at 28 weeks of gestation (left) and after 1 week (right) in the middle cerebral artery. The loss of vasodilatation can be seen

Color plate 39 Fetal hemodynamic changes in severe intrauterine growth retardation at 28 weeks of gestation (left) and after 1 week (right) in the umbilical vein. Dicrotic pulsation can be seen. Color plates 1–4 show observations of the same fetus. Fetal death occurred 12 h after the last Doppler observation

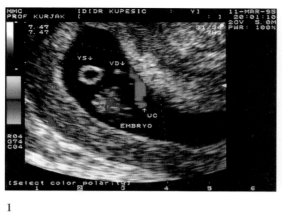

1

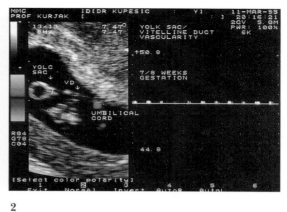

2

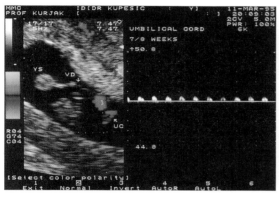

3

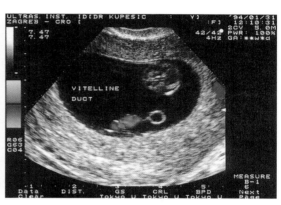

4

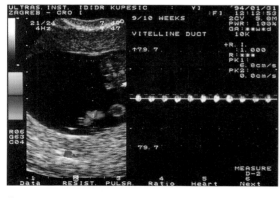

5

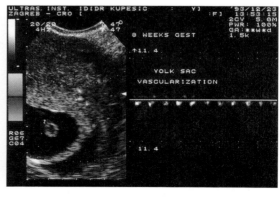

6

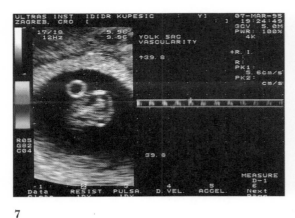

7

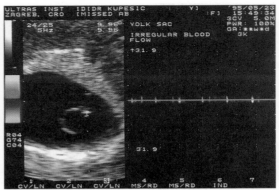

8

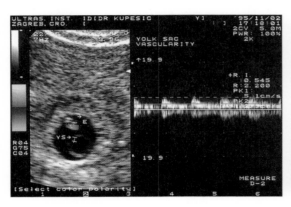

9

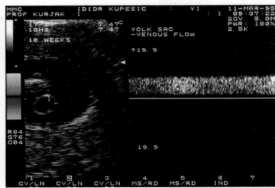

10

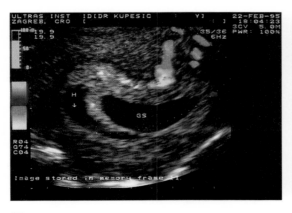

11

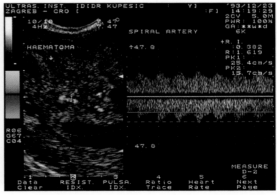

12

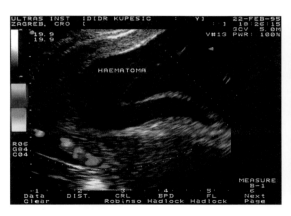

13

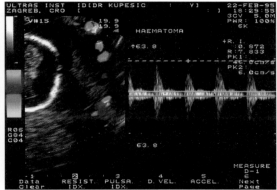

14

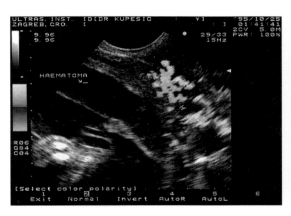

15

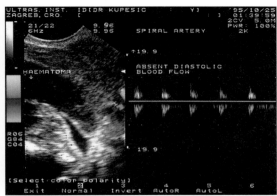

16

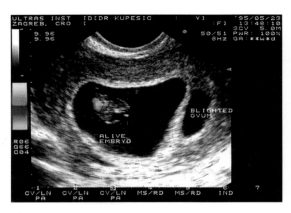

17

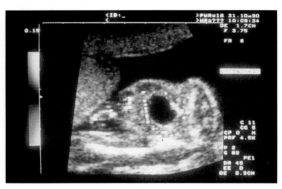

18

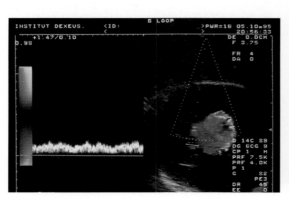

19

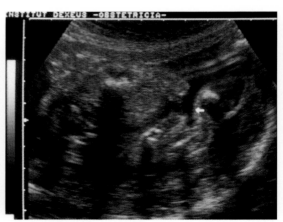

20a

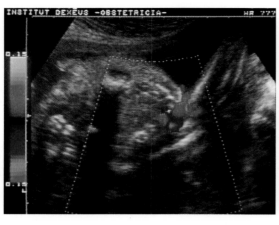

20b

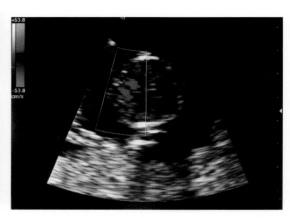

21

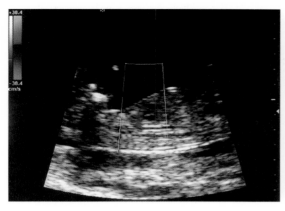

22

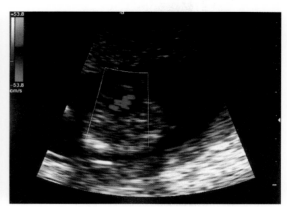

23

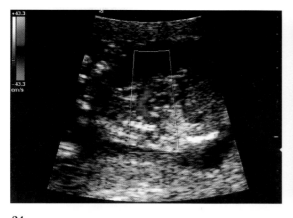

24

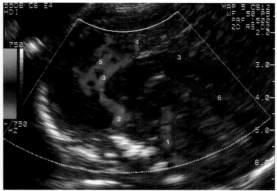

25

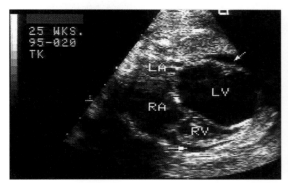

26a

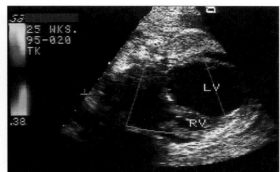

26b

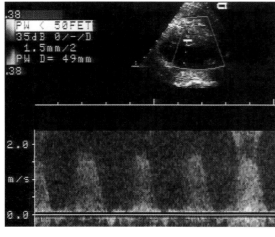

26c

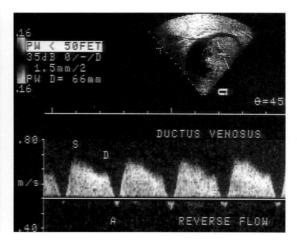

26d

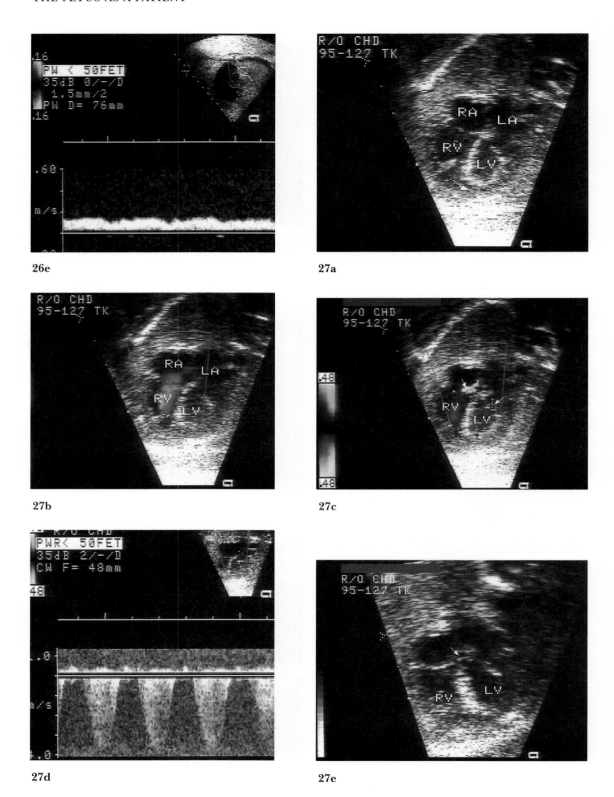

26e

27a

27b

27c

27d

27e

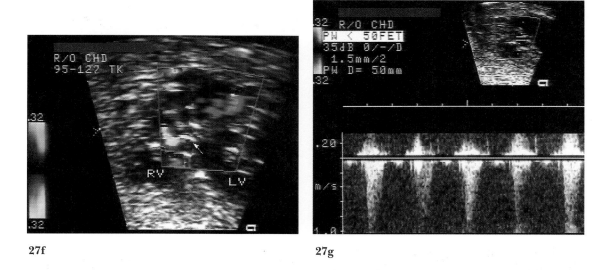

27f   27g

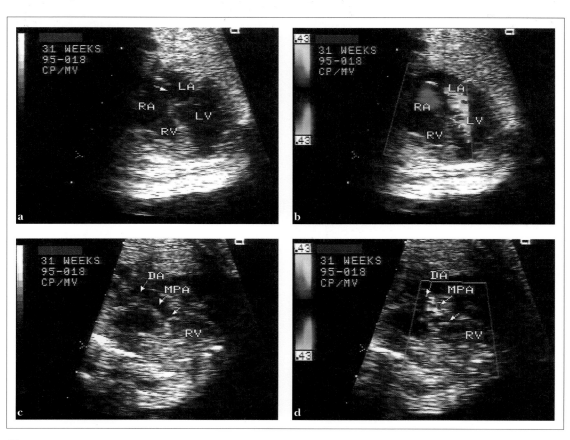

28

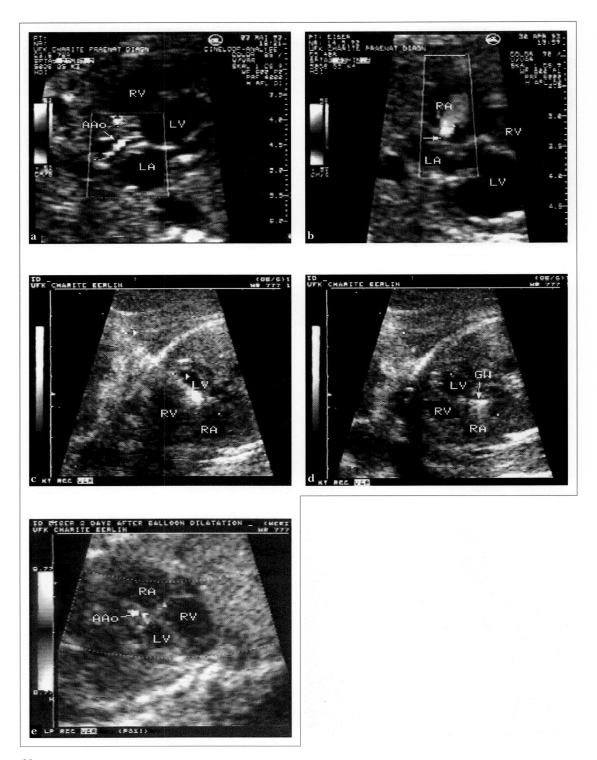

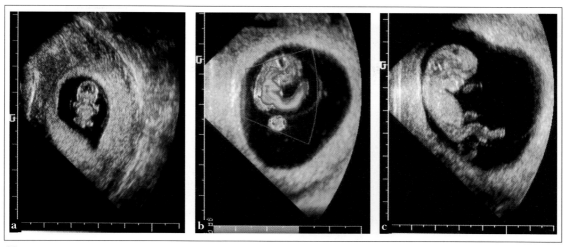

30

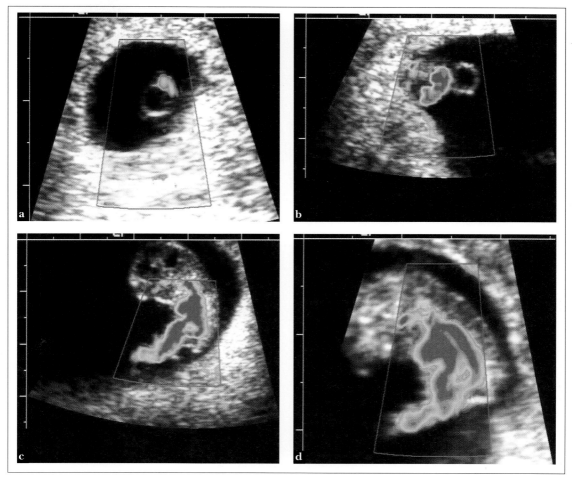

31

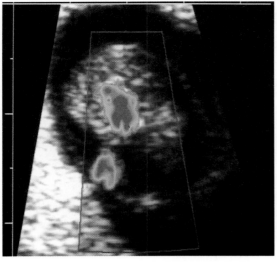

32

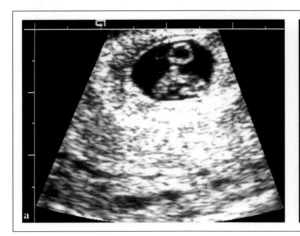 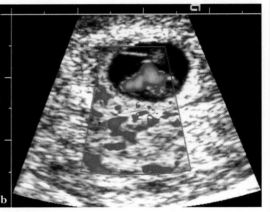

33

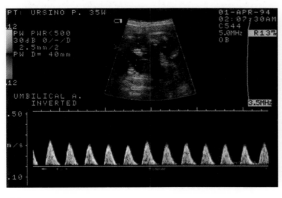 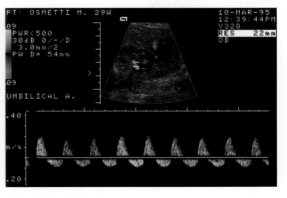

34   35

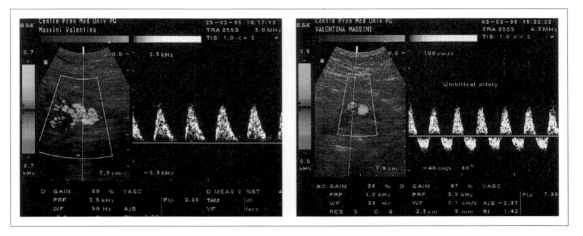

36

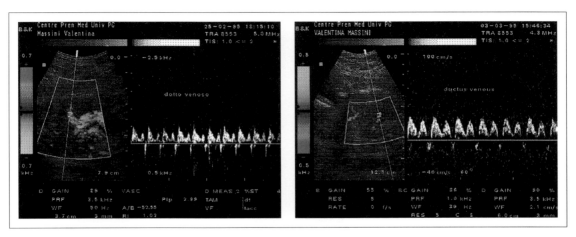

37

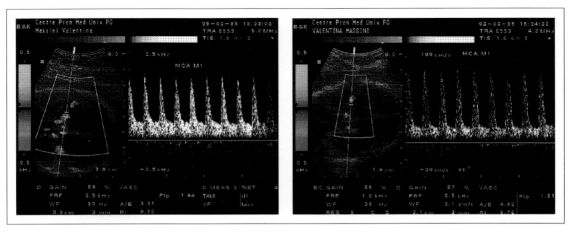

38

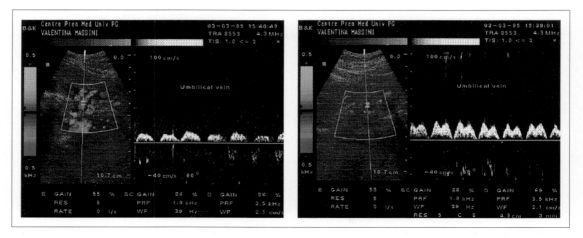

38

An essential clinical ethical concept

F. A. Chervenak, L. B. McCullough and A. Kurjak

1

This book is devoted to the fetus as a patient. An understanding of the ethical dimensions of this concept is essential for full appreciation of the clinical dimensions of the fetus as a patient. In this chapter we elucidate this concept and its major clinical applications. First, we review the role of ethics in clinical judgement and practice. Second, on the basis of this review, we analyze the ethical concept of the fetus as a patient. Third, we identify the clinical implications of this concept for fetal medicine. Fourth, we provide criteria for ethical analysis and argument in the ethics of fetal medicine.

ETHICS IN CLINICAL JUDGEMENT AND PRACTICE

Ethics is the disciplined study of morality. Ethics, therefore, concerns both right and wrong conduct, what one ought and ought not to do, and good and bad character, virtues and vices. The fundamental question of ethics is, 'What ought morality to be?' Because ethics concerns both behavior and character, this question involves two further questions, 'What ought our behavior to be?', and 'What virtues ought to be cultivated in our moral lives?' Ethics in fetal medicine deals with these same questions, focusing on what morality ought to be for specialists in fetal medicine.

For centuries the starting point for what morality ought to be in clinical practice has been the obligation to protect and promote the interests of the patient. This obligation is quite general and therefore needs to be made more specific if it is to be clinically useful. This can be accomplished by developing two perspectives, in terms of which the patient's interests can be understood: that of the physician and that of the patient[1].

The older of the two perspectives on the interests of patients in the history of medical ethics is that of medicine. On the basis of scientific knowledge, shared clinical experience and a careful, unbiased evaluation of the patient, the physician identifies clinical strategies that are reasonably expected to protect and promote the health-related interests of the patient and those that are not. The health-related interests of the patient include preventing premature death and preventing, curing, or at least managing disease, injury, handicap, or unnecessary pain and suffering[1]. The identification of a patient's interests is not a function of the personal or subjective outlook of a particular physician, but rather of rigorous clinical judgement, a point that cannot be overemphasized.

The ethical principle of beneficence gives structure to this rigorous clinical perspective on the interests of the patient, because it obliges the physician to seek the greater balance of goods over harms for the patient in the consequences of the behaviors of the physician and the patient[1]. On the basis of rigorous clinical judgement, physicians should identify those clinical strategies that are expected to result in the greater balance of goods over harms for the patient.

The principle of beneficence in the ethics of fetal medicine should be distinguished from the principle of non-maleficence, commonly known as *primum non nocere* or 'first, do no harm'. It is important to note that *primum non nocere* does not appear anywhere in the Hippocratic texts, including the famous Oath of Hippocrates. Instead, the principle of beneficence was the primary consideration of the Hippocratic writers. For example, in *Epidemics*, the text reads, 'As to diseases, make a habit of two things – to help or to at least do no harm'[2]. In fact, the historical origins of *primum non nocere* remain obscure.

There is a powerful conceptual and clinical justification for rejecting *primum non nocere* as the primary principle of ethics in fetal medicine: virtually all medical and surgical interventions on the fetus involve unavoidable risks of harm. If *primum non nocere* were to be made the primary principle of the ethics of fetal medicine, many of the interventions described in this book, e.g. amniocentesis and fetal surgery, would be unethical.

A rigorous clinical perspective on the interests of the patient is not the only legitimate perspective on those interests. The patient's perspectives on her interests is equally important for the physician[1]. This is because the patient has developed a set of values and beliefs according to which she should be assumed to be capable of making judgements about what will and will not protect and promote her interests.

In making her judgements, the patient may utilize values and beliefs that range far beyond the scope of health-related interests, e.g. religious beliefs or beliefs about how many children she wants to have. Beneficence-based clinical judgement, because it is limited by the competencies of medicine, denies the physician the authority to assess the worth or meaning to the patient of the patient's non-health-related interests. These are matters solely for the patient to determine.

The ethical significance of this patient-based perspective is captured by the ethical principle of respect for autonomy. This principle obliges the physician to respect the integrity of the patient's values and beliefs, to respect her perspective on her interests, and to implement only those clinical strategies authorized by her as the result of the informed consent process.

Respect for autonomy is put into clinical practice by the informed consent process. This process is usually understood to have three elements:

(1) Disclosure by the physician to the patient of adequate information about the patient's condition and its management;

(2) Understanding of that information by the patient; and

(3) A voluntary decision by the patient to authorize or refuse clinical management[1,3].

THE ETHICAL CONCEPT OF THE FETUS AS A PATIENT

There are obviously beneficence-based and autonomy-based obligations to the pregnant patient[1]. The obstetrician's rigorous clinical perspective on the pregnant woman's interests provides the basis for beneficence-based obligations owed to her. Her perspective on those interests is the basis for autonomy-based obligations owed to her. Because the fetus has an insufficiently developed central nervous system, it cannot meaningfully be said to possess values and beliefs. Thus, there is no basis for saying that a fetus has a perspective on its interests. There can therefore be no autonomy-based obligations to any fetus[1]. Therefore, the language of fetal rights has no meaning and no application to the concept of the fetus as a patient in the ethics of fetal medicine, despite the popularity of this language in public and political discourse in the United States and other countries. Obviously, the physician has a perspective on the fetus's health-related interests and the physician can have beneficence-based obligations to the fetus, but only when the fetus is a patient.

The concept of the fetus as a patient has recently come to prominence, principally because of developments in fetal diagnosis and management strategies to optimize fetal outcome[4-6], and has become widely accepted. This concept has considerable clinical significance for maternal–fetal medicine, because, when the fetus is a patient, directive counselling, i.e. recommending a form of management for fetal benefit, would be ethically justified and, when the fetus is not a patient, non-directive counselling, i.e. offering but not recommending a form of management, would be ethically justified[1,7]. However, these apparently straightforward roles for directive and non-directive counselling are often difficult to apply in maternal–fetal medicine, because of uncertainty about when the fetus is a patient.

One approach to resolving this uncertainty would be to argue that the fetus is or is not a patient in virtue of personhood[8], or some other form of independent moral status[9,10]. We begin our account of the ethical concept of the fetus as a patient, therefore, by arguing that this approach fails to resolve the uncertainty and we will therefore defend an alternative approach that does resolve the uncertainty.

A prominent approach for establishing whether or not the fetus is a patient has involved attempts to show whether or not the fetus has independent moral status. Independent moral status for the fetus means that one or more characteristics that the fetus possesses in and of itself and, therefore, independently of the pregnant woman or any other factor, ground obligations to the fetus on the part of the pregnant woman and her physician.

A striking variety of characteristics has been nominated for this role, e.g. conception, implantation, central nervous system development, quickening and birth[11]. Given the variability of proposed characteristics, there is marked variation among ethical arguments about when the fetus is thought to acquire independent moral status. Some take the view that the fetus has independent moral status from the moment of conception or implantation[12]. Others believe that independent moral status is acquired by degrees, thus resulting in 'graded' moral status[10,13]. Still others hold, at least by implication, that the fetus never has independent moral status so long as it is *in utero*[9].

Despite an ever-expanding literature on this subject, there has been no closure on a single authoritative account of the independent moral status of the fetus[14]. Given the absence of a single methodology that would be authoritative for all of the markedly diverse theological and philosophical schools of thought involved in this endless debate, closure is impossible. For closure ever to be possible, debates about such a final authority within and between theological and philosophical traditions would have to be resolved in a way satisfactory to all; however, this is simply an inconceivable intellectual

and cultural event. We therefore abandon futile attempts to understand the fetus as a patient in terms of independent moral status of the fetus and turn to an alternative approach that makes it possible to analyze the ethical concept of the fetus as a patient and the clinical implications of this concept for maternal–fetal medicine.

Our analysis of the ethical concept of the fetus as a patient begins with the recognition that being a patient does not require that one possesses independent moral status[15]. Instead, being a patient means that one can benefit from the application of the clinical skills of the physician. Put more precisely, a human being without independent moral status should be regarded as a patient when two conditions are met: (1) that that human being is presented to the physician; and (2) that there exist clinical interventions that are reliably expected to be efficacious, in that they are reliably expected to result in a greater balance of goods over harms for the human being in question[1]. We call this the dependent moral status of the fetus.

The authors have argued elsewhere that beneficence-based obligations to the fetus exist when the fetus is reliably expected later to achieve independent moral status (some time during the second year postpartum)[1]. That is, the fetus is a patient when the fetus is presented for medical interventions, whether diagnostic or therapeutic, that reasonably can be expected to result in a greater balance of goods over harms for the person the fetus can later become during early childhood. The ethical significance of the concept of the fetus as a patient, therefore, depends on links that can be established between the fetus and the child later achieving independent moral status.

One such link is viability. Viability is not, however, an intrinsic property of the fetus, because viability should be understood in terms of both biological and technological factors[16] (See also Roe vs. Wade 1973, United States). It is only in virtue of both factors that a viable fetus can exist *ex utero* and thus later achieve independent moral status. Moreover, these two factors do not exist as a function of the autonomy of the pregnant woman. When a fetus is viable, i.e. when it is of sufficient maturity so that it can survive into the neonatal period and later achieve independent moral status, given the availability of the requisite technological support, and when it is presented to the physician, the fetus is a patient.

Viability exists as a function of biomedical and technological capacities, which are different in different parts of the world. As a consequence there is, at the present time, no worldwide, uniform gestational age that defines viability. At present, in the United States, the authors believe, viability occurs at approximately 24 weeks of gestational age[17,18].

IMPLICATIONS FOR DIRECTIVE VS. NON-DIRECTIVE COUNSELLING

When the fetus is a patient, directive counselling for fetal benefit is ethically justified. In maternal–fetal medicine, directive counselling for fetal benefit involves one or more of the following: recommending against termination of pregnancy; recommending against non-aggressive management; or recommending aggressive management. Aggressive obstetric management includes interventions such as fetal surveillance, tocolysis, Cesarean delivery, or delivery in a tertiary-care center when indicated. Non-aggressive obstetric management excludes such interventions. Directive counselling for fetal benefit, however, must take account of the presence and severity of fetal anomalies, extreme prematurity and obligations to the pregnant woman.

In fetal medicine the strength of directive counselling for fetal benefit varies according to the presence and severity of anomalies. As a rule, the more severe the fetal anomaly, the less directive counselling should be for fetal benefit[1,19,20]. In particular, when there is '(1) a very high probability of a correct diagnosis and (2) either (a) a very high probability of death as an outcome of the anomaly diagnosed or (b) a very high probability of severe irreversible deficit of cognitive developmental capacity as a result of the anomaly diagnosed'[21], counselling should be non-directive in recommending between aggressive and non-aggressive management, but directive in recommending against termination

of the viable fetus. This is because minimal beneficence-based obligations to such fetuses exist to provide aggressive obstetric management[1,19,21]. In contrast, when lethal anomalies can be diagnosed with certainty, there are no beneficence-based obligations to provide aggressive management[1,19,22]. Such fetuses are not patients; they are appropriately regarded as dying fetuses and the counselling should be non-directive in recommending between non-aggressive management and termination of pregnancy, but directive in recommending against aggressive management, for the sake of maternal benefit[1,19].

The strength of directive counselling for fetal benefit in cases of extreme prematurity of viable fetuses does not vary. In particular, this is the case for what we term just-viable fetuses[1], those with a gestational age of 24–26 weeks, for which there are significant rates of survival but high rates of mortality and morbidity[17,18]. These rates of morbidity and mortality can be increased by non-aggressive obstetric management while aggressive obstetric management may favorably influence outcome. Thus it would appear that there are substantial beneficence-based obligations to just-viable fetuses to provide aggressive obstetric management. This is all the more the case in pregnancies beyond 26 weeks' gestational age[17,18]. Therefore, directive counselling for fetal benefit is justified in all cases of extreme prematurity of viable fetuses, considered by itself. Of course, such directive counselling is only appropriate when it is based on documented efficacy of aggressive obstetric management for each fetal indication. For example, such efficacy has not been demonstrated for routine Cesarean delivery to manage extreme prematurity[17].

Any directive counselling for fetal benefit should occur in the context of balancing beneficence-based obligations to the fetal patient against beneficence-based and autonomy-based obligations to the pregnant woman[1]. Any such balancing must recognize that a pregnant woman is obliged only to take reasonable risks of medical interventions that are reliably expected to benefit the viable fetus or child later. The unique feature of ethics in fetal medicine is that whether, in a particular case, the viable fetus ought to be regarded as presented to the physician is, in part, a function of the pregnant woman's autonomy.

Obviously, any strategy for directive counselling for fetal benefit that takes account of obligations to the pregnant woman must be open to the possibility of conflict between the physician's recommendation and a pregnant woman's autonomous decision to the contrary. Such conflict is best managed preventively through informed consent as an ongoing dialogue throughout the pregnancy, augmented as necessary by negotiation and respectful persuasion[1,23].

The only possible link between the pre-viable fetus and the child it can become is the pregnant woman's autonomy. This is because technological factors cannot result in the pre-viable fetus becoming a child. This is simply what pre-viable means. The link, therefore, between a fetus and the child it can become, when the fetus is pre-viable, can be established only by the pregnant woman's decision to confer the status of being a patient on her pre-viable fetus. The pre-viable fetus, therefore, has no claim to the status of being a patient independently of the pregnant woman's autonomy. The pregnant woman is free to withhold, confer, or, having once conferred, withdraw the status of being a patient on or from her pre-viable fetus according to her own values and beliefs. The pre-viable fetus is presented to the physician solely as a function of the pregnant woman's autonomy.

Counselling the pregnant woman regarding the management of her pregnancy when the fetus is pre-viable should be non-directive in terms of continuing the pregnancy or having an abortion, if she refuses to confer the status of being a patient on her fetus. If she does confer such status in a settled way, then at that point beneficence-based obligations to her fetus come into existence and directive counselling for fetal benefit becomes appropriate. Just as for viable fetuses, such counselling must take account of the presence and severity of fetal anomalies, extreme prematurity and obligations owed to the pregnant woman.

For pregnancies in which the woman in uncertain about whether to confer such status, the authors propose that the fetus be provisionally regarded as a patient[1]. This justifies directive counselling against behavior that can harm a fetus in significant and irreversible ways, e.g. substance abuse, until the woman settles on whether to confer the status of being a patient on the fetus.

In particular, non-directive counselling is appropriate in cases of what we term near-viable fetuses[1], i.e. those which are of 22–24 weeks' gestational age, and for which there are anecdotal reports of survival[17]. Aggressive obstetric and neonatal management should be regarded as clinical investigation, i.e. a form of medical experimentation – not a standard of care[1]. There is no obligation on the part of a pregnant woman to confer the status of being a patient on a near-viable fetus, because the efficacy of aggressive obstetric and neonatal management has yet to be proven.

CRITERIA FOR RIGOROUS ETHICAL ANALYSIS AND ARGUMENT IN THE ETHICS OF FETAL MEDICINE

Ethical analysis and argument are the basic tools of clinical ethics, including ethics in fetal medicine[24]. Ethical analysis identifies component elements of ethical issues in terms of ethical principles such as beneficence and respect for autonomy and virtues such as compassion and integrity. Ethical argument utilizes ethical principles and virtues as premises from which conclusions can reliably be drawn, as we have done above. Throughout the centuries, philosophical ethics has developed a number of criteria for intellectually rigorous ethical analysis and argument in normative ethics. Our reading of that history is that six criteria are relevant for evaluating ethical analysis and argument for their intellectual rigor.

Clarity

The first of these is clarity, which requires that terms and concepts have precise meanings. Consider, for example, the popular phrase, 'right to life'[12]. Clarifying this phrase leads in our view to the recognition that 'right to life' does not refer to a single right but to at least three. These are (1) the right not to be killed unjustly; (2) the right not to have technological or biological supports discontinued unjustly; and (3) the right to have such supports continued for as long as it is reasonable to do so. These rights, however, make different demands upon the pregnant woman. For example, the first version seems limited by very few exceptions, whereas the third version must admit of many exceptions, because no human being has an overriding right to the property or body of another human being. Yet another clarification can be made about the 'right to life'. In the first two senses just identified, the right is a negative right, i.e. a right to non-interference. In the third sense identified above, the right to life is a positive right, i.e. a claim to the resources of others. There is a temptation to trivialize the criterion of clarity as a definition of terms. As the preceding example illustrates, clarity involves much more than mere definition, e.g. careful explanation and the introduction of relevant distinctions.

Consistency

A second criterion is consistency. Consistency makes two requirements of ethical analysis and argument. First, once we have clarified key terms and phrases, such as the fetus as a patient, they should always be used with the same meaning. Second, consistency requires that arguments be free of contradiction. That is, a conclusion of an argument should logically follow from its premises. For example, an inconsistent argument about abortion might be one in which different senses of the 'right to life' are introduced into either the premises or the conclusion of an argument. An example would be asserting the first version of the right to life as the sole premise of an argument and concluding that abortion in the case of rape or incest is permissible because the fetus does not have an overriding right to continue to exist under those circumstances. The problem is that this conclusion does not follow from a premise that asserts the right of the fetus not to be killed unjustly. This is because such a right stands independently of how the fetus is conceived. Therefore, the exceptions claimed in the conclusion, rape and incest, are inconsistent with the first sense of a fetal right to life. The argument fails because of a lack of consistency.

Coherence

A third criterion is coherence. Coherence requires the premises of an argument to connect together into a meaningful whole. For example, simply listing ethical principles without demonstrating their connection to each other fails to satisfy the criterion of coherence. Thus, if one were to say that fetal surgery was ethically justified on the grounds of the principles of autonomy and beneficence, without showing how the two principles complement each other, such a stringing together of principles would fail the criterion of coherence.

Clinical applicability

A fourth criterion is clinical applicability. Applicability requires that normative obstetric ethics can actually be used to guide and direct clinical judgement and behavior in obstetrics. That is, normative obstetric ethics worthy of the name is never an 'ivory tower' enterprise. In particular, normative obstetric ethics should be solidly grounded in clinical reality. We demonstrated clinical applicability above in our discussion of directive vs. non-directive counselling for fetal benefit.

Clinical adequacy

A fifth and related criterion is clinical adequacy. Applicability means that normative obstetric ethics applies to present clinical realities. Adequacy means that normative obstetric ethics will be applicable in future, as yet unforeseen, clinical situations. This is surely relevant to the rapidly developing field of fetal medicine.

Completeness

Finally, all of the preceding criteria presuppose a well known criterion of scholarship, namely, completeness. Just as in clinical research so, too, in normative ethics, no ethical analysis and argument in obstetric ethics is complete unless it takes account of and responds to the existing literature on the subject being addressed, as we have done above in our analysis of claims for and against the independent moral status of the fetus.

PITFALLS TO BE AVOIDED

Critical evaluation of positions on the ethics of fetal medicine involves the identification of pitfalls to be avoided. These pitfalls occur when the inherent limitations in the several disciplines that contribute to normative obstetric ethics are ignored. Because of their prominence, we will consider law, religion, professional consensus, uses of authority and philosophy.

The main limitations of the law – common, statutory, regulatory and administrative – are its incomprehensiveness and possible inconsistency. While the law is surely clinically applicable and clinically adequate to many areas of obstetric practice, it is silent or virtually silent in many other areas. For example, some state courts in the United States have issued court orders for Cesarean delivery for fetal distress or placenta previa. However, no court has addressed, or is likely to address, a pregnant woman's disinclination to appear for prenatal care until she is in labor, although there would be justified ethical doubts about such a practice. Moreover, the law is largely silent on the virtues that physicians in obstetric practice ought to cultivate. Yet, attention to virtues such as integrity and compassion is critical for any adequate response to society's concerns about the dehumanization of obstetric practice.

The law is also at risk for internal conflict and thus possible inconsistency. On the one hand, statutory and regulatory law governing publicly funded health care seems to oblige physicians to do less for their patients. On the other hand, the common law of malpractice seems to oblige physicians to do more. Ignoring the incomprehensiveness or possible inconsistency of the law involves a pitfall.

The main limitations of religion are its potential lack of clinical applicability and clinical adequacy. This is because obstetric ethics based on religious belief requires all to accept (1) the existence of a deity or some transcendent reality and (2) a particular interpretation within a faith community of what the deity or transcendent reality deems to be the ultimate good of human beings – two conditions that can never be satisfied in a pluralistic society that includes atheists or agnostics[8]. In addition, because the intellectual warrant of medicine, the biomedical sciences, and because the legal warrant of medicine, licensure by the state, are secular in character, obstetric ethics based on religion cannot be presumed to be clinically applicable or clinically adequate. To suggest otherwise involves a serious pitfall.

The main limitation of consensus[25] concerns the distinction drawn earlier between descriptive and normative ethics. The limitation of consensus is that it is a version of descriptive ethics. Taking consensus to be normative obstetric ethics involves a serious pitfall.

Uses of authorities are also subject to limitations[26]. The problem here is that the intellectual authority of any expert view in obstetric ethics depends on the quality of the analysis and argument that supports the view and not the prestige of an individual, an academic institution, professional association, or government commission or agency. These individuals or institutions may well have produced well-reasoned analysis and argument. The pitfall of inappropriate uses of authorities occurs when one overlooks the need for critical evaluation of the statements of authorities according to the criteria discussed just above. Such statements, therefore, should not be taken at face value.

The main limitation of philosophical ethics is a function of its subject matter. Aristotle noted centuries ago that a science or area of knowledge can only be as exact as its subject matter[27]. The subject matter of philosophical ethics comprises beliefs and behaviors, which are notoriously inexact. From this fact Aristotle correctly concluded that philosophical argument in ethics cannot ever be exact in the sense that geometric proofs are exact. The lesson of Aristotle for us is that the aims of any endeavor in normative obstetric ethics should be intellectually rigorous ethical analysis and argument that acknowledge intellectually rigorous competing ethical analysis and argument. This should not be a disabling shortcoming, provided that the ethical analysis and argument in question satisfy the criteria discussed above. The pitfall of philosophical ethics is to treat one's ethical analysis as final and irrefutable and thus above the necessity to acknowledge competing ethical analysis and argument.

Accepting this limitation of philosophical ethics has great value, because doing so obliges one to be willing to receive, and respond in a thoughtful way to, the critical evaluation of others. Every experienced clinician knows that failure to be open to critical evaluation of one's clinical judgement and practice in scientific matters more often than not leads to preventable problems in the care of patients. The same is true for clinical judgement and practice in ethical matters. In other words, the lack of finality that at first appears to be a serious limitation turns out on closer consideration to be an intellectual and clinical virtue and thus a powerful antidote to narrow-mindedness and inflexibility.

Competing ethical analyses and arguments should be expected in the ethics of fetal medicine, which is one of the most complex areas of contemporary medicine. Not all analyses and arguments are equal, however. That is, any one position is not necessarily as good as another. Only intellectually rigorous ethical analyses and arguments deserve the reader's serious attention. It is indeed possible to distinguish intellectually rigorous from non-rigorous ethical analysis and argument, by utilizing the tools described in this chapter.

CONCLUSION

In conclusion, every specialist in fetal medicine appreciates that the practice of fetal medicine is filled with ethical challenges. In this chapter we have argued that understanding the ethical concept of the fetus as a patient is essential for addressing these clinical ethical challenges effectively in daily clinical practice. We have provided the tools for critical evaluation of claims about what the ethics of fetal medicine ought to be.

References

1. McCullough, L. B. and Chervenak, F. A. (1994). *Ethics in Obstetrics and Gynecology*. (New York: Oxford University Press)
2. Hippocrates. *Epidemics*, i:xi, trans. Jones, W. H. S. (1923). *Loeb Classical Library*, vol. 147. (Cambridge: Harvard University Press)
3. Faden, R. R. and Beauchamp, T. L. (1986). *A History and Theory of Informed Consent*. (New York: Oxford University Press)
4. Liley, A. W. (1972). The foetus as a personality. *Aust. NZ. J. Psychiatry*, **6**, 99–105
5. Fletcher, J. C. (1981). The fetus as patient; ethical issues. *J. Am. Med. Assoc.*, **246**, 772–3
6. Harrison, M. R., Golbus, M. S. and Filly, R. A. (1984). *The Unborn Patient*. (New York: Grune & Stratton)
7. Chervenak, F. A. and McCullough, L. B. (1991). The fetus as patient: implications for directive versus non-directive counseling for fetal benefit. *Fetal Diagn. Ther.*, **6**, 93–100
8. Engelhardt, H. T. Jr (1995). *The Foundations of Bioethics*, 2nd edn. (New York: Oxford University Press)
9. Elias, S. and Annas, G. J. (1987). *Reproductive Genetics and the Law*. (Chicago: Year Book Medical Publishers)
10. Evans, M. I., Fletcher, J. C., Zador, I. E. *et al.* (1988). Selective first-trimester termination in octuplet and quadruplet pregnancies: clinical and ethical issues. *Obstet. Gynecol.*, **71**, 289–96
11. Noonan, J. T. (ed.) (1970). *The Morality of Abortion*. (Cambridge, Massachusetts: Harvard University Press)

12. Bopp, J. (ed.) (1985). *Human Life and Health Care Ethics.* (Frederick, Maryland: University Publications of America)

13. Dunstan, G. R. (1984). The moral status of the human embryo. A tradition recalled. *J. Med. Ethics,* **10**, 38–44

14. Callahan, S. and Callahan, D. (eds.) (1984). *Abortion: Understanding Differences.* (New York: Plenum Press)

15. Ruddick, W. and Wilcox, W. (1982). Operating on the fetus. *Hastings Cent. Rep.,* **12**, 10–14

16. Mahowald, M. (1989). Beyond abortion: refusal of cesarean section. *Bioethics,* **3**, 106–21

17. Hack, M. and Fanaroff, A. A. (1989). Outcomes of extremely-low-birth-weight infants between 1982 and 1988. *N. Engl. J. Med.,* **321**, 1642–7

18. Whyte, H. E., Fitzhardinge, P. M. *et al.* (1993). External immaturity: outline of 568 pregnancies of 23–26 weeks' gestation. *Obstet. Gynecol.,* **82**, 1–7

19. Chervenak, F. A. and McCullough, L. B. (1990). An ethically justified, clinically comprehensive management strategy for third-trimester pregnancies complicated by fetal anomalies. *Obstet. Gynecol.,* **75**, 311–16

20. Chervenak, F. A. and McCullough, L. B. (1990). Does obstetric ethics have any role in the obstetrician's response to the abortion controversy? *Am. J. Obstet. Gynecol.,* **163**, 1425–9

21. Chervenak, F. A. and McCullough, L. B. (1989). Nonaggressive obstetric management: an option for some fetal anomalies during the third trimester. *J. Am. Med. Assoc.,* **261**, 3439–40

22. Chervenak, F. A., Farley, M. A., Walters, L. *et al.* (1984). When is termination of pregnancy during the third trimester morally justifiable? *N. Engl. J. Med.,* **310**, 501–4

23. Chervenak, F. A. and McCullough, L. B. (1990). Clinical guides to preventing ethical conflicts between pregnant women and their physicians. *Am. J. Obstet. Gynecol.,* **162**, 303–7

24. Chervenak, F. A. and McCullough, L. B. (1993). How to critically evaluate positions on obstetric ethics. *J. Reprod. Med.,* **38**, 281–4

25. Moreno, J. (1995). *Deciding Together. Bioethics and Moral Consensus.* (New York: Oxford University Press)

26. Rachels, J. (1991). When philosophers shoot from the hip. *Bioethics,* **5**, 67

27. Aristotle. *Nichomachean Ethics* (1984). Translated by Ross, W.D. In Barnes, J. (ed.) *The Complete Works of Aristotle,* pp. 1729–867. (Princeton, NJ: Princeton University Press)

Section 1

New dimensions in fetal imaging

Safety of obstetric ultrasound

2

G. Kossoff and S. B. Barnett

INTRODUCTION

Several recent studies have shown that, at acoustic levels generated by modern diagnostic equipment, ultrasound affects biological tissue. Also, changes in international standards and regulations are being developed that may allow increased levels of acoustic output to be used in fetal examinations, provided that the equipment incorporates a form of output display that operates in real-time. Because of these developments, the safety of obstetric ultrasound is a high-priority issue.

The international interest in research into the bioeffects of ultrasound is illustrated by the fact that the World Federation for Ultrasound in Medicine and Biology (WFUMB) has sponsored three symposia on Safety and Standardization in Medical Ultrasound[1-3]. The published proceedings of the latest Symposium contains recommendations which are endorsed by the WFUMB as its official policy statements on safety relating to ultrasonically induced thermal bioeffects. Barnett and colleagues[4] recently reviewed international consensus on the safety of ultrasound in medicine with regard to the thermal mechanisms.

WFUMB RECOMMENDATIONS ON THERMAL EFFECTS

Safe temperature rise

Based solely on a thermal criterion, a diagnostic exposure that produces a maximum temperature rise of 1.5 °C above normal physiological levels (37 °C) may be used without reservation in clinical examinations.

B-mode imaging

Known diagnostic ultrasound equipment, as used today for simple B-mode imaging, operates at acoustic levels that are not capable of producing harmful temperature rises. Its use in medicine is therefore not contraindicated on thermal grounds; this includes endoscopic, transvaginal and transcutaneous applications.

Doppler

It has been demonstrated in experiments with unperfused tissue that some pulsed Doppler diagnostic equipment has the potential to produce biologically significant temperature rises, specifically at the bone/soft tissue interface. The effects of temperature rise can be reduced by shortening the dwell-time exposure to any single point in the tissue. Where the output power can be controlled, the lowest power level required to obtain the necessary diagnostic information should be used.

Transducer heating

A substantial source of heating may be the transducer itself. Tissue heating from this source is localized to the volume in contact with the transducer.

RECENT IMPORTANT ISSUES

In recent years a number of publications have described some effects in animals and in children exposed, *in utero*, to diagnostic ultrasound. To date, mechanisms have not been clearly established to explain the observed results.

HUMAN STUDIES

Two studies have indicated a possible association between routine obstetric ultrasound examinations and subsequent increased incidence of non-right handedness[5] and of delayed speech[6], implying disturbance of fetal neurological development. Epidemiological studies are difficult to set up when the end-point is a subtle, relatively infrequent effect that can also occur spontaneously. The studies require a large number of matched control patients and strict adherence to a pre-defined, pre-tested research protocol. This is frequently difficult to implement when patients may need a different form of clinical management. As an example of these difficulties, a subsequent analysis of data from a larger population concluded that routine ultrasound was not contraindicated by the evidence that was available with the larger data set[7].

A study by Newnham and co-workers[8] has had a major impact on the debate. They compared the effect of frequent (five times) B-mode and continuous Doppler examinations (intensive group) throughout pregnancy on a large, randomized, matched group of patients (1400) with that of a single scan at 18 weeks on a similar number of patients. The study protocol was originally set up to test whether frequent examinations improve the perinatal outcome in a low-risk group of patients. Results showed that frequent examinations did not alter the mortality, the morbidity, or the average birth weight. However, when the intensive group was compared with the regular, single-scan group, the proportion of liveborn infants with birth weight less than the tenth centile was 35% (179 vs. 132) greater in those frequently examined by ultrasound. A 65% increase (58 vs. 35) in the proportion of infants from the frequently examined group were below the third centile.

The American Institute of Ultrasound in Medicine (AIUM) Bioeffects Committee has reviewed this study and concluded that the protocol did not allow conclusive assessment of the results, as they could have been influenced by statistical variability[9]. Nevertheless, it is important that sonologists/sonographers are aware of these results and that further work, using protocols designed to assess birth weight as an end point, be conducted to determine if the results can be replicated.

Reports of low birth weight in infants following multiple exposures *in utero* cannot be explained by current knowledge of the mechanisms of these bioeffects.

ANIMAL STUDIES

Several transient developmental and hematological effects were reported in monkeys (11 exposed, 11 sham) exposed frequently to B-mode examination throughout pregnancy[10]. The birth weights of the offspring were reported to have been reduced by 10%. White blood cell development was depressed by 20% in late gestation and at birth. Full recovery was noted in 4 months.

A significant bioeffect occurring at relatively low intensities manifests itself as hemorrhage in the lung and the intestine[11–14]. The effect has been observed in tissues that contain air cavities. Lung lesions have been described in newborn and adult animals exposed to acoustic outputs at the maximum level achievable from some commercial diagnostic equipment, using combined imaging and pulsed Doppler. The formation of the hemorrhage in the lungs is related to the peak pressure in the acoustic pulse and is more readily obtained at higher outputs and in newborn animals. This topic is a major part of the deliberations in the current WFUMB Symposium on non-thermal bioeffects and safety of diagnostic ultrasound.

The clinical significance and likelihood of ultrasound-induced hemorrhage occurring in humans is not known. Nevertheless, the potential risk of causing lung hemorrhage, particularly in a premature neonate, by an inappropriately conducted cardiographic examination performed at maximum pulsed Doppler output levels cannot be excluded.

These publications reinforce the WFUMB recommendation to use the lowest power output and the shortest dwell time consistent with obtaining the required diagnostic information. This policy is commonly referred to as the ALARA principle (As Low As Reasonably Achievable).

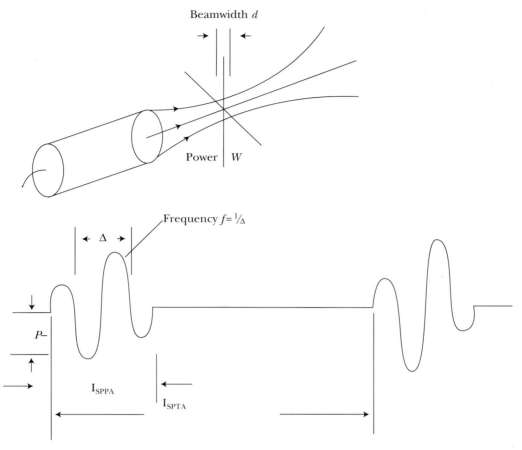

Figure 1 *Acoustic pulse generated by diagnostic equipment. The parameters of the pulse are specified. W is the total power output as measured by a radiation pressure balance; d is the −6 DB beamwidth; P− is the peak negative pressure; f is the center frequency, defined as the inverse of the duration Δ of the maximum amplitude cycle of the waveform. Intensity is defined as power divided by the beamwidth. I$_{SPPA}$ is the spatial peak pulse-average intensity within the pulse, I$_{SPTA}$ the spatial peak temporal average intensity*

REGULATIONS AND THERMAL AND MECHANICAL INDICES

It is essential to study the mechanisms whereby ultrasound interacts with tissue to provide useful insight into the effect of ultrasonic exposure and the risk of significant associated bioeffects.

Thermally and cavitationally induced events are the major causes of bioeffects induced by acoustic levels generated by diagnostic equipment. The degree of temperature rise in tissue is determined by the average power output and the beamwidth, and is related to the average intensity. Cavitation, on the other hand, is most influenced by the peak negative pressure in the

pulse and is related to the spatial peak, pulse-average intensity. Some data on bioeffects show a frequency relationship, where the threshold for cavitation-induced bioeffects increases with increasing frequency. The relevant acoustic parameters are illustrated in Figure 1.

To date, the Food and Drug Administration in the United States has been the only regulatory authority to specify permissible 'safe' maximum intensity outputs for four classes of diagnostic ultrasound application. The 'safe' levels, as measured in water, and their corresponding derated values estimated in tissue, are given in Table 1.

Table 1 *Maximum allowable intensity as specified by the United States Food and Drug Administration for the four listed areas of application*

	Vascular		Cardiac		Fetal		Eye	
	Water	Tissue	Water	Tissue	Water	Tissue	Water	Tissue
I_{SPTA} (mW/cm^2)	1500	720	730	430	180	94	70	17
I_{SPPA} (W/cm^2)	350	190	350	190	350	190	110	28

I_{SPTA}, spatial peak temporal average intensity; I_{SPPA}, spatial peak pulse average intensity

The intensity parameters listed in Table 1 are insufficient to predict when an ultrasonically induced bioeffect may occur. The scientific community, in general, agrees that it is more appropriate to classify risk on the basis of known biophysical events. This has been described in detail in a recent review of the status of biophysical effects of ultrasound[15].

The AIUM, in conjunction with the National Electrical Manufacturers Association (NEMA) has formulated a scheme that allows real-time display of a risk indicator which estimates the likelihood of producing a thermal or cavitation effect. This AIUM/NEMA output display standard[16] has been adopted by some manufacturers in the USA, although it is not yet accepted internationally. The International Electrotechnical Commission (IEC) is taking a different approach by developing an international standard for classifying the output of, and labelling, ultrasound medical equipment on the basis of its capability to produce significant biological effects.

The AIUM/NEMA output display standard specifies displaying a thermal and a mechanical index. The thermal index (TI) is defined as the power output of the equipment divided by the power required to produce a temperature elevation of 1 °C in tissue. The intent is to provide a device to indicate the relative risk of producing a temperature-related biological effect.

The mechanical index (MI) is defined as the derated (i.e. estimated value in tissue) peak rarefaction pressure divided by the square root of frequency. Thus, if the peak rarefaction pressure is 2 MPa and the frequency is 4 MHz, the MI is equal to 1. This is intended to predict cavitation events.

THERMAL BIOEFFECTS – SOME BACKGROUND DATA

The data from studies on animals with hyperthermia indicate that damage to tissue is a function of the temperature rise, the duration of exposure and the type and sensitivity of tissue. Rapidly dividing embryonic tissue is most susceptible to damage. The smallest prolonged temperature increase that has produced neural tube developmental abnormalities is 2 °C. No significant teratogenic effects have been reported at lower levels and it is assumed that a temperature elevation of 1.5 °C can be applied indefinitely (i.e. it is safe)[3]. A temperature rise of 4 °C is hazardous to the embryo or fetus if it is maintained for 15 min.

As an example of ultrasound-induced heating, Figure 2 illustrates some results of research in the Ultrasonics Laboratory on the temperature elevation *in vitro* near the bone/brain interface of the fetal guinea pig. The acoustic power level used was within the range available in modern equipment functioning in the pulsed spectral Doppler mode. The exposure was applied for a period of 120 s. As illustrated, the resulting temperature rise is a function of the gestational age of the fetus[17] and correlates with the development of bone. A temperature rise of approximately 5 °C was obtained in the 60-day, near-term fetus. The temperature rise occurred quickly, with half the temperature elevation being achieved within 20 s. The fall in temperature following cessation of irradiation had a similar rapid time constant. A temperature rise of 2.6 °C was observed in the brain of 60-day fetuses when the skull layer was removed. The ossification of the skull has a significant influence on the ultrasound-induced

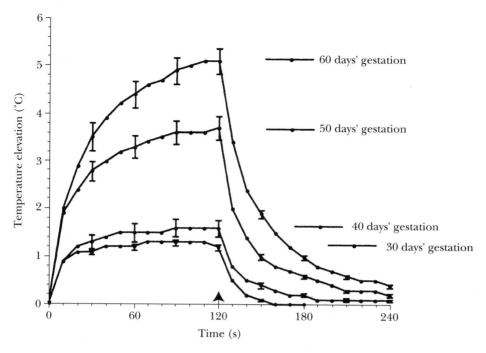

Figure 2 *Temperature elevation measured in vitro in the brain of the fetal guinea pig exposed to pulsed ultrasound*

temperature elevation produced in fetal development.

CAVITATION BIOEFFECTS – SOME BACKGROUND DATA

To date, cavitation-induced bioeffects have not been reported in the fetus. The lungs of the fetus do not contain air and there are no ready nuclei present to assist the development of cavitation-induced bioeffects during ultrasound obstetric examinations. For example, Carstensen and associates[18] found no evidence of damage to the kidney of a mouse when they used pulsed ultrasound at peak negative p_- pressures of 5 MPa and a frequency of 4 MHz. This is equivalent to the maximum levels used by current diagnostic equipment. Studies on the effects of lithotripsy irradiation (typically using high-peak positive p_+ pressures) of the fetal mouse reported minimal effects in the early stage of pregnancy, but increased fetal damage and death following insonation in the later

stages of gestation[19]. Another study reported fetal weight reduction in rats following exposure in early pregnancy to an ultrasound-guided lithotripsy device[20].

In animal studies significant biological effects, associated with gas–body interaction, have been consistently observed in lung tissues, containing air cavities, from different species of mammal. Figure 3 summarizes the collected data. The exposure conditions were within the range of those available in spectral Doppler examinations and most studies used commercially available equipment.

As shown, hemorrhage was most easily obtained in the mouse. In the adult mouse it was obtained at output settings above a MI of 0.5 and this remained constant in the frequency range of 1–4 MHz. In the neonate mouse hemorrhage was reported at 1 MHz with an MI of 0.3, and in the monkey the effect was observed at 4 MHz with an MI of 1.8. In a study on dose–response, a threshold for hemorrhage in neonatal swine was found to be above an MI of

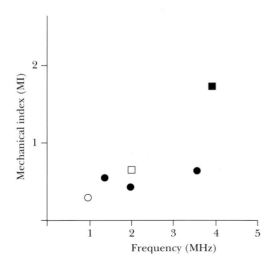

Figure 3 *Mechanical index values at which lung hemorrhage has been reported in animals insonated with 10-μs pulses. Filled circles, adult mouse; open circle, neonatal mouse; filled square, monkey; open square, neonatal swine*

0.6, at 2 MHz frequency[21]. The data suggest a species- or size-dependency, and the effect occurred more readily in the neonate.

In some clinical procedures, such as saline flushing of the ovary to assist oocyte recovery, air bubbles are inadvertently introduced into the patient. There is also growing interest in the application of ultrasonic contrast agents that introduce nuclei, not normally present, into tissues. The potential for causing a cavitationally induced bioeffect under these conditions is enhanced. More research is required into bioeffect studies when contrast agents are present, to determine the output threshold levels for cavitation-induced bioeffects in human tissues.

CONCLUSIONS

The following conclusions can be drawn at our current level of knowledge on ultrasonically induced bioeffects.

(1) B-mode gray-scale imaging is safe from the point of view of thermally induced bioeffects. This applies to transcutaneous as well as intracavitory scanning.

(2) Pulsed Doppler exposures can cause significant temperature rises, particularly at soft tissue/bone interfaces.

(3) In pulsed spectral Doppler the beam is kept stationary, but in color Doppler it is scanned to produce the color image. Therefore, spectral Doppler causes higher local temperature elevation.

(4) A diagnostic exposure that produces a maximum temperature rise in tissue of 1.5 °C above normal physiological levels does not impose a risk to embryonic and fetal development.

(5) An *in situ* temperature rise of 4 °C for 15 min is hazardous for embryonic and fetal development.

(6) The mechanical index values at which lung hemorrhage has been observed in animals is 0.3 in rodents and 1.8 in primates. At present it is not known whether this effect would occur in humans at levels generated by current diagnostic equipment.

(7) Cavitationally induced bioeffects have not been studied in the fetus at acoustic levels generated by diagnostic equipment.

(8) Sonologists/sonographers should become familiar with issues concerning bioeffects and dosimetry, and the definitions and concepts of output display equipment.

(9) All ultrasonic examinations should be performed on the basis of the ALARA principle (as low as reasonably achievable), i.e. the lowest power output and shortest examination time should be used that are consistent with obtaining the required diagnostic information.

References

1. Kossoff, G. and Barnett, S. B. (eds.) (1986). First WFUMB Symposium on Safety and Standardisation of Ultrasound in Obstetrics. *Ultrasound Med. Biol.*, **12**, 9

2. Kossoff, G. and Nyborg, W. L. (eds.) (1989). Second WFUMB Symposium on Safety and Standardisation in Medical Ultrasound. *Ultrasound Med. Biol.*, **15** (Suppl.) 1–115

3. Barnett, S. B. and Kossoff, G. (eds.) (1992). WFUMB Symposium on Safety and Standardisation in Medical Ultrasound: issues and recommendations regarding thermal mechanisms for biological effects of ultrasound. *Ultrasound Med. Biol.*, **18**, 9

4. Barnett, S. B., Kossoff, G. and Edwards, M. J. (1994). Is diagnostic ultrasound safe? Current international consensus on the thermal mechanism. *Med. J. Aust.*, **160**, 33–7

5. Salvesen, K. A., Vatten, L. J., Eik-Nes, S. H., Hugdahl, K. and Bakketeig, L. S. (1993). Routine ultrasonography *in utero* and subsequent handedness and neurological development. *Br. Med. J.*, **307**, 159–64

6. Campbell, J. D., Elford, R. W. and Brant, R. F. (1993). Case–control study of prenatal ultrasonography exposure in children with delayed speech. *Can. Med. Assoc. J.*, **149**, 1435–40

7. Salvesen, K. A., Vatten, L. J., Bakketeig, L. S. and Eik-Nes, S. H. (1994). Routine ultrasonography *in utero* and speech development. *Ultrasound Obstet. Gynecol.*, **4**, 101–3

8. Newnham, J. P., Evans, S. F., Michael, C. A., Stanley, F. J. and Landau, L. I. (1993). Effects of frequent ultrasound during pregnancy: a randomised controlled trial. *Lancet*, **342**, 887–91

9. AIUM Bioeffects Committee (1994). Bioeffects literature review. *J. Ultrasound Med.*, **13**, 731–4

10. Tarantal, A. F., O'Brien, W. D. and Hendrickx, A. G. (1993). Evaluation of the bioeffects of prenatal ultrasound exposure in the cynomolgus macaque (*Macaca fascicularis*): III. Developmental and hematologic studies. *Teratology*, **47**, 159–70

11. Child, S. Z., Hartman, C. L., Schery, L. A. and Carstensen, E. L. (1990). Lung damage from exposure to pulsed ultrasound. *Ultrasound Med. Biol.*, **16**, 817–25

12. Frizzell, L. A., Chen, E. and Lee, C. (1994). Effects of pulsed ultrasound on the mouse neonate: hind limb paralysis and lung hemorrhage. *Ultrasound Med. Biol.*, **20**, 53–63

13. Tarantal, A. F. and Canfield, D. R. (1994). Ultrasound induced lung hemorrhage in the monkey. *Ultrasound Med. Biol.*, **20**, 65–72

14. Dalecki, D., Raeman, C. H., Child, S. Z., Penney, D. P. and Carstensen, E. L. (1995). Thresholds for intestinal hemorrhage in mice from exposures to pulsed ultrasound. *Ultrasound Med. Biol.*, **21**, 1067–72

15. Barnett, S. B., ter Haar, G. R., Ziskin, M. C., Nyborg, W. L., Maeda, K. and Bang, J. (1994). Current status of research on biophysical effects of ultrasound. *Ultrasound Med. Biol.*, **20**, 205–18

16. AIUM/NEMA (1992). *Standard for Real-Time Display of Thermal and Mechanical Acoustic Output Indices on Diagnostic Ultrasound Equipment.* (American Institute of Ultrasound in Medicine/National Electrical Manufacturers Association)

17. Bosward, K. L., Barnett, S. B., Wood, A. K. W., Edwards, M. J. and Kossoff, G. (1993). Heating of guinea pig fetal brain during exposure to pulsed ultrasound. *Ultrasound Med. Biol.*, **19**, 415–24

18. Carstensen, E. L., Hartman, C., Child, S. Z., Cox, C. A., Mayer, R. and Schenk, K. (1990). Test for kidney hemorrhage following exposures to intense, pulsed ultrasound. *Ultrasound Med. Biol.*, **16**, 681–5

19. Ohmori, K., Matsuda, T., Horii, Y. and Yoshida, O. (1994). Effects of shock waves on the mouse fetus. *J. Urol.*, **151**, 255–8

20. Smith, D. P., Graham, J. B., Prystowksy, J. B., Dalkin, B. L. and Nemcek, A. A. (1992). The effect of ultrasound-guided shock waves during early pregnancy in sprague-Dawley rats. *J. Urol.*, **147**, 231–4

21. Baggs, R., Penny, D. P., Cox, C., Child, S. Z., Raeman, C. H., Dalecki, D. and Carstensen, E. L. (1996). Thresholds for ultrasonically induced lung hemorrhage in neonatal swine. *Ultrasound Med. Biol.*, in press

Ultrasonic and Doppler studies of the human yolk sac

3

A. Kurjak, S. Kupesic, M. Kos, V. Latin and M. Kos

INTRODUCTION

Development and function of the human yolk sac

The yolk sac is a structure that develops simultaneously with the embryo. In describing its development it is therefore impossible to avoid mentioning embryonal development as well. The development of the human embryo from fertilization until it has reached a crown–rump length of 30 mm is divided into 23 stages. Each stage is characterized by external morphology, or by somite development during the early stages. This staging permits accurate evaluation of human embryonic specimens[1,2].

Embryonic development begins with fertilization (stage 1), leading to the formation of a diploid zygote. The cleavage process is repeated in the following 4 days, during which time the conceptus travels along the Fallopian tube, still encircled by a zona pellucida. On the 4th day after fertilization, the conceptus consists of 16–20 cells and is called a morula (stage 2). Within 1 day of its arrival in the uterus, the zona pellucida is digested by uterine secretions and the fluid accumulates in the tiny spaces between the peripheral and central cells of the morula. When these spaces coalesce into the larger, fluid-containing space (the blastocele), the blastocyst is formed. The blastocele space divides the mass of cells into the outer layer of flattened cells (the trophoblast), and the conceptus begins to implant in the endometrium. The blastocyst makes contact at a point overlying the embryoblast[3,4]. The pre-villous implantation stage is stage 5. It is further subdivided into stages 5a, 5b and 5c. In stage 5a (7–8 days after fertilization) the trophoblast is a solid mass without lacunae. The conceptus still consists only of the blastocele cavity and the embryoblast mass of cells. The embryoblast begins to resolve into two cell plates – the epiblast, composed of tall columnar epithelium; and the hypoblast, composed of low cuboidal epithelium – forming the bilaminar embryonic disc. The margins of the epiblast give rise to a thin epithelial layer, the amnion, which together with the epiblast forms the amniotic sac. The innermost cells, a flattened layer of epithelium (Heuser's membrane), enclose the central cavity forming the primary yolk sac. However, certain observations on human blastocysts derived from *in vitro* fertilization[5] and animal blastocysts[6] indicate that the complete primary yolk sac might already be formed at the time of implantation[7]. The primary yolk sac largely fills the blastocyst and chorionic cavity, its diameter increasing to about 0.4 mm in stage 5c[1]. In stage 5b (8–9 days after fertilization), lacunae begin to appear within the trophoblastic layer, and in stage 5c (9–12 days after fertilization) lacunae form an almost complete sphere around the conceptus. From the margins of the hypoblast, branched cells invade the cavity of the blastocyst. These cells constitute the extraembryonic mesoderm. Spaces developing within the mesoderm coalesce, creating the extraembryonic celom. This splits the mesoderm into a visceral layer, investing the amniotic sac and yolk sac, and a parietal layer, which contributes to the chorion. The visceral and parietal layers are connected by the connecting stalk (the forerunner of the umbilical cord). During this stage, the primary yolk sac loses its ability to maintain turgor and collapses. The collapse most likely occurs repeatedly, leading to fragmentation, establishment of several small vesicles and formation

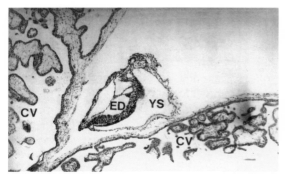

Figure 1 *Secondary yolk sac (YS) and embryonic disc (ED) surrounded by chorionic villi (CV). (Hematoxylin & eosin, × 28)*

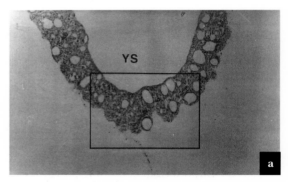

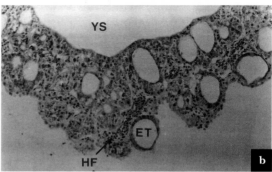

Figure 2 *Secondary yolk sac (YS) wall, at 7 weeks and 4 days. Hematoxylin & eosin (a) × 28; and detail (b) showing endodermal tubules (ET) and hemopoietic foci (HF) × 71*

of the secondary yolk sac (called simply the yolk sac) (Figure 1). Fragmentation of the primary yolk sac and formation of the secondary yolk sac during stages 5c and 6 is connected with the events that take place during stage 6 (gastrulation). The hypoblast is displaced by the endoderm that migrates inside the wall of the primary yolk sac. The vitelline stalk is a finger-like projection from the yolk sac into the connecting stalk.

Chorionic villi appear in stage 6a (12–15 days after fertilization) and the primitive streak becomes clearly visible in stage 6b (day 16 after fertilization). The linear primitive streak appears in the caudal end of the epiblast. Epiblastic cells invaginate through the streak and migrate laterally beneath it. Some of these cells displace the underlying hypoblast and form the embryonic endoderm, while the remainder form the embryonic mesoderm. Those epiblastic cells that do not migrate form the embryonic ectoderm. This process is called gastrulation and results in the formation of the three germ layers. Approximately 16 days after ovulation, the notochordal process is present, this being stage 7.

The secondary yolk sac is initially smaller than the primary, and flattened, composed of the visceral endoderm together with some parietal endoderm and a few associated mesoblasts from the primary yolk sac. It rapidly expands to form a large sac extending beyond the embryo in stages 7 (16–17 days) and 8 (18–19 days after fertilization), its diameter being up to

2 mm. At the end of the 10th week of pregnancy the diameter of the secondary yolk sac reaches 6.0–6.5 mm[8]. After formation, the secondary yolk sac undergoes a number of developmental changes, connected with its function, and finally with its cessation. One of the earliest morphological changes is the increase in thickness of the yolk sac wall (Figure 2a). Histologically, the thickness of the human yolk sac is about 200–700 μm and it consists of three layers: endoderm facing the yolk sac cavity, mesothelium facing the chorionic cavity and mesenchyme between them. The mesothelial cells are flat and arranged in one layer, covering the yolk sac and vitelline stalk. The endoderm consists of cuboidal cells with narrow intercellular spaces. Several endodermal cells are arranged to form tubular structures (endodermal tubules) (Figure 2b). In the early stages of pregnancy, the endodermal layer occupies the major part of the yolk sac wall, but the area that it covers decreases as the pregnancy progresses. Within a few days after the formation of the secondary yolk sac,

hemopoietic foci appear and the mesenchymal layer becomes more prominent, together with the endodermal layer. The mechanism by which the endodermal layer develops a thickened and stratified appearance is still unclear[9]. The mesenchyme consists of loose connective tissue and its proportion increase so that it occupies more than half of the yolk sac wall by the 7–8th week of pregnancy[8,9].

Human yolk sac carries out several important functions. Endodermal cells contain abundant protein synthesizing apparatus and they can synthesize a variety of proteins at approximately 12 weeks of gestation. Some of these proteins are albumin, prealbumin, α-1-antitrypsin and α-fetoprotein[10–12]. Evidence for an absorptive function of the human yolk sac is at this time only circumstantial. It is probable that the yolk sac has a transient nutritive function during organogenesis, and that interference with its function may result in malformations[13–15]. The yolk sac is also the site where primordial germ cells first appear in the embryo and from where they migrate through the mesentery to the developing gonads. The hemopoietic function of the human yolk sac has been known for a long time. Blood cells and blood islands are observed in the endodermal layer and also between the endodermal layer and mesothelial layers at about the middle of the 3rd week of embryogenesis[8,16]. The central cells of each blood island are hemocytoblasts; they acquire hemoglobin and become primitive, nucleated blood cells. The peripheral cells are angioblasts, which form a capillary endothelium around each blood island. The endothelial cells sprout branches, grow and fuse with one another, forming larger vascular channels. In this way, a rich capillary bed develops on the surface of the yolk sac. Angioblasts also differentiate from the extraembryonic mesoderm of the connective stalk and chorion. The endothelial channels extend into the embryo and link up with similar vessels in the yolk sac.

The vitelline stalk contains vitelline vessels (arteries and veins) and a vitelline duct. The vitelline duct develops with progressive constriction of the wide communication between the yolk sac and primitive embryonic gut cavity.

Regression of the yolk sac begins at about days 45–50 of gestation[16,18]. By the end of the first trimester the exocelomic fluid is absorbed, the amnion has fused with the chorion and the yolk sac degenerates. By the 12th week of pregnancy it can no longer be visualized with abdominal ultrasound[18]. Its remains are usually clearly visible on the chorionic plate of the placenta as a yellowish-white nodule with a diameter of 3–4 mm.

Pathological examination and histopathological changes of the yolk sac

Although the complete physiological role of the yolk sac is still poorly understood, its importance during the first few weeks of embryonic development cannot be disputed. Pathological study of the yolk sac could improve the understanding of the mechanisms of early spontaneous abortion and teratogenesis. It is therefore necessary to examine material from early pregnancy wastage and to correlate pathological findings with clinical data and ultrasound findings. Because of the fact that the yolk sac regresses and degenerates by the end of the first trimester of pregnancy, pathological examination of the yolk sac is restricted only to the products of early spontaneous or artificial abortions (or ectopic pregnancies). There is a wide variety of classifications of (early and late) spontaneous abortions by different authors, reflecting a wide variety of specimens received for examination in a pathology laboratory[19–21]. Products of conception in early spontaneous abortion should be submitted to the pathologist fresh (not fixed in formalin) in a sterile or at least clean and tightly closed (to avoid drying out) plastic container. Small specimens should be kept moist with gauze soaked in sterile saline. Such specimens are best examined in a sterile petri dish with sterile instruments (allowing samples to be taken for tissue culture and chromosomal analysis) under a dissecting microscope. For the examination and assessment of the yolk sac the ideal specimen is the intact chorionic sac, measuring from 10 to 80 mm, that is usually found in a pear-shaped decidual cast of the uterine cavity. Regrettably, the pathologist usually receives ruptured or, even more often, fragmented chorionic tissue (with or without embryonic tissue) as a result of vacuum aspiration or uterine curettage, sometimes even pre-selected by the clinician. The yolk sac is a very delicate structure that bursts or fragments during the procedure of uterine evacuation. Furthermore, it is also easily overlooked, because it floats away or adheres to membranes, and it is indeed difficult to find, even if especially sought for. In the ideal case of receiving the intact chorionic sac, this has to be opened very carefully along its smoothest area (chorion laeve). After the opening, the presence or absence of an amniotic sac, yolk sac, body stalk or cord and embryo can be accurately described. The yolk sac can be found free floating as a delicate vesicle with transparent wall if preserved, or opacified if macerated. It should be measured and transferred to a wire mesh capsule, where it should be floated in a drop of fixative to avoid damage[22]. Sometimes, the yolk sac is found adherent to the wall of the gestational sac near the umbilical cord insertion, its color being yellow or white. In that case a square of the surrounding membranes should also be cut and processed. In normal pregnancy, adhesion of the yolk sac may occur during the 11th or 12th week. One publication reported that in specimens from spontaneous abortion, at least 10% of yolk sacs had previously adhered to the amniotic membrane[22].

The proposed morphological classification of the secondary yolk sac contains two categories: (1) cases with preserved structure, the measures of the yolk sac being normal or showing altered expansion (whether shrunken or overly distended); and (2) cases in which the normal structure has been distorted, by retrogressive changes such as coagulative necrosis, calcification, fibrosis, edema or inflammatory changes[23] (Figure 3). The largest series, of 200 grossly and histopathologically examined yolk sacs, is that of Nogales and associates[22]. In their study, secondary yolk sacs in spontaneous abortions with altered expansion changes were subdivided into the categories of hypoplastic yolk sacs and cystic yolk sacs (each category comprising 6.7% of the examined material).

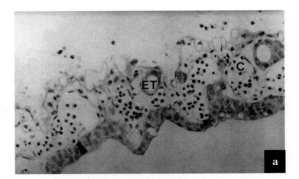

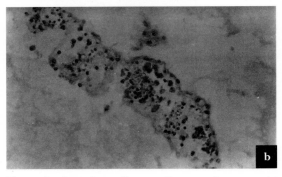

Figure 3 *Secondary yolk sac wall – normal structure (a) with primitive capillaries (C) and endodermal tubules (ET), at 7 weeks' gestational age. For comparison, (b) shows degenerative changes, necrosis in wall structure and degeneration of hemopoietic cells. Hematoxylin & eosin, × 71*

Hypoplastic yolk sacs had an average diameter of 3 mm, the average gestation in abortion with these changes being 8 weeks + 3 days. Two-thirds of them were free floating, and the rest were found adhering to the amniotic membrane. Cystic yolk sacs had an average diameter of 5.5 mm, some of them even up to 10 mm. The mean gestational age in pregnancy showing a cystic yolk sac was 10 weeks + 3 days. Half of the cystic yolk sacs had adhered to the amniotic membrane.

Yolk sacs showing retrogressive changes were found either free floating or adhering to the amniotic membrane, with no consistency in findings. These accounted for 75% of the pathological yolk sacs in the same study. They were also subdivided into two groups: those with the triad of necrosis, fibrosis and calcification (seen in 62% of all material), and those showing edema (6% of all material). In only one case were signs of infection found. These took the form of an intraluminal abscess in a fibrotic yolk sac, coexisting with acute villitis.

Fibrosis and calcification may occur during the normal regression of the yolk sac[24] and should only be considered of pathological significance if found before the 11th week[22]. Total coagulative necrosis and complete infarction of the yolk sac most probably result from acute ischemia. Partial necrosis involves only the endoderm, while the intervening connective tissue remains able to proliferate and form fibrosis. The damaged tissue eventually becomes dystrophically calcified. Although retrogressive changes probably represent involutive phenomena secondary to embryonal death, necrosis of the yolk sac can occur prior to the necrosis of the embryonal tissues. Edematous yolk sacs showed preserved architecture, with flattened endodermal cells, marked edema in the intervening mesenchyme and macrophages within the edema fluid[22].

Yolk sacs whose structure was normal for the gestational age and the stage of their development were seen in 18.5% of the cases in the series of Nogales and co-workers[22], the average gestational age in these cases being 8 weeks (range 6–11 weeks). They were usually found floating freely in the chorionic cavity. The majority of these findings were associated with normally formed fresh embryos, and the chorionic villi were well vascularized[22]. These findings suggest that the pregnancy wastage was most probably due to environmental rather than genetic causes.

However, pathologically changed yolk sacs were usually associated with retention of the conceptus and abnormally formed embryos. In all of these cases placentas showed poorly developed vascularization, changes being the most pronounced when an edematous yolk sac was found. Edematous yolk sacs were associated with the most marked placental and embryonic abnormalities. Altered expansion changes seemed to reflect the earlier pathological processes involving the yolk sac, whereas retrogressive changes were noted at a later gestational age[22]. The clinical significance of these findings is not yet fully understood and remains to be clarified.

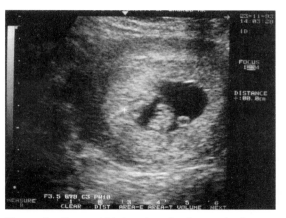

Figure 4 *Sonographic imaging of embryo and yolk sac at 7 weeks' gestational age. Transabdominal scan at 3.5 MHz*

ULTRASONIC STUDIES

The yolk sac in normal pregnancy

During the last decade, few authors confirmed the secondary yolk sac as the earliest visible embryonic landmark within the gestational sac[25–28]. With the use of transabdominal sonography, the overall visualization rate ranged from 69 to 100% (Figure 4). Yolk sac is often recognizable when the mean gestational sac diameter is approximately 10–15 mm and should always be seen with a mean gestational sac diameter of 20 mm[29]. According to the various investigators, transvaginal studies show that the yolk sac should be consistently visible when the gestational sac diameter exceeds 6–10 mm[30–32]. Moreover, Lindsay and colleagues[33] were able to visualize the yolk sac in normal pregnancy within the gestational sac diameter of 3.2 mm. In normal intrauterine pregnancy it is always characteristic that the yolk sac is visible before the viable embryo[33]. In our study, consisting of 105 patients with a normal pregnancy, the yolk sac measured 4.0–5.0 mm in diameter until 7–8 weeks of gestation, reaching 6.0–6.5 mm by the end of the 9th week[34].

The yolk sac in abnormal early pregnancy

The sonographic detection of abnormal yolk sac morphology may predict abnormal fetal outcome. Attempts have been made to characterize the normal sonographic appearance of the yolk sac and to identify abnormal parameters. For example, it has been confirmed that yolk sac malformations occur in diabetic mothers during the first trimester of pregnancy, but prior to 9 weeks' menstrual age[35]. Absence of yolk sac, and its abnormal size, shape and number are predictive indicators of early pregnancy failure. All of these parameters should be defined and assessed prior to 10 gestational weeks. Visualization of the yolk sac may serve also as an additional marker that helps clarify the developmental status of the aborted conceptus and provides useful information for counselling regarding future reproduction[28].

Abnormal yolk sac size may be the first sonographic indicator of associated failure. Primarily, the presence of an embryo without the visible yolk sac before the 10th gestational week is mostly an abnormal finding[36]. The fetus may still be abnormal, even if it survives the first trimester. A yolk sac with an abnormal sonographic appearance that persists has frequently been associated with fetal pathology, including chromosomal abnormalities[28,33]. Lyons and Lindsay have reported that the average sensitivity of yolk sac size as a predictor of pregnancy outcome is only about 16%, because many abnormal pregnancies have a normal yolk sac diameter which is not necessarily indicative of normal outcome[33,37].

According to Lyons, the inner diameter of the yolk sac is always less than 5.6 mm in a normal pregnancy before the 10th week of gestational age[37]. The same author has also established that for a mean gestational sac diameter of less than 10 mm, the yolk sac diameter should be less than 4 mm. In 15 patients who had abnormally large sacs, six had no embryo, five aborted spontaneously and only one conceptus survived. Out of nine others with embryo and large yolk sac, eight patients aborted and in one patient trisomy 21 was detected at the 24th gestational week[37]. The predictive value for abnormal outcome seemed to be 60% in that sample. However, this occurred in only a small number of all the following pregnancies.

The yolk sac can be too small, and this is accepted as a marker of poor pregnancy outcome[33,38]. Green and Hobbins[38] reported a group of patients distributed between 8 and 12 weeks' gestational age, with a yolk sac diameter less than 2 mm associated with an adverse outcome. The yolk sac diameter of more than two standard deviations below the mean allowed prediction of an abnormal outcome with a sensitivity of 15.6%, specificity of 95.3% and positive predictive value of 44.4%[33]. When the group with yolk sacs that were too large was combined with the group with yolk sacs that were too small, the sensitivity of predicting an abnormal pregnancy outcome increased to 26.9%, the specificity to 92.7%, and the positive predictive value to 51.1%[33,37].

Most often, the shape of the yolk sac is changed when compressed by an enlarging fetus after the 10th gestational week. The normal spherical shape of the yolk sac can be distorted even earlier, requiring intensive follow-up within the next few weeks. If abnormality persists, the outcome is doubtful, but if it reverts to normal, then the outcome is usually normal, too[37]. The most difficult diagnostic puzzle is the double yolk sac. Each singleton pregnancy should have a single yolk sac. A double yolk sac is an extremely rare finding. The diagnostic puzzle includes the morphological differentiation of a retarded disappearance of physiological midgut herniation or an early abdominal wall defect.

The first calcified yolk sac, with a diameter of only 2.0 mm, was reported in 1985[39]. Two more cases were described[40], associated with intrauterine embryonic demise, in which the same appearance was demonstrated. The calcification of the yolk sac in these two cases was connected with *in utero* embryonic demise of relatively long-standing duration (2 weeks or longer). These findings were possibly due to the dystrophic changes that occur in non-viable cellular material.

It is unknown whether abnormalities of the yolk sac are related primarily to the yolk sac or secondary to embryonic maldevelopment. According to the present data it seems that the yolk sac plays an important role in maternofetal transportation in early pregnancy. Changes in size and shape could indicate or reflect the significant dysfunction of this system, and therefore could influence early embryonic development. Regardless of the possible role of the yolk sac, clinical findings have confirmed the association between the abnormal size and persistent irregular shape and abnormal outcome of pregnancy: spontaneous abortion, missed abortion and the higher incidence of chromosomal and structural anomalies. On the basis of these findings the routine measurements of yolk sac diameter and the assessment of yolk sac shape are recommended in all pregnancies until the 10th week of gestation. In patients with an ultrasonographically abnormal yolk sac in whom the pregnancy continues, further ultrasound examinations are necessary to exclude fetal anomalies.

Currently, the major benefits of the sonographic evaluation of the yolk sac are:

(1) Differentiation of potentially viable and non-viable gestations;

(2) Confirmation of the presence of an intrauterine pregnancy vs. a decidual cast; and

(3) Indication of a possible fetal abnormality[37].

Color Doppler studies of the yolk sac and vitelline stalk

Recently, interesting results have been published on the assessment of yolk sac vascularization in normal pregnancy. Kurjak and associates[34] performed a transvaginal color Doppler study on 105 patients whose gestational age ranged from 6 to 10 weeks from the last menstrual period. Transvaginal color and pulsed Doppler examination was performed before the termination of pregnancy for psychosocial reasons.

The overall visualization rate for yolk sac vessels was 72.38%. The highest visualization rates were obtained in the 7th and 8th weeks of gestation, reaching the value of 85.71%. In the same period the visualization rates of the vitelline stalk arteries were 85.71% and 89.28%, respectively (Color plate 1). A characteristic waveform profile included low velocity (5.8 ± 1.7 cm/s), and the absence of diastolic flow was found in all examined yolk sacs (Color plate 2). The

Table 1 Visualization rate of yolk sac vascularity between 6 and 10 weeks' gestation. The pulsatility index (PI) is shown $\pm$ SD

Gestational age (weeks)	n	Visualization rate		PI
		n	%	
6	15	5	33.3	3.42 ± 0.58
7	21	18	85.7	3.14 ± 0.82
8	28	24	85.7	3.10 ± 0.94
9	23	18	78.3	3.12 ± 0.85
10	18	11	61.1	3.45 ± 0.72
Total	105	76	72.4	3.24 ± 0.94

Table 2 Visualization rate of the vitelline stalk vascularity between 6 and 10 weeks' gestation. The pulsatility index (PI) is shown $\pm$ SD

Gestational age (weeks)	n	Visualization rate		PI
		n	%	
6	15	—	—	—
7	21	18	85.7	3.02 ± 0.92
8	28	25	89.3	3.05 ± 0.89
9	23	17	73.9	3.08 ± 0.91
10	18	10	55.6	3.38 ± 0.82
Total	105	70	66.7	3.14 ± 0.92

pulsatility index (PI) showed a mean value of 3.24 ± 0.94 without significant changes between subgroups ($p > 0.05$). The distribution of mean PI values for yolk sac vascularity is shown in Table 1. Pulsed Doppler signals derived from the umbilical cord demonstrated different PI values in the same patients analyzed (Color plate 3).

Vitelline stalk vessels showed similar peak systolic velocity (5.4 ± 1.8 cm/s) and PI values (3.14 ± 0.91) ($p > 0.05$) to those obtained from the yolk sac. The distribution of the vitelline artery PI values is shown in Table 2. Transvaginal color Doppler ultrasound and spectral analysis at 9–10 weeks' gestation of the vitelline artery is shown in Color plates 4 and 5.

The vascularization of the yolk sac wall (Color plate 6) takes place in the mesoderm surrounding the vitelline duct and communicates with the primitive cardiovascular system of the embryo by means of paired vitelline veins and arteries. The vitelline stalk wall is considered to be of the same embryological origin as the yolk sac wall. Blood vessels are seen in the vitelline stalk, but the mesenchyme usually seen in the yolk sac wall at all stages cannot be observed between the mesothelium and the vitelline duct. It is suggested that blood cells and blood vessels develop earlier than the mesenchyme, i.e. hemopoiesis could occur before the formation of mesenchyme in the yolk sac wall. With subsequent growth of the amniotic sac and elongation of the vitelline stalk, the yolk sac is removed from the body wall. The embryonic celom is gradually obliterated and the amnion sheaths the connecting stalk, forming the epithelial covering of the definitive umbilical cord[41].

In our own study the first color and pulsed signals from the yolk sac were obtained between 5 and 6 weeks of gestation. The visualization rate of the yolk sac vessels in the 6th week of gestation was 33.33%, and it increased to a value of 85.71% during the 7th and 8th weeks of gestation. As the functional activity of the yolk sac progressively declined, the visualization rate of 78.26% for 9 weeks' gestation and 61.11% for 10 weeks' gestation paralleled this process (Color plate 7).

The overall visualization rate for vitelline arteries was 66.67%. Color and pulsed Doppler signals could be obtained from the vitelline duct during the 7th week of gestation in 85.71% of patients. The peak of visualization (89.28%) occurred during the 8th week of gestation.

The process of elongation of the vitelline duct together with the removal of the yolk sac from the body wall was paralleled with a decreased rate of vitelline duct visualization during the 9th (73.91%) and 10th (55.55%) weeks of gestation. All of these findings may help in better understanding the early development of both blood cells and blood vessels.

Hemopoiesis in human embryos begins in the yolk sac at about the middle of the 3rd week of embryogenesis. Later it appears in the liver and bone marrow at the 4–5th week and the 8th week, respectively[42,43]. At about the 10–12th week, hemopoietic tissues are found distributed evenly in bone marrow throughout the body[42,44,45]. The hemopoietic function of the human yolk sac, in evidence by 17–18 days of gestation, has long been appreciated[18,24,46–48], and modern studies have better defined the origin and stages of development of various types of blood cells[49–52].

Maturation of blood cells is considered to take place extravascularly. With occasional exceptions, the blood cells in the endodermal layers are the most immature, and maturation appears to proceed as the cells migrate to the mesenchymal layers and, further, into the blood vessels. Furthermore, biochemical and immunocytochemical studies have shown that the human yolk sac can synthesize a variety of proteins during approximately the first 12 weeks of gestation. Some of these proteins include albumin, prealbumin, α-1-antitrypsin, α-fetoprotein, apolipoproteins, insulin-like growth factor and transferrin[12,53–55].

The yolk sac also has another critical function, namely that it is the site where primordial germ cells first appear in the embryo[56,57].

There are several papers published on the ultrasonic assessment of the morphology of the secondary yolk sac[27–29,33,35,38,40,58–60]. This report is the first systematic study on vascularization of both the secondary yolk sac and the vitelline duct. It is part of our continuing interest in early fetomaternal circulation[61–63].

Vascularization of the yolk sac in abnormal pregnancies

Three types of abnormal vascular signals were derived from the yolk sac in patients with missed abortion: irregular blood flow (Color plate 8), permanent diastolic flow (Color plate 9) and venous blood flow signals (Color plate 10).

The prognostic significance of these circulatory changes is not clearly established. Only a small proportion of abnormal early pregnancies presented changes in vascularity. It seems that changes in both yolk sac appearance (size, shape and echogenicity) and vascularization are probably a consequence of poor embryonic development or even embryonic death, rather than being the primary cause of an early pregnancy failure.

The fact that blood vessels first develop in the secondary yolk sac may be related to the important role of this structure in the process of early embryonic nutrition.

Further Doppler studies analyzing a large cohort of patients with both normal and abnormal pregnancies will probably answer some of the numerous questions on the role of yolk sac vascularity in early embryonic development. Doppler studies of the yolk sac and vitelline stalk are in their infancy. It is exciting research, but its clinical significance for the time being should be neither underestimated nor overestimated.

References

1. O'Rahilly, R. and Muller, F. (1987). *Developmental Stages in Human Embryos*, Publication 637 (Washington, DC: Carnegie Institution)
2. Streeter, G. L. (1951). *Developmental Horizons in Human Embryos*. (Washington DC: Carnegie Institute of Embryology)
3. Kalousek, D. K., Lau, A. E. and Baldwin, V. J. (1992). Development of the embryo, fetus and placenta. In Dimmick, J. E. and Kalousek, D. K. (eds.) *Developmental Pathology of the Embryo and Fetus*, pp. 1–25. (Philadelphia: J.B. Lippincott)
4. FitzGerald, M. J. T. and FitzGerald, M. (1994). *Human Embryology*. (London: Baillière Tindall)
5. Lopata, A., Kohlman, D. J. and Kellow, G. N. (1982). The fine structure of human blastocysts developed in culture. In Burger, M. M. and Weber, R. (eds.) *Embryonic Development*, pp. 69–85. (New York: Liss)
6. Enders, A. C., Lantz, K. C. and Schlafke, S. (1990). Differentiation of the inner cell mass of the baboon blastocyst. *Anat. Rec.*, **226**, 237–48
7. Luckett, W. P. (1978). Origin and differentiation of the yolk sac and extraembryonic mesoderm in presomite human and rhesus monkey embryos. *Am. J. Anat.*, **152**, 59–98
8. Takashina, T. (1993). Histology of the secondary human yolk sac with special reference to hematopoiesis. In Nogales, F. F. (ed.) *The Human Yolk Sac and Yolk Sac Tumors*, pp. 48–69. (Berlin: Springer-Verlag)
9. Enders, A. C. and King, B. F. (1993). Development of the human yolk sac. In Nogales, F. F. (ed.) *The Human Yolk Sac and Yolk Sac Tumors*, pp. 33–47. (Berlin: Springer-Verlag)
10. Nogales-Fernandez, F., Siverberg, S. G., Bloustein, P. A., Martinez-Hernandez, A. and Pierce, G. B. (1977). Yolk sac carcinoma (endodermal sinus tumor). Ultrastructure and histogenesis of gonadal and extragonadal tumors in comparison with normal human yolk sac. *Cancer*, **39**, 1462–74
11. Topilko, A. and Pisarski, T. (1971). Ultrastructure of the human yolk sac. *Acta Med. Pol.*, **12**, 127–32
12. Gitlin, D. and Perricelli, A. (1970). Synthesis of serum albumin, prealbumin, alpha-fetoprotein, alpha-1-antitrypsin and transferrin by the human yolk sac. *Nature (London)*, **228**, 995–7
13. Naftolin, F., Diamond, M. P., Pinter, E., Reece, E. A. and Sanyal, M. K. (1987). A hypothesis concerning the general basis of organogenetic congenital anomalies. *Am. J. Obstet. Gynecol.*, **157**, 1–4
14. Reece, E. A., Scioscia, A. L., Pinter, E., Hobbins, J. C., Green, J., Mahoney, M. J. and Naftolin, F. (1988). Prognostic significance of the human yolk sac assessed by ultrasonography. *Am. J. Obstet. Gynecol.*, **159**, 1191–4
15. Brent, R. L., Beckman, D. A., Jensen, M. and Koszalka, T. R. (1990). Experimental yolk sac disfunction as a model for studying nutritional disturbances in the embryo during early embryogenesis. *Teratology*, **41**, 405–13
16. Exalto, N. (1993). Yolk sac abnormalities: a clinical review. In Nogales, F. F. (ed.) *The Human Yolk Sac and Yolk Sac Tumors*, pp. 126–34. (Berlin: Springer-Verlag)
17. Johnson, K. E. (1988). *Human Developmental Anatomy*. (Baltimore: Williams and Wilkins)
18. Branca, A. (1912). Sur l'histogenese de la vesicule ombilicale humaine. *C. R. Assoc. Anat.*, **14**, 15–21
19. Fujikura, T., Froehlich, L. A. and Driscoll, S. G. (1966). A simplified anatomic classification of abortions. *Am. J. Obstet. Gynecol.*, **95**, 902–5
20. Geneva Conference (1966). Standardisation of procedures for chromosome studies in abortion. *Cytogenetics*, **5**, 963–4
21. Rushton, D. I. (1978). Simplified classification of spontaneous abortions. *J. Med. Genet.*, **15**, 1–9
22. Nogales, F. F., Beltran, E. and Gonzales, F. (1993). Morphological changes of the secondary human yolk sac in early pregnancy wastage.

In Nogales, F. F. (ed.) *The Human Yolk Sac and Yolk Sac Tumors*, pp. 175–94. (Berlin: Springer-Verlag)

23. Nogales, F. F., Beltran, E. and Fernandez, P. L. (1992). The pathology of secondary human yolk sac in spontaneous abortion: findings in 103 cases. In Fenoglio, C. and Rilke, F. (eds.) *Progress in Surgical Pathology*, vol. 12, pp. 291–303. (New York: Fild and Wood)

24. Branca, A. (1913). Recherches sur la structure, l'evolution et le role de la vesicule ombilicale de l'homme. *J. Anat. Physiol.*, **49**, 171–211

25. Mantoni, F. and Pedersen, J. F. (1979). Ultrasound visualization of the human yolk sac. *J. Clin. Ultrasound*, **7**, 459–60

26. Sauerbrei, E., Cooperberg, P. L. and Poland, B. J. (1980). Ultrasound demonstration of the normal fetal yolk sac. *J. Clin. Ultrasound*, **8**, 217–20

27. Crooij, M. J., Westhuis, M., Schoemaker, J. and Exalto, N. (1982). Ultrasonographic measurements of the yolk sac. *Br. J. Obstet. Gynaecol.*, **89**, 931–4

28. Ferrazzi, E., Brambati, B., Lanzani, A., Oldrini, A., Stripparo, L., Guerneri, S. and Makowsky, E. L. (1988). The yolk sac in early pregnancy failure. *Am. J. Obstet. Gynecol.*, **1**, 137–42

29. Nyberg, D. A., Laing, F. C. and Filly, R. A. (1986). Threatened abortion: sonographic distinction of normal and abnormal gestation sac. *Radiology*, **158**, 397–400

30. Bree, R. L., Edwards, M. and Bohm-Velez, M. (1989). Transvaginal sonography in the evaluation of normal early pregnancy: correlation with HCG level. *Am. J. Roentgenol.*, **153**, 75–9

31. Levi, C. S., Lyons, E. A. and Lindsay, D. J. (1988). Early diagnosis of nonviable pregnancy with endovaginal US. *Radiology*, **167**, 383–5

32. Cacciatore, B., Titinen, A., Stenman, U. H. and Ylostalo, P. (1990). Normal early pregnancy: serum HCG levels and vaginal ultrasonography findings. *Br. J. Obstet. Gynaecol.*, **97**, 889–903

33. Lindsay, D. J., Lovett, I. S., Lyons, E. A., Levi, C. S., Zheng, X. H., Holt, S. C. and Dashefsky, S. M. (1992). Endovaginal appearance of the yolk sac in pregnancy: normal growth and usefulness as a predictor of abnormal pregnancy outcome. *Radiology*, **183**, 115–18

34. Kurjak, A., Kupesic, S. and Kostovic, Lj. (1994). Vascularization of yolk sac and vitelline duct in normal pregnancies studied by transvaginal color and pulsed Doppler. *J. Perinat. Med.*, **22**, 433–40

35. Pedersen, J. F., Molsted-Pedersen, L. and Mortensen, H. B. (1984). Fetal growth delay and maternal hemoglobin A1C in early diabetic pregnancy. *Obstet. Gynecol.*, **64**, 351–2

36. Levi, C. S., Lyons, E. A., Zheng, X. H., Lindsay, D. J. and Holt, S. C. (1990). Endovaginal US:
demonstration of cardiac activity in embryos of less than 5.0 mm in crown–rump length. *Radiology*, **176**, 71–4

37. Lyons, E. A. (1994). Endovaginal sonography of the first trimester of pregnancy. *Proceedings of the 3rd International Perinatal and Gynecological Ultrasound Symposium*, Ottawa, Ontario, pp. 1–25

38. Green, J. J. and Hobbins, J. C. (1988). Abdominal ultrasound examination of the first trimester fetus. *Am. J. Obstet. Gynecol.*, **159**, 165–75

39. Ferrazzi, E., Brambati, B., Lanzani, A. and Oldrini, A. (1985). New sonographic criteria in monitoring the first trimester pregnancy. In Fraccaro, M., Simoni, G. and Brambati, B. (eds.) *First Trimester Fetal Diagnosis*, pp. 92–8. (Berlin: Springer-Verlag)

40. Harris, R. D., Vincent, L. M. and Askin, F. B. (1988). Yolk sac calcification: a sonographic finding associated with intrauterine embryonic demise in the first trimester. *Radiology*, **166**, 109–10

41. Jauniaux, E., Jurkovic, D., Henriet, Y. *et al.* (1991). Development of the secondary yolk sac: correlation of sonographic and anatomic features. *Hum. Reprod.*, **6**, 1160–6

42. Fukuda, T. (1973). Fetal hemopoiesis – electron microscopic studies on human yolk sac hemopoiesis. *Virchows Arch. (B).*, **14**, 197–200

43. Zamboni, L. (1965). Electron microscopic studies of human blood embryogenesis in human. II. The hemopoietic activity in the fetal liver. *J. Ultrastruct. Res.*, **12**, 525–8

44. Fukuda, T. (1974). Fetal hemopoiesis. II. Electron microscopic studies on human hepatic hemopoiesis. *Virchows Arch. (B)*, **16**, 249–52

45. Fukuda, T. (1978). Ultrastructure of fetal hemopoiesis. *Acta Haematol. Jpn.*, **41**, 1204–6

46. Bloom, W. and Bartelmez, G. W. (1940). Hematopoiesis in young human embryos. *Am. J. Anat.*, **67**, 21–5

47. Gladstone, R. J. and Hamilton, W. J. (1941). A presomite human embryo (Shaw) with primitive streak and chorda canal, with special reference to the development of the vascular system. *J. Anat.*, **76**, 9–12

48. Jordan, H. E. (1910). A microscopic study of the umbilical vesicle of a 13 mm human embryo, with special reference to the entodermal tubulus and the flood islands. *Anat. Anz.*, **37**, 12–16

49. Enzan, H. (1986). Electron microscopic studies of macrophages in early human yolk sacs. *Acta Pathol. Jpn.*, **36**, 49–51

50. Hesseldahl, H. and Falck-Larsen, J. F. (1971). Hemopoiesis and blood vessels in human yolk sac. An electron microscopic study. *Acta Anat. (Basel)*, **78**, 274–9

51. Hoyes, A. D. (1969). The human foetal yolk sac. An ultrastructural study of four specimens. *Z. Zellforsch*, **99**, 469–74

52. Janossy, G., Bofill, M., Poulter, L. W., Rawlings, E., Burford, G. D., Navarrete, C., Ziegler, A. and Kelemen, E. (1986). Separate ontogeny of two macrophage-like accessory cell populations in the human fetus. *J. Immunol.*, **136**, 4354–9

53. Gitlin, D., Perricelli, A. and Gotlin, G. M. (1972). Synthesis of alpha-fetoprotein by liver, yolk sac, and gastrointestinal tract of the human conceptus. *Cancer Res.*, **32**, 979–88

54. Hopkins, B., Sharpe, C. R., Barelle, F. E. and Graham, C. F. (1986). Organ distribution of apolipoprotein gene transcripts in 6–12 week postfertilization human embryos. *J. Embryol. Exp. Morphol.*, **97**, 177–83

55. Takashina, T., Kanda, Y., Hazakawa, O., Kudo, R. and Ito, E. (1987). Yolk sac tumors of the ovary and the human yolk sac. *Am. J. Obstet. Gynecol.*, **156**, 223–8

56. Hamilton, W. J. and Mossman, H. W. (1972). *Human Embryology. Prenatal Development of Form and Function*, 4th edn, pp. 162–88. (Baltimore: Williams and Wilkins)

57. Langman, J. (1969). *Medical Embryology, Human Development – Normal and Abnormal*, 2nd edn, pp. 183–98. (Baltimore: Williams and Wilkins)

58. Barzilai, M., Lyons, E. A., Levi, C. S. and Lindsay, D. J. (1989). Vitelline duct cyst or double yolk sac. *J. Ultrasound Med.*, **8**, 523–6

59. Nyberg, D. A., Mack, L. A., Harvey, D. *et al.* (1988). Value of the yolk sac in evaluating early pregnancies. *J. Ultrasound Med.*, **7**, 129–33

60. Reece, E. A., Pinter, E., Green, J. *et al.* (1987). Significance of isolated yolk sac visualized by ultrasonography. *Lancet*, **1**, 269–71

61. Kurjak, A., Crvenkovic, G., Salihagic, A., Zalud, I. and Miljan, M. (1993). The assessment of normal early pregnancy by transvaginal color Doppler ultrasonography. *J. Clin. Ultrasound*, **21**, 3–7

62. Kurjak, A., Zudenigo, D., Funduk-Kurjak, B., Shalan, H., Predanic, M. and Sosic, A. (1993). Transvaginal color Doppler in the assessment of uteroplacental circulation in normal early pregnancy. *J. Perinat. Med.*, **21**, 25–31

63. Kurjak, A., Zudenigo, D., Predanic, M. and Kupesic, S. (1994). Recent advances in the Doppler study of early fetomaternal circulation. *J Perinat. Med.*, **22**, 419–23

Doppler studies of subchorionic hematomas in early pregnancy

4

S. Kupesic, A. Kurjak and F. A. Chervenak

INTRODUCTION

Most of the emergency admissions to obstetrics departments are due to vaginal bleeding before 28 weeks' gestation. According to data in the literature these symptoms occur in up to 25% of all pregnancies[1-22]. Sometimes bleeding is found with intrauterine hematomas, closely associated with early spontaneous abortion. Since the clinical observation and history are frequently inconclusive, it is obligatory to perform further non-invasive diagnostic procedures such as ultrasonography and biochemical investigations. Considerable progress in sonographic techniques and the introduction of transvaginal sonography in particular have enabled detailed studies to be carried out on early embryonic development. Moreover, Doppler techniques can provide a wealth of information on the physiology and pathology of both the embryonic and the maternal circulation. Our group has been particularly interested in color Doppler studies of blood flow in the maternal part of the placental circulation in pregnancies complicated by intrauterine hematoma.

SONOGRAPHIC STUDIES

Subchorionic hematoma is defined sonographically as an echo-free area located between the membranes and the uterine wall (Color plate 11). Physiologically this represents a separation of the chorionic plate from the underlying decidua. In such a complicated early pregnancy the decidua surrounding the gestational sac demonstrates irregular echogenicity, subdecidual bleeding and fragmentation. The gestational sac may be detached from the decidual wall and chorion, or appears crumpled and flat[1]. The pathological mechanism is probably placental abruption, in which retroplacental clots are located between the placenta and myometrium, and pre-placental clots are found between the amniotic fluid and the placenta later in the second trimester[2].

The first reported sonographic observation of an intrauterine hematoma was made by Mantoni and Pedersen[3] in women with viable pregnancies at the 12–20th week of gestation. Other reports[4-6] have confirmed these findings.

In the study of Ylöstalo and colleagues[7], hematoma was identified in 62% of patients with uterine bleeding during pregnancy. In this cohort of patients, placental abruption was confirmed after the delivery.

Mantoni and Pedersen[3] analyzed three patients with hematomas with volumes of more than 50 ml. Two of these aborted and one had a premature delivery. The remaining pregnancies with hematomas of 35 ml or less continued uneventfully until term. The same observation was made by Stabile and Grudzinskas[2], since none of the patients with small hematoma (< 16 ml) aborted. Furthermore, they found that repeated episodes of painless bleeding was followed by ultrasonic evidence of diminution of the clot size.

Numerous studies have been performed on this topic. Most of them examined the volume or site of the hematoma. Table 1 shows the summarized results of different investigators[3-17].

The precise cause of subchorionic hematoma is unknown. Postulated associative factors

Table 1 *Clinical outcome of pregnancies complicated by subchorionic hematomas (SCH)*

Authors	n	Outcome of pregnancy	Comments
Abu-Yousef et al. (1987)[10]	21	7 spontaneous abortions 3 preterm deliveries 5 severe bleeding, therapeutic abortion	larger SCH associated with increased risk of poor outcome
Baxi and Pearlstone (1991)[8]	5	1 preterm delivery at 24 weeks	selected group of patients with autoantibodies
Bloch et al. (1989)[11]	31	3 spontaneous abortions 2 preterm deliveries 26 full-term deliveries	size of SCH unrelated to pregnancy outcome
Borlum et al. (1989)[12]	86	19 spontaneous abortions	volume of SCH was < 30 ml in 85% of patients
Goldstein et al. (1983)[5]	10	2 spontaneous abortions	size of SCH unrelated to pregnancy outcome
Jakab et al. (1994)[13]	35	8 spontaneous abortions	size of hematoma unrelated to pregnancy outcome
Jouppila (1985)[6]	33	6 spontaneous abortions 3 preterm deliveries	size of SCH unrelated to pregnancy outcome
Mantoni and Pedersen (1981)[3]	12	2 spontaneous abortions 1 preterm delivery	larger SCH associated with increased risk of poor outcome
Nyberg et al. (1987)[14]	46	3 fetal mortalities 6 terminations of pregnancy 12 preterm deliveries	size of SCH unrelated to pregnancy outcome
Pedersen and Mantoni (1990)[15]	23	1 spontaneous abortion 2 preterm deliveries	large SCH (> 50 ml) not associated with increased risk of poor outcome
Saurbrei and Pham (1986)[16]	30	3 spontaneous abortions 4 stillbirths 7 preterm deliveries	large SCH (> 60 ml) associated with increased risk of poor outcome
Spirit et al. (1979)[17]	4	2 preterm deliveries 2 full-term deliveries	
Stabile et al. (1989)[4]	20	0 spontaneous abortions	volume of SCH in all study patients < 16 ml
Ylöstalo et al. (1984)[7]	16	5 placental abruptions	median duration of pregnancy shorter in patients with a hematoma

include autoimmune reactions[3], coumarin drugs, or deficiency of a hematological factor[9].

Most investigators agree that subchorionic hematoma is a risk factor for spontaneous abortion. However, differences in the obtained results are a possible consequence of different study designs, in which the distinction between supracervical hematomas and fundal corporeal collections was not made.

As can be seen from Table 1, much emphasis has been put on the volume of the hematoma[19,20], but not on the location of the hemor-rhage. It is likely, if the bleeding occurs at the level of the definitive placenta (under the cord insertion), that it may result in placental separation and subsequent hematoma[21,22]. Conversely, a subchorionic hematoma only detaching the membrane opposite to the cord insertion can probably reach a significant volume before it affects normal pregnancy development.

Perigestational hemorrhage appears similar to placental abruption later in pregnancy[23]. The prognosis of this event depends on numerous factors, among which the most important are the dissecting capacity of the decidua and the existence of decidual necrosis.

DOPPLER STUDIES – THE ZAGREB EXPERIENCE

Recently our group analyzed 59 women with vaginal bleeding, closed cervix, and ultrasonic findings of a living embryo and subchorionic hematoma[24]. The gestational ages in this case–control study ranged from 6 to 14 weeks. A total of 135 matched controls were randomly selected from a pool of 941 women who were studied at the same time.

Subchorionic hematoma was diagnosed when B-mode sonography showed an echo-poor or echo-free crescent-shaped collection between the chorionic membrane and the myometrium. The hematoma was measured in three diameters and the volume calculated by multiplying the three diameters and then dividing by 2. The hematoma size was categorized as small or large, according to whether it was more or less than 20 ml in a range of 8.4–72.5 ml.

Color flow Doppler was used to visualize the spiral arteries (Color plate 12). In general, these vessels are located in the present or future placental site. Blood flow velocity waveforms were analyzed by means of pulsed Doppler. Indices used in the study were the resistance index (RI) – peak systole minus end-diastole/systole – and the peak-systolic velocity (PSV).

Women with subchorionic hematomas received no drug therapy, only bedrest and observation until the bleeding stopped. Those with hematomas and continuing pregnancies were seen at intervals of 2 weeks, at least three times, for follow-up and Doppler studies.

Table 2 lists the statistical data for the study when the dependent variable was gestational weeks. All parameters showed correlation. The RI slowly declined during the 8-week observation period, whereas the flow, as expressed by peak-systolic velocity, rose at a faster rate. The hematoma volume showed a weak positive correlation.

Table 3 summarizes the correlation among all the variables. The RI and PSV had a correlation of -0.791, reflecting the reciprocal relationship between resistance and flow (Color plates 13 and 14). This also validates the concept of using an absolute measurement for small vessels when the angle of insonation is unknown. The hematoma volume had a weak negative correlation with PSV, suggesting that flow decreases as the hematoma enlarges (Color plates 15 and 16).

Table 4 shows the data for spontaneous abortions and preterm deliveries. More spontaneous abortions occurred when there were subchorionic hematomas, 17% vs. 6.5%. A significant difference was documented.

Table 5 analyzes the effect of the location of the subchorionic hematoma on the pregnancy outcome. The significant factor was the presence of the hematoma in the corpus or fundus of the uterus. Since this is the region of the placental site in most cases, it suggests a possible disruption of placental function.

In 23 women, the volume of the hematoma was < 20 ml. In this group there were three spontaneous abortions. In the remaining 36 women with larger hematomas, there were seven abortions. This was not a significant difference.

Table 2 *Correlation of gestational age with other parameters*

Variable	Correlation	t	p
Resistance index	−0.304	3.42	0.0012
Peak systolic velocity	0.702	9.05	0.0001
Volume	0.157	2.36	0.0219

Table 3 *Correlation among variables*

Variable	Gestational weeks	Resistance index	Peak systolic velocity	Volume
Gestational weeks	1.000			
Resistance index	−0.304	1.000		
Peak systolic velocity	0.702	−0.791	1.000	
Volume	0.157	0.527	−0.276	1.000

Table 4 *Frequency of spontaneous abortions and preterm deliveries*

Group	n	Spontaneous abortions		Preterm deliveries	
		n	%	n	%
Control	135	8	5.9	9	6.7
Subchorionic hematoma	59	10	17.0*	3	5.1
Total	194	19	9.8	12	6.2

*p-value vs. controls; Fisher exact test: one-tail, 0.06; two-tail, 0.02

Table 5 *Hematoma site and pregnancy outcome**

Site	n	Spontaneous abortion		Preterm delivery	
		n	%	n	%
Supracervical	30	2	6.7	2	6.7
Fundus–corpus	29	8	27.6	1	3.4
Total	59	10	17.0	3	5.1

*p-value; Fisher exact test: one-tail, 0.01; two-tail, 0.03

The essential finding of our study is that in the presence of hematomas, resistance was increased and flow was decreased. When pregnancy continued, these indices returned to normal values. This statistical relationship suggests that the changes in flow velocity are secondary, and not the cause of subchorionic hematoma[25].

Occasionally, subchorionic hematoma can be mistaken for a blighted twin. A blighted twin may be a cause of vaginal bleeding in women whose ultrasound examination reveals a living co-twin[23].

Using transabdominal sonography Stabile and associates[4] observed an empty second sac in 8.5% of patients who were bleeding but who had a live embryo (3.9% of total patients). A perigestational hemorrhage was found in an additional 8.6% of cases. The sonographic appearance of a blighted twin is typically a well-defined rounded or oval fluid collection, surrounded by an echogenic ring (Color plate 17).

This appearance contrasts with that of a perigestational hemorrhage, which tends to conform in shape to the gestational sac and frequently demonstrates internal echoes[23]. Furthermore, the presence of an internal embryo or yolk sac confirms that the fluid is a second gestational sac.

Contrary to the case of subchorionic hematoma, at the periphery of the gestational sac of the vanishing twin one can detect low impedance to blood flow typical of spiral arteries. Sometimes color flow is helpful in distinguishing the echo-free black-and-white image that can represent perigestational hemorrhage, venous sinus or a highly vascularized placental site.

CONCLUSION

The prognostic significance of identifying perigestational hemorrhage still remains uncertain. Some studies have reported a higher risk of spontaneous abortion when subchorionic hematoma was identified, while other studies have found greater risk only if the hemorrhage was large. We believe that transvaginal color and pulsed Doppler have the potential to detect the patients with altered spiral artery blood flow who are at increased risk for spontaneous abortion. Furthermore, serial examination may have a prognostic significance, since it gives us a direct insight into the pathophysiology of a perigestational hemorrhage. In the presence of hematoma, resistance is increased and blood flow is decreased. With continuation of the pregnancy and reabsorption of the hematoma, impedance to blood flow returns to normal values. Improvement of blood flow is predictive for normal pregnancy outcome, while decreased spiral artery perfusion indicates increased risk of first- and early second-trimester loss. Since no increased risk for preterm delivery was found in patient with subchorionic hematoma, it is expected that the elevated impedance to blood flow is a transitory consequence of a compression of the arterial walls by the hemorrhage itself.

These observations seem to be helpful in clinical management and follow-up of the patients with vaginal bleeding in early pregnancy.

References

1. Timor-Tritsch, I. E., Rottem, S. and Blumenfeld, Z. (1987). Pathology of the early intrauterine pregnancy. In Timor-Tritsch, I. E. and Rottem, S. (eds.) *Transvaginal Sonography*, pp. 109–23. (New York: Elsevier)
2. Stabile, I. and Grudzinskas, J. G. (1993). Early pregnancy wastage. In Chervenak, F. A., Isaacson, G. C. and Campbell, S. (eds.) *Ultrasound in Obstetrics and Gynecology*, pp. 1417–28. (Boston; Little, Brown)
3. Mantoni, M. and Pedersen, J. F. (1981). Intrauterine hematoma: an ultrasound study of threatened abortion. *Br. J. Obstet. Gynaecol.*, **88**, 47–50
4. Stabile, I., Campbell, S. and Grudzinskas, J. G. (1989). Ultrasound assessment in complications of first trimester pregnancy. *Lancet*, **2**, 1237–9
5. Goldstein, S. R., Subramanyam, B. M., Raghavendra, B. N., Horii, S. C. and Hilton, S. (1983). Subchorionic bleeding in threatened abortion: sonographic findings and clinical significance. *Am. J. Radiol.*, **141**, 975–8
6. Jouppila, P. (1985). Clinical consequences after ultrasound diagnosis of intrauterine hematoma in threatened abortion. *J. Clin. Ultrasound*, **13**, 107–10
7. Ylöstalo, P., Ammala, P. and Seppala, M. (1984). Intrauterine hematoma and placental protein 5 in patients with uterine bleeding during pregnancy. *Br. J. Obstet. Gynaecol.*, **91**, 353–6
8. Baxi, L. and Pearlstone, M. (1991). Subchorionic hematomas and the presence of autoantibodies. *Am. J. Obstet. Gynecol.*, **165**, 1423–6
9. Guy, G., Baxi, L. and Chao, C. (1992). An unusual complication in a patient with factor IX deficiency. *Obstet. Gynecol.*, **80**, 502–4
10. Abu-Yousef, M. M., Bleicher, J. J. and Williamson, R. A. (1987). Subchorionic hemorrhage: sonographic diagnosis and clinical significance. *Am. J. Roentgenol.*, **149**, 737–40
11. Bloch, C., Altchek, A. and Levy-Ravetch, M. (1989). Sonography in early pregnancy: the significance of subchorionic hemorrhage. *M. Sinai J. Med.*, **56**, 290–3
12. Borlum, K. G., Thomsen, A., Clausen, I. and Eriksen, G. (1989). Long-term prognosis of pregnancies in women with intrauterine hematomas. *Obstet. Gynecol.*, **74**, 231–4
13. Jakab, A. Jr, Juhasz, B. and Toth, Z. (1994). Outcome of the first trimester subchorial hematomas. In *Tenth International Congress, The Fetus as a Patient*, Brijuni, Croatia, p. 54 (abstr.)
14. Nyberg, D. A., Laurence, A. M., Benedetti, T. J., Cyr, D. R. and Schulman, W. P. (1987). Placental abruption and placental hemorrhage: correlation of sonographic findings with fetal outcome. *Radiology*, **164**, 457–60
15. Pedersen, J. F. and Mantoni, N. (1990). Large intrauterine hematoma in threatened miscarriage. Frequency and clinical consequences. *Br. J. Obstet. Gynaecol.*, **97**, 75–8
16. Saurbrei, E. E. and Pham, D. H. (1986). Placental abruption and subchorionic hemorrhage in the first half of pregnancy: US appearance and clinical outcome. *Radiology*, **160**, 109–11
17. Spirit, B. A., Kagan, E. H. and Rozanski, R. M. (1979). Abruptio placentae: sonographic and pathologic correlation. *Am. J. Roentgenol.*, **133**, 877–80
18. Nyberg, D. A., Filly, R. A. and Mahoney, B. S. (1985). Early gestation: correlation of HCG levels and sonographic identification. *Am. J. Radiol.*, **144**, 951–4
19. Mandruzzato, G. P., D'Ottavio, G., Rustico, M. A., Fontana, A. and Bogalti, P. (1989). The intrauterine hematoma: diagnostic and clinical aspects. *J. Clin. Ultrasound*, **17**, 503–10
20. Dickey, R. P., Olar, T. T., Curole, D. N., Taylor, S. N. and Matulich, F. M. (1992). Relationship of first-trimester subchorionic bleeding detected by color Doppler ultrasound to subchorionic fluid, clinical bleeding and pregnancy outcome. *Obstet. Gynecol.*, **80**, 415–20
21. Jauniaux, E., Garrii, P. and Nicolaides, K. H. (1995). Ultrasonographic assessment of early pregnancy complications. In Jurkovic, D. and Jauniaux, E. (eds.) *Ultrasound and Early Pregnancy*, pp. 53–64. (Carnforth, UK: Parthenon Publishing)

22. Pearlstone, M. and Baxi, L. (1993). Sub-chorionic hematoma; a review. *Obstet. Gynaecol. Surv.*, **48**, 65–8

23. Nyberg, D. and Laing, F. C. (1992). Threatened abortion and abnormal first trimester intrauterine pregnancy. In Nyberg, D. A., Hill, L. M., Bohm-Velez, M. and Mendelson, E. B. (eds.) *Transvaginal Ultrasound*, pp. 85–104. (St Louis: Mosby Year Book)

24. Kurjak, A., Schulman, H., Zudenigo, D., Kupesic, S., Kos, M. and Goldenberg, M. (1996). Subchorionic hematomas in early pregnancy: clinical outcome and blood flow patterns. *J. Matern. Fetal Med.*, in press

25. Kurjak, A., Chervenak, F., Zudenigo, D. and Kupesic, S. (1994). Early pregnancy hemodynamics assessed by transvaginal color Doppler. In Kurjak, A. and Chervenak, F. A. (eds.) *The Fetus as a Patient*, pp. 435–55. (Carnforth, UK: Parthenon Publishing)

Color Doppler in prenatal diagnosis 5

J. M. Carrera, R. Devesa, M. Torrents, C. Mortera, C. Comas and A. Muñoz

INTRODUCTION

The introduction of color Doppler in obstetrics and gynecology has allowed the precise evaluation of the fetal cardiovascular system, not only anatomically, but also physiologically. The evaluation of fetal hemodynamics, begun with continuous and pulsed Doppler, is improved substantially with this new technique, allowing us to learn much about fetal physiology and pathophysiology.

In recent years, the interest of research investigators has been directed towards the developing embryo, and because of transvaginal color Doppler, our knowledge and understanding of the uteroplacental and embryonal circulation has improved tremendously. As such, at 7–8 weeks of gestation, it is possible to obtain images not only of the umbilical artery, but also of the aorta and intracranial arteries. However, except in cases of congenital cardiopathies, very little work has been done to evaluate the use of color Doppler in the field of prenatal diagnosis.

In this chapter, in an attempt to define the role of color Doppler in prenatal diagnosis, we will discuss color Doppler as an adjunct to invasive techniques, in the diagnosis of malformations, in general, in the diagnosis of congenital cardiopathies and in the evaluation of possible chromosomal defects.

COLOR DOPPLER AS AN ADJUNCT TO INVASIVE TECHNIQUES

The advantage of the use of color Doppler in invasive procedures in prenatal diagnosis (chorionic villus sampling, amniocentesis, funiculocentesis) resides fundamentally in the excellent vision provided of the placenta, the cord, and, in general, the integrity of the mater-

nofetal circulation. It allows greater safety, in some cases, while performing these procedures.

However, the procedure that probably benefits most from color Doppler is funiculocentesis. This system permits the identification and differentiation of the umbilical arteries and vein, facilitating remarkably, the advancement of the needle whether it is done through the placenta (anterior placenta) or through the amniotic sac (posterior placenta). Naturally, the use of color Doppler becomes even more important when it is necessary to perform, for justified indications, procedures such as the collection of fetal blood from the intrahepatic umbilical vein or the cardiac ventricles.

In spite of these undisputed advantages, we have to accept that most current invasive procedures can be performed adequately without the use of color Doppler.

COLOR DOPPLER IN THE DIAGNOSIS OF MALFORMATIONS

Color Doppler provides information that can contribute to the improved diagnosis of structural abnormalities in basically three situations:

(1) As an aid to establish the topography or origin of a structure that is poorly identified with conventional echography.
  (a) This is the case, for example, in differentiating the urinary bladder from other cystic images (Color plate 18). The bladder is always surrounded by the two fetal hypogastric arteries that are easily identified by color Doppler. As such, the visualization in this image of only one hypogastric artery would prompt confirmation of the existence

of a single hypogastric artery. If the missing artery is the right one, cytogenetic studies of the fetus are indicated since the incidence of chromosomal anomalies is multiplied by four.

(b) The anomalous localization of the intrahepatic umbilical vein may be an indication of an aberrant hepatic condition.

(c) In difficult cases, e.g. oligohydramnios, the identification of the renal vessels may be used to locate the kidney, even if it is in an ectopic location.

(2) In all defects which involve fetal circulation, especially in malformations of the central nervous system, thorax and abdomen.

(a) Malformations of the central nervous system.

(i) In hydrocephaly, compression of the cerebral circulation increases vascular resistance causing hypoxia and progressive degeneration of the cerebral parenchyma. In cases of unilateral hydrocephalus, a precocious difference may be noted in the cerebral vascular flow between the affected hemisphere and the contralateral side thus facilitating early diagnosis[1].

(ii) In cases of exencephaly, the cephalic mass may demonstrate vascular images originating from the circle of Willis in an abnormal fashion.

(iii) In encephalocoele, the visualization of vascular structures within the herniated cerebral mass permits a differential diagnosis from cystic hygroma.

(iv) In cerebral areas that appear anechogenic of hypoechogenic, color Doppler permits the differentiation between cystic or vascular origin. As such, in the aneurysm of the vein of Galen, the color Doppler study demonstrates a turbulent blood flow that is easy to identify[2,3] that permits, for example, a differential diagnosis from an arachnoid cyst (Color plate 19).

(b) Malformations of the thorax.

(i) In pulmonary sequestration, color Doppler permits the identification of the aberrant origin of the systemic vascularization of the pulmonary parenchyma, allowing it to be differentiated from an adenomatoid cystic malformation.

(ii) Similarly, color Doppler improves the diagnosis of all intra- or extracardiac malformations that are accompanied by an anomalous venous return (inferior or superior vena cava, portal vein, etc.) that can be located early on with this technique.

(c) Malformations of the abdomen.

(i) Color Doppler informs us whether vascular structures exist, or not, in abdominal cystic masses (intestinal obstruction, enteric cysts, ovarian cysts, hydrometrocolpos, obstructive uropathy, abdominal lyphangioma, etc.) in addition to helping to locate certain structures, because of their vascular relationships.

(ii) Color Doppler also permits confirmation of the absence of renal arteries in cases of bilateral renal agenesis, or in displacement of these arteries in cases of ectopic kidneys[4].

(iii) The increased vascularization in certain organs, such as the liver, permits suspicion of a hemangioma.

(iv) Additionally, color Doppler permits the confirmation of early diagnosis in cases of structural pathologies that are difficult to diagnose early. As such, in the differential diagnosis of anterior abdominal wall defects, color Doppler can demonstrate hepatic vascular displacement in the herniated mass in cases of gastroschisis and the absence of umbilical circulation with visualization of the mesenteric vessels in the base of the defect in cases of omphalocoele.

(d) Other possible contributions.

(i) Detection of a fissure of the palate, in the absence of a harelip, is possible

with color Doppler due to an abnormal oronasopharyngeal flow[5]. Color Doppler is not only capable of visualizing blood flow, but also of other liquids, such as amniotic fluid (entering and leaving the digestive and respiratory systems) and uterine (Color plate 20).
(ii) Sacrococcygeal teratoma. The great vascularity of these tumors, with a characteristic low-resistance blood flow, helps to differentiate these tumors from other diagnoses such as myelomeningocoeles.
(iii) Early diagnosis of an acardiac twin.

(3) Prenatal diagnosis of cardiopathies. The use of color Doppler in this pathology will be addressed later in this chapter.

COLOR DOPPLER IN THE DIAGNOSIS OF CONGENITAL CARDIOPATHIES

Prenatal diagnosis of congenital cardiopathies was a difficult area in echographic diagnosis until the development of special equipment for echocardiography (two-dimensional echo, time motion, pulsed and continuous Doppler, etc.) and the availability of exceptionally skilled and experienced operators. The possibility of this diagnosis is important since these pathologies can be serious and are relatively frequent (affecting eight of every 1000 live newborns), and their identification *in utero* permits adequate evaluation and follow-up after the delivery.

The development of color Doppler signified an important milestone in our diagnostic capabilities in this specific field. Currently, the sensitivity of echocardiography and color Doppler together in diagnosing a congenital cardiopathy easily exceeds 90%.

Advantages and inconveniences of color Doppler

The use of color Doppler provides additional *advantages* compared to conventional Doppler echography[6]. It improves the definition, be-

cause of opacification of color, of both vascular canals and cardiac chambers. In contrast to 2-dimensional echography, color Doppler does not leave any spaces echo free. It permits the rapid identification of communications between the different chambers, both normal and those produced by septal defects. It immediately defines turbulent flow (mosaic effect) and/or high velocity (shunting effect) drawing rapid attention towards areas of abnormal circulation. Color Doppler allows the rapid recognition of valvular regurgitation. It facilitates the positioning of the sampling volume of pulsed Doppler, thus shortening the examining time, and thus, exposure to the Doppler. Finally, it is safer than pulsed Doppler since it necessitates a lower maximum intensity. The power necessary in color Doppler, (spatial peak temporal average < 100 mW/cm^2) has been accepted to be within established limits in diagnostic ultrasound.

Color Doppler also has *limitations*[7]. Its use in fetal echocardiography is limited by the depth of the structures being evaluated and by its poor penetration. The fetal heart is normally situated at 5–10 cm from the transducer, but in some cases this distance is increased considerably (maternal obesity, polyhydramnios, placenta previa, etc.) which means that color Doppler is of little use. Increasing the emission frequency (5–7.5 MHz) may improve the situation, but results are often inadequate and unreliable. Interpretation of the images is not always easy. A skilled expert is necessary, preferably one who dedicates himself exclusively to prenatal echocardiography. Sometimes, normal patterns of flow are erroneously considered to be pathological because of the phenomenon of shunting. This effect, which generally accompanies high velocities, can appear with normal velocities when transducers of high frequency are used. Finally, its cost is considered a limitation since its use is inaccessible to many services.

Practical use of color Doppler in prenatal diagnosis

Color Doppler is very useful in the first phase of the echocardiographic examination since it provides rapid identification of the great vessels, such as the aorta and the pulmonary artery, allowing for immediate orientation by the examiner.

In a *normal fetus*, color Doppler allows the studying of cardiovascular hemodynamics with great simplicity[8]. Venous circulation is easily observed by identifying blood flow in the superior vena cava and inferior to the right atrium, as well as blood flow through the foramen ovale to the left atrium. It is also easy to define both afferent and efferent vessels of both ventricles. The aortic arch is also identified without difficulty and the presence of an 'aliasing' phenomenon in the region of the ductus often facilitates the identification of this structure. In the same manner, it is possible to clearly observe the turbulent flow of the pulmonary artery and its branches. The fact that color Doppler completely opacifies these vessels greatly facilitates the measurement of their diameters.

In *fetuses with congenital cardiopathies*, the additional information provided by color Doppler facilitates the identification and documentation of a certain number of anomalies, especially septi, valvular regurgitation and complex lesions. According to Copel and colleagues[9] 20% of cardiopathies can be diagnosed *in utero* only with the use of color Doppler, therefore this technique is considered essential in these cases. In 47% of cardiopathies, the contribution of color Doppler is considered useful but not essential, and in 24%, color Doppler does not provide any additional diagnostic information than that provided by conventional echocardiography.

In general, we can say that color Doppler is essential to determine the course and direction of blood flow in the great vessels, is helpful but not essential in identifying the tiny 'jets' in areas of regurgitation from the atrioventricular valves, and, finally, it is not essential in diagnosing the majority of anatomic congenital cardiopathies which are generally readily identified with two dimensional ultrasound[9]. The congenital cardiopathies that are diagnosed much more readily with color Doppler, or those cases in which color Doppler is essential, are listed in Table 1. However, as already mentioned, the

Table 1 *Congenital cardiopathies diagnosed more readily with color Doppler and cases in which color Doppler is essential*

Transposition of the great vessels
Truncous arteriosis
Ebstein's anomaly
Hypoplastic left heart
Aortic stenosis and coarctation of the aorta
Pulmonary stenosis
Right ventricle with double outlet
Tetralogy of Fallot

contribution of color Doppler is not essential in septal defects of the ventricles, atria, or atrialventricular defects, or in other pathologies such as dextrocardia.

COLOR DOPPLER IN EVALUATING THE RISK OF CHROMOSOMAL DEFECTS

Besides the morphological examination of the fetus to exclude any type of structural anomaly, this examination, performed between weeks 16 and 18 of gestation, should search for the indirect signs of chromosomal defects, phenotypic markers of aneuploidy and cardiopathies commonly associated with chromosomal defects.

Diagnosis of indirect signs of chromosomal defects

A *single umbilical artery* is a sign associated with a large number of syndromes, perinatal complications, intrauterine growth retardation and fetal malformations. Between 12 and 47% of these disorders are associated with chromosomal defects. The incidence of this sign is around 1% in singleton pregnancies and 4.6% in twin gestations. The incidence is estimated to be higher when the diagnosis is made during the first trimester. Early detection is aided by the use of transvaginal color Doppler. Prenatal diagnosis by color Doppler during the course of the first trimester has recently been described. However, early diagnosis is accompanied by a higher rate of false positives, and this is why confirmation of the diagnosis during the second half of gestation is recommended.

Pseudocysts of the umbilical cord have recently been associated with chromosomal defects of the fetus, especially trisomies 18 and 13. Unlike true cysts, these pseudocysts display focal degeneration of the Wharton's jelly without involving embryonic vestigial structures of the omphalomesenteric or alantoid canals. Detection of isolated umbilical pseudocysts is considered to be an indication for further cytogenetic studies of the fetus. Even though the published literature refers to diagnosis in the second half of gestation, the introduction of transvaginal ultrasound testing and color Doppler means that prenatal diagnosis can be made earlier.

Increased resistance in umbilical circulation without simultaneous alteration of uterine flow is a warning sign commonly described in the second half of gestation associated with the manifestation of perinatal complications and chromosomal defects[10]. Application of this measurement for predicting aneuploid and/or imminent fetal death in the early stages of gestation have recently been described. Color Doppler is very useful during early gestation as it facilitates the localization of the umbilical cord and improves the measurement of the indices by completely opacifying the vessel.

Shortening of the length of the umbilical cord has recently been associated with several malformations and chromosomal defects[11]. Color Doppler is very useful when performing this measurement during the first trimester of gestation as it allows the tracing of the umbilical cord all the way from the placenta insertion to the fetal insertion.

Persistence of the choroidal artery, a branch of the ophthalmic artery, beyond week 25 (under normal circumstances it is not apparent during the last 3 months), is associated with trisomies and central nervous system anomalies[2,3].

Detection of markers of aneuploidy by ultrasound

Although the use of color Doppler improves the imaging of some markers (choroidal plexus cysts, signs of nuchal translucency, hyperechogenicity of the intestine, etc.), according to some reports[12], it does not increase the sensitivity of ultrasound in identifying fetuses with chromosomal abnormalities (Table 2) in a statistically significant way, except for pyelectasis where the differences are very noticeable (Tables 3 and 4).

Finding these markers and, in general, detection of the characteristic morphological profile of each trisomy depend more on the skills and experience of the operator than the availability of color Doppler, even though the sensitivity of finding one or more echographic abnormalities to identify fetuses with chromosomal anomalies seems to increase for both trisomy 21 and chromosomal anomalies in general when color Doppler is added in real-time imaging (Table 5). The literature quotes sensitivity figures ranging from 19 to 75%[13-15].

Identification of heart defects

The examination of the heart is particularly important given that between 16 and 20% of fetuses with congenital heart defects are carriers of chromosomal anomalies[12,16] and between 50 and 52% of the chromosomal

Table 2 *Chromosomal defects: incidence and positive predictive value (PPV) of the echographic findings*

Finding	Incidence (%)		PPV (%)	
	Literature	Color Doppler	Literature	Color Doppler
≥ 1 Abnormal findings*	NA	10.7	11–14.7	16
≥ 2 Abnormal findings*	NA	2.9	26–29	39
Choroid plexus cysts*	1.9	2.8	10	17
Nuchal translucency**	0.7	0.78	28	31
Intestinal hyperechogenicity*	0.81	2.3	21.8	17
Pyelectasis**	2.2–2.8	1.6	17.25	33

*All abnormal chromosomes; **only trisomy 21; NA, not available

defects (trisomies 13, 18 and 21, triploids, unbalanced translocations, etc.) indicate complex heart defects[12,15,17]. The most important problem associated with examination of the fetal heart is improper recognition of congenital defects before week 18 of gestation[18].

In the study carried out by DeVore and Alfi[12], the results of ultrasound examinations are clearly very different depending on whether conventional echography is done in real time or whether color Doppler is added. In the first case only 12% of trisomy 21 cases would have been

Table 3 *Sensitivity of abnormal ultrasound findings for identification of fetuses with trisomy 21. Reprinted with permission from the American College of Obstetricians and Gynecologists (Obstet. Gynecol., 1995, 85, 378–86)*

Abnormal ultrasound finding	Real-time imaging (n = 17)		Real-time imaging and color Doppler (n = 15)	
	%	n	%	n
Central nervous system*	0	0	20.0	3
Choroid plexus cysts	0	0	6.6	1
Nuchal translucency	12.0	2	13.0	2
Intestinal hyperechogenicity	12.0	2	13.0	2
Pyelectasis	6.0	1	33.0	5

*Including any malformation other than choroid plexus cysts

Table 4 *Sensitivity of abnormal ultrasound finding for identification of fetuses with all chromosomal abnormalities. Reprinted with permission from the American College of Obstetricians and Gynecologists (Obstet. Gynecol., 1995, 85, 378–86)*

Abnormal ultrasound finding	Real-time imaging (n = 28)		Real-time imaging and color Doppler (n = 28)	
	%	n	%	n
Central nervous system*	3.6	1	25.0	7
Choroid plexus cysts	7.0	7	18	5
Nuchal translucency	11.0	3	11.0	3
Intestinal hyperechogenicity	25.0	2	18.0	5
Pyelectasis	3.5	1	18.0	5

*Including any malformation other than choroid plexus cysts

Table 5 *Sensitivity of one or more echographic findings for the identification of fetuses with abnormal chromosomes*

Chromosomal abnormality	Sensitivity			
	Real-time imaging		Real-time imaging and color Doppler	
	%	n	%	n
Trisomy 13	0	0/0	100	1/1
Trisomy 18	50	1/2	100	7/7
Trisomy 21	29	5/17*	87	13/15
Abnormality of the sex chromosomes	25	1/4	0	0/2
Mosaicism	100	1/1	100	1/1
Triploidy	50	1/2	0	0/0
Unbalanced translocation	50	1/2	0	0/2
All chromosomal abnormalities	36	10/28**	75	21/28**

*$p < 0.002$, odds ratio = 15.6, 95% confidence interval (CI) (range 2–173); **$p < 0.006$, odds ratio = 5.4, 95% CI (range 1.5–2.0)

suspected, the percentage increased to 47% using color Doppler ($p < 0.05$ and $R = 6.1$) (Table 6). The differences are even more significant if all chromosomal abnormalities are grouped together: 7% sensitivity in real time as compared to 43% with color Doppler ($p < 0.004$ and $R = 9.7$).

The incidence of isolated ventricular septal defects diagnosed by color Doppler is clearly higher than the incidence confirmed in the newborn, in both the normal population and carriers of trisomy 21. Moe and Gunteroth[19] stated that the detection rate for this finding during gestation in fetuses without chromosomal alterations was 6.8-times greater than the figure reported at birth (6.4 vs. 0.39%) and, according to DeVore and Alfi[12], the figure was 2.1-times greater in trisomic fetuses (13 vs. 6%).

These discrepancies may be explained in several ways: possible echographic error, spontaneous abortions of some fetuses with congenital defects and closure of the defects *in utero* communication during the second half of gestation. The latter would explain the greater frequency of defects of this nature in premature babies (twice the usual number). This is also related to the progressive closure during the first year of life of a large number of the intraventricular defects. Most of these defects are located at the entry tracts or the membranous septum.

If a chromosomal abnormality is not confirmed and in the absence of any other cardiac or extracardiac structural anomaly, termination of the pregnancy must be advised against because of all the reasons given above.

Amniocentesis and detection rates by primary screening

The study of DeVore and Alfi[12] carried out on 2056 consecutive pregnant women having a theoretical trisomy 21 risk equal to or greater than 1/270 (age, biochemical screening, etc.) allows us to deduce that in patients aged 35 years or over, the trisomy 21 detection index provided by biochemical 'triple screening' gradually increases from 71% at the age of 35 to 99% at the age of 44. However, this implies a high amniocentesis rate varying between 13% at the age of 35 and 99% at the age of 46 (Figure 1).

Conversely, if a decision is made routinely to perform echocardiography using color Doppler beyond the stated age, the trisomy 21 detection rate remains invariable with a sensitivity of 87%. The need to proceed with amniocentesis in cases where one or more suspicious echographic findings are apparent will therefore be reduced to 13% (Figure 2). This alternative also has the advantage of identifying a considerable number of other malformations at that time (especially cardiovascular and nervous system ones) that are not associated with an abnormal karyotype.

Evaluation of the risk of trisomy 21 using color Doppler ultrasound

In pregnant women aged 35 or over, echographic examination using color Doppler considerably alters the theoretical risk of trisomy 21[12]. If we accept that the potential risk of this trisomy is 1/270 at the age of 35 and 1/134 for any chromosomal anomaly, these indices are only reached at the age of 42 if a color Doppler

Table 6 *Sensitivity of the echographic findings of congenital cardiac defects for the identification of fetuses with abnormal chromosomes. Reprinted with permission from the American College of Obstetricians and Gynecologists (Obstet. Gynecol., 1995, **85**, 378–86)*

	Trisomy 21		All chromosomal defects	
Echographic findings	RT ($n = 17$)	RT + color Doppler ($n = 15$)	RT ($n = 28$)	RT + color Doppler ($n = 28$)
Complex cardiac defects	12% (2)*	47% (7)*	7% (2)**	43% (12)**
Interventricular septal defects	6% (1)	13% (2)	11% (3)	14% (4)

RT, echographic real-time imaging; *$p < 0.05$, odds ratio = 6.1, 95% CI 0.82–69; ** $p < 0.004$, odds ratio = 9.7, 95% CI 1.7–42

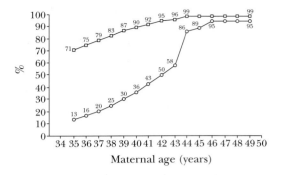

Figure 1 *The indices of detection of trisomy 21 by 'biochemical screening' beyond the age of 35 (□——□) and rate of amniocentesis (○——○) necessary to confirm the diagnosis. Reprinted with permission from the American College of Obstetricians and Gynecologists (Obstet. Gynecol., 1995, 85, 378–86)*

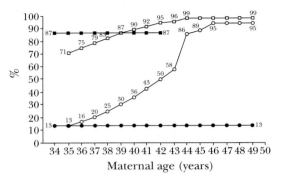

Figure 2 *The indices of detection of trisomy 21 by 'biochemical screening' beyond the age of 35 (□——□) and rate of amniocentesis (○——○) necessary to confirm the diagnosis. The performance of a color Doppler ultrasound examination concomitantly achieves a similar sensitivity rate for detecting trisomy 21 (■——■) with a reduction in the indication for amniocentesis (●——●). Reprinted with permission from the American College of Obstetricians and Gynecologists (Obstet. Gynecol., 1995, 85, 378–86)*

examination is performed to exclude anomalies. Beyond that age, the risk of trisomy 21 or any other anomaly increases as it usually does beyond the age of 35 (Figures 3 and 4). Therefore, if the color Doppler study is normal, no cytogenetic study needs to be carried out until after the age of 42.

ALTERNATIVES TO PRESENT STANDARD POLICIES

Some possible alternatives to present standards could be:

(1) To subject pregnant women under the age of 35 to an ultrasound–biochemical aneuploid screening (UBA-I screening) performed between weeks 12 and 14 of gestation. This would allow a combined risk factor index to be calculated, improving both the sensitivity and the positive predictive value (PPV) from that provided by the tests individually. It goes without saying that this examination should be done at a suitable ultrasound facility (level II/III) and vaginal probes should be used, allowing the ultrasound trisomy markers to be recognized, especially nuchal translucency (nuchal edema, cystic hygroma, etc.). Color Doppler could improve the results. The main drawback of this program would be its higher cost.

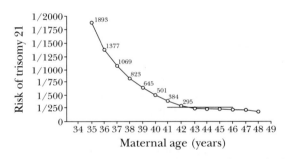

Figure 3 *When color Doppler study is normal, the risk of 1/270 for trisomy 21 (expected age 35) is reached only after age 42. Reprinted with permission from the American College of Obstetricians and Gynecologists (Obstet. Gynecol., 1995, 85, 378–86)*

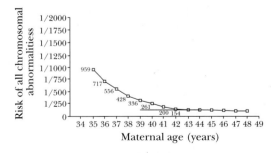

Figure 4 *When all chromosomal abnormalities are considered, the risk of 1/134 for any chromosomal anomaly, expected at age 35, is only reached at age 42, when color Doppler study excludes the presence of anomalies*

(2) To set up a specific program for pregnant women over the age of 35 involving biochemical screening and an echographic examination using color Doppler, paying special attention to the examination of the heart. This screening (UBA-II) should be performed between weeks 16 and 18 of gestation[29,30], and color Doppler would be a fundamental element in achieving good results. This examination could be an alternative for patients who reject amniocentesis. It should be done at level III facility.

(3) To design an action plan including both proposals: echographic examinations between weeks 12 and 14 (vaginal probe) and at 18 weeks (color Doppler) together with biochemical screening in all pregnant women. The high cost of this strategy probably makes it an unlikely possibility.

CONCLUSIONS

The gradual introduction of color Doppler in the field of embryonal medicine strengthens the role and capabilities of ultrasound in prenatal diagnosis. Some of the most significant contributions of this technique are:

(1) Greater safety for invasive techniques, especially funiculocentesis.

(2) Greater ease of diagnosing malformation involving the circulation, allowing a differential diagnosis to be made with other entities. Recognition of the vascular elements makes the topographical diagnosis of the different anatomical structures considerably easier.

(3) The identification of kinetic patterns of different fluids like the amniotic fluid or fetal urine. Abnormal movements or channels of these fluids leads to the suspicion of some type of malformation that is difficult to diagnose by conventional echography (pharyngeal anomalies, cleft palate, etc.)

(4) A clear increase in the diagnostic sensitivity of echocardiography. At around 20–25 weeks heart defects can only be diagnosed by color Doppler. The technique proves particularly useful in cardiopathies that alter the course and direction of the flow in the great vessels.

(5) An improvement in the value of echography in detection of chromosomal defects. Color Doppler allows better imaging of some indirect signs, especially those involving the umbilical cord (single umbilical artery, cord pseudocysts, shortening of the cord, etc.) as well as some 'phenotypic markers' such as pyelectasia.

(6) Beyond the age of 35 years performing echocardiography using color Doppler between weeks 16 and 18 of gestation attains an apparently high rate of trisomy 21 detection (87%) with an indication for amniocentesis of 13%. If this information is confirmed by a greater number of cases, this diagnostic procedure could become a valid alternative to the current standard protocols. Amniocentesis, if color Doppler echocardiographic examination is normal, would only be necessary beyond the age of 42.

References

1. Bronshtein, M. and Shlovino, B. (1991). Choroid plexus dysmorphism detected by transvaginal sonography: the earliest sign of fetal hydrocephalus. *J. Clin. Ultrasound*, **19**, 547–53

2. Bonilla-Musoles, F., Ballester, M. J. and Raga, F. (1994). Transvaginal color Doppler in early embryonic malformations. In Kurjak, A. (ed.) *An Atlas of Transvaginal Color Doppler*, pp. 105–23. (Casterton, UK: Parthenon Publishing)

3. Kurjak, A., Takeuchi, H. and Matijevic, R. (1994). Color Doppler in the second and third trimester of pregnancy. In Kurjak, A. (ed.) *An Atlas of Transvaginal Color Doppler*, pp. 139–48.(Casterton, UK: Parthenon Publishing)

4. Hecher, K., Spernol, R. and Szalay, S. (1989). Doppler blood flow velocity waveforms in the fetal renal artery. *Arch. Gynecol. Obstet.*, **246**, 133–7

5. Sherer, D. M., Abramowicz, J. S., Jaffe, R. and Woods, J. R. Jr (1993). Cleft palate: confirmation of prenatal diagnosis by colour Doppler ultrasound. *Prenat. Diagn.*, **13**, 953–6

6. Colloridi, V., Pizzuto, F., Ventriglia, F., Giglioni, E., Formigiari, R. and Pachi, A. (1992). Valoración con Doppler color del flujo sanguíneo intracardiaco y en los grandes vasos. In Carrera, J. M. (ed.) *Ecografía Obstétrica*, p. 177–84. (Barcelona: Salvat)

7. Sharland, G. K. (1992). Papel del Doppler en la ecocardiografía fetal. In Carrera, J. M. (ed.) *Doppler en Obstetricia*, p. 167–70. (Barcelona: Salvat-Masson)

8. Mortera, C., Carrera, J. M. and Torrents, M. (1992). Doppler pulsado codificado en color. Mapa Doppler color de la circulación fetal. In Carrera, J. M. (ed.) *Doppler en Obstetricia*, p. 185–98. (Barcelona: Salvat-Masson)

9. Copel, J. A., Morotti, R., Hobbins, J. C. and Kleinman, C. H. S. (1991). The antenatal diagnosis of congenital heart disease using fetal echocardiography: is color flow mapping necessary? *Obstet. Gynecol.*, **78**, 1–8

10. Carrera, J. M. and Mortera, C. (1991). Estudio Doppler de los Defectos Congénitos. Presented at *I Congreso Mundial de Obstetricia y Ginecología*, January, London

11. Szabó J., Gellén, J. and Szemere, G. (1992). Nuchal edema as an ultrasonic sign of trisomy 21 during the first trimester of pregnancy. *Orv. Hetil.*, **133**, 3167–8

12. DeVore, G. R. and Alfi, O. (1995). The use of color Doppler ultrasound to identify fetuses at increased risk for trisomy 21: an alternative for high-risk patients who decline genetic amniocentesis. *Obstet. Gynecol.*, **85**, 378–86

13. Nyberg, D. A., Resta, R. G., Luthy, D. A., Hickok, D. E., Mahoney, B. S. and Hirsch, J. H. (1990). Prenatal sonographic findings in Down syndrome. A review of 94 cases. *Obstet. Gynecol.*, **76**, 370–7

14. Benacerraf, B. R., Neuberg, D., Bromley, B. and Frigoletto, F. D. (1992). Sonographic scoring index for prenatal detection of chromosomal abnormalities. *J. Ultrasound Med.*, **11**, 449–58

15. Stoll, C., Dott, B., Alembik, Y. and Roth, M. P. (1993). Evaluation of routine prenatal ultrasound examination in detecting fetal chromosomal abnormalities in a low risk population. *Hum. Genet.*, **91**, 37–41

16. Allan, L. D., Sharland, G. K., Chita, S. K., Lockhart, S. and Maxwell, D. J. (1991). Chromosomal anomalies in fetal congenital heart disease. *Ultrasound Obstet. Gynecol.*, **1**, 8–11

17. Dicke, J. M. and Crane, J. P. (1991). Sonographic recognition of major malformations and aberrant fetal growth in trisomic fetuses. *J. Ultrasound Med.*, **10**, 433–8

18. Bromley, B., Estroff, J. A., Sanders, S. P., Parad, R., Roberts, D. and Frigoletto, F. D. Jr (1992). Fetal echocardiography: accuracy and limitations in a population at high and low risk for heart defects. *Am. J. Obstet. Gynecol.*, **166**, 1473–81

19. Moe, D. G. and Gunteroth, W. G. (1987). Spontaneous closure of uncomplicated ventricular septal defect. *Am. J. Cardiol.*, **60**, 674–8

20. DeVore, G. R., Horenstein, J., Siass, B. and Platt, L. D. (1987). Fetal echocardiography. VII. Doppler color flow mapping: a new technique for the diagnosis of congenital heart disease. *Am. J. Obstet. Gynecol.*, **156**, 1054–64

21. DeVore, G. R. (1992). The aortic and pulmonary outflow tract screening examination in the human fetus. *J. Ultrasound Med.*, **11**, 345–8

Current perspective on the evaluation of suspected intrauterine growth retardation

6

W. J. Ott

INTRODUCTION

The antenatal recognition of altered fetal growth should be an important goal for every obstetrician, since significant neonatal complications may be associated with both ends of the spectrum of altered growth. This review is a summary of the recent literature and the author's experience with the diagnosis and evaluation of altered fetal growth over the past 15 years. In addition, data from current on-going research projects will also be presented.

Our understanding of the significance of altered growth, especially intrauterine growth retardation (IUGR), is undergoing constant revision. There are significant problems in defining and diagnosing altered fetal growth, both in the antenatal and postpartum periods. This article will discuss the problems associated with the diagnosis and management of altered fetal growth.

DEFINING ALTERED GROWTH: DEFINITIONS AND ASSOCIATIONS

Intrauterine growth retardation

One of the difficulties in the evaluation, treatment and follow-up of suspected IUGR is its imprecise definition. The most commonly utilized definition of IUGR equates it with the small-for-gestational age (SGA) infant; that is, an infant with a birth weight less than a specific cut-off point based on birth weight for gestational age derived from a series of live born infants. A number of problems, however, are inherent in this definition of IUGR.

Although the most commonly used definition of IUGR equates it with those infants less than the 10th centile for gestational age, there is no uniform agreement as to the use of this cut-off point; and other centile values, such as the 5th or 3rd centile, or two or more standard deviations from the mean, have been used[1-3]. However, there are multiple non-pathological determinants of neonatal size at birth. Maternal demographic and anthropometric factors, socioeconomic conditions and environmental factors all play a role in determining neonatal size at birth[4-7]. Most importantly, the intrinsic growth potential of each fetus may result in an infant who is smaller than standard cut-off values but totally normal[8,9]. IUGR implies a pathological process which affects normal fetal growth and results in an infant whose growth is less than its inherent potential[2]. A number of chronic maternal medical conditions, such as the hemoglobinopathies or significant heart disease, result in decreased oxygen delivery leading to diminished fetal growth[3,6,10]. Other maternal diseases, especially those in which hypertension is a component, can also cause IUGR[3,6,10]. Abnormalities of placentation have also been associated with IUGR[3,6,10,11]. Other problems such as congenital anomalies or intrauterine infection damage the developing fetus and decrease its growth. These pathological processes can diminish the normal inherent growth potential of the fetus.

Villar and Belizan[12] have divided IUGR into three categories based on both etiology and timing. Type 1 are those infants with proportional growth retardation which began early in gestation (*symmetrical* IUGR). Type 2 are disproportionately growth-retarded infants who were subjected to negative growth factors around the 30th week of gestation (may be symmetrical or asymmetrical IUGR). Type 3 are those infants who suffered from decreased substrate supply in the last 4–6 weeks of pregnancy which caused a depletion of fetal fat stores. These infants are disproportionately small for their length (*asymmetrical* IUGR).

Numerous studies have reported a 5–27% incidence of congenital abnormalities associated with IUGR, as compared to a 0.1–4% anomaly rate in control groups of normally-grown neonates[13,14]. Our own experience in a series of patients scanned for suspected IUGR showed a 10% incidence of structural anomalies.

The incidence of chromosomal abnormalities in IUGR infants is 4–5 times that of average for gestational age (AGA) infants (2 vs. 0.4%)[13]. Intrauterine infection, especially cytomegalovirus which has a high incidence of severe neonatal neurological complications, has been reported in 0.3–3.5% of IUGR infants[13,14].

Significant problems also occur in IUGR infants not suffering from congenital abnormalities, intrauterine infection or other severe intrauterine complications. Growth retarded infants have up to an 8–10-fold increase in stillbirth and neonatal mortality[15–17]. This, in part, is related to a higher incidence of hypoxia, asphyxia, meconium aspiration and a generally poorer ability to tolerate labor that is seen in IUGR infants[13,14,16,18,19]. Other developmental problems, such as necrotizing enterocolitis, intraventricular hemorrhage or other complications, can also be related to IUGR. Those infants who survive the immediate perinatal period are still at risk for hypothermia, hypoglycemia, polycythemia and other neonatal complications[13,16,20].

Follow-up evaluations of IUGR infants have been hampered by the heterogeneous nature of the infants studied. As discussed later in this chapter, the imprecise nature of the definition of IUGR has frequently led to the inclusion of non-growth retarded (but SGA) infants or small, premature (neither IUGR nor SGA) infants in follow-up studies of low birth weight (and presumably growth retarded) neonates. Recent review articles by Allen[13], Taylor[14] and Jones and Roberton[16] have discussed the problems inherent in follow-up studies of suspected growth-retarded infants.

Obviously, the etiology of the IUGR also has a significant bearing on neonatal outcome. Keeping these restrictions in mind, some follow-up studies of growth-retarded infants who did not have structural, chromosomal, or infections complications have shown catch-up somatic growth in IUGR infants[16,20–22], while other studies have shown these infants to be significantly smaller than their AGA cohorts[23–25]. A follow-up study of infant somatic growth by Holmes and colleagues[26] divided infants into SGA, AGA and LGS (large-for-gestational-age) groups, and further subdivided SGA infants into two subgroups based on their ponderal index. Infants with low ponderal indices ('true' IUGR) showed significant catch-up growth, while infants with normal ponderal indices (constitutionally small infants not actually growth retarded) did not show catch-up growth.

Follow-up neurodevelopmental studies of IUGR infants suffer from the same problems as somatic growth studies[27]. However, early evidence seemed to indicate that, when corrected for socioeconomic and etiological factors, most IUGR infants have normal neurological and developmental evaluation by the age of 2 years[23–28]. A recent study by Spinillo and co-workers[29] followed 236 singleton pregnancies with idiopathic IUGR and found a direct correlation between the severity of the growth retardation and neurodevelopmental outcome by age of 2 years. Paz and associates[30] compared the cognitive performance and schooling achievements at the age of 17 years of 64 children born at term whose weights were less than the third centile, but otherwise normal, to 1643 matched AGA controls; and found small, but significant decreases in intellectual testing scores and academic achievement in the SGA group[30]. These differences appeared to be unrelated to their intranatal course. Whether or not these small but significant differences between AGA and idiopathic IUGR infants will be diminished or eliminated by current methods of diagnosis and treatment of IUGR has yet to be determined.

Additional definitions of altered fetal growth

Many investigators feel that the use of other neonatal morphometric measurements, such as the neonatal ponderal index (the neonatal weight in grams divided by the cube of the crown–heel length in centimeters, times 100) or skin-fold thickness avoids the problems associated with birth weight for gestational age and is a more accurate method of diagnosing altered fetal growth[31–35].

Neonatal ponderal index is a measurement of soft-tissue and muscle mass[6,31,33–37]. Asymmetrically growth retarded infants will have low ponderal index, while symmetrically growth retarded infants will have normal ponderal indices. LGA infants will have elevated ponderal indices. Although there appears to be some change in ponderal index with gestational age, most investigators use a lower level of 2.2 and an upper level of 3.0 in defining normal growth and proportionality[6,33].

This measurement of neonatal proportions gives more information on the nutritional status of the neonate and is relatively independent of race, sex or gestational age[37]. This has led many investigators to advocate its use for defining altered fetal growth[6,10,38–43]. However, recent research on SGA infants delivering at term has cast doubt on the validity of the ponderal index.

SGA vs. IUGR

Although IUGR and SGA are not synonymous terms, most methods of diagnosis involve the identification of the SGA infant. All SGA infants may not weight less than an arbitrary cut-off value for birth weight when compared to their cohorts because of a pathological process.

Recent studies have cast doubt on the concept of IUGR in the term infant[44], while other studies have questioned the value of the neonatal ponderal index, especially in term infants[43–45]. Catalano and colleagues[43] studied a group of 188 normal neonates from uncompli-

cated singleton term pregnancies and found an extremely poor correlation between ponderal index and percentage body fat. In a recent review, Chard and co-workers[44] argued that rather than identifying asymmetrical growth retardation, low ponderal indices represent a continuum of weight and body proportion rather than a distinct subgroup of asymmetrically retarded infants. They hypothesised that, at least in term infants, the concept of asymmetric and symmetric growth retardation is an artefact, and that true intrauterine growth retardation does not exist in term infants.

A recent study at this author's institution retrospectively evaluated the significance of low birth weight for gestational age, neonatal ponderal index and the presence of maternal risk factors in predicting neonatal outcome, during the years 1990 and 1991. The following information was tabulated: the presence of maternal risk factors, gestational age at delivery, birth weight, neonatal ponderal index, perinatal mortality, significant congenital anomalies, significant neonatal morbidity, Apgar score < 7 at 5 min and length of stay in the neonatal intensive care unit. SGA infants were defined as those infants with a birth weight of less than the 10th centile for gestational age from the combined fetal weight for gestational age curves of Ott[46] and Hadlock and associates[47,48] (Table 1 and Figure 1).

A total of 1316 neonates were studied. Table 2 shows the types and frequency of indications

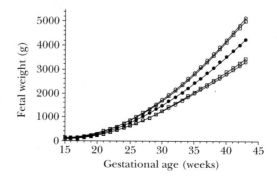

Figure 1 *Combined fetal weight for gestational age curve from the Hadlock and co-workers[48] and Ott[46] curves. Open circles, 5th and 95th centiles; open squares, 10th and 90th centiles; closed circles, 50th centile*

Table 1 *Fetal weight (g) for gestational age data*

Gestational age (weeks)	5th centile	10th centile	50th centile	90th centile	95th centile
15	115	119	139	158	162
16	127	131	152	174	178
17	150	155	180	205	210
18	184	190	221	251	257
19	229	237	274	312	319
20	285	294	340	386	395
21	350	362	418	474	486
22	426	439	508	576	589
23	510	526	608	690	706
24	603	622	720	817	837
25	704	727	842	957	979
26	813	840	974	1108	1134
27	930	960	1115	1270	1301
28	1053	1088	1266	1444	1479
29	1183	1223	1426	1628	1668
30	1318	1364	1594	1823	1869
31	1460	1511	1770	2028	2079
32	1606	1663	1953	2243	2300
33	1757	1821	2144	2467	2531
34	1912	1983	2342	2700	2771
35	2071	2149	2546	2942	3020
36	2233	2320	2756	3192	3278
37	2399	2493	2971	3449	3544
38	2566	2669	3192	3715	3818
39	2736	2848	3418	3987	4099
40	2907	3029	3648	4266	4388
41	3079	3211	3882	4552	4684
42	3252	3395	4119	4844	4987

Table 2 *Indications for ultrasound examination*

	Frequency (%)
Genetic amniocentesis	30.5
Fetal well-being	17.6
Maternal hypertension	20.2*
Maternal diabetes	14.2*
Poor obstetric history	7.7*
Fetal viability	6.4*
Antiphospholipid antibody	1.3*
Not stated	51.2*
Rule out fetal anomaly	14.3
Evaluation of fetal growth	10.8
Amniotic fluid abnormality	6.5
Placental abnormality	4.4
Multiple gestation	4.2
Preterm labor	3.8
Premature rupture of membranes	3.4
Maternal indications	1.5
Isoimmunization	0.8
Other	2.2

*Percentage distribution of complications associated with evaluation of fetal well-being

for ultrasound examination that were present or developed later in pregnancy. The types and frequency of significant neonatal morbidity that occurred are shown in Table 3.

Neonatal outcome for the entire group, stratified as to whether or not infants were SGA, is shown in Table 4. There were significant differences in all outcome parameters when SGA and non-SGA infants were compared. There were no significant differences in the distribution of the types of anomalies seen in SGA or non-SGA infants.

Because of the possible interrelated effects of gestational age at delivery, maternal risk factors, birth weight and ponderal indices, the data were subdivided into three gestational age groupings (delivery at or beyond 37 weeks, between 34 and 36 completed weeks and at < 34 weeks' gestation). The infants with normal or abnormal occurrence of the three classifications to be evaluated (birth weight for gestational age, maternal risk factors and ponderal index) were then compared within each gestational age group. Table 5 shows the results of this analysis for infants without significant congenital anomalies.

For all gestational age groups there were significant differences in ponderal index when

Table 3 *Significant neonatal morbidity*

	Frequency (n)
Respiratory distress syndrome*	40
Sepsis	16
CNS anomalies[†]	13
Persistent fetal circulation	11
Pneumothorax	9
Intraventricular/cranial hemorrhagia	8
Extreme immaturity	5
Hypoglycemia	4
Necrotizing enterocolitis	2
Neonatal hydrops	2
Retinopathy	1
Severe arrhythmia	1
Multiple[‡]	14
Total	128

CNS, central nervous system; *requiring intubation or continuous positive pressure ventilation, also includes pulmonary hypoplasia; [†]includes seizures, encephalopathy, or abnormal neurological examination; [‡]multiple physical or physiological abnormalities requiring intensive care

Table 4 *Neonatal outcome in total patient population* (n = 1316)

	SGA by birth weight centile	Not SGA	Significance
n	255 (19.4%)	1061 (80.6%)	
Maternal high risk	86 (33.7%)	247 (23.3%)	< 0.001
Gestational age at delivery (weeks)	36.6 ± 4.9	38.2 ± 3.1	< 0.0001
Birth weight (g)	2150 ± 753	3334 ± 686	< 0.001
Apgar < 7 at 5 min	9.3%	3.5%	< 0.01
Ponderal index	2.1528 ± 0.4041	2.4548 ± 0.8967	< 0.001
Days in ICU	14.2 ± 27.3	3.3 ± 13.1	< 0.0001
Mortality	24 (9.4%)	17 (1.6%)	< 0.0001
Morbidity	27.6%	7.0%	< 0.0001
Significant anomalies	24 (9.4%)	44 (4.1%)	< 0.001

SGA, small for gestational age

infants were classified by birth weight, and significant differences in birth weight when infants were classified by ponderal index. When infants were classified by maternal risk factors, the only significant differences in birth weight (lower birth weight in the high-risk group) were seen in the infants who delivered at or beyond 37 weeks' gestational age. There were no differences in ponderal index for any gestational age group when infants were classified by maternal risk factors.

Neonatal outcome parameters

Infants delivering at or beyond 37 weeks' gestation
Although SGA infants spent on average 4 more days in the intensive care unit than non-SGA infants, this was not a statistically significant difference. Because there were only three perinatal deaths, the difference in perinatal mortality between SGA and non-SGA infants could not be evaluated. The two deaths in the SGA group, not attributable to congenital anomalies, were a stillbirth where no diagnosis was made, and a SGA neonate delivered of a mother with disseminated herpes infection with evidence of chronic abruption. The infant died from severe intraventricular hemorrhage. Except for these two infants, there were no essential differences in outcome between SGA and non-SGA infants.

Classification by ponderal index showed no differences in neonatal outcome parameters or maternal risk factors.

Classification by maternal risk showed an increased incidence of low Apgar scores and a higher incidence of significant neonatal morbidity in infants delivered of mothers with risk factors.

Infants delivering between 34 and 36 weeks' gestation
Classification by birth weight showed a significant increase in the number of days spent in the neonatal intensive care unit when infants were SGA. Classification by ponderal index and by maternal risk showed no significant differences in neonatal outcome.

Infants delivering at less than 34 weeks' gestation
Classification by birth weight showed both a significant increase in the number of days spent in the neonatal intensive care unit and an increased incidence of significant neonatal morbidity in SGA infants.

Classification by ponderal index showed no significant differences in neonatal outcome.

Classification by maternal risk showed a significant increased number of days spent in the neonatal intensive care unit for infants delivered of mothers with risk factors.

Logistic regression analysis

The logistic regression analysis of infants without congenital anomalies indicates even less of an association between birth weight for gestational age, ponderal index or maternal risk with the three parameters of neonatal outcome evaluated (mortality, morbidity and low 5 min Apgar scores) than did the univariate analysis.

Table 5 Significant outcome parameters stratified by gestational age at delivery and excluding congenital anomalies

	SGA	Not SGA	PI < 2.2	PI > 2.2	High risk	Not high risk
> 37 weeks						
n	150 (15.7%)	807 (84.3%)	66 (25.0%)	198 (75.0%)	194 (20.3%)	763 (79.7%)
Maternal high risk	38 (25%)*	152 (18.8%)	19 (28.8%)*	38 (19.2%)	194 (100%)**	0
Gestational age at delivery (weeks)	39.5 ± 1.6*	39.5 ± 1.2	39.3 ± 1.4*	39.3 ± 1.3	39.2 ± 1.3*	39.5 ± 1.2
Birth weight (g)	2464 ± 472**	3565 ± 457	2867 ± 567**	3381 ± 644	3289 ± 699**	3448 ± 526
Apgar < 7 at 5 min	1.8%*	1.9%	1.9%*	1.9%	7.1%**	0.6%
Ponderal index	2.1264 ± 0.2163**	2.4287 ± 0.2749	2.0411 ± 0.1382**	2.4836 ± 0.2366	2.3598 ± 0.3256*	2.3685 ± 0.2292
Days in ICU	3.8 ± 18.0*	0.6 ± 8.6	1.0 ± 3.2*	4.7 ± 23.2	2.2 ± 13.3*	0.6 ± 9.0
Mortality	2 (1.3%)***	0	0*	0	1 (0.5%)*	1 (0.1%)
Morbidity	5.8%*	2.1%	4.8%*	11.6%	6.8%**	1.7%
Significant anomalies	4 (2.6%)*	24 (3.0%)	4 (6.1%)*	24 (12.1%)	5 (2.6%)*	23 (3.0%)
34–36 weeks						
n	47 (24.5%)	145 (75.5%)	45 (37.5%)	75 (62.5%)	61 (33.5%)	121 (66.5%)
Maternal high risk	17 (36.1%)*	44 (30.3%)	25 (55.6%)**	20 (26.7%)	61 (100%)**	0
Gestational age at delivery (weeks)	35.7 ± 0.9*	35.9 ± 0.8	35.7 ± 0.9*	35.8 ± 0.8	35.9 ± 0.7*	35.9 ± 0.8
Birth weight (g)	1953 ± 254**	2902 ± 447	2316 ± 486**	2681 ± 582	2650 ± 622*	2693 ± 553
Apgar < 7 at 5 min	0*	0	0*	0	0*	0
Ponderal index	2.2331 ± 0.2971**	2.4050 ± 0.3188	2.0369 ± 0.1125**	2.5311 ± 0.2578	2.3184 ± 0.3837*	2.3639 ± 0.228
Days in ICU	12.1 ± 9.1**	3.1 ± 6.2	8.3 ± 8.9*	6.6 ± 8.3	6.5 ± 8.7*	4.1 ± 7.1
Mortality	0	0	0*	0	0*	0
Morbidity	8.5%*	11.7%	11.1%*	13.3%	11.5%*	6.6%
Significant anomalies	6 (12.8%)**	0	4 (8.8%)*	7 (9.3%)	5 (8.2%)*	12 (9.9%)
< 34 weeks						
n	42 (37.2%)	71 (62.8%)	45 (50.6%)	44 (49.4%)	61 (54%)	52 (46%)
Maternal high risk	27 (64.3%)*	34 (47.9%)	26 (57.8%)*	24 (54.5%)	61 (100%)**	0
Gestational age at delivery (weeks)	28.3 ± 4.7*	30.2 ± 4.2	29.9 ± 4.3*	30.9 ± 2.7	29.4 ± 4.1*	29.6 ± 4.9
Birth weight (g)	1028 ± 540**	1846 ± 627	1425 ± 627**	1820 ± 666	1481 ± 791*	1613 ± 720
Apgar < 7 at 5 min	48.1%*	33.8%	23.3%*	23%	25%*	27.1%
Ponderal index	1.9912 ± 0.4624**	2.5185 ± 2.1352	1.8905 ± 0.3353**	2.7553 ± 2.3505	2.4670 ± 2.2614*	2.1247 ± 0.3950*
Days in ICU	59.1 ± 37.4**	29.3 ± 25.9	43.0 ± 33.0*	37.1 ± 29.4	45.5 ± 36.3**	26.6 ± 21.6
Mortality	12 (28.6%)*	13 (18.3%)	7 (15.6%)*	1 (2.3%)	12 (19.7%)*	1 (1.9%)
Morbidity	61.9%*	32.3%	48.9%*	45.6%	55.7%*	59.6%
Significant anomalies	6 (14.3%)*	14 (19.7%)	8 (17.8%)*	8 (18.2%)	8 (13.1%)*	12 (23.1%)

SGA, small for gestational age; PI, ponderal index. 'Significant anomalies' indicates the number of patients with anomalies that were excluded from the study. Comparisons were performed by t-test for numerical data and χ^2 analysis for distributional data. *Non-significant difference ($p > 0.01$); **significant difference ($p < 0.01$); ***too few deaths to analyse

Only the presence of maternal risk factors in infants delivering at or beyond 37 weeks showed a significant association with outcome; and infants classified as SGA delivering at < 34 weeks also showed a significant association with poor outcome.

This analysis shows the complex relationships between birth weight, gestational age and maternal risk factors as they relate to neonatal outcome. Our interpretation of the results suggests that the hypothesis of Chard and associates[44] may be correct, that intrauterine growth retardation, as a pathological process leading to poor neonatal outcome and based on low birth weight for gestational age in the infant delivered at or beyond 37 weeks, may be a myth. Stratifying term infants as SGA by birth weight or ponderal index showed no differences in neonatal outcome parameters. Stratification by maternal risk factors, however, did. This is also consistent with Chard's hypothesis that suggested that classification of infants delivering at term as IUGR is only of value in cases where there is specific evidence of maternal complications.

In preterm infants, especially those infants delivering at < 34 weeks' gestational age, both classification of infants as SGA and the presence of maternal risk factors did predict poor neonatal outcome. This is consistent with the theory proposed by Ott[46] and Hadlock and colleagues[48] that suggests there is a strong relationship between preterm delivery and intrauterine growth retardation, and that these IUGR infants are at increased risk.

Classifying infants as symmetrically or asymmetrically growth retarded by using neonatal ponderal index showed no prognostic significance[47]. This is also consistent with the statement of Chard and co-workers who felt that there was a continuum of weight and body proportion rather than a distinct subgroup of asymmetrically growth retarded infants.

Caution should be used in the evaluation of these results, however, because of a number of hidden biases in the study:

(1) Multiple gestations were included in the study. The majority of previous studies on IUGR have excluded multiple gestations from the analysis. However, multiple gestation itself is a risk factor for IUGR. A comparison of neonatal outcome parameters between single and multiple gestation showed no significant differences.

(2) Infants in the study with significant risk factors or who developed signs of fetal compromise during the pregnancy were serially evaluated using biophysical testing and the information was available to the attending physician. This may have led to earlier delivery of SGA infants with a resultant biased decrease in IUGR infants at term. An alternative interpretation, however, would be that infants with abnormal biophysical parameters requiring earlier delivery were true IUGR infants, while SGA infants delivering at term (and having normal biophysical parameters) were not growth retarded but only SGA.

(3) Only 37% of the infants studied had ponderal indices available for analysis, and this certainly may have introduced bias into the results. However, proportionally as many high-risk SGA preterm infants were without ponderal indices as were low-risk non-SGA term infants.

Although firm conclusions cannot be made from this analysis, the data do support the hypothesis of Chard and associates that suggests that true IUGR at term does not exist. In addition, it confirms that IUGR (as equated with the SGA infant) and maternal risk factors are associated with increased neonatal morbidity in the preterm infants. Additional prospective studies of this type may further clarify the complex topic of intrauterine growth retardation.

Intrauterine growth retardation and preterm delivery

An additional problem in defining SGA or IUGR infants involves the birth weight standards themselves. A number of birth weight standards exist and vary from one another because of differences in patient population, time and location[49–52]. As Wilcox[53] has pointed out, birth weight for gestational age standards are an over simplification of a complex relationship between weight, gestational age and other factors influencing size at birth.

A problem inherent in all birth weight standards is the inclusion of premature infants. By definition, premature delivery (< 37 weeks' gestation) is an abnormal occurrence. Current understanding of the etiology of premature labor is at best incomplete, and one possible explanation for its occurrence may be altered fetal growth. Recent studies have shown a disproportionately large number of growth retarded infants delivered from mothers in premature labor[54], and ultrasonographic studies of fetal growth suggest that prematurely delivered infants weigh less than their normal intrauterine cohorts[55,56]. These data suggest that standards based on birth weight data may be too low.

Since preterm infants may have a significantly higher incidence of SGA than that of infants born at term, a study was recently undertaken at the author's institution designed to evaluate the rate of SGA in infants born prior to the 37th completed week of gestation and compare it to the rate of SGA at term[46]. Computerized discharge data from all live-born infants delivered at the author's institution for the years 1990 and 1991 were used for analysis. Data from the computerized discharge summaries for the year 1990 were used to construct a postnatal birth weight for gestational age curve for that patient population. This curve was then used to analyze the 1991 birth weight data and determine the incidence of SGA infants at each week of gestation, defined as an infant less than the 10th centile of birth weight for gestational age based on the 1990 birth weight curve.

In addition, 1991 infants were also classified as SGA based on the 10th centile values of three other curves: one additional postnatal birth weight for gestational age curve (Brenner and associates[57]), and two antenatal ultrasonic estimated fetal weight for gestational age curves: an estimated fetal weight curve derived from normal singleton pregnancies scanned from 1987 to 1990; and the fetal growth curve of Hadlock and co-workers[48].

The percentage of infants at each gestational age from the 1991 data that were below the 10th centile value of each curve was calculated. In addition, infants were divided into two larger groups: those who delivered at < 37 weeks (preterm), and those who delivered after 37 weeks (term). The number of infants classified as SGA by each of the four curves was then determined for the preterm and term groups.

During 1991 there were 5908 live-born infants. The percentage of infants classified as SGA by each weight curve is listed in Table 6. Linear regression analysis showed that both ultrasound curves had a significant decrease in the incidence of SGA with advancing gestational age while the postnatal 1990 birth weight and Brenner and colleagues' curve did not. Logarithmic transformation of the data gave similar results.

Table 7 shows the percentage of infants, classified as SGA by each of the curves, that delivered before the 37th completed week (preterm) or after the 37th week (term). Both ultrasound curves showed a significant increase in the incidence of SGA in preterm infants (< 37 weeks) when compared to term infants. The Brenner and colleagues' curve also showed a significant difference, but not as strongly as the ultrasound curves. Classification by the 1990 birth weight curve did not show a significant difference.

Results of this analysis give full support to previous reports that suggested that SGA infants

Table 6 *Percentage of infants diagnosed as small for gestational age*

Gestational age (weeks)	Weight curves			
	Hadlock et al.[48]	SJMMC-BW	SJMMC-US	Brenner et al.[57]
31	14.3	14.3	33.3	14.3
32	11.1	11.1	27.8	11.1
33	17.6	5.9	26.5	2.9
34	8.5	4.3	23.4	4.3
35	7.0	7.0	11.6	7.0
36	6.3	5.8	14.7	6.3
37	3.1	3.4	8.0	3.4
38	1.1	1.9	4.3	2.3
39	1.5	2.7	4.4	2.3
40	1.5	6.2	7.2	1.8

SJMMC-BW, birthweight for gestational age curve from 1990; SJMMC-US, ultrasonic fetal weight curve

Table 7 *Preterm delivery and small-for-gestational-age infants*

Weight curve	IUGR (%)		Significance	
	< 37 weeks	> 37 weeks	χ^2	p
Hadlock et al.[48]	7.9	1.5	79.14	< 0.00001
SJMMC-US	23.1	8.3	111.3	< 0.00001
SJMMC-BW	6.3	4.0	4.691	NS
Brenner et al.[57]	6.3	2.1	27.46	< 0.0001

SJMMC-BW, birthweight for gestational age curve from 1990; SJMMC-US, ultrasonic fetal weight curve

occur more commonly in preterm than in term deliveries[51,58–61]. A recent prospective study of Hediger and associates[62] has confirmed the author's findings. They followed 290 primigravidae and compared fetal growth characteristics between fetuses that delivered prematurely and those that delivered at term. By 32 weeks' gestation, fetuses that later delivered preterm were significantly smaller than fetuses that delivered at term. Infants that were delivered prematurely for medical or obstetric indications were asymmetrically small, while infants that delivered preterm after premature rupture of the membranes or failed tocolyis for idiopathic preterm labor were symmetrically small. These authors also felt that current birth weight for gestational age standards under estimate the proportion of preterm infants who are actually growth retarded.

These studies are all consistent with the basic hypothesis that SGA (and probably IUGR) is significantly related to preterm birth, and that population specific postnatal birth weight for gestational age curves under estimate its incidence.

Despite improved understanding of the pathophysiological mechanisms involved in preterm labor and the development of a variety of drugs to combat preterm uterine contractions, there appears to be little, if any, reduction in the overall incidence of preterm deliveries in the United States[63]. Intrauterine infection, fetal congenital anomalies and others problems appear to be significantly related to preterm birth. The above studies also suggest that SGA is also associated with preterm delivery. This is consistent with the findings of Salafia and co-workers[64,65] who have shown a high rate of placental and decidual vascular abnormalities in preterm births. These findings suggest a possible interrelated cause for SGA infants and preterm delivery and point to the need for careful evaluation of patients in preterm labor to rule out underlying associations, such as IUGR, that may contribute to or cause preterm labor.

Ultrasonic fetal weight curves

An additional factor complicating the use of birth weight standards to define SGA/IUGR is the accuracy of gestational age estimation. Even under ideal clinical situations, the use of historical (last menstrual period, LMP) or clinical data to calculate gestational age has an inherent 2-week error[66–68]. In an attempt to minimize this error most birth weight for gestational age studies have used large numbers of patients for developing their curves[57,69–71]. Examination of the data in these studies suggests that there is still unintentional bias because of the inclusion of large numbers of patients with uncertain or erroneous LMPs, especially at both extremes of gestational age. A recent study of Secher and associates[72] showed a more linear relationship between gestational age and birth weight than previous studies, and the authors attributed this to the use of ultrasound for more accurate gestational dating in their study population.

One attempt at overcoming some of the above mentioned problems is the use of ultrasonic measurements to calculate an estimated fetal weight and develop intrauterine fetal weight curves[34,73]. Although the accuracy of gestational age estimation is improved in these studies, the small numbers of patients analyzed and the inherent error in the ultrasonic formulas for weight estimation make even these curves somewhat suspect.

Large for gestational age infants

Macrosomic, or LGA infants can have different, but equally as serious perinatal problems as SGA infants. Traumatic delivery with clavicular, humeral or other fractures; dystocia;

neurological complications, such as fascial or brachial palsies; and meconium aspiration are all known complications of the delivery of an LGA infant[74–77]. Lazer and colleagues[78] reported the complications of 525 infants weighing > 4500 g that delivered at a single institution in Israel between 1972 and 1982. Table 8 compares labor and delivery complications of these macrosomic infants to a control group of infants weighing between 2500 and 4000 g.

In the neonatal period these infants, especially if they are delivered of a mother with glucose intolerance, are prone to hypoglycemia, hypocalcemia and other metabolic complications[77]. In addition, although size and proportionality are important in the evaluation of LGA infants, it is the relationship of fetal size to maternal pelvic and soft tissue characteristics that is the important determinant for the prediction of dystocia and birth trauma.

ANTENATAL DIAGNOSIS OF ALTERED FETAL GROWTH

Intrauterine growth retardation

Clinical screening for IUGR

The diagnosis of IUGR begins with the identification of those patients at significant risk for delivering a growth retarded infant. Many socioeconomic and medical complications can lead to IUGR. Table 9 lists some of the common risk factors frequently associated with IUGR[6,10,38–42].

The two most significant historical factors related to IUGR are maternal smoking and a history of a previous growth-retarded infant. Numerous maternal constitutional and socioeconomic factors have been related to increased risk for IUGR, but the most consistent factor appears to be short interpregnancy interval, with a duration between pregnancies of < 9 months showing a strong correlation with both IUGR and preterm delivery[79,80]. The most common maternal medical complication associated with IUGR is hypertensive disease, and a recent study of Duvekot and co-workers[81] suggested a possible mechanism: early defective volume adaption to pregnancy. Mounting evidence in-

dicates that both preterm labor and IUGR are also related to chronic placental inflammation[82]. An additional important obstetric risk for IUGR is multiple gestation. Placental discordance, with one twin having a significantly larger placental mass than the other, can occur in any type of placentation and lead to IUGR in the twin with the smaller placenta. In diamniotic monochorionic placentation twin–twin transfusion syndrome may occur leading to IUGR in the donor twin. Other medical conditions, such as cardiac or hematological diseases, are significant, but much less common causes of IUGR.

Screening for these risk factors will identify about half of the growth retarded infants. Using an antenatal-risk scoring system, Wennergren and colleagues[41] were able to identify prior to delivery all mothers who delivered growth

Table 8 *Labor and delivery complications of macrosomic infants*[80]

Complication	Macrosomic (%)	Control (%)
Oxytocin augmentation	20.4	11.9
Postpartum bleeding	8.8	1.2
Shoulder dystocia	18.5	0.2
Maternal trauma	8.6	1.7
Postpartum fever	17.7	6.7

All values are statistically different at $p < 0.05$

Table 9 *Maternal risk factors for intrauterine growth retardation*

Social history
Poor weight gain in pregnancy
Smoking
Poor socioeconomic history

Obstetric history
Previous growth retarded infant
History of stillbirth or neonatal death
History of multiple abortions

Medical history
Hypertensive disease
  pregnancy induced hypertension
  essential hypertension
Renal disease
  chronic renal disease
  multiple urinary tract infections
Chronic liver disease
Significant cardiac disease
Hemoglobinopathies

Table 10 *Diagnostic value of ultrasound in detecting intrauterine growth retardation[88] ***

Parameter	Sensitivity (%)	Specificity (%)	Positive predictive value (%)	Negative predictive value (%)
Placental grade	62	64	16	94
Amniotic fluid volume	24–80	72–98	21–55	92–97
BPD				
small	24–88	62–94	21–44	92–98
poor growth	75	84	35	97
FL/AC ratio	34–49	78–83	18–20	92–93
HC/AC ratio	82	94	62	98
Distal femoral epiphysis	83	97	76	98
Fetal weight estimation	89	88	45	99

*Estimated values if a 10% prevalence of SGA is assumed (Bayes theorem); BPD, biparietal diameter; FL, fetal femur length; AC, abdominal circumference; HC, head circumference

retarded infants[41]. Their high-risk group comprised 7% of the total population screened, but only 34% of the high-risk group of patients delivered IUGR infants. Other investigators have found similar results[38–40].

Although patients at risk for IUGR can be identified, additional methods must be used to diagnose actual IUGR. In addition, 20–30% of IUGR infants will be born from mothers with no identifiable risk factors.

The most common clinical method of diagnosing suspected IUGR is the measurement of symphysis-fundal height[83–87]. Belizan and associates[83] found a sensitivity of 86% and a specificity of 90% for the prediction of IUGR. However, other investigators have not found as high a sensitivity and specificity for this technique[84–86], and Calvert and co-workers[84] found a false positive rate of 71%.

Ultrasonic diagnosis of SGA and suspected IUGR

Currently, one of the most common methods of screening for and identification of the SGA and suspected IUGR infant is the measurement of various fetal parameters by real-time ultrasound. Table 10, based on the work of Benson and colleagues[88] (who reviewed the predictive value of ultrasonic criteria for antenatal diagnosis of IUGR) and other more recent studies, shows the sensitivity, specificity and predictive values for some of the ultrasonic parameters currently in use for the diagnosis of IUGR[2,88–95].

Table 11 *Predictive values of selected ultrasonic tests for detection of altered fetal growth*

Test	Sensitivity (%) SGA	Sensitivity (%) LGA	Specificity (%)	Predictive value (%) SGA	Predictive value (%) AGA	Predictive value (%) LGA
Fetal weight estimation	90	74	79	60	93	63
FL/AC	37	—	75	29	81	—

SGA, small for gestational age; LGA, large for gestational age; AGA, average for gestational age; FL, fetal femur length; AC, abdominal circumference

Since predictive values are dependent on sensitivity, specificity and the prevalence rate of the process under investigation in the study population, Bayesian analysis was used to calculate the positive and negative predictive value of each test based on an assumed prevalence of IUGR in a general population of 10%[88,98]. The author's experience with two of these tests (fetal femur length/abdominal circumference ratio (FL/AC) and estimated fetal weight) for the diagnosis of both IUGR and LGA is shown in Table 11[34,95].

Although most of these tests give reasonable negative predictive values, with the exception of the head circumference (HC)/AC ratio and the distal femoral epiphysis, they all have less than ideal positive predictive values. In addition, with the exception of the FL/AC ratio and amniotic fluid volume, all of these parameters depend on an accurate estimation of gestational age. In many clinical situations this may not be possible.

Table 12 *Fetal weight estimation formulas*

	Formula $\log_{10} BW$	R^2	Percentage error
Hadlock *et al.*[109]	$1.5622 - 0.01080\,HC + 0.04680\,AC + 0.171\,FL + 0.00034\,HC^2 - 0.003685\,AC \times FL$	0.965	0.3 (7.6)
Ott *et al.*[112]	$2.0660 + 0.04355\,HC + 0.05394\,AC - 0.000858\,HC \times AC + 1.2594\,FL/AC$	0.956	0.3 (8.8)
Shepard *et al.*[111]	$-1.7492 + 0.166\,BPD + 0.046\,AC - 0.00246 \times BPD \times AC$	—	-1.1 (9.1)*
		—	1.9 (13.5)†

BW, birthweight (g); HC, head circumference (cm); AC, abdominal circumference (cm); FL, femur length (cm); BPD, biparietal diameter (cm); *evaluated by Hadlock *et al.*[109]; †evaluated by Ott *et al.*[112]. Figures in parentheses are standard deviations

Sholl and associates[96] evaluated the use of serial measurements of biparietal diameter for the diagnosis of IUGR and felt this technique to be highly advantageous in patients where an accurate estimation of gestational age could not be made. Other investigators have also suggested that serial evaluation of fetal growth is a more appropriate way to diagnose IUGR[91–94]. However, in cases of significant IUGR, especially if associated with severe maternal disease, it is frequently unsafe to wait the necessary time required to evaluate serial changes in ultrasonic parameters.

Fetal weight estimation and intrauterine growth curves

The accurate estimation of fetal weight is important in many clinical situations[100,101]. A variety of ultrasonic parameters have been evaluated in order to develop a formula to accurately estimate fetal weight.

Campbell and Wilkin[102] were one of the first to publish a series comparing ultrasonic estimated weight and birth weight. The accuracy of weight estimation calculated from an abdominal circumference at the level of the umbilical vein as it passed through the fetal liver was evaluated in 140 fetuses that had been examined by ultrasonic compound B-scan within 48 h of delivery. The overall error was approximately 13%. Since then, numerous studies have been published using various ultrasonic parameters, alone and in combination, in order to improve the accuracy of fetal weight estimation[100,103–124]. The accuracy of these techniques has also been evaluated by a number of studies.

Table 13 *Simplified method of fetal weight estimation*[115]

Parameters	LnFW
BPD + AD + FL	$0.143x + 4.198$
BPD + AD	$0.193x + 4.2581$
AD + FL	$0.2053x + 4.3726$

BPD, biparietal diameter (cm); AD, mean abdominal diameter (cm); FL, femur length (cm); LnFW, natural log of the estimated fetal weight (g); x, the sum of parameter measurements

The lowest error obtained appears to be about 8%, which is clinically insignificant in lower weight ranges (< 2500 g), but may cause significant clinical error in large infants (> 3800 g). The most accurate methods of fetal weight estimation use two or more measurements, usually the HC, AC and FL.

Table 12 lists the three most accurate formulas (in this author's opinion) for fetal weight estimation. Table 13, taken from the study of Rose and McCallum[115], is a slightly less accurate simplified method of fetal weight estimation that can be used when it is possible to measure only two parameters.

A number of other more complex methods of fetal weight estimation involving volume determinations are also available. In general, however, these methods appear to obtain only minimal improvements in accuracy[125–128]. With recent advances in real-time ultrasound, such as three-dimensional scanning, additional techniques may be developed that may improve the accuracy of weight estimation.

A logical extension of fetal weight estimation is to use it to define normal fetal growth. There is strong evidence that a significant percentage of infants that deliver preterm may be SGA or IUGR. Therefore, the use of delivery data to define altered growth may underestimate its true incidence. This has led many investigators to advocate the use of fetal weight for gestational age curves to define altered fetal growth.

Over 10 years ago, we reported one of the first intrauterine fetal weight for gestational age curves[55], and, subsequently, published the results of the use of this curve for the diagnosis of altered fetal growth[34]. As illustrated in Tables 10 and 11 estimated fetal weight has a high degree of sensitivity for the diagnosis of altered growth.

Figure 2 shows a comparison of the Hadlock/Ott intrauterine fetal weight for gestational age curve to a recent birth weight for gestational age curve from Canada. Of particular note is the comparison of the lower 10th centiles of each curve between 25 and 35 weeks' gestational age. The ultrasound intrauterine curve (Hadlock/Ott) values are significantly higher than the birth weight values (Canada), confirming the hypothesis that preterm babies weigh less than their intrauterine cohorts.

Other studies have developed and used a variety of fetal growth curves for the evaluation of fetal growth. Table 1 lists the data for the fetal weight for gestational age curve that is currently in use at our own institution: a composite fetal

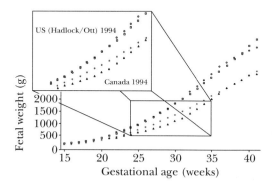

Figure 2 *Comparison of the 10th and 90th centile values of the Hadlock/Ott fetal weight for gestational age curve (Figure 1) and a recent birth weight for gestational age curve from Canada (unpublished data). The insert compares the Canadian 10th centiles (triangles) with the ultrasound 10th centiles (asterisks) between 24 and 35 weeks' gestational age, showing that birth weight curves underestimate SGA infants in this gestational age range*

weight curve derived from the work of Ott and Hadlock[46,48].

Fetal dysanthropometry

Abnormal fetal ratios have been used to screen for chromosomal, structural and growth abnormalities. Hadlock and colleagues[129] have recently reviewed the use of a variety of fetal body ratios in identifying chromosomally abnormal fetuses (biparietal diameter/femur length ratio (BPD/FL), femur length/head circumference ratio (FL/HC), femur length/abdominal circumference ratio (FL/AC), and head circumference/abdominal circumference ratio (HC/AC)). They found that many of these ratios provided important information concerning the risk of chromosomal abnormalities, but felt that their sensitivity was too low to recommend that patients with an abnormal ratio undergo genetic amniocentesis. An additional finding of the Hadlock study was that the ratios were also helpful in identifying other forms of abnormal fetal growth not necessarily associated with chromosomal abnormalities. David and co-workers[130] evaluated the utility of the HC/AC ratio in 134 otherwise normal SGA fetuses and found that an elevated ratio was associated with an increased perinatal mortality (odds ratio 3.27) but felt that this parameter had weak prognostic significance, especially when compared to umbilical artery Doppler velocity waveform analysis.

The author has recently undertaken a study to evaluate the utility of abnormal fetal body ratios (dysanthropometry) for the prediction of chromosomal, structural or growth abnormalities. The computerized ultrasound data base from 1988 to 1992 at the author's institution was searched for patients who met the following criteria:

(1) Singleton pregnancy;

(2) At least two scans performed during the pregnancy; the first, at or before the 28th week, and the gestational age calculated from multiple parameters within 10 days of the gestational age calculated from the patient's last menstrual period;

(3) No obstetric or medical complications; and

(4) Delivered live-born infants at, or beyond, 37 completed weeks of gestation without evidence of structural or chromosomal abnormalities.

The following normal fetal ratios were then calculated from each scan:

(1) AC/FL;

(2) BPD/FL;

(3) HC/AC;

(4) HC/FL; and

(5) Two fetal ponderal indices[131]:
    (a) [Estimated fetal weight (g)/femur length cubed] times 100 $(100\ FWT/FL^3)$;
    (b) Abdominal circumference squared/femur length cubed (AC^2/FL^3).

Linear and non-linear regression analysis was used to determine the best fit relationship between each ratio and gestational age. This information was then used to construct the smoothed 10th and 90th centile values vs. gestational age for these ratios (Tables 14–17).

The 10th and 90th centile values of each of the above ratios were then applied to a second study group of patients with singleton pregnancies who had been referred for comprehensive ultrasound examination because of suspected maternal or fetal complications of pregnancy during the years 1990–92. The number of infants with chromosomal abnormalities, structural anomalies not associated with chromosomal abnormalities, and the number of infants that were SGA at delivery were determined for the study group. SGA was defined as birth weight below the 10th centile value for weight for gestational age taken from the combined

Table 14 *10th and 90th centile values for abdominal circumference/femur length ratio*

Gestational age (weeks)	Centile	
	10th	*90th*
14	4.959	6.72
15	4.665	6.122
16	4.441	5.654
17	4.288	5.315
18	4.206	5.105
19	4.194	5.024
20	4.156	4.918
21	4.139	4.882
22	4.126	4.851
23	4.115	4.825
24	4.107	4.804
25	4.102	4.787
26	4.1	4.776
27	4.1	4.769
28	4.104	4.766
29	4.111	4.769
30	4.12	4.777
31	4.133	4.789
32	4.148	4.806
33	4.166	4.828
34	4.187	4.854
35	4.211	4.886
36	4.238	4.922
37	4.268	4.963
38	4.3	5.009
39	4.336	5.06
40	4.374	5.115

Table 15 *10th and 90th centile values for biparietal diameter/femur length ratio*

Gestational age (weeks)	Centile	
	10th	*90th*
14	1.632	2.301
15	1.533	2.057
16	1.452	1.865
17	1.389	1.726
18	1.344	1.64
19	1.316	1.608
20	1.29	1.511
21	1.283	1.502
22	1.277	1.493
23	1.271	1.484
24	1.265	1.475
25	1.259	1.466
26	1.253	1.457
27	1.247	1.448
28	1.241	1.439
29	1.234	1.43
30	1.228	1.421
31	1.222	1.412
32	1.216	1.403
33	1.21	1.395
34	1.204	1.386
35	1.198	1.377
36	1.191	1.368
37	1.185	1.359
38	1.179	1.35
39	1.173	1.341
40	1.167	1.332

Table 16 *10th and 90th centile values for fetal weight/femur length cubed ratio*

Gestational age (weeks)	Centile	
	10th	90th
14	2.128	6.909
15	1.639	4.503
16	1.268	2.759
17	1.014	1.677
18	0.878	1.257
19	0.859	1.5
20	0.61	1.001
21	0.609	0.998
22	0.607	0.996
23	0.606	0.993
24	0.604	0.991
25	0.602	0.989
26	0.601	0.986
27	0.599	0.984
28	0.597	0.981
29	0.596	0.979
30	0.594	0.976
31	0.592	0.974
32	0.591	0.971
33	0.589	0.969
34	0.588	0.967
35	0.586	0.964
36	0.584	0.962
37	0.583	0.959
38	0.581	0.957
39	0.579	0.954
40	0.578	0.952

Table 17 *10th and 90th centile values for head circumference/abdominal circumference ratio*

Gestational age (weeks)	Centile	
	10th	90th
14	1.109	1.311
15	1.101	1.294
16	1.093	1.277
17	1.085	1.261
18	1.077	1.244
19	1.068	1.227
20	1.051	1.194
21	1.05	1.192
22	1.048	1.189
23	1.046	1.186
24	1.042	1.181
25	1.037	1.176
26	1.032	1.17
27	1.025	1.163
28	1.018	1.156
29	1.01	1.147
30	1.0	1.138
31	0.99	1.128
32	0.979	1.118
33	0.967	1.106
34	0.954	1.094
35	0.94	1.081
36	0.925	1.067
37	0.91	1.052
38	0.893	1.037
39	0.875	1.021
40	0.857	1.003

ultrasonic weight for gestational age curves of Ott and Hadlock (Table 1 and Figure 1)[42,54].

The ratio(s) that showed significant correlations with the above mentioned fetal abnormalities were then used to calculate the sensitivity, specificity, positive and negative predictive values, and false positive rates for these ratio(s), or combination of ratios for the prediction of chromosomal, structural or IUGR anomalies in the study group.

A total of 2544 normal patients were utilized to generate 5088 data points for analysis for each of the fetal ratios studied. Scatter plots of each ratio against gestational age for most ratios showed a distinct change in slope at 20 weeks. Figure 3, a plot of the BPD/FL ratio vs. gestational age, illustrates these findings. Inspection of Figure 3 shows that the range of the BPD/FL ratio is significantly wider prior to 20

weeks' gestation than it is in the second half of pregnancy. All the other ratios, with the exception of the HC/AC ratio, showed an identical relationship with gestational age. The HC/AC ratio showed a constant small but significant negative correlation with advancing gestational age and relatively similar widths for the ratio ranges across gestational ages. The 10th and 90th centile values for these ratios were then used in the second part of the study to define normal or abnormal ratios, and these values are listed in Tables 14–17.

In all 1196 patients were evaluated in the study group. There were 18 fetuses with chromosomal abnormalities (1.5%), eight of which were trisomy 21. Three of the infants with trisomy 21 (37.5%) had no structural anomalies seen on ultrasound examination. Two (25%) had only dysmorphic features and one had an

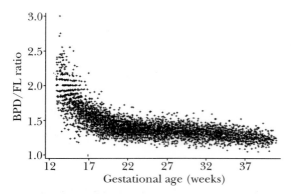

Figure 3 *Graph of the BPD/FL (biparietal diameter/femur length) ratio for gestational age compiled from over 2500 normal obstetric patients*

atrioventricular canal defect that was missed on antenatal ultrasound. Two of the remaining infants with chromosomal anomalies had no structural anomalies seen on ultrasound: one who had mild hydrocephaly at delivery that was not present at the time of antenatal ultrasound examination, and one who had only dysmorphic features. Therefore, four of the 18 fetuses with chromosomal abnormalities (22.2%) were without structural anomalies that could have been seen on ultrasound examination.

Eighty-two fetuses in the study group had structural anomalies not associated with chromosomal abnormalities (6.9%), and 204 (17.1%) of the total study group were classified as SGA. As would be expected, there was a strong relationship between chromosomal anomalies, structural anomalies and SGA infants. Seventy-eight per cent of infants with chromosomal aneuploidy also had structural anomalies and 61% of the total infants with chromosomal anomalies were SGA. Twenty-four per cent of the infants with structural anomalies without chromosomal anomalies were also SGA. Ten per cent of the infants who were SGA had structural anomalies not associated with chromosomal anomalies and 5.4% of the SGA infants had chromosomal anomalies. Table 18 shows the statistical correlations between the ratios studied and the occurrence of chromosomal anomalies, structural anomalies and SGA. For each fetal complication analyzed, there were two ratios that showed significant statistical cor-

relation: elevated BPD/FL and elevated HC/AC for chromosomal anomalies; elevated AC/FL and elevated HC/AC for structural anomalies; and low FWT/FL^3 and elevated HC/AC for SGA.

Table 19 shows the predictive values for these ratios in screening for the presence of SGA, structural anomalies or a fetus with either of these two complications or a chromosomal anomaly. Since the predictive value of a test is dependent not only on the sensitivity and specificity but also on the prevalence of the abnormality in the population studied[132,133], the positive and negative predictive values were recalculated assuming an incidence of chromosomal abnormalities in the general fetal population greater than 14 weeks' gestation of 1.2%[122,123]. The combined use of HC/AC and AC^2/FL^3 ratios showed a corrected positive and negative predictive value of 73.6% and 88.2%, respectively; and a false-positive rate of 2.2% for the prediction of IUGR, chromosomal anomalies, structural anomalies, or any combination of these three problems.

Although controversy exists, the use of these ratios appears to be a useful screening tool for the identification of not only SGA infants but also infants with chromosomal or structural anomalies.

Other ultrasonic methods of identifying growth retardation

Cerebellar diameter Measurements of the transverse diameter of the cerebellar hemispheres in the posterior fossa is one of the alternative methods of ultrasonic calculation of gestational age[134]. Reece and associates[135] evaluated multiple ultrasonic parameters in 19 documented growth retarded infants and found that the growth of the transverse cerebellar diameter was unaffected. Campbell and colleagues[136] prospectively studied 162 patients, measuring the transverse cerebellar diameter (TCD) and abdominal circumference and calculated a ratio between the two (TCD/AC ratio). The authors found that this ratio was gestational age-independent and suggested that it may be a method for screening for fetal growth

Table 18 *Statistical correlations – fetal dysanthropometry*

Condition	Ratio	Value	χ	$\chi\, p$	Logistic regression odds ratio*
Chromosomal anomaly	AC/FL	—	5.70	0.0578	2.54 (0.38–16.95)
	BPD/FL	elevated	17.54	0.0002	5.18 (1.45–18.54)
	FWT/FL^3	—	2.89	0.3356	2.36 (0.29–19.29)
	HC/AC	elevated	22.64	0.0001	5.46 (1.89–15.78)
	HC/FL	—	0.42	0.8125	0.19 (0.02–1.49)
	AC^2/FL^3	—	4.54	0.1050	1.82 (0.51–6.52)
Small for gestational age	AC/FL	—	18.15	0.0001	1.75 (0.71–4.33)
	BPD/FL	—	1.52	0.4673	1.22 (0.83–1.81)
	FWT/FL^3	low	18.67	0.0001	3.87 (1.59–9.45)
	HC/AC	elevated	38.91	0.0001	2.88 (1.97–4.25)
	HC/FL	—	3.11	0.2108	1.19 (0.51–2.76)
	AC^2/FL^3	—	7.94	0.0189	0.42 (0.15–1.14)
Structural anomaly	AC/FL	elevated	13.48	0.0009	3.13 (1.48–6.60)
	BPD/FL	—	12.96	0.0015	1.24 (0.66–2.34)
	FWT/FL^3	—	3.30	0.1919	1.31 (0.71–2.39)
	HC/AC	elevated	24.96	0.0001	3.10 (1.75–5.50)
	HC/FL	—	1.59	0.4506	0.28 (0.10–0.75)
	AC^2/FL^3	—	10.74	0.0047	0.90 (0.40–1.98)

AC, abdominal circumference; FL, femur length; BPD, biparietal diameter; FWT, fetal weight; FL^3, femur length cubed; HC, head circumference.
*Statistical significance present if the odds ratio greater than one and the 5th centile for the odds ratio also greater than one

Table 19 *Use of fetal ratios to screen for anomalies*

	Sensitivity (%)	Specificity (%)	Positive predictive value (%)	Negative predictive value (%)	False positives (%)
Presence of SGA					
FWT/FL^3	9.3	97.1	39.6 (26.3)*	83.9 (90.6)	2.9
HC/AC	27.5	88.9	33.7 (21.6)	85.6 (91.7)	11.1
Combined	2.9	99.5	54.5 (39.2)	83.3 (90.2)	0.3
Presence of a structural anomaly					
AC/FL	36.5	80.3	12.4 (5.4)	94.3 (97.6)	19.6
HC/AC	24.7	86.9	12.7 (5.5)	93.8 (97.4)	13.1
Combined	2.4	99.5	28.6 (11.0)	93.0 (97.1)	2.4
Any (SGA, chromosomal or structural) anomaly					
HC/AC	25.1	89.5	41.6 (28.0)	80.0 (88.0)	10.5
AC^2/FL^3	29.5	78.2	28.7 (18.1)	78.8 (87.2)	21.8
Combined	18.8	98.9	31.6 (73.6)	97.8 (88.2)	2.2

SGA, small for gestational age; FWT, fetal weight; FL^3, femur length cubed; HC, head circumference; AC, abdominal circumference; FL, femur length.
Figures in parentheses are predictive values recalculated by Bayesian analysis, assuming a prevalence of intrauterine growth retardation (IUGR) of 10%, an incidence of significant structural anomalies of 3% and an incidence of either IUGR or a structural anomaly or chromosomal anomaly of 14%

abnormalities (both IUGR and macrosomia): TCD/AC = 0.137 ± 0.012(SD). Meyer and co-workers[137] evaluated the TCD/AC ratio in 825 low-risk patients and 250 patients at risk for either IUGR or macrosomia. They also found that the TCD/AC ratio was independent of gestational age in normal patients $(0.136 \pm 0.0093(SD))$. They found that a ratio greater than 2 standard deviations from the mean was significantly associated with IUGR: 98% of asymmetrically and 71% of symmetrically growth retarded infants.

However, Hill and associates[138,139] found that cerebellar diameter measurements were more than two standard deviations below the mean in only 60% of growth retarded infants, and that abnormal TCD/AC ratios were only 53% and 47% sensitive in predicting IUGR or macrosomic infants, respectively. This finding was also confirmed by a study of Cabbad and colleagues[140]. The status of cerebellar measurements in screening for altered fetal growth, therefore, is still controversial.

Evaluation of subcutaneous adipose tissue and other soft tissues Abramowicz and co-workers[141] evaluated fetal subcutaneous adipose tissue by measuring cheek-to-cheek diameters from a coronal view of the fetal face at the level of the nostrils and lips. They found significant differences in cheek-to-cheek diameters between IUGR, normal and macrosomic infants. Additional studies, however, are necessary to determine the usefulness of this measurement in screening for IUGR or macrosomia.

A number of other measurements of fetal adipose tissues have been studied, such as subcutaneous tissue thickness at the level of the fetal mid-calf, mid-thigh or abdominal wall[142]. Hill and associates[143] have recently evaluated these measurements and felt that the degree of overlap in subcutaneous tissue thickness between normal, IUGR and macrosomic fetuses was too great to be reliable in predicting abnormal growth.

Gimondo and colleagues[144] estimated fetal liver weight using the formula: $D1 \times D2 \times D3 \times 0.42$, where D1 equals the longitudinal, D2 the anteroposterior and D3 the cephalocaudal liver dimensions, respectively. They found good correlation between ultrasonically estimated fetal liver weights and published norms, and postulated that estimated fetal liver weight may be an excellent method of diagnosing IUGR. Further research in this area is needed to determine the utility of this measurement.

Placental measurements Evaluation of placenta growth theoretically should be important in the evaluation of fetal growth. Naeye[145] studied the relationship between placental weight and neonatal outcome in over 38 000 cases. He found a strong association between small placentas and low birth weight, increased neonatal hemoglobin concentration, and lower than expected body size in later childhood. Increased placental size (usually due to villous edema) was associated with poor neonatal outcome. Composite values of placental weights for gestational age from Naeye's study and from a study of Hendricks are presented in Table 20[145,146].

A number of ultrasonic methods of estimating placental volume (and, therefore, weight) have been developed[147,148]. Geirsson and associates[148] longitudinally studied 147 normal singleton pregnancies and measured placental volume using a parallel planimetric area method. Table 21 shows the results of this study. Figure 4 illustrates a comparison between placental weight and ultrasonically determined placental volume. There is an

Table 20 *Placental weight (g) for gestational age*[145,146]

Gestational age (weeks)	10th centile	Mean	90th centile
24	187	281	375
25	203	305	407
26	220	329	438
27	236	353	470
28	253	378	503
29	268	402	536
30	286	426	566
31	301	450	599
32	317	474	631
33	334	498	662
34	350	522	694
35	366	546	726
36	381	570	759
37	400	595	790
38	415	619	823
39	431	643	855
40	448	667	886

almost one to one correlation between the estimated mean placental volume by ultrasound measurement and the mean placental weight for gestational age: placental volume (ml) − 110 = placental weight (g). Wolf and co-workers[149,150] have shown good correlation between poor placental growth and subsequent IUGR and poor perinatal outcome, with poor placental growth preceding IUGR by at least 3 weeks and having over 90% sensitivity in predicting IUGR. Jauniaux and colleagues[151] used a different method of estimating placental volume combined with Doppler ultrasound and maternal serum α-fetoprotein levels and showed a strong association between these measurements and neonatal outcome.

Although these techniques appear to provide sufficient accuracy to be useful in identifying and evaluating IUGR, they are somewhat complicated to perform and, to date, have not been fully evaluated.

Two formulas for estimation of placental volume, using a prolated ellipsoid method, are listed below:

(1) Volume = $0.3491 \times [T1 \times (3 \times R1^2 + T1^2) + T2 \times (3 \times R2^2 + T2^2)]$[152];

(2) Volume = $0.5233 \times (T1 + T2)/2 \times (2 \times R1) \times (2 \times R2)$[153];

where T1 and T2 are the greatest thicknesses of the placenta in two slices at right angles to each other through the mid-portion of the placenta (usually at the cord insertion), and R1 and R2 are half the diameter of the base of each slice, respectively.

Table 21 *Placental volume (ml) for gestational age*[148]

Gestational age (weeks)	10th centile	Mean	90th centile
24	261	396	531
25	279	423	567
26	298	450	602
27	314	476	638
28	333	503	673
29	351	530	709
30	370	557	744
31	387	584	781
32	405	610	815
33	423	637	851
34	440	664	888
35	459	691	923
36	477	717	957
37	494	744	995
38	512	771	1030
39	531	798	1065
40	549	825	1101

Summary: defining IUGR

From the above discussion it can be seen that there is a great deal of confusion concerning the definition of IUGR. The most common definitions of IUGR equate it with the SGA infant; but, as has been shown, this definition (especially in term infants) is not truly accurate. A more appropriate definition of IUGR might be: *a fetus that fails to attain or maintain its inherent growth potential.* This definition would exclude infants who are SGA at term, but otherwise entirely normal, assuming that no other underlying pathological conditions (such as a placental abnormality, infection, etc.) exist and that there were no maternal risk factors present. Infants with chromosomal abnormalities might also be considered to be included in this definition, unless we broaden the term 'inherent' to mean that potential that would exist if the chromosomal abnormality was not present.

Determination of the inherent growth potential of a fetus may be difficult, but not impossible. Evaluation of the mother's family history, especially her birth weight, the weight of her siblings, and the weight of any previous

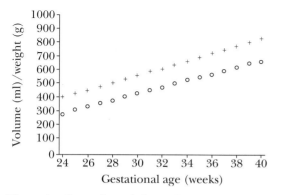

Figure 4 *Comparison of placental weight (circles) to ultrasonically determined placental volume (crosses)*

children, together with the use of projected ideal fetal weight for the current pregnancy will give good insight into the growth potential of her fetus.

Our current knowledge of fetal growth is, at best, incomplete. Hopefully, with further observation and research we will be able to improve our understanding of the complex issues of fetal growth; and, therefore, be better able to diagnosed altered fetal growth. The combined use of fetal weight estimation, fetal ratios and Doppler velocity flow studies appears to be the best available method of diagnosis and surveillance in suspected IUGR.

References

1. Keirse, M. J. N. C. (1984). Epidemiology and aetiology of the growth retarded baby. *Clin. Obstet. Gynecol.*, **11**, 415–22
2. Seeds, J. W. (1984). Impaired fetal growth: definition and clinical diagnosis. *Obstet. Gynecol.*, **64**, 303–30
3. Varma, T. R. (1984). Low birth weight babies. The small for gestational age. A review of current management. *Obstet. Gynecol. Surv.*, **39**, 616–31
4. Anderson, G. D., Blidner, I. N., McClemont, S. *et al.*, (1984). Determinants of size at birth in a Canadian population. *Am. J. Obstet. Gynecol.*, **150**, 236–45
5. Khoury, M. J. and Cohen, B. H. (1987). Genetic heterogeneity of prematurity and intrauterine growth retardation: clues from the old order Amish. *Am. J. Obstet. Gynecol.*, **157**, 400–9
6. Miller, H. C. (1988). Prenatal factors affecting intrauterine growth retardation. *Clin. Perinatol.*, **12**, 307–15
7. Peters, T. J., Golding, J., Butler, N. R. *et al.* (1983). Predictors of birth weight in two national studies. *Br. J. Obstet. Gynaecol.*, **90**, 107–12
8. Bakketeig, L. S., Hoffman, H. J. and Harley, E. E. (1979). The tendency to repeat gestational age and birth weight in successive births. *Am. J. Obstet. Gynecol.*, **135**, 1086–99
9. Jones, O. W. (1978). Genetic factors in the determination of fetal size. *J. Reprod. Med.*, **21**, 305–10
10. Resnik, R. (1978). Maternal diseases associated with abnormal fetal growth. *J. Reprod. Med.*, **21**, 315–20
11. DeWolf, F., Brosens, I. and Ranaer, M. (1980). Fetal growth retardation and the maternal arterial supply of the human placenta in the absence of sustained hypertension. *Br. J. Obstet. Gynaecol.*, **87**, 678–82
12. Villar, J. and Belizan, J. M. (1982). The timing factor in the pathophysiology of the intrauterine growth retardation syndrome. *Obstet. Gynecol. Surv.*, **137**, 499–510
13. Allen, M. C. (1984). Developmental outcome and follow-up of the small for gestational age infant. *Semin. Perinatol.*, **8**, 123–9
14. Taylor, D. J. (1984). Low birth weight and neurodevelopmental handicap. *Clin. Obstet. Gynecol.*, **11**, 525–31
15. Edouard, L. and Alberman, E. (1980). National trends in the identified causes of perinatal mortality 1960–1978. *Br. J. Obstet. Gynaecol.*, **87**, 833–41
16. Jones, R. A. K. and Roberton, N. R. C. (1984). Problems of the small-for-dates baby. *Clin. Obstet. Gynecol.*, **11**, 499–519
17. Tejani, N. and Mann, L. I. (1977). Diagnosis and management of the small for gestational age fetus. *Clin. Obstet. Gynecol.*, **20**, 943–50
18. Cefalo, R. C. (1978). The hazards of labor and delivery for the intrauteirne-growth-retarded fetus. *J. Reprod. Med.*, **21**, 300–14
19. Lin, C., Moawad, A. H., Rosenow, P. J. *et al.* (1980). Acid-base characteristics of fetuses with intrauterine growth retardation during labor and dleivery. *Am. J. Obstet. Gynecol.*, **137**, 353–61
20. Neligan, G. A., Kolvin, I., Scott, D. *et al.* (1978). *Born too Soon or Born too Small. A Follow-up Study to Seven Years of Age. Spastic International Medical Publications*, p. 66. (London: William Heinemann Medical Books)
21. Hill, D. E. (1978). Physical growth and development after intrauterine growth retardation. *J. Reprod. Med.*, **21**, 335–45
22. Vohr, B. R., Oh, W., Rosenfield, A. G. *et al.* (1979). The preterm small-for-gestational age infant: a two-year follow-up study. *Am. J. Obstet. Gynecol.*, **133**, 425–32
23. Low, J. A., Galbraith, R. S., Muir, D. *et al.* (1978). Intrauterine growth retardation: a preliminary report of long-term morbidity. *Am. J. Obstet. Gynecol.*, **130**, 534–9

24. Low, J. A., Galbraith, R. S., Muir, D. *et al.* (1982). Intrauterine growth retardation: a study of long-term morbidity. *Am. J. Obstet. Gynecol.*, **142**, 670–82

25. Westwood, M., Kramer, M. S., Munz, D. *et al.* (1983). Growth and development of full term nonasphyxiated small-for-gestational-age newborns: follow-up through adolescence. *Pediatrics*, **71**, 376–83

26. Holmes, G. E., Miller, H. C., Hassanein, K. *et al.* (1977). Postnatal somatic growth in infants with atypical fetal growth patterns. *Am. J. Dis. Child.*, **131**, 1078–85

27. Teberg, A. J., Walther, F. J. and Pena, I. C. (1988). Mortality, morbidity and outcome of the small-for-gestational age infant. *Semin. Perinatol.*, **12**, 84–94

28. Winer, E. K., Tejani, N. A., Atluru, V. J. *et al.* (1982). Four to seven-year evaluation in two groups of small-for-gestational age infants. *Am. J. Obstet. Gynecol.*, **143**, 425–35

29. Spinillo, A., Capuzzo, E., Egbe, T. O. *et al.* (1995). Pregnancies complicated by idiopathic intrauterine growth retardation. Severity of growth failure, neonatal morbidity and two-year infant neurodevelopmental outcome. *J. Reprod. Med.*, **40**, 209–15

30. Paz, I., Gale, R., Laor, A. *et al.* (1995). The cognitive outcome of full-term small for gestational age infants at adolescence. *Obstet. Gynecol.*, **85**, 452–6

31. Hays, D. and Patterson, R. M. (1987). A comparison of fetal biometric ratios to neonatal morphometries. *J. Ultrasound Med.*, **6**, 71–82

32. Miller, H. C. and Hassanein, K. (1971). Diagnosis of impaired fetal growth in newborn infants. *Pediatrics*, **48**, 511–19

33. Miller, H. C. (1981). Intrauterine growth retardation: an unmet challenge. *Am. J. Dis. Child.*, **135**, 944–52

34. Ott, W. J. and Doyle, S. (1984). Ultrasonic diagnosis of altered fetal growth by use of a normal ultrasonic fetal weight curve. *Obstet. Gynecol.*, **63**, 201–7

35. Patterson, R. M. and Pouliot, M. R. (1987). Neonatal morphometries and perinatal outcome: who is growth retarded? *Am. J. Obstet. Gynecol.*, **157**, 861–9

36. Miller, J. M., Korndorffer, F. A., Kissling, G. E. *et al.* (1987). Recognition of the overgrown fetus: *in utero* ponderal indices. *Am. J. Perinatol.*, **4**, 86–93

37. Walther, F. J. and Ramaekers, L. H. J. (1982). The ponderal index as a measure of the nutritional status at birth and its relation to some aspects of neonatal morbidity. *J. Perinat. Med.*, **10**, 42–57

38. Adelstein, P. and Fedrick, J. (1987). Antenatal identification of women at increased risk of being delivered of a low birth weight infant at term. *Br. J. Obstet. Gynaecol.*, **85**, 8–19

39. Ounsted, M., Moar, V. A. and Scott, A. (1985). Risk factors associated with small-for-dates and large-for-dates infants. *Br. J. Obstet. Gynaecol.*, **92**, 226–32

40. Visser, G. H. A., Huisman, A., Saathof, P. W. F. *et al.* (1986). Early fetal growth retardation: obstetric background and recurrence rate. *Obstet. Gynecol.*, **67**, 40–6

41. Wennergren, M., Karlsson, K. and Olsson, T. (1982). A scoring system for antenatal identification of fetal growth retardation. *Br. J. Obstet. Gynaecol.*, **89**, 520–9

42. Wolfe, H. M., Gross, T. L. and Sokol, R. J. (1987). Recurrent small for gestational age birth. Perinatal risks and outcomes. *Am. J. Obstet. Gynecol.*, **157**, 288–97

43. Catalano, P. M., Tyzbir, E. D., Allen, S. R. *et al.* (1992). Evaluation of fetal growth by estimation of neonatal body composition. *Obstet. Gynecol.*, **79**, 46–50

44. Chard, T., Yoong, A. and Macintosh, M. (1993). The myth of fetal growth retardation at term. *Br. J. Obstet. Gynaecol.*, **100**, 1076–81

45. Chard, T., Costeloe, K. and Leaf, A. (1992). Evidence of growth retardation in neonates of apparently normal weight. *Eur. J. Gynecol. Reprod. Biol.*, **45**, 59–62

46. Ott, W. J. (1993). Intrauterine growth retardation and preterm delivery. *Am. J. Obstet. Gynecol.*, **168**, 1710–17

47. Wolf, E. J., Vintzileos, A. M., Rosenkrantz, T. S. *et al.* (1993). Do survival and morbidity of very-low-birth-weight infants vary according to the primary pregnancy complication that results in preterm delivery? *Am. J. Obstet. Gynecol.*, **169**, 1233–9

48. Hadlock, F. P., Harrist, R. B. and Martinez-Poyer, J. (1991). *In utero* analysis of fetal growth: a sonographic weight standard. *Radiology*, **181**, 129–33

49. Carr-Hill, R. A. and Pritchard, C. W. (1983). Reviewing birth weight standards. *Br. J. Obstet. Gynaecol.*, **90**, 718–23

50. Forbes, J. F. (1983). A comparative analysis of birth weight for gestational age standards. *Br. J. Obstet. Gynaecol.*, **99**, 297–308

51. Naeye, R. L. and Dixon, J. B. (1979). Distortions in fetal growth standards. *Pediatr. Res.*, **12**, 987–1008

52. Raju, T. N. K., Winegar, A., Seifert, L. *et al.* (1987). Birth weight and gestational age standards based on regional perinatal network data: an analysis of risk factors. *Am. J. Perinatol.*, **4**, 253–67

53. Wilcox, A. J. (1981). Birth weight, gestation, and fetal growth curve. *Am. J. Obstet. Gynecol.*, **139**, 863–71

54. Goldenberg, R. L., Nelson, K. G., Koski, J. F. *et al.* (1985). Low birth weight, intrauterine growth retardation, and preterm delivery. *Am. J. Obstet. Gynecol.*, **152**, 980–5

55. Ott, W. J. and Doyle, S. (1982). Normal ultrasonic fetal weight curve. *Obstet. Gynecol.*, **59**, 603–7

56. Secher, N. J., Hansen, P. K., Thomsen, B. L. *et al.* (1987). Growth retardation in preterm infants. *Br. J. Obstet. Gynaecol.*, **94**, 115–21

57. Brenner, W. E., Edelman, D. A. and Hendricks, C. H. (1976). A standard of fetal growth for the United States of America. *Am. J. Obstet. Gynecol.*, **126**, 555–64

58. Ott, W. J. (1988). The diagnosis of altered fetal growth. *Obstet. Gynecol. Clin. North Am.*, **15**, 237–63

59. Goldenberg, A. L., Cutter, G. R., Hoffman, H. J. *et al.* (1989). Intrauterine growth retardation: standards for diagnosis. *Am. J. Obstet. Gynecol.*, **161**, 271–7

60. Goldenberg, R. L., Nelson, K. G., Koski, J. F. *et al.* (1985). Low birth weight, intrauterine growth retardation, and preterm delivery. *Am. J. Obstet. Gynecol.*., **152**, 980–4

61. Tamura, R. K., Sabbagha, R. E., Depp, R. *et al.* (1984). Diminished growth in fetuses born preterm after spontaneous labor or rupture of membranes. *Am. J. Obstet. Gynecol.*, **148**, 1105–10

62. Hediger, M. L., Scholl, T. O., Schall, J. I. *et al.* (1995). Fetal growth and the etiology of preterm delivery. *Obstet. Gynecol.*, **85**, 175–82

63. Leveno, K. J., Little, B. B. and Cunningham, F. G. (1990). The national impact of ritodrine hydrochloride for inhibition of preterm labor. *Obstet. Gynecol.*, **76**, 12–15

64. Salafia, C. M., Vintzileos, A. M., Bantham, K. F. *et al.* (1991). Placental pathologic findings in preterm birth. *Am. J. Obstet. Gynecol.*, **165**, 934–8

65. Salafia, C. M., Vogel, C. A., Bantham, K. F. *et al.* (1992). Preterm delivery: correlation of fetal growth and placental pathology. *Am. J. Perinatol.*, **9**, 190–3

66. Deter, R. L., Rossavik, I. K., Harrist, R. B. *et al.* (1986). Mathematical modeling of fetal growth: development of individual growth curve standards. *Obstet. Gynecol.*, **68**, 156–64

67. Johnson, T. R. B. (1986). Clinical estimation of gestational age. *Cont. Obstet. Gynecol.*, **11**, 55–66

68. Ott, W. J. (1984). Routine prenatal care and identification of the high-risk patient. In Arias, F. A. (ed.) *High-Risk Pregnancy and Delivery*, pp. 1–17. (St Louis: CV Mosby)

69. Babson, S. G., Bearhman, R. E. and Lessel, R. (1970). Live born birth weights for gestational age of white middle-class infants. *Pediatrics*, **45**, 937–49

70. Lubchenco, L. O., Hansman, C., Dressler, M. *et al.* (1963). Intrauterine growth as estimated from live-born weight data at 24–42 weeks of gestation. *Pediatrics*, **32**, 793–801

71. Williams, R. L., Creasy, R. K., Cunningham, G. C. *et al.* (1982). Fetal growth and perinatal viability in California. *Obstet. Gynecol.*, **59**, 624–32

72. Secher, N. J., Hansen, P. K., Lenstrup, C. *et al.* (1986). Birth weight-for-gestational age charts based on early ultrasound estimation of gestational age. *Br. J. Obstet. Gynaecol.*, **93**, 128–36

73. Jeanty, P., Cantraine, F., Romero, R. *et al.* (1984). A longitudinal study of fetal weight growth. *J. Ultrasound Med.*, **3**, 321–34

74. Boyd, M. E., Usher, R. J. and McLean, F. H. (1983). Fetal macrosomia: prediction, risks, proposed management. *Obstet. Gynecol.*, **61**, 715–23

75. Curran, J. S. (1981). Birth-associated injury. *Clin. Perinat.*, **8**, 111–21

76. Golditch, I. M. and Kirkman, K. (1978). The large fetus: management and outcome. *Obstet. Gynecol.*, **52**, 26

77. Modanlou, H. C., Komatsu, G., Dorchester, W. *et al.* (1982). Large for gestational age neonates: anthropometric reasons for shoulder dystocia. *Obstet. Gynecol.*, **60**, 417–22

78. Lazer, S., Hiale, Y., Mozor, M. *et al.* (1987). Complications associated with the macrosomic fetus. *J. Reprod. Med.*, **31**, 501–5

79. Lieberman, E., Lang, J. M., Ryan, K. J. *et al.* (1989). The association of inter-pregnancy interval with small for gestational age births. *Obstet. Gynecol.*, **74**, 1–5

80. Rawlings, J. S., Rawlings, V. B. and Read, J. A. (1995). Prevalence of low birth weight and preterm delivery in relation to the interval between pregnancies among white and black women. *N. Engl. J. Med.*, **332**, 69–74

81. Duverot, J. J., Cheriex, E., Pieters, F. A. A. *et al.* (1995). Maternal volume homeostasis in early pregnancy in relation to fetal growth restriction. *Obstet. Gynecol.*, **85**, 361–7

82. Salafia, C. M., Ernst, L. M., Pezzullo, J. C. *et al.* (1995). The very low birthweight infant: maternal complications leading to preterm birth, placental lesions, and intrauterine growth. *Am. J. Perinatol.*, **12**, 106–10

83. Belizan, J. M., Villar, J., Nardin, J. C. *et al.* (1978). Diagnosis of intrauterine growth retardation by a simple clinical method: measurement of uterine height. *Am. J. Obstet. Gynecol.*, **131**, 643–58

84. Calvert, J. P., Crean, E. E. and Newcombe, R. G. (1982). Antenatal screening by measurement

of symphysis-fundus height. *Br. Med. J.*, **285**, 846–53

85. Mathai, M., Jairaj, P. and Muthurathnam, S. (1987). Screening of light-for-gestational age infants: a comparison of three simple measurements. *Br. J. Obstet. Gynaecol.*, **94**, 217–27

86. Pearce, J. M. and Campbell, S. (1987). A comparison of symphysis-fundal height and ultrasound as screening tests for light-for-gestational age infants. *Br. J. Obstet. Gynaecol.*, **94**, 100–7

87. Quaranta, P., Currell, R. and Robinson, J. S. (1981). Prediction of small-for-dates infants by measurement of symphysial-fundal-height. *Br. J. Obstet. Gynaecol.*, **88**, 115–21

88. Benson, C. B., Doubilet, P. M. and Saltzman, D. H. (1986). Intrauterine growth retardation: predictive value of US criteria for antenatal diagnosis. *Radiology*, **160**, 415–26

89. Brown, H. L., Miller, J. M., Gabert, H. A. *et al.* (1987). Ultrasonic recognition of the small-for-gestational-age fetus. *Obstet. Gynecol.*, **69**, 631–47

90. Crane, J. P., Lopta, M. M., Welt, S. I. *et al.* (1977). Abnormal fetal growth patterns: ultrasonic diagnosis and management. *Obstet. Gynecol.*, **50**, 205–9

91. Deter, R. L., Harrist, R. B., Hadlock, F. P. *et al.* (1982). The use of ultrasound in the detection of intrauterine growth retardation: a review. *J. Clin. Ultrasound*, **10**, 9–22

92. Deter, R. L., Hadlock, F. P. and Harrist, R. B. (1983). Evaluation of normal fetal growth and the detection of intrauterine growth retardation. In Callen, P. W. (ed.) *Ultrasonography in Obstetrics and Gynecology*, pp. 113–40. (Philadelphia: W. B. Saunders)

93. Hadlock, F. P., Deter, R. L., Harrist, R. B. *et al.* (1983). Sonographic detection of fetal intrauterine growth retardation. *Perinatol. Neonatol.*, **7**, 21–32

94. Little, D. and Campbell, S. (1982). Ultrasound evaluation of intrauterine growth retardation. *Radiol. Clin. North Am.*, **20**, 335–42

95. Ott, W. J. (1985). Fetal femur length, neonatal crown–heel length and screening for IUGR. *Obstet. Gynecol.*, **65**, 460–5

96. Sholl, J. S., Woo, D., Rubin, J. M. *et al.* (1982). Intrauterine growth retardation risk detection for fetuses of unknown gestational age. *Am. J. Obstet. Gynecol.*, **144**, 709–12

97. Zilianti, M., Fernandez, S., Azuaga, A. *et al.* (1987). Ultrasound evaluation of the distal femoral epiphyseal ossification center as a screening test for intrauterine growth retardation. *Obstet. Gynecol.*, **70**, 361–9

98. Arora, S. S. (1984). Predictive value of test results. *Am. J. Obstet. Gynecol.*, **149**, 104–9

99. Stemple, L. E. (1982). Eenie, meenie, minie, mo... What do the data really show? *Am. J. Obstet. Gynecol.*, **144**, 745–8

100. Ott, W. J. (1981). Clinical application of fetal weight determination by real-time ultrasound measurements. *Obstet. Gynecol.*, **57**, 758–62

101. Timor-Tritsch, I. E., Itskoviz, J. and Brandes, J. M. (1981). Estimation of fetal weight by real time sonography. *Obstet. Gynecol.*, **57**, 653–7

102. Campbell, S. and Wilkin, D. (1975). Ultrasonic measurement of fetal abdomen circumference in the estimation of fetal weight. *Br. J. Obstet. Gynaecol.*, **82**, 689–97

103. Robson, S. C., Galivan, S., Walkinshaw, S. A. *et al.* (1993). Ultrasonic estimation of fetal weight: use of targeted formulas in small for gestational age fetuses. *Obstet. Gynecol.*, **82**, 359–64

104. Mills, M. D., Nageotte, M. P., Elliott, J. P. *et al.* (1990). Reliability of ultrasonographic formulary in the prediction of fetal weight and survival of very-low-birth-weight infants. *Am. J. Obstet. Gynecol.*, **163**, 1568–74

105. Guidetti, D. A., Divon, M. Y., Braverman, J. J. *et al.* (1990). Sonographic estimates of fetal weight in the intrauterine growth retardation population. *Am. J. Perinatol.*, **7**, 5–7

106. Tahilramaney, M. P., Platt, L. D., Yeh, S. Y. *et al.* (1985). Ultrasonic estimation of weight in the very low-birth weight fetus: a resident versus staff physician comparison. *Am. J. Obstet. Gynecol.*, **151**, 90–1

107. Townsend, R. R., Filly, R. A., Callen, P. W. *et al.* (1988). Factors affection prenatal sonographic estimation of weight in extremely low birth weight infants. *J. Ultrasound Med.*, **7**, 183–7

108. Medchill, M. T., Peterson, C. M., Kreinick, C. *et al.* (1991). Prediction of estimated fetal weight in extremely low birth weight neonates (500–1000 g). *Obstet. Gynecol.*, **78**, 286–90

109. Hadlock, F. P., Harrist, R. B., Carpenter, R. J. *et al.* (1984). Sonographic estimation of fetal weight. *Radiology*, **150**, 553–540

110. Warsof, S. L., Gohari, P., Berkowitz, R. L. *et al.* (1977). The estimation of fetal weight by computer-assisted analysis. *Am. J. Obstet. Gynecol.*, **128**, 881–92

111. Shepard, M. J., Richards, V. A., Berkowitz, R. L. *et al.* (1982). An evaluation of two equations for predicting fetal weight by ultrasound. *Am. J. Obstet. Gynecol.*, **142**, 47–54

112. Ott, W. J., Doyle, S., Flamm, S. *et al.* (1986). Accurate ultrasonic estimation of fetal weight: prospective analysis of new ultrasonic formulae. *Am. J. Perinatol.*, **3**, 307–10

113. Ott, W. J., Doyle, S., Flamm, S. and Wittman, J. (1986). Accurate ultrasonic estimation of fetal

weight. III. Prospective analysis of new ultrasonic formulae. *Am. J. Perinatol.*, **3**, 307–11

114. Winn, H. N., Rauk, P. N. and Petrie, R. H. (1992). Use of the fetal chest in estimating fetal weight. *Am. J. Obstet. Gynecol.*, **167**, 448–50

115. Rose, B. I. and McCallum, W. D. (1987). A simplified method for estimating fetal weight using ultrasound measurements. *Obstet. Gynecol.*, **69**, 671–5

116. Vintzileos, A. M., Campbell, W. A., Rodis, J. F. *et al.* (1987). Fetal weight estimation formulas with head, abdominal, femur, and thigh circumference measurements. *Am. J. Obstet. Gynecol.*, **157**, 410–14

117. Ott, W. J., Doyle, S. and Flamm, S. (1985). Accurate ultrasonic estimation of fetal weight. *Am. J. Perinatol.*, **2**, 178–82

118. Thompson, H. O., Casaceli, C. and Woods, J. R. (1990). Ultrasonographic fetal weight estimation by an integrated computer-assisted system: can each laboratory improve its accuracy? *Am. J. Obstet. Gynecol.*, **163**, 986–95

119. Chauhan, S. P., Lutton, T. C., Bailey, K. J. *et al.* (1993). Intrapartum prediction of birth weight: clinical versus sonographic estimation based on femur length alone. *Obstet. Gynecol.*, **81**, 695–7

120. Timor-Tritsch, I. E., Itskovitz, J. and Brandes, J. M. (1981). Estimation of fetal weight by real-time sonography. *Obstet. Gynecol.*, **57**, 653–6

121. Chang, T. C., Robson, S., Spencer, J. A. D. *et al.* (1993). Ultrasonic fetal weight estimation: analysis of inter- and intra-observer variability. *J. Clin. Ultrasound*, **21**, 515–19

122. Platek, D. N., Divon, M. Y., Anyaegbunam, A. *et al.* (1991). Intrapartum ultrasonographic estimates of fetal weight by the house staff. *Am. J. Obstet. Gynecol.*, **165**, 842–5

123. Catanzarite, V. A. and Rose, B. I. (1987). Ultrasound in obstetric decision making: how accurate are late ultrasound scans in gestational age and fetal weight assessment? *Am. J. Perinatol.*, **4**, 147–51

124. Hill, L. M., Breckle, R., Wolfgram, K. R. *et al.* (1986). Evaluation of three methods for estimating fetal weight. *J. Clin. Ultrasound*, **14**, 171–8

125. Favre, R., Nisand, G., Bettahar, K. *et al.* (1993). Measurement of limb circumferences with three-dimensional ultrasound for fetal weight estimation. *Ultrasound Obstet. Gynecol.*, **3**, 176–9

126. Farmer, R. M., Medearis, A. L., Hirata, G. I. *et al.* (1992). The use of a neural network for the ultrasonographic estimation of fetal weight in the macrosomic fetus. *Am. J. Obstet. Gynecol.*, **166**, 1467–72

127. Combs, C. A., Jaekle, R. K., Rosenn, B. *et al.* (1993). Sonographic estimation of fetal weight based on a model of fetal volume. *Obstet. Gynecol.*, **82**, 365–70

128. Dudley, N. J., Lamb, M. P. and Copping, C. (1987). A new method for fetal weight estimation using real-time ultrasound. *Br. J. Obstet. Gynaecol.*, **94**, 110–14

129. Hadlock, F. P., Harrist, R. B. and Martinez-Poyer, J. (1992). Fetal body ratios in second trimester: a useful tool for identifying chromosomal abnormalities? *J. Ultrasound Med.*, **11**, 81–5

130. David, C., Gabrielli, S., Pilu, G. *et al.* (1995). The head-to-abdomen circumference ratio: a reappraisal. *Ultrasound Obstet. Gynecol.*, **5**, 256–9

131. Ott, W. J. (1988). The diagnosis of altered fetal growth. *Obstet. Gynecol. Clin. North Am.*, **15**, 237–63

132. Emery, A. E. H. and Rimoin, D. L. (1990). Nature and incidence of genetic disease. In Emery, A. E. H. and Rimoin, D. L. (eds.) *Principles and Practice of Medical Genetics*, pp. 3–6. (Edinburgh: Churchill Livingstone)

133. Schauer, G. M., Kalousek, D. K. and Magee, J. F. (1992). Genetic causes of stillbirth. *Semin. Perinatol.*, **16**, 341–51

134. Goldstein, I., Reece, E. A.., Pulu, G. *et al.* (1987). Cerebellar measurements with ultrasonography in the evaluation of fetal growth and development. *Am. J. Obstet. Gynecol.*, **157**, 632–8

135. Reece, E. A., Goldstein, I., Puli, G. *et al.* (1987). Fetal cerebellar growth unaffected by intrauterine growth retardation: a new parameter for prenatal diagnosis. *Am. J. Obstet. Gynecol.*, **157**, 632–8

136. Campbell, W. A., Nardi, D., Vintzileos, A. M. *et al.* (1991). Transverse cerebellar diameter/abdominal circumference ratio throughout pregnancy: a gestational age-independent method to assess fetal growth. *Obstet. Gynecol.*, **77**, 893–6

137. Meyer, W. J., Gauthier, D., Ramakrishnan, V. *et al.* (1994). Ultrasonographic detection of abnormal fetal growth with the gestational age-independent, transverse cerebellar diameter/abdominal circumference ratio. *Am. J. Obstet. Gynecol.*, **171**, 1057–63

138. Hill, L. M., Guzick, D., Rivello, D. *et al.* (1990). The transverse cerebellar diameter cannot be used to assess gestational age in the small for gestational age fetus. *Obstet. Gynecol.*, **75**, 329–33

139. Hill, L. M., Guzick, D., DiNofrio, D. *et al.* (1994). Ratios between the abdominal circumference, head circumference, or femur length and the transverse cerebellar diameter of the growth-retarded and macrosomic fetus. *Am. J. Perinatol.*, **11**, 144–8

140. Cabbad, M., Kofinas, A., Simon, N. *et al.* (1992). Fetal weight-cerebellar diameter discordance as an indicator of asymmetrical fetal growth impairment. *J.. Reprod. Med.*, **37**, 794–8

141. Abramowicz, J. S., Sherer, D. M., Bar-Tov, E. *et al.* (1991). The *cheek-to-cheek diameter* in the ultrasonographic assessment of fetal growth. *Am. J. Obstet. Gynecol.*, **165**, 846–52

142. Hill, L. M., Guzick, D., Thomas, M. L. *et al.* (1989). Thigh circumference in the detection of intrauterine growth retardation. *Am. J. Perinatol.*, **6**, 349–52

143. Hill, L. M., Guzick, D., Doyles, D., *et al.* (1992). Subcutaneous tissue thickness cannot be used to distinguish abnormalities of fetal growth. *Obstet. Gynecol.*, **80**, 268–71

144. Gimondo, P., Mirk, P., LaBella, A. *et al.* (1995). Sonographic estimation of fetal liver weight: an additional biometric parameter for assessment of fetal growth. *J. Ultrasound Med.*, **14**, 327–33

145. Naeye, R. L. (1987). Do placental weights have clinical significance? *Hum. Pathol.*, **18**, 387–91

146. Hendricks, C. H. (1964). Patterns of fetal and placental growth: the second half of normal pregnancy. *Obstet. Gynecol.*, **24**, 357–65

147. Wolf, H., Oosting, H. and Treffers, P. E. (1987). Placental volume measurement by ultrasonography: evaluation of the method. *Am. J. Obstet. Gynecol.*, **156**, 1191–4

148. Geirsson, R. T., Ogston, S. A., Patel, N. B. *et al.* (1985). Growth of total intrauterine, intra-amniotic and placental volume in normal singleton pregnancy measured by ultrasound. *Br. J. Obstet. Gynaecol.*, **92**, 46–53

149. Wolf, H., Oosting, H. and Treffers, P. E. (1989). Second-trimester placental volume measurement by ultrasound: prediction of fetal outcome. *Am. J. Obstet. Gynecol.*, **160**, 121–6

150. Wolf, H., Oosting, H. and Treffers, P. E. (1989). A longitudinal study of the relationship between placental and fetal growth as measured by ultrasonography. *Am. J. Obstet. Gynecol.*, **161**, 1140–5

151. Jauniaux, E., Ramsay, B. and Campbell, S. (1994). Ultrasonographic investigation of placental morphologic characteristics and size during the second trimester of pregnancy. *Am. J. Obstet. Gynecol.*, **170**, 130–70

152. Hellman, L. M., Kobayashi, M., Tolles, W. E. *et al.* (1970). Ultrasonic studies on the volumetric growth of the human placenta. *Am. J. Obstet. Gynecol.*, **108**, 740–50

153. Geirsson, R. T., Christie, A. D. and Patel, N. (1982). Ultrasound volume measurements comparing a prolated ellipsoid method with a parallel planimetric area method against a known volume. *J. Clin. Ultrasound*, **10**, 329–32

Three-dimensional ultrasound in the evaluation of fetal anatomy and fetal malformations

7

E. Merz

INTRODUCTION

The evaluation of fetal structures and fetal abnormalities has made great strides in recent years owing to the development of high-performance ultrasound instruments. The fact remains, however, that conventional ultrasound technology can provide only two-dimensional sectional views of three-dimensional structures. It is true that two-dimensional ultrasound can define and document the sectional planes of interest for prenatal diagnosis in the majority of cases. Also, an experienced examiner can readily piece together the two-dimensional planes to create a three-dimensional mental image. Problems arise, however, when individual sectional planes cannot be achieved in the two-dimensional image because of fetal position, or in fetuses with complex anomalies that must be evaluated in multiple planes. Another disadvantage of conventional two-dimensional ultrasound technology is that, once the examiner has gained a three-dimensional impression of a fetal anomaly, this can be communicated to the parents only in descriptive terms.

Today, not only can three-dimensional ultrasonography portray individual image planes, like two-dimensional ultrasound, but it can also store complete tissue volumes. These stored volumes can be digitally manipulated to display all mutually perpendicular image planes in rotated or translated views, allowing a systematic tomographic survey of a particular fetal region. This same technology can also display surface-rendered and transparent views to provide a realistic, three-dimensional portrayal of fetal structures.

METHODS OF VOLUME DATA ACQUISITION

The first results of *in vitro* three-dimensional ultrasound imaging experiments were reported in the early 1980s[1,2], but various technical difficulties delayed the clinical application of the technology for several years[3–15].

Two main techniques are currently available for the acquisition of volume data:

(1) The localization of manual transducer movements in space with the use of a position sensor[6,7,13,16]. In this technique individual two-dimensional image planes are spatially correlated with the momentary transducer position, and the digitized data are stored at corresponding sites in a volume image memory. A computer program is then used to generate three-dimensional images from the stored volume data. The advantage of this technique is that it can be used with any type of ultrasound imager. Its disadvantage is that it does not yet provide satisfactory image quality, so at present it is unsuitable for routine clinical use.

(2) The use of a special three-dimensional transducer[17–27] connected to a two-dimensional ultrasound scanner with an integrated three-dimensional control and storage unit. The basic principle of this technique is that a scanner-specific three-dimensional transducer is swept through a designated volume comprised of many separate planes of section whose intervals are precisely known. This is done automatically

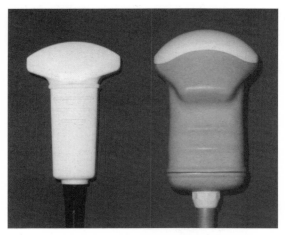

Figure 1 *Mechanical three-dimensional annular phased volume transducer (5 MHz) (right-hand side) for abdominal imaging (Kretztechnik, Austria) compared with a conventional cured-array transducer*

with a motor-driven transducer mounted inside the probe casing. With the endovaginal probe, a rotary transducer movement is used for data acquisition[26,27]. With the abdominal probe, the transducer is swept through a designated arc[19,24,25] (Figures 1 and 2).

In transvaginal as well as abdominal volume scanning, all echoes are processed and stored as digital signals at correlative sites in a volume memory. This memory can then be accessed for computing, simultaneously displaying all sectional planes within the scanned volume along with the corresponding perpendicular planes. The volume data can also be processed to generate three-dimensional surface and transparent views.

Examination technique

Three-dimensional data acquisition and rendering consists of five basic steps:

(1) Volume data acquisition and checking of the data set;

(2) Tomographic analysis of the sectional images (simultaneous display of all three orthogonal planes);

(3) Processing of the volume data;

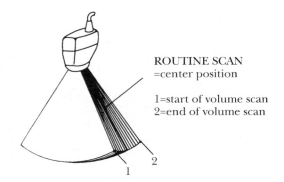

ROUTINE SCAN
=center position

1=start of volume scan
2=end of volume scan

Figure 2 *For abdominal volume data acquisition, the transducer element is automatically swept from point 1 to point 2. An arc of 30–70 ° gives the scanned volume the shape of a truncated pyramid. (Reproduced with permission of Kretztechnik, Austria)*

(4) Generation of a surface, transparent or X-ray view; and

(5) Optimization of the image and display of rotated views.

Volume data acquisition

The examination starts like a conventional two-dimensional ultrasound examination, except that a three-dimensional probe is used. First, the fetal region of interest is surveyed, and the B-mode image settings are optimized. A volume box of adjustable size is superimposed on the B-mode image to outline the volume that will be stored. The scanning speed and angle of arc are selected, and volume storage is initiated. Within about 4 s the outlined volume is automatically scanned and stored in memory.

Care is taken to hold the transducer stationary while the volume data are being fed into the volume memory. Also, the scan should be initiated at a time when there is little or no fetal movement. This avoids motion artifacts that could lead to misinterpretation or interfere with three-dimensional image reconstruction (Figure 3).

Orthogonal image display

After the volume data have been collected and stored, all three mutually perpendicular

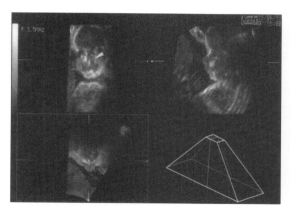

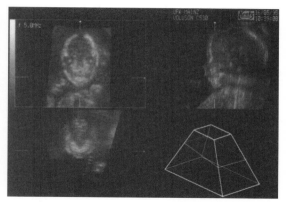

Figure 3 *Motion artifact mimicking cleft lip and palate in coronal view (arrowhead) at 20 weeks*

Figure 4 *Display of all three mutually perpendicular sectional planes (orthogonal image planes), illustrated here for a fetal face at 20 weeks. A volume model can be inserted at lower right to indicate the position of the active, outlined image plane within the stored volume*

(orthogonal) image planes are displayed simultaneously on the monitor (Figures 3 and 4). The corresponding scan planes are marked by lines at the periphery of the field. A fourth, graphic model image can be superimposed to indicate the position of the outlined reference plane within the stored volume (Figures 3 and 4). By manipulating three rotation controls, the user can conduct a highly detailed, slice-by-slice on-line survey of fetal structures. This can be done on conventional scan planes as well as planes that are not accessible to traditional two-dimensional abdominal ultrasound, such as coronal and oblique sections. Additionally, the entire volume can be rotated so that the region of interest can be viewed on the plane that allows the best evaluation. This means that conventional terms of orientation such as cranial, caudal, left and right can be applied only to the object being examined. They are no longer applicable to the monitor, as in conventional two-dimensional ultrasound, because the only views of interest to the examiner are those that most clearly portray the abnormal finding. This may be seen most clearly in longitudinal section, transverse section, or any of a number of oblique sections[24].

This technique is advantageous for the accurate portrayal of a specific plane of section, such as the mid-sagittal plane for defining the fetal head and facial profile. It must be absolutely certain that the plane displayed is actually the desired plane before the examiner can confi-

dently diagnose the presence of an abnormality such as retrognathism (Figures 5 and 6). Undesired obliquity of the section could easily mimic such an anomaly. Similar considerations apply to defining the fetal profile in severe oligohydramnios (Figure 7) and accurately demonstrating the absence of a fetal brain structure (Figure 8).

As various groups have pointed out, the simultaneous display of all three sectional planes is also advantageous in terms of making accurate volume determinations[28,29].

Surface view

For a surface-rendered view, the stored volume data are retrieved and processed to display a three-dimensional view of a designated portion of the fetal body surface. The necessary calculations are performed with a desktop computer integrated into the ultrasound unit, eliminating the need for a separate and costly workstation.

Good surface rendering requires optimum visualization of the object in the two-dimensional images (Figure 9) as well as a sufficiently large amniotic fluid collection in front of the surface to be rendered. Adjacent or superimposed structures such as placental tissue, the umbilical cord, or a fetal limb can interfere with rendering and should first be eliminated by

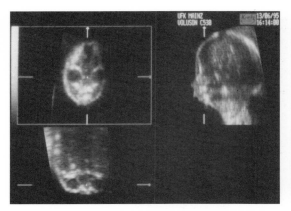

Figure 5 *Face of a fetus with trisomy 18 (orthogonal display) at 23 weeks. Marked retrognathism is noted in this accurately positioned profile view*

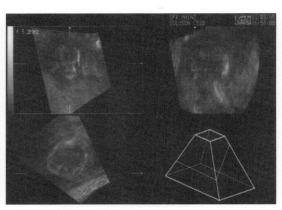

Figure 7 *Face of a fetus with trisomy 21 in severe oligohydramnios (orthogonal view). Note the abnormal facial profile and brachycephaly (17 weeks)*

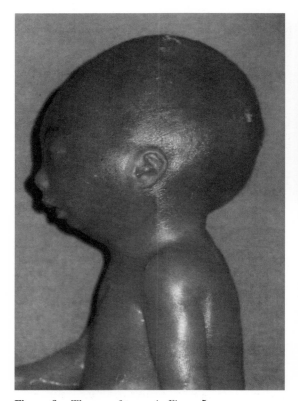

Figure 6 *The same fetus as in Figure 5*

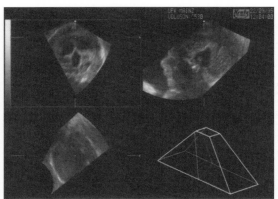

Figure 8 *Orthogonal view of hydrocephalus with agenesis of the corpus callosum in a fetus with trisomy 18 (32 weeks)*

'Cartesian storage', in which only the relevant partial volume is stored[25] (Figure 9). Small extraneous echoes can be eliminated by adjusting the threshold control (Figure 10). After the desired volume has been outlined in all three orthogonal image planes and the three-dimensional switch has been activated, it takes about 20 s for the computer to generate and display the first sculpture-like image on the monitor (Figure 11). The image can then be fine–adjusted to obtain optimum brightness and contrast. By rendering several images in sequence, i.e. from different viewing angles, the user can rotate the rendered surface structure on the monitor. This creates a more realistic impression that the object is actually being viewed in three dimensions (Figure 12).

The three-dimensional surface view of the fetal body opens up entirely new possibilities in the evaluation of normal fetal anatomy (Figures 11–15) and in the detection of subtle

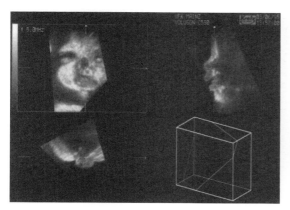

Figure 9 *Orthogonal view of a normal fetal face (32 weeks) after elimination of extraneous structures by Cartesian storage*

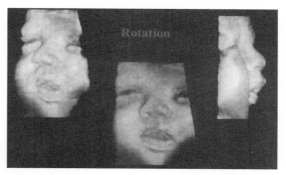

Figure 12 *The fetal face can be viewed from various angles by rotating the volume. Same fetus as in Figures 9–11*

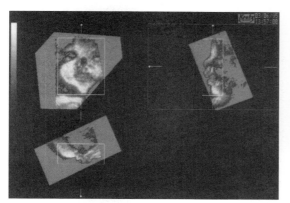

Figure 10 *Unwanted echoes are eliminated by adjusting the threshold control (gray area). Same fetus as in Figure 9*

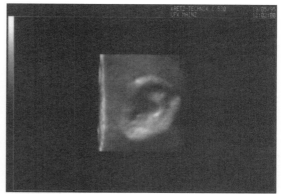

Figure 13 *Surface view of a normal left ear (23 weeks)*

anomalies[20,22–25,30]. Abnormalities of the fetal body surface can be selectively visualized, and the extent of a defect can be accurately assessed in all three planes. This is particularly useful in the diagnosis of anomalies such as facial deformities, cleft lip and palate, low-set ears, auricular dysplasia, spina bifida, ventral clefts, and malformations of the hands and feet (Figures 16–30). Rotating the surface view not only strengthens the three-dimensional impression of an abnormality but also clearly demonstrates anomalies that are associated with angular deformity (e.g. clubfoot).

Transparent and X-ray views

This mode differs from the surface-rendered view by displaying the object as if it were made of a translucent material. Echogenic features

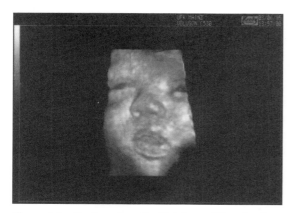

Figure 11 *Surface view of a fetal face at 28 weeks. Same fetus as in Figures 9 and 10*

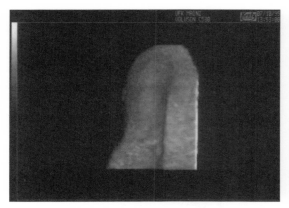

Figure 14 *Surface view of a normal left upper arm (27 weeks)*

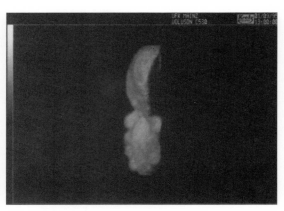

Figure 17 *Surface view of an abnormal facial profile with frontal bossing and depressed nasal root in thanatophoric dysplasia (24 weeks)*

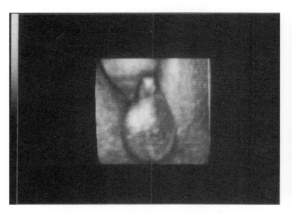

Figure 15 *Surface view of normal male genitalia (29 weeks)*

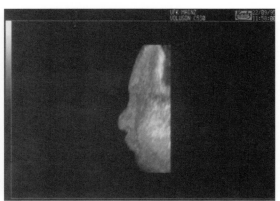

Figure 18 *Surface view of an abnormally flat facial profile in trisomy 18 (28 weeks)*

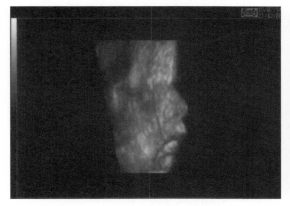

Figure 16 *Surface view of facial dysmorphism and right orbital hypoplasia in a fetus with trisomy 13 (28 weeks)*

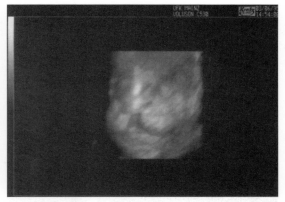

Figure 19 *Surface view of cleft lip and palate (23 weeks)*

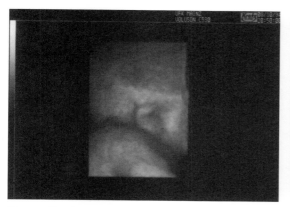

Figure 20 *Surface view of low-set ears in a fetus with arthrogryposis multiplex congenita (28 weeks)*

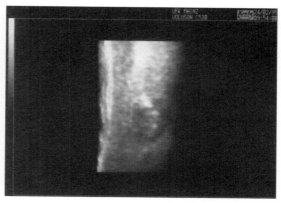

Figure 23 *Surface view of a lumbar myelomeningocele (22 weeks)*

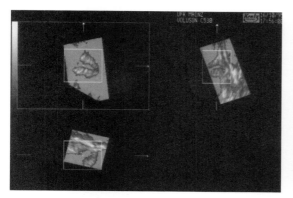

Figure 21 *Orthogonal view of left-sided auricular dysplasia in trisomy 18 (29 weeks). Extraneous echoes were eliminated with the threshold control (gray area)*

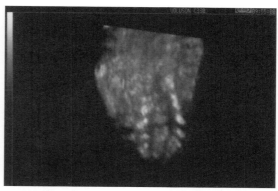

Figure 24 *Surface view of open spina bifida in the lumbar region (21 weeks)*

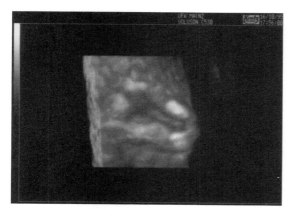

Figure 22 *Surface view of left-sided auricular dysplasia in trisomy 18 (29 weeks). Same fetus as in Figure 21*

can be displayed in isolation by filtering out hypoechoic structures. This provides a complete survey view of the fetal skeleton, similar to the appearance of an X-ray film (Figures 31–34)[23–25,31]. Extraneous echoes are unimportant in the transparent view, where they are automatically eliminated. As in the surface view, multiple image planes can be processed to generate rotated views of the transparent object, again reinforcing the impression of viewing a three-dimensional object in space.

Volume data storage

Because of the large storage requirements, we store the volume data and three-dimensional

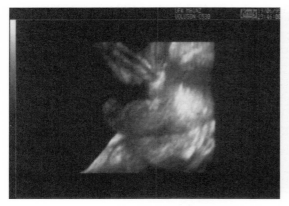

Figure 25 *Surface view of a small omphalocele, viewed from the left side (23 weeks)*

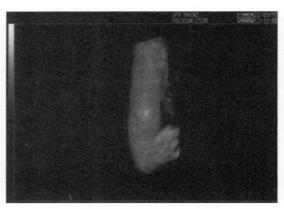

Figure 28 *Surface view of the fetus in Figure 27 clearly demonstrates the cephalad angulation of the four-fingered hand*

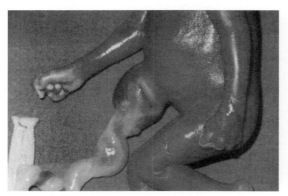

Figure 26 *Small omphalocele (23 weeks). Same fetus as in Figure 25*

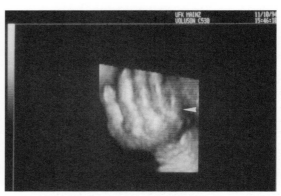

Figure 29 *Surface view of a right hand with hexadactyly (arrowhead, digit VI) (36 weeks). The thumb is located behind the five visible fingers*

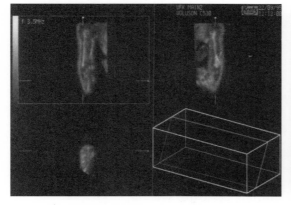

Figure 27 *Orthogonal view of a malformed hand and forearm (32 weeks)*

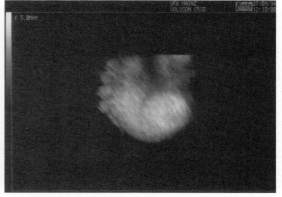

Figure 30 *Surface view of clubfoot, seen from the plantar aspect (24 weeks)*

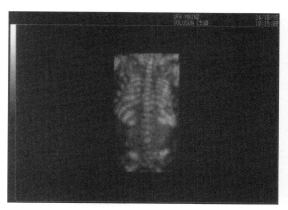

Figure 31 *Transparent view provides an X-ray-like display of the normal spinal column and ribs, viewed from the posterior aspect (20 weeks)*

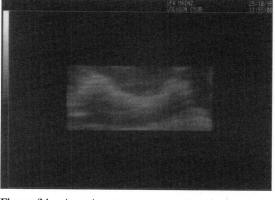

Figure 34 *Anterior transparent view demonstrates marked bowing of the short femur in osteochondrodysplasia (21 weeks)*

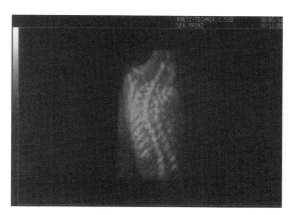

Figure 32 *Orthogonal view of severe scoliosis (23 weeks)*

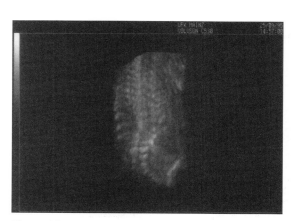

Figure 33 *Lateral transparent view demonstrates severe bowing of the spinal column in the lumbosacral region (26 weeks)*

images on a hard disk drive (Syquest) with removable 88 MB cartridges.

ADVANTAGES OF THREE-DIMENSIONAL ULTRASONOGRAPHY IN PRENATAL DIAGNOSIS

The advantages of three-dimensional ultrasonography over traditional two-dimensional imaging[24] are as follows:

(1) Capabilities for storage and retrieval of a complete volume

    (a) The stored volume is accessible for a detailed, slice-by-slice on-line review in all three planes;

    (b) Patient examination time can be reduced; the stored volumes can be reviewed off-line after the patient has left;

    (c) The volume can be permanently stored on hard disk without degradation, allowing for multiple analysis (including fetal biometry) as well as a retrospective analysis of the stored volume, even after a period of weeks, months, or years;

    (d) The volume can be mailed in the form of a removable hard disk cartridge for independent analysis by a second examiner; and

    (e) Multiple copies of the stored volume provide an excellent medium for education and training (e.g. group practice in locating biometry planes and detecting specific fetal anomalies).

(2) Simultaneous image display

  (a) Demonstration of the third plane, which cannot be displayed by conventional means;

  (b) Unique identification of the displayed anatomic plane (facial profile, biometry planes); and

  (c) Improved volumetric precision.

(3) Surface view for the examiner

  (a) Realistic depiction of fetal surface anatomy;

  (b) Detailed scrutiny of surface structures (e.g. facial evaluation);

  (c) Reliable detection or exclusion of surface defects;

  (d) Visualization of complex anomalies or anomalies that are associated with angular deformity; and

  (e) Ability to view the fetus from various angles by rotating the surface image.

(4) Surface view for the parents

  (a) Entirely new visual experience for parents, owing to near-photographic depiction of fetal structures;

  (b) Potential strengthening of parent–child bond;

  (c) Better assessment of the severity of a fetal anomaly; and

  (d) Greater reassurance for parents in cases where fetal anomalies have been excluded.

(5) Transparent view

  (a) Demonstration of the fetal skeleton provides a prenatal 'babygram'.

Compared with conventional two-dimensional ultrasound, three-dimensional ultrasonography with the capacity for orthogonal, surface and transparent displays opens up entirely new visual possibilities for the examiner and the patient in the evaluation of fetal abnormalities[23–25]. Once the desired volume has been stored, it can be accessed for an accurate and minutely detailed on-line review in conventional scan planes as well as planes not accessible to conventional two-dimensional ultrasound, such as coronal and oblique views. Also, the entire volume can be rotated to give the examiner an optimum view of the investigated region. This ensures unique plane selection for biometry and also allows more accurate volume determinations[28,29] than can be achieved with conventional two-dimensional ultrasound. This also creates new opportunities for the estimation of fetal body weight[32].

In the diagnosis of fetal malformations, three-dimensional ultrasound is advantageous for accurately defining a specific fetal plane, detecting or excluding small surface defects (e.g. cleft lip and palate, spina bifida) and demonstrating facial deformities[23–25]. Three-dimensional ultrasound also permits an accurate tomographic examination of complex organ regions such as the fetal central nervous system[33]. The capacity for the selective visualization of subtle fetal abnormalities opens up new vistas in the diagnosis of chromosomal abnormalities and various syndromic conditions in which it is essential to be able to recognize fine details.

Moreover, the X-ray-like portrayal of the fetal skeleton in the transparent mode offers an entirely new approach to studies of fetal ossification and the diagnosis of ossification defects[23–25,31].

Surface rendering of the fetal face offers a dramatic new visual experience for the parents, who for the first time can see their child with near-photographic clarity. This can contribute significantly to maternofetal bonding[24].

When applied to the diagnosis of fetal anomalies, three-dimensional ultrasound not only can help parents better appreciate the nature and severity of a fetal defect, but in negative cases it can demonstrate the normal condition of the fetus more convincingly than traditional two-dimensional sonograms[24].

In a study comparing two-dimensional and three-dimensional ultrasound findings in 458 fetuses, Merz and colleagues[24] were able to show that three-dimensional ultrasound provided a significant diagnostic gain in a large percentage of the cases (294/458, 64.2%). This gain was recorded in 46.2% of the cases examined by orthogonal imaging alone, owing to the accurate topographic display of the desired plane and the ability to recognize off-axis planes. When the surface and transparent views were added to the orthogonal view, a diagnostic gain was recorded in 71.5% (233/326) of the cases. This higher percentage resulted from the sculpture-like surface view of the fetus, the ability to scrutinize the object from various angles, the accurate size determination of a defect, the skeletal display obtained in the transparent mode and the clearer portrayal of complex malformations.

Further advantages of three-dimensional ultrasonography result from the capacity for volume data storage. The ability to store and retrieve a complete volume rather than a two-dimensional image makes it possible to conduct multiple off-line readings after the patient has left the examination suite. The stored volume can be repeatedly accessed and reviewed millimeter-by-millimeter by the same examiner or a different examiner. The stored volume is also accessible to retrospective analysis after a period of weeks or months. Finally, stored volumes illustrating specific fetal anomalies can be utilized in the training of sonographers.

PROBLEMS WITH THREE-DIMENSIONAL ULTRASONOGRAPHY

The following problems have been identified with three-dimensional ultrasonography[24].

(1) The examiner must get accustomed to the unfamiliar size and shape of the three-dimensional probe;

(2) Movements during the storage process lead to motion artifacts;

(3) Orientation can be difficult in the stored volume;

(4) Three-dimensional reconstruction is relatively time-consuming if the computed image sequence contains a large number of individual images;

(5) Oligohydramnios prevents satisfactory surface reconstruction;

(6) Overlying or adjacent structures interfere with surface rendering and must be eliminated by 'Cartesian storage' prior to surface reconstruction;

(7) If the threshold is set too high, it can mimic structural defects; and

(8) Storage of the three-dimensional images requires a high storage capacity (one abdominal three-dimensional volume requires 5–10 MB of storage).

An initial difficulty of three-dimensional ultrasound is the inevitable learning curve involved in mastering the technique. The routine use of three-dimensional ultrasound requires an ability for good spatial visualization on the part of the examiner and a correspondingly intense learning phase in which the examiner learns how a volume must be acquired and processed so that the object of interest is rendered as quickly as possible with an acceptable image quality. The image quality depends directly on the quality of the ultrasound signals that are produced.

Other problems relate to the presence of oligohydramnios, which prevents satisfactory surface rendering, and to the imaging of moving objects (e.g. the fetal heart), which cause motion artifacts. While a faster scanning speed can be used to store moving objects and reduce artifacts, this tends to degrade the image quality, due to the acquisition of fewer sectional planes.

Another problem is the rendering of image sequences composed of many separate three-dimensional surface images. While surface rendering with a few images can be accomplished in 1–2 min, an image sequence composed of 40 images takes more than 10 min to compute.

Finally, the volumes require a relatively large data storage capacity (about 5–10 MB for an abdominal volume), so the costs of storing numerous volumes can be high.

CRITICAL APPRAISAL AND OUTLOOK

Despite the problems that still exist with three-dimensional ultrasonography, it is already apparent that this technology has evolved into a useful adjunct to conventional two-dimensional ultrasound, and that an examiner experienced in diagnosing fetal anomalies can profitably apply the technology for the selective investigation of suspicious findings.

There is a definite need for further technical refinements that will speed up three-dimensional image computation and allow a more cost-effective storage of volume data. Considering the very rapid pace at which three-dimensional technology has evolved thus far, it is reasonable to expect that many current problems will be solved in the near future, bringing us ever closer to the goal of real-time three-dimensional ultrasound imaging. It remains to be seen whether this goal will be achieved more quickly through refinements in existing technology or by developing improved optical lens systems that are placed in front of the transducer[34,35].

References

1. Brinkley, J. F., Muramatsu, S. K., McCallum, W. D. and Popp, R. L. (1982). *In vitro* evaluation of ultrasonic three dimensional imaging and volume system. *Ultrasonic Imaging*, **4**, 126–39
2. Fredfelt, K. E., Holm, H. H. and Pedersen, J. F. (1984). Three dimensional ultrasonic scanning. *Acta Radiol. Diagn.*, **25**, 237–41
3. Sohn, C., Grotepaß, J., Schneider, W., Funk, A., Sohn, G., Jensch, P., Fendel, H., Ameling, W. and Jung, H. (1988). Erste Untersuchungen zur dreidimensionalen Darstellung mittels Ultraschall. *Z. Geburtsh. Perinat.*, **192**, 241–8
4. Baba, K., Satch, K., Sakamoto, S., Okal, T. and Shiego, I. (1989). Development of an ultrasonic system for three-dimensional reconstruction of the fetus. *J. Perinat. Med.*, **17**, 19–24
5. Sohn, C., Grotepaß, J. and Swobodnik, W. (1989). Möglichkeiten der 3-Dimensionalen Ultraschalluntersuchung. *Ultraschall*, **10**, 307–13
6. King, D. L., King, D. L. Jr and Shao, M. Y. (1990). Three dimensional spatial registration and interactive display of position and orientation of real-time ultrasound images. *J. Ultrasound Med.*, **9**, 525–32
7. Rotten, D., Levaillant, J. M., Constancis, E., Billon, A. C., Le Guerinel, Y. and Rua, P. (1991). Three-dimensional imaging of solid breast tumors with ultrasound: preliminary data and analysis of its possible contribution to the understanding of the standard two-dimensional sonographic images. *Ultrasound Obstet. Gynecol.*, **1**, 384–90
8. Pretorius, D. H. and Nelson, T. R. (1991). Three-dimensional ultrasound imaging in patient diagnosis and management: the future. *Ultrasound Obstet. Gynecol.*, **1**, 381–3
9. Kratochwil, A. (1992). Versuch der 3-Dimensionalen Darstellung in der Geburtshilfe. *Ultraschall Med.*, **13**, 183–6
10. Sohn, C., Stolz, W., Nuber, B., Hesse, A. and Hornung, B. (1991). Die dreidimensionale Ultraschalldiagnostik in Gynäkologie und Geburtshilfe. *Geburtsh. Frauenheilkd.*, **51**, 335–40
11. Lees, W. R., Gardener, J. E. and Gillams, A. (1991). Three-dimensional ultrasound of the fetus. *Radiology*, **181**, 132
12. Merz, E., Macchiella, D., Bahlmann, F. and Weber, G. (1991). Fetale Fehlbildungsdiagnostik mit Hilfe der 3-D-Sonographie. *Ultraschall Klin. Prax.*, **6**, 147
13. Kelly, I. M. G., Gardener, J. E. and Lees, W. R. (1992). Three-dimensional fetal ultrasound. *Lancet*, **339**, 1062–4
14. Kuo, H. C., Chang, F. M., Wu, C. H., Yao, B. L. and Liu, C. H. (1992). The primary application of three-dimensional ultrasonography in obstetrics. *Am. J. Obstet. Gynecol.*, **166**, 880–6
15. Nelson, T. R. and Pretorius, D. H. (1992). Three-dimensional ultrasound of fetal surface features. *Ultrasound Obstet. Gynecol.*, **2**, 166–74
16. Watkin, K. L., Khalifé, S., Nuwayhid, B., Baer, L., Mathur, S., El-Hakim, S. and Diouf, I. (1993). Three dimensional reconstruction of freehand abdominal and vaginal ultrasonic images. *Ultrasound Obstet. Gynecol.*, **3** (Suppl. 2), 185
17. Bernaschek, G. and Deutinger, J. (1993). Voluvision fetaler Fehlbildungen. *Ultraschall Klin. Prax.*, **8**, 154
18. Steiner, H., Staudach, A., Spitzer, D., Graf, A. H. and Wienerroither, H. (1993). Bietet die 3-D-Sonographie neue Perspektiven in der Gynäkologie und Geburtshilfe? *Geburtsh. Frauenheilkd.*, **53**, 779–82

19. Kirbach, D. and Whittingham, T. A. (1994). 3-D ultrasound – the Kretztechnik Voluson® approach. *Eur. J. Ultrasound*, **1**, 85–9

20. Lee, A., Deutinger, J. and Bernaschek, G. (1994). Voluvision: three-dimensional ultrasonography of fetal malformations. *Am. J. Obstet. Gynecol.*, **170**, 1312–14

21. Merz, E. (1994). Volume (3-D) scanning in the evaluation of fetal malformation. *Ultrasound Obstet. Gynecol.*, **4** (Suppl. 1), 196

22. Steiner, H., Staudach, A., Spitzer, D. and Schaffer, H. (1994). Three-dimensional ultrasound in obstetrics and gynaecology; technique, possibilities and limitations. *Hum. Reprod.*, **9**, 1773–8

23. Merz, E., Bahlmann, F. and Weber, G. (1995). Volume (3-D)-scanning in the evaluation of fetal malformations – a new dimension in prenatal diagnosis. *Ultrasound Obstet. Gynecol.*, **5**, 222–7

24. Merz, E., Bahlmann, F., Weber, G. and Macchiella, D. (1995). Three-dimensional ultrasonography in prenatal diagnosis. *J. Perinatal Med.*, **23**, 213–22

25. Merz, E. (1995). Einsatz der 3-D-Ultraschalltechnik in der pränatalen Diagnostik. *Ultraschall Med.*, **16**, 154–61

26. Feichtinger, W. (1993). Transvaginal three-dimensional imaging. *Ultrasound Obstet. Gynecol.*, **3**, 375–8

27. Merz, E., Weber, G., Bahlmann, F. and Macchiella, D. (1995). Transvaginale 3-D-Sonographie in der Gynäkologie. *Gynäkologie*, **28**, 270–5

28. Gregg, A., Steiner, H., Staudach, A. and Weiner, C. P. (1993). Accuracy of 3 D sonographic volume measurements. *Am. J. Obstet. Gynecol.*, **168**, 348

29. Gilja, O. H., Thune, N., Matre, K., Hausken, T., Odegaard, S. and Berstad, A. (1994). *In vitro* evaluation of three-dimensional ultrasonography in volume estimation of abdominal organs. *Ultrasound Med. Biol.*, **20**, 157–65

30. Steiner, H., Merz, E. and Staudach, A. (1995). 3-D Facing (video). *Hum. Reprod.*, Update (CD-Rom)

31. Steiner, H., Spitzer, D., Weiss-Wichert, P. H., Graf, A. H. and Staudach, A. (1995). Three-dimensional ultrasound in prenatal diagnosis of skeletal dysplasia. *Prenat. Diagn.*, **15**, 373–7

32. Favre, R., Nisand, G., Bettahar, K., Grange, G. and Nisand, I. (1993). Measurement of limb circumferences with three-dimensional ultrasound for fetal weight estimation. *Ultrasound Obstet. Gynecol.*, **3**, 176–9

33. Pilu, G. (1994). Sonography of fetal ventriculomegaly: the never-ending story. *Ultrasound Obstet. Gynecol.*, **4**, 180–1

34. Chiba, Y., Hayashi, K., Yamazaki, S., Takamizawa, K. and Sasaki, H. (1994). New technique of ultrasound, thick slicing 3-D imaging and the clinical aspects in the perinatal field. *Ultrasound Obstet. Gynecol.*, **4** (Suppl. 1), 337

35. Kossoff, G., Griffiths, K. A. and Warren, P. S. (1994). Real-time quasi-three-dimensional viewing in sonography, with conventional, gray-scale volume imaging. *Ultrasound Obstet. Gynecol.*, **4**, 211–16

Tissue echogenicity
8

M. Smith-Levitin, I. Blickstein and E. Gurewitsch

INTRODUCTION

Modern imaging techniques provide accurate representations of human tissues that often require little subjective interpretation. With improved quality of sonographic images, quantitative measurements can now be obtained, further objectifying the information acquired. An aspect of diagnostic ultrasound that remains controversial, however, is the assessment of tissue echogenicity.

Tissue echogenicity results from the interplay between ultrasound beams and a given tissue. The image obtained by ultrasound is an electronic interpretation of this interaction of tissue with sound. The image itself has a specific optical density, which the observer subjectively uses to assess the echogenic properties of the tissue. Assessment of tissue echogenicity could potentially serve as a means of tissue characterization, because it represents the acoustic nature of the scanned tissue. The cluster of white-on-black spots that appears as the image output has a unique echo pattern, or image density, that could be used to differentiate normal from abnormal tissue.

Each tissue, because of its unique properties, should have only one echogenicity value when scanned at a specific point in time, using specific sonographic settings. It follows that an objective method for assessing image density should be able to provide this tissue echogenicity value. To be objective, a method must yield the same interpretation of a tissue's echogenicity by different observers. Repeated images of the same tissue must have the same density value, provided that the tissue's characteristics have not changed. Furthermore, echogenicities assessed from images of different tissues must be able to be compared. Before this can be done, however, impediments to accurate tissue echogenicity assessment must be overcome.

IMPEDIMENTS TO ASSESSMENT OF TISSUE ECHOGENICITY

The subject being imaged, the equipment used to generate the image and the observer interpreting that image, each influence the density of a given sonographic output and thus its interpretation. These impediments to accurate assessment of tissue echogenicity, which are outlined in Table 1, are considered separately below.

The subject

Molecular composition of tissues

Tissues with different histological compositions may or may not produce images with different

Table 1 *Impediments to echogenicity assessment*

The subject
Molecular composition of tissues
Intervening tissues
Beam inclination

The equipment
Transducer
  configuration
  frequency
Time gain compensation
Zooming
Log compression
Pre-processing
Persistence
Post-processing
Visual output

The observer
Resolution acuity
Personal preference

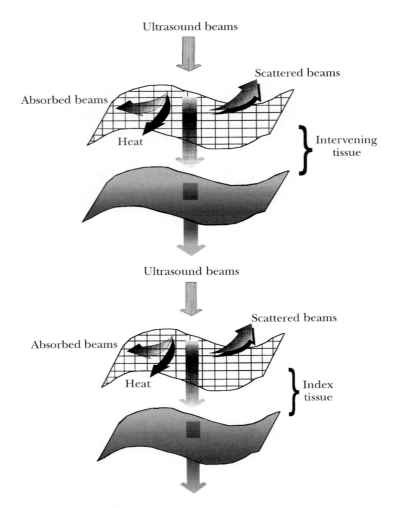

Figure 1 *Attenuation of the ultrasound beam*

echotextures, depending on the way a particular beam interacts with the molecules in the tissue. Ultrasound beams are initially absorbed or scattered when they interact with tissues. The absorption is dependent on the molecular make-up of the tissue, and some molecules will reflect sound waves, while other molecules will convert more of the mechanical energy into heat[1]. Heterogeneities in the tissue cause scatter phenomenon[2]. The machine creates an image by interpreting sound waves that have already been attenuated and backscattered by the tissue under investigation.

Intervening tissues

Intervening tissues attenuate the ultrasound beam even before it interacts with the structure being scanned. This is always a problem in real-time sonography of fetuses, for example, where the transducer is never placed directly on the scanned tissue. The degree of attenuation of energy depends on the attenuation characteristics of the intervening tissue, as depicted in Figure 1. Haberkorn and associates[3] used a tissue-mimicking phantom to simulate differences in abdominal wall thickness and composition and found than an increasing fat

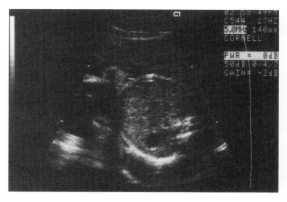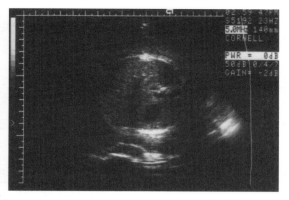

Figure 2 *Effect of transducer configuration on apparent echogenicity: left, sector; right, curvilinear*

path caused a decrease in ultrasound brightness and microtexture. Hence, a mass that is located deep in a voluminous organ, such as the breast, may produce images of differing densities when viewed from different locations on the breast. Furthermore, when two distinctly echogenic structures appear on the same visual output, the attenuation of the ultrasound beam will be different as the beam crosses the two structures. The image will reflect this difference[4].

Beam inclination

Beam inclination is a related problem caused by the subject, and it is also best exemplified by fetal sonography. Since the fetus is a moving target, the same tissue may be scanned at different angles, leading to different transducer-to-target distances, ultimately producing different echo patterns.

Any method that assesses echogenicity should take these subject-related variables into account.

The equipment

Different aspects of the equipment used to image a given tissue affect the energy that is transmitted and received by the machine even before an image is generated.

Modern sonography, which is digital, can also cosmetically change the sonographic output of a subject after the image is generated. Indeed, many features of modern sonographic equip-

ment *purposely* alter the image density in order to improve image quality. However, these pre- and post-image computer manipulations of the final image density can potentially interfere with assessment of tissue echogenicity. For images of different subjects to be compared, a method of echogenicity assessment must either control or correct for the effect produced by these alterations.

The transducer

The field and frequency of sound produced by a transducer influence the apparent echogenicity of the tissue being imaged. As shown in Figure 2, different configurations of the transducer, such as sector or curvilinear, used on the same tissue will produce images of differing density. As the frequency of the individual transducer increases, the penetration depth decreases due to increased absorption and scattering of the beam. This leads to changes in the attenuation of the beam and, consequently, in the echotexture of the image[2] (Figure 3).

The time gain compensation

The time gain compensation control (TGC) of the ultrasound machine compensates for the loss of energy that otherwise occurs as the ultrasound beam passes deeper into a homogeneous tissue. At full compensation, the TGC will produce an evenly echogenic pattern of the homogeneous tissue. Any change of this control will

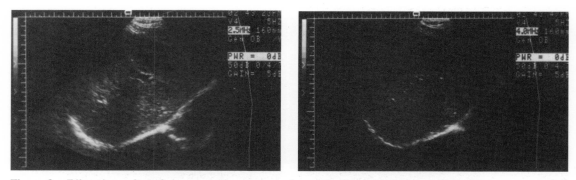

Figure 3   *Effect of transducer frequency on the apparent echogenicity: left, 2.5 MHz; right, 4.0 MHz*

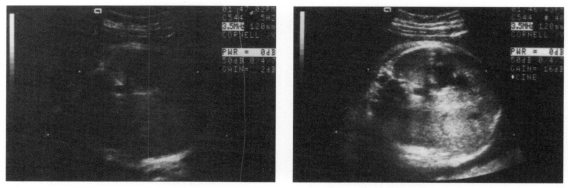

Figure 4   *Effect of gain setting on the apparent echogenicity of a fetal liver: left, gain = 2 dB; right, gain = 16 dB*

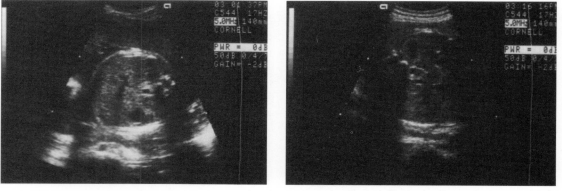

Figure 5   *Effect of different subjects on the apparent echogenicity when scanning fetal livers at the same gain setting. Note that all sonographic parameters have been held constant. Left, subject 1; right, subject 2*

significantly change the pattern[5]. Adding further complexity to this influence is the fact that some of today's advanced equipment includes automatic or differential far vs. near gain adjustments. Figure 4 illustrates the effect of using different gain settings on scans of the same tissue in the same subject. Figure 5 shows the effect of using the identical gain setting when scanning the same tissue in different subjects.

When two distinctly echogenic structures appear on the same visual output, as discussed

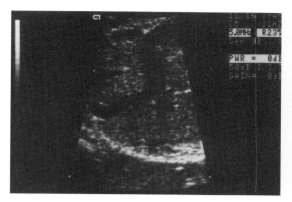 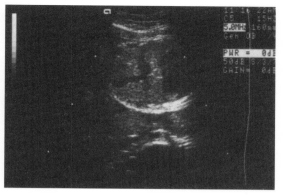

Figure 6 *The effect of 'zooming' on the apparent echogenicity. The only difference in these two images is that the left image is magnified*

above, the reduction or enhancement of their respective image densities that will occur when there is a change in the gain setting may not produce the same effect on each structure. This phenomenon is more pronounced when the differences in echogenicities are relatively small, such as with fetal lung and liver. In such instances, a slight change in the gain setting in one direction will result in an almost isoechoic image, while a slight change in the opposite direction will result in an image in which the two structures appear to have significantly different echogenicities. This effect has been demonstrated in a breast model, where a solid mass is surrounded by normal breast tissue[4]. Many investigators have failed to take the TGC setup into account when reporting on their experimental outcomes in assessing tissue echogenicity[5]. Some standardization of the system gain is needed.

The zoom feature

Image magnification, or zooming, will also affect image density. As shown in Figure 6, the same tissue will appear less echogenic under magnification.

Manipulations of the gray scale

Once the image is achieved, advanced systems, such as the Acuson 128XP (Mountainview, CA), have additional functions that affect the gray scale of the image. These include log compression, pre-processing, persistence and post-processing – all of which contribute to the final density of a sonographic image. Log compression controls the gray scale of the image by compressing or expanding the displayed shades of gray. If the log compression is increased, the image appears smoother or more gray; whereas, if the log compression is decreased, the image has greater contrast (appears more black and white). Pre-processing acts to enhance the interfaces between areas of different echogenicity. Similarly, adaptive speckle reduction, designed to improve image contrast, dramatically alters the familiar appearance of scans and enhances the textural information[6]. Persistence adds 'history' from previous frames to the present image by averaging changes in echogenicity that occur with movement of the subject. The visual output can also be manipulated with the use of built-in two-dimensional post-processing curves[7]. These procedures interpolate and fill in information that is lost when the reflected echos return from the tissue to the transducer to create a smoother, more continuous image. Particular curves can be chosen by the operator, and, as illustrated in Figure 7, each curve may produce a different image density for a given tissue.

Transfer to hard copy

Images that appear on the screen are transient, making it difficult to compare current images

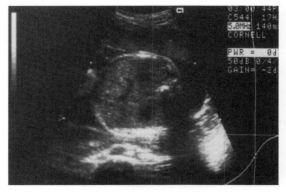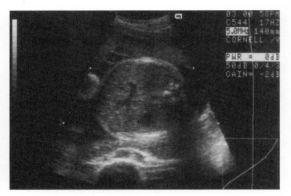

Figure 7 *The effect of different post-processing curves on the apparent echogenicity: left, post-processing level 7; right, post-processing level 3*

with either prior images or future images. Transfer of sonographic images to either paper or transparent film is necessary, but it adds additional variations to the final image density, depending on the processing technique. X-ray film has its own optical density, and, although usually considered as 'fast', is prone to the spurious effects of the development conditions, such as solarization. Therefore, in order to compare scans using X-ray film hard copy, only one type of film must be used, and a correction of the gray-scale range for each film must be applied.

The observer

Perceived image density is affected by the observer who interprets the image because of a unique optical ability to distinguish detail, known as resolution acuity, and a personal preference. Image resolution by the human eye is rather complicated[8], and many factors affect it. Some factors may directly interfere with the assessment of echogenicity. For example, the examination of photographic positives will differ from that of negatives, because the resolvability of bright-on-dark images is not the same as that of dark-on-bright. Acuity is also influenced by the general illumination falling on the retina and will be altered in the setting of a semi-dark examination room. Glare from the ultrasound screen lowers the contrast in the retinal image and lowers acuity accordingly.

Inter-observer differences in pupil size and refractive state may affect acuity considerably. Aging lowers acuity as a function of lens density. Eye color also affects resolution acuity, whereby darker eyes have superior acuity. Performance also improves with practice and deteriorates with reduced attention, suggesting that experience and fatigue may both influence resolution acuity.

It is not surprising, then, that inter-observer differences in the assessment of image density are quite large. Nyberg's group found inter-observer differences in the grading of bowel echogenicity in approximately 10% of cases[9]. Our group (unpublished data) recently found more than a 50% inconsistency between observers attempting to discern differences in echogenicity, particularly between images with the same density or with only slight density differences. Lamont and colleagues[10] asked 20 observers to estimate renal cortical echogenicity from sonographic images and found significant inter- as well as intra-observer variation. Eggert and co-workers[11] demonstrated that evaluation by the naked eye does not permit consistent assessment of echogenicity, also showing that repeated assessments by an individual examiner differ considerably.

In addition to the differences in their resolution acuity, observers may have different preferences for contrast and brightness settings, resulting in images with different echo patterns. A sonographer may wish to use a special transducer frequency at a special system gain setting for the fetal liver of one patient and a different frequency and gain for the fetal liver of another patient. Accurate, reliable and reproducible assessment of echogenicity, therefore, requires technology that controls for human variation.

The different factors that impede echogenicity assessment are not independent of each other. The transducer frequency, the distance from the tissue, and the unique characteristics of the tissue all influence the attenuation of the ultrasound beam. Observers having different preferences for gray-scale contrast may choose different settings, resulting in images with different echo patterns. A simple visual assessment of echogenicity is just not possible because of these subject-, equipment-, and observer-related variables.

QUALITATIVE ASSESSMENT OF TISSUE ECHOGENICITY

Several qualitative methods for increasing reproducibility and accuracy of echogenicity assessment from sonographic images have been proposed. One method simply compares the index tissue to a control tissue. Bromley and associates[12] compared the appearance of the bowel in over 8000 fetuses to the surrounding bone. Caspi and co-workers[13] refined this technique by comparing the index tissue to an internal scale of echogenicities. Their group used the following four internal fetal standards: fluid (grade 0), liver (grade 2), lung (grade 4), and bone (grade 6), which they objectively showed by densitometry to be of consistently different echogenicities from each other, irrespective of the gain setting. Slotnick and associates[14] suggested a more dynamic method, using a contiguous view of fetal bowel with iliac crest while linearly reducing the system gain. Sonodense fetal bowel that became unidentifiable before the loss of the iliac crest image was assigned a score of 1. Fetal bowel whose image was lost at the same gain setting at which the image of the iliac crest was lost was assigned a score of 2, and bowel that sustained echogenicity after the loss of the iliac crest was assigned a score of 3. This

yielded a more accurate assessment of fetal echogenic bowel compared to other published methods[9,15–18].

A selected list of such methods is given in Table 2. All had limitations: most involved several observers, many used at least two transducer frequencies, and only two compared the results to objective densitometry[10,11]. Table 3 summarizes the differences in the reported prevalences of chromosomal abnormalities in those studies assessing the outcomes of pregnancies in which echogenic fetal bowel was found in mid-gestation. Most have found an increased incidence of aneuploidy and adverse perinatal outcomes, but to different degrees. The differences are probably due, in large part, to variations in the way that 'echogenic' bowel was defined, which further exemplifies the limitations of qualitative echogenicity assessment.

QUANTITATIVE ASSESSMENT OF TISSUE ECHOGENICITY

Densitometry

Densitometry is a quantitative method that bypasses subjective visual impediments. It measures the 'crowdedness' and 'darkness' of the dots known as pixels that comprise a screen image. Some sonographic equipment has the capacity for on-screen densitometry as part of ultrasound screen resolution. Of course, limited storage of screen images makes comparison between images difficult. Another way to quantify image density, shown in Figure 8, is by transmission densitometry, in which light transmitted through the hard-copy transparent films is measured using an electro-optical densitometer such as the Gretag D200 (Regensdorf/Zurich, Switzerland)[19]. The relationship between transmission and density is logarithmic and can be expressed as $D = (-)\log_{10} T$, where D is density and T is transmission (Figure 9). T varies between 0, where no light is transmitted, and 1, where all light is transmitted. Thus, the more light that is transmitted, the lower the measured image density will be. Because white-on-black (negative) images are generally used, it is important to realize that more echogenic tissues

Table 2 *Studies comparing echogenicity of the index tissue to a nearby control tissue*

Investigators	Index tissue/control tissue	Purpose
Liao et al.[21]	renal cortex/adjacent liver	estimate renal maturation
Gershen et al.[22]	renal cortex/adjacent liver	renal echogenicity as a prognostic indicator in childhood nephrotic syndrome
Lamont et al.[10]	renal cortex/liver	reliability of human assessment of renal parenchymal echogenicity in infants
Eggert et al.[11]	renal parenchyma/liver	reliability of human assessment of renal parenchymal echogenicity in infants
Platt et al.[23]	renal parenchyma/liver	renal echogenicity as an indicator of kidney disease
Fried et al.[24]	lung/liver	fetal lung echogenicity as it relates to fetal lung maturity
Murao[25]	liver/bowel	relationship between fetal liver echogenicity and fetal growth
Nyberg et al.[9]	bowel/liver	clinical importance of fetal echogenic bowel
Sepulveda et al.[15]	bowel/iliac crest	intra-amniotic bleeding as a cause for fetal echogenic bowel
Scioscia et al.[18]	bowel/iliac wing	outcome of pregnancies in which echogenic bowel was detected
Dicke and Crane[16]	bowel/bone	clinical significance of fetal echogenic bowel
Ewer et al.[17]	bowel/vertebrae	fetal echogenic bowel as a marker for ischemia
Bromley et al.[12]	bowel/bone	clinical significance of fetal echogenic bowel
Hill et al.[26]	bowel/liver and bone	association of fetal echogenic bowel with adverse perinatal outcome
Slotnick et al.[14]	bowel/bone	clinical significance of echogenic bowel
Caspi et al.[13]	bowel/fluid, liver, lung and bone	human vs. densitometry assessment of normal fetal bowel echogenicity

Table 3 *Prevalence of chromosomal abnormalities with echogenic bowel*

Investigator	Percentage of fetuses with echogenic bowel that had a karyotypic abnormality
Nyberg et al.[9]	25
Scioscia et al.[18]	27
Hill et al.[26]	6
Dicke and Crane[16]	3
Redwine et al.[27]	2.9
Gollin et al.[28]	13
Bromley et al.[12]	16
Slotnick et al.[14]	6.6

produce whiter images that actually transmit more light and, therefore, register lower density values by transmission densitometry.

There are many problems with simple densitometry that make it an ill-suited replacement for the human eye. As shown in Figure 9, there is a sharp drop in density with small increments in transmitted light at the lower range (between 0 and 30% transmission) and small, almost linear, decreases in density with increased transmission. This important relationship, which also exists in human vision, makes it difficult for transmission densitometry to ascertain slight differences in the echogenicities of hyperechoic structures. Furthermore, densitometry is subject to many of the factors discussed above that impede echogenicity assessment since it only measures the image density, whether on-screen or by transmission of light through hard-copy films. One recent study (M. Smith-Levitin and colleagues, unpublished data) found that 87% of images that were identical except for the post-processing curve had different mean image densities as measured by transmission densitometry. Even if an image density were a true representation of a tissue's echogenicity, densitometry would only allow for evaluation of that singular image. Comparison of multiple images could not be made, because of all the factors

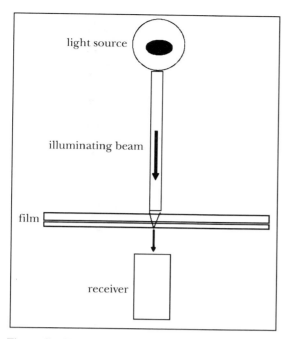

Figure 8 *Transmission densitometer*

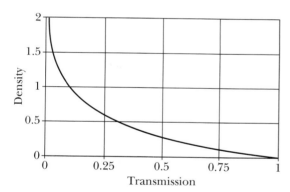

Figure 9 *The logarithmic relationship between transmission and densitometry.* $D = -\log_{10} T$

discussed above that affect the comparability of density values derived from different images.

Gain-assisted densitometric evaluation of sonograms

If one could correct the density value of an image obtained by transmission densitometry for the pre-image and post-image processing variables discussed above, the method would be more valid in assessing tissue echogenicity. Gain-assisted densitometric evaluation of sonograms (GADES) is a first attempt at such standardization. In a two-step process that will be outlined in detail below, GADES initially corrects the density values obtained from different images by transmission densitometry for the gray-scale differences between the different hard-copy transparent films on which those images are printed. Mathematical transformations are then applied to the corrected densitometric values of a given image obtained at different gain settings in order to arrive at a constant density value for that tissue[19,20].

The GADES method is only valid if several prerequisites are met first. All scans must be obtained with the same transducer and the same frequency to control for the ultrasound energy. In addition, transparent film of only one type must be used with the gray scale displayed on each scan to eliminate the effects of different processing on different film types. Finally, the scanned structures should be relatively homogeneous, having relatively few intra-object density differences.

Within the limits of these prerequisites, the transmission density of a specific image of a given tissue, D_{sp}, will be a density value that lies somewhere between the density value of the black end of that specific image's gray scale, denoted as B_{sp}, and the density value of the white end of the same gray scale, W_{sp}. $B_{sp} - W_{sp}$ denotes the specific gray-scale range, or R_{sp}, for a sonographic image. In a large number of images (≥ 100) taken of the same tissue, a maximal range of densities, R_{max}, can be calculated, extending from the lowest density corresponding to the lowest W_{sp}, or W_{max}, to the highest density, B_{max}, the highest B_{sp} in the group of images. The specific optical density of the index tissue, D_{sp}, can then be related to the maximal gray scale, thereby standardizing the films to one scale. The corrected density value (D_{cor}) relates to R_{max} as follows:

$$\frac{D_{sp} - W_{sp}}{R_{sp}} = \frac{D_{cor} - W_{max}}{R_{max}}$$

By solving for D_{cor}, the following mathematical formula is derived:

$$D_{cor} = [(D_{sp} - W_{sp}) \times (R_{max}/R_{sp})] + W_{max}$$

Since R_{max} and W_{max} are constants for any given sample of images, D_{cor} may change as a function of the other variables. D_{cor} increases linearly as D_{sp} increases, decreases linearly as W_{sp} increases, and decreases as an inverse function of R_{sp}.

Once densitometric values of images printed on different transparent films are corrected, the next step of GADES attempts to control for the pre-imaging variables that further confound comparison of density values of different images. The second step of GADES is based on the premise that a given tissue will cause a specific change in acoustic energy. Since time gain compensation is a linear manipulation of the energy returning to the transducer, a difference in image density will correlate with the difference in system gain. In other words, a change in the system's overall time gain compensation will change the density of the sonographic output by a constant, as long as linear system electronics are used (i.e. the General Electric RT-3000 scanner, Milwaukee, WI), and all other variables used in generating the image remain constant. Therefore, the differences between three image density values generated from transmission densitometry of three scans of the same tissue taken at three different gains can be related as follows:

$$\frac{D_c - D_a}{G_c - G_a} = \frac{D_c - D_b}{G_c - G_b}$$

where $D_{a,b,c}$ are the densities of the three images obtained by transmission densitometry and $G_{a,b,c}$ are the three gain settings.

This assumption enables a standardization of the system gain setting to an arbitrary gain, such as the subjectively optimal gain for scanning a particular image, G_{opt}. Thus, after substituting the corrected density values from the previous step of the GADES method, the corrected density value of the image obtained at the optimal gain, $D_{cor}opt$, can be calculated as follows: $D_{cor}opt = [G_{opt} (D_{cor}a - D_{cor}b) + G_a (D_{cor}b) - G_b (D_{cor}a)]/(G_a - G_b)$.

This formula corrects the measured image density to an arbitrary optimal gain setting. As a result, two images of the same structure scanned at different G numbers will have essentially the same $D_{cor}opt$ with only tiny differences attributable to the measurement technique. The advantage of this gain-assisted method is that the prerequisites for generating the images for GADES analysis allow free choice of the preferred gain setting, bypassing the need for an otherwise obligatory, and highly complicated, standardized processing of films. In addition, the use of different gains for assessment of echogenicity of one structure controls for the influence of intervening tissue, since a different optimal gain will be necessary for either deeper structures or for structures located behind a beam-attenuating tissue.

The first attempt at using the GADES method employed the fetal liver model[19]. Using the same sonographic equipment and the same films, the fetal liver was scanned at three different gains corresponding to the optimal, minimal, and maximal gains that allowed a clear image to be obtained. The densities of these fetal liver images were measured using visible panchromatic light transmitted through different round transmission holes. The transmitted light was electro-optically measured, giving a digitalized reading (reproducibility of ± 0.01 D). Each of the two extremes of the gray scale (B_{sp} and W_{sp}) was measured three times through a 0.5-mm hole, and a mean value was calculated. The fetal liver area was measured five times at random locations through a 3-mm (7.1 mm^2) hole, and a mean specific density (D_{sp}) was calculated. The variance of these five measurements was used to establish homogeneity ($< 20\%$ variance). Although the entire surface density of the fetal liver was not measured, several random densitometries through a large measuring hole adequately represent the mean surface transmission density[13]. After the mathematical transformations were carried out, two initially different echogenicities (and densities) of the same liver had the same corrected density value.

A subsequent study showed a significant linear correlation between the film-corrected density and eight gain intervals from the optimal gain, and a predicted gain-dependent decrease in density[20]. After standardization of

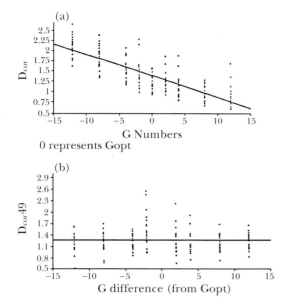

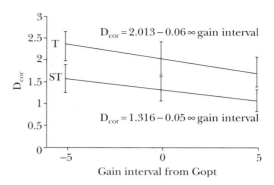

Figure 11 *Film-corrected density (D_{cor}) of two distinct echogenic structures appearing on the same scan, as a function of different gain intervals (dB) from the optimal gain (0). T, tumor; ST, surrounding tissue. Vertical bars represent SD of the mean. Reprinted from Journal of Ultrasound in Medicine[4] with permission*

Figure 10 *(a) Film-corrected density (D_{cor}) as a function of different gain intervals. Note the linear relationship; r = 0.81; p < 0.000001. (b) Standardized density to G = 49 (D_{cor}49) as a function of the G differences used for standardization. Note the gain-independent convergence of the values. Reprinted from Journal of Ultrasound in Medicine[20] with permission*

the values to an arbitrary gain setting, a gain-independent convergence of the values was found (Figure 10). These two studies provided a highly reproducible estimate of tissue echogenicity, thereby setting the stage for clinical trials of the method.

In order for quantitative image density evaluation to be a means of tissue characterization, it must be able to distinguish normal from abnormal tissue in the same subject. The first clinical application of the GADES method used a breast model in order to establish that two distinctly echogenic structures appearing on the same image, such as a breast mass and its surrounding normal breast tissue, produce density-to-gain-setting lines for each structure that have similar slopes, which can then be reliably compared[4] (Figure 11). This study found that the slight differences in the structures' respective slopes were negligible within the gain intervals used in GADES, and comparison of two structures by GADES was as accurate as the assessment of a single echogenic structure.

The second clinical application of GADES focused on the question of whether the method could be used to compare images of the same organ from different patients (I. Blickstein and associates, unpublished data). This study used the fetal liver model to establish that the density-to-gain lines of relatively hyperechogenic and hypoechogenic livers have similar slopes within the gain intervals used in GADES. The results suggested that liver images representing even the two extremes of density distribution may indeed be compared by using GADES.

The full clinical utility of GADES has yet to be established. GADES only standardizes for the differences in the gray scales of different transparent film images and for the system gain, but it otherwise requires that other variables that manipulate the image be held constant. There are still some confounders to tissue echogenicity assessment, such as the effect of different transducer frequencies, and the various manipulators of the gray scale, such as log compression, that need to be considered.

CONCLUSIONS

Clearly, simple assessments of tissue echogenicity by the human eye, or even by densitometry, are not accurate unless the many factors that impede them are taken into account. The majority of advances made in the last 5 years have been mostly in understanding these problems. GADES, on the other hand, is a first attempt to solve these problems. The assessment of breast masses and multiple fetal organs by GADES is currently under investigation, as is the comparison of the method to other imaging modalities such as magnetic resonance imaging. If the results confirm the early GADES studies and further refine the technique, it may be possible to develop standard density nomograms of

various tissues. Such quantitative measurements have the potential to be extremely useful in clinical practice. Having a range of normal echogenicities for fetal tissues across gestational age would make the determination of abnormally echogenic structures more accurate, thereby improving the positive predictive value and specificity of such findings. Unnecessary interventions, such as amniocentesis or early delivery, might then be avoided.

References

1. Jongen, H. A., Thijssen, J. M. and van den Aarssen, M. (1986). A general model for the absorption of ultrasound by biological tissues and experimental verifications. *J. Acoust. Soc. Am.*, **79**, 535–40
2. Thijssen, J. M. and Ooterveld, B. J. (1990). Texture in tissue echograms: speckle or information? *J. Ultrasound Med.*, **9**, 215–29
3. Haberkorn, U., Layer, G., Rudat, V., Zuna, I., Lorenz, A. and van Kaick, G. (1993). Ultrasound image properties influenced by abdominal wall thickness and composition. *J. Clin. Ultrasound*, **21**, 423–9
4. Blickstein, I., Goldschmit, R., Strano, S. D. and Goldman, R. D. (1995). Quantitative comparison of two distinct echogenicities appearing on the same image using gain-assisted densitometric evaluation of sonograms (GADES). *J. Ultrasound Med.*, **14**, 509–13
5. Carson, P. L., Meyer, C. R. and Bowerman, R. A. (1985). Prediction of fetal lung maturity with ultrasound. *Radiology*, **155**, 533
6. Crawford, D. C., Cosgrove, D. O., Tohno, E., Svensson, W. E., Al-Murrani, B., Bell, D. S., Stepniewska, K. and Bamber, J. C. (1992). Visual impact of adaptive speckle reduction on US B-mode images. *Radiology*, **183**, 555–61
7. Goldstein, A. (1993). Instrumentation of digital gray scale ultrasound. *Radiographics*, **13**, 1389–95
8. Rubin, M. L. (1972). Visual acuity. In Potts, A. M. (ed.) *The Assessment of Visual Function*, p. 3. (St Louis: C. V. Mosby)
9. Nyberg, D. A., Dubinsky, T., Resta, R. G., Mahony, J. B. S., Hickok, D. E. and Luthy, D. A. (1993). Echogenic fetal bowel during the second trimester: clinical importance. *Radiology*, **188**, 527–31
10. Lamont, A. C., Graebe, A. C., Pelmore, J. M. and Thompson, J. R. (1990). Ultrasound assessment of renal cortical brightness in infants: is naked eye evaluation reliable? *Invest. Radiol.*, **25**, 250–3
11. Eggert, P., Debus, F., Kreller-Laugwitz, G. and Oppermann, H. C. (1991). Densitometric measurements of renal echogenicity in infants and naked eye evaluation: a comparison. *Pediatr. Radiol.*, **21**, 111–13
12. Bromley, B., Doubilet, P., Frigoletto, F. D., Krauss, C., Estroff, J. A. and Benacerraf, B. R. (1994). Is fetal hyperechoic bowel on second-trimester sonogram an indication for amniocentesis? *Obstet. Gynecol.*, **83**, 647–51
13. Caspi, B., Blickstein, I. and Appelman, Z. (1992). The accuracy of the assessment of normal fetal intestinal echogenicity-electro-optical densitometry versus the ultrasonographer's eye. *Gynecol. Invest.*, **33**, 26–30
14. Slotnick, R. N. and Abuhamad, A. Z. (1996). Prognostic analysis of fetal echogenic bowel. *Lancet*, **347**, 85–7
15. Sepulveda, W., Hollingsworth, J., Bower, S., Vaughan, J. I. and Fisk, N. M. (1994). Fetal hyperechogenic bowel following intra-amniotic bleeding. *Obstet. Gynecol.*, **83**, 947–50
16. Dicke, J. M. and Crane, J. P. (1992). Sonographically detected hyperechoic fetal bowel: significance and implications for pregnancy management. *Obstet. Gynecol.*, **80**, 778–82
17. Ewer, A. K., Mchugo, J. M., Chapman, S. and Newell, S. J. (1993). Fetal echogenic gut: a marker of intrauterine ischemia? *Arch. Dis. Child.*, **69**, 510–13
18. Scioscia, A. L., Pretorius, D. H., Budorick, N. E., Cahill, T. C., Axelrod, F. T. and Leopold, G. R. (1992). Second trimester echogenic bowel and chromosomal abnormalities. *Am. J. Obstet. Gynecol.*, **167**, 889–94
19. Blickstein, I. (1993). Quantitative assessment of sonographic image echogenicity by transmission

densitometry: fetal liver model. *J. Ultrasound Med.*, **12**, 567–71

20. Blickstein, I. and Goldman, R. D. (1994). The relation between different system gain settings and the accuracy of densitometric assessment of echogenicity. *J. Ultrasound Med.*, **13**, 675–8

21. Liao, M. H., Tsau, Y. K. and Chu, J. M. (1993). Using quantitative ultrasound to estimate renal maturation. *Acta. Pediatr. Sin.*, **34**, 367–71

22. Gershen, R. S., Brody, A. S., Duffy, L. C. and Springate, J. E. (1994). Prognostic value of sonography in childhood nephrotic syndrome. *Pediatr. Nephrol.*, **8**, 76–8

23. Platt, J. F., Rubin, J. M., Bowerman, R. A. and Marn, C. S. (1988). The inability to detect kidney disease on the basis of echogenicity. *Am. J. Roentgenol.*, **151**, 317–19

24. Fried, A. M., Loh, F. K., Umer, M. A., Dillon, K. P. and Kryscio, R. (1985). Echogenicity of fetal lung: relation to fetal age and maturity. *Am. J. Roentgenol.*, **145**, 591–3

25. Murao, F. (1991). Relationship between fetal growth and echogenicity of the fetal liver. *Gynecol. Obstet. Invest.*, **32**, 20–3

26. Hill, L. M., Fries, J., Hecker, J. and Grzybek, P. (1994). Second-trimester echogenic small bowel: an increased risk for adverse perinatal outcome. *Prenat. Diagn.*, **14**, 845–50

27. Redwine, F. D., Vanner, L. and Hays, P. (1993). The significance of very echogenic fetal bowel. Abstracts of the 13th annual meeting of the Society of Perinatal Obstetricians. *Am. J. Obstet. Gynecol.*, **168**, 352

28. Gollin, Y. G., Gollin, G., Shaffer, W. and Copel, J. (1993). Increased abdominal echogenicity *in utero*: a marker of intestinal obstruction? Abstract 3063. AIUM Convention. *J. Ultrasound Med.*, **12**, S72

Fetal radiology

9

B. R. Elejalde, M.-M. de Elejalde, R. R. Lebel, J. M. Acuna, J. Gomez and R. A. Elejalde

INTRODUCTION

The use of radiographic imaging of the fetus has been limited, due to the effects of X-rays in the developing human. The most common application of fetal analysis by X-rays has been the analysis of deceased fetuses who are known or presumed to have a skeletal dysplasia. Before the advent of ultrasonography, fetography was used to image the fetus *in utero*. Contrast medium was injected into the amniotic fluid, to delineate the fetal external structures with the lipid-soluble solution, and the gastrointestinal tract with water-soluble contrast media. Occasionally, maternal abdominal radiographs were used in the diagnosis of fetuses suspected to have severe malformations and skeletal dysplasias. The excellent imaging produced by ultrasonography and its lack of harmful effects on fetuses has completely replaced the use of radiography in the analysis of the fetus *in utero*.

It is widely recommended that X-ray images be obtained from all fetuses subjected to postmortem analysis, but this is very seldom done with fetuses which do not show an abnormality that is going to be proven or described in more detail by X-rays.

The most common X-ray approach uses standard techniques with or without intensifying screens. The quality of this image is good, but it does not reveal the structures of the fetus with the great detail needed for the appropriate analysis. As a component of the fetal medicine program that we have developed between the institutions where we work, we have used fetal radiographic images extensively in the analysis of fetal disease, because of their unique contribution to the assessment of the pathogenesis of fetal disease. In 1985, we reported the adaptation of xeroradiography using contrast media to the analysis of the fetus[1], for the examination of the skeleton, the soft tissues, the ventricular system of the brain, and the pulmonary, gastrointestinal, urinary and cardiovascular systems.

The basis of fetal medicine is the analysis of fetal disease. The physical examination of the fetus occurs in two main modalities, the examination of the fetus *in utero* by ultrasonography, and the direct physical examination after delivery. If the fetus is born alive, standard radiologic studies are performed according to the indications; fetuses born dead sometimes undergo autopsies. The radiographic analysis produces detailed information on fetal disease which cannot be obtained otherwise.

Most radiology and pediatric pathology books make reference to the importance and the need to perform radiographic studies to the fetus; books and papers usually refer to single simple applications of this diagnostic technique. Most of the larger studies have been focused on congenital malformations and skeletal dysplasias, but very few on the manifestations of acquired disease[1-6]. A concerted effort to examine one of the aspects of fetal radiology was made by Ornoy and colleagues[7], illustrating some aspects of the normal chondro-osseous development and normal fetal skeletal radiology, and describing the radiographic characteristics of fetuses with various skeletal dysplasias.

During the last 20 years we have been examining fetuses that are born prematurely, both alive and dead. In those in which we perform postmortem examinations, we include extensive radiographic analysis. In this chapter, we will describe the methodology, applications and results of this technique in the diagnosis of fetal disease.

METHODS

All fetuses received for postmortem examination after spontaneous or induced abortion were subjected to radiographic analysis. Anterior–posterior, posterior–anterior and lateral views were taken from each one. One or several of the following procedures using contrast media were performed: ventriculogram with descending and ascending myelograms, analysis of the gastrointestinal tract, upper respiratory tract and bronchogram, and visualization of the renal pelves, ureters, bladder and urethra. In addition, the analysis of the cardiovascular system included full body arteriogram, venogram, coronary angiography and visualization of the heart chambers. The pleural and peritoneal cavities were imaged using contrast media.

The contrast media used contained 20% sodium diatriazoate (Sigma Chemical Company) in water. This preparation is a lot less expensive than commercial preparations for clinical use and produces results of very high quality with very fine definition of details.

GENERAL EXAMINATION

Anterior–posterior, posterior–anterior and lateral views often reveal normal soft tissues and skeleton. This is a common observation, and is important, because it excludes the abnormalities that can be recognized. By this method, we have observed a wide variety of abnormalities, which may be considered under several categories.

Soft tissues

Subdermic edema

The most commonly seen abnormality is subdermic edema. This alteration can be seen in a particular anatomic region or may involve the entire fetal body. The measurements of the thickness of the skin and of the subdermic tissues are useful in determining the severity of the edema. It is also useful when determining areas where trauma caused edema, as in the case in prolonged labor, with subdermic edema of the skull.

Constriction rings

The severity and compromise of the lesion can be identified and quantified by the direct analysis of these views. Specifically, they help to determine the involvement of the skeleton and the disruption of muscular and skeletal tissues.

Severity of maceration

The degree of dermic laceration, displacement of the bones of the skull and dislocation of other bones can be documented. The loss of tissue mass, which occurs as the processes of necrosis and decomposition take place, can also be documented. It is useful in determining the approximate time of death, on the basis of the stage of maceration. It integrates the external and the internal changes, in order to produce a more complete evaluation of the stage of decomposition.

Figure 1 shows a severely macerated fetus which had been dead for 4 weeks. It shows the disintegration of the soft tissues, the abnormal position and dislocation of the cranial bones, the phalanges of the fingers, the decreased echogenicity of all the bones and mild bowing of the femora. The size of the bones helps to identify the age at which this fetus died.

Accumulation of gas

One of the most common causes of fetal death is infection. Some of the pathogenic bacteria that cause the fetal infection, septicemia and death produce gas that accumulates in the arteries and veins, and that is seen in the simple views delineating the fetal vasculature without contrast media. This observation is of great diagnostic value, because it adds evidence to the diagnosis of the infectious cause of the fetal death, and because when the infectious process has not been suspected, it points to this etiology. When a simple radiography of the fetus shows gas in the vascular system, samples should be taken for microbiological study. It is for this reason that

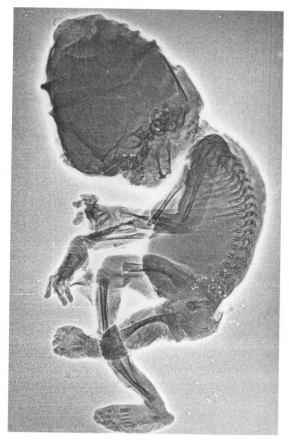

Figure 1 *Severely macerated fetus which had been dead for 4 weeks*

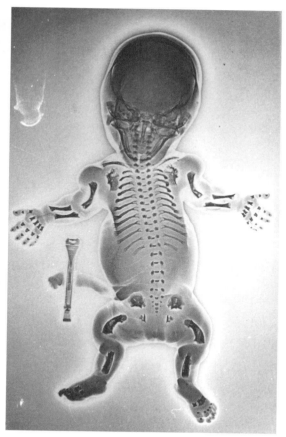

Figure 2 *Fetus affected by thanatophoric dysplasia*

the X-rays of the fetus should be taken as soon as the fetus is received.

Analysis of the fetal skeleton

General characteristics

The anterior–posterior and lateral views of the fetal body allow for a very detailed analysis of the skeleton. They should include the detailed examination of the structure of the bones. Their internal and external appearance should be examined. Xeroradiography produces a clear differentiation of the perichondral and endochondral bone. The epiphyseal process and the metaphyseal plates, as well as the specific landmarks of each bone should be examined and noted specifically.

The fetus shown in Figure 2 was affected by thanatophoric dysplasia. This condition was diagnosed by ultrasonography at 20 weeks, the pregnancy was terminated 1 week later, and a complete radiographic study was carried out. The picture shows an abnormal skull with incipient craniosynostosis (accentuated lambdoidal suture, completely fused; partially fused sagittal suture), severely hypoplastic mid-face, and clavicles lacking the normal strong S-shape and in a horizontal position. The vertebrae are short, and the intervertebral space is wider than normal; the interpeduncular distance is longer than normal and the lateral processes of the vertebrae show the formation of spiculae, which extend cephalically. The rib cage is abnormally shaped and small. The ribs are hypomineralized for this age. They are wider and thinner than normal, with a wide head and very thin bone formation; they are further apart than normal from the vertebrae, their neck is accentuated and they lack their normal curvature. Their most anterior aspect is also wider than normal and thin. The scapulae have abnormal shape, mineralization and structure. All of the long bones are abnormal. They are smaller than expected for age (below the 3rd centile). The humeri, ulnae, radii, tibiae and fibulae are externally concave and the femur is externally convex; all of them are bowed. The perichondral and the endochondral bone of the long bones is abnormal in distribution, position and modelling. The metaphyseal plates of all the bones are abnormal. They are irregular, with recognizable spiculae, with indentations and with lower mineralization than normal for age. The ilia are very abnormal, showing irregular bone formation, smallness of size and lower than normal mineralization. The ischia are also severely abnormal: small, with an abnormal pattern of ossification with formation of spiculae. The metacarpals and metatarsals are severely shortened; their metaphyses are irregular and concave. The phalanges are triangular, shorter than normal and have concave metaphyses. The soft tissues are redundant, due to the fact that while they grew at the normal pace, the bones did not. The details of each bone and structure can be noted.

Ossification centers

A pattern of ossification center development in the human fetus was established long ago[8]. We present a modified list (Table 1). We used the original list by Cruickshank and co-workers and validated it by the radiographic analysis of 1856 fetuses of different ages and by 13 210 ultrasonographic examinations. The fetal ossification centers are seen similarly by X-rays and by ultrasound, with the only exception that the ossification centers of the face are visible by ultrasound several weeks before they are seen by X-rays. The analysis of the ossification centers is useful in determining:

(1) The pattern of osteochondral development;

(2) The age of gestation, since they appear at specific ages; and

(3) Abnormalities that affect the development of some of them, with specific patterns.

In the estimation of the fetal age at the time of death, the ossification centers are informative about the process preceding the fetal death. A fetus whose measurements correspond to 30 weeks of gestation but which has the ossification centers for the distal epiphyses of the femora, which appear at 34 weeks of gestation, is clearly a 34-week-old fetus with severe intrauterine growth retardation, equivalent to a delay of growth of 4 weeks.

Anthropometric analysis

Each and every one of the bones should be measured; this is useful in determining several aspects of fetal development.

Gestational age The size of each bone can be compared with tables obtained from the analysis of normal fetuses[9]. These measurements were obtained by ultrasonography and they were validated by comparison with those obtained from radiographs. The centiles of growth for each bone measured are obtained from the normative data. The size of the bones helps to estimate the age when the bones stopped growing (at the time of death). It is common that one may receive a severely macerated fetus that has lost a great deal of its mass due to maceration and thus its age is difficult to determine, but with the bone measurements the time of death can be determined with great precision.

Symmetry The measurement of the bones helps to determine whether growth was symmetric; in cases such as the ulnar radial hypoplasia syndrome, growth is asymmetric. The measurements document the severity.

Table 1 *Ossification centers, and the week of detection by X-rays*

Center	Week	Center	Week	Center	Week
Head					
Mandible	7	Temporal	9	Nasal bone	10
Occipital (squamous portion)	8	Sphenoid (inner lamella of pterygoid process)	9	Frontal bone	9–10
Occipital (lateral and basilar portions)	9–10	Sphenoid (greater wings)	10	Bony labyrinth	17–20
		Sphenoid (lesser wings)	13	Milk teeth	17–20
Superior maxilla	8	Sphenoid (anterior body)	13–14	Hyoid bone (greater cornua)	28–32
Thorax, spine, and abdomen					
Clavicle (diaphysis)	7	Ribs (2nd, 3rd, 4th, 8th, 9th, 10th and 11th)	9	Rib (12th)	10
Scapula	8–9			Sternum	21–24
Ribs (5th, 6th and 7th)	8–9	Rib (1st)	10		
Vertebral arches					
All cervical and 1st or 2nd dorsal	9	All dorsal and 1st or 2nd lumbar	10	Upper sacral	12
		Lower lumbar	11	4th sacral	19–25
Bodies					
From 2nd dorsal to last lumbar	10	From upper cervical to upper sacral	12	Structural arrangement	13–16
From lower cervical to upper sacral	11	5th sacral	13–28	Odontoid process of axis	17–20
		1st coccygeal	37–40		
Costal process					
6th and 7th cervical	21–32	5th cervical	32–36	4th, 3rd and 2nd cervical	37–40
Transverse processes					
Cervical and dorsal	21–24	Pelvic girdle		os pubis (horizontal ramus)	21–28
Lumbar	25–28	ischium (descending ramus)	16–17	ilium	9
Upper extremity					
Humerus (diaphysis)	8	Phalanges		middle 3rd, 4th and 2nd	12
Radius (diaphysis)	8	terminal	9	Metacarpals	
Ulna (diaphysis)	8	basal 3rd and 2nd	9	2nd and 3rd	9
		basal 4th and 1st	10	4th, 5th and 1st	10–12
		basal 5th	13–16		
Lower extremity					
Femur (diaphysis)	8–9	Tibia (proximal epiphysis)	40	Astragalus	24–32
Femur (distal epiphysis)	35–40	Fibula	9	Cuboid	40
Tibia (diaphysis)	8–9	Os calcis	21–29		
Metatarsals					
2nd and 3rd	9				
4th, 5th and 1st	10–12				
Phalanges					
Terminal 1st	9	Basal 1st, 2nd, 3rd, 4th and 5th	13–14	Middle 4th	29–32
Terminal 2nd, 3rd and 4th	10–12			Middle 5th	33–36
Terminal 5th	13–14	Middle 2nd	20–25		
		Middle 3rd	21–26		

Abnormality The bones may be shorter or longer than expected for age. They are abnormally large in cases of overgrowth. This occurs in cases of primary acceleration, as in the overgrowth syndromes, and in families who have very long bones. Growth acceleration can be secondary to fetal–maternal conditions such as diabetes, in which they are longer than expected for the age of the gestation. Shortening of the bones is seen in skeletal dysplasias. The bones may only be shorter, or they may not only be short but also have abnormal shape and structure, depending upon the specific abnormality. Some of the patterns are very specific and allow for a very precise diagnosis of the disease. The patterns for different diseases have been described in the literature[7,9–13]: achondrogenesis Houston–Harris (type 1A), achondrogenesis Fraccaro (type 1B), achondrogenesis–hypochondrogenesis Langer–Saldino (type II), achondrogenesis–hypochondrogenesis Langer–Saldino type milder form (type II), atelosteogenesis (spondylohumerofemoral hypoplasia), Schneckenbecken dysplasia, short rib polydactyly type I (Saldino–Noonan), short rib polydactyly type II (Majewski type), classic campomelic dysplasia, dyastrophic dysplasia, chondroectodermal dysplasia (Ellis–van Creveld syndrome), osteogenesis imperfecta type II[10], asphyxiating thoracic dystrophy (Jeune syndrome)[11], Melnick–Needles syndrome, dyssegmental dysplasia (Silverman–Handmaker type), hypophosphatasia, mucopolysaccharidosis type II (MPS II, Hunter disease), mucolipidosis II (I-cell disease), Weyers syndrome (deficient ulnar and fibular rays with bilateral hydronephrosis[12]), and thanatophoric dysplasia[13]. The radiographic delineation of the fetal manifestations of these conditions is required for their prenatal diagnosis by ultrasonography. The anatomic, histological, biochemical and molecular analysis of the affected fetuses helps to delineate the pathophysiology of skeletal dysplasias *in utero*.

It is very common that the ultrasonographic examination of a given fetus indicates that the fetus has a skeletal dysplasia, but the precise diagnosis is not possible until the radiographic analysis is carried out. On other occasions, the diagnosis is correctly made by ultrasonography and it is confirmed and further documented by the radiological analysis. This type of analysis is also important because it helps to obtain information about the fetal manifestations and about the natural history of fetal skeletal disease.

The size of the bones can be altered by a non-genetic delay of growth, as occurs in many cases of fetal growth retardation secondary to placental failure. In these cases, the analysis of the size of the bones is of great importance, because it allows determination of the severity of the growth retardation and helps to quantify it. In the examination of a fetus which died with a well known gestational age, the measurement of the bones quantifies the effect of the growth retardation on the fetal development.

Figure 3 is an anterior–posterior view of a set of twins affected by growth retardation, more severe in the one on the left. They both had a deformed chest, with subdermic edema. The heads are of about the same size and are an

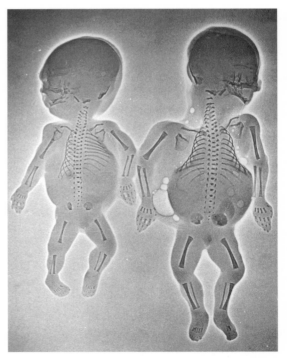

Figure 3 *Anterior–posterior view of a set of twins affected by growth retardation*

example of the cephalic protection common to most cases of progressive secondary growth retardation. This pregnancy was affected by twin-to-twin transfusion syndrome. The degree of bone maturation was different for each of the twins, also reflecting the growth retardation–restriction.

Analysis with contrast media

The central nervous system

The analysis described above reveals very few characteristics of the brain and of the spine. The injection of contrast media prepared as previously described allows for the analysis of these organs in great detail. The number and type of structures visualized is greatly dependent on the fetal age. The best method to analyze the ventricular system is the injection of the contrast medium inside the lateral ventricles. This is done by positioning the needle over the anterior fontanel and introducing it at a 45° angle to a distance equivalent to one-third of the skull height. The volume injected varies with age: at 8 weeks, 1 ml is enough; at 20 weeks, 10 ml; at 30 weeks, 15 ml; and at 40 weeks, 20 ml. After the contrast medium is injected, the fetal body is turned upside down a couple of times to allow for the contrast medium to mix with the cerebrospinal fluid. When there are no obstructions, this method will allow for the visualization of the lateral ventricles, the subarachnoid space and the cisternal system, and will produce a descending myelogram. The presence of contrast medium in the spine excludes obstruction of the drainage system of the cerebrospinal fluid. When there is an obstruction, the myelogram is not produced. The contrast medium will delineate with great precision the site of the obstruction. This type of information is very difficult if not impossible to obtain by other means, especially by the direct examination of the nervous system. When an obstruction is diagnosed, then an ascending myelogram is performed by the spinal injection of the contrast medium.

The delineation of the nervous system and especially of the brain and of the lateral ventricles demonstrates the severity of a lesion such as hydrocephaly, which alters the thickness of the cortex, the architecture of the brain and the distortion caused to other organs and tissues.

The same method can be used to examine cysts of the central nervous system, especially subarachnoid cysts. The contrast medium delineates the cyst, its communication with the cisternal system of the brain, and the distortion that it may have caused to the structures of the brain. This method of analysis is particularly important in the differentiation of hydrocephaly caused by obstruction, and communicating hydrocephaly, where the abnormally large ventricular system is produced by the inability of the dysplastic and dystrophic brain to grow and produce a ventricular system of normal size.

Figure 4 is a lateral view of a fetus with two subarachnoid cysts, medially located, that indent into the cortex. Note the excellent resoluting of the normal bones.

The ventriculogram is especially useful in the precise diagnosis of the different varieties of holoprosencephaly, as the contrast medium delineates the internal structure of the ventricular system.

The injection of contrast media into the central nervous system also helps to determine the structure and the anatomic relationships of other intracranial lesions. Intrathecal injection of contrast media delineates the giri and the sulci in great detail.

The injection of contrast media into the spine in cases of spina bifida determines whether the lesion is open or closed, and in cases of anencephaly it determines whether the cephalic sac commonly found in these cases is open or closed; and the amount and type of nervous tissue present.

Figure 5 shows a contrast medium study of the central nervous system and the spine of a 21-week-old fetus. Note the structure of the ventricular system and consequently the cortex, the cerebellum and the cisternal system, and the ability of the contrast medium to migrate and delineate the spine. Note the structure of the spine, especially the cauda equina. This picture also shows the normal appearance of the skeleton and soft tissues for a 21-week-old fetus.

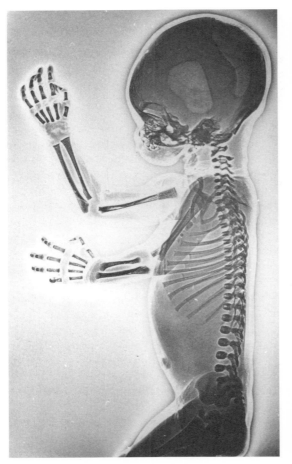

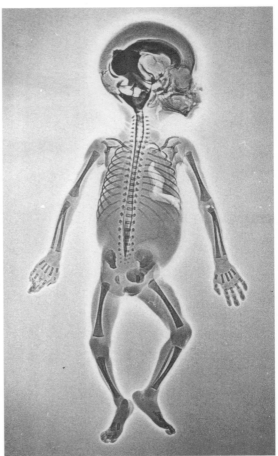

Figure 4 *Lateral view of a fetus with two subarachnoid cysts, medially located, that indent into the cortex. Note the resolution of the skeleton*

Figure 5 *Contrast medium study of the central nervous system and the spine of a 21-week-old fetus*

The gastrointestinal tract

X-ray views of the fetus taken after the injection of contrast media allow for the visualization of all of the major gastrointestinal components, revealing normal and abnormal variants. They also help to determine the anatomic relationship with other organs and tissues of the abdomen. When this technique is combined with other contrast medium analyses of the fetal body, one can gather information very difficult to obtain by other means. The injection of contrast media into the upper tract may delineate the esophagus and the trachea. When there is a tracheoesophageal fistula, the injection into the esophagus shows the anatomic defect. Obstruc-

tions are particularly well delineated by this method. The medium is injected by means of a catheter that is introduced progressively as the contrast medium is injected. The volume of medium needed to delineate the full tract varies with age.

The catheter can be introduced rectally when the obstruction is complete and does not allow for passage of the medium through the entire intestine.

Figure 6 shows a 20-week-old fetus with trisomy 18 which had severe growth retardation–restriction. The ventriculogram shows normal thickness of the cerebral cortex, except for the occipital lobe, which is abnormally thin, a flat tentorium cerebelli with a smaller than normal

110

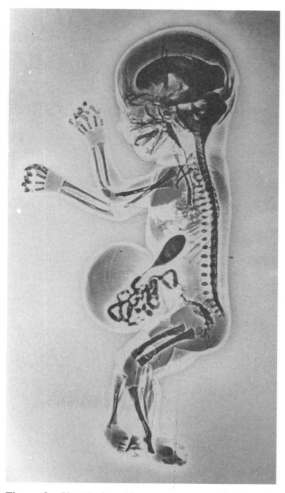

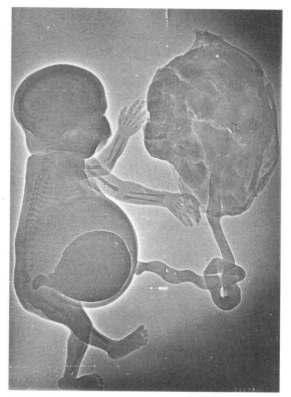

Figure 7 *A 19-week-old fetus with a megacystis produced by an obstructed urethra*

Figure 6 *Ventriculography, gastroenterography, bronchography and descending myelography of a 20-week-old fetus with trisomy 18*

cerebellum and cisterna magna. The descending myelogram is normal. This fetus had a large omphalocele containing a portion of the stomach and most of the intestine, as is demonstrated by the gastroenterogram. The abnormal hands, the positioning of the fingers and the abnormal feet can be noted. The contrast medium also delineates the trachea and larger bronchi.

Urogenital tract

The injection of contrast media into the urinary tract is done either by passing a catheter through the urethra or by suprapubic or intrapelvic injection. This type of analysis delineates the anatomic landmarks and gives information about their function. It clearly delineates abnormalities of the ureters, urethra and bladder. In cases of polycystic disease of the kidney, and of hydronephrosis, it provides the information required to differentiate one from the other. In the former, the contrast media, if injected intrarenally, will delineate a single cyst (most commonly they are not connected). In hydronephrosis, the injection at one site will delineate all the dilated cavities of the kidney. In cases of obstruction, the ascending or descending migration of the contrast media will be impeded by the obstruction, localizing it.

Figure 7 shows a lateral view of a 19-week-old fetus with a large abdominal mass, corresponding to a megacystis, produced by an obstructed urethra.

Cavities

It is common that the fetus has multiple effusions that are related to the cause of death. They are usually documented by measuring the volume of the fluid at the time of the autopsy, or by paracentesis. The injection of contrast media into the pleural, pericardial and peritoneal cavities illustrates with great clarity the internal organs and the anatomic effects of the accumulated fluid.

Cysts

The injection of contrast media into cystic cavities helps to determine their connections to normal and abnormal structures, and to determine whether the cyst has a drainage or is completely closed.

Arteriogram and venogram

The injection of contrast media into the vascular system is one of the most dramatic radiographic analyses of the fetus. The contrast medium is injected through catheters that are inserted into the umbilical vein and arteries. We use two different approaches: a large volume of contrast medium is injected at once and the complete vascular system is delineated; or one can inject smaller volumes in sequence to delineate the vascular tree in sections. When this latter approach is used, X-rays are taken after each injection.

The large arteries and veins are the first to be visualized, followed by medium, small and very small vessels. As the perfusion with the contrast medium advances, one can see many of the organs clearly delineated by their vascular system.

The brain, heart, lungs, liver, kidneys and intestine are commonly visualized by this method. The view of the vascular system and central nervous system has the same utility as the central nervous system arteriogram in children and adults; it helps to delineate the normal and the abnormal structures of the brain and the associated structures. In cases of severe malformations of the brain, it shows the severely abnor-

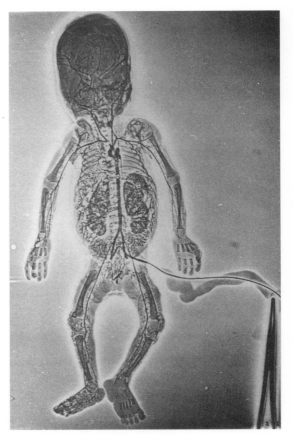

Figure 8 *Detailed arteriogram, which includes all the areas of the fetal body. Note the kidneys*

mal patterns that help to elucidate the process leading to the malformation. The combination of the analysis of the vascular system with other imaging techniques, such as the ventriculogram, adds to the amount of information rendered.

Figure 8 shows a fetus with a very detailed arteriogram, which includes all the areas of the fetal body. This picture shows the kidneys and the adrenals particularly well delineated by the perfusion of their arterial system. Note the exquisite detail of the arteriogram.

Figure 9 shows a fetus whose head was fused to the placenta. This fetus had acrania but not anencephaly. A significant portion of the brain was formed, but it was difficult by inspection or anatomic dissection to determine the precise site where the placenta and brain fused.

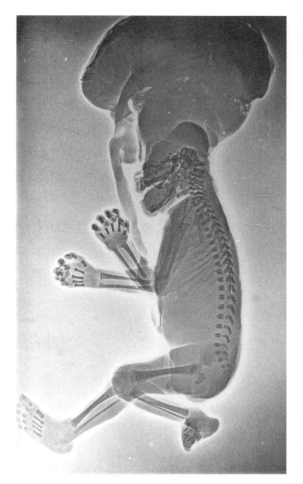

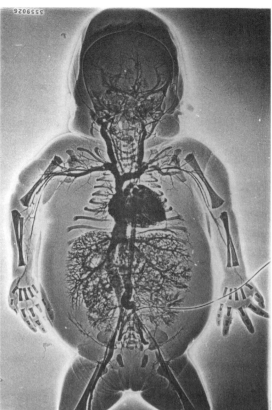

Figure 10 *A 31-week stillborn, with severe generalized subdermic edema. Note the detailed venogram and the syphilitic metaphysitis*

Figure 9 *Fetus whose brain was fused to the placenta (the cephalic mass). This fetus had acrania but not anencephaly*

Contrast medium was injected into the fetal venous system and, as shown in this picture, the precise site where an abnormal brain venous system ended and where the placenta began can clearly be seen. Perfusion of the placental vessels with contrast medium also showed that the placental circulation stopped at the same site where the fetal circulation ended. There were neither placental nor fetal vessels that crossed over. This analysis greatly contributed to the analysis of the abnormality affecting this fetus.

The view of the heart is particularly impressive. The inflows and outflows are clearly delineated. The serial perfusion imaged the vascular system in great detail, including the chambers and the coronary circulation. Malformations and deformations of the heart are clearly demonstrated.

The delineation of the hepatic circulation, as with the other organs, helps to demonstrate malformations and to localize a lesion with great precision; it also helps in determining abnormalities of the size of the organ.

The perfusion of the renal vascular system demonstrates in great detail the position and structure of these organs. This analysis, combined with what was described before for the urogenital tract, increases the resolution of anatomic variants and abnormalities.

Figure 10 shows the radiographic study of a 31-week stillborn, who had severe generalized subdermic edema. This fetus also had pleural, pericardial and peritoneal effusions.

The anterior–posterior xeroradiography show the edema involving the entire body. The ribs are abnormal in shape and position, they are broad, acutely angled anteriorly and the rib cage is bell-shaped.

A catheter was placed inside the umbilical vein and contrast medium was injected. It delineated the cerebral circulation, both jugulars and venous cardiac inflows, the venous circulation of the myocardium, a dilated inferior vena cava, a very large liver and a well delineated intestinal circulation. The long bones were normal in size, but the metaphyses were abnormal and show incipient syphilitic metaphysitis (more noticeable at the proximal end of the humeri, the distal ends of the ulnae and radii and proximal ends of the proximal phalanges).

The placenta

The xeroradiographic analysis of the placenta with and without contrast media provides a great deal of information not obtainable by other mean. Calcifications and severe fibrosis are clearly demonstrated by this method. The visualization of the placental arteries and veins demonstrates the internal structure of the placental. In cases of thrombosis or infarction, it identifies the areas of the placenta that are occluded as a consequence of the vascular accident. It also demonstrates the anatomy, cystic formations and other malformations and abnormalities of the placenta.

The vascular analysis of the placenta is of particular interest and utility when placentas from twin gestations are examined. The combined venogram and arteriogram identify the vascular pattern for each twin. The injection of the contrast medium should be done on one side at a time. If there are vascular anastomoses (as occurs in cases leading to the twin-to-twin transfusion syndrome), the contrast medium on one side will transfer to the other and will delineate the arteries and veins of the opposite side. When the circulations for each twin are completely separated, the vascular imaging of the placenta with contrast medium identifies each circulation separately, with a clear avascular zone between the placental regions for each twin.

CONCLUSION

In summary, it can be stated that the use of the radiographic analysis of the fetus and the placenta provides information that cannot be obtained by any other means, with great detail and precision, contributing to the diagnostic analysis of fetal and neonatal death, and to increased knowledge of the manifestations of fetal disease. Many of the radiographically diagnosable abnormalities can be diagnosed by ultrasonography and vice versa. Using both methods, the radiographic analysis and correlation with the results of any prenatal ultrasonographic examinations constitutes a method of diagnostic validation, measuring the outcome (in this case the accuracy of the ultrasonographic diagnosis). The process of comparison between the prenatal and postnatal imaging procedures should be an integral part of any quality assurance–management–maintenance program in any unit dedicated to fetal medicine, high-risk perinatal medicine and obstetrics. Fetal radiology is also an integral part of the progress of one of the most important branches of fetal medicine and clinical genetics, fetal clinical genetics, because of the great number of abnormalities identified by the radiographic analysis of the human fetus and stillborn.

ACKNOWLEDGEMENTS

To Mr Mark Woodford for this help in the preparation of this manuscript and for the photographic work.

References

1. Elejalde, B. R., de Elejalde, M. M. and Gilman, M. (1985). Analysis of the human skeleton and organs with xeroradiography. *Am. J. Obstet. Gynecol.*, **151**, 666–70
2. Winter, R. M., Knowles, S. A. S., Bieber, F. R. and Baraitser, M. (1988). *The Malformed Fetus and Stillbirth, a Diagnostic Approach*, pp. 30–5. (Chichester: John Wiley & Sons)
3. Cremmin, B. J. and Draper, R. (1981). The value of radiology in perinatal deaths. *Pediatr. Radiol.*, **11**, 143–6
4. Foote, G. A., Wilson, A. J. and Stewart, J. H. (1978). Perinatal postmortem radiography – experience of 2500 cases. *Br. J. Radiol.*, **51**, 351–6
5. Graham, J. M., Crow, H. C., Rownsley, E. F., Simmons, J. M. and Hoefnagel, D. (1984). Enhanced visualization of soft tissues in the study of aborted fetuses through the use of xeroradiography. *Teratology*, **30**, 11–24
6. Keeling, J. W. (ed.) *Fetal and Neonatal Pathology*, p. 11. (London: Springer-Verlag)
7. Ornoy, A., Borochowitz, Z., Lachman, R. and Rimoin, D. L. (1988). *Atlas of Fetal Skeletal Radiology*. (Chicago: Year Book Medical Publishers)
8. Cruickshank, J. N., Miller, M. J. and Browne, F. J. (1924). *The Estimation of Foetal Age, the Weight and Length of Normal Foetuses, and the Weights of Foetal Organs*, Medical Research Council special series no. 86. (London: His Majesty's Stationery Office)
9. Elejalde, B. R. and de Elejalde, M. M. (1985). The prenatal growth of the human body determined by the measurement of bones and organs by ultrasonography. *Am. J. Med. Genet.*, **24**, 575–98
10. Elejalde, B. R. and de Elejalde, M. M. (1983). Prenatal diagnosis of perinatally lethal osteogenesis imperfecta. *Am. J. Med. Genet.*, **14**, 353–9
11. Elejalde, B. R., de Elejalde, M. M. and Pansch, D. (1985). Prenatal diagnosis of Jeune syndrome. *Am. J. Med. Genet.*, **21**, 433–8
12. Elejalde, B. R., de Elejalde, M. M., Booth, C., Kaye, C. and Hollison, L. (1985). Prenatal diagnosis of Weyers syndrome (Deficient ulnar and fibular rays with bilateral hydronephrosis. *Am. J. Med. Genet.*, **21**, 439–44
13. Elejalde, B. R. and de Elejalde, M. M. (1985). Thanatophoric dysplasia with cloverleaf skull: fetal manifestations and prenatal diagnosis. *Am. J. Med. Genet.*, **22**, 669–83

Section 2

Advances in prenatal screening and diagnosis

Molecular genetics in fetal medicine 10

B. R. Elejalde and M. M. de Elejalde

INTRODUCTION

In the last ten years, the astonishing development of molecular genetics has led to the identification of gene mutations that cause many diseases. The diseases selected for such analysis are characterized by their severity in postnatal life. The search for such genes and their mutations has been undertaken to identify the cause, to understand the pathogenesis of the disease, in order to develop more precise diagnostic methods, and, hopefully, to design successful treatments and eventually a cure. Two fields have benefitted greatly from the advances in molecular genetics: prenatal diagnosis and molecular embryology.

To date, more than 6000 autosomal dominant, recessive and X-linked conditions in humans are known. More than 2100 genetic syndromes have been described. They have been found in newborns, infants and adults, and in a more limited fashion, in fetuses. A very large number of human fecundations die before birth, and the precise cause of embryonic and fetal death is not known in most cases. Both genetic and acquired diseases seem to play a very important role. It seems possible that there are many more abnormal embryos than fetuses, and many more fetuses than children and adults affected by diseases due to mutations. It is, therefore, likely that there are many more genetic diseases affecting the fetus, which have not been recognized yet, and many which may be incorrectly diagnosed.

Molecular genetics has also made major inroads into the identification of the causes of some acquired and multifactorial diseases as well as in the understanding of their pathophysiology and in the development of diagnostic methods. Initially, prenatal diagnosis was limited to the analysis of amniotic fluid to diagnose neural tube defects and chromosomal abnormalities. The identification of biochemical markers allows for the diagnosis of other metabolic diseases. With the use of ultrasonography, physicians are able to diagnose many more diseases and malformations in the fetus. The use of molecular genetics increases the number of diseases that can be diagnosed with more precision than before. It is the purpose of this chapter to describe the applications of molecular genetics to fetal medicine and to explore the possibilities for future developments, highlighting the role of the practitioners of fetal medicine. We will discuss a few diseases that illustrate the molecular characteristics of disease, the diagnostic approaches, the benefits, risks, and the clinical, ethical, moral and legal implications.

FETAL MOLECULAR MEDICINE

Fetal medicine has emerged from the practice of prenatal diagnosis for genetic defects, and has evolved to include the diagnosis of acquired, fetal and maternal diseases. The progress and future developments of fetal medicine depend upon the development of prenatal diagnosis and its integration with fetal therapy and fetal pathology. For prenatal diagnosis to be appropriate, of good quality and accurate, detailed knowledge of genetic and acquired fetal disease is necessary.

Prenatal diagnosis has its roots in the hope and desire to improve perinatal outcomes, to reduce perinatal mortality, to reduce the familial suffering and pain caused by fetal and neonatal death and to reduce the burden of disease that is inherited or begins *in utero*. The obstetric prenatal care is geared at discovering signs of maternal and fetal disease and, hopefully, developing treatments to cure and prevent undesirable pregnancy outcomes. The knowledge of fetal disease, genetic and acquired, is quite limited. The tools to study normal and abnormal fetal development have been limited by the biological and cultural limitations of the maternal fetal environment.

In the last 30 years, however, two principal tools have dramatically changed the methods of acquiring knowledge of fetal disease: amniocentesis and ultrasonography. The former allows for the cytogenetic, biochemical, molecular and immunological analysis of the fetus. The latter allows for a detailed morphological, functional, behavioral and developmental analysis of the fetus. Other fetal sampling techniques have also been used including: chorionic villus sampling, fetal biopsies (skin, muscle and liver), percutaneous fetal blood sampling, placental biopsies and analysis of other fetal fluids (cystic and urine). Previously, the fetal cells obtained by these methods required culturing before they were used for diagnostic testing. Now, polymerase chain reaction (PCR) has removed the need for tissue culturing, shortening the time to complete the diagnostic testing and increasing accuracy.

As a result of the increased knowledge of DNA chemistry, and the detailed understanding of the cellular mechanisms controlling the genetic material, molecular genetics has evolved as a powerful diagnostic technique. The application of this knowledge to the analysis of human disease is probably the most powerful tool ever used in diagnosis. The localization and characterization of human genes has explained the etiology, pathogenesis and prognosis of a large growing number of conditions, making their diagnosis and prognosis more accurate and, in some cases, possible for the first time.

The expansion of the accuracy, range and timing of disease diagnosis by the introduction of molecular diagnosis has special impact on fetal medicine. Prenatal diagnosis had been limited to a number of diseases that are lethal *in utero*, after birth, or some time soon afterwards. It has been practiced for conditions that are compatible with a significantly long life, associated with severe handicaps and/or mental retardation. The identification of the genes and mutations producing diseases that are characterized by having a period of life when the individual is normal for some time, usually with a normal productive life, before developing the disease, has created the possibility of:

(1) Presymptomatic diagnosis, pre- and postnatal in the cases where the identification of a mutation predicts with almost complete certainty that the individual will develop a disease later in life. A good example of this case is Huntington disease; once the mutation is identified, one can predict with great certainty that the individual will develop the disease.

(2) Predisposition diagnosis, also before and after birth. Certain mutations such as the ones of the BRCA1 gene once found in one individual will indicate a high risk of developing cancer of the breast and/or the ovary. This type of diagnosis also can be used in the diagnosis of predisposition to many diseases at the present time (coronary heart disease, colorectal carcinoma, medullary carcinoma of the thyroid, multiple endocrine neoplasia type II and others) and many more in the future.

The prenatal use of these two new diagnostic modalities has opened many medical, moral, ethical and legal questions that should be addressed and answered appropriately to allow and support the development of these disciplines. Humanity should use the same creativity and serendipity that has allowed the gathering of the amazing knowledge on the human genome, to develop the medical, social, ethical, moral and political strategies for the acceptable application of this technology for the benefit of humanity and of the world.

DIAGNOSTIC MODALITIES

Molecular diagnosis is performed in three different situations: (1) when a member of the family has the condition, (2) when an individual is at higher risk because of ethnic origin, and (3) when the mother or fetus has shown signs of abnormality diagnosed by the standard obstetric and genetic explorations. These three categories can be subclassified according to the time of onset of the disease, to incorporate the concepts of symptomatic, presymptomatic and predisposition fetal diagnosis.

Diagnosis when there is an affected family member

When there is an affected family member, it is of utmost importance to have precise knowledge and characterization of the condition. If the clinical diagnosis is wrong, the molecular testing will seek a condition different from that which is present in the family. Several abnormal hemoglobins produce sickling; however, if one assumes that a sickling test is diagnostic of hemoglobin S (Hb S), and the prenatal diagnosis is undertaken for Hb S, it may be said that the fetus is normal, when indeed it is affected by hemoglobin C (Hb C). For genetic prenatal diagnosis to be successful, a precise and accurate clinical diagnosis is of absolute necessity.

Diagnosis of individuals at higher risk because of ethnic origin

In these cases, families seek prenatal diagnosis once they become familiar with the complications of genetic disease common among members of their ethnic group. For example, the diagnosis of Hb S *in utero* in its homozygous state has been done on a large number of patients. Blacks have been screened for Hb S because of complications of the disease and the possibility of treatment that may reduce the complications of the disease and its long-term prognosis. Ashkenazic Jews have a higher frequency of Tay–Sachs (1 : 27) than other Caucasians (1 : 150) except French Canadians (1 : 18). Couples at risk because of their ethnic origin have been tested prenatally. When both parents are carriers of the mutant gene, the fetus is tested. Two families may make completely different decisions facing the same diagnosis, that the fetus is affected. Some choose to continue the pregnancy while others decide to terminate it. When they choose to continue the pregnancy, pre-

natal diagnosis allows for the prompt initiation of preventive therapy which can be successful in reducing the complications of the condition in the case of Hb S, and in cases of fetuses with Tay–Sachs disease to be prepared for the birth of an affected child.

Diagnosis when the mother or fetus has shown signs of abnormality diagnosed by the standard obstetric and genetic explorations

Ultrasound is the prenatal diagnostic method that detects the largest number of fetal defects. For example, a highly echogenic intestinal loop is suggestive that the fetus may have cystic fibrosis (CF). Five per cent of highly echogenic intestinal loops are caused by fetal cystic fibrosis[1]. The CFTR (cystic fibrosis transconductance receptor) gene, the one that prevents the development of CF when normal, and the one that causes CF when mutated (over 450 mutations have been recognized), can be analyzed by PCR analysis leading to the diagnosis of the condition if the fetus has one of the known mutations.

SYMPTOMATIC DIAGNOSIS FOR DISEASES WITH FETAL MANIFESTATIONS

For the illustration of this type of disease, we have chosen three groups; skeletal dysplasias, syndromes with craniosynostosis and congenital adrenal hyperplasia.

Skeletal dysplasias

The prenatal diagnosis of achondroplasia, thanatophoric dysplasia and hypochondroplasia has been based on the ultrasonographic analysis of the fetal bones. While the ultrasonographic characteristics of thanatophoric dysplasia are present before 20 weeks of gestation, achondroplasia and hypochondroplasia do not show any ultrasonographically recognizable abnormalities before this age. The differential diagnosis between thanatophoric dysplasia and the other two is easier due to the severe alterations of the fetal size and modelling abnormalities characterizing it[2–5].

These three skeletal dysplasias are caused by mutations of the fibroblast growth factor receptor 3 (FGFR3) gene which is located on chromosome 4p[6–8].

The recognition of the mutations causing these skeletal dysplasias allows for their precise diagnosis. Most (95%) achondroplasias (inherited and new mutations) are caused by a single amino acid substitution, glycine for arginine at position 380 (G380R)[6]. When a family is at risk, with one or both parents affected, the fetus can be tested as early as fetal cells can be sampled. In cases where the ultrasonographic pattern of achondroplasia[4] is detected, the molecular testing makes the diagnosis with precision and excludes other dysplasias which may have similar manifestations *in utero*. One of these conditions is hypochondroplasia, which has very similar manifestations *in utero* to achondroplasia. While the sonographic differential diagnosis between the two is possible but quite difficult, the molecular diagnosis is not only more precise but simpler, as it differentiates between the conditions with clarity. The precise diagnosis *in utero* is important because the natural history, complications, long-term prognosis and quality of life are different in achondroplasia and hypochondroplasia. Most of the cases of hypochondroplasia seem to be caused by mutations that cause an amino acid substitution at position 540 from asparagine to lysine (N540K)[8]. The recognition of the mutation will make the diagnosis precise.

The molecular genetics of these three skeletal dysplasias is an exquisite example of the effects of mutations at different domains of a protein. The FGFR3 has three extracellular immunoglobulin-like domains, a transmembrane, a juxtamembrane domain, a proximal and a distal tyrosine kinase domain that are separated by the spacer region. Mutations affecting the transmembrane domain produce achondroplasia, those affecting the proximal region of the tyrosine kinase domain produce hypochondroplasia. Thanatophoric dysplasia is produced at several sites[7], more commonly in regions between the immunoglobulin like domains 2 and 3 (extracellular) and also the distal region of the tyrosine kinase domain (intracellular).

This example is probably the first one to illustrate the complementarity of molecular genetic diagnosis and ultrasonography. That is, the use of both expands the diagnostic range and preciseness of skeletal dysplasias *in utero* and makes it more accurate.

Craniosynostosis syndromes

Apert, Crouzon, Pfeiffer and Jackson–Weiss syndromes have craniosynostosis, facial and other malformations as their manifestations. These three conditions are caused by mutations of the fibroblast growth factor receptor 2 (FGFR2) which is located on chromosome 10q[9–12].

The prenatal diagnosis of these conditions is difficult. In many cases, the diagnosis was missed until the discovery of the responsible mutations made it more precise. The diagnosis of Apert syndrome was dependent upon the ultrasonographic diagnosis of syndactyly. The craniosynostosis and the facial abnormalities are difficult to recognize by ultrasound, partly because they are not severe enough until late in the pregnancy. Since most of these syndromes are due to new mutations, the diagnosis still depends upon the ultrasonographic recognition of one or more of the abnormalities characteristic of these conditions, except for those families with a history of the condition. The molecular diagnosis of these syndromes is of great utility in families with affected individuals and pregnancies at risk, and in fetuses who are found to have ultrasonographic abnormalities compatible with the diagnosis, who do not have a family history of the condition.

Syndactyly is diagnosable by ultrasonography more easily than the facial defects of these syndromes. Once this malformation is diagnosed, molecular testing for mutations of the FGFR2 can be undertaken to either prove or exclude the diagnosis of Apert syndrome. If craniofacial defects are recognized by ultrasonography that are suggestive of a craniosynostosis syndrome, testing for the FGFR2 mutation will determine if the condition is one of those caused by this gene.

Congenital adrenal hyperplasia

This disease is an example of a disease with severe fetal manifestations that will have serious postnatal consequences that can be prevented. Several disorders are grouped under this name. All of them interfere with normal steroidogenesis to form cortisol. The most common type (90%) of the disease is caused by mutations in the 21-hydroxylase gene. The others are produced by mutations of the genes coding for 11β-hydroxylase (5%), 17α-hydroxylase, 17,20-lyase, 3β-hydroxysteroid dehydrogenase and 11α-hydroxylase[13]. The importance of prenatal diagnosis for this condition is that the embryo who is at risk of developing the condition (because it has two mutations of the 21-hydroxylase gene, and is a female) can be successfully treated *in utero* to prevent the manifestations of the disease with dexamethasone, 20 μg/kg of body weight/24 h. The treatment has to be started before 5–6 weeks of gestation since the masculinization of the female genitalia takes place between the 5th and 12th weeks of gestation. The most commonly used protocol starts treating the mother with dexamethasone by the 5th week and is continued until genetic prenatal diagnosis indicates that the fetus is a male, or that it is a female heterozygote or normal homozygote. This is an important example of the role of molecular genetics in the diagnosis and management of disease that produces severe long-term consequences, physical and psychological.

There are two 21-hydroxylase genes that map within the class III major histocompatibility complex on chromosome 6p. There is an active gene CYP21 and a pseudo gene CYP21P. Mutations producing the disease include deletions, large conversions, duplications and point mutations. Contrary to the mutations producing achondroplasia and hypochondroplasia, there are many mutations producing congenital adrenal hyperplasia. The prenatal diagnosis of this autosomal recessive disease requires the parental mutations to be identified precisely, allowing for specific fetal testing. If the parental mutations are not known, fetal testing is not possible.

PRESYMPTOMATIC DIAGNOSIS OF DISEASES WITH MANIFESTATIONS AFTER BIRTH AND IN CHILDHOOD

Abnormal hemoglobins

Hemoglobin S (Hb S) does not produce any fetal signs of disease, these only appear in the first years of life. While sickle cell disease can have very serious complication and shorter life, it can be treated. This was the first condition to be diagnosed prenatally through the use of recombinant DNA technology[14]. This development was possible due to the knowledge of the amino acid sequence for the normal hemoglobin A and for the amino acid change producing Hb S.

Two methods have been used: restriction fragment length polymorphism (RFLP) and polymerase chain reaction (PCR). Initially, it was discovered that, if the DNA extracted from an individual's amniotic cells or chorionic villi contains the normal sequence cutting with Mst II, it will produce a 1.15 kb (kilobase) fragment and a 1.35 kb fragment if the mutation for Hb S is present[14]. This is due to the mutation destroying the site recognized by the enzyme, and thus not cutting the Hb S sample but cutting in the Hb A sample (Figure 1).

The second method is the use of PCR. DNA polymerase has the ability to copy DNA using one of the strands to produce a new one which is a complementary copy. It does not initiate the

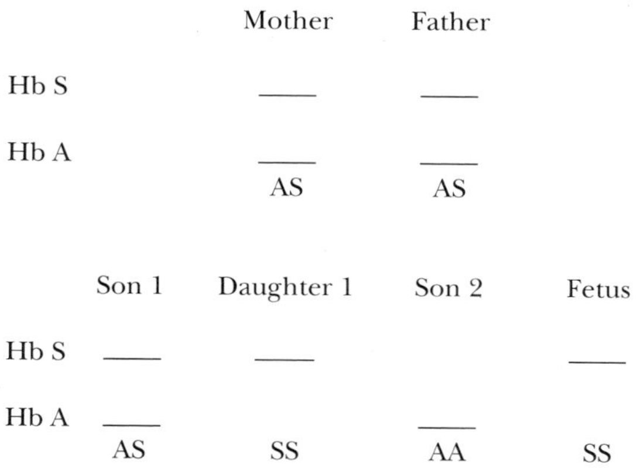

Figure 1 *A representation of an autoradiograph of a restriction fragment length polymorphism study for hemoglobin S (Hb S). Hemoglobin A (Hb A)*

copy unless it is 'primed' by a stretch of DNA bound to its 5′ end. PCR takes advantage of this requirement and the primers needed to initiate the polymerase activity are also used to delimitate the region to be copied. Two primers are needed, one in each complementary strand at the 5′ end of the region to be amplified. Human genomic DNA is mixed with the primers, four single nucleotides, a DNA polymerase and the reaction buffer. The mixture is heated at 95 °C to break the complementary bonds between the two strands, producing single stranded DNA. The reaction is allowed to cool to the specific annealing temperature for the primers (around 55 °C). The great excess of primers favors the preferential annealing of the primer to the template, over the reannealing of the template strands. Then the temperature is raised to optimal for the polymerase (about 75 °C) to synthesize the new strand beginning at the primer site. After the first cycle, the number of molecules containing the selected sequence has doubled. The repetition of the cycle several times, commonly between 20 and 30 times produces an exponential increase in the number of molecules containing the target sequence. This amplification of the target sequence is an incredibly powerful tool in molecular genetics that has opened unexpected avenues in the exploration of the human genome.

In the case of Hb S, primers have been designed to copy the region where the Hb S mutation occurred in the β-globin gene. Two to three million copies of this region are produced in a period of 3 h. The PCR product is subject to restriction digestion using Mst II. The PCR reaction copies a segment that contains 230 base pairs. The site of the Hb S mutation is located at position 100. If the gene has the normal mutation, the enzyme cuts and produces two fragments, one of 100 base pairs (bp) and the other of 130 bp. If the gene has the Hb S mutation, the enzyme does not cut. Consequently, individuals who are normal homozygotes have two fragments (represented by two bands in the electrophoretic gel) one 100 bp long and the other 130 bp. Individuals who are homozygous for the mutation (affected by Hb S disease) have only one fragment (one single band in the elec-

trophoretic gel) of 230 base pairs. Individuals who have a normal and a mutant gene have three fragments (three bands in the electrophoretic gel), 100, 130 and 230 bp, and are carriers for Hb S disease. A similar technology can be used for the diagnosis of many other diseases.

Two situations have made this diagnosis possible: the abundance of messenger RNA for the β-globin gene in reticulocytes allowed the development of testing strategies for the diagnosis of Hb S, and the availability of a restriction endonuclease (Mst II) that cuts the normal sequence, but does not cut if the gene has the mutation producing Hb S (Figure 2).

Initially, cells needed to be cultured until enough were obtained for DNA extraction and for molecular analysis. We have developed and used the PCR analysis for Hb S using the cells contained in 1 ml of amniotic fluid. This method reduces the time needed for the testing, the cost of the test and the amount of work.

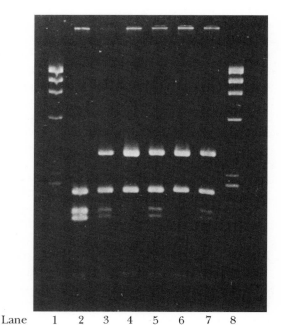

Lane   1   2   3   4   5   6   7   8

Figure 2 *The first lane is a 'ladder' of DNA molecules of known weight, the second is the pattern of the amplified β-globin region containing the S mutation and showing the normal pattern produced by homozygote AA, the third is the pattern for heterozygote AS, the fourth is for SS and the fifth for AS, the sixth SS and the seventh AS*

In the past, the parents were tested to determine if they were carriers of Hb S, and if both were carriers, the fetus would be tested. Most couples at risk are not tested prenatally for many different reasons, including denial by health care organizations to pay for parental testing, making prenatal diagnosis very difficult for Hb S. This situation has caused several states to develop mandatory neonatal testing for abnormal hemoglobins. We have developed a program for prenatal testing in which we test all fetuses at risk because of their ethnicity using uncultured amniotic cells and polymerase chain reaction products digested with CvnI.

Cystic fibrosis

Most of the manifestations of this disease occur after birth, and most of the children affected by cystic fibrosis are born to families not known to be at risk. Occasionally, the fetus shows highly echogenic intestine and meconium peritonitis. The gene causing this autosomal recessive condition is located on chromosome 7q, over 450 mutations have been discovered and they still do not account for all the cases of CF[1]. The prenatal diagnosis of this condition is simple in cases where a family at risk has been studied prior to the fetal diagnosis, and the parental mutations have been identified. In this case, the fetus is tested specifically for them. If the fetus has the two parental mutations, it is affected. If it has only one mutation, the fetus is a carrier, as are its parents, and if it does not have either of them, it will be a non-carrier for those particular mutations.

When a family is at risk, the first diagnostic step should be the determination of the mutations present in the affected individual. Once identified, the parents should be tested. If both are carriers, the fetus should be tested. There are families where one or two mutations cannot be identified; however, with the use of RFLP and linkage analysis, it is possible to determine the haplotype that is linked with the disease. In these cases the diagnosis is done by linkage analysis, rather than by direct mutation analysis.

The diagnosis is much more difficult when the mutations that may produce the disease are not known. This situation is particularly common in families with an affected family member who is deceased. The diagnostic situation is equally difficult when the family is not known to be at risk, and it is the ultrasonographic examination which shows a highly echogenic intestine or meconium peritonitis. The diagnostic problem is further compounded because the frequency of the different mutations varies greatly between populations and ethnic groups. The most common mutation is ΔF508 (the deletion of three base pairs), it is found in 68–76% of cases in Caucasians (mixed European ancestry), 71% of Hispanics, 69% of Louisiana French Acadians, 54–69% of French Canadians, 26–50% of Ashkenazic Jews, 37% of African Americans and 35% of Hutterites[15]. The difference between the noted percentages and 100% is caused by the other more than 450 mutations. The detection of such a large number of mutations is technically impossible within the time that is normally allowed for prenatal diagnosis as well as extremely expensive. Different approaches have been undertaken to deal with this problem. One is the detection of a group of mutations that explain a large number of cases.

The mutations ΔF508 and W1228X account for about 75% of the cases in individuals of European ancestry including Ashkenazic Jews. Six other mutations (G551D, R553X, 621+1T, G542X, N1303K and 3849+10T) account for 97% of the Ashkenazic Jews cases and about 82% of the American whites. The addition of 16 other mutations to the test increases the number of cases in American whites (mixed European ancestry) to 89.1%[16]. Amniotic fluid can be tested using the cells from 1 ml of uncultured amniotic fluid, similarly to the method that we use for sickle cell disease. This approach resolves some of the problems of fetal testing for cystic fibrosis. By not requiring that the cells be cultured, the time and expense of the test are significantly reduced. If the fetus has one or two of the 16 mutations tested by this method, one would have the diagnosis. For the detection of the other mutations one needs to analyze all the regions of the CFTR gene and do PCR reactions for different regions. The PCR product is subjected to single stranded conformational polymorphism (SSCP) or heteroduplex analysis. These procedures detect differences in the DNA strands produced by PCR. Normal products produce electrophoretic patterns that are different from those with mutations. Those products that produce abnormal heteroduplexes, homoduplexes or SSCPs are subjected to DNA sequence analysis for the identification of the specific mutation. While 100% of the cases of Hb S can be diagnosed prenatally by molecular fetal analysis, some cystic fibrosis cases cannot be diagnosed because the mutations cannot be identified. It is not practical, at the present time, to examine the complete CFTR gene for each and every fetus, if one were to take the same approach that we have taken with Hb S. Sickle cell disease occurs in 1 : 655 African Americans, cystic fibrosis in 1 : 2500 Caucasians, 1 : 9600 Hispanics, 1 : 18 000 African Americans and 1 : 90 000 Asians in the United States[17].

Duchenne and Becker muscular dystrophies

Duchenne and Becker muscular dystrophies (D and BMD) are X-linked conditions that are produced by abnormalities of a very large gene (2 million base pairs)[18]. The clinical manifestations of these diseases appear in childhood, usually around the 5th year of life. One-third of those affected are new mutations, while the other two-thirds inherit the defective gene from their mother through the X chromosome. The mutations producing DMD alter the protein in a more severe form than those producing BMD. These conditions are good examples of two methods of molecular genetic prenatal diagnosis: direct detection of the mutation and linkage analysis.

Of all the cases of DMD, 60% are due to deletions[19] and 6% to duplications[20] of different parts of the gene that code for a muscular protein known as dystrophin. Most of the deletions cluster at 14 gene regions that can be tested by PCR[21,22]. This is a method designed to copy 14 regions of the gene and to amplify them many times. Several millions copies of each region can be made in a few hours. If the region is deleted, it cannot be copied and the product will be absent. This reaction is known as multiplex PCR. It is designed to produce 14 pieces of DNA of different sizes. The DNA product of this reaction is subjected to electrophoresis to separate the DNA fragments by size. To recognize them, they are stained with ethidium bromide which produces fluorescence at the site where DNA is observed. The absence of a band is indicative of a deletion of the gene region corresponding to the selected region (Figure 3).

The remaining 34% of the cases of DMD are caused by other types of mutations, including point mutations and duplications. The precise characterization is difficult, in many cases requiring the use of linkage analysis for prenatal diagnosis. A recent study by Prior and colleagues[23], showed that extensive analysis failed to detect small mutations producing either DMD or BMD. They found mutations in 29/159 patients tested who did not have a deletion or a duplication. The authors concluded that it is not possible at the present time to perform direct carrier and prenatal diagnosis for many families without deletions or duplications. The only method in these families is linkage analysis. Linkage is based on the recognition of a chromosome by the characterization of the markers that are closely linked to the disease in question. The classical example is the linkage between the nail patella syndrome and the ABO groups.

DNA fragments have been analyzed to determine the chromosomes and where they come from; a few have been found to be linked with certain genetic disease by linkage analysis. Linked DNA is easily obtained from cDNA (complementary DNA) which is synthesized from the mRNA by the use of reverse transcriptase into cDNA. It contains the part of the gene that is transcribed into RNA. It normally represents the exons, and it lacks a significant part of the gene, its introns (intervening sequences), which are not translated into the protein sequence. DNA fragments known to be part of or close to the gene in question are used to identify the chromosome carrying the normal or abnormal gene.

By typing the DNA of the affected individual, mother and normal members of the family,

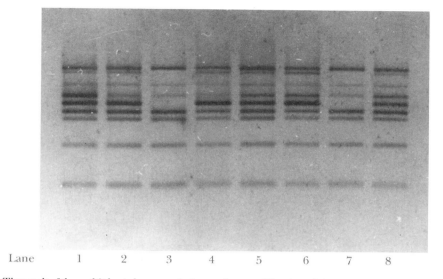

Figure 3 *The result of the multiplex polymerase chain reaction amplification of nine regions of the dystrophin gene. Lanes 1, 2, 4, 5, 6 are normal members of the family. Lanes 3 and 7 are two brothers affected by Duchenne muscular dystrophy (DMD) caused by a double deletion where two bands are missing: the second and the fourth from the top. Lane 8 is the fetal DNA, which shows a normal pattern, indicating that this male fetus is not affected by DMD*

it is possible to track the chromosome that carries the defective gene and determine if the fetus will or will not be affected. This is depicted in Figure 3.

Linkage analysis is not as precise as mutation detection because several factors may produce false results. The most important is recombination, which occurs commonly in human chromosomes. The closer the marker is to the gene, the less likely that recombination will occur. In genes as large as the DMD gene, intragenic recombination has been reported. It is recommended that when using linkage for DNA-based diagnosis, one should use markers flanking the gene at each of its ends and one located inside the gene (Figure 4).

The most common type of markers are known as restriction fragment length polymorphism (RFLP). They are pieces of DNA obtained from cDNA or by other methods that are determined to be closely linked to a given chromosome, gene, or genetic marker. The method most commonly used in the analysis of RFLP consists of extracting DNA from lymphocytes, amniocytes, or other cells. The DNA is digested (cut) with a restriction endonuclease to produce DNA fragments of many different sizes.

They are subjected to electrophoresis to separate them by size. The larger fragments are closer to the point of initiation of migration, and the smaller migrate the longest distances. Once separated, the product of the electrophoresis is transferred to a nylon or nitrocellulose membrane to immobilize the DNA fragments at the position they had at the end of the electrophoresis. The membrane containing the DNA is exposed to a mixture containing the DNA that is either linked or is the gene for the condition being tested. This DNA or probe has been marked (labelled) with radioactive phosphorus to identify the site where it finds complementary sequences in the membrane. The membrane is then exposed to an X-ray film and the site where the complementary sequences hybridize produces a dark band on the X-ray film.

Most probes when used in DNA digested with a restriction nuclease produce two bands (dimorphic RFLP); some produce more than two bands (polymorphic RFLP). A probe that produces two bands can have four combinations: 1/1, 2/2, 1/2 and 2/1 as seen in Figure 4. When several probes are used, they produce a pattern (haplotype) as noted, in the above example, for probes a, b, c and d.

Probe (RFLP)	Mother X	X	Father X	Y
a	1	2	1	
b	2	1	1	
c	1	1	2	
d	2	2	1	
Chromosome	A	N1	N2	

	Daughter 1		Son 1		Son 2		Daughter 2		Fetus has or			
	X	X	X	Y	X	Y	X	X	X	Y	X	Y
	1	1	1		2		2	1	2		1	
	2	1	2		1	1	1		1		2	
	1	2	1		1		1	2	1		1	
	2	1	2		2		2	1	2		2	
	A	N2	A		N1		N1	N2	N1		A	

Figure 4 *The mother has two X chromosomes, one of them marked A (affected), is present in son 1 and absent in son 2. This observation identifies the chromosome carrying the defective gene producing Duchenne muscular dystrophy (DMD) in this family, since the markers are linked to the dystrophin gene. Based on the typing (haplotypes) of this family, daughter 1 is a carrier, she inherited chromosome A from the mother (with the defective gene) and chromosome N2 (normal) from the father. Daughter 2 inherited normal chromosomes from the mother (N1) and from the father (N2), thus she is not a carrier. The fetus is a male, thus he has only one chromosome X, necessarily inherited from his mother; if he inherits N1 he will be normal, if he inherits A he will suffer DMD*

The prenatal diagnosis of DMD is not possible when the affected individual is dead or when the mutation cannot be characterized by the deletion and duplication detection methods.

PRESYMPTOMATIC DIAGNOSIS OF DISEASES WITH MANIFESTATIONS AFTER BIRTH AND IN ADULTHOOD

Precise presymptomatic diagnosis of disease is a growing reality. A significant number of diseases of adulthood can be diagnosed prenatally, many years before the individual shows even minor signs of the condition. A telling example is Huntington disease. The gene was localized by linkage to chromosome 4. For many years, pre- and postnatal diagnosis has been done by linkage analysis requiring at least one affected and non-affected member of the family.

Recently, the gene and mutation producing the disease were characterized. The mutation consists of having more than 38 copies of a CAG triplet repeat[24]. Normal individuals have fewer than 38. The diagnosis is done by the use of PCR, amplifying the region near the mutation. A normal individual with 18 repeats produces a frag-ment of 247 base pairs; if the fragment is larger than 313 base pairs (over 40 repeats) the patient is affected by Huntington disease (Figure 5). The age of onset varies greatly, but it occurs commonly during the third and the fourth decades of life. The age of onset is directly related to the number of repeats, the larger the number, the earlier the onset of Huntington disease. Many families with this condition had chosen not to reproduce in the past because of their fear that their children might be affected, but with testing available, they now have the chance to get tested. Although the recognition of the mutation opens the possibility of prenatal diagnosis, it is troublesome because these individuals have 30–40 years of normal productive life.

There is a group of neurological diseases of adulthood that are due to expanded repeats and that can be diagnosed prenatally by the same methods in use for Huntington disease, but the same concerns apply to them. They are myotonic dystrophy, cerebrospinal muscular atrophy, spinocerebellar ataxia type I, dentatorubral and pallidoluysian atrophy, and Machado–Joseph disease. When these diseases do not show anticipation, the affected individuals have a life span of 30–40 years in which they have normal

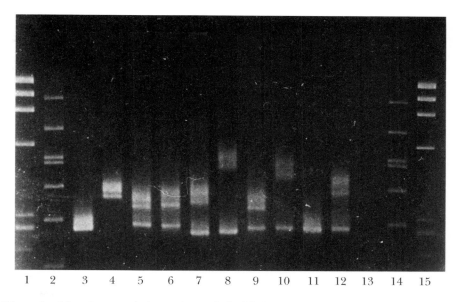

Figure 5 *The results of the polymerase chain reaction analysis of the huntingtin gene. Lanes 1, 2, 14 and 15 are molecular weight markers. Lane 3 is the product of a normal gene containing 18 repeats, lane 4 is the product of a mutated gene containing 48 repeats, lanes 5, 6, 9 and 11 are normal individuals, the last is a homozygote for 17 repeats. Lanes 7, 8 and 10 show the expanded repeats of two affected individuals, the expanded repeat is larger in 8 than in 10*

or near normal life, and in which they develop and perform as individuals who do not have the mutation. Prenatal diagnosis has been performed a few times for some of these conditions, based on the parents' right to request testing and the precedent that prenatal diagnosis has been widely accepted and practised for the detection of Down syndrome. Individuals with Down syndrome can live as long as 50 years and through education they achieve and have a better life than they had before.

Perhaps a better comparison is that prenatal diagnosis and selective termination of pregnancies have been used for hemophilia and for some of the thalassemias. These individuals have severe conditions that do not impair intellectual function and that are compatible with long lives. Thus, one may conclude that the prenatal diagnosis for neurodegenerative conditions of adulthood is permissible in some selected cases and after extensive counselling and analysis of the motivations and purposes.

The low density lipoprotein receptor gene has mutations that produce severe coronary heart disease at predictable ages[25]. It is possible to determine if a fetus has one of the more than

150 mutations known in this gene, and consequently predict the type and severity of the coronary heart disease that in time the individual will develop.

Many other diseases can be included in this group. Some among this growing group are: Alzheimer disease, long Q–T syndrome, hypertrophic cardiomyopathy and other cardiomyopathies, Charcot–Marie–Tooth, familial amyotrophic lateral sclerosis and a growing spectrum of neoplastic diseases. The availability of precise presymptomatic testing begs the question: when, by whom and how will the fetal testing be done?

GENETIC PRENATAL DIAGNOSIS OF ACQUIRED DISEASE

Other aspects of DNA molecular diagnosis at the present time include the diagnosis of infectious disease. DNA probes for many bacteria and viruses have been characterized. The molecular diagnosis of infectious disease *in utero* permits diagnosis when only a few organisms are present and in a shorter period of time than traditional methods since culture, isolation and characterization methods are not required. The faster diagnosis allows for the initiation of the treatment (in the cases where it is possible) sooner than when traditional methods are used.

Some infectious diseases, such as parvovirus B19[26], are particularly important because they allow the diagnosis of a condition which can be treated successfully by intrauterine transfusions and thus prevent a fetus from developing severe aplastic anemia. A similar case can be made for listeria[27], HIV, cytomegalovirus, chlamydia, gonorrhea and many more[28].

GENETIC MOLECULAR DIAGNOSIS OF MATERNAL FETAL ACQUIRED DISEASE: THE CASES OF Rh ISOIMMUNE DISEASE AND CONGENITAL THROMBO-CYTOPENIC PURPURA

The molecular typing of the blood groups and Rh in amniotic cells and in chorionic villus sampling (CVS) allows the diagnosis of the fetal blood typing very early in the pregnancy. The use of this technology avoids the uncertainty of waiting for the fetus to show ultrasonographic signs of isoimmune disease. The molecular blood typing can be done as early as the time when CVS and early amniocentesis are done. This testing will divide the population at risk into two groups with great certainty, those at risk and those not at risk. This approach avoids having to perform repeated amniocenteses to determine the concentration of bilirubin, or to have a percutaneous umbilical blood sampling for blood typing.

A similar approach is being used for the diagnosis of individuals at risk of developing congenital thrombocytopenic purpura. The molecular diagnosis of the platelet antigens that determine fetal thrombocytopenic purpura allows for the selection of fetuses at risk because they bear the antigen. In these cases, the total population at risk does not have to undergo an intensive diagnostic and management program and only those at risk of the disease will require testing.

GENETIC MOLECULAR DIAGNOSIS OF COMPATIBLE STEM CELLS FOR TRANSPLANTATION

Certain families who have individuals affected by a given genetic disease may benefit from a bone marrow transplant, because some of the manifestations of the condition can be corrected with bone marrow with normal genes. The cord blood of neonates is very rich in stem cells and it has been shown that the transplant of stem cells obtained from the umbilical cord at the time of birth can be used successfully for transplantation. We have used this approach for the treatment of a girl who was affected by Chediak–Higashi disease. The mother became pregnant, the fetus was diagnosed as not affected by Chediak–Higashi. A sample of fetal blood was obtained at 20 weeks of gestation and was subjected to typing studies for transplantation. The studies showed that the fetus and her sister were compatible. The stem cells were separated from the cord blood and transplanted to the affected sister who has been free of immune and hematological manifestations of the disease for more than 3 years. HLA typing is done by DNA molecular methods using allele specific oligonucleotides and by DNA sequencing.

The application of this approach combines molecular and biochemical diagnosis, immunological typing and the use of non-affected cells for treatment of affected family members, using cells that are commonly discarded.

GENETIC PRENATAL DIAGNOSIS OF PATERNITY

All the genetic markers analyzed by molecular DNA analysis are inherited from the parents, most of them in a Mendelian fashion. This characteristic allows for the analysis of paternity *in utero*.

Paternity can be questioned *in utero* in two different situations, when the mother requests the test because she wants to know which one of her sexual partners is the father of the fetus, and when in the process of doing genetic diagnostic analysis it is found that the individual alleged to be the father cannot be the father.

Both cases are common. The latter occurs in situations such as in a family who requests to be tested for CF, because the mother has one affected brother. The molecular testing of the mother and her family shows that the mutation causing cystic fibrosis in her family is ΔF508. The mother carries the mutation, but the father does not have any of the mutations tested. The fetus is heterozygote N/G542X. This finding clearly excludes paternity for the mother's husband since he does not have the mutation G542X. This is one of the risks of molecular genetic prenatal diagnosis.

The ability of DNA molecular analysis to determine the DNA fingerprint (the analysis of the characteristics of many genes that produce a pattern exclusive to a single individual) of the fetus and of his or her parents is the most accurate method of determining paternity *in utero* (Figure 6).

CORRELATION OF GENOTYPE–PHENOTYPE AND CONSEQUENCES OF MOLECULAR FETAL DIAGNOSIS

The analysis of many genes producing human disease has shown that in many cases a particular mutation produces a very specific disease. Different mutations can produce different ages of onset, a more severe disease, or a more severe involvement of a given organ or tissue. The prenatal detection not only of the certainty of the disease, but of its characteristics, adds power to fetal molecular diagnosis by helping to have a more precise prognosis on the course and evolution of the disease. For a given family it may be acceptable to have a child who will develop Huntington disease at 30–40 years of age because he or she has 44 CAG repeats in the huntingtin gene, which is the same count in another affected member of the family, including the father, but it may not be acceptable to have a child who will develop Huntington disease in childhood because she/he has 200 CAG repeats in the huntingtin gene.

A fetus who has two mutations for cystic fibrosis, ΔF508 and R117H, will have a different disease from individuals who are homozygous for ΔF508. The former have a milder disease and

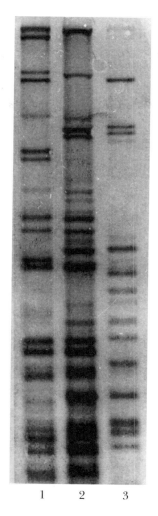

Figure 6 *A DNA fingerprint obtained by a multi-locus probe for the core sequence of the minisatellite of the human myoglobin gene. Lane 1 is the maternal DNA, lane 2 is the fetal DNA, and lane 3 is the alleged father's DNA. Note that all the fetal bands can be assigned either to the father or to the mother, indicating that the alleged father is the biological father*

congenital absence of the vas deferens (CAVD), while the latter have a very severe form of CF. Commonly, this combination of CF mutations produces CAVD in males and chronic sinusitis in females, because the R117H mutation is a class IV mutation with normal channel regulation but altered conduction properties[29].

Mutations of the dystrophin gene can produce either Duchenne or Becker muscular dystrophy. When the mutation disturbs the reading frame of the gene, it either produces an abnormal protein or does not produce the protein, causing the Duchenne type, which is a severe disease. If the mutation does not alter the reading frame allowing for the production of shorter protein, or one containing a point mutation, it causes a milder disease, Becker muscular dystrophy.

In the case of Tay–Sachs and Gaucher diseases, the type of mutation/s is correlated with the type and severity of the condition. The homozygotes for a mutation have a severe congenital form, homozygotes for another mutation have a mild adult form, and compound heterozygotes (with two different mutations) have intermediate forms in some cases.

The ability to correlate specific mutations to the manifestations and severity of the condition brings a new dimension of preciseness to genetic prenatal diagnosis.

SOURCES OF ERROR IN MOLECULAR GENETIC PRENATAL DIAGNOSIS

The knowledge and technology that we have described here is so powerful, that it can make us forget that it is another human activity and, consequently, it has all the good and bad human actions. One cannot lose sight of the fact that this technology has many reasons to have errors that may severely alter the diagnosis or that it may be missed. Special consideration should be given to these aspects when practicing genetic molecular fetal diagnosis. Molecular genetic prenatal diagnosis has several sources of error.

False family relationships

Both direct mutation and RFLP analysis can produce false results if the biological relationship of the family is not real. Some of the most common situations are false paternity, false maternity and children changed during the neonatal period, which can produce false results. If the affected child in the Duchenne muscular dystrophy example pre-sented above is not the child of that family, and he was accidentally switched at birth, the whole study is false because the mother is very probably not a carrier and the fetal haplotype apparently linked to the mutant dystrophin gene is normal. Thus, the fetus will be normal regardless of which chromosome he inherited from his mother.

Diagnostic error in the index case

If the condition affecting son 1 in Figure 4 is not DMD, but limb girdle muscular dystrophy, which is autosomal dominant or recessive depending upon the case, testing for linked markers on chromosome X will produce false results leading to a false diagnosis.

Contamination of DNA samples and other technical difficulties producing false results

Extreme care should be undertaken to prevent these and other causes of false positive and false negative results. Contamination can occur at different stages when obtaining the sample and during its processing and analysis. One needs to take account of the fact that there is human DNA almost everywhere and that if it is mixed with the sample it may change the test results. The following are a few examples.

If the amniotic fluid, fetal blood, or chorionic villus samples are contaminated with maternal blood, the test may show that the fetus is affected by a disease for which it does not have the mutation/s. A mother is a carrier for Duchenne muscular dystrophy, the fetus inherits her chromosome X with the deletion and, consequently, he will develop DMD after birth. The multiplex PCR reaction shows 14 normal bands and no evidence of the deletion. Based on this finding, the fetus is diagnosed as normal. The deletion was not discovered because the normal maternal chromosome contained in the contaminating maternal blood contributed with the needed DNA for the amplification of the involved region that is deleted in the fetus and will cause him to be affected.

Another example of contamination in the laboratory can happen when a fetus at risk for cystic fibrosis due to both parents being carriers of the ΔF508 mutation is tested by PCR. The fetal DNA shows him to be a heterozygote N/ΔF508 and is predicted to be a carrier as his parents. At birth, the child is an affected homozygote for ΔF508. The error occurred when droplets of saliva from the technologist doing the test, who is a normal homozygote introduced the normal sequence in the sample, creating a false heterozygote.

Diagnosis of the condition at risk is correct in general but not the precise type

One example would be, the family is told that they are at risk of hemophilia due to deficiency of factor 8, the fetus is tested and shows to be normal. The family was at risk of hemophilia due to a mutation in the factor IX gene, and the newborn is affected. The prevention of this problem is done by testing the affected family member, or obtaining the test results that were done by a reputable laboratory. The parent or parents (according to the specific situation) should be tested to determine if they carry the mutation/s at risk.

Testing of the wrong sample

While most laboratories are extremely careful in the handling of samples, mislabelling and exchange of samples may occur. If the sample is not the one of the fetus at risk the results will be wrong. This is particularly possible when a sample is obtained at one site, processed at another, and at times at a third site, to be finally referred to the testing laboratory. To prevent this risk, one should reduce the number of individuals involved in the processing of the sample to a minimum and one must exercise extreme caution in handling and labelling.

Other laboratory errors that have been noted in the practice of laboratory medicine can equally alter the results of DNA molecular diagnosis.

RISKS OF GENETIC MOLECULAR FETAL DIAGNOSIS

As with all other medical intervention, fetal diagnosis has specific risks. One of the more serious risks is the practice of this branch of medicine by individuals who do not have appropriate knowledge about genetic and acquired fetal disease, who do not have the appropriate training for the assessment, diagnosis and counselling in this very complex field of medicine and of human psychological, emotional, ethical, moral, legal and medical problems. The patient must be informed of the known risks including the sources of error discussed above, and of the possibility that unknown ones may endanger the quality of the diagnostic process leading to a wrong diagnosis and management.

The best preventive measure is full disclosure followed by the process of written informed consent. It should include the benefits, risks, complications and limitations of fetal diagnosis. In dealing with these issues that are frequently featured in the lay press and on radio and television, it is wise to make an extra effort to explain the limitations and causes of error, since this type of testing is commonly pictured as incredibly powerful and precise.

Prenatal diagnosis is the foundation for the application of fetal medicine. Since many of the fetal diseases are genetic, vigorous training in genetics, fetal pathology and acquired diseases of the fetus must be the minimal training of individuals doing prenatal diagnosis. The introduction of DNA molecular technology has made the field more complicated rather than simpler, calling for more specific detailed training of individuals involved in fetal diagnosis.

One of the most serious risks of fetal diagnosis is the exclusion of paternity by the diagnostic testing. It is not uncommon that the test done to diagnose a certain disease may indicate that the alleged father is not the biological father. In a case of diagnosis for Hb S, the fetus is found to be homozygous for the mutation, the mother is a proven carrier by the same test but the alleged father does not have the mutation. The biological father should have the mutation for the fetus to be homozygous for the Hb S

Table 1 *Partial list of conditions that can be tested prenatally*

Aarskog syndrome	Isovaleric acidemia
Achondroplasia	Jackson–Weiss
Achondrogenesis II/hypochondrogenesis	Kennedy syndrome
Adrenoleukodystrophy, X-linked	Lesch–Nyhan syndrome
Albinism, ocular, autosomal recessive	Machado–Joseph Disease
Albinism, oculocutaneous, brown (OCA3)	Maple syrup urine disease
Albinism, oculocutaneous, tyrosinase-negative (OCA1)	Marfan syndrome
Albinism, oculocutaneous, tyrosinase-positive (OCA2)	Medium chain Acyl-CoA dehydrogenase deficiency
Albinism, oculocutaneous, yellow	Medullary thyroid carcinoma, familial
α-1-antitrypsin deficiency	Miller–Dieker syndrome
Alport syndrome	Mitochodrial disorders
Amyloidosis, familial	Multiple endocrine neoplasia, Type 1
Amyloidosis, type I	Multiple endocrine neoplasia, Type 2 + 2A
Angelman syndrome	Multiple endocrine neoplasia, Type 2B
Aniridia	Muscular dystrophy, Duchenne/Becker
Apert Syndrome	Muscular dystrophy, Emery Dreifuss
Arachnodactyly, congenital contractural	Muscular dystrophy, Fukuyama congenital
Branchio-oto-renal syndrome	Muscular dystrophy, limb-girdle
Carbamyl phosphate synthetase deficiency	Myotonia congenita, autosomal dominant (Thomsen
Cerebro-spinal muscular atrophy type 1	disease)
Charcot–Marie–Tooth (MIM 118200)	Myotonia congenita, autosomal recessive (Becker disease)
Charcot–Marie–Tooth, X-linked neuropathy (MIM 302800)	Myotonic dystrophy
Chronic granulomatous disease, X-linked	Nail-patella syndrome
Citrullinemia	Narcolepsy
Color blindness	Nemaline rod myopathy
Congenital adrenal hyperplasia	Neurofibromatosis, Type I
Cranio-frontonasal dysplasia	Ornithine transcarbamylase deficiency
Crouzon syndrome	Osteogenesis imperfecta
Cystic fibrosis	Paramyotonia congenita
Dentatorubral and pallydolusyian atrophy	Paternity
Diabetes insipidus, nephrogenic	Pfeiffer syndrome
Diabetes mellitus, maturity onset of diabetes of the young	Phenylketonuria
Diabetes mellitus, non-insulin dependent (NIDDM)	Polycystic kidney disease, adult onset
Disorganization mutation in mice, human homologue of	Polyposis, adenomatous, intestinal
Ectrodactyly	Prader–Willi syndrome
Ehlers–Danlos syndrome, Type IV	Retinitis pigmentosa, autosomal dominant
Ehlers–Danlos syndrome, Type VII	Retinitis pigmentosa, autosomal recessive
Endocardial fibroelastosis	Retinoblastoma
Epidermolysis bullosa dystrophica	Saethre–Chotzen syndrome
Epidermolysis bullosa simplex	Schizophrenia
Epidermolytic hyperkeratosis	Sickle cell anemia/disease
Fibrosis of extraocular muscles, congenital	Smith–Magenis syndrome
Fragile X syndrome	Spastic paraplegia, X-linked
Friedreich's ataxia	Spinal muscular atrophy
Galactosemia	Spondyloepiphyseal dysplasia
Gaucher disease	Steroid sulfatase deficiency
Glucose-6-phosphate dehydrogenase deficiency	Stickler syndrome
Glycerol kinase deficiency	Tay–Sachs disease
Glycogen storage disease, Type III	Thalassemia
Glycoprotein 1A deficiency	Thalassemia, α
Hemochromatosis	Thalassemia, β
Hemoglobinopathies (A, S, C, D, E)	Thanatophoric dysplasia
Hemophilia A	Treacher–Collins syndrome
Hemophilia B	Tyrosinemia, Type I, hereditary
Hermansky–Pudlak syndrome	Usher syndrome
Hunter syndrome	Vas deferens, congenital bilateral absent
Huntington disease	von Hippel–Lindau disease
Hydrocephalus, X-linked	von Willebrand disease
Hyperkalemic periodic paralysis	Waardenburg syndrome
Hypochondroplasia	Wilms' tumor
Hypohidrotic ectodermal dysplasia, X-linked	Wilson's disease
Incontinentia pigmenti	Wiskott–Aldrich syndrome
	X-linked lymphoproliferative disease (MIM 308240)

mutation. The disclosure of this information can in many cases cause severe familial, personal and psychological complications. The best way to prevent this complication is by having comprehensive genetic counselling prior to the DNA testing disclosing to the mother that the test may exclude that the individual she is presenting as the father is not the biological father. The patients must be informed about this risk before consenting to be tested as part of the process of full disclosure needed to protect patients' rights.

Table 1 shows an incomplete list of conditions that can be tested prenatally by DNA analysis. The list of diseases that can be tested changes from day to day due to the incredibly fast analysis of the human genome.

CONCLUSION

Fetal molecular diagnosis has developed in the last 30 years from a very limited practice of fetal medicine, to a broader and more complex discipline. It has been the foundation of the analysis of fetal disease. Initially used to diagnose malformations associated with high levels of α-fetoprotein and chromosomal abnormalities, it has progressed to include ultrasonography and lately DNA molecular diagnostic analysis. In this chapter, we have reviewed a few diseases as examples of many others that can be similarly diagnosed and many more that will be diagnosable in the future. But the most important aspect of this analysis is the need for properly trained individuals to properly use this amazingly powerful technology.

ACKNOWLEDGEMENTS

We would like to acknowledge Mrs Colleen Townsend MT ASCP and Mrs Michelle Luhm MT ASCP, for their contribution to fetal molecular genetic testing, and Mr Mark Woodford for his help in preparing this manuscript and the photographic work.

References

1. Welsh, M. J., Tsui, L. C., Boat, T. F. and Beaudet, A. L. (1995). Cystic fibrosis. In Scriver, C. R., Beaudet, A. L., Sly, W. S. and Valle, D. (eds.) *The Metabolic and Molecular Bases of Inherited Disease*, p. 3851. (New York: McGraw-Hill)
2. Mladinov, G. and Krzisnik, Z. (1977). Achondroplasia revealed by ultrasound *in utero. Jugosl. Ginekol. Opstet.*, **17**, 239–41
3. Elejalde, B. R., de Elejalde, M. M., Hamilton, P. R. and Lombardi, J. M. (1983). Prenatal diagnosis in two pregnancies of an achondroplastic woman. *Am. J. Med. Genet.*, **15**, 437–9
4. Kurtz, A. B., Filly, R. A. and Wapner, R. J. (1986). *In utero* analysis of heterozygous achondroplasia: variable time of onset as detected by femur length measurements. *J. Ultrasound Med.*, **5**, 137–45
5. Elejalde, B. R. and de Elejalde, M. M. (1985). Thanatophoric dysplasia with cloverleaf skull: fetal manifestations and prenatal diagnosis. *Am. J. Med. Genet.*, **22**, 669–83
6. Shiang, R., Thompson, L. M., Ya-Zhen, Z., Church, D. M., Fileder, T. J., Bocian, M., Winokur, S. T. and Wasmuth, J. J. (1994). Mutations in the transmembrane domain of the FGFR3 cause the most common genetic form of dwarfism, achondroplasia. *Cell*, **78**, 335–42
7. Tavormina, P. L., Shiang, R., Thompson, L. M., Zhu, Y. Z., Wilkin, D. J., Lachman, R. S., Wilcox, W. R., Rimoin, D. L., Cohn, D. H. and Wasmuth, J. J. (1995). Thanatophoric dysplasia (types I and II) caused by distinct mutations in fibroblast growth factor receptor 3. *Nature Genet.*, **9**, 321–8
8. Bellus, G. A., McInstosh, I., Smith, E. A., Aylsworth, A. S., Kaitila, I., Horton, W. A., Greenhaw, G. A., Hecht, J. T. and Francomano, C. (1995). A recurrent mutation in the tyrosine kinase domain of fibroblast growth factor receptor 3 causes hypochondroplasia. *Nature Genet.*, **10**, 357–9
9. Wilkie, A. O. M., Slaney, S. F., Oldridge, M., Poole, M. D., Ashworth, G. J., Hockley, A. D., Hayword, R. D., David, D. J., Pulleyn, L. J., Rutland, P., Malcolm, S., Winter, R. M. and Reardon, W. (1995). Apert syndrome results from localized mutations of FGFR2 and are allelic with Crouzon syndrome. *Nature Genet.*, **9**, 165–72

10. Reardon, W., Winter, R. M., Pulleyn, L. J., Jones, B. M. and Malcolm, S. (1994). Mutations in the fibroblast growth factor 2 gene cause Crouzon syndrome. *Nature Genet.*, **8**, 98–103

11. Lajeunie, E., Ma, H. W., Bonaventure, J., Munnich, A. and Merrer, M. L. (1995). FGFR2 Mutation in Pfeiffer syndrome. *Nature Genet.*, **9**, 108

12. Jabs, E. W., Li, X., Scott, A. F., Meyers, G., Chen, W., Eccles, M., Mao, J., Charnas, L. R., Jackson, C. E. and Jaye, M. (1994). Jackson–Weiss and Crouzon syndromes are allelic with mutations in fibroblast growth factor receptor 2. *Nature Genet.*, **8**, 275–9

13. Donohoue, P. A., Parker, K. and Migeon, C. (1995). Congenital adrenal hyperplasia. In Scriver, C. R., Beaudet, A. L., Sly, W. S. and Valle, D. (eds.) *The Metabolic and Molecular Bases of Inherited Disease*, p. 2929–61. (New York: McGraw-Hill)

14. Chang, J. C. and Kahn, Y. W. (1982). A sensitive new prenatal test for sickle cell anemia. *N. Engl. J. Med.*, **307**, 30–32

15. Congress of the United States, Office of Technology Assessment (1994). *Cystic Fibrosis and DNA tests: Implications of Carrier Screening*, p. 247–53. (Washington: US Government Printing Office)

16. Welsh, M. J., Tsui, L. C., Boat, T. F. and Beaudet, A. L. (1995). Cystic fibrosis. In Scriver, C. R., Beaudet, A. L., Sly, W. S. and Valle, D. (eds.) *The Metabolic and Molecular Bases of Inherited Disease*, p. 3850. (New York: McGraw-Hill)

17. Congress of the United States, Office of Technology Assessment (1994). *Cystic Fibrosis and DNA tests: Implications of Carrier Screening*, p. 5. (Washington: US Government Printing Office)

18. Kunkel, L. M., Monaco, A. P., Middlesworth, W., Ochs, H. D. and Latt, S. A. (1985). Specific cloning of DNA fragments absent from the DNA of a male patient with an X chromosome deletion. *Proc. Natl. Acad. Sci. USA*, **82**, 4778–82

19. Koenig, M., Hoffman, E. P., Berterlson, C. J., Monaco, A. P., Feener, C. and Kunkel, L. M. (1987). Complete cloning of the Duchenne muscular dystrophy (DMD) cDNA and preliminary organization of the DMD gene in normal and affected individuals. *Cell*, **50**, 509–15

20. Hu, X. Y., Ray, P. N., Murphy, E. G., Thompson, M. W. and Worton, R. G. (1990). Duplicational mutation at the Duchenne muscular dystrophy locus: its frequency, distribution, origin and phenotype-genotype correlation. *Am. J. Hum. Genet.*, **46**, 682–99

21. Chamberlain, J. S., Gibbs, R. A., Ranier, J. E., Nguyen, P. N. and Caskey, C. T. (1988). Deletion screening of the Duchenne muscular dystrophy locus via multiplex DNA amplification. *Nucleic Acid Res.*, **16**, 11141–50

22. Beggs, A. H., Koenig, M., Boyce, F. M. and Kunkel, L. M. (1990). Detection of 98% of DMD/BMD gene deletions by polymerase chain reaction. *Hum. Genet.*, **86**, 45–51

23. Prior, T. W., Bartolo, C., Pearl, D. K., Papp, A. C., Snyder, P. J., Sedra, M. S., Burghes, A. H. M. and Mendel, J. R. (1995). Spectrum of small mutations in the dystrophin coding region. *Am. J. Hum. Genet.*, **57**, 22–33

24. Huntington Disease Collaborative Research Group (1993). A novel gene containing a trinucleotide repeat that is expanded and unstable on Huntington's disease chromosomes. *Cell*, **72**, 971–93

25. Goldstein, J. L., Hobbs, H. H. and Brown, M. S. (1995). Familial hypercholesterolemia. In Scriver, C. R., Beaudet, A. L., Sly, W. S. and Valle, D. (eds.) *The Metabolic and Molecular Bases of Inherited Disease*, p. 1997–2000. (New York: McGraw-Hill)

26. Salimans, M. M. M. (1989). Detection of parvovirus B19 DNA in fetal tissues by *in situ* hybridization and polymerase chain reaction. *J. Clin. Path.*, **42**, 525–30

27. Nocera, D. (1990). Characterization by DNA restriction endonuclease analysis of listeria monocytogenes strains related to the Swiss epidemic of listeriosis. *J. Clin. Microbiol.*, **28**, 2259–63

28. Bernstam, V. A. (1992). *Handbook of Gene Level Diagnosis in Clinical Practice*, p. 509–48. (Boca Raton: CRC Press)

29. Welsh, M. J., Tsui, L. C., Boat, T. F. and Beaudet, A. L. (1995). Cystic fibrosis. In Scriver, C. R., Beaudet, A. L., Sly, W. S. and Valle, D. (eds.) *The Metabolic and Molecular Bases of Inherited Disease*, p. 3846. (New York: McGraw-Hill)

Fetal echocardiography in the late first trimester of pregnancy

11

I. A. L. Groenenberg, J. M. G. van Vugt and H. P. van Geijn

INTRODUCTION

In 1980 the first reports were published on two-dimensional real-time echography of the fetal heart[1-3]. Technical advances in two-dimensional echocardiography as well as the introduction of pulsed wave Doppler echocardiography, color flow imaging techniques and color-coded M-mode Doppler echocardiography have led to major improvements in the diagnostic capabilities of ultrasound.

To date, there is still debate on the efficacy of routine ultrasound screening for congenital heart disease in the second trimester[4-10]. However, the sensitivity in detecting cardiac malformations for extended echocardiography in specialized referral centers reaches 78–86%[6,7]. Because of the clinical significance of congenital heart disease, a mid-trimester in-depth cardiac scan offering detailed assessment of the fetal heart is recommended in high-risk pregnancies.

The introduction of the high-frequency, high-resolution transvaginal transducers enables early detection of structural anomalies. Gembruch and colleagues[11] reported the diagnosis of a complete atrioventricular canal defect and complete heart block as early as 11 weeks of gestation. Assessment of the fetal cardiac anatomy and fetal cardiovascular performance under both normal and pathological circumstances has been performed in the late first trimester with a combination of two-dimensional transvaginal, Doppler and color Doppler techniques.

This chapter presents an overview on normal heart development and ultrasonic heart anatomy in the late first trimester and early second trimester of pregnancy. Aspects of fetal cardiovascular performance are discussed using Doppler ultrasonography. In addition, attention is focused on the role of early transvaginal sonography in the assessment of fetal congenital heart disease.

SONOEMBRYOLOGY

The cardiovascular system is the first system to function in the embryo, with blood beginning to circulate in the 22nd day after conception[12]. Development of the heart starts with the aggregation of splanchnic mesenchymal cells ventral to the pericardial celom to form a pair of elongated strands called cardiogenic cords at 18 or 19 days. Canalization and fusion of the cardiogenic cords takes place at 20–21 days. By day 22 ($\pm$ 1 day) a single heart tube has formed. At this time cardiac activity begins. The contractions of the heart tube result in a unidirectional flow by the end of the 4th week[12].

The 22nd day after conception corresponds to 36 menstrual days, or a crown–rump length (CRL) of 1.5–3 mm. High-frequency transvaginal ultrasonography enables visualization of the embryonic pole when it measures about 2–3 mm[13]. The earliest detection of fetal heart beats by transvaginal ultrasound is at 5 weeks and 4 days[14]. Fetal heart activity can be quantitated in the 3-mm embryo when two-dimensional transvaginal ultrasonography is combined with pulsed Doppler[15]. There is a progressive rise in fetal heart rate from a mean of 110 bpm at 3 mm CRL to a mean of 170 bpm at 15 mm CRL. When the CRL is about 5 mm (6–6.5 weeks menstrual age), cardiac pulsations should be clearly seen if the embryo is alive[13,14].

Formation of the heart is completed by the end of the 8th week. As the heart tube grows, it bends upon itself to the right. Partitioning into four chambers of the thus-formed atrioventricular canal begins in the 4th week and is completed by the 7th week. In this period the truncus arteriosus is divided into the aorta and pulmonary trunk. During weeks 6–8, the primitive aortic arch pattern is transformed into the basic adult arterial arrangement[12].

The sequence of events resulting in the formation of the heart is a complex process and therefore, congenital malformations are relatively common. One study[16] on cardiac malformations in spontaneously aborted fetuses reported an overall incidence of 15.4% with the incidence of cardiac malformations in fetuses less than 25 mm being as high as 68%. No information was given on the incidence of chromosomal abnormalities, which are responsible for a significant proportion of cardiac malformations.

Whereas first-trimester transvaginal ultrasonography allows the visualization of developmental changes of extracardiac organs such as those of the central nervous system, a detailed developmental survey of the heart is beyond the performance of high-resolution transvaginal probes. Only several weeks after major embryological development of cardiac structure is completed, is detailed assessment of full cardiac anatomy possible, as is described below.

VISUALIZATION OF NORMAL CARDIAC ANATOMY

Several reports have been published on normal fetal cardiac anatomy and cardiac dimensions in the first trimester[14,17–23]. D'Amelio and colleagues[17] compared the resolution of transabdominal vs. transvaginal probes in assessing cardiac morphology. The transvaginal probe provided the highest resolution between the 11th and 14th weeks. It is noteworthy that nearly similar results were obtained for M-mode recording as compared to two-dimensional real-time echocardiography in visualizing the cardiac chambers[14]. The movement of the

interventricular septum can be seen as early as 9 weeks of gestation on M-mode recordings.

Cardiac dimensions showed a linear increase with gestational age between 11 and 17 weeks of gestation, as determined by two-dimensional real-time transvaginal echocardiography[18]. The structures measured were the total transverse diameter of the heart, the inner diameters of the right and left ventricles and the aorta root dimension. In the 12th week of gestation, when the transverse diameter of the heart is about 5 mm, the four-chamber view can be visualized by transvaginal ultrasound in the majority of fetuses[19] (Figure 1).

Dolkart and Reimers[19] provided normative data on detailed cardiac anatomy between 10 and 14 weeks of gestation, using a 7.5 MHz transvaginal probe. The earliest cardiac structures visible in the first trimester were the mitral and tricuspid valves. In 25% of cases each atrioventricular valve was individually discernible by 10 weeks of gestation. By week 12, the complete four-chamber view could be visualized in 90% of cases. The aorta in short axis, the pulmonary trunk and the long parasagittal left ventricular view could be visualized in 70%, 40% and 40% of cases, respectively. At 13 and 14 weeks of gestation, the four-chamber view was successfully obtained in 100% of cases, whereas the origin and crossing of the aorta and pulmonary

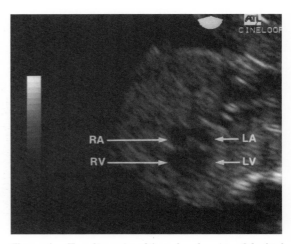

Figure 1 *Two-dimensional four-chamber view of the fetal heart at 13 weeks. LA, left atrium; LV, left ventricle; RA, right atrium; RV, right.ventricle*

trunk was demonstrated in approximately 40% of cases (Figures 1 and 2).

Johnson and colleagues[20] visualized the four-chamber view in over 70% of cases at 13 and 14 weeks of gestation, using a 5-MHz transvaginal probe. Identification and origin of the great arteries was possible in 43% and 46% of cases, respectively. A maximum of 10 min of scanning time per patient was allowed.

Gembruch and colleagues[21] reported a success rate of 100% in obtaining full cardiac anatomy using color Doppler flow imaging in addition to two-dimensional ultrasound (Color plates 21 and 22). The four-chamber view, origin and crossing of the great vessels was always demonstrated at 13 and 14 weeks of gestation. It was suggested that the combined use of two-dimensional echocardiography and color Doppler flow imaging resulted in an increased success rate in identifying the great arteries. These two techniques complement each other, because the most favorable insonation angle for B-mode ultrasound is 90° and for Doppler methods 0° or 180°[22]. Similar results were obtained by Achiron and colleagues[23]. Extended fetal echocardiography was completed in 98% of cases between 13 and 15 weeks' gestation, with the use of 6.5 and 7.5-MHz transvaginal probes.

These studies demonstrate that, in expert hands, detailed examination of full cardiac anatomy can be successfully performed from 12 weeks' gestation, when high-frequency transvaginal probes are used.

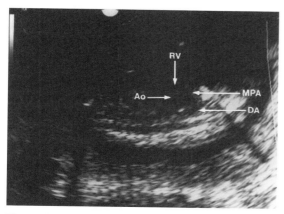

Figure 2 *Short-axis view of the fetal heart parallel to the fetal spine at 13 weeks, showing the main pulmonary artery (MPA) and ductus arteriosus (DA). Ao, ascending aorta; RV, right ventricle*

CARDIOVASCULAR HEMODYNAMICS AND DOPPLER ULTRASOUND

Doppler measurements have been performed to assess cardiovascular performance in the late first trimester of pregnancy. The fetal heart rate decreased significantly from 170–180 bpm at 11 weeks to 140–150 bpm at 16 weeks' gestation[24]. This has been associated with maturation of the parasympathetic system[25].

At atrioventricular level, there is a marked rise in peak E-wave velocities (early ventricular filling), whereas peak A-wave velocities (atrial contraction) do not change significantly between 11 and 16 weeks' gestation[26]. As a result, E/A ratios, representing ventricular diastolic function, increase with advancing gestational age from approximately 0.5 at 11–12 weeks to values ranging between 0.8 and 0.9 in late pregnancy[26–28] (Figure 3). At the same time, there is a marked decrease in the percentage of retrograde flow in the inferior vena cava during this period[24]. The increase in peak E-wave velocity and E/A ratio suggests a shift of blood flow from late towards early diastole, which may result from increased ventricular compliance and/or a raised ventricular relaxation rate or a reduced afterload with advancing gestational age[29]. Tulzer and colleagues[30] found that the proportion of ventricular filling as a contribution of

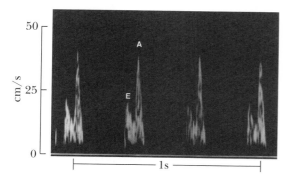

Figure 3 *Doppler flow velocity waveform tracing from the tricuspid valve at 12 weeks. E, E-wave (early diastolic filling); A, A-wave (atrial contraction)*

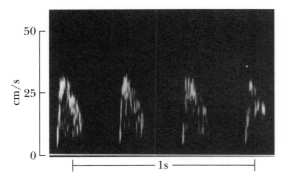

Figure 4 *Doppler flow velocity waveform tracing from the pulmonary artery at 14 weeks*

atrial contraction remained constant, indicating unchanged ventricular compliance or constant diastolic function, despite the significant increase in E/A ratio from 14 weeks' gestation until term. Moreover, the isovolemic relaxation time corrected for the decrease in fetal heart rate during gestation remained unchanged. Therefore, it was suggested that an increasing atrioventricular pressure gradient with increasing blood flow in the growing heart is responsible for the increase in E-wave velocities with unchanged isovolemic relaxation time.

At cardiac outflow tract level, flow velocity waveforms have been obtained from the ascending aorta and pulmonary artery as early as 11 weeks' gestation[26,28,29] (Figure 4). Peak systolic velocities in both cardiac vessels increase with advancing gestational age, with velocities in the ascending aorta being higher than those in the pulmonary artery. Documented peak systolic velocities at outflow tract level are in the same range, with values of approximately 30 cm/s at the end of the first trimester of pregnancy[26,28,31]. Peak systolic values in the ductus arteriosus also depict an increase with gestational age[32]. The gestational age-related changes in peak systolic velocities in the ascending aorta and pulmonary artery may be accounted for by increased volume flow through the semilunar valves, raised contractility, or reduced afterload[33]. Age-related reduction in afterload may occur in the human fetus as a result of the decrease in placental vascular resistance[34,35]. The appearance of end-diastolic velocities in the umbilical and descending aorta after 12 weeks' gestation

suggest a drop in fetal placental vascular resistance[24,28,36–38]. This coincides with secondary trophoblast invasion of the spiral arteries during the early second trimester of pregnancy, resulting in low-resistance uteroplacental vessels[39].

Products of time velocity integrals and fetal heart rate may reflect volume flow. At atrioventricular and outflow tract level, these values show an increase with advancing gestational age, suggesting an increase in cardiac output[28]. Documented mean, peak E-wave and A-wave velocities at tricuspid valve level are higher than those at mitral valve level. Since volume flow is equal to mean velocity multiplied by vessel area, the higher transtricuspid mean velocities may reflect the presence of *in utero* right heart dominance at the end of the first trimester[40].

The above-mentioned studies demonstrate significant changes in cardiovascular hemodynamics in the first half of pregnancy, as determined by Doppler ultrasound. However, interpretation of Doppler data is hampered by the lack of data on blood pressure and venous and arterial volume flow in the late first trimester.

DIAGNOSIS OF CARDIAC MALFORMATIONS

An increasing number of cardiac malformations have been detected in the late first trimester of pregnancy by transvaginal ultrasonography[11,41,42]. The first report, on a case of non-immune hydrops fetalis, complete atrioventricular canal defect, insufficiency of the atrioventricular valves and a complete heart block diagnosed by transvaginal two-dimensional ultrasound and Doppler echocardiography at 11 weeks' gestation, originated from Gembruch and colleagues[11].

Cardiac malformations in the first trimester tend to be more severe and complex than those detected later in pregnancy[21,22,42–44]. In the first trimester the presence of fluid accumulation is often associated with congenital heart disease. It was suggested that hemodynamic disturbances such as accumulation of fluid in the nuchal region, ascites and pleural–pericardial effusion in the 11- and 12-week-old fetus are the result of the severity of cardiac disease in this early stage of pregnancy[44].

Cardiac malformations are commonly associated with structural anomalies of other organ systems and/or chromosomal abnormalities. In the second trimester the incidence of associated chromosomal abnormalities has been estimated to be as high as 16–32%[7,45,46]. The high incidence of chromosomal abnormalities (65%) reported in one study[22] on first- and early second-trimester echocardiography may be explained by referral criteria. The reason for referral was the presence of a nuchal translucency or the presence of ascites or fluid accumulation elsewhere in the fetus. First-trimester nuchal translucency of 3 mm or more is strongly associated with a chromosomal anomaly of the fetus, in particular trisomy 21[47–49]. One large study[43] on early second-trimester fetal echocardiography in a mainly low-risk population reported a rate of associated chromosomal anomaly of 36% in fetuses with congenital heart disease. The prevalence of congenital heart disease in this study was 0.36%. This is in accordance with the reported prevalence varying between three and ten per 1000 live births[4,50,51].

The overall results of early extensive fetal echocardiography appear to be promising. Several screening studies[20–23,43,52] have been performed to assess the potential of transvaginal echocardiography in the detection of congenital heart disease in the late first trimester and/or early second trimester. Most of the early-diagnosed cardiac malformations reported by these studies were severe, including single ventricle, hypoplastic left heart, complete atrioventricular canal, double outlet right ventricle, and coarctation of the aorta (Color plates 23 and 24).

Bronshtein and colleagues[43] performed extended transvaginal fetal echocardiography in a mixed population of 12 793 patients at 12–16 weeks' gestation. In 24 of the 47 cardiac malformations, the diagnosis was confirmed on postmortem examination or after birth. Nine out of 24 detected cardiac abnormalities were correctly diagnosed. In three cases, postmortem examination revealed a completely different, although severe, cardiac malformation. Slightly different results were obtained for the remaining 12 cases. Cardiac malformations were often diagnosed in combination with extracardiac anomalies (62%). The sensitivity for detection of fetal congenital heart disease was 77%, whereas the sensitivity for isolated congenital heart defects was 55%. There were three cases of a false-positive diagnosis: one case of hypoplastic left heart syndrome, one case of tetralogy of Fallot and one case of a small left ventricle. Ten cases of isolated ventricular septal defect, four cases of mild pulmonary stenosis and one case of an interrupted arch were missed.

Achiron and colleagues[23] conducted a pilot study of early fetal heart assessment by transvaginal ultrasonography in 660 low-risk patients at 13–15 weeks' gestation. Three cases of major cardiac malformation were diagnosed: one case of persistent truncus arteriosus, one case of tetralogy of Fallot and one case of aortic atresia, detected at 13, 14 and 15 weeks' gestation, respectively. Twice, a small ventricular septal defect was missed. At 34 weeks' gestation, one case of multiple rhabdomyoma was detected after referral because of fetal arrhythmia.

Gembruch and colleagues[21,22] reported fetal echocardiography in 309 fetuses, with 81 fetuses being referred because of extracardiac anomalies found at routine scanning. Two-dimensional transvaginal ultrasound in combination with color Doppler and pulsed wave Doppler techniques was used to evaluate the fetal heart. Twenty-two cases of cardiac malformations were diagnosed, the greater number being detected between 11 and 14 weeks. The combined use of ultrasound techniques resulted in the first-trimester diagnosis of six cases of atrioventricular valve regurgitation. In four out of 22 cases, an atrioventricular block was demonstrated. Two cases of ventricular septal defect and one case of atrial septal defect II were missed. A delayed diagnosis of complete atrioventricular canal and double outlet ventricle was made at 20 weeks, with the heart appearing normal at 12 weeks' gestation. In several cases the main cardiac malformation was correctly diagnosed, but additional cardiovascular anomalies were overlooked. It was concluded that early transvaginal echocardiography should be restricted to the high-risk fetus.

Yagel and colleagues[52] evaluated the effectiveness of an early second-trimester scan as compared to a mid-trimester scan for detection of congenital anomalies in high-risk pregnancies. It was strongly recommended that early transvaginal ultrasonography should be followed by a mid-trimester scan, as a significant number of congenital anomalies were not detected by early second-trimester ultrasonography. Both Gembruch and Johnson support this point of view. Of the 16 cases of cardiac malformations, 11 cases were detected by the first scan, whereas one case of tetralogy of Fallot and one case of total anomalous pulmonary venous drainage were detected by the second scan. One case of moderate pulmonary stenosis and two cases of a mild ventricular septal defect were missed.

According to one report by Johnson and colleagues[20] it was not possible to make a firm diagnosis at the time of the initial early scan in all three cases of congenital heart disease; the diagnosis was not confirmed until 18 weeks. Early transvaginal echocardiography was not recommended for routine screening for congenital heart disease. In contrast, Bronshtein and colleagues[43] considered extended transvaginal echocardiography to be a valuable tool in both high-risk and low-risk patients. In their study, the majority of cardiac malformations were diagnosed in the low-risk group. This was also supported by the study of Achiron and colleagues[23].

With regard to the accuracy of early transvaginal echocardiography, the above-mentioned studies clearly demonstrate that the accuracy is less compared to that of a mid-trimester scan. Diagnostic accuracy of early transvaginal echocardiography is determined by several factors. Gembruch and colleagues[21] enumerated these: limitation of imaging planes, spatial orientation, limited resolution relative to the small size of the heart, relatively low spatial resolution of Doppler techniques and later manifestation of structural and functional changes in some congenital heart diseases. Also, the technique of transvaginal echocardiography requires considerable experience[23]. Early fetal echocardiography may not detect left and right ventricular outflow tract lesions, including coarctation, aortic stenosis, hypoplastic left heart and pulmonary atresia or stenosis[21,23,53]. These forms of congenital heart disease progress *in utero*, since a normal flow pattern is essential for the normal growth and development of the fetal heart[54]. Consequently, some cardiac anomalies may not become apparent until the second or third trimester[52,55–57]. This also accounts for endocardial fibroelastosis[21]. This is a major limitation of early fetal echocardiography. Due to the above-mentioned limitations of early fetal echocardiography, a second mid-trimester scan is strongly recommended in high-risk patients[20,21,23,52,58].

There are advantages to early diagnosis of congenital heart disease. There is less time pressure while awaiting the results of fetal karyotyping. Also, termination of pregnancy can be performed at an earlier stage of pregnancy. For high-risk patients, early exclusion of some major cardiac malformations may relieve anxiety.

CONCLUSION

Many severe cardiac malformations are detected by early transvaginal extended echocardiography from 11 weeks' gestation. However, highly skilled sonographers are a prerequisite for obtaining an acceptable level of detection of cardiac malformations. To date, only patients who have an increased risk for a cardiac malformation in their offspring should be offered early transvaginal echocardiographic examination. A follow-up mid-trimester scan is recommended. The early results of this technique, although promising, do not justify routine early screening of the population. Further studies are needed to evaluate the efficacy of this technique.

References

1. Allan, L. D., Tynan, M. J., Campbell, S., Wilkinson, J. L. and Anderson, R. H. (1980). Echocardiographic and anatomical correlates in fetal congenital heart disease. *Br. Heart J.*, **44**, 444–51
2. Kleinman, C. S., Hobbins, J. C., Jaffe, C. C., Lynch, D. C. and Talner, N. S. (1980). Echocardiographic studies of the human fetus, prenatal diagnosis of congenital heart disease and cardiac dysrhythmias. *Pediatrics*, **65**, 1059–67
3. Sahn, D. J., Lange, L. W., Allen, H. D., Goldberg, S. J., Anderson, C., Giles, H. and Haber, K. (1980). Quantitative real-time cross-sectional echocardiography in the developing normal human fetus and newborn. *Circulation*, **62**, 588–97
4. Allan, L. D., Crawford, D. C., Chita, S. K. and Tynan, M. J. (1986). Prenatal screening for congenital heart disease. *Br. Med. J.*, **292**, 1717–19
5. Sharland, G. K. and Allan, L. D. (1992). Screening for congenital heart disease prenatally. Results of a 2 1/2-year study in the South East Thames region. *Br. J. Obstet. Gynaecol.*, **99**, 220–5
6. Achiron, R., Glaser, J., Gelernter, I., Hegesh, J. and Yagel, S. (1992). Extended fetal echocardiographic examination for detecting cardiac malformations in low risk pregnancies. *Br. Med. J.*, **304**, 671–4
7. Bromley, B., Estroff, J. A., Sanders, S., Parad, R., Roberts, D., Frigoletto, F. D. Jr and Benacerraf, B. R. (1992). Fetal echocardiography: accuracy and limitations in a population at high and low risk for heart defects. *Am. J. Obstet. Gynecol.*, **166**, 1473–81
8. Crane, J. P., LeFevre, M. L., Winborn, R. C., Evans, J. K., Ewigman, B. G., Bain, R. P., Frigoletto, F. D. and McNellis, D. (1994). A randomized trial of prenatal ultrasonographic screening: impact on the detection, management, and outcome of anomalous fetuses. *Am. J. Obstet. Gynecol.*, **171**, 392–9
9. Ott, W. (1995). The accuracy of antenatal fetal echocardiography screening in high- and low-risk patients. *Am. J. Obstet. Gynecol.*, **172**, 1741–9
10. Stoll, C., Alembik, Y., Dott, B., Roth, P. M. and De Geeter, B. (1993). Evaluation of prenatal diagnosis of congenital heart disease. *Prenat. Diagn.*, **13**, 453–61
11. Gembruch, U., Knöpfle, G., Chatterjee, M., Bald, R. and Hansmann, M. (1990). First-trimester diagnosis of fetal congenital heart disease by transvaginal two-dimensional and Doppler echocardiography. *Obstet. Gynecol.*, **75**, 469–79
12. Moore, K. L. (1982). *The Developing Human*, 2nd edn, pp. 259–300. (New York: WB Saunders)
13. Levi, C. S., Lyons, E. A., Zheng, X. H., Lindsay, D. J. and Holt, S. C. (1990). Endovaginal US: demonstration of cardiac activity in embryos of less than 5.0 mm in crown–rump length. *Radiology*, **176**, 71–4
14. Timor-Tritsch, I. E., Peisner, D. B. and Raju, S. (1990). Sonoembryology: an organ oriented approach using a high-frequency vaginal probe. *J. Clin. Ultrasound*, **18**, 286–98
15. Achiron, R., Tadmor, O. and Mashiach, S. (1991). Heart rate as a predictor of first-trimester spontaneous abortion after ultrasound-proven viability. *Obstet. Gynecol.*, **78**, 330–3
16. Gerlis, L. M. (1985). Cardiac malformations in spontaneous abortions. *Int. J. Cardiol.*, **7**, 29–43
17. D'Amelio, R., Giorlandino, G., Masala, L., Garofalo, M., Martinelli, M., Anelli, G. and Zichella, L. (1991). Fetal echocardiography using transvaginal and transabdominal probes during the first period of pregnancy: a comparative study. *Prenat. Diagn.*, **11**, 69–75
18. Bronshtein, M., Siegler, E., Eshcoli, Z. and Zimmer, E. Z. (1992). Transvaginal ultrasound measurements of the fetal heart at 11 to 17 weeks of gestation. *Am. J. Perinatol.*, **9**, 38–42
19. Dolkart, L. A. and Reimers, F. T. (1991). Transvaginal fetal echocardiography in early pregnancy: normative data. *Am. J. Obstet. Gynecol.*, **165**, 688–91
20. Johnson, P., Sharland, G., Maxwell, D. and Allan, L. (1992). The role of transvaginal sonography in the early detection of congenital heart disease. *Ultrasound Obstet. Gynecol.*, **2**, 248–51
21. Gembruch, U., Knöpfle, G., Bald, R. and Hansmann, M. (1993). Early diagnosis of fetal congenital heart disease by transvaginal echocardiography. *Ultrasound Obstet. Gynecol.*, **3**, 310–17
22. Gembruch, U., Knöpfle, G. and Lettau, R. (1994). Diagnosis of fetal heart disease in early pregnancy by transvaginal echocardiography. *Ultrasonoor Bull.*, jaargang 22, Special issue 3, pp. 13–18
23. Achiron, R., Weissman, A., Rotstein, Z., Lipitz, S., Mashiach, S. and Hegesh, J. (1994). Transvaginal echocardiographic examination of the fetal heart between 13 and 15 weeks' gestation in a low-risk population. *J. Ultrasound Med.*, **13**, 783–9
24. Wladimiroff, J. W., Huisman, T. W. A., Stewart, P. A. and Stijnen, T. (1992). Normal fetal Doppler vena cava, transtricuspid and umbilical artery flow velocity waveforms between 11 and 16 weeks' gestation. *Am. J. Obstet. Gynecol.*, **166**, 921–4

25. Wladimiroff, J. W. and Seelen, J. C. (1972). Doppler tachometry in early pregnancy. Development of fetal vagal function. *Eur. J. Obstet. Gynaecol. Reprod. Biol.*, **2**, 55–63

26. Wladimiroff, J. W., Huisman, T. W. A. and Stewart, P. A. (1991). Cardiac Doppler flow velocities in the late first trimester fetus; a transvaginal Doppler study. *J. Am. Coll. Cardiol.*, **17**, 1357–9

27. van der Mooren, K., Barendregt, L. G. and Wladimiroff, J. W. (1991). Fetal atrioventricular and outflow tract flow velocity waveforms during the normal second half of pregnancy. *Am. J. Obstet. Gynecol.*, **165**, 668–74

28. Rizzo, G., Arduini, D. and Romanini, C. (1991). Fetal cardiac and extra cardiac circulation in early gestation. *J. Matern. Fetal Invest.*, **1**, 73–8

29. Wladimiroff, J. W., Stewart, P. A., Burghouwt, M. T. and Stijnen, T. (1992). Normal fetal cardiac flow velocity waveforms between 11 and 16 weeks' gestation. *Am. J. Obstet. Gynecol.*, **167**, 736–9

30. Tulzer, G., Khowsathit, P., Gudmundsson, S., Wood, D. C., Tian, Z., Schmitt, K. and Huhta, J. C. (1994). Diastolic function of the fetal heart during second and third trimester: a prospective longitudinal Doppler-echocardiography study. *Eur. J. Pediatr.*, **153**, 151–4

31. Sharkey, A., Tulzer, G. and Huhta, J. (1991). Doppler blood flow velocities in the first trimester of pregnancy (Abstr. 312). *Am. J. Obstet. Gynecol.*, **164**, 331

32. Brezinka, C., Huisman, T. W. A., Stijnen, T. and Wladimiroff, J. W. (1992). Flow velocity waveforms in the fetal ductus arteriosus in the first half of pregnancy. *Ultrasound Obstet. Gynecol.*, **2**, 397–401

33. Groenenberg, I. A. L., Stijnen, T. and Wladimiroff, J. W. (1990). Flow velocity waveforms in the fetal cardiac outflow tract as a measure of fetal well-being in intrauterine growth retardation. *Pediatr. Res.*, **27**, 379–82

34. Griffin, D. R., Bilardo, K., Masini, L., Diaz-Recasens, J., Pearce, J. M., Willson, K. and Campbell, S. (1984). Doppler blood flow waveforms in the descending aorta of the human fetus. *Br. J. Obstet. Gynaecol.*, **91**, 997–1006

35. Trudinger, B. J., Giles, W. B. and Cook, C. M. (1985). Flow velocity waveforms in the maternal uteroplacental and fetal umbilical placental circulation. *Am. J. Obstet. Gynecol.*, **152**, 155–63

36. Loquet, P., Broughton Pipkin, F., Symonds, E. M. and Rubin, P. C. (1988). Blood velocity waveforms and placental vascular formation (letter). *Lancet*, **2**, 1252–3

37. Wladimiroff, J. W., Huisman, T. W. A. and Stewart, P. A. (1992). Intracerebral, aortic and umbilical artery flow velocity waveforms in the late first trimester fetus. *Am. J. Obstet. Gynecol.*, **166**, 46–9

38. Van Zalen-Sprock, M. M., van Vugt, J. M. G. and van Geijn, H. P. (1994). First-trimester uteroplacental and fetal blood flow velocity waveforms in normally developing fetuses: a longitudinal study. *Ultrasound Obstet. Gynecol.*, **4**, 284–8

39. Pijnenburg, R., Dixon, G., Robertson, W. B. and Brosens, I. (1980). Trophoblastic invasion of human decidua from 8 to 18 weeks of pregnancy. *Placenta*, **1**, 3–19

40. Huisman, T. W. A., Stewart, P. A. and Wladimiroff, J. W. (1992). Doppler assessment of the normal early fetal circulation. *Ultrasound Obstet. Gynecol.*, **2**, 300–5

41. Bronshtein, M., Siegler, E., Yoffe, N. and Zimmer, E. Z. (1990). Prenatal diagnosis of ventricular septal defect and overriding aorta at 14 weeks' gestation, using transvaginal sonography. *Prenat. Diagn.*, **10**, 697–702

42. Bronshtein, M., Zimmer, E. Z., Milo, S., Ho, S. Y., Lorber, A. and Gerlis, L. M. (1991). Fetal cardiac abnormalities detected by transvaginal sonography at 12–16 weeks' gestation. *Obstet. Gynecol.*, **78**, 374–8

43. Bronshtein, M., Zimmer, E. Z., Gerlis, L. M., Lorber, A. and Drugan, A. (1993). Early ultrasound diagnosis of fetal congenital heart defects in high-risk and low-risk pregnancies. *Obstet. Gynecol.*, **82**, 225–9

44. Achiron, R., Rotstein, Z., Lipitz, S., Mashiach, S. and Hegesh, J. (1994). First-trimester diagnosis of fetal congenital heart disease by transvaginal ultrasonography. *Obstet. Gynecol.*, **84**, 69–72

45. Copel, J. A., Cullen, M., Green, J. J., Mahoney, M. J., Hobbins, J. C. and Kleinman, C. S. (1988). The frequency of aneuploidy in prenatally diagnosed congenital heart disease, an indication for fetal karyotyping. *Am. J. Obstet. Gynecol.*, **158**, 409–13

46. Allan, L. D., Sharland, G. K., Chita, S. K., Lockhart, S. and Maxwell, D. J. (1991). Chromosomal anomalies in fetal congenital heart disease. *Ultrasound Obstet. Gynecol.*, **1**, 8–11

47. Nicolaides, K. H., Azar, G., Byrne, D., Mansur, C. and Marks, K. (1992). Fetal nuchal translucency: ultrasound screening for chromosomal defects in first trimester of pregnancy. *Br. Med. J.*, **304**, 867–9

48. Van Zalen-Sprock, M. M., van Vugt, J. M. G. and van Geijn, H. P. (1992). First-trimester diagnosis of cystic hygroma – course and outcome. *Am. J. Obstet. Gynecol.*, **167**, 94–8

49. Van Zalen-Sprock, M. M., van Vugt, J. M. G. and van Geijn, H. P. (1992). Non-echogenic nuchal oedema as a marker in trisomy 21 screening. *Lancet*, **339**, 1480–1

50. Romero, R., Pilu, G., Jeanty, P., Chidini, A. and Hobbins, J. C. (1988). *Perinatal Diagnosis of Congenital Anomalies*, pp. 125–94. (Norwalk: Appleton Lange)

51. Hoffman, J. I. E. (1990). Congenital heart disease: incidence and inheritance. *Pediatr. Clin. North Am.*, **37**, 25–43

52. Yagel, S., Achiron, R., Ron, M., Revel, A. and Anteby, E. (1995). Transvaginal ultrasonography at early pregnancy cannot be used alone for targeted organ ultrasonographic examination in a high-risk population. *Am. J. Obstet. Gynecol.*, **172**, 971–5

53. Hornberger, L. K., Sanders, S. P., Sahn, D. J., Rice, M. J., Spevak, P. J., Benacerraf, B. R., McDonald, R. W. and Colan, S. D. (1995). *In utero* pulmonary artery and aortic growth and potential for progression of pulmonary outflow tract obstruction in tetralogy of Fallot. *J. Am. Coll. Cardiol.*, **25**, 739–45

54. Reller, M. D., McDonald, R. W., Gerlis, L. M. and Thornburg, K. L. (1991). Cardiac embry-ology: basic review and clinical correlations. *J. Am. Soc. Echocardiol.*, **4**, 519–32

55. Allan, L. D., Chita, S. K., Anderson, R. H., Fagg, N., Crawford, D. C. and Tynan, M. J. (1988). Coarctation of the aorta in prenatal life: an echocardiographic, anatomical, and functional study. *Br. Heart J.*, **59**, 356–60

56. Allan, L. D., Sharland, G. K. and Tynan, M. J. (1989). The natural history of the hypoplastic left heart syndrome. *Int. J. Cardiol.*, **25**, 341–3

57. Todros, T., Presbitero, P., Gaglioto, P. and Demarie, D. (1989). Pulmonary stenosis with intact ventricular septum: documentation of development of the lesion echocardiographically during fetal life. *Int. J. Cardiol.*, **19**, 355–60

58. Cullen, M. T., Green, J., Whetham, J., Salafia, C., Gabrielli, S. and Hobbins, J. C. (1990). Transvaginal ultrasonographic detection of congenital anomalies in the first trimester. *Am. J. Obstet. Gynecol.*, **163**, 466–76

Fetal heart screening: a diagnostic challenge

12

E. Tegnander and S. H. Eik-Nes

INTRODUCTION

Congenital heart defect is the most common of all birth defects[1]. The ultrasound technique has become a valuable tool for the prenatal diagnosis of congenital anomalies. Despite this new diagnostic technique, heart defects have been difficult to detect prenatally due to the complexity of this organ. The introduction of the four-chamber view of the fetal heart[2,3] was a significant step forward in the improvement of prenatal definition of defects. Another important event for the detection of heart defects was the integration of the second-trimester fetal ultrasound examination as part of the prenatal care in several countries. As most of the pregnant population accept this ultrasound scan, including the heart evaluation, we now are able to examine the majority of fetuses for this specific purpose.

Congenital heart defects are responsible for more than half the deaths from lethal malformations in childhood[4]. The prenatal detection of a heart defect will ensure appropriate care for the parents and the fetus during the rest of the pregnancy and prepare the postnatal staff in cases of specific problems. Prenatal diagnosis is therefore of great importance for all involved in fetal and neonatal care.

EPIDEMIOLOGY

Congenital heart defect is one of the most common structural anomalies. The incidence varies in different studies; the lowest rates (3.3–5.5/1000 live births) are from studies that follow the children for only a short time period after birth or when certain types of minor diseases, e.g. mild pulmonary stenosis, small atrial and ventricular septal defects, are underrepresented[5–7]. Longitudinal studies with a long follow-up period allowing later identification of congenital heart defects report an incidence of 8/1000 live births[8–10].

Heart defects may be classified as critical and non-critical with an incidence of 4/1000 in each group[8,11,12]. Following the classification by Mitchell and Korones[8], a defect is critical when a surgical repair most probably is required because of gross structural complexity having functional significance, e.g. transposition of the great arteries, hypoplastic left heart syndrome, atrioventricular septal defect, coarctation of the aorta, large ventricular septal defect. A defect is non-critical when no intervention is likely to be required, e.g. mild pulmonary stenosis, mild aortic stenosis, small ventricular septal defect, small atrial septal defect. Recent studies report an increase of the incidence up to 11 and 12/1000[11,13,14]. In these studies the incidence of critical congenital heart defects has remained unchanged, 4/1000, while the incidence of non-critical congenital heart defects has increased in comparison to the previous studies. One reason for this increase might be that minor congenital heart defects not diagnosed earlier, such as small atrial and ventricular septal defects, are now being detected postnatally due to improved diagnostic techniques such as color Doppler[11,14,15]. Interestingly, Martin and colleagues[15] found that the increase in the prevalence of congenital heart defect (from 3.6 to 4.5 per 1000 live births) in the period of 1981–1984 was due to the increase in the prevalence of small isolated ventricular septal defects. There was no increase when a ventricular septal defect was found in association with other cardiac defects, or among ventricular septal defects requiring catheterization or surgery, or when detected by autopsy. The increase in the prevalence was found among isolated ventricular septal defects diagnosed by echocardiography, only. These findings were also demonstrated by Anderson and colleagues[16] and confirm the improved postnatal diagnosis of isolated minor ventricular septal defects.

Several investigators suggest that most trabecular septal defects in the neonatal period are a result of incomplete trabecular coalescence of interventricular channels, and that the closure of these small defects towards the end of the pregnancy and during the first months of life may be a delay of a normal process[13,14,17]. Results from a study by Hiraishi and co-workers[13] showed that of those trabecular ventricular septal defects with a diameter ranging from 1.4 to 6.6 mm, 76% had closed spontaneously by 12 months of age, most commonly during the first 6 months. Other recent studies confirm these data[11,14]. This indicates that we will have to revise the traditionally accepted incidence (8/1000) of congenital heart defects.

In selected populations, the incidence of congenital heart defects has been found to be between 6 and 15%[18-20]. It is well known that specific maternal and fetal conditions and a family history of congenital heart defect increase the risk of recurrence[21,22]. At most centers these pregnant women are offered a fetal echocardiography[23]. The detection rate in such studies is then high because the incidence of heart defects is increased and because the high-risk nature of the pregnancies has alerted the operator prior to the scan. Some cases are even referred because of a suspected cardiac defect. However, only a small percentage of the total congenital heat defects (1–3%) that are present in the population are found among these selected high-risk groups[2,19,20,24]. The majority of the cases with congenital heart defect are found among the pregnant women with normal risk. Data from selected populations with an incidence higher than normal, therefore, are of limited value in relating our ability to detect congenital heart defects in the normal-risk population.

Since most of the congenital heart defects are of multifactoral origin, the majority of children born with heart defects are born to mothers at no increased risk at all[24-28]. As an ultrasound examination has become a part of the prenatal care, and a detailed visualization of the fetal heart is a standard procedure, the potential for detecting congenital heart defects prenatally has been increased. The second-trimester fetal examination with ultrasound then becomes of great importance since this scan is offered to all pregnant women, with or without risk factors. A standard procedure for fetal heart evaluation should therefore be included in the protocol for this scan.

THE SECOND-TRIMESTER FETAL EXAMINATION

Initially, the fetal examination with ultrasound in the second trimester was performed to assess the fetal age, detect multiple pregnancy and locate the placenta. As the technique improved, we were able to obtain a detailed view of the fetal anatomy. More and more developmental disorders previously not detected, could then be diagnosed, some even treated, *in utero*. The sick fetus became a patient.

The detection rate of congenital developmental disorders during the second-trimester ultrasound examination has been reported in several studies[29-33]. The sensitivity of the prenatal detection increases with improved technique and more skilled operators. Major developmental disorders, such as those in the central nervous system, the renal and gastrointestinal system, thorax and skeleton, have a high detection rate, while minor disorders, such as facial, hand and feet anomalies still are mostly in the non-detected group. Although critical congenital heart defects are detected prenatally, there are still too many left undetected. The detection rate of congenital heart defect does not seem to increase at the same rate as for the other organs.

The published data show that congenital heart defects are detected prenatally, but at a low rate. At the second-trimester ultrasound examination 9–43% (mean 25%) of the critical

148

heart defects were detected[29–33]. Improving this figure probably means including visualization of detailed structures of the fetal heart. Improved technique and training are important issues. The cardiovascular system seems to be a greater challenge than the other major anatomical structures.

THE FETAL HEART EXAMINATION

For several reasons the fetal heart is difficult to examine. At 18 weeks the heart is a tiny structure, approximately one centimeter in diameter. In addition, it is an organ in movement; this influences the image and makes it more difficult to interpret. At a time when other anatomical structures can be imaged well, the fetal heart still is difficult to examine. Additionally, the heart has been looked at as a complicated organ too difficult for prenatal examination. As the technique and the knowledge about the fetal heart have improved, the attitude towards fetal heart diagnosis has changed.

A major breakthrough in the prenatal diagnosis of heart defects came with the introduction of the four-chamber view by Fermont and associates[2] and Allan and colleagues[3] (Figure 1).

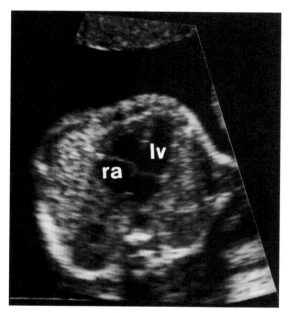

Figure 1 *An apical four-chamber view of the fetal heart. ra, right atrium; lv, left ventricle*

Today we know that a skilled operator can obtain images of detailed structures of the fetal heart and detect critical heart defects at 18–20 weeks in the pregnancy. There is also reason to believe that this can be done as part of the routinely-performed fetal examination[11].

The critical congenital heart defects with an abnormal four-chamber view can be detected when the technique of the four-chamber view is applied. These are defects such as hypoplastic left heart syndrome, mitral or tricuspid atresia, severe Ebstein anomaly, atrioventricular septal defect, double inlet ventricle, large ventricular septal defect, aortic or pulmonary atresia, critical pulmonary or aortic stenosis and severe coarctation of the aorta. Some critical congenital heart defects appear with a normal four-chamber view and the defects are not detected before the great arteries are examined. These are defects such as transposition of the great arteries, tetralogy of Fallot, double outlet right ventricle and truncus arteriosus. Non-critical heart defects, usually not detectable prenatally, include mild–moderate coarctation of the aorta, mild–moderate pulmonary and aortic stenosis and small ventricular septal defects[34]. To detect as many critical congenital heart defects as possible prenatally, the second-trimester ultrasound examination should include images of both the four-chamber view and the great vessels.

A good image is dependent on many factors. Since the heart is tiny at 18–20 weeks, it is important to obtain the best image possible. Factors that influence the quality of the scan are fetal position, gestational age, obesity, oligohydramnios, polyhydramnios, extra cardiac malformations, quality of the equipment and experience of the operator[34,35].

Prenatal detection of congenital heart defects requires basic knowledge about the normal fetal heart. One has to know the normal anatomy to be able to identify the abnormal. The best way to learn this is by systematically going through the heart step-by-step[36]. Initially, only the atrioventricular junction with the four-chamber view should be imaged. Interpretation and evaluation of all the details obtained from different views should be focused on

Table 1 *The normal fetal heart examination. Details from the four-chamber view, the great vessels and the venous return*

The atrioventricular junction – the four-chamber view	
Position, size and rhythm	located in the middle of the fetal thorax apex pointing towards the left anterior chest wall fills approximately 1/3 of the thorax regular rhythm (120–160 beats/min) bradycardia for a short period a normal finding
Atria and foramen ovale	two atria equal in size flap of the foramen ovale into the left atrium apical view: visualize two pulmonary veins connecting to the left atrium
Ventricles	two ventricles equal in size, contract equally left ventricle to be followed to the apex right ventricle has an echogenic thickening towards apex (moderator band) intact ventricular septum (be aware of dropout) ventricle walls equal in thickness
Atrioventricular valves	tricuspid valve more towards the apex than the mitral valve on the interventricular septum atrial and ventricular septa and atrioventricular valves meet at the crux (center) of the heart
The ventriculoarterial junction – the great vessels	
Aorta and the aortic arch	aorta from the left ventricle, sweeps to the right continuity between the anterior wall of the ascending aorta and the interventricular septum; between the posterior wall of the ascending aorta and the anterior leaflet of the mitral valve the aortic arch a tight hook (candy cane shape) giving rise to the head and neck vessels
Pulmonary artery and the ductal arch	pulmonary artery from the right ventricle slightly greater than the aorta in size branches into the left and the right pulmonary artery and ductus arteriosus ductal arch from the right ventricle straight back to the descending aorta (hockey stick shape) no head and neck vessels
The venous atrial junction – the venous return	
Abdominal aorta, inferior and superior vena cavae	cross-section of the fetal abdomen: aorta anterior, on the left side of the spine inferior vena cava anterior, on the right side of the abdominal aorta sagittal view: the two vena cavae connect to the right atrium

(Table 1)[37]. When the four-chamber view is easily obtained, the same learning process should be followed to view the great vessels and later the venous return. Over time, the total fetal heart examination will be incorporated in the second-trimester scan[38].

Table 1 shows the details one should consider when obtaining the different views of the fetal heart. The easiest way to start the fetal heart examination is to obtain the four-chamber view in a cross-section of the fetal thorax, just above the diaphragm (Figure 1)[36,39,40]. One entire rib should be seen to make sure that the cross-section is not oblique. The ultrasound beam should be positioned perpendicular to the structure of interest to obtain the best image. An apical view should provide information about the position of the heart, the size, the rhythm, the four chambers, the atrioventricular valves and the pulmonary veins. The transducer should be moved around the fetal thorax to obtain a subcostal view where the septa and the foramen ovale flap can be seen (Figure 2)[36,41]. Disproportion between the chambers should not be present in the second trimester. In the third trimester the right side of the heart is normally slightly larger than the left side. Thus, disproportion that is an abnormal finding in the second trimester might be a normal finding in the third trimester.

The next step is to examine the great vessels (Table 1). From the four-chamber view, the ascending aorta can be imaged by slowly rotating the transducer towards the fetus's right shoulder (Figure 3a). Angling the transducer slightly more cranially the pulmonary artery appears (Figure 3b). The two great arteries should be at right angles to each other at their origin ('crossing great arteries')[36,39,42]. The aortic arch and the ductal arch are obtained in a sagittal view through the fetus (Figure 4).

During the second-trimester fetal examination (18–20 weeks), the four-chamber view and the views of the great vessels are the most important views to obtain since these structures are usually involved when a critical heart defect is

present. Identification of the atrial situs is also an important step when looking for congenital heart defects (Table 1). Anomalous venous return can be the first suspicion of a congenital heart defect[43]. The views used to image the veins are often the same views used when examining or measuring other anatomical structures; the

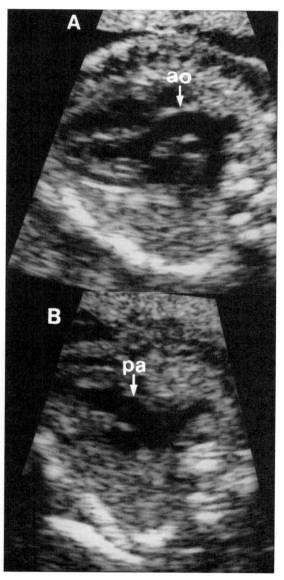

Figure 3 *The fetal heart viewed in a cross-section through the thorax showing the crossing great arteries. The ascending aorta arising from the left ventricle (A) and the main pulmonary artery arising from the right ventricle (B)*

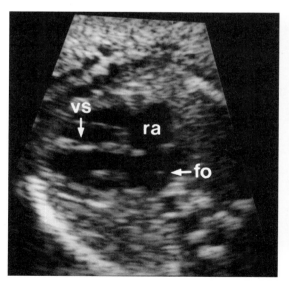

Figure 2 *A subcostal view of the fetal heart. vs, ventricle septum; ra, right atrium; fo, foramen ovale flap*

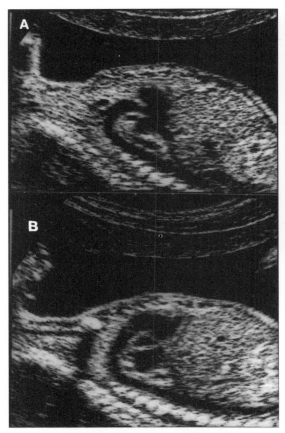

Figure 4   *A sagittal view through the fetus: A, aortic arch with head and neck vessels; B, ductal arch*

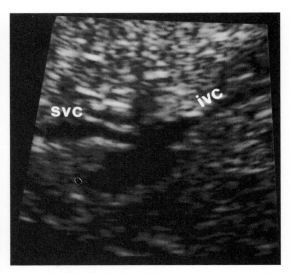

Figure 5   *The fetal heart obtained in a parasagittal view showing the right atrium with the vena cavae connections. svc, superior vena cava; ivc, inferior vena cava*

cross-section of the fetal abdomen at the level of the abdominal measurements will, for example, reveal the relationship between the abdominal aorta and the inferior vena cava where left or right atrial isomerism can be detected. When imaging the fetus in a long-axis parasagittal view, for example when examining the spine or the diaphragm, a view of the inferior and superior vena cavae connecting to the right atrium can be obtained (Figure 5)[36,39].

The fetal heart structures can be imaged from different views[44]. The images and structures are there; it is the operator's responsibility to draw all the possible information from the image. If the operator lacks knowledge about the fetal heart, information might be missed. The learning curve is long, but it is certainly possible to include the fetal heart examination

into the routine scan[11]. The keywords are knowledge, practice and skill!

REVIEW OF THE LITERATURE

In recent years, studies from non-selected populations focusing on the fetal heart have been published. Table 2 summarizes the sensitivity of prenatal detection of congenital heart defect from various studies[11,12,29,30,34,45,46]. Common for the studies are: the prospective approach in non-selected or low-risk populations, an offer of routine ultrasound examination in the second trimester of the pregnancy to all pregnant women and an incidence of critical congenital heart defects of 3–4/1000 births.

The studies show that the four-chamber view is easy to obtain. It is possible to image this view in 90–98% of fetuses. It has also been shown that it is more difficult to obtain the four-chamber view prior to 18 weeks because the fetal heart structures are then too small for optimal imaging[34,47]. The same studies show that the skill of the operator is another important factor influencing the demonstration of the four chambers. The best time to perform the fetal heart examination in a routine setting is between 18 and 20 weeks[34,47]. In the third trimester it might

Table 2 Sensitivity of prenatally-detected congenital heart defects and karyotype at second-trimester ultrasound screening programs

Author	Study years	n	Gestational age (weeks)	Heart examination	4-chamber view obtained (%)	No attention* (%)	4-chamber (%)	Great arteries (%)	Abnormal karyotype (%)
						Sensitivity			
Achiron et al., 1992[46]	88–90	5347	21 (18–24)	4-chamber + great arteries	98	—	48	78	9
Luck, 1992[29]	88–91	8523	19	4-chamber, great arteries as more experienced	—	—	33	—	—
Sharland et al., 1992[34]	88–90	23 861	not specified	4-chamber, rescan when not obtained	90	—	69	—	—
Vergani et al., 1992[45]	85–89	9016	19 (18–20)	no attention* + 4-chamber	95	47	81	—	45
Levi et al., 1995[30]	84–92	25 046	14–23	4-chamber	—	—	21	—	—
Rustico et al., 1995[12]	86–92	7024	20–22	4-chamber + great arteries + venous return, rescan when not obtained	—	—	—	61	29
Tegnander et al., 1995[11]	86–90	11 894	18	no attention* + 4-chamber	96	18	26	—	9

*No attention, indicating that a systematic evaluation of the heart was not performed

be difficult to image the heart because of increased shadowing from the bone structures, normally decreased amount of amniotic fluid and decreased fetal movements.

The equipment used is an important factor when performing the ultrasound scan. Comparing the 3.5- and 5-MHz transducers, the results were significantly better with the 5-MHz transducer in obtaining the four-chamber view[47]. Sharland and Allan[34] confirmed these data by comparing two machines which provided images of different quality. A higher percentage of four-chamber views could be obtained by using the machine with both a 3.5- and 5-MHz transducers than by using the machine with a 3.5-MHz transducer only.

It has been suggested that by obtaining the four-chamber view, 50% of the critical congenital heart defects should be detected[2,3]. This suggestion was received with some scepticism a few years ago because the four-chamber view was not yet a part of the routine scan. As the technique and our knowledge have improved, the results from several studies have confirmed this assertion, as shown in Table 2. Vergani and associates[45] found a high detection rate (81%) with the four-chamber view. Since the theoretical estimates suggest that only 2/1000 congenital heart defects could be detected by obtaining the four chambers[3], the findings by Vergani and co-workers[45] need to be verified. Sharland and Allan[34] excluded the congenital heart defects that had a normal four-chamber view when reporting the sensitivity of prenatally detected heart defects (69%); the exclusion may have improved the sensitivity. Advanced gestational age[12,30,46] and a repeat scan if the first failed[12,34] are also likely to increase the sensitivity. Table 2 confirms that approximately half of the critical heart defects may be detected by obtaining the four-chamber view at the 18–20 week ultrasound examination. To improve that figure, the great vessels need to be included in the ultrasound examination[12,46].

THE TEAM APPROACH

When a congenital heart defect is suspected, a second opinion is always important, either made by another ultrasound specialist in the same department or by referral to another and preferably a tertiary center. A congenital heart defect may be an isolated finding, but is often associated with other disorders and/or abnormal karyotype. Table 2 shows that when a heart defect is present, the percentage of fetuses with an abnormal karyotype is high. In our series, 32% of the critical congenital heart defects, and 16% of the non-critical ones, were associated with extracardiac malformations including abnormal karyotype[11]. When a congenital heart defect is diagnosed one should therefore always perform a detailed anatomical survey to look for other anomalies, or vice versa: when extracardiac anomalies are found, fetal echocardiography should always be performed. The fetal karyotype should be determined routinely since this might significantly affect the management of the pregnancy.

When the prenatal diagnosis of a congenital heart defect is certain, this information has to be given to the parents. This is a very important part of the process, since the parents' decisions will be based on that information. Caring for the parents and the fetus with a congenital heart defect requires a close collaboration between different professionals. A perinatal team, including the ultrasound operator, obstetrician, perinatal cardiologist and neonatologist, should counsel the parents. Depending on the needs of the parents, the team might also include a neonatal nurse, a social worker and a clergyman. It is of importance that the couple get the best information possible for their special situation and their needs.

The obstetrician

When a heart defect is detected prenatally, the prenatal care and follow up during the pregnancy is organized by the obstetrician. A pediatric cardiologist and other professionals may be contacted to ensure a correct diagnosis. We have experienced that some couples appreciate contact with other couples who have experienced the same situation. The obstetrician organizes the information given to the parents and supports them in whatever their decision may be following the prenatal diagnosis. Close follow up of the fetus and preparation for the delivery will make this difficult situation easier for everyone involved.

The perinatal cardiologist

The perinatal cardiologist plays an important role in the diagnostic process and follow up of prenatally-diagnosed heart defects. Thorough evaluation of the defect is crucial for information about the prognosis given to the parents. The perinatal cardiologist should therefore be involved as early as possible following a suspected or final diagnosis. Some children with congenital heart defect need treatment immediately after birth, these include ductus dependent congenital heart defects (hypoplastic left heart syndrome, pulmonary atresia, complete transposition of the great arteries). The life of such a child may depend on rapid and correct treatment. Thus, for some children the delivery should take place in a hospital where the necessary expertise in cardiology and/or cardiac surgical treatment is available. In some ultrasound units the perinatal cardiologist is involved in such decisions. One of the most important advantages with prenatal diagnosis in general is the option of transporting the fetus *in utero* to the delivery hospital rather than transferring a sick neonate. The issue of 'maternal transport' is of particular importance in the field of prenatal diagnosis of heart defects[48].

The parents

Learning about their child's serious condition is a psychological trauma in itself for parents-to-be. Prenatal diagnosis allows them time to prepare for what will come. Prior to the delivery they get to know the personnel who will take care of their baby after birth. This might moderate some of their anxiety. By knowing the condition of their baby they can take part in the discussion about where and when to deliver, to some extent discuss the treatment options and make necessary practical arrangements. For parents confronted with the critical condition of their newborn, being prepared gives more precious time together with the baby during the first important days of life.

For some parents termination of the pregnancy might be considered when a critical and/or lethal heart defect is found at an early gestational age. A correct diagnosis is a prerequisite for the counselling and follow up of the parents; this emphasizes the necessity of the team approach for the diagnosis and evaluation of congenital heart defects.

The geneticist and the perinatal pathologist

Genetic counselling is of importance when the couple considers a new pregnancy. The geneticist has information available to estimate the recurrence risk for the various defects; consequences of genetic counselling is one of the primary methods for preventing congenital heart diseases in future pregnancies[27]. To ensure an optimal diagnosis in the cases when a fetus or a child dies, a close collaboration with a perinatal pathologist is of great value.

PRENATAL DETECTION OF HEART DEFECTS IS STILL A CHALLENGE

A few years ago it was suggested that most congenital heart defects could be detected prenatally by examining the four-chamber view of the fetal heart[49]. Today, we know that the reported high detection rate was based on targeted examination on selected populations and not representative for the general population. The detection rate of congenital heart defects during the second-trimester fetal examination of the general population remained low due to the low incidence in such populations combined with the technical problems in general that existed with detection of heart defects.

This challenge was met by the introduction of the four-chamber view and brought us a step forward towards a higher detection rate. In addition, the recent inclusion of the great vessels in ultrasound examinations has been another big step forward. Based on data from specialized centers, the results now are improving and there is reason to believe that these anatomical sections are sufficient for the diagnosis of fetal heart defects[11,34]. There is no scientific work indicating that the addition of the Doppler technique will further improve the results in a screening situation.

The heart remains the organ with the lowest detection rate of anomalies in non-selected populations. We therefore must accept that fetal heart diagnosis is difficult and that we must pay special attention to this organ in order to increase the detection rate to the same level we have obtained for other organs. In order to make this work in large populations outside the specialized centers there must be a special focus on the fetal heart. This can only be done through extensive education and training. The ultrasound equipment available today can provide detailed images of the fetal heart. During the last 10 years we have learned that the correct anatomical views for optimal fetal heart examination are the four-chamber view and the presentation of the great vessels. Now the real challenge before us is to teach those involved in the fetal ultrasound examination offered in the second trimester to master this technique!

References

1. Campbell, M. (1973). Incidence of cardiac malformations at birth and later, and neonatal mortality. *Br. Heart J.*, **35**, 189–200
2. Fermont, L., De Geeter, B., Aubry, M. C., Kachaner, J. and Sidi, D. (1985). A close collaboration between obstetricians and pediatric cardiologists allows antenatal detection of severe cardiac malformations by 2D echocardiography. Presented at the *2nd World Congress of Paediatric Cardiology*, New York, June, abstr. p. 10
3. Allan, L. D., Crawford, D. C., Chita, S. K. and Tynan, M. J. (1986). Prenatal screening for congenital heart disease. *Br. Med. J.*, **292**, 1717–19
4. Keith, J. D. (1978). Prevalence, incidence and epidemiology. In Keith, J. D., Rowe, R. D. and Vlad, P. (eds.) *Heart Disease in Infancy and Childhood*, p. 3–13. (New York: MacMillan Publishing Co.)
5. Ferencz, C., Rubin, J. D., McCarter, R. J., Brenner, J. I., Neill, C. A., Perry, L. W., Hepner, S. I. and Sowning, J. W. (1985). Congenital heart disease: prevalence at livebirth. *Am. J. Epidemiol.*, **121**, 31–6
6. Dickinson, D. F., Arnold, R. and Wilkinson, J. L. (1981). Congenital heart disease among 160 480 liveborn children in Liverpool 1960 to 1969. *Br. Heart J.*, **46**, 55–62
7. Hoffman, J. I. E. (1990). Congenital heart disease: incidence and inheritance. *Pediatr. Clin. North Am.*, **37**, 25–43
8. Mitchell, S. C. and Korones, S. B. (1971). Congenital heart disease in 56 109 births. Incidence and natural history. *Circulation*, **43**, 323–32
9. Stoll, C., Alembik, Y., Roth, M. P., Dott, B. and De Geeter, B. (1989). Risk factors in congenital heart disease. *Eur. J. Epidemiol.*, **5**, 382–91
10. Hoffman, J. I. E. and Christianson, R. (1978). Congenital heart disease in a cohort of 19 502 births with long-term follow-up. *Am. J. Cardiol.*, **42**, 641–7
11. Tegnander, E., Eik-Nes, S. H., Johansen, O. J. and Linker, D. T. (1995). Prenatal detection of heart defects at the routine fetal examination at 18 weeks in non-selected population. *Ultrasound Obstet. Gynecol.*, **5**, 372–80
12. Rustico, M. A., Benettoni, A., D'Ottavio, G., Maieron, A., Fischer-Tamaro, I., Conoscenti, G., Meir, Y., Montesano, M., Cattaneo, A. and Mandruzzato, G. (1995). Fetal heart screening in low-risk pregnancies. *Ultrasound Obstet. Gynecol.*, **6**, 313–19
13. Hiraishi, S., Agata, Y., Nowatari, M., Oguchi, K., Misawa, H., Hirota, H., Fujino, N., Horiguchi, Y., Yashiro, K. and Nakae, S. (1992). Incidence and natural course of trabecular ventricular septal defect: two-dimensional echocardiography and color Doppler flow imaging study. *J. Pediatr.*, **120**, 409–15
14. Meberg, A., Otterstad, J. E., Frøland, G., Sørland, S. and Nitter-Hauge, S. (1994). Increasing incidence of ventricular septal defects caused by improved detection rate. *Acta Pædiatr.*, **83**, 653–7
15. Martin, G. R., Perry, L. W. and Ferencz, C. (1989). Increased prevalence of ventricular septal defect: epidemic or improved diagnosis. *Pediatrics*, **83**, 200–3
16. Anderson, C. E., Edmonds, L. D. and Erickson, J. D. (1978). Patent ductus arteriosus and ventricular septal defect: trends in reported frequency. *Am. J. Epidemiol.*, **107**, 281–9
17. Ben-Shachar, G., Arcilla, R. A., Lucas, R. V. and Manasek, F. J. (1985). Ventricular trabeculations

in the chick embryo heart and their contribution to ventricular and muscular septal development. *Circ. Res.*, **57**, 759–66

18. Copel, J. A. and Kleinman, C. S. (1986). The impact of fetal echocardiography on perinatal outcome. *Ultrasound Med. Biol.*, **12**, 327–35

19. Stewart, P. A., Wladimiroff, J. W., Reuss, A. and Sachs, E. S. (1987). Fetal echocardiography: a review of six years experience. *Fetal Ther.*, **2**, 222–31

20. Wheller, J. J., Reiss, R. and Allen, H. D. (1990). Clinical experience with fetal echocardiography. *Am. J. Dis. Child.*, **144**, 49–53

21. Nora, J. J. and Nora, A. H. (1988). Update on counseling the family with a first-degree relative with a congenital heart defect. *Am. J. Med. Genet.*, **29**, 137–42

22. Pradat, P. (1994). Recurrence risk for major congenital heart defects in Sweden: a registry study. *Genet. Epidemiol.*, **11**, 131–40

23. Benacerraf, B. R. and Sanders, S. P. (1990). Fetal echocardiography. *Radiol. Clin. North Am.*, **28**, 131–47

24. Allan, L. D., Sharland, G. K., Milburn, A., Lockhart, S. M., Groves, A. M. M., Anderson, R. H., Cook, A. C. and Fagg, N. L. K. (1994). Prospective diagnosis of 1006 consecutive cases of congenital heart disease in the fetus. *J. Am. Coll. Cardiol.*, **23**, 1452–8

25. Callan, N. A., Maggio, M., Stegar, S. and Kan, J. S. (1991). Fetal echocardiography: indications for referral, prenatal diagnoses, and outcomes. *Am. J. Perinat.*, **8**, 390–4

26. Davis, G. K., Farquhar, C. M., Allan, L. D., Crawford, D. C. and Chapman, M. G. (1990). Structural cardiac abnormalities in the fetus: reliability of prenatal diagnosis and outcome. *Br. J. Obstet. Gynaecol.*, **97**, 27–31

27. Nora, J. J. and Nora, A. H. (1984). The genetic contribution to congenital heart diseases. In Nora, J. J. and Takao, A. (eds.) *Congenital Heart Diseases: Causes and Processes*, p. 3–13. (New York: Futura Publishing Co.)

28. Cullen, S., Sharland, G. K., Allan, L. D. and Sullivan, I. D. (1992). Potential impact of population screening for prenatal diagnosis of congenital heart disease. *Arch. Dis. Child.*, **67**, 775–8

29. Luck, C. A. (1992). Value of routine ultrasound screening at 19 weeks: a four year study of 8849 deliveries. *Br. Med. J.*, **304**, 1474–8

30. Levi, S., Schaaps, J.-P., De Havay, P., Coulon, R. and Defoort, P. (1995). End-result of routine ultrasound screening for congenital anomalies: the Belgian multicentric study 1984–92. *Ultrasound Obstet. Gynecol.*, **5**, 366–71

31. Rosendahl, H. and Kivinen, S. (1989). Antenatal detection of congenital malformations by routine ultrasonography. *Obstet. Gynecol.*, **73**, 947–51

32. Brocks, V. and Bang, J. (1991). Routine examination by ultrasound for the detection of fetal malformations in a low risk population. *Fetal Diagn. Ther.*, **6**, 37–45

33. Crane, J. P., LeFevre, M. L., Winborn, R. C., Evans, J. K., Ewigman, B. G., Bain, R. P., Frigoletto, F. D., McNellis, D. and the RADIUS study group (1994). A randomized trial of prenatal ultrasonographic screening: impact on the detection, management, and outcome of anomalous fetuses. *Am. J. Obstet. Gynecol.*, **171**, 392–9

34. Sharland, G. K. and Allan, L. D. (1992). Screening for congenital heart disease prenatally. Results of a 2½-year study in the South East Thames Region. *Br. J. Obstet. Gynaecol.*, **99**, 220–5

35. De Vore, G. R., Medearis, A. L., Bear, M. B., Horenstein, J. and Platt, L. D. (1993). Fetal echocardiography: factors that influence imaging of the fetal heart during the second trimester of pregnancy. *J. Ultrasound Med.*, **12**, 659–63

36. Allan, L. D. (1986). *Manual of Fetal Echocardiography* (Lancaster: MTP Press Ltd.)

37. Brown, D. L., DiSalvo, D. N., Frates, M. C., Doubilet, P. M., Benson, C. B., Laing, F. C. and Parness, A. (1993). Sonography of the fetal heart: normal variants and pitfalls. *Am. J. Roentgenol.*, **160**, 1251–5

38. DeVore, G. R. (1985). The prenatal diagnosis of congenital heart disease – a practical approach for the fetal sonographer. *J. Clin. Ultrasound*, **13**, 229–45

39. Reed, K. L., Anderson, C. F. and Shenker, L. (1988). *Fetal Echocardiography. An Atlas.* (New York: Alan R. Liss Inc.)

40. McGahan, J. P. (1991). Sonography of the fetal heart: findings on the four-chamber view. *Am. J. Roentgenol.*, **156**, 547–53

41. Wladimiroff, J. W., Stewart, P. A. and Vosters, R. P. L. (1984). Fetal cardiac structures and function as studied by ultrasound. *Clin. Cardiol.*, **7**, 239–53

42. DeVore, G. R. (1992). The aortic and pulmonary outflow tract screening examination in the human fetus. *J. Ultrasound Med.*, **11**, 345–8

43. Yeager, S. B., Parness, I. A., Spevak, P. J., Hornberger, L. K. and Sanders, S. P. (1994). Prenatal echocardiographic diagnosis of pulmonary and systemic venous anomalies. *Am. Heart J.*, **128**, 397–405

44. Allan, L. D., Tynan, M. J., Campbell, S., Wilkinson, J. L. and Anderson, R. H. (1980). Echocardiographic and anatomical correlates in the fetus. *Br. Heart J.*, **44**, 444–51

45. Vergani, P., Mariani, S., Ghidini, A., Schiavina, R., Cavallone, M., Locatelli, A., Strobelt, N. and

Cerruti, P. (1992). Screening for congenital heart disease with the four-chamber view of the fetal heart. *Am. J. Obstet. Gynecol.*, **167**, 1000–3

46. Achiron, R., Glaser, J., Gelernter, I., Hegesh, J. and Yagel, S. (1992). Extended fetal echocardiographic examination for detecting cardiac malformations in low risk pregnancies. *Br. Med. J.*, **304**, 671–4

47. Tegnander, E., Eik-Nes, S. H. and Linker, D. T. (1994). Incorporating the four-chamber view of the fetal heart into the second-trimester routine fetal examination. *Ultrasound Obstet. Gynecol.*, **4**, 24–8

48. Chang, A. C., Huhta, J. C., Yoon, G. Y., Wood, D. C., Tulzer, G., Cohen, A., Mennuti, M. and Norwood, W. I. (1991). Diagnosis, transport, and outcome in fetuses with left ventricular outflow tract obstruction. *J. Thorac. Cardiovasc. Surg.*, **102**, 841–8

49. Copel, J. A., Pilu, G., Green, J., Hobbins, J. C. and Kleinman, C. S. (1987). Fetal echocardiographic screening for congenital heart disease: the importance of the four-chamber view. *Am. J. Obstet. Gynecol.*, **157**, 648–55

New dimensions in fetal neuroscanning

13

A. Monteagudo and I. E. Timor-Tritsch

INTRODUCTION

The fetal brain, along with the fetal heart and skeletal system, is considered to be among the most 'difficult' organs to scan. This difficulty arises from a variety of sources. The anatomy of these organs is complex and may not be easily imaged with the standard transabdominal sonographic approach. Although, performing transvaginal sonography enables better image resolution, it creates a 'new problem', namely a somewhat unusual set of images, since the anatomy is presented in two different and less-used planes, the sagittal and coronal planes. The continuously changing developmental anatomy poses further problems. Certain features of the fetal brain (e.g. shape of the lateral ventricles) change their sonographic appearance and, in addition, with the advancing gestational age new structures such as the corpus callosum become evident. A large variety of anomalies, some subtle and others more obvious, may disrupt the normal anatomy of this important organ.

Fetal neuroscanning is an integral part of every malformation work-up regardless of the age. At 9–11 weeks we look at a few structures, such as the tortuous sonolucent ventricular system, the basic symmetry of the hemispheres on the two sides of the falx cerebri and the hyperechoic choroid plexus. At 16 weeks it is possible to detect a much larger number of structures, however, those parts of the fetal brain which have not completed their normal development would not be expected to be seen. Finally, at 22–23 weeks, the fetal brain is close to its final anatomy, with the exception of gyri and sulci.

Standardization of scanning technique is important in order not to miss or forget to scan certain structures. The aim of this chapter is to delineate a scanning approach which allows the sonologist or sonographer to be consistent from patient to patient. Standardization of the scan allows subsequent brain images of the neonate to be compared to those taken during gestation.

The first part of this chapter will review the normal fetal brain anatomy using the main sections in each of the scanning planes (axial, coronal and sagittal). The second part will describe a variety of commonly occurring congenital brain malformations and their sonographic appearance. However, before dealing with the normal anatomy of the prenatal brain, the scanning technique should be considered.

ULTRASOUND EQUIPMENT

It is our belief that for an effective and targeted neuroscan of the fetus, a transabdominal, as well as a high-frequency transvaginal scan, is required. It is beyond the scope of this article to expand on all the physical properties of these transducers. It is well known that the penetration of the transabdominal transducer using a 3.5–5-MHz transducer crystal is adequate to image fetal brain structures. However, the resolution at times is less than optimal. Although the high-frequency transducer probes penetrate to a lesser degree, we are able to take advantage of their much higher resolution and imaging properties due to the closer proximity to the fetal head through the vagina[1]. It is therefore important to understand that for complete and exhaustive, as well as accurate, neuroscanning of the fetal brain after 18 weeks, at times two probes (i.e. transabdominal and transvaginal) are required; this, of course, if the fetus is in a vertex presentation. The transvaginal approach provides valuable and extremely high resolution images in as much that at times when a suspicion of an undetermined or otherwise difficult-to-image lesion is found, version of the fetus may become a real necessity, or at least an option.

THE SCANNING CONCEPT

In addition to describing a possible pathology of the prenatal brain, we have to be able to relate this to the pediatric neurologists, neonatologists and neonatal brain surgeons, who will counsel the pregnant woman and take care of the neonate after birth. These specialists will require sonographic or other radiological studies to pinpoint the lesion. It is extremely important to be able to relate to these specialists and describe the location, as well as the nature of the pathology, using coordinates, sections and planes that they are familiar with. It is fortunate, therefore, that the transvaginal approach emulates the neonatal brain scanning performed through the bone-free area of the neonatal anterior fontanelle. Transvaginal scanning, using the very same window to the fetal brain, is able to generate pictures using the same scanning angles and directions[2–8].

One issue that we find important in fetal neuroimaging is the use of an end-firing, symmetrical, inactive or in-line transvaginal probe. Such a probe is easier to use when maneuvering and orientation is required. The final issue for those who would like to engage in fetal neuroimaging is the importance of refreshing their memory regarding brain anatomy.

SCANNING TECHNIQUE

The scanning technique is relatively simple, but requires a different approach for fetuses up to 12 weeks than for fetuses over 12 weeks. First-trimester embryos/fetuses can be scanned with a transvaginal probe no matter what their position.

After 12 weeks, it is important to have the fetus in a vertex presentation. However, at this gestational age this is easily accomplished by very slightly maneuvering the fetus using the abdominal hand and vaginal probe. Up to 16 weeks, in the case of singleton pregnancies, the transvaginal approach should be the first-line approach to fetal neuroscanning. Over 16–17 weeks, the transabdominal and transvaginal approach should be used individually or in combination as required and mandated by fetal position. It should always be remembered that if the fetus is in the vertex presentation, the transvaginal approach yields images of higher quality and resolution.

NORMAL PRENATAL BRAIN ANATOMY

Ultrasound of the fetal brain before 12 weeks

Fetuses less than 13 postmenstrual weeks should be scanned primarily with high-frequency transvaginal probes. Although impressive descriptions of the developing embryonic brain have been published by us and others[2-4,6,9–11], the practical clinical information at this time is limited to observing the normal-appearing embryo and to ruling out major structural anomalies. The largest sonolucent structures at around 7–8 postmenstrual weeks are in the area of the rhombencephalon (Figures 1 and 2). At around 9 postmenstrual weeks, the falx is clearly visible, partitioning the brain into the two hemispheres. At this time, the hyperechoic choroid plexus is prominent. From the 9th and 10th postmenstrual weeks, using a high-frequency transvaginal probe, it is possible to obtain several sections in the coronal, axial and sagittal planes. From 9 postmenstrual weeks on, the tortuous fluid-filled ventricular system imaged in the median sagittal plane is evident and should be considered normal (Figure 2).

Blaas and colleagues[10,11] performed not only interesting and extensive imaging studies of the developing embryonic and early fetal brain, but they also were able to create a computer-generated 'cast' of the well-delineated ventricular system closely to study the change in shape of these structures from 8 to 12 postmenstrual weeks.

From 11 to 12 postmenstrual weeks, there is a relative increase in the anterior horns of the lateral ventricles and for the next 2–3 weeks they

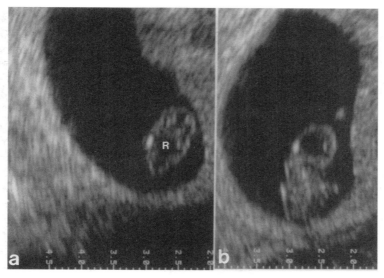

Figure 1 *Two coronal sections of an embryo of 8 postmenstrual weeks and 3 days. The posterior coronal section (a) shows the rhombencephalon (R). A more anterior coronal section (b) shows the large sonolucent structure which is not yet partitioned by the later-developing falx cerebri*

will remain relatively large. After 12 weeks, the choroid plexus is seen literally to move back on top of the thalamus into its final position, which is the body and atrium of the lateral ventricle (Figure 3).

Scanning the fetal brain after 15 weeks

At about 15–16 postmenstrual weeks, there is significant thickening of the skull bones. This thickened skull bone presents a relative obstacle for the high-frequency sound waves to penetrate and image the brain. To circumvent this problem the anterior fontanelle is used as a sound window allowing continued scanning of the fetal brain with high accuracy and resolution (Figure 4). However, this solution comes at the price of being unable to scan the fetal brain in the customary and classical parallel sections of each of the three major planes, i.e. the sagittal, coronal and axial planes (Figures 5). Because of the single point of access, which, as previously stated, is the anterior fontanelle, the obtained sections in the sagittal and coronal planes diverge in a radial fan-shaped fashion. This particular scanning technique has been long

known and used in the neonatal brain scanning which is done in a similar fashion, i.e. through the same anterior fontanelle (Figures 6 and 7).

We have developed and propose a new standardized way to examine the fetal brain using the transvaginal ultrasound probe. In the sagittal section, we propose two sections in addition to the customary and well-known median sagittal section (Figure 8). These two sections are the right and left oblique-1 and oblique-2 sections. In the coronal plane, we propose a frontal, mid-coronal and occipital sections (Figure 9). The frontal sections contain the frontal-1 and frontal-2. The mid-coronal group contains the mid-coronal-1, -2 and -3 sections, and finally the occipital group contains the occipital-1 and 2. Using these sections, the entire brain can be scanned in an orderly and standardized fashion. Each of these sections, in the two general planes, contains a unique combination of structures that define only that one particular section. Using these sagittal and coronal sections, not only a precise location of structures and possible lesions can be achieved, but it is simple to convey this information to the neonatologist, pediatric neurologist and pediatric neurosurgeon for an easy understanding.

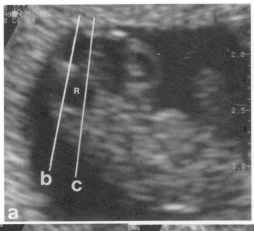

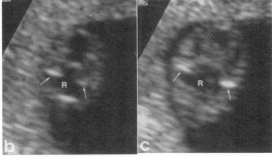

Figure 2 *An embryo at 9 postmenstrual weeks and 5 days. Median section (a), showing the tortuous ventricular system (R, rhombencephalon). The two white lines represent the sections at which Figures 2b and 2c were obtained. Posterior coronal section (b) (R, rhombencephalon). The small arrows point to the developing choroid plexus. Coronal section (c) which shows the rhombencephalon (R); the small arrows point to the choroid plexus*

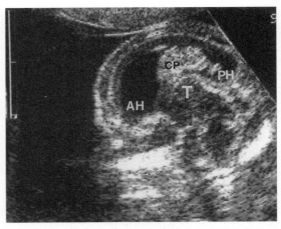

Figure 3 *Paramedian section of a fetal head at 13 postmenstrual weeks and 3 days. Note the relatively large anterior horn (AH). The choroid plexus (CP) is seen on top of the thalamus (T). The posterior horn (PH) is relatively small at this gestational age*

For easier reference, the *sagittal* plane contains the following structures as far as each section is concerned:

(1) *The median section* contains the corpus callosum, cavum septum pellucidum, caudate nucleus, thalamus, tela choroidea, tectum, corpora quadrigemina, vermis, fourth ventricle and cisterna magna (Figure 10a and b).

(2) *The oblique-1 section* contains the lateral ventricle with its anterior horn, posterior horn, atrium and choroid plexus of the lateral ventricle and the thalami (Figure 11).

(3) *The oblique-2 section* contains the insula (Figure 8), parietal operculum, temporal operculum and the lateral sulcus.

The sections in the *coronal plane* (Figure 9) contain the following structures:

(1) *The frontal-1 section* contains white matter only, as well as the falx.

(2) *The frontal-2 section* contains the orbit, the anterior horn of the lateral ventricle and the falx.

(3) *The mid-coronal-1 section* contains the body of the lateral ventricle, the cavum septum pellucidum, the cross-section of the corpus callosum (mainly its anterior part), the caudate nucleus and the falx.

(4) *The mid-coronal-2 section* contains the body of the lateral ventricle – this time containing the choroid plexus and the tela choroidea covering the thalamus, the cross-section of the trunk of the corpus callosum and the falx.

(5) *The mid-coronal-3 section* contains the atrium with the choroid plexus, the splenium or the posterior part of the corpus callosum, the thalamus and the falx.

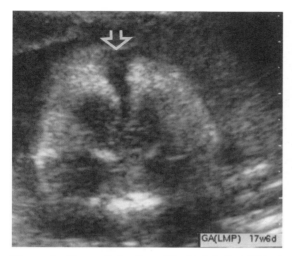

Figure 4 *Tangential section of the fetal skull at 17 post-menstrual weeks and 6 days, showing the anterior fontanelle (open arrow) through which most of the images of the fetal brain are obtained in the second and third trimesters*

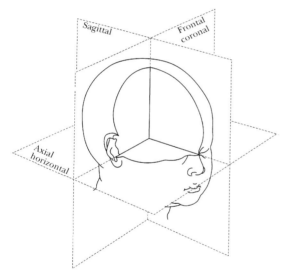

Figure 5 *The three main classical planes of the head. The mid-sagittal section is usually called 'median', and the sections lateral to it are also called 'parasagittal sections'*

(6) *The occipital-1 section* contains the posterior horns, two hemispheres of the cerebellum, at times the fourth ventricle, the falx, the tentorium and maybe a small sliver of the cisterna magna (Figure 12).

(7) *The occipital-2 section* contains the hemispheres of the cerebellum, the vermis which

is hyperechoic, the falx cerebri, the tentorium and the cisterna magna.

The axial planes are equally important in neuroimaging of the fetal brain. They typically cannot be obtained by transvaginal scanning and therefore transabdominal scanning still maintains its extremely important role in the diagnostic algorithm. It is not within the scope of this review to describe the structures seen on the axial planes, since these are sufficiently well known.

The ventricular system

The fetal cerebral ventricular system consists of the lateral ventricles with anterior, posterior and inferior horns, and the atrium (hosting the choroid plexus). The intraventricular foramina on both sides of the lateral ventricles lead into the third ventricle, which is connected to the fourth ventricle by way of the cerebral aqueduct. The fourth ventricle connects in the median plane with the cisterna magna through the median and lateral apertures.

It is important to understand the flow of the cerebrospinal fluid since any obstruction at the various levels would result in a very specific clinical picture. It is also important to be able to measure the normal, as well as abnormal sizes of this ventricular system, to be able to detect deviation from the normal. Several nomograms of the entire ventricular system exist. The classical tables and graphs are based on the measurements of the axial section. Our group has developed more refined and accurate measurements of the entire lateral ventricular system which enable the detection of ventriculomegaly even in its incipient stages[8].

The corpus callosum

Even though the corpus callosum is part of the mid-brain, it should be mentioned separately because it connects the right and left hemispheres and its development is completed only at around 20–22 postmenstrual weeks. It forms the roof of the cavum pellucidum and the cavum vergae and develops from the anterior to

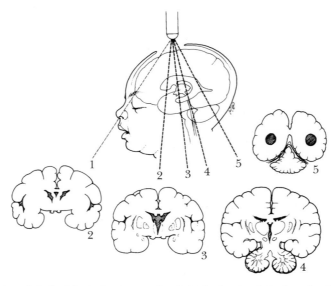

Figure 6 *Neuroscanning of the fetal brain in the second and third trimesters is performed using the anterior fontanelle. Note that several coronal sections can be obtained in a fan-shape through this acoustic window to the brain*

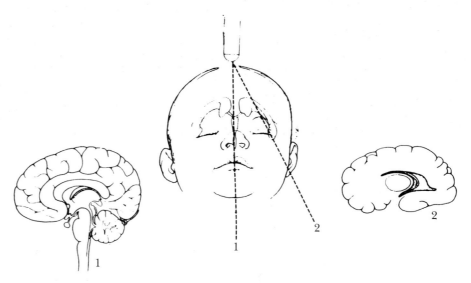

Figure 7 *If the transducer is turned 90° from the position through which the images in Figure 6 were obtained, sagittal images of the brain can be obtained. 1, median plane; 2, parasagittal/oblique-1 section*

the posterior part creating first the knee, then the trunk and, finally, the tail of this structure (Figure 10).

Subarachnoid spaces and cisterns

Between the cortex and the skull bones, subarachnoid spaces and cisterns are found con-

taining fine cords of the arachnoid, crossing blood vessels, and arachnoid granulations. These spaces are filled with cerebral spinal fluid (Figure 13).

Some of these spaces and cisterns can easily be recognized on ultrasonography. The largest of them is the cisterna magna, below the cerebellum. Measurements of the normal cisterna

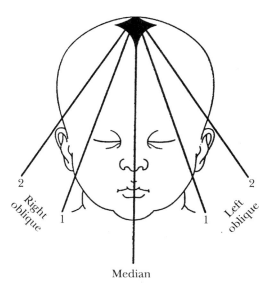

Median

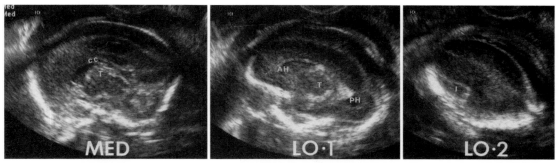

Figure 8 *The sections in the sagittal plane are shown. The median (MED) is the only plane which shows among other structures, the corpus callosum (CC). Below the CC is the sonolucent cavum septum pellucidum which is not marked, and the thalamus (T). The oblique-1 (O-1) section can be obtained on the left (L) or the right side and reveals the anterior horn (AH), hyperechoic choroid plexus and posterior horn (PH), which are behind the thalamus (T). The oblique-2 (O-2) plane is at times hard to obtain and its hallmark is the gaping insula (I)*

magna are important and are usually taken at the time of neuroscanning. The subarachnoid space along the sagittal sinus between and on top of the two hemispheres is also an easily-detected space and becomes important when growth pathologies of the brain, as well as faulty gyrations and sulcations, are investigated.

The posterior fossa

The easiest way to investigate the posterior fossa is by using the posterior coronal sections such as the occipital-1 and 2 sections, or the median sagittal section. It is also feasible and easy to scan the posterior fossa on an axial scan, if the oc-

ciput is close to the probing transducer. The main structures in this anatomical area are the two cerebral hemispheres connected by the hyperechoic vermis on top of which the tentorium is seen and the posteriorly situated cisterna magna (Figure 14).

Gyri, sulci and fissures

The sonographic appearance of the sulci and fissures is dependent upon the echogenicity of the pia matter and the pia arachnoid complex, called soft-brain coverings. These are of high echogenicity and are highly visible appearing as bright echoes on ultrasonography. Duplications

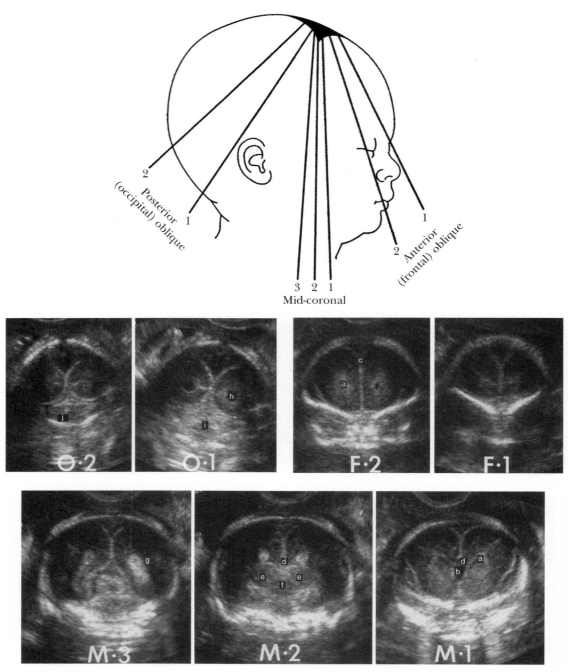

Figure 9 *The seven main sections in the coronal plane are shown. Anteriorly, the frontal-1 (F-1) shows only the white matter. Frontal-2 (F-2), the anterior horn (a) and falx (c) are seen on this image that resembles the steer's head configuration. Mid-coronal-1 (M-1), the anterior horn (a), the cavum septi pellucidum (b) and the corpus callosum (d) are seen. Mid-coronal-2 (M-2), the corpus callosum below which the hyperechoic lines of the choroid plexus are seen to dip into the third ventricle (f), which is situated between the thalami (e). Mid-coronal-3 (M-3), this section reveals the atrium in which the hyperechoic bulk of the choroid plexus (g) is seen. Occipital-1 (O-1), this image is called 'the owl's eye configuration' because of the prominent posterior horn (h). The cerebellum is also seen on this section (i). Occipital-2 (O-2), the main features of this section are the vermis and the cisterna magna (j)*

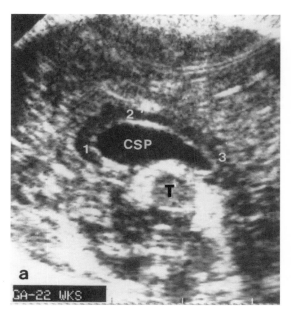
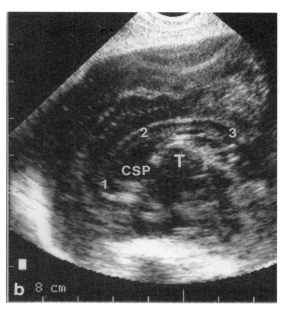

Figure 10 *Median sections of the brain at 22 postmenstrual weeks (a), and at 31 postmenstrual weeks (b). The three parts of the corpus callosum are marked: 1 is the knee, 2 is the trunk and 3 is the tail of the corpus callosum. The thalamus (T) is also seen, covered with a hyperechoic choroid plexus.*

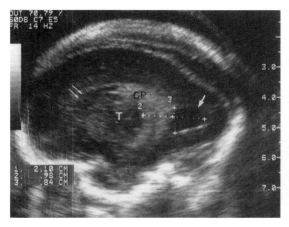

Figure 11 *This is an oblique-1 image of the normal fetal brain at 18 weeks' gestation. The small white arrow points to the posterior horn; the two double arrows point to the anterior horn; the choroid plexus (CP) is seen in the atrium of the lateral ventricle, above and behind the thalamus (T). The measurements seen were performed to study the size of the posterior horn*

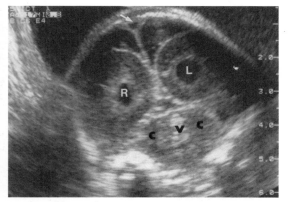

Figure 12 *The occipital-1 section reveals the right (R) and left (L) posterior horns. They are uneven in their size in spite of the fact that this is a perfectly symmetrical section. The infratentorial structures such as the two cerebellar hemispheres (c) and hyperechoic vermis (v) are seen. A horizontal (axial) image of the posterior fossa approached from the area of the occiput, the cisterna magna is seen behind the cerebellar hemispheres, the small arrow points to the fourth ventricle*

of the dura such as the falx and the tentorium are easily recognized. The detection of sulci and gyri is highly dependent upon the temporal development of the cerebral hemispheres, and up to 32–35 weeks only several early-developing and relatively deep sulci and prominent gyri can be detected sonographically. It is also important to state that it is easier to detect these structures

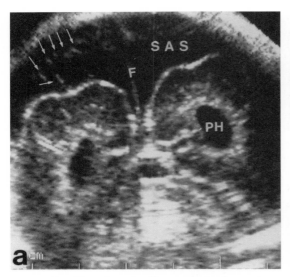

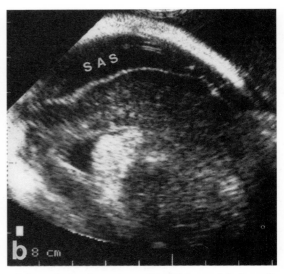

Figure 13 *The subarachnoid space is clearly seen in tangential or other sections. An occipital-1 image (a) shows the occipital or posterior horn (PH), above the brain tissue the falx (F) is seen, partitioning the subarachnoid space (SAS), the transection of arachnoid vessels is marked by multiple small white arrows. Paramedian section (b) highlighting the subarachnoid space (SAS)*

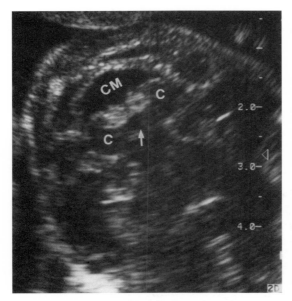

Figure 14 *An occipital-axial approach to the posterior fossa. The cisterna magna (CM) and the cerebellar hemispheres (C) are seen. The arrow points to the fourth ventricle*

sulci, gyri and fissures, this area is still relatively neglected.

Blood vessels of the fetal brain

The blood supply to the brain is well understood and documented. Sonographic studies of blood supply to the brain became feasible when Doppler imaging was developed. The introduction of color Doppler evaluation of vessels and lately the angio-capabilities of the modern ultrasound machines enable the studying of blood vessels with relative ease (Color plate 25).

It is beyond the scope of this review to describe the blood supply to the fetal brain, however, it should be stressed that almost every large vessel supplying the brain, such as the circle of villus at the base of the brain, surrounding the midbrain and its main suppliers such as the anterior, medial and posterior cerebral arteries, and at times their branches, can be imaged. The study of these vessels may become important when space-occupying lesions or vascular malformations are suspected. Only selected and relatively common sonographic fetal brain pathologies will be discussed in this chapter.

on a median section than on any other approach since it is hard to scan the convexity of the hemispheres. Although significant work has been invested in studying the development of

ANOMALIES OF THE FETAL BRAIN

Choroid plexus cysts

Probably the most common and controversial intracranial finding during pregnancy is the fetal choroid plexus cyst (CPC). Their reported incidence ranges from 0.18 to 3.6% of all fetuses scanned during the second trimester. Choroid plexus cysts are fluid-filled cystic spaces. Their sonographic appearance is that of a hypoechoic or sonolucent area(s) within the echogenic choroid plexus[12–20]. They are asymptomatic and benign lesions which usually measure between 3 and 20 mm. They may be unilateral, bilateral or multicystic and as a rule resolve by the mid-trimester (23–24 weeks) of pregnancy[21–26] (Figure 15).

Choroid plexus cysts are usually an isolated finding, but once one is detected a targeted scan should be performed to look for other malformations. Malformations which have been associated with CPC include bowel containing omphalocele, congenital heart disease (ventricular septal defect, hypoplastic left heart, etc.), renal abnormalities (hydronephrosis, multicystic kidneys, etc.), nuchal thickening, cystic hygroma, cleft palate, micrognathia and hydrocephalus[12,20,27]. Some of these malformations can also be associated with chromosomal trisomies (trisomy 18 and 21).

The literature seems to agree that fetuses with a CPC and an associated malformation should undergo genetic counselling and fetal karyotyping[12,20,21]. However, controversy exists in cases of an isolated CPC. Some authors recommend that all pregnant women with a fetal CPC should be offered genetic testing. Others argue that a good structural evaluation in these fetuses can successfully exclude chromosomal aneuploidy. The argument for genetic testing is that the experience, equipment and/or ability of all sonographers or sonologists scanning these patients may not be equally good. Therefore, in some less-experienced hands an associated malformation heralding a possible chromosomal problem may be missed[13,14,19,23,26–30].

Several recent publications have dealt with the risk of a chromosomal abnormality in cases of isolated CPCs. Kupferminc and co-workers[27] reported a series of 98 case of isolated CPC in which four abnormal karyotypes were found among 75 women who elected to have amniocentesis. The abnormal karyotypes were trisomy 21 (three cases) and trisomy 18 (one case). In their study the risk of chromosomal abnormality in cases of isolated choroid plexus cyst was 1 : 25. Gross and associates[20] using a meta-analysis and their own cases calculated the risk of trisomy 18 in cases of isolated choroid plexus to be 1/374. Gonen and colleagues[31] in a study performed to determine the incidence of abnormal karyotypes among fetuses with anomalies detected by sonography found no chromosomal abnormalities among 108 cases of isolated CPC.

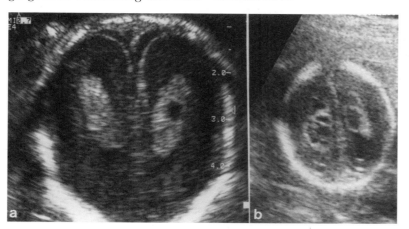

Figure 15 *The choroid plexus. Mid-coronal-3 section (a) at 21 postmenstrual weeks showing a small 3–4 mm choroid plexus cyst on the left side. (b) Bilateral and multiple choroid plexus cyst at 19 postmenstrual weeks*

In conclusion, to date there is no consensus regarding the need for chromosomal studies in cases of an isolated CPC. But in the event of detecting a CPC as well as another anomaly, the literature supports the need to perform a fetal karyotype.

Neural tube defects

Neural tube defects are relatively common anomalies of the central nervous system. In the United States pregnant women are routinely offered screening for neural tube defects using maternal serum α-fetoprotein during the second trimester of pregnancy. As a consequence most neural tube defects are diagnosed as a result of an abnormally elevated α-fetoprotein level during the second trimester of pregnancy. Among the neural tube defects anencephaly and spinal dysraphism are the most common.

Anencephaly

Anencephaly is a lethal condition in which there is complete or partial absence of the fetal cranium. The reported incidence is about 1 case per 1000 births[32–34]. Anencephaly and related disorders are theorized to be complex developmental malformations that primarily affect the production of mesenchyme. This then results in skeletal defects and imperfect fusion of the neural folds[35,36].

Using experimental animals exposed to high doses of Vitamin A the developmental sequence of events leading to anencephaly was first elucidated. Three phases in the development of anencephaly have been described:

(1) *Dysraphia* or a failure of the neural groove to close in the rostral region;

(2) *Exencephaly* or exposure of a well-developed and differentiated brain outside the skull;

(3) Disintegration of the exposed brain during intrauterine development resulting in *anencephaly*[35,37–39].

From studies in human embryos it appears that anencephaly progresses in a similar fashion in humans. The progression of anencephaly from exencephaly has been observed in human fetuses using prenatal sonography[40].

The sonographic appearance of the first-trimester fetus with exencephaly is that of a fetus with an abnormally-wide fetal head. In addition, the exposed brain may contain sonolucent spaces giving the fetal head an appearance similar to that of 'Mickey Mouse'[41]. At the time of delivery the majority of the cases of exencephaly will have the typical anencephalic appearance.

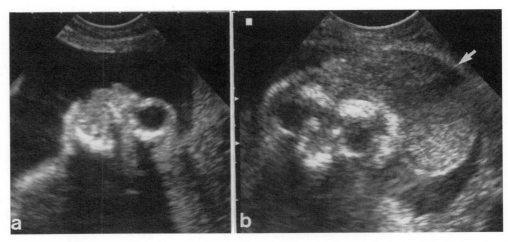

Figure 16 *Anencephalus at 17 postmenstrual weeks. Median section (a) through the face, above the prominent orbits, there is no calvarium. Coronal section (b) showing the orbits above which a soft tissue mass is seen (white arrow), without surrounding bony structure*

The prenatal sonographic appearance of anencephaly during the second and third trimesters is that of a symmetrical, total or partial absence of the cranium above the orbits. There may be variable amounts of 'disintegrating' brain tissue present (Figure 16). The fetal eyes appear prominent giving the anencephalic fetus its typical 'frog's face'. If anencephaly or exencephaly is the result of *amniotic bands* the defect is asymmetric. In addition, multiple amputations of the fingers or toes, as well as defects of the abdominal wall, may also be present. In amniotic bands, the most important sonographic finding is the presence of a band between the fetal defect and the placenta[42,43].

Polyhydramnios may be present in up to 50% of anencephalic pregnancies. Polyhydramnios usually develops during the second half of the pregnancy, probably as a result of decreased fetal swallowing[44-47].

Cephalocele

Cephalocele is a defect of the cranial bones usually along the sutures, through which brain and/or meninges herniate. Encephalocele is the term used when the cephalocele sac contains brain tissue, and meningocele when cerebral spinal fluid (CSF) is present. The reported incidence ranges from 1/3500 to 1/5000 live births[48]. Cephaloceles may involve the occipital, frontal, temporal and parietal regions of the fetal head and their location shows a geographical variation. In Europe and North America, approximately 66–89% of all cephalocele are occipital with the rest distributed equally among the other types. While in Thailand and countries of southern Asia the frontal location is the more common type of cephalocele[49-52].

Occipital cephalocele have been diagnosed as early as 12 weeks' gestation using transvaginal sonography[53,54]. The prenatal sonographic appearance of an occipital cephalocele is that of a sac-like structure adjacent to the fetal head (Figure 17). In approximately 5–24% of cases the fetus may show microcephaly with the biparietal and head circumference significantly smaller than expected[55]. The size of the cephalocele sac may range from a few millimeters to a mass

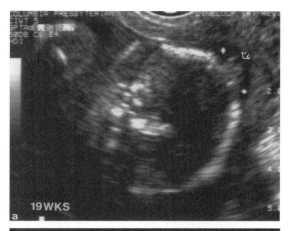

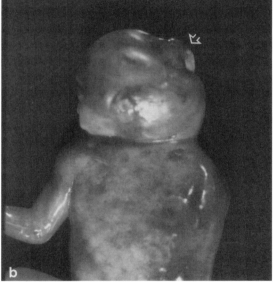

Figure 17 *Occipital cephalocele. Note the protruding brain tissue (open arrow), through the opening created by the bony tissue marked by the solid arrow (a). Specimen showing the posterior cephalocele (b) (open arrow)*

exceeding the size of the normal cranial vault[50]. The brain tissue most often present in the encephalocele sac are the occipital lobes which exhibit a normal gyral pattern.

Other intracranial findings in cases of cephalocele include: hydrocephalus in 20–65% of the cases as a result of aqueductal stenosis or Chiari III malformation; total or partial agenesis of the corpus callosum; agenesis of the septum pellucidum; and cerebellar dysplasia[55-58].

Cephaloceles usually occur as isolated lesions, but in a small percentage of cases may be a part of a non-chromosomal or chromosomal syndrome[59]. Chromosomal syndromes associated with cephaloceles are trisomy 13, 18; mosaic trisomy 20; deletion (13q), (2) (q21→q24); monosomy X; duplication (6) (q21→qter), (7) (pter→p11) and (8) (q23→qter). The non-chromosomal syndromes most commonly associated with a cephalocele are the Meckel–Gruber syndrome (occipital cephalocele, polycystic kidneys and postaxial polydactyly) and Walker–Warburg syndrome (hydrocephalus, agyria, retinal dysplasia, encephalocele).

The prognosis for fetuses with a cephalocele depends on the location, size, content of the lesion and on the concurrent intracranial, as well as extracranial, malformations. Small defects can be easily corrected with surgery, but larger lesions are usually not compatible with life or may result in a neurologically impaired infant[60]. The reported survival for infants with posterior cephalocele ranges from 40 to 75%[58,61–63]. Mortality is most commonly due to the severity of other associated malformation(s) or inability to repair the defect. Meningocele has a lower mortality rate which ranges from 10 to 25%[64]. Disabilities occur in the surviving children.

Spinal dysraphism

Spinal dysraphism is an open lesion with protrusion of the spinal contents through a bony defect. Approximately 10–15% of spinal dysraphic defects are closed and normal skin covers the bony defect. Therefore, in these skin-covered defects the maternal α-fetoprotein level will be normal.

The incidence of spinal dysraphism in the United States is estimated to be between 0.2 and 0.4 per 1000 live births. This reflects a downward trend from the 1970s when the incidence was reported to be of 0.5–0.6 per 1000 live births[65]. The most common site of lesion is in the lumbar region accounting for approximately 80% of the spinal defects, and the least common sites are the cervical and sacral areas[66] (Figure 18).

The 'lemon' and 'banana' signs are two well-established cranial findings, which may aid or facilitate the diagnosis of spinal dysraphism[67,68]. The 'lemon sign' refers to the pressure changes resulting in the deformity of the frontal bones which results in a lemon-shaped axial section of the fetal head (Figure 19). The 'banana sign' refers to the abnormal shape of the cerebellum as it herniates into the foramen magnum obliterating the cisterna magna. Blumenfeld and colleagues[69] reported on the diagnosis of neural tube defects between 12 and 17 weeks by using the 'banana' and 'lemon' signs. In their report they found that the 'lemon' and 'banana' signs may be imaged as early as the 14th week of gestation. But is important to remember that at this early gestational age the findings may be subtle and therefore a follow-up scan later on in the second trimester may be indicated in suspicious or at risk cases.

The 'lemon sign' is present in almost all cases of early developing spinal defects, i.e. 16–24 postmenstrual weeks. After 24 weeks of gestation this sign is a less-reliable marker, and is present in only 13–50% of the fetuses[70–73]. In contrast, the 'banana sign' with obliteration of the cisterna magna is present throughout gestation in 95–100% of the cases[70,73–75]. After 24 weeks cerebellar absence is more commonly seen than the 'banana sign'[73].

The 'normal' fetal spine can be scanned in three planes (sagittal, coronal and transverse planes) from the early second trimester. In the sagittal view the spine appears as two echogenic, parallel lines, flaring towards the upper cervical spine and converging towards the sacrum. Scanning in the coronal plane it appears as two or three parallel bands of echoes corresponding to the body and one in each side of the posterior neural arch. In the transverse plane the intact vertebral arch is represented by a triangular configuration of three echoes, forming a closed circle around the spinal canal[76].

On a transverse section the open or dysraphic spine has a U-shape. On the coronal section the affected bony segment shows a divergent configuration replacing the subsequent normal parallel lines of the normal vertebral arches. The sensitivities for the prenatal sonographic

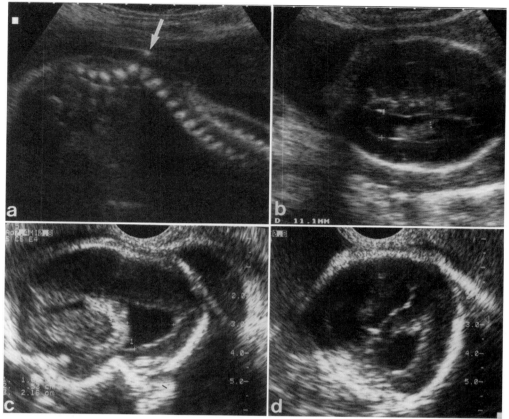

Figure 18 *Lumbosacral spina bifida and meningomyelocele associated with kyphosis and Arnold–Chiari type II malformation. Image (a), the white arrow points to the kyphotic deformity of the spine and the cystic bulge through the area without the vertebral arches. Typical axial image (b) of the brain obtained by transabdominal sonography. Note that hemisphere close to the transducer is blurred. The far hemisphere shows a dilatation of the posterior horn of 11.1 mm. The floating hyperechoic choroid plexus within the ventricle is also seen. Transvaginal oblique-1 section (c) showing the colpocephaly or the dilatation of the posterior horn. The measurements taken clearly show signs of dilatation of the posterior horn. Occipital-1 section (d) depicts the dilatation of the posterior horns*

detection of myelomeningocele are reported to be between 80 and 90% even without having the benefit of knowing that the results of the maternal serum α-fetoprotein are elevated[77–79].

Hydrocephalus is commonly present in cases of spinal dysraphism (i.e. Arnold–Chiari malformation), but other anomalies or malformations, such as microcephaly and agenesis of the corpus callosum, may also be present. In addition, non-central nervous system anomalies, such as congenital scoliosis or kyphosis and hip deformities, may also be present[73,80].

Management of a pregnancy with myelomeningocele should include genetic counselling and karyotyping. Controversy exists regard-ing the best method to deliver fetuses with spinal defects. Luthy and co-workers[81] published a retrospective review of 160 cases of myelomeningocele. Their results showed that those infants delivered by Cesarean section before the onset of labor had a better motor function when compared to infants that were delivered vaginally, or if the Cesarean section was performed after the onset of labor.

Hydrocephalus and ventriculomegaly

Hydrocephalus is defined as a dilatation of the lateral ventricles as a result of an increased amount of CSF. Ventriculomegaly refers to

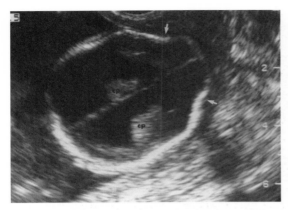

Figure 19 *Arnold–Chiari type II malformation detected early, at around 18 weeks. Note the marked ventriculomegaly and the dangling choroid plexus (cp). Note also the depression of the frontal bones, marked bilaterally by the white arrows. This typical image is called the 'lemon sign'*

dilatation of the fetal lateral ventricles in the presence of normal fetal intraventricular pressures. Since there is no increase in pressure there is no increase in the size of the fetal head. These two terms are (mistakenly) used interchangeably by many sonologists or sonographers.

The reported incidence of hydrocephalus ranges from 0.5 to 3 per 1000 live births[82]. Ventriculomegaly as well as hydrocephalus is usually bilateral, although unilateral hydrocephalus can rarely affect the fetus[83,84].

Fetal or neonatal hydrocephalus may be *non-communicating* or *communicating*. In communicating hydrocephalus the obstruction to the flow of CSF is extraventricular, at the level of the subarachnoid space. In the non-communicating form the obstruction to the flow of CSF occurs outside the ventricular system. The most common etiologies of hydrocephalus are aqueductal stenosis (33–43% of all cases), myelomeningocele with Arnold–Chiari malformation (approximately 28%), communicating hydrocephalus (22–38%), Dandy–Walker malformation (7–13%) and other pathologies such as agenesis of the corpus callosum (6–10%)[85–88].

Aqueductal stenosis is characterized by a lesion obstructing the flow of CSF through the cerebral aqueduct. Approximately 1–2% of all cases

may be inherited as an X-linked disorder affecting males and transmitted through female carriers[89,90]. The prenatal diagnosis of X-linked hydrocephalus has been made based on the presence of ventriculomegaly (lateral and third ventricle) in male fetuses in women who are suspected to be carriers. In addition, adducted thumb(s) have been found to be present in up to 44% of cases of X-linked hydrocephaly[91]. Prenatal diagnosis of aqueductal stenosis may not be possible early in the second trimester due to the fact that ventriculomegaly and/or hydrocephalus may only become evident later on in pregnancy or early infancy[90]. In cases of X-linked aqueductal stenosis the hydrocephalus is severe, there is a high rate of stillbirths and perinatal mortality, and the survivors show significant neurological impairment[92].

The fetal lateral ventricles can be assessed by sonography in a quantitative as well as a qualitative way. Several nomograms to assess the degree of ventriculomegaly by transabdominal sonography employing an axial plane, have been published and widely accepted[93–99]. Using transvaginal sonography, we have developed and published nomograms of the fetal lateral ventricles. In these nomograms the measurements were obtained from sections in the sagittal or coronal plane[100,101].

During the development of ventriculomegaly or hydrocephalus two changes in the shape of the lateral ventricles occur early: dilatation of the posterior horn of the lateral ventricle and compression of the choroid plexus[97,101–107]. Using the transvaginal sonography derived nomograms these changes can be quantified.

Qualitatively the presence of hydrocephalus or ventriculomegaly can be determined by visual observation of the lateral ventricles. This usually entails sonographer and/or sonologist experience; a less-experienced operator may miss a subtle case. Morphological changes suggestive of hydrocephalus are:

(1) The presence of dilated anterior horns in a 'frontal-1' section;

(2) Progressive rounding and bulging of the superior and lateral aspects of the frontal

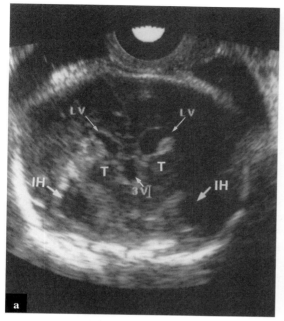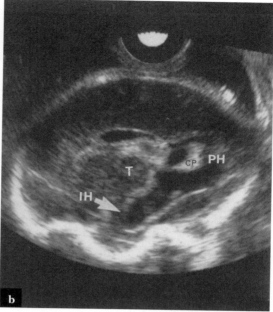

Figure 20 *Ventriculomegaly. Mid-coronal-2 section (a) through the lateral ventricles (LV), within which the hyperechoic choroid plexus is seen. Between the thalami (T) the unusually dilated third ventricle is evident. The ventriculomegaly is significant enough to dilate the inferior horns (IH). Oblique-1 section (b) through the lateral ventricular system. The posterior and inferior horns (PH and IH) are evident. The choroid plexus (CP) is also seen in the atrium, behind the thalamus (T). Note that this section contains the anterior (AH), posterior and inferior horns, attesting to a true ventriculomegaly. On the normal oblique-1 image, the inferior horn is not visible*

horns (resembling an inverted 'teardrop') in the 'mid-coronal-1' section;

(3) On an oblique-1 section imaging all three parts of the lateral ventricle;

(4) A 'dangling' and compressed choroid plexus within the dilated ventricle; and

(5) Dilated third ventricle (Figure 20).

Prenatal diagnosis of hydrocephalus should trigger a careful search for associates anomalies. In approximately 70–83% of the cases presenting with fetal hydrocephalus other anomalies are present[107–111]. Of these anomalies approximately 40% are intracranial, the balance being extracranial[107,112]. In addition, chromosomal abnormalities, such as trisomies 13 and 18, have been reported in 4.2–28.6% of cases of fetal hydrocephalus[108,109,111,112]. Fetuses with isolated ventriculomegaly have a good prognosis with up to 63% being normal and the rest having mild to severe mental and motor developmental delay[113]. In summary, the prognosis for the fetus with hydrocephalus depends on the presence or absence of associated anomalies or abnormal karyotype. A worse outcome can be expected for those fetuses with other and more severe associated anomalies[96]. Abnormal amniotic fluid volume may complicate the pregnancy with fetal hydrocephalus. Polyhydramnios may be present in up to 30% of cases[114] and oligohydramnios in 21–23% of cases[96,97].

Holoprosencephaly

Holoprosencephaly is a malformation sequence which results from failure of the prosencephalon to differentiate into the cerebral hemispheres and lateral ventricles. It occurs between the 4th and 8th weeks of gestation. The incidence of holoprosencephaly in abortuses has been reported to be 0.4 per 1000 with a lower incidence in live births of 0.06 per 1000[115]. Holoprosencephaly can be further divided into

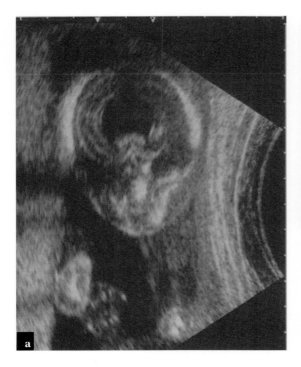

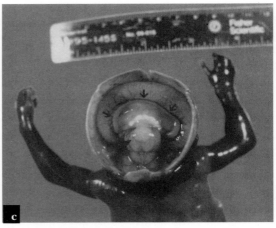

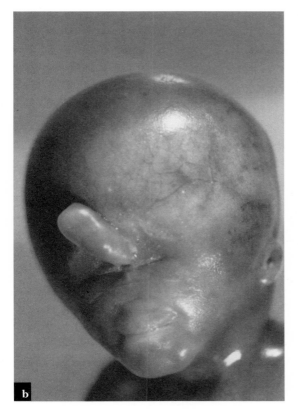

Figure 21 *Alobar holoprosencephaly is relatively easy to detect since there is a single ventricular cavity and absence of the midline structures and fused thalami. Coronal section (a) showing the lack of falx and the fused thalami on top of which the choroid plexus is seen. A close-up (b) of the specimen showing cyclopia. Note that the proboscis is located above the almost fused orbits. The calvarium is removed (c) demonstrating alobar holoprosencephaly. Note there is a single ventricular cavity (arrows), fused thalami (arrowhead), and no falx, corpus callosum or cavum septum pellucidum is seen*

three types: *alobar, semilobar* and *lobar*, depending on the degree of failed differentiation. In conjunction with the brain malformation, variable degrees of facial dysmorphism such as cyclopia, ethmocephaly, cebocephaly, hypertelorism and other midline facial defects may be present[33,115–117].

Alobar holoprosencephaly is the most severe type of the holoprosencephalies. In this anomaly there is a single lateral ventricle, small cerebrum, fused thalami, agenesis of the corpus callosum and falx cerebri[118]. Sonographic findings of alobar holoprosencephaly in the mid-coronal plane include absence of midline structures (falx cerebri, interhemispheric fissure, agenesis of the corpus callosum and cavum septum pellucidum), monoventricular cavity with communicating dorsal cyst, fused thalami and facial dysmorphism. The most severe facial dysmorphism occurs with alobar holoprosencephaly[119] (Figure 21).

In semilobar holoprosencephaly, some degree of cleavage of the brain has occurred. The ventricles and the cerebral hemispheres are partially separated posteriorly, there is incomplete separation of the thalami, but anteriorly a single ventricular cavity is present[118]. The prenatal sonographic findings in the mid-coronal section include the presence of the interhemispheric fissure, and fused frontal horns with a flat roof which communicate freely with the third ventricle; agenesis of the septum pellucidum is a consistent finding, but the corpus callosum may or may not be present, and there may be midline fusion of the cingulate gyrus.

In lobar holoprosencephaly the hemispheres are separated, except in the anterior portion. There is agenesis of the cavum septum pellucidum, although the corpus callosum may be present, hypoplastic or absent. Pilu and co-workers[120] have described an echogenic linear structure running within the third ventricle as a specific sign of fetal lobar holoprosencephaly. This echogenic structure in the mid-coronal plane appears as a small round solid structure approximately in the mid-portion of the third ventricle. This structure is believed to demonstrate abnormally fused fornices in the midline.

Infections affecting the CNS: cytomegalovirus and toxoplasmosis

Cytomegalovirus (CMV) infection is the most common infection affecting the developing human fetus. It is estimated that approximately 3000–4000 infants are born each year with the symptomatic disease and an additional 30 000–40 000 with the asymptomatic disease[121]. Fetal infection can result from a primary maternal infection, reinfection or from a reactivation of a latent infection. Maternal primary infection during pregnancy may be asymptomatic, but it results in a 30–40% risk of intrauterine transmission. The prognosis for the fetus is worse if infection occurs in the first trimester[122]. Diagnosis of primary disease during pregnancy can be made by documenting seroconversion or the presence of CMV specific IgM antibodies[123].

The typical sonographic findings in fetuses with CMV are bilateral periventricular hyperechogenicities (calcifications)[124,125] (Figure 22). Although these 'calcifications' or hyperechoic foci can be highly reflective they may not cast an acoustic shadow[126]. Estroff and associates[127] first reported on branching linear echogenic areas in the thalami of a fetus with CMV (Figure 22b). These branching echogenic structures correspond to arteries in the basal ganglia and thalamus[128]. Other cranial sonographic findings in fetal CMV include microcephaly, hydrocephalus, cerebellar hypoplasia, large cisterna magna, lissencephaly, paraventricular cysts and ischemic destructive lesions such as porencephaly, hydranencephaly and polymicrogyria[129–137].

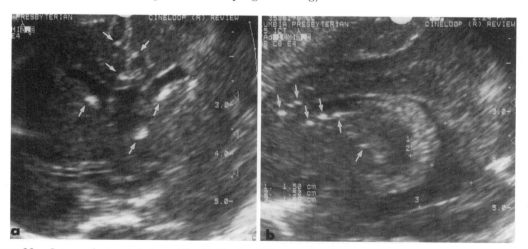

Figure 22 *Cytomegalovirus infection of the fetal brain. Mid-coronal section (a) showing highly-echogenic foci (arrows) around the ventricles and the cavum septum pellucidum. An oblique-1 section (b) with the same highly echogenic foci (arrows) attributed to cytomegalovirus infection*

The prognosis for the infant relates to the severity of the intracranial abnormalities. Approximately 95% of the infants with microcephaly and intracranial 'calcifications' will either die or exhibit major neurological sequelae such as developmental delay, seizures, deafness and motor deficits. Infants with 'milder' neurological signs have a better prognosis[138,139].

Prenatal diagnosis of fetal cytomegalovirus infection relies on a combination of diagnostic tests. Sonography may pick up fetuses with intracranial 'calcifications', hydrocephalus, microcephaly, ascites and intrauterine growth retardation. Amniotic fluid studies for either viral culture or a polymerase chain reaction (PCR) to amplify CMV DNA are, at present, the best methods used to make the diagnosis[140]. Unfortunately, at present no drug therapy is available to treat fetal cytomegalovirus infection.

Toxoplasmosis is the result of a transplacental infection with the parasite *Toxoplasma gondii*. The most common source of infection in the human is the domesticated cat, or the ingestion or handling of contaminated meat. The incidence of congenital toxoplasmosis ranges from 0.5 to 2.0 per 1000 live births[141–143]. The risk of fetal infection is dependent upon when during the pregnancy the primary maternal infection took place. The overall risk of transmission to the fetus is approximately 40%[144]. Similarly to CMV the severity of the fetal disease is dependent upon when in gestation the primary maternal infection takes place. Infection during the first and second trimester results in approximately 20–25% of fetuses becoming infected while infection during the third trimester results in infection in up to 65%[145–147]. However, the severity of the disease decreases from approximately 75% severe infection in the first trimester to 0% in the third trimester[148]. The diagnosis of maternal primary disease is made based upon documentation of seroconversion, a marked increase in antibody titers, or the presence of toxoplasmosis specific IgM[129].

The intracranial sonographic findings of fetal toxoplasmosis include intracranial hyperechogenic foci or 'calcifications', hydro-cephalus, microcephaly, brain atrophy and hydranencephaly[149]. The intracranial 'calcifications' in fetal toxoplasmosis are multifocal and are present in many areas of the brain such as the basal ganglia, periventricular area, and white matter and cerebral cortex[149,150]. Prenatal diagnosis of fetal toxoplasmosis has relied on sonography to look for intracranial 'calcifications' and hydrocephalus as well as on amniocentesis. Amniotic fluid is obtained for tissue culture, and inoculation of mice or for testing using polymerase chain reaction and fetal-blood sampling for the determination of toxoplasmosis specific IgM[151].

Fetal therapy includes the treatment of the mother with spiramycin in cases of primary infection during the pregnancy. But once fetal infection has been documented a combination of pyrimethamine, sulfadiazine and folinic acid is recommended[145,152–156].

The prognosis for the fetus and subsequent neonate affected with toxoplasmosis relates to the severity of the neuropathology. Only 9% of neonates with severe neurological features are normal on follow-up. The remainder suffer from mental retardation, seizures, spastic motor deficits and severe visual impairment[145].

For a more comprehensive description of the normal and abnormal prenatal brain the interested reader is referred to other texts dedicated to this matter[157,158].

SUMMARY

Fetal neurosonography is based upon the knowledge of the appearance of the normal and developing fetal brain. As technology improves, our understanding of the neuroanatomy of the fetal and neonatal brain widens and the distinction between normal and abnormal becomes increasingly feasible.

It is, therefore, our view that neuroscanning should rely on the liberal use of the high-frequency transvaginal probes as well as the newly-proposed scanning planes which emulate the neonatal scan.

References

1. Kossoff, G., Griffith, K. A. and Dixon, C. E. (1991). Is the quality of transvaginal images superior to transabdominal ones under matched conditions? *Ultrasound Obstet. Gynecol.*, **1**, 29–35

2. Timor-Tritsch, I. E., Farine, D. and Rosen, M. G. (1988). A close look at early embryonic development with the high-frequency transvaginal transducer. *Am. J. Obstet. Gynecol.*, **159**, 676–81

3. Timor-Tritsch, I. E., Monteagudo, A. and Warren, W. B. (1991) Transvaginal ultrasonographic definition of the central nervous system in the first and early second trimesters. *Am. J. Obstet. Gynecol.*, **164**, 747–53

4. Monteagudo, A., Reuss, M. L. and Timor-Tritsch, I. E. (1991). Imaging the fetal brain in the second and third trimesters using transvaginal sonography. *Obstet. Gynecol.*, **77**, 27–32

5. Timor-Tritsch, I. E. and Monteagudo, A. (1991). Transvaginal sonographic evaluation of the fetal central nervous system. *Obstet. Gynecol. Clin. North Am.*, **18**, 713–48

6. Achiron, R. and Achiron, A. (1991). Transvaginal ultrasonic assessment of the early fetal brain. *Ultrasound Obstet. Gynecol.*, **1**, 336–44

7. Monteagudo, A., Timor-Tritsch, I. E., Reuss, M. L. and Rosen, M. G. (1990). Transvaginal sonography of the second- and third-trimester fetal brain. In Timor-Tritsch, I. E. and Rottem, S., (eds.) *Transvaginal Sonography*, 2nd edn., pp. 393–425. (New York: Elsevier)

8. Monteagudo, A., Timor-Tritsch, I. E. and Moomjy, M. (1993). Nomograms of the fetal lateral ventricles using transvaginal sonography. *J. Ultrasound Med.*, **5**, 265–9

9. Kushnir, U., Shalev, J., Bronshtein, M. *et al.* (1989). Fetal intracranial anatomy in the first trimester of pregnancy: transvaginal ultrasonographic evaluation. *Neuroradiology*, **32**, 222–5

10. Blaas, H. G., Eik-Nes, S. H., Kiserud, T. *et al.* (1994). Early development of the forebrain and midbrain: a longitudinal ultrasound study from 7 to 12 postmenstrual weeks of gestation. *Ultrasound Obstet. Gynecol.*, **4**, 183–92

11. Blaas, H. G., Eik-Nes, S. H., Kiserud, T. *et al.* (1995). Early development of the hindbrain: a longitudinal ultrasound study from 7 to 12 weeks of gestation. *Ultrasound Obstet. Gynecol.*, **5**, 151–60

12. Nadel, A. S., Bromley, B. S., Frigoletto, F. D., Estroff, J. A. and Benacerraf, B. R. (1992). Isolated choroid plexus cysts in the second-

trimester fetus: is amniocentesis really indicated? *Radiology*, **185**, 545–8

13. Gabrielli, S., Reece, E. A., Pilu, G. *et al.* (1989). The clinical significance of prenatally diagnosed choroid plexus cysts. *Am. J. Obstet. Gynecol.*, **160**, 1207–10

14. Achiron, R., Barkai, G., Katznelson, B. and Mashiach, S. (1991). Fetal lateral ventricle choroid plexus cysts: the dilemma of amniocentesis. *Obstet. Gynecol.*, **78**, 815–18

15. Chinn, D. H., Miller, E. I., Worthy, L. M. and Towers, C. V. (1991). Sonographically detected fetal choroid plexus cysts: frequency and association with aneuploidy. *J. Ultrasound Med.*, **10**, 255–8

16. Clark, S. L., De Vore, G. R. and Sabey, P. L. (1988). Prenatal diagnosis of cysts of the fetal choroid plexus. *Obstet. Gynecol.*, **72**, 585–7

17. Chan, L., Hixson, J. L., Laifer, S. A. *et al.* (1989). A sonographic and karyotypic study of second-trimester fetal choroid plexus cysts. *Obstet. Gynecol.*, **73**, 703–6

18. De Roo, T. R., Harris, R. D., Sargent, S. K., Denholm, T. A. and Crow, H. C. (1988). Fetal choroid plexus cysts: prevalence, clinical significance, and sonographic appearance. *Am. J. Roentgenol.* **151**, 1179–81

19. Chitkara, U., Cogswell, C., Norton, K., Wilkins, I. A., Mehalek, K. and Berkowitz, R. L. (1988). Choroid plexus cysts in the fetus: a benign anatomic variant or pathologic entity? *Obstet. Gynecol.*, **72**, 185–9

20. Gross, S. J., Shulman, L. P., Tolley, E. A., Emerson, D. S., Felker, R. E., Simpson, J L. and Elias, S. (1995). Isolated fetal choroid plexus cysts and trisomy 18: a review and meta-analysis. *Am. J. Obstet. Gynecol.*, **172**, 83–7

21. Benacerraf, B. R., Harlow, B. and Frigoletto, F. D. (1990). Are choroid plexus cysts an indication for second-trimester amniocentesis? *Am. J. Obstet. Gynecol.*, **162**, 1001–6

22. Benacerraf, B. R. and Laboda, A. (1989). Cyst of the fetal choroid plexus: a normal variant? *Am. J. Obstet. Gynecol.*, **160**, 319–21

23. Hertzberg, B. S., Kay, H. H. and Bowie, J. D. (1989). Fetal choroid plexus lesions. Relationship of antenatal sonographic appearance to clinical outcome. *J. Ultrasound Med.*, **8**, 77–82

24. Farhood, A. I., Morris, J. H. and Bieber, F. R. (1987). Transient cysts of the fetal choroid plexus: morphology and histogenesis. *Am. J. Med. Genet.*, **27**, 977–82

25. Nicolaides, K. H., Rodeck, C. H. and Godsen, C. M. (1986). Rapid karyotyping in non-lethal fetal malformations. *Lancet*, **1**, 283–6

26. Fitzsimmons, J., Wilson, D., Pascoe-Mason, J. *et al.* (1989). Choroid plexus cysts in fetuses with trisomy 18. *Obstet. Gynecol*, **73**, 257–60

27. Kuperminc, M. J., Tamura, R. K., Sabbagha, R. E. *et al.* (1994). Isolated choroid plexus cyst(s): an indication for amniocentesis. *Am. J. Obstet. Gynecol.*, **171**, 1068–71

28. Porto, M., Murata, Y., Warneke, L. A. *et al.* (1993). Fetal choroid plexus cysts: an independent risk factor for chromosomal anomalies. *J. Clin. Ultrasound*, **21**, 103–8

29. Perpignano, M. C., Cohen, H. L., Klein, V. R. *et al.* (1992). Fetal choroid plexus cysts: beware the smaller cyst. *Radiology*, **182**, 715–17

30. Platt, L. D., Carlson, D. E., Medearis, A. L. and Walla, C. A. (1991). Fetal choroid plexus in the second trimester of pregnancy: a cause for concern. *Am. J. Obstet. Gynecol.*, **164**, 1652–6

31. Gonen, R., Dar, H. and Degani, S. (1995). The karyotype of fetuses with anomalies detected by second trimester ultrasonography. *Eur. J. Obstet. Gynecol. Biol.*, **58**, 153–5

32. Cunningham, M. E. and Walls, W. J. (1976). Ultrasound in the evaluation of anencephaly. *Radiology*, **118**, 165–7

33. Icenogle, D. A. and Kaplan, A. M. (1981). A review of congenital neurologic malformations. *Clin. Pediatr.*, **9**, 565–76

34. Limb, J. and Holmes, L. B. (1994). Anencephaly: changes in prenatal detection and birth status, 1972 through 1990. *Am. J. Obstet. Gynecol.*, **170**, 1333–8

35. O'Rahilly, R. and Müller, F. (1992). The nervous system. In *Human Embryology and Teratology*, pp.285–6. (New York: Wiley-Liss)

36. Marin-Padilla, M. (1991). Cephalic axial skeletal-neural dysraphia disorders: embryology and pathology. *Can. J. Neurol. Sci.*, **18**, 153–69

37. O'Rahilly, R. and Müller, F. (1994). *The Embryonic Human Brain. An Atlas of Developmental Stages.* (New York: Wiley-Liss)

38. Müller, F. and O'Rahilly, R. (1984). Cerebral dysraphia (future anencephaly) in a human twin embryo at stage 13. *Teratology*, **30**, 167–77

39. Müller, F. and O'Rahilly, R. (1991). Development of anencephaly and its variants. *Am. J. Anat.*, **190**, 193–218

40. Bronshtein, M. and Ornoy, A. (1991). Acrania: anencephaly resulting from secondary degeneration of a closed neural tube: two cases in the same family. *J. Clin. Ultrasound*, **19**, 230–4

41. Nishi, T. and Nakano, R. (1994). First-trimester diagnosis of exencephaly by transvaginal ultrasonography. *J. Ultrasound Med.*, **13**, 149–51

42. Mahoney, B. S., Filly, R., Callem, P. W. and Golbus, M. S. (1985). The amniotic band syndrome: antenatal sonographic diagnosis and potential pitfall. *Am. J. Obstet. Gynecol.*, **152**, 63–8

43. Casellas, M., Ferrer, M., Rovira, M., Pla, F., Marinez, M. A. and Cabero, L. (1991). Prenatal diagnosis of exencephaly. *Prenat. Diagn.*, **13**, 417–22

44. Johnson, A., Losure, T. A. and Weiner, S. (1985). Early diagnosis of fetal anencephaly. *J. Clin. Ultrasound*, **13**, 503

45. Pretorius, D. H., Reuss, P. D., Rumack, C. M. and Manco-Johnson, M. L. (1986). Diagnosis of brain neuropathology *in utero*. *Neuroradiology*, **28**, 386–97

46. Moore, K. L. (1988). *The Developing Human. Clinically Oriented Embryology*, pp.364–401. (Philadelphia: WB Saunders Company)

47. Salamanca, A., Gonzalez-Gomez, F., Padilla, M. S., Sabatel, R. M., Camra, M. and Cuadros, J. L. (1992). Prenatal ultrasound semiography of anencephaly: sonographic-pathological correlations. *Ultrasound Obstet. Gynecol.*, **2**, 95–100

48. Harley, E. H. (1991). Pediatric nasal masses. *Ear-Nose-Throat J.*, **70**, 28–32

49. Chervenak, F. A., Isaacson, G., Mahoney, M. J. *et al.* (1984). Diagnosis and management of fetal cephalocele. *Obstet. Gynecol.*, **64**, 86–90

50. McLaurin, R. L. (1987). Encephalocele and cranium bifidum. In *Handbook of Clinical Neurology. Malformations*, Vol. 6 (50), pp.97–111. (Amsterdam: Elsevier Science Publishers)

51. Nyberg, D. A., Hallesy, D., Mahoney, B. S. *et al.* (1990). Meckel–Gruber syndrome. Importance of prenatal diagnosis. *J. Ultrasound Med.*, **9**, 691–6

52. Monteagudo, A. and Timor-Tritsch, I. E. (1992). Cephalocele, anterior. *Fetus*, **2**, 1–4

53. Fleming, A. D., Vintzileos, A. M. and Scorza, W. E. (1991). Prenatal diagnosis of occipital encephalocele with transvaginal sonography. *J. Ultrasound Med.*, **10**, 285–6

54. Bronshtein, M., Timor-Tritsch, I. E. and Rottem, S. (1991). Early detection of fetal anomalies. In Timor-Tritsch, I. E. and Rottem, S. (eds.) *Transvaginal Sonography*, pp.327–71. (New York: Chapman & Hall)

55. Naidich, T. P., Altman, N. R., Braffman, B. H., McLone, D. G. and Zimmerman, R. A. (1992). Cephaloceles and related malformations. *Am. J. Neuroradiology*, **13**, 655–90

56. Pretorius, D. H., Reuss, P. D., Rumack, C. M. and Manco-Johnson, M. L. (1986). Diagnosis of brain neuropathology *in utero*. *Neuroradiology*, **28**, 386–97

57. Fiske, E. C. and Filly, R. A. (1982). Ultrasound evaluation of the abnormal fetal neural axis. *Radiol. Clin. North Am.*, **20**, 285–96

58. Simpson, D. A., David, D. J. and White, J. (1984). Cephalocele: treatment, outcome and antenatal diagnosis. *Neurosurgery*, **15**, 14–21

59. Hunter, A. G. (1993). Brain and spinal cord. In Stevenson, R. E., Hall, J. G. and Goodman, R. M. (eds.) *Human Malformations and Related Anomalies*, Vol. II, pp.109–37. (New York: Oxford University Press)

60. Sarnat, H. B. and Mueller, D. L. (1990). Fetal neurology. In Eden, R. D., Boehm, F. H. and Haire, M. (eds.) *Assessment and Care of the Fetus. Physiological, Clinical, and Medicolegal Principles*, pp.43–67. (Norwalk: Appleton & Lange)

61. Lorber, J. (1967). The prognosis of occipital encephalocele. *Dev. Med. Child Neurol.*, **9** (Suppl. b), 75–86

62. Lorber, J. and Schofield, J. K. (1979). The prognosis of occipital encephalocele. *Z. Kinderchir.*, **28**, 347–51

63. Mealey, J., Dzenitis, A. J. and Hockey, A. A. (1970). The prognosis of encephalocele. *J. Neurosurg.*, **32**, 209–18

64. Brown, M. S. and Sheridan-Pereira, M. (1992). Outlook for the child with a cephalocele. *Pediatrics*, 90, 914–19

65. Yen, I. H., Khoury, M. J., Erickson, J. D. *et al.* (1992). The changing epidemiology of neural tube defects – United States, 1968–1989. *Am. J. Dis. Child.*, **146**, 857–61

66. Welch, K. and Winston, K. R. (1987). Spina bifida. In Myrianthopoulos, N. C. (ed.) *Handbook of Clinical Neurology*. Malformations. Vol. 6. (50), pp. 477–508 (Amsterdam: Elsevier Science)

67. Nicolaides, K. H., Gabbe, S. G., Guidetti, R. *et al.* (1986). Ultrasound screening for spina bifida: cranial and cerebellar signs. *Lancet*, **2**, 72–4

68. Campbell, J., Gilbert, W. M., Nicolaides, K. H. and Campbell, S. (1987). Ultrasound screening for spina bifida: cranial and cerebellar signs in a high risk population. *Obstet. Gynecol.*, **70**, 247–50

69. Blumenfeld, Z., Siegler, E. and Bronshtein, M. (1993). The early diagnosis of neural tube defects. *Prenat. Diagn.*, **13**, 863–71

70. Thiagarajah, S., Henke, J., Hogge, W. A., Abbitt, P. L., Breeden, N. and Ferguson, J. E. (1990). Early diagnosis of spina bifida: the value of cranial ultrasound markers. *Obstet. Gynecol.*, **76** 54–7

71. Nyberg, D. A., Mack, L. A., Hirsch, J. and Mahoney, B. S. (1988). Abnormalities of fetal cranial contour in sonographic detection of spina bifida: evaluation of the 'lemon' sign. *Radiology*, **167**, 387–92

72. Penso, C., Redline, R. W. and Benacerraf, B. R. (1987). A sonographic sign which predicts which fetuses with hydrocephalus have an associated neural tube defect. *J. Ultrasound Med.*, **6**, 307–11

73. Van den Hof, M. C., Nicolaides, K. H., Campbell, J. and Campbell, S. (1990). Evaluation of the lemon and banana signs in one hundred thirty fetuses with open spina bifida. *Am. J. Obstet. Gynecol.*, **162**, 322–7

74. Goldstein, R. B., Podrasky, A. E., Filly, R. A. and Callen, P. A. (1989). Effacement of the fetal cisterna magna in association with myelomeningocele. *Radiology*, 172, 409–13

75. Pilu, G., Romero, R., Reece, A., Goldstein, I., Hobbins, J. and Bovicelli, L. (1988). Subnormal cerebellum in fetuses with spina bifida. *Am. J. Obstet. Gynecol.*, **158**, 1052–6

76. Sarnat, H. B. and Mueller, D. L. (1990). Fetal neurology. In Eden, R. D. and Boehm, F. H. (eds.) *Assessment and Care of the Fetus. Physiological, Clinical, and Medicolegal Principles.* pp.43–67. (Norwalk: Appleton & Lange)

77. Main, D. M. and Mennuti, M. T. (1986). Neural tube defects: issues in prenatal diagnosis and counseling. *Obstet. Gynecol.*, **67**, 1–16

78. Thornton, J. G., Lilford, R. J. and Newcomb, R. G. (1991). Tables for estimation of individual risks of fetal neural tube and ventral wall defects, incorporating prior probability, maternal serum alpha-fetoprotein levels, and ultrasonographic examination results. *Am. J. Obstet. Gynecol.*, **164**, 154–60

79. Hogge, W. A., Thiagarajah, S., Fergunson, J. E., Schnatterly, P. T. and Harbert, G. M. Jr (1989). The role of ultrasonography and amniocentesis in the evaluation of pregnancies at risk of neural tube defects. *Am. J. Obstet. Gynecol.*, **161**, 520–4

80. Osborn, A. G. (1994). *Diagnostic Neuroradiology. Normal Anatomy and Congenital Anomalies of the Spine and Spinal Cord.* pp.799–807. (St Louis:Mosby-Year Book)

81. Luthy, D. A., Wardinsky, T., Shurtleff, D. B. *et al.* (1991). Cesarean section before the onset of labor and subsequent motor function in infants with myelomeningocele diagnosed antenatally. *N. Engl. J. Med.*, **324**, 662–6

82. Habib, Z. (1981). Genetics and genetic counselling in neonatal hydrocephalus. *Obstet. Gynecol. Surv.*, **36**, 529

83. Patten, R. M., Mack, L. A. and Finberg, H. J. (1991). Unilateral hydrocephalus: prenatal sonographic diagnosis. *Am. J. Roentgenol.*, **156**, 359–63

84. Chari, R., Bhargava, R., Hammond, I. *et al.* (1993). Antenatal unilateral hydrocephalus. *Can. Assoc. Radiol. J.*, **44**, 57–9

85. Volpe, J. J. (1995). *Neurology of the Newborn*, 3rd edn. pp.3–42. (Philadelphia:W. B. Saunders Company)

86. Mealy, J. Jr, Gilmor, R. L. and Bubb, M. P. (1973). The prognosis of hydrocephalus overt at birth. *J. Neurosurg.*, **39**, 348–55

87. McCollough, D. C. and Balzer-Martin, L. A. (1982). Current prognosis in overt neonatal hydrocephalus. *J. Neurosurg.*, **57**, 378–83

88. Burton, B. K. (1979). Recurrence risks for congenital hydrocephalus. *Clin. Genet.*, **16**, 47

89. Milhorat, T. H. (1987). Hydrocephaly. In Myrianthopoulos, N. C. (ed.) *Handbook of Clinical Neurology. Malformations*, Vol.50 (6), pp.285–300. (Amsterdam: Elsevier Science)

90. Bickers, D. S. and Adams, R. D. (1949). Hereditary stenosis of the aqueduct of Sylvius as a cause of congenital hydrocephalus. *Brain*, **72**, 246–62

91. Brocard, O., Ragage, C., Vilbert, M., Cassier, T., Kowalski, S. and Ragage, J. P. (1993). Prenatal diagnosis of X-linked hydrocephalus. *J. Clin. Ultrasound*, **21**, 211–14

92. Hunter, A. G. (1993). Brain: hydrocephalus. In Stevenson, R. E., Hall, J. G. and Goodman, R. M. (eds.) *Human Malformations and Related Anomalies*, Vol. II, pp.62–73. (New York: Oxford University Press)

93. Jeanty, P., Dramaix-Wilmet, M., Delbeke, D. *et al.* (1981). Ultrasonic evaluation of fetal ventricular growth. *Neuroradiology*, **21**, 127–31

94. Pretorius, D. H., Drose, J. A. and Manco-Johnson, M. L. (1986). Fetal lateral ventricular ratio determination during the second trimester. *J. Ultrasound Med.*, **5**, 121–4

95. Cardoza, J. D., Goldstein, R. B. and Filly, R. A. (1988). Exclusion of fetal ventriculomegaly with a single measurement of the width of the lateral ventricular atrium. *Radiologu*, **169**, 711–14

96. Pilu, G., Reece, E. A., Goldstein, I. *et al.* (1989). Sonographic evaluation of the normal development anatomy of the fetal cerebral ventricles. II. The atria. *Obstet. Gynecol.*, **73**, 250–5

97. Siedler, D. E. and Filly, R. A. (1987). Relative growth of higher fetal brain structures. *J. Ultrasound Med.*, **6**, 573–6

98. Denkhaus, H. and Winsberg, F. (1979). Ultrasonic measurement of the fetal ventricular system. *Radiolgy*, **131**, 781–7

99. Johnson, M. L., Dunne, M. G., Mack, L. A. *et al.* (1980). Evaluation of fetal intracranial anatomy by static and real-time ultrasound. *J. Clin. Ultrasound*, **8**, 311–18

100. Monteagudo, A., Timor-Tritsch, I. E. and Moomjy, M. (1993). Nomograms of the fetal lateral ventricles using transvaginal sonography. *J. Ultrasound Med.*, **5**, 265–9

101. Monteagudo, A., Timor-Tritsch, I. E. and Moomjy, M. (1994). *In utero* detection of ventriculomegaly during the second and third trimesters by transvaginal sonography. *Ultrasound Obstet. Gynecol.*, **4**, 193–8

102. Epstein, F., Naidich, T., Kricheff, I. *et al.* (1977). Role of computerized axial tomography in diagnosis, treatment and follow-up of hydrocephalus. *Child's Brain*, **3**, 91–100

103. Fiske, E. C. and Filly, R. A. (1982). Ultrasound evaluation of the abnormal fetal neural axis. *Radiol. Clin. North Am.*, **20**, 285–96

104. Benacerraf, B. R. and Birnholz, J. C. (1987). The diagnosis of fetal hydrocephalus prior to 22 weeks. *J. Clin. Ultrasound*, **15**, 531–6

105. Bronshtein, M. and Ben-Shlomo, I. (1991). Choroid plexus dysmorphism: a sonographic sign of fetal hydrocephalus. *J. Clin. Ultrasound*, **19**, 547–53

106. Chinn, D. H., Callen, P. W. and Filly, R. A. (1983). The lateral cerebral ventricle in early second trimester. *Radiology*, **148**, 529–31

107. Drugan, A., Krause, B., Canady, A., Zador, I. E., Sacks, A. J. and Evans, M. I. (1989). The natural history of prenatally diagnosed cerebral ventriculomegaly. *J. Am. Med. Assoc.*, **261**, 1785–8

108. Pretorius, D. H., Davis, K., Manco-Johnson, M. L. *et al.* (1985). Clinical course of fetal hydrocephalus: 40 cases. *Am. J. Roentgenol.*, **144**, 827–31

109. Nyberg, D. A., Mack, L. A., Hirch, J. *et al.* (1987). Fetal hydrocephalus: sonographic detection and clinical significance of associated anomalies. *Radiology*, **163**, 187–91

110. Hudgins, R. J., Edwards, M. S. B., Goldstein, R. *et al.* (1988). Natural history of fetal ventriculomegaly. *Pediatrics*, **82**, 692–7

111. Chervenak, F. A., Berkowitz, R. L., Tortora, M. and Hobbins, J. C. (1985). The management of fetal hydrocephalus. *Am. J. Obstet. Gynecol.*, **151**, 933–42

112. Glick, P. L., Harrison, M. R., Nakayama, K. D. *et al.* (1984). Management of ventriculomegaly in the fetus. *J. Pediatr.*, **105**, 97–105

113. Gupta, J. K., Bryce, F. C. and Lilford, R. J. (1994). Management of apparently isolated fetal ventriculomegaly. *Obstet. Gynecol. Surv.*, **49**, 716–21

114. Vintzileos, A. M., Ingardia, C. J. and Nochimson, D. J. (1983). Congenital hydrocephalus: a review and protocol for perinatal management. *Obstet. Gynecol.*, **62**, 539–49

115. Filly, R. A., Chinn, D. H. and Callen, P. W. (1984). Alobar Holoprosencephaly: ultrasonographic prenatal diagnosis. *Radiology*, **151**, 455

116. Babcock, D. S. (1986). Sonography of congenital malformations of the brain. *Neuroradiology*, **28**, 428

117. Cohen, M. M. Jr and Sulik, K. K. (1992). Perspectives on holoprosencephaly. II. Central nervous system, craniofacial anatomy,

syndrome commentary, diagnostic approach, and experimental studies. *J. Craniofac. Genet. Dev. Biol.*, **12**, 196–244

118. Nyberg, D. A., Mahoney, B. S. and Pretorius, D. H. (1990). *Diagnostic Ultrasound of Fetal Anomalies Text and Atlas*, pp.83–202. (Littleton:Year Book Medical Publishers)

119. DeMyer, W., Zeman, W. and Palmer, C. G. (1964). The face predicts the brain: diagnostic significance of medial facial anomaliess for holoprosencephaly (arrhinencephaly) *Pediatrics*, **34**, 256–62

120. Pilu, G., Ambrosetto, P., Sandri, F. *et al.* (1994). Intraventricular fused fornices: a specific sign of fetal lobar holoprosencephaly. *Ultrasound Obstet. Gynecol.*, **4**, 65–7

121. Yow, M. D. (1989). Congenital cytomegalovirus disease: A NOW problem. *J. Infect. Dis.*, **159**, 163–7

122. Stagno, S., Pass, R. F., Cloud, G., Britt, W. J., Henderson, R. E., Walton, P. D., Veren, D. A., Page, F. and Alford, C. A. (1986). Primary cytomegalovirus infection during pregnancy. *J. Am. Med. Assoc.*, **256**, 1904–8

123. Griffiths, P. D., Stagno, S., Pass, R. F. *et al.* (1982). Infection with cytomegalovirus during pregnancy: specific IgM antibodies as a marker of recent primary infection. *J. Infect. Dis.*, **145**, 647–53

124. Graham, D., Guide, S. M. and Saunders, R. C. (1982). Sonographic features of *in-utero* periventricular calcification due to cytomegalovirus infection. *J. Ultrasound Med.*, **1**, 171–2

125. Ghidini, A., Sirtori, M., Vergani, P., Mariani, S., Tucci, E. and Scola, G. C. (1989). Fetal intracranial calcifications. *Am. J. Obstet. Gynecol.*, **160**, 86–7

126. Fakhry, J. and Khoury, A. (1991). Fetal intracranial calcifications. The importance of periventricular hyperechoic foci without shadowing. *J. Ultrasound Med.*, **10**, 51–4

127. Estroff, J. A., Parad, R. B., Teele, R. L. and Benacerraf, B. R. (1992). Echogenic vessels in the fetal thalami and basal ganglia associated with cytomegalovirus infection. *J. Ultrasound. Med.*, **11**, 686–8

128. Teele, R. L., Hernaz-Schulman, M. and Sotrel, A. (1988). Echogenic vasculature in the basal ganglia of neonates: a sonographic sign of vasculopathy. *Radiology*, **169**, 423–7

129. Mittlemann-Handwerker, S., Pardes, J. G., Post, R. C., Sumal, M., Rosenberg, J. and Chervenak, F. A. (1986). Fetal ventriculomegaly and brain atrophy in a woman with intrauterine cytomegalovirus infection. A case report. *J. Reprod. Med.*, **11**, 1061–4

130. Ceballos, R., Ch'ien, L. T., Whitley, R. J. *et al.* (1976). Cerebellar hypoplasia in an infant with congenital cytomegalovirus infection. *Pediatrics*, **57**, 155–7

131. Shackelford, G. D., Fulling, K. H. and Glasies, C. M. (1983). Cysts of the subependedymal germinal matrix: sonographic demonstration with pathologic correlation. *Radiology*, **149**, 117–21

132. Butt, W., Mackay, R. J., de Crespigny, L. C., Murton, L. J. and Ray, R. N. D. (1984). Intracranial lesions of congenital cytomegalovirus infection detected by ultrasound scanning. *Pediatrics*, **73**, 611–14

133. Marques-Dias, M. J. M., van Rijckevorsel, G. H., Landriue, P. and Lyon, G. (1984). Prenatal cytomegalovirus disease and cerebral microgyria: evidence for perfusion failure, not disturbance of histogenesis, as a major cause of fetal cytomegalovirus encephalopathy. *Neuropediatrics*, **15**, 18–24

134. Friede, R. L. and Mikolasek, J. (1978). Postencephalic porencephaly, hydranencephaly or polymicrogyria. A review. *Acta Neuropathol. (Berlin)*, **43**, 161–8

135. Perlman, J. M. and Argyle, C. (1992). Lethal cytomegalovirus infection in preterm infants: clinical, radiological, and neuropathological findings. *Ann. Neurol.*, **31**, 64–8

136. Drose, J. A., Dennis, M. A. and Thickman, D. (1991). Infection *in utero*: US findings in 19 cases. *Radiology*, **178**, 369–74

137. Twickler, D. M., Pearlman, J. and Maberry, M. C. (1993). Congenital cytomegalovirus infection presenting as cerebral ventriculomegaly on antenatal sonography. *Am. J. Perinat.*, **10**, 404–6

138. MacDonald, H. and Tobin, H. O. (1978). Congenital cytomegalovirus infection: a collaborative study on epidemiological, clinical and laboratory findings. *Dev. Med. Child. Neurol.*, **20**, 471–82

139. Volpe, J. J. (1995). Viral, protozoan and related intracranial infections. In *Neurology of the Newborn*, pp.675–729. (Philadelphia: W. B. Saunders)

140. Donner, C., Liesnard, C., Content, J., Busine, A., Aderca, J. and Rodesch, F. (1993). Prenatal diagnosis of 52 pregnancies at risk for congenital cytomegalovirus infection. *Obstet. Gynecol.*, **82**, 481–6

141. Gordon, N. (1993). Toxoplasmosis: a preventable cause of brain damage (review article). *Dev. Med. Child. Neurol.*, **35**, 567–73

142. Stagno, S. (1980). Congenital toxoplasmosis. *Am. J. Dis. Child.*, **134**, 635–7

143. Walpole, I. R., Hodgen, N. and Bower, C. (1991). Congenital toxoplasmosis: a large survey in western Australia. *Med. J. Aust.*, **154**, 720–4

144. Peckham, C. S. and Logan, S. (1993). Screening for toxoplasmosis during pregnancy. *Arch. Dis. Child.*, **68**, 3–5

145. Desmonts, G. and Couvreur, J. (1974). Toxoplasmosis in pregnancy and its transmission to the fetus. *Bull. NY Acad. Med.*, **50**, 146–59

146. Desmonts, G. and Couvreur, J. (1974). Congenital toxoplasmosis. A prospective study of 378 pregnancies. *N. Engl. J. Med.*, **290**, 1110–16

147. Lee, R. V. (1988). Parasites and pregnancy: the problems of malaria and toxoplasmosis. *Clin. Perinatol.*, **15**, 351–63

148. Carter, A. O. and Frank, J. W. (1986). Congenital toxoplasmosis: epidemiological features and control. *Can. Med. Assoc. J.*, **135**, 618–23

149. Becker, L. E. (1992). Infections of the developing brain. *Am. J. Neuroradiol.*, **13**, 537–49

150. Fitz, C. R. (1992). Inflammatory diseases of the brain in childhood. *Am. J. Neuroradiol.*, **13**, 551–7

151. Hohlfeld, P., Daffos, F., Costa, J. M., Thulliez, P., Forestier, F. and Vidaud, M. (1994). Prenatal diagnosis of congenital toxoplasmosis with polymerase-chain-reaction test on amniotic fluid. *N. Engl. J. Med.*, **331**, 605–9

152. Couvreur, J. (1988). Prophylaxis of congenital toxoplasmosis: effects of spiramycin on placental infection. *J. Antimicrob. Chemother.*, **22** (Suppl. B), 193–200

153. Daffos, F., Forestier, F., Capella-Pavlovsky, M. *et al.* (1988). Prenatal management of 746 pregnancies at risk for congenital toxoplasmosis. *N. Engl. J. Med.*, **318**, 271–5

154. Couvreur, J., Thulliez, P. H., Daffos, F. *et al.* (1993). *In utero* treatment of toxoplasmic fetopathy with the combination pyrimethamine-sulfadiazine. *Fetal Diagn. Ther.*, **8**, 45–50

155. Georgiev, V. S. (1994). Management of toxoplasmosis. *Drugs*, **48**, 178–88

156. Matsui, D. (1994). Prevention, diagnosis, and treatment of fetal toxoplasmosis. *Clin. Perinatol.*, **21**, 675–89

157. Chervenak, F. A., Kurjak, A. and Comstock, C. H. (eds.) (1995). *Ultrasound and the Fetal Brain.* (Carnforth, UK: Parthenon Publishing)

158. Timor-Tritsch, I. E., Monteagudo, A. and Cohen, H. L. (eds.) (1996). *Ultrasonography of the Prenatal and Neonatal Brain.* (Stamford: Appleton & Lange)

Congenital cerebral infections

14

G. Nigro and E. V. Cosmi

INTRODUCTION

During intrauterine development, the central nervous system (CNS) may be infected by numerous micro-organisms, in particular by a number of viruses, a protozoan (*Toxoplasma gondii*) and a spirochete (*Treponema pallidum*). These infections are commonly designated by the term TORCH syndrome, in which T indicates toxoplasmosis, O others, i.e. syphilis and human immunodeficiency virus (HIV), R rubella, C cytomegalovirus (CMV) and H herpes simplex virus (HSV). The epidemiology of TORCH infections has dramatically changed during the last two decades, due to the decreased prevalence of congenital rubella as a consequence of vaccination programs, the appearance of new agents such as HIV and the re-emergence of old infections such as syphilis (Table 1). The introduction of new diagnostic procedures, such as enzyme immunoassay and nucleic acid detection systems, and new therapeutic means, such as acyclovir and ganciclovir, may have contributed to these changes[1].

The majority of TORCH infections occur by transplacental transmission, however, occasionally they occur by the ascending route. Congenital infections are generally asymptomatic at birth, but dramatic neurological syndromes may occur, and late neurological sequelae may also follow asymptomatic infections. The neuropathological processes generally consist of two different types of lesions: the inflammatory or destructive and the developmental or teratogenic (predominantly due to altered neuronal proliferation and migration). However, destructive processes frequently cause developmental lesions[2].

CYTOMEGALOVIRUS

Microbiology

Human CMV is a large (150–200 nm) enveloped DNA virus which shows several biological and epidemiological properties of the herpesvirus family, including the persistence in human cells with alternate periods of latency and viral activity[3].

Epidemiology

Cytomegalovirus infection is usually transmitted by direct human-to-human contact, as infected persons are capable of excreting CMV in urine, saliva, semen, cervical secretions and breast milk[4]. Blood products and solid organs are also important sources of infection. Cytomegalovirus is the most common and serious congenital infection as it is associated with important neurological sequelae, although the majority of infants are asymptomatic at birth[5]. Approximately 0.5–2.5% of infants show cytomegaloviruria in the neonatal period[4].

Table 1 *Neurological involvement at birth in major congenital infections*

Etiological agent	Maternal–fetal transmission (trimester of infection)	Symptomatology at birth	
		Present (%)	Absent (%)
Cytomegalovirus	I–II	0–25	76–100
HIV	II–III	0–25	76–100
Toxoplasmosis	I–II	0–25	76–100
Rubella	I	26–50	51–75
Syphilis	II–III	0–25	76–100
Varicella	I–II	51–75	25–50
Herpes simplex	III	76–100	0–25

HIV, human immunodeficiency virus; I, first trimester; II, second trimester; III, third trimester

Pathogenesis

Active maternal CMV infection is very common being present in 3–6% of pregnant women[5]. Cytomegalovirus is transmitted to the fetus following viremia with placentitis during a primary maternal infection. Recurrent infections could also be transmitted after CMV reactivation in the cervix. Congenital CMV infection may occur in approximately 40% of infants born to mothers with primary infection; of these, 10–12% are symptomatic at birth[4]. Intrapartum and immediately postpartum transmission (through the breast milk or other sources) account for an additional 10–15% of infants acquiring CMV infection in the first 4–8 weeks of life[3]. In low birth weight infants, blood transfusions are an important source of infection[6]. Prominent neuropathological processes are meningoencephalitis, periventricular calcifications, microcephaly, polymicrogiria and other migrational alterations[2]. Meningoencephalitis is characterized by the presence of meningeal and perivascular inflammatory cells, necrotic neuronal cells often associated with calcifications (particularly in the periventricular areas), enlarged neuronal and glial cells containing intranuclear CMV inclusions and glial proliferation. Viral predilection for the periventricular area may relate to the proximity to the cerebrospinal fluid (CSF) pathway, through which CMV probably spreads, and to the actively proliferating subependymal germinal matrix cells, which are particularly vulnerable to CMV[2].

Microcephaly is associated with encephaloclastic viral effects and possible neuro-proliferative disturbances which are a consequence of CMV predilection for actively proliferating cells. Alterations in neuronal migration include polymicrogyria, which occurs in approximately 65% of reported cases and may involve both cerebral and cerebellar cortex, lissencephaly, pachygiria and neuronal heterotopias[7]. These manifestations show that the teratogenic effects of CMV may also occur in the second trimester of pregnancy, when neuronal migration takes place[8]. In fact, CMV is the only congenitally transmitted pathogen to cause altered gyral development, the pathogenesis of which includes both teratogenic and encephaloclastic mechanisms[2]. Porencephaly, hydranencephaly, hydrocephalus, cerebellar hypoplasia and diffuse cerebral calcifications are less frequent neurological manifestations of congenital CMV infection.

Clinical manifestations

Symptomatic congenital CMV infection predominantly includes signs of reticuloendothelial involvement (hepatosplenomegaly, jaundice, thrombocytopenia). Although fatal cirrhosis can occur, liver abnormalities generally disappear completely, sometimes after several months. Pneumonia and a purpuric rash may also be present. Intrauterine growth retardation (IUGR) is frequent and about one-third of infected infants have a gestational age of less than 38 weeks. Ocular manifestations include chorioretinitis, which is prevalent in premature infants, microphthalmia and cataract. Approximately 25% of infants show inguinal hernia[4].

The neurological syndrome, including seizures, microcephaly and periventricular calcifications, is the most serious consequence of congenital CMV infection and occurs in 30–50% of symptomatic infants[9]. Approximately 20% of these also develop sensorineural hearing loss. The majority of patients have CSF signs of encephalitis (e.g. pleocytosis, elevated protein concentration); diabetes insipidus may also occur. Neuroimaging studies show a variety of neurological abnormalities, ranging from lissencephaly to multicystic encephalomalacia. The clinical course is generally slow, but progressive encephaloclastic disease or hearing loss may occur[10]. In fact, viruria still persists in about 50% of patients at 5 years of age[3].

Diagnosis

Prenatal diagnosis of CMV infection may be obtained by viral detection in the amniotic fluid which, however, does not predict an adverse fetal outcome. Fetal CMV infection should be closely monitored for evidence of growth retardation, intracranial calcifications or microcephaly.

Congenital CMV infection is diagnosed by viral isolation or CMV DNA detection by polymerase chain reaction (PCR) from urine or blood. Demonstration by electron microscopy of viral particles and detection of CMV antigens by immunofluorescence may occur in over 90% of cases and provide diagnostic information in 1–3 days[11]. Neurological involvement is clearly demonstrated by viral presence in the CSF, but this is only occasionally possible.

Cytomegalovirus infection can also be diagnosed by detecting specific IgM antibodies in cord or neonatal blood specimens, but false positive or particularly false negative results may occur[11]. Cytomegalovirus-specific IgA antibodies appear to be a useful complementary tool for the serodiagnosis of congenital or perinatally-acquired CMV infection[12].

Periventricular calcifications as well as precise definition of the cerebral damage can be obtained by computerized tomography (CT) scanning which is more sensitive than radiography, magnetic resonance imaging (MRI) or ultrasonography[2]. Cranial ultrasound scans can also demonstrate abnormalities including periventricular cysts, ventriculomegaly, periventricular echolucencies due to leukomalacia and thalamic echodensities representing arteries. Magnetic resonance imaging is very useful in revealing altered neuronal migration, parenchymal loss, delayed myelination and cerebellar hypoplasia[2]. In symptomatic as well as asymptomatic infants, testing of brain stem auditory evoked potentials could reveal abnormalities[1].

Prognosis

In children with symptomatic congenital CMV infection, the outcome is closely related to the severity of the neurological syndrome. In fact, approximately 95% of the infants with microcephaly, periventricular calcifications or chorioretinitis may have major neurological sequelae, such as mental retardation (frequently with IQ < 50), seizures, deafness, spasticity[6,8,9]. Children with microcephaly without calcifications may not have mental retardation. Among children with asymptomatic

congenital infections, approximately 10% have been reported to develop bilateral hearing loss, which may not be diagnosed until serious language impairment occurs. However, hearing loss may not be detectable before the first year of life, being related to a direct and progressive lesion of the cochlear cells and of the neurons of the eighth cranial nerve[10]. Late onset and reactivation of chorioretinitis in children with congenital CMV infection may also occur[13]. Therefore, clinical and laboratory follow-up is very important (Table 2).

Prevention

A subunit vaccine consisting of recombinant-derived CMV glycoprotein B (UL55) combined with an adjuvant derived from saponin, QS-21, appeared to be potentially useful for the immunoprophylaxis of CMV disease[14]. However, a suitable CMV vaccine, particularly for women of childbearing age, has not yet been developed. Appropriate hygienic measures (e.g. handwashing, avoidance of contact with oral secretions) can prevent CMV transmission.

Table 2 *Scheme of clinical and laboratory follow-up for children with congenital cerebral infections*

At birth
Neuroimaging studies
CSF examination
Ophthalmoscopy (syphilis: long-bone radiographs)
Audiogram
EEG (if seizures occur)

At 3, 6 and 12 months
Developmental evaluation
Audiogram (CMV, rubella)
Serological tests (syphilis)

Annually (after 1 year)
Growth and developmental evaluation
Audiogram (CMV, rubella)

Preschool assessment
Audiogram
Ophthalmoscopy
Developmental evaluation
EEG (if seizures occur)
Dental and orthopedic evaluations (syphilis)

CSF, cerebral spinal fluid; EEG, electrocardiogram; CMV, cytomegalovirus

Primary maternal infections can be treated with hyperimmune immunoglobulins, but data from large-scale studies are lacking probably due to the difficulty in detecting these infections. For prevention of transfusion-acquired CMV infections, fewer units of blood, red blood cells or CMV-seronegative blood should be used[4].

Therapy

Antiviral therapy for infants with severe CMV disease can be attempted with ganciclovir or foscarnet, which are capable of inhibiting CMV replication by inactivating its DNA polymerase by different mechanisms. Clinical benefit (e.g. loss of hepatosplenomegaly, improvement in tone) has been associated with a ganciclovir regimen based on an initial course with a high dosage and a long maintenance course, to inhibit CMV replication for as long as possible[15].

TOXOPLASMOSIS

Microbiology

Toxoplasma gondii is a ubiquitous intracellular protozoan parasite infecting, among other mammals, domestic cats which excrete considerable quantities of oocysts. These oocysts may also be harbored by meat-producing animals such as pigs. Humans acquire toxoplasmosis after ingestion of oocysts or consumption of undercooked infected meat[16].

Epidemiology

Congenital toxoplasmosis is probably second only to congenital CMV infection in terms of frequency and clinical importance. The prevalence of infection depends on several factors, such as age, geographic area and dietary regimens. In women of childbearing age, the rate of infection varies from 1 per 1000 in the USA or Italy to 10 per 1000 in France. The annual number of infants with congenital toxoplasmosis in the USA is approximately 3000[17].

Pathogenesis

During pregnancy, the transmission rate is approximately 40%, with the highest prevalence in the third trimester (approximately 65%). Early first-trimester toxoplasmosis may lead to abortion. Infections during the second trimester frequently cause fetal death or severe disease, and those during the third trimester are generally asymptomatic[1]. As with CMV infections, pregnant women with toxoplasmosis generally are asymptomatic, although they can sometimes show lymphadenopathy, mild fever and other signs of mononucleosis-like syndrome. Congenital toxoplasmosis is characterized by:

(1) Primary maternal infection;

(2) Maternal parasitemia;

(3) Placentitis;

(4) Fetal parasitemia[2].

T. gondii does not show teratogenicity such as that shown in CMV infection, and neuropathological processes are limited to tissue inflammation and destruction. Meningoencephalitis is multifocal, necrotizing and granulomatous, being characterized by the presence of inflammatory cells in the meninges, perivascular infiltrates, parenchymal necroses with possible calcifications, glial proliferation and miliary granulomas with free or encysted organisms[17]. The predilection of *T. gondii* for periventricular areas with invasion of the ventricular system, possible thrombosis and periventricular infarction by immunocomplexes may account for the frequent occurrence of aqueductal block and consequent hydrocephalus in congenital toxoplasmosis[18]. When cerebral destructive disease is particularly severe and diffuse, and intraventricular pressure is elevated, porencephalic cysts and hydranencephaly can occur[2]. However, brain alterations, such as those in CMV infection, are unlikely. Microcephaly, which may develop in about 15% of patients, is a result of multifocal necrotizing encephalitis.

Clinical manifestations

The majority of infants with congenital toxoplasmosis are asymptomatic at birth, as are the majority of infants with CMV. The rate of toxoplasmosis infection however is generally higher than that of patients with symptomatic congenital CMV infection. Clinical manifestations, which occur in about 10% of the infected infants, mainly include signs of systemic infection attributable to reticuloendothelial involvement (hepatosplenomegaly, jaundice and anemia). The presence of a petechial rash is less common than in CMV infection[17]. The neurological syndrome, which occurs in approximately two-thirds of infants with symptomatic toxoplasmosis, consists of abnormal CSF and other signs of meningoencephalitis, seizures, hydrocephalus or microcephaly, intracranial calcifications and encephaloclastic lesions[19]. At least 90% of the patients exhibit chorioretinitis, which is the only lesion in approximately 15% of congenitally infected infants and is typically bilateral and prominent in the macular regions as yellowish-white cotton-like patches with indistinct margins[2]. In some children who are asymptomatic at birth, ocular involvement can develop later[20]. The severity of clinical manifestations appears to be related to inadequate cellular defenses, mostly including mononuclear macrophages[21].

Diagnosis

T. gondii can be isolated from placenta, CSF and blood, but diagnosis of toxoplasmosis depends principally on serological tests. The Sabin–Feldman dye test, which is performed by mixing the parasites with patient serum, and IgM-fluorescent antibody assay have been the most commonly used tests. Recently, specificity and sensitivity of serodiagnosis have been increased using enzyme immunoassays for detection of IgM and IgA antibodies. Moreover, promising results have been obtained by detection of *T. gondii* DNA by PCR[22].

Of particular interest in congenital toxoplasmosis is the detection of increased protein content in the ventricular fluid, this being related to aqueductal obstruction. Cerebral ultrasonography can show calcifications or echogenic thalamic vasculature as observed in congenital CMV infection[2].

Prognosis

In contrast to CMV infection, the majority of children with systemic toxoplasmosis, if untreated, have a poor neurological outcome, and severe visual impairment occurs in approximately 40% of these. A relatively high frequency of chorioretinitis and intellectual impairment have also been reported in children with congenital subclinical toxoplasmosis. Only 9% of the infants with the neurological syndrome are normal on follow-up (Table 2). Mortality rates range from 1–6%[23].

Prevention

Avoidance of primary maternal infection is the first important approach, which can be obtained by avoiding ingestion of undercooked meat (infective cysts) and contact with cat feces (sporulating oocysts). The second step for prevention is treatment of primary maternal infection. Finally, abortion can be performed in women who acquire toxoplasmosis during early pregnancy. Prenatal diagnosis of congenital toxoplasmosis may be obtained by detection of specific IgM antibodies, or more accurately, by identification of parasitic DNA by PCR in fetal blood.

Therapy

Some neurological lesions may be successfully treated or prevented by giving pyrimethamine (1 mg/kg/day) and sulfadiazine (100 mg/kg/day), with the addition of folinic acid, spiramycin and corticosteroids for 1 year, with an initial duration of pyrimethamine and sulfadiazine lower in asymptomatic than in symptomatic patients[23].

Fetal infection may also be treated by giving the mother alternative 3-week courses of spiramycin, pyrimethamine, sulfadiazine and folinic acid[1].

RUBELLA

Microbiology and epidemiology

Rubella virus is a 60–80 nm non-arthropod-borne togavirus which infects human beings endemically during winter and spring. Transmission occurs by the respiratory route, through direct or droplet contact with nasopharyngeal sections. In the USA, the incidence of rubella has declined by more than 99% in the last two decades, although an increased number of cases, with occasional occurrence of congenital rubella syndrome, has been reported since 1988. Moreover, rubella remains a common illness in many parts of the world[24].

Pathogenesis

Viremia occurs a week prior to the onset of clinical manifestations, which include fever, cervical adenopathy and a maculopapular rash lasting for about 3 days. The occurrence and the severity of fetal infection depends on the time of maternal infection: the earlier rubella occurs, the greater the frequency of fetal transmission and the severity of the clinical disease are[1]. Although hearing loss is still found in approximately half of infants infected in the fourth month, neurological, ocular and cardiac defects do not occur after the first trimester[25].

As with CMV infection, neuropathological processes in congenital rubella involve inflammation, necrosis and cell replication disturbances. Meningoencephalitis, which is similar to that of other forms of neonatal encephalitis, is the most frequent neurological feature of congenital rubella. Additional features are vasculopathy, with concomitant focal areas of ischemic necrosis particularly in the cerebral white matter and basal ganglia; microcephaly, which is not conspicuous until months after birth, and impaired myelinization, which may relate to viral effect on cell replication[2].

Clinical manifestations

Approximately two-thirds of infants are asymptomatic at birth, but the majority of these will develop overt disease in the first years of life, because of prolonged viral replication[1]. Clinical features include IUGR, reticuloendothelial involvement (hepatosplenomegaly, thrombocytopenia with or without purpura), cardiovascular disease (pulmonary artery stenosis, patent ductus arteriosus), metaphyseal radiolucency of the long bones and interstitial pneumonia[24]. The most common neurological manifestations (lethargy and hypotonia followed by irritability and occasional seizures), which occur in approximately 50–75% of infected infants, are due to a meningoencephalitis[26]. Ocular lesions include cataracts, usually white or pearly, chorioretinitis, with a 'salt-and-pepper' appearance, and microphtalmia[25]. The auditory lesions, which can lead to hearing loss, are due to cochlear inflammatory and destructive lesions, but may also follow neuronal lesions[27]. The CSF may show lymphocytic pleocytosis and high protein content[2].

Diagnosis

Laboratory diagnosis is based on virus isolation, or more likely genome detection by PCR, from urine, CSF, nasopharyngeal secretions or blood, and demonstration of specific IgM antibodies by enzyme immunoassays[24]. Prenatal diagnosis can be obtained by fetal blood sampling in the 20th week of pregnancy. In congenital rubella as well as rubella reinfection, the detection of rubella-specific IgA antibodies may have a diagnostic role, supplementing IgM detection[28]. Computerized tomography and MRI scans may show ischemic lesions secondary to vasculopathy and impaired myelinization. Cerebral ultrasound may detect focal areas of calcification, subependymal cysts and vascular echodensities in the basal ganglia and thalamus[2].

Prognosis

The outcome is not so clearly related to the neonatal clinical features, as with congenital CMV or toxoplasmosis. In fact, even some infants who appear to be less severely affected at birth may develop severe neurological deficits

(Table 2). The outcome of cognitive development is generally related to linear growth: children with normal growth had good cognitive outcome[29]. Rarely, a progressive encephalitis, which is probably due to a persistent viral infection or an immune-mediated mechanism, may become apparent in the second decade[30].

Prevention and therapy

Vaccination with a live attenuated vaccine has been utilized to limit the spread of infection in the pregnant woman, although it is unclear how long immunization is effective or whether asymptomatic maternal reinfection can cause fetal involvement. Hyperimmune immunoglobulins may be useful for susceptible pregnant women. No effective chemotherapeutic agents are available[24].

HERPES SIMPLEX VIRUSES

Microbiology

Herpes simplex virus types 1 and 2 are ubiquitous DNA viruses of 180–200 nm in diameter, which exhibit approximately 50% nucleotide homology and share several important biological properties, notably the capacity to cause latent infections with periodic reactivations associated with mucocutaneous or neurological disease[31].

Epidemiology

In contrast to HSV-2, HSV-1 is usually transmitted sexually; however, either virus can infect the neonate following both primary and, less frequently, recurrent maternal infection. The incidence of neonatal HSV infection ranges from approximately 1 per 2500 to 1 per 20 000 live births. Of these cases, approximately two-thirds are due to HSV-2[32].

Pathogenesis

Herpes simplex virus infection can be transmitted *in utero* (by primary/transplacental or reactivated/ascending infection), intrapartum or postnatally, but the great majority of cases of vertical transmission occur perinatally. Only a few of the mothers of HSV-infected infants show genital lesions at delivery, and less than one-half have a history of genital herpes; however, about 25% of mothers have fever[33]. Host factors, mostly concerning natural killer cytotoxicity, interferon and antibody production, T-cell proliferation and activity, may have a role in the vertical transmission[34].

Significant neurological involvement in neonatal HSV infection is frequent and includes predominantly signs of inflammation and destruction[35]. The few infants with intrauterine infection by transplacental transmission may also have developmental alterations (e.g. early intrauterine infection is associated with microcephaly)[36]. Meningoencephalitis is the typical neuropathological process, and is characterized by the occurrence of meningeal inflammatory cells, perivascular infiltrates, multifocal neuronal necrosis, reactive glial proliferation and Cowdry type A intranuclear inclusions in neuronal and glial cells[2]. Brain swelling and hemorrhage in the necrotic areas, in part due to endothelitis, may also occur[35]. Neonatal HSV infection is generally followed by destructive effects on the neurons, with subsequent microcephaly, multicystic encephalomalacia or even hydranencephaly[36]. The frequent occurrence of neurological involvement (31%) in infants with localized ocular disease may relate to direct viral transmission from the eye to CNS[35].

Clinical manifestations

Three clinical aspects are distinguishable: mucocutaneous and ocular lesions; encephalitis; and systemic illness (fever, lethargy, liver dysfunction, pneumonitis, disseminated intravascular coagulopathy and shock). The incidence of these different manifestations is approximately 42%, 35% and 23%, respectively[33]. Infants with encephalitis have fever, irritability or lethargy within the first 2 weeks after birth. In infants with progressive disease, alterations in the muscle tone with partial or generalized seizures occur. Other organs, particularly the liver, may also be involved. In premature infants, there are some additional complications, such as respiratory distress syndrome[1].

Infants who are infected *in utero* (approximately 5%) show numerous abnormalities including cutaneous lesions, chorioretinitis or microphtalmia, and severe neurological involvement (i.e. microcephaly or hydranencephaly)[36].

Diagnosis

Laboratory abnormalities include anemia, thrombocytopenia, increased transaminase and bilirubin levels, and signs of coagulopathy, such as prolongation of the prothrombin time or reduced fibrinogen time. Neurological involvement is frequently associated with mixed or lymphocytic pleocytosis and high protein content. Computerized tomography or MRI may reveal cerebral swelling or focal hypodensities in perinatal HSV infections and calcifications or severe cystic encephalomalacia in congenital infections[2]. Abnormal background rhythms and patterns of slow or sharp waves may be revealed by the electroencephalogram[1].

The virological diagnosis of HSV infection is based on viral isolation from the oropharynx, CSF, vesicles, conjunctiva or rectum[33]. However, viral isolation from CSF is difficult to obtain, and brain biopsy should be considered when encephalitis is suspected. Cytopathic effects are usually detectable in cell cultures within 1–3 days. Cytological examinations from mucocutaneous or conjunctival manifestations may be performed using immunochemistry and monoclonal antibodies. Polymerase chain reaction assays have been shown to be highly sensitive and specific in CSF examination[37].

Prognosis

Several factors, predominantly including early antiviral therapy, influence the outcome in infants with neonatal HSV infection. In the past, the mortality rate was highest with systemic disease (approximately 80%), and survivors exhibited severe neurological sequelae (Table 2). Recently, due to earlier diagnosis and antiviral therapy, there has been a decrease in the rate of

systemic HSV infection and an increased number of localized infections to skin, eye and mouth. However, mortality rates are still high (50–65%) for infants with disseminated disease or with neurological involvement (15%). The most favorable outcome is with mucocutaneous-ocular disease (90–100% normal)[2]. In infants with congenital HSV infection, the outcome is poor with severe sequelae[36].

Prevention

Since neonatal HSV infection generally occurs during delivery, identification of infected pregnant women, particularly those with a first episode of genital infection is essential[33]. The management of delivery is controversial, mostly dependent on the status of the amniotic membranes because the risk of ascending infection increases when rupture of the membranes occurs. However, although the rise of neonatal infection increases considerably with duration of rupture membranes, the preventive value of Cesarean section is apparent[38]. Development of a safe non-oncogenic vaccine has not yet been obtained.

Therapy

The institution of antiviral therapy mostly concerns which patients to treat, since the benefits of therapy are related to an early initiation and previous collection of samples for virological diagnosis. Four drugs, idoxuridine (IDU), cytosine arabinoside (Ara-C), adenine arabinoside (Ara-A or vidarabine), and acyclovir, are capable of inhibiting HSV by blocking DNA synthesis. IDU and Ara-C can be toxic to rapidly-dividing cells, such as gastrointestinal and hematopoietic cells. Vidarabine and acyclovir appear to be equally efficient, achieving viricidal levels in the CNS without or with few adverse effects[39]. However, acyclovir is preferable since it can be given more easily, with the regimen of 30 mg/kg/day in three doses i.v. for at least 10 days. Fluid and electrolyte balance, respiratory status, clotting and liver function tests have to be monitored during treatment[39].

CONGENITAL SYPHILIS

Microbiology and epidemiology

Treponema pallidum is a spirochete which enters through abraded skin or mucosal sites where its replication causes the characteristic primary lesion or chancre. Secondary and tertiary disease may develop in patients who are not appropriately treated. Humans are the only natural host and transmit the microorganism by intimate contact[40]. The incidence of syphilis in developed countries as demonstrated by seropositivity rates, ranges from 0.02% to 0.08%, in contrast the rate may be extremely high in developing countries (in Zambia 12.8% of pregnant women)[41]. However, in some developed nations such as the USA, the incidence of congenital syphilis rose dramatically during the 1980s in relation to several factors, such as prostitution, cocaine use, HIV infection, limited access to medical care, and changes in the definition of congenital syphilis[1].

Pathogenesis

The fetus is infected during maternal spirochetemia following placentitis and fetal spirochetemia[41]. Two main factors determine fetal outcome: the stage of maternal infection and the time of fetal exposure: the longer the time for maternal primary stage, the better the fetal outcome is, probably by development of an efficient immunity[42]. Vertical transmission rarely occurs before 16–20 weeks of gestation, and it is most likely after 24 weeks when complete atrophy of the Langhans' cell layer of the early placenta takes place[42].

Congenital syphilis affects the CNS in the majority of cases, although the involvement is generally limited to the meningeal membranes[43]. Syphilitic meningitis, which may be acute or subacute, often occurs at 4–5 months of age and is characterized by inflammatory infiltration of the leptomeninges with mononuclear cells. Superficial cortical layers may also be involved[2]. Chronic meningovascular syphilis may follow acute/subacute meningitis and is characterized by marked involvement of basilar meninges with two predominant consequences:

cranial nerve abnormalities (i.e. optic atrophy) and hydrocephalus, by chronic arachnoiditis (with onset between 4th and 9th month)[43]. After 1–2 years of age, persistent vasculitis can produce cerebral infarction. At the age of 10–15 years, in addition to optic atrophy and auditory nerve lesion, juvenile general paresis and tabes dorsalis may occur[2].

Clinical manifestations

Approximately one-third of infected live-born infants have signs of syphilis at birth, mostly involving skin and reticuloendothelial/skeletal systems, which are not usually apparent before the first 2 weeks[41]. The early features are caused by disseminated infection and consist of low birth weight, hepatosplenomegaly, jaundice, skin rash (particularly of palms and soles), condylomata lata, persistent rhinitis with a mucopurulent discharge ('snuffles'), lymphadenopathy, meningitis, periostitis or osteochondritis. Skeletal abnormalities, which are the most typical clinical features of congenital syphilis (particularly if early acquired), involve the long bones and may inhibit limb movement (pseudoparalysis). Bone changes may also be observed in asymptomatic infants[44]. Late consequences, which appear after 2 years of age, include saddle nose, peg-shaped upper incisors (Hutchinson teeth), mulberry molars, perioral rhagades, interstitial keratitis, sensorineural deafness, visual loss, hydrocephalus, mental retardation, general paresis or tabes dorsalis[1]. Neurological involvement is manifested by CSF pleocytosis and increased protein content.

Diagnosis

Serological assays include non-treponemal (e.g. venereal disease research laboratory or VDRL) and treponemal (e.g. fluorescent treponemal antibody adsorption of FTA-ABS) tests. The FTA-ABS IgM test has been shown to be highly sensitive as an indicator of neonatal syphilitic infection[42]. In general, the detection of specific IgM antibodies by Western blot together with immunofluorescent antigen detection of *T. pallidum* is most useful[41]. Infants or mothers with syphilis should also be investigated for HIV infection

According to Centers for Disease Control (CDC) criteria, congenital syphilis is confirmed when *T. pallidum* is identified in tissues. Presumptive cases include any infant whose mother had untreated or inadequately treated syphilis at delivery or with a positive treponemal test together with any physical sign of congenital syphilis or long-bone abnormality[45]. Polymerase chain reaction assays for the amplification of parasitic DNA in cytobrushings of umbilical cord appear to be a valid diagnostic tool[42]. The most important neurodiagnostic study is the examination of the CSF, particularly in view of CSF VDRL or PCR testing; a positive result is considered diagnostic of CNS involvement.

Prognosis

The earlier therapy is initiated, the more likely a satisfactory response will be obtained and neurological sequelae prevented[2]. A longitudinal clinical assessment and diagnostic examinations should be performed 3, 6 and 12 months after initial treatment (Table 2). In infants with stable antibody levels, retreatment with penicillin should be considered. Moreover, infants with neurosyphilis require serial CSF examinations at 6-month intervals until 3 years of age or until the CSF VDRL or PCR becomes negative[1]. Numerous congenitally infected infants (approximately 40%) are stillborn or die in the perinatal period[44].

Prevention

Preventive measures include three approaches: avoidance of infection in pregnancy, early diagnosis and treatment of maternal and fetal infection. Within the first 16 weeks of pregnancy, the syphilitic woman should be treated with 2.4 million units of benzathine penicillin; after the 16th week, a second dose of benzathine penicillin or a 10–14-day course of procaine penicillin G (600 000 U/day) are recommended[45].

Therapy

Infants with confirmed or presumptive congenital syphilis require i.v. or i.m. administration of 50 000 U/kg (divided every 12 h) of crystalline penicillin G within the first week of life or 150 000 U/kg (divided every 8 h) between 1 and 4 weeks or 200 000 U/kg (divided every 6 h). Administration of 50 000 U/day of procaine penicillin G has also been suggested[41]. Penicillin should be given for 10–14 days. A single dose of 50 000 U/kg of benzathine penicillin i.m. may be used if maternal treatment is uncertain or it was initiated during the last month of pregnancy (provided that the infant is asymptomatic and CSF and long bones are normal)[45].

HUMAN IMMUNODEFICIENCY VIRUS

Microbiology and epidemiology

Human immunodeficiency virus types 1 and 2 are retroviruses of about 100 nm in diameter, belonging to the lentivirus family. At present, HIV-2 is restricted to countries in west Africa, while HIV-1 is distributed worldwide[46].

HIV infection of the fetus and newborn is a great public health problem, and its impact on the CNS is enormous, relating in part to the high prevalence of HIV-infected women of childbearing age in many areas of the world. In the USA, the seroprevalence is 1.5 per 1000, whilst it is as high as 30% in some regions of Africa and Haiti[46]. Vertical transmission accounts for the great majority of pediatric AIDS, ranging from 10 to 40% with lowest rates in Europe, intermediate in the USA and highest in Africa[46]. Although neurological disorders are rare at birth, subsequent development of encephalopathy, justifies the consideration of HIV among the causes of cerebral fetal infection[47].

Pathogenesis

Transplacental HIV transmission occurs predominantly in the second trimester, relating to high plasma HIV levels[48]. Placentitis with disruption of the trophoblastic barrier (e.g.

by CMV or syphilis) is an important predisposing factor. Intrapartum HIV transmission is probably the most important vertical route, as shown by the higher incidence of infections in first-born twins and vaginally-delivered infants than second-born twins and infants delivered by Cesarean section[49]. Possible mechanisms are ingestion of maternal blood, maternal–fetal placental transfusion or direct fetal exposure to infected cervico-vaginal secretions[50].

Human immunodeficiency virus encephalopathy is predominantly related to the immune response without conventional inflammatory signs, although cerebral infection is demonstrated by the recovery of HIV or HIV-DNA from brain and CSF, or detection of HIV-specific antibodies in CSF (as an indicator of synthesis within the blood-brain barrier)[47,51]. Cerebral atrophy is the most prominent feature, secondary to neuronal death and myelinic loss probably caused by viral and immunological products (i.e. cytokines)[52]. Cellular findings include numerous multinucleated giant cells, frequently in syncitial formations, and macrophages often containing the virus[53]. A crucial role may be played by the coat protein of HIV, gp120, as it has been shown in transgenic mice, in which the production of gp120 was associated with neuronal and glial changes similar to those typical of HIV encephalopathy[54]. However, HIV encephalopathy has several steps including: HIV infection of brain macrophages; gp120-induced release of 'neurotoxins' (e.g. cytokines, glutamate, arachidonic acid metabolites) which act synergistically with endogenous glutamate to activate glutamate receptors; and entry of calcium, activation of nitric oxide synthesis, and neuronal death caused by free radical generation from nitric oxide[55–58]. In fact, inhibitors of nitric oxide synthetase prevent the neurotoxicity of gp120 suggesting that calcium activation of nitric oxide synthetase and production of nitric oxide is probably the final common pathway to neuronal death[59]. Cortico-cerebral atrophy may also be related to dendritic abnormalities, which could be particularly important in infants, in view of the active dendritic development that

occurs in infancy[60]. Myelin loss may be marked, both diffuse and multifocal, probably consequent to a destructive process as shown by reactive astrocytosis[61].

Calcific vasculopathy, mostly in basal ganglia, is a striking feature of HIV encephalopathy which is manifested later by the occurrence of hemorrhagic or ischemic stroke[2]. The spinal cord frequently has myelin loss, particularly of the lateral cortical-spinal tracts[47]. At autopsy, approximately 25% of HIV-infected infants show evidence of cerebrovascular disease, and 20% exhibit neoplastic or infectious complications[51]. A rare occurrence in the relative absence of meningeal inflammatory signs is that of CSF pleocytosis[2].

Clinical manifestations

Although single case reports of infants with neonatal meningoencephalitis or seizures with brain atrophy have been reported, neurological manifestations are generally clinically evident at 2–5 months of age[52]. Most infants present with non-neurological disease including failure to thrive, generalized lymphadenopathy, hepatosplenomegaly, recurrent diarrhea, parotitis and persistent oral candidiasis[62]. Clinical presentation as progressive neurological disease occurs in approximately 12% of infants, at a median age of 9 months[51]. Neurological disease may be differentiated into progressive encephalopathy, static encephalopathy and no neurological abnormalities[47]. Progressive encephalopathy occurs in 30–75% of cases and includes a dementing process, decreasing rate of head growth, microcephaly, spastic motor deficits and extrapyramidal or cerebellar signs[2]. Seizures are not frequent, being generally related to opportunistic infections (e.g. CMV, HSV). Static encephalopathy occurs in approximately 30–40% of infants, and is characterized by the delay of cognitive and motor development[2]. The proportion of neurologically normal infants varies in relation to different studies, and ranges from 10–30% in the USA to 60–85% in Africa[52].

Diagnosis

The major diagnostic approaches for neonatal HIV infection are viral culture and detection of HIV DNA by PCR or p24 antigen. While the sensitivity of culture is approximately 50%, that of PCR approaches 100%[63]. The detection of p24 antigen may relate to severity of disease; in fact, it is positive in the CSF of infants with progressive encephalopathy but negative in those with static encephalopathy or asymptomatic[2]. Since maternal HIV-specific IgG antibodies can persist as long as 15 months, early serodiagnosis may be performed by detection of specific IgA antibodies, which are more frequently detectable than IgM[64]. A CT scan is most useful for detection of basal ganglia and cerebral calcifications, whilst MRI is preferable for revealing cerebral atrophy and myelinic abnormalities[2].

Prognosis

The age of diagnosis and clinical evolution are important prognostic factors. Infants younger than 1 year at diagnosis or with encephalopathy have a mean survival time lower than those who are asymptomatic in the first period of life[46].

Prevention

Vertical HIV transmission may be stopped by preventing maternal infection, detecting maternal infection and treating the infected mothers. Conner and colleagues[65] showed that the rate of HIV transmission can be reduced from 26 to 8% in pregnant women who are treated with zidovudine (AZT).

Therapy

Zidovudine therapy has been associated with improvement of cognition and auditory brain stem responses, reduced brain atrophy and immunological improvement[46]. The potential effectiveness of other antiretroviral drugs such as didanosine, dideoxycytidine and zalcitabene is under evaluation[66].

VARICELLA

Varicella-zoster virus (VZV) is a member of the herpesvirus family, averaging 200 nm in diameter, which produces chicken pox during primary infection and shingles during reactivation. The occurrence of VZV infection during pregnancy is rare (0.7 per 1000 pregnancies), mainly because most women are already seropositive[67]. Although the risk of fetal involvement is small, congenital VZV infection can occur[68]. The two syndromes caused by intrauterine VZV infection should be distinguished: congenital and perinatal varicella[2].

Congenital varicella

Congenital varicella syndrome generally follows maternal varicella with transplacental transmission during the first 20 weeks of pregnancy. Unlike CMV infection, fetal VZV infection is due to an acute process, including inflammation and tissue destruction[68]. Neuropathological processes include meningoencephalitis, myelitis, dorsal root ganglionitis and segmental muscle denervation with hypoplasia. The involvement of dorsal root ganglia is particularly interesting in view of the alternating phases of latency and reactivation of VZV in these sites[2]. In fact, in infants with intrauterine exposure to VZV, herpes zoster has been observed at 2 weeks and at 17 months[69,70]. In several other children, CT scan revealed microcephaly, ventriculomegalia and cerebral calcification[68,71]. Clinical features include typical cutaneous scars in a segmental distribution, limb abnormalities (muscle atrophy or hypoplasia and deformities), bulbar signs (particularly difficulty in swallowing), cerebral involvement (seizures, retarded neurological development) and ocular abnormalities (chorioretinitis, microphtalmia, cataracts, optic atrophy, anisocoria, Horner's syndrome)[68,71–73].

Perinatal varicella

Perinatal varicella is the result of VZV transmission near the time of delivery and is clinically apparent within the first 10 postnatal days.

Approximately 25% of infants born to mothers with varicella during the last 31 days of pregnancy will develop the disease[68]. The incubation period (interval between maternal–fetal/neonatal disease) is 9–15 days. Infants with early onset of disease (within 4 days of life) have milder disease than those with later onset, probably because several days are needed before maternal VZV-specific IgG antibodies cross the placenta and equilibrate with the fetal circulation[2]. The pathological processes include inflammation and necrosis (associated with calcifications) of the lungs, liver, adrenal glands, gastrointestinal system, kidneys and spleen. Clinical features include a vesicular rash that may become hemorrhagic[68].

Diagnosis

Viral culture from cutaneous lesions and detection of viral antigens by immunofluorescence of VZV DNA by PCR are the principal diagnostic procedures. Serodiagnosis may be obtained by detection of specific IgM antibodies or seroconversion. In congenital varicella, attempts to isolate VZV from CSF, eye and other tissues have not been successful, and serodiagnosis appears to be compatible with fetal infection in 75% of cases[71,73].

Prognosis

Differences in prognosis depend on the time of maternal infection. Approximately 20% of infants with congenital varicella have normal development in the first year of life[67,68].

Prevention

Prevention of infection is difficult. Although the risk of fetal involvement is low (approximately 2% in the first 20 weeks of pregnancy), the outcome for the affected infants is so serious that both an accurate prenatal diagnosis and the prevention of maternal varicella with a safe and effective vaccine should be considered[72–74]. It is not known if the administration of VZV immunoglobulins decreases the risk of fetal infection[71].

Therapy

Varicella-zoster virus immunoglobulins should be given to infants delivered less than 5 days after the onset of maternal varicella or born to mothers with varicella in the first days after delivery (the infant might have acquired varicella transplacentally during maternal viremia). Passive immunization may modify neonatal disease[68,71]. Acyclovir appears to be useful and well tolerated, but its derivative famciclovir is more effective at a lower dosage[75].

ENTEROVIRUSES

Infections caused by enteroviruses and echoviruses may occur prenatally, intrapartum (approximately 4% of women at delivery excrete enteroviruses in the feces) or postnatally following human-to-human contact. Non-polio enteroviruses are relatively common causes of such infections, which have a seasonal prevalence (late summer, early autumn) and may be epidemic, particularly in nurseries. Symptomatic enteroviral infections are more frequent in neonates whose mother developed the illness within a week or less from delivery. The most common neurological presentation for enteroviral infections in the neonatal as well as late period is meningitis. This is frequently caused by intrauterine or perinatal Coxsackie B infections, with or without encephalitis. Myocarditis is another prominent clinical feature of Coxsackie B infections. Echovirus infections are relatively common in the neonatal period[76]. Clinical syndromes include asymptomatic infection, febrile illness, gastroenteritis, pneumonia, liver disease and meningitis. The most prominent systemic signs are fever and diarrhea (enteroviruses are transmitted by the fecal–oral route). Indeed, the clinical presentation of enteroviral infections is so diverse that it is difficult to distinguish indicative features. Therefore, it should be suspected in any patient with 'aseptic meningitis' (CSF pleocytosis and high protein content)[77]. Diagnosis is based on viral isolation and detection of enteroviral RNA by PCR in CSF from infants with meningitis[78]. The prognosis is generally good.

OTHER INFECTIONS

Adenovirus type II has been isolated from the brain of a neonate with fatal encephalitis, characterized by perivascular mononuclear infiltrates, edema and reactive astrocytosis were noted[79]. Parvovirus B19, which can cause fetal hydrops by maternal–fetal infection, has also been reported to cause congenital ocular defects and convulsions following prenatal infection[80,81]. Infants whose mothers were infected near delivery with the Western equine encephalitis virus, a mosquito-borne α-virus, may have fever and signs of meningoencephalitis including seizures, lethargy, bulging fontanels and altered muscle tone[82]. Venezuelan equine encephalitis virus is another α-virus, which can induce fetal cerebral abnormalities including necrosis, hemorrhage and hydranencephaly[83]. Lymphocytic choriomeningitis virus, an arenavirus that chronically infects rodents, has been associated with congenital chorioretinitis, hydrocephalus and microcephaly[84].

Lyme disease, caused by the spirochete *Borrelia burgdorferi*, during pregnancy has been associated with neonatal death and heart disease, but the agent has also been detected in the brain[85].

Infants congenitally infected with *Trypanosoma cruzi*, the agent of American trypanosomiasis or Chagas disease, may have multisystem involvement with hepatosplenomegaly, anemia, jaundice, edema, petechiae and neurological signs such as tremors or convulsions[86].

ACKNOWLEDGEMENT

This work has been supported in part by the National Research Council (CNR), Rome, Italy.

References

1. Bale, F. B. and Murph, J. R. (1992). Congenital infections and the nervous system. *Pediatr. Clin. North Am.*, **39**, 669
2. Volpe, J. J. (1995). Viral, protozan, and related intracranial infections. In *Neurology of the Newborn*, 3rd edn., pp. 685–729. (Philadelphia: WB Saunders)
3. Naraqi, S. (1991). Cytomegaloviruses. In R. B. Belshe (ed.) *Textbook of Human Virology*, 2nd edn. (St Louis: Mosby Year Book)
4. Ho, M. (1991). *Cytomegalovirus: Biology and Infection.* (New York: Plenum Press)
5. Yow, M. D. and Demmler, G. J. (1992). Congenital cytomegalovirus infection disease – 20 years is long enough. *N. Engl. J. Med.*, **326**, 702
6. Stagno, S., Pass, R. F., Sworsky, M. E. *et al.* (1983). Congenital and perinatal cytomegalovirus infection. *Semin. Perinatol.*, **7**, 31
7. Hayward, J. C., Titelbaum, D. S., Clancy, R. R. and Zimmerman, R. A. (1991). Lissencephaly-pachygyria associated with congenital cytomegalovirus infection. *J. Child. Neurol.*, **6**, 109
8. Baskar, J. F., Furnari, B. and Huang, E. S. (1993). Demonstration of developmental anomalies in mouse fetuses by transfer of murine cytomegalovirus DNA-injected eggs to surrogate mothers. *J. Infect. Dis.*, **167**, 1288
9. Boppana, S. B., Pass, R. F., Britt, W. J., Stagno, S. and Alford, C. A. (1992). Symptomatic congenital cytomegalovirus infection: neonatal morbidity and mortality. *Pediatr. J. Infect. Dis.*, **11**, 93
10. Williamson, W. D., Demmler, G. J., Percy, A. K. and Catlin, F. I. (1992). Progressive hearing loss in infants with asymptomatic congenital cytomegalovirus infection. *Pediatrics*, **90**, 862
11. Chou, S. (1990). Newer methods for diagnosis of cytomegalovirus infection. *Rev. Infect. Dis.*, **12**, S727
12. Nigro, G., Mattia, S. and Midulla, M. (1989). Simultaneous detection of specific serum IgM and IgA antibodies for rapid serodiagnosis of congenital or acquired cytomegalovirus infection. *Serodiagn. Immunother. Infect. Dis.*, **3**, 355
13. Boppana, S., Amos, C., Britt, W. *et al.* (1994). Late onset and reactivation of chorioretinitis in children with congenital cytomegalovirus infection. *Pediatr. Infect. Dis.*, **13**, 1139
14. Britt, W., Fay, J., Seals, J. and Kensil, C. (1995). Formulation of an immunogenic human cytomegalovirus vaccine: responses in mice. *J. Infect. Dis.*, **171**, 18
15. Nigro, G., Scholz, H. and Bartmann, U. (1994). Ganciclovir therapy for symptomatic congenital cytomegalovirus infection in infants: a two-regimen experience. *J. Pediatr.*, **124**, 318

16. Beaman, M. H., McCabe, R. E., Wong, S.-Y. and Remington, J. S. (1995). *Toxoplasma gondii*. In Mandell, G. L., Bennett, J. E. and Dolin, R. (1995). *Principles and Practise of Infectious Diseases*, 4th edn. (New York: Churchill Livingstone)

17. Remington, G. S. and Desmonts, G. (1990). Toxoplasmosis. In Remington, J. S. and Klein, J. O. (eds.) *Infectious Diseases of the Fetus and Newborn Infant*. (Philadelphia: WB Saunders)

18. Frenkel, J. K. (1974). Pathology and pathogenesis of congenital toxoplasmosis. *Bull. NY Acad. Med.*, **50**, 182

19. Diebler, C., Dusser, A. and Dulac, O. (1985). Congenital toxoplasmosis: clinical and neuroradiological evaluation of the cerebral lesions. *Neuroradiology*, **27**, 125

20. Robinson, R. O. and Baumann, R. J. (1980). Later cerebral relapse of congenital toxoplasmosis. *Arch. Dis. Child.*, **55**, 231

21. Wilson, C. B. and Haas, J. E. (1984). Cellular defenses against *Toxoplasma gondii* in newborns. *J. Clin. Invest.*, **73**, 1606

22. Thulliez, P., Daffos, F. and Forestier, F. (1992). Diagnosis of toxoplasma infection in the pregnant woman and the unborn child: current problems. *Scand. J. Infect. Dis.*, **84**, 18

23. Hohlfeld, D., Daffos, F., Thulliez, P. *et al.* (1989). Fetal toxoplasmosis: outcome of pregnancy and infant follow-up after *in utero* treatment. *J. Pediatr.*, **115**, 765

24. Lamprecht, C. L. (1991). Rubella virus. In Belshe, R. B. (ed.) *Textbook of Human Virology*, 2nd edn. (St Louis: Mosby Year Book)

25. Enders, G., Miller, E., Nickeri-Pacher, U. *et al.* (1988). Outcome of confirmed periconceptional maternal rubella. *Lancet*, **1**, 1445

26. Desmond, M. M., Fisher, E. S. and Vorderman, A. L. (1978). The longitudinal course of congenital rubella encephalitis in nonretarded children. *J. Pediatr.*, **93**, 584

27. Wild, N. J., Sheppard, S., Smithells, R. W. *et al.* (1989). Onset and severity of hearing loss due to congenital rubella infection. *Arch. Dis. Child.*, **64**, 1280

28. Nigro, G., Nanni, F. and Midulla, M. (1985). Rubella reinfection and the fetus. *Lancet*, **1**, 1040

29. Chirboga-Klein, S., Oberfield, S. E., Casullo, A. M. *et al.* (1989). Growth in congenital rubella syndrome and correlation with clinical manifestations. *J. Pediatr.*, **115**, 251

30. Weil, M. L., Itabashi, H. H. and Carnay, L. (1975). Chronic progressive panencephalitis due to rubella virus simulating subacute sclerosing panencephalitis. *N. Engl. J. Med.*, **292**, 994

31. Mattison, H. R., Eisenberg, R. J. and Reichman, R. C. (1991). Herpes simplex virus. In Belshe, R. B. (ed.) *Textbook of Human Virology*, 2nd edn. (St Louis: Mosby Year Book)

32. McIntosh, D. and Isaacs, D. (1992). Herpes simplex virus infection in pregnancy. *Arch. Dis. Child.*, **67**, 1137

33. Whitley, R. J. (1990). Herpes simplex. In Remington, J. S. and Klein, J. O. (eds.) *Infectious Diseases of the Fetus and Newborn Infant*. (Philadelphia: WB Saunders)

34. Kohl, S. (1989). The neonatal human's immune response to herpes simplex virus infection: a critical review. *Pediatr. Infect. Dis. J.*, **8**, 67

35. Corey, L. and Spear, P. G. (1986). Infections with herpes simplex viruses (two parts). *N. Engl. J. Med.*, **314**, 686 and 749

36. Hutto, C., Arvin, A., Jacobs, R. *et al.* (1987). Intrauterine herpes simplex virus infections. *J. Pediatr.*, **110**, 97

37. Rowley, A. H., Whitley, R. J., Lakeman, F. D. and Wolinsky, S. M. (1990). Rapid detection of herpes-simplex-virus DNA in cerebrospinal fluid of patients with herpes simplex encephalitis. *Lancet*, **335**, 440

38. Randolph, A. G., Washington, A. E. and Prober, C. G. (1993). Cesarean delivery for women presenting with genital herpes lesions. Efficacy, risks, and costs. *J. Am. Med. Assoc.*, **270**, 77

39. Whitley, R., Arvin, A., Prober, C. *et al.* (1991). A controlled trial comparing vidarabine with acyclovir in neonatal herpes simplex virus infection. *N. Engl. J. Med.*, **324**, 444

40. Tramont, E. C. (1995). *Treponema pallidum* (syphilis). In Mandell, G. L., Bennett, J. E. and Dolin, R. (eds.) *Principles and Practise of Infectious Diseases*, 4th edn. (New York: Churchill Livingstone)

41. Ingall, D., Dobson, S. R. M. and Musher, D. (1990). Syphilis. In Remington, J. S. and Klein, J. O. (eds.) *Infectious Diseases of the Fetus and Newborn Infant*. (Philadelphia: WB Saunders)

42. Rawstron, S. A., Jenkins, S., Blanchard, S. *et al.* (1993). Maternal and congenital syphilis in Brooklyn, NY. Epidemiology, transmission, and diagnosis. *Am. J. Dis. Child.*, **147**, 727

43. Wolf, B. and Kalangu, K. (1993). Congenital neurosyphilis revisited. *Eur. J. Pediatr.*, **152**, 493

44. Dorfmann, D. H. and Glaser, J. H. (1990). Congenital syphilis presenting in infants after the newborn period. *N. Engl. J. Med.*, **323**, 1299

45. Ikeda, M. K. and Jenson, H. B. (1990). Evaluation and treatment of congenital syphilis. *J. Pediatr.*, **117**, 843

46. Cosmi, E. V., Falcinelli, C., Anceschi, M. M. and Di Renzo, G. C. (1992). Perinatal AIDS: a review. *Eur. J. Obstet. Gynecol. Biol. Reprod.*, **44**, 165

47. Epstein, L. G. and Gendelmann, H. E. (1993). Human immunodeficiency virus type I infection of the nervous system: pathogenetic mechanisms. *Ann. Neurol.*, **33**, 429

48. Husson, R. H., Lan, Y., Kojima, E. *et al.* (1995). Vertical transmission of human immunodeficiency virus type 1: autologous neutralizing antibody, virus load, and virus phenotype. *J. Pediatr.*, **126**, 865

49. European Collaborative Study (1992). Risk factors for mother-to-child transmission of HIV-1. *Lancet*, **339**, 1007

50. Newell, M. L. and Peckham, C. (1993). Risk factors for vertical transmission of HIV-1 and early markers of HIV-1 infection in children. *AIDS*, **7**, S91

51. Masliah, E., Achim, C. L., Ge, N. *et al.* (1992). Spectrum of human immunodeficiency virus-associated neocortical damage. *Ann. Neurol.*, **32**, 321

52. Tyor, W. R., Glass, J. D., Griffin, J. W. *et al.* (1992). Cytokine expression in the brain during the acquired immunodeficiency syndrome. *Ann. Neurol.*, **31**, 349

53. Belman, A. L. (1992). Acquired immunodeficiency syndrome and the child's central nervous system. *Pediatr. Neurol.*, **39**, 691

54. Toggas, S. M., Masliash, E., Rockenstein, E. M. *et al.* (1994). Central nervous system damage produced by expression of the HIV-1 coat protein gp120 in transgenic mice. *Nature*, **367**, 188

55. Barks, J. D., Nair, M. P., Schwartz, S. A. *et al.* (1993). Potentiation of N-methyl-D-aspartate-mediated brain injury by a human immunodeficiency virus-1-derived peptide in perinatal rodents. *Pediatr. Res.*, **34**, 192

56. Lipton, S. A., Sucher, N. J., Kaiser, P. K. *et al.* (1991). Synergistic effects of HIV coat protein and NMDA receptor-mediated neurotoxicity. *Neuron*, **7**, 111

57. Dreyer, E. B., Kaiser, P. K., Offermann, J. T. *et al.* (1990). HIV-1 coat protein neurotoxicity prevented by calcium channel antagonists. *Science*, **248**, 364

58. Lipton, S. A. (1992). Memantine prevents HIV coat protein-induced neuronal injury *in vitro*. *Neurology*, **42**, 1403

59. Dawson, V. L., Dawson, T. M., Uhl, G. R. *et al.* (1993). Human immunodeficiency virus type 1 coat protein neurotoxicity mediated by nitric oxide in primary cortical cultures. *Neurobiology*, **90**, 3256

60. Masliah, E., Ge, N., Morey, M. *et al.* (1992). Cortical dendritic pathology in human immunodeficiency virus encephalitis. *Lab. Invest.*, **66**, 285

61. Kaufmann, W. E. (1992). Cerebrocortical changes in AIDS. *Lab. Invest.*, **66**, 261

62. Tovo, P. A., De Martino, M., Gabiano, C. *et al.* (1992). Prognostic factors and survival in children with perinatal HIV-1 infection. *Lancet*, **339**, 1249

63. Italian Multicentre Study (1988). Epidemiology, clinical features and prognostic factors of paediatric HIV infection. *Lancet*, **2**, 1043

64. Martin, N. L., Levy, J. A., Legg, H. *et al.* (1991). Detection of infection with human immunodeficiency virus (HIV) infection type 1 in infants by an anti-HIV immunoglobin A assay using recombinant proteins. *J. Pediatr.*, **118**, 354

65. Connor, E. M., Sperling, R. S., Gelber, R. *et al.* (1994). Reduction of maternal-infant transmission of human immunodeficiency virus type 1 with zidovudine treatment. *N. Engl. J. Med.*, **331**, 1173

66. Husson, R. N., Mueller, B. U., Farley, M. *et al.* (1994). Zidovudine and didanosine combination therapy in children with human immunodeficiency virus infection. *Pediatrics*, **93**, 316

67. Schauf, V. and Salo, R. J. (1991). Varicella-zoster virus. In Belshe, R. B. (ed.) *Textbook of Human Virology*, 2nd edn. (St Louis: Mosby Year Book)

68. Brunell, P. A. (1992). Varicella in pregnancy, the fetus, and the newborn – problems in management. *J. Infect. Dis.*, **166**, S42

69. Bennet, R., Forsgren, M. and Herin, P. (1985). Herpes zoster in a 2-week-old premature infant with possible congenital varicella encephalitis. *Acta Paediatr. Scand.*, **74**, 979

70. Leis, A. A. and Butler, I. J. (1987). Infantile herpes zoster ophthalmicus and acute hemiparesis following intrautiner chickenpox. *Neurology*, **37**, 1537

71. McIntosh, D. and Isaacs, D. (1993). Varicella zoster virus infection in pregnancy. *Arch. Dis. Child.*, **68**, 1

72. Pastuszak, A. L., Levy, M., Schick, B. *et al.* (1994). Outcome after maternal varicella infection in the first 20 weeks of pregnancy. *N. Engl. J. Med.*, **330**, 901

73. Enders, G., Miller, E., Cradock-Watson, J. *et al.* (1994). Consequences of varicella and herpes zoster in pregnancy: prospective study of 1739 cases. *Lancet*, **343**, 1547

74. Watson, B. A. and Starr, S. E. (1994). Varicella vaccine for healthy children. *Lancet*, **343**, 928

75. Vere Hodge, R. A. (1993). Review: antiviral portraits series, number 3. Famciclovir and penciclovir. The mode of action of famciclovir including its conversion to penciclovir. *Antiviral Chem. Chemother.*, **4**, 67

76. Cherry, J. D. (1990). Enteroviruses. In Remington, J. S. and Klein, J. O. (eds.) *Infectious Diseases of the Fetus and Newborn Infant.* (Philadelphia: WB Saunders)

77. Rorabaugh, M. L., Berlin, L. E., Heldrich, F. *et al.* (1993). Aseptic meningitis in infants younger than 2 years of age: acute illness and neurologic complications. *Pediatrics*, **92**, 206

78. Glimaker, M., Johansson, B., Olcen, P. *et al.* (1993). Detection of enteroviral RNA by polymerase chain reaction in cerebrospinal fluid from patients with aseptic meningitis. *Scand. H. Infect. Dis.*, **25**, 547

79. Osamura, T., Mizuta, R., Yoshioka, H. *et al.* (1993). Isolation of adenovirus type 11 from the brain of a neonate with pneumonia and encephalitis. *Eur. J. Pediatr.*, **152**, 496

80. Weiland, H. T., Vermey-Keers, C., Salimans, M. M. *et al.* (1987). Parvovirus B19 associated with fetal abnormality. *Lancet*, **1**, 682

81. Nigro, G., D'Eufemia, P., Zerbini, M. *et al.* (1994). Parvovirus B19 infection in a hypogammaglobulinemic infant with neurologic disorders and anemia: successful immunoglobulin therapy. *Pediatr. Infect. Dis.*, **13**, 1019

82. Shinefield, H. R. and Townsend, T. E. (1953). Transplacental transmission of Western equine encephalomyelitis. *J. Pediatr.*, **43**, 21

83. Wenger, F. (1977). Venezuelan equine encephalitis. *Teratology*, **16**, 359

84. Sheinbergas, M. M. (1976). Hydrocephalus due to prenatal infection with the lymphocytic choriomeningitis virus. *Infection*, **4**, 185

85. Weber, K., Bratzke, H. J., Neubert, U. *et al.* (1988). *Borrelia burgdorferi* in a newborn despite oral penicillin for Lyme borreliosis during pregnancy. *Pediatr. Infect. Dis. J.*, **7**, 286

86. Bittencourt, A. L. (1976). Congenital Chagas disease. *Am. J. Dis. Child.*, **130**, 97

Routine obstetric ultrasound examination: a clinical and ethical evaluation

15

D. W. Skupski, F. A. Chervenak and L. B. McCullough

Routine ultrasound examination is defined as a screening procedure that is carried out on low-risk patients (i.e. those without a clinical indication for ultrasound scanning). This procedure should ideally be performed at about 18–20 weeks' gestation. Because the indications for ultrasonography during pregnancy are quite extensive, it must be understood that it is actually the majority of patients who have a clinical indication for ultrasound, and thus are not the group of which we are speaking when we discuss routine ultrasound examinations. It is also important for the clinician to realize that, in addition to fetal biometry for dating of the pregnancy, a comprehensive examination of fetal anatomy is an *essential* part of the routine examination, i.e. not optional. The value of routine obstetric ultrasound screening in pregnancy has long been debated[1,2]. The recent RADIUS[3,4] study has exacerbated this controversy.

This chapter reviews the safety of routine (or screening) ultrasound, ultrasound's ability to detect fetal anomalies, randomized clinical trials and the ethical dimensions of routine ultrasound screening.

SAFETY

Several long-term studies of the safety of ultrasonography during pregnancy have been completed, showing no adverse effects of exposure to prenatal ultrasound waves. Stark and co-workers[5] found no decrease in birth weight or impairment of neurological function. Salvensen and associates[6], in a group of 2000 children at ages 8 and 9, found no difference in school performance as rated by their teachers (who

were blinded to which of the children had been exposed to ultrasound and which had not), and no difference in dyslexia between the ultrasound and control groups. In addition, a recent study specifically designed to address the issue of safety in a large cohort of low-risk patients in Winterhaven, Florida showed no measurable effect of ultrasound on Bayley scales of infant development, the mental development index and psychomotor development index[7]. This study also showed that higher education of the mother led to higher infant scores on the neurological and psychomotor tests (an internal control).

The American Institute of Ultrasound in Medicine (AIUM) states: '. . . current data indicate that the benefits to patients of the prudent use of diagnostic ultrasound outweigh the risks, if any, that may be present'[8].

STUDIES ON THE DETECTION OF FETAL ANOMALIES

Central to consideration of the clinical value of routine ultrasound scanning is its ability to detect fetal anomalies. We have chosen for review several large studies conducted in Europe that have evaluated the detection of fetal anomalies by ultrasound.

In Finland, Rosendahl and Kivinen[9] performed ultrasound examinations routinely at 18 weeks' gestation in 9012 patients. Anomalous infants were discovered in 93 cases (1.03%). The sensitivity and specificity for the detection of any anomalies were 52.8% and 99.9%, respectively. When a second scan was added at 34 weeks' gestation, the sensitivity rose to 63.8%. The authors emphasized the necessity of ultrasound examinations for all pregnant patients.

The results of a Belgian multicenter trial were published by Levi and colleagues[10]. Ultrasound scanning was performed between 12 and 20 weeks' gestation in 16 370 patients. A total of 381 fetuses (2.3%) were found to have malformations after birth. A total of 154 fetuses were correctly diagnosed by prenatal ultrasound. The sensitivity for the detection of fetal malformations in this study was 21%. When an additional scan was added later in pregnancy, the sensitivity rose to 40.4%. The specificity for the diagnosis of fetal malformations was 99.9%. There were eight false-positive diagnoses (0.05%); aggressive therapy was neither offered nor used in these cases. A comprehensive list of criteria which justify the use of routine ultrasound screening for the detection of fetal malformations was provided by the authors.

In a low-risk population of 8785 fetuses, Chitty and co-workers[11] studied the efficacy of routine ultrasound screening prior to 24 weeks' gestation for the detection of fetal structural anomalies. Sensitivity for the detection of fetal malformations was 74.4%. Fifteen infants with abnormal karyotypes, but who did not have structural anomalies, were not included in these data. Inclusion of these infants lowered the sensitivity for the detection of anomalies to 66%. There were two false-positive diagnoses not affecting outcome. No therapy was attempted for either case and both infants were normal at birth. Chitty and colleagues pointed out that ultrasound will never be perfect in the detection of anomalies, for several reasons: (1) technical problems such as maternal obesity, multiple pregnancy and fetal position; (2) uncertain outcomes of recognizable malformations; (3) late development of some anomalies; (4) inability to detect certain anomalies; (5) inadequate data on the long-term outcome of minor changes such as mild pyelectasis and choroid plexus cysts; and (6) late presentation of patients for prenatal care or non-compliance with recommendations for ultrasound screening.

Luck[12] studied routine ultrasound screening at 19 weeks' gestation in 8523 pregnancies. The prevalence of anomalies was 1.95%. Prenatal ultrasound examinations detected anomalies in 140 of 166 cases discovered after birth, for a sensitivity of 84.3%; the specificity was 99.9%. Esophageal atresia and diaphragmatic hernia were the only two false-positive diagnoses (both infants were normal at birth). Routine ultrasound scanning by trained, experienced ultrasonographers at 19 weeks' gestation was recommended to all obstetric departments.

Shirley and associates[13] studied 6183 pregnancies by second-trimester ultrasound examination in a combined prospective and retrospective study in England. Abnormalities were discovered in 89 fetuses either at delivery or at induced termination of pregnancy, and of these, 84 had been scanned in the second trimester. The sensitivity for the detection of any anomaly prior to 22 weeks' gestation was 60.7% (51/84). The sensitivity and specificity for the detection of major anomalies were 73% and 99.8%, respectively. There was one false-positive diagnosis not affecting outcome; the infant was normal at birth. The authors concluded that all pregnant women would benefit from routine ultrasound screening for congenital malformations.

Romero, in an excellent review[14], has analyzed the above five[9–13] studies together with the results available from the Helsinki trial (see below)[15]. He found that of the 52 295 patients screened, ultrasound had an overall sensitivity of 50.9% (393/772), a specificity of 99.9% (43 366/43 381), a positive predictive value of 95.9% (356/371), and a negative predictive value of 99.26% (43 366/43 689).

RANDOMIZED CONTROLLED CLINICAL TRIALS

Six prospective, randomized trials of routine ultrasound scanning have been performed in Europe. In London, Bennett and colleagues[16] performed a randomized controlled trial of the predictive value of ultrasound measurement at about 16 weeks' gestation. The results showed no difference in fetal outcome (birth weight centile, Apgar score at 1 min or perinatal mortality). However, a significantly larger number of labors were induced for suspected growth retardation when the gestational age was known. Of the group screened by ultrasound, the findings provided valuable obstetric information in 25%.

Randomization to either an ultrasound screening group or a control group took place in 877 women in a study in Glasgow by Neilson and co-workers[17]. The screened group had two scans. They found a sensitivity and specificity of 94% and 90%, respectively, for identifying infants who were small for dates at birth. They stated that there did not appear to be any benefits from a routine two-stage ultrasound screening procedure in low-risk pregnancies.

The Trondheim trial was conducted in Norway[18], and included 1009 women randomly allocated to either routine ultrasound screening at 19 and 32 weeks' gestation or no routine ultrasound screening (510 screened vs. 499 controls). Neither perinatal mortality nor the number of inductions for presumed postterm pregnancies were altered by routine ultrasound screening. Five of six twin gestations in the screened group were diagnosed before 20 weeks' gestation; the sixth patient never attended for her ultrasound examination. In the control group, three of four twin gestations were diagnosed before 24 weeks' gestation, but the fourth set of twins went undiagnosed until the time of labor. In the ultrasound-screened group, there were slightly fewer post-term inductions (non-significant reduction) and twins were diagnosed earlier. The authors concluded that the observed differences were suggestive of marginal benefits from ultrasound screening.

In Alesund, Eik-Nes and colleagues[19] conducted a trial of routine ultrasound screening vs. 'indicated only' ultrasound examinations on 1628 patients (809 screened, 819 controls). There was a significant reduction in induction of labor for presumed post-term pregnancy in the screened group (1.9%) compared to the control group (7.8%). There was also a significant decrease in perinatal morbidity in those infants who had induction of labor for pre-

sumed post-term pregnancy (fewer hospital days – 15 days among the screened group vs. 55 days in controls). Severe intrauterine growth retardation (IUGR) was recognized in the ultrasound-screened group, but not in the control group. Therefore, there were fewer deaths due to IUGR in the group screened by ultrasound.

The previous four[16–19] randomized, controlled trials of routine obstetric ultrasound screening were reviewed by Thacker[20]. He concluded that a pooled analysis of data from all four trials failed to demonstrate adequately the usefulness of screening ultrasound for all pregnant women, but he did detect a significant reduction in the rate of induction of labor, which he stated was *very suggestive* that ultrasound screening does actually decrease the rate of induction.

The Stockholm trial[21] was a Swedish study of 4997 women who were randomized to either a routine ultrasound group (at 15 weeks; 2482 patients) or a control group (no routine ultrasound; 2515 patients). In the screened group there were significantly fewer inductions for post-term pregnancies, an earlier detection of twins, and fewer infants with low birth weight (< 2500 g). The authors concluded that ultrasound provided a significant benefit in decreasing unnecessary inductions of labor for presumed post-term gestation.

The largest of the European randomized controlled trials was the Helsinki trial[15]. Randomization of 9310 women took place. The screened group received routine ultrasound screening at 16–20 weeks' gestation and the control group received follow-up only (4691 screened vs. 4619 controls). There were fewer hospitalizations, an improved detection of twins (100% vs. 76.3%), and a decrease in the perinatal mortality rate (4.6/1000 vs. 9.0/1000) – all in the group screened by ultrasound. Women in the screened group who underwent termination of pregnancy after the discovery of lethal fetal anomalies were responsible for the decrease in perinatal mortality. After postnatal ascertainment of anomalies, the sensitivity of prenatal ultrasound (for the detection of fetal anomalies) was 36.0% at the City Hospital and 76.9% at the University Hospital.

Meta-analysis

In the *British Medical Journal* in July 1993[22], four clinical trials[15,18,21,23] of routine ultrasound scanning were included in a meta-analysis. Each of the studies met two criteria for inclusion: (1) randomization occurred before the first ultrasound examination; and (2) the perinatal mortality rate and the number of pregnancies were reported. A total of 15 935 pregnancies (7992 screened and 7943 controls) were included. The main outcome measures were perinatal mortality rate, Apgar score at 1 min < 7, the number of induced labors, and the live birth rate (defined as the number of live births per pregnancy). There was no difference in the live birth rate, but there was a significantly lower perinatal mortality rate in the screened group, mostly due to the influence of the Helsinki trial, which not only had the largest number of patients, but also had a highly significant reduction in perinatal mortality. The authors of the meta-analysis thus concluded that routine ultrasound examination may be effective and useful as a screening tool for malformations.

The RADIUS study

The Routine Antenatal Diagnostic Imaging with Ultrasound (RADIUS) study[3,4] was a prospective, randomized clinical trial designed to answer the following question. Is there a significant reduction in adverse perinatal outcome with the use of routine ultrasound in low-risk pregnancies? A large multicenter clinical trial conducted in the United States at five major centers and 109 clinical practices in six states, the RADIUS study was sponsored by the National Institute for Child Health and Human Development. Pregnant women ($n = 15\ 530$) were randomized into two groups: routine ultrasound examinations (two scans, one in the second and one in the third trimester) and controls (indicated ultrasound scans only). The primary outcome measure was adverse perinatal outcome, defined as fetal or neonatal death, and severe or moderate neonatal morbidity. The investigators performed power calculations to determine the number of patients needed for the primary outcome measure. Secondary outcome measures included: (1) the incidence of small-for-gestational-age births; (2) the incidence of post-term pregnancies; (3) the need for induction of labor in presumed post-term pregnancies; and, for the patients discovered to have multiple gestation, (4) birth weight; and (5) the incidence of premature delivery.

There was no difference in adverse perinatal outcome between the routinely scanned and control pregnancies. There was a threefold increase in the detection of fetal anomalies prior to 24 weeks' gestation, from 4.9% (8/163) in the control group to 16.6% (31/187) in the screened group. All but one patient in the screened group (who did not appear for her ultrasound appointment) had the diagnosis of multiple pregnancy established before 26 weeks' gestation. In contrast, 23 women (37%) with multiple gestation in the control group were not identified until after 26 weeks' gestation, and in eight of these cases not until the time of delivery. Significant differences were also found in the incidence of post-date pregnancy, defined as > 42 weeks' gestation, and in the rate of tocolytic usage. With both these findings, there was a decreased rate in the group screened by ultrasound.

The RADIUS study group concluded that routine ultrasound screening does not improve perinatal outcome among low-risk pregnant women, and would result in excessive cost[3]. They also stated, 'screening ultrasonography resulted in no clinically significant benefit'[4].

Critical analysis

The authors of the RADIUS study should be commended for their efforts in performing the largest randomized clinical trial of routine ultrasound scanning. However, at least four important points must be considered by any fair-minded reviewer before concluding, as the RADIUS authors did, that routine ultrasound screening would result in no improvement in perinatal outcome and would result in excessive cost.

Applicability of RADIUS study results to the general population   It has become known that doctors involved in the RADIUS study would not waste time even attempting to recruit a patient who expressed interest in ultrasound. Thus, in addition to receiving private obstetric care, patients also had to be indifferent to the possibility of termination of pregnancy if an anomaly were diagnosed by obstetric ultrasound examination, in order to be considered for entry into the RADIUS study. This low-risk population, indifferent to the option of termination of pregnancy for fetal anomalies, is the starting point of the RADIUS trial. It needs to be emphasized that 60% of *this population* was subsequently found to be at high risk by study criteria. So, in reality, the RADIUS study conclusions are applicable *at best* to only 40% of women who present for private obstetric care. Because many women are not indifferent to the option of termination of pregnancy for fetal anomalies, the RADIUS conclusions are actually applicable to much, much less of the population. It also needs to be remembered that of the 40% of the women who were at low risk, 45% of these still required an indicated ultrasound examination.

Appropriateness of outcome parameters   The RADIUS study concluded that routine ultrasound screening was without clinical value, because it did not result in a significant decrease in perinatal mortality or morbidity or in maternal morbidity. The RADIUS authors did not emphasize the four significant findings of the study: (1) increased detection of fetal anomalies; (2) improvement in diagnosis of twin gestations; (3) decreased use of tocolysis; and (4) improved diagnosis of post-date pregnancy. We believe that this emphasis is wrong. The RADIUS study clearly showed that routine ultrasound screening was successful in doing what routine ultrasound would reasonably be expected to do, i.e. improve gestational age estimation, detect twins and detect fetal anomalies. To require a decrease in maternal morbidity and in perinatal mortality and morbidity from the use of routine ultrasound screening would require standard management

protocols[24], which the RADIUS study did not incorporate.

It also needs to be emphasized that the statistical power in the RADIUS trial is lacking in the secondary outcome measures. With a large enough population, significant improvements in gestational age assessment, early detection of twins and detection of poor fetal growth would clearly improve perinatal outcome. A comparison would be the evaluation of the value of maternal serum α-fetoprotein by its ability to improve perinatal mortality and morbidity, without emphasizing its ability to detect fetal anomalies such as neural tube defects. In addition, this evaluation would be carried out in a setting in which women were indifferent to the option of termination of pregnancy. Clearly this would not represent a fair trial.

Quality of ultrasound   The RADIUS authors made a reasonable attempt to assure the quality of the ultrasound examinations performed in the trial. Nonetheless, it is a misrepresentation of modern ultrasound capabilities to suggest that only 16.6% of fetal anomalies are diagnosable prior to 24 weeks of gestation, given the results of the European studies described above[9-13]. In addition, the quality of the ultrasound examinations was heterogeneous, in that three times the rate of fetal anomalies were detected in tertiary centers than in doctors' offices.

Excessive cost   The initial points discussed under our section on applicability need to be emphasized when cost is considered. The authors of the RADIUS study stated, 'The routine use of screening ultrasonography in this study added, on average, 1.6 scans per pregnancy. Screening more than 4 million pregnant women annually in the United States at $200 per scan would increase costs by more than $1 billion. Confining the estimate of increased cost to 40 per cent of all pregnancies on the basis of eligibility for this study would still result in an increase of over $500 million'[3]. In reality, *much less* than 40% of all pregnancies would incur the increased cost of routine ultrasound examinations, because a large portion of the general population would have an indicated ultrasound scan. When clinic populations were examined in the RADIUS study, 95% of the patients had an indication for obstetric ultrasound examination. In addition, the cost of lifetime care for infants with anomalies is extremely high and the cost saved when women choose abortion for serious fetal anomalies must be part of any cost–benefit analysis. The cost per anomaly detected in the RADIUS study, even with the low anomaly detection rate, was less than that for the California maternal serum α-fetoprotein screening program or for genetic amniocentesis after the age of 35 years[25].

ETHICAL DIMENSIONS OF ROUTINE OBSTETRIC ULTRASOUND SCREENING

In addition to complex technical, epidemiological and clinical questions, the current controversy about routine obstetric ultrasound screening also has ethical dimensions[26]. Objections to routine ultrasound scanning fail to adequately address the implications of the central ethical principle of respect for autonomy.

Implications of respect for autonomy

Providing patients with information about diagnostic and therapeutic alternatives is an essential component of respect for the patient's autonomy[27]. Non-disclosure of diagnostic alternatives impairs the exercise of the patient's autonomy. Respect for autonomy obliges the physician to acknowledge and respect the patient's values, to elicit the patient's preferences, and in the absence of compelling constraints to implement these preferences[28]. Because there is restriction of access to the diagnosis of serious fetal anomalies and, therefore, restriction of access to abortion for anomalies[26], not routinely offering obstetric ultrasound examinations shows disrespect of the autonomy of pregnant women and routinely offering obstetric ultrasound examinations systematically respects that autonomy[29]. Such

matters are not ethically and clinically trivial, either regarding respect for the autonomy of pregnant women or regarding modern obstetric practice[30].

A practice of discussing ultrasound only when women initiate inquiries makes a sham of respect for autonomy, because many women are ignorant of this modality and its abilities[3,31]. Thus, the physician's initiative in routinely offering obstetric ultrasound scanning bases the physician–patient relationship in the principle of respect for autonomy[29].

The informed consent process is the means for implementing the clinical strategy of prenatal informed consent for sonogram (PICS) with every pregnant woman[29]. First, every pregnant woman should be provided with information about the known and theoretical benefits and harms of obstetric ultrasound scanning (early in the course of the pregnancy). Second, in terms of her own values, the pregnant woman should evaluate this information, something every autonomous patient is qualified to do. Deciding whether to elect obstetric ultrasound examination is less complex than complex personal descisions the patient makes routinely, e.g. writing wills of property or writing advance directives in medical matters. The third stage in PICS is for the pregnant woman to articulate her preference regarding the use of ultrasound. The fourth stage is for the physician to provide the pregnant woman with the physician's own recommendation, if he or she has one. The fifth stage is a thoughtful and sensitive discussion of any disagreement that may emerge. Lastly, the woman makes her final decision. This decision should then determine the use of obstetric ultrasound for that pregnant woman. This process provides a significant role for the physician's clinical judgement and experience, as well as any recommendation he or she thinks is in the patient's interest. Professional integrity requires an up-to-date knowledge of the current literature as the basis for any such recommendation.

The entire process of PICS is dependent on the needs of patients, which vary widely. That the physician can respond knowledgeably and meaningfully to each patient's needs is what is important and this is part of the principle of respect for autonomy. This does not create unreasonable burdens on the physician.

The informed consent process described above emphasizes eliciting the patient's preference before the physician makes a recommendation. Thus, PICS does *not* lead to a slippery slope in which the physician is free to manipulate the patient's decision, particularly to promote the possible financial interest of the physician in performing the examination. Only a perversion of the informed consent process would create a slippery slope of manipulating the patient, and this is a violation of the virtue of professional integrity. Only a willful departure from this well understood virtue produces patient manipulation. It is a moral failure on the part of the physician, not a risk of the process of informed consent, that produces a willful undermining of the process of informed consent.

Routinely offering obstetric ultrasound scanning counteracts practices that have much more important clinical ramifications. Doctors who have strong personal convictions against abortion are disinclined to offer ultrasound, because abortion of an anomalous fetus may follow. PICS is a powerful antidote to the slippery slope of physicians cloaking personal convictions in the guise of professional judgement. Women may 'opt in' for routine ultrasound examination in centers where this practice is not advocated, but also women may 'opt out' of routine ultrasound examination in centers that favor the practice. PICS is thus a powerful anti-paternalistic check on physician preference.

Limitations on respect for autonomy

The authors do not accept that respect for autonomy is an absolute ethical principle. Instead, it is a prima facie ethical principle[32]. By this we mean that the demands of respect for autonomy hold only when there are no over-riding considerations to the contrary. Two such considerations have been advanced against routine ultrasound examination: lack of benefit and excessive cost. We will show how each of these objections fails in any reasonable ethical and, therefore, clinical analysis.

Lack of benefit

The RADIUS authors assumed that any possible benefits of secondary outcome measures (detection of fetal anomalies and twin pregnancies, decreased use of tocolysis and reduction of postdatism) would be truly clinical benefits only if they had a documented improvement in the primary outcome measures, maternal morbidity and adverse perinatal outcome. This is a beneficence-based conclusion. Arguing for a lack of benefit of routine obstetric ultrasound scanning is thus equivalent to stating that beneficence-based considerations over-ride autonomy-based considerations. Since the RADIUS trial lacked the statistical power to detect the effect of routine obstetric ultrasound screening on perinatal mortality and morbidity for secondary outcome measures[13], the beneficence-based conclusion of RADIUS that routine ultrasound screening lacks clinical benefit loses a great deal of its force.

Beneficence-based clinical judgement should not narrow itself to consideration only of outcomes research end points such as adverse perinatal outcome, but should also include the prevention of harm in important subsets of patients. RADIUS was captured by an unjustifiably narrow concept of beneficence, because it ignored other clinical realities, such as prevention of unnecessary tocolysis, prevention of undiagnosed twin gestations, ignorance of the presence of fetal anomalies and inappropriate assignment of postdatism. These other clinical realities are also significant *in and of themselves* in any adequate beneficence-based clinical judgement. The correction to the unacceptable narrowness adopted by the RADIUS trial is to expand beneficence-based clinical judgement to its proper scope, provided that the benefits outweigh the possibility of harm from erroneous ultrasound diagnoses. In well formed beneficence-based clinical judgement, the physician justifiably offers obstetric ultrasound scanning as a matter of prudence, to avoid adverse outcomes such as unnecessary tocolysis. Given the seriousness of the adverse outcomes due to undetected clinical complications, such an unexpected twins at the time of delivery, it is justifiable to attempt to prevent those outcomes when in beneficence-based clinical judgement the risks of not performing the ultrasound examination outweigh the risks of performing it. In our view, high-quality ultrasound, which is required as a matter of professional integrity[26], tips the balance in favor of this prudential judgement because the high quality reduces the risk of harm from erroneous ultrasound findings.

An ethical analysis of routine ultrasound examination based on beneficence reaches two conclusions: (1) endpoints of overall perinatal mortality and morbidity are only a part of, and not equivalent to, well formed beneficence-based clinical judgement; and (2) prudential beneficence-based clinical judgement supports offering high-quality ultrasound. The first is neutral in the beneficence-based judgement of PICS; the second supports PICS in beneficence-based clinical judgement. Therefore, objection to PICS on the ground that it provides no benefit fails. Moreover, since allowing the patient to make an informed choice about the management of her pregnancy is a benefit of PICS, central matters of respect for autonomy are at stake. On balance, autonomy-based obligations should clearly be the physician's primary guide in response to objections based on lack of benefit.

Excessive cost

Suggesting that routine obstetric ultrasound examination is excessively costly asserts that justice-based considerations over-ride autonomy-based considerations. Central justice-based considerations are cost-effectiveness and cost-benefit. An important goal of obstetric ultrasound scanning is to detect fetal anomalies. De Vore has shown that the cost per detected case of an anomaly in the RADIUS trial was less than the cost per detected anomaly in the California maternal serum α-fetoprotein screening program[25]. If this screening program is a reliable marker for cost-effectiveness, then routine obstetric ultrasound scanning is surely cost-effective. We suggest that routine ultrasound examination is not just cost-effective because of its reasonable cost comparison to the California maternal serum α-fetoprotein screening program, but also cost-beneficial because the cost per anomaly detected with quality ultrasound is far below the neonatal and lifetime costs of those anomalies. This, of course, assumes that for many pregnancies in which serious anomalies are detected women will elect abortion.

At the very least, cost-based arguments must show that the cost per detected anomaly is so excessive as to establish conclusively that this excessive cost violates accepted theories of justice. Simply subordinating respect for autonomy to ill-defined considerations of cost, as some have done[3,31,33], falls far below this demanding intellectual standard.

CONCLUSION

The routine offering of obstetric ultrasound screening is the central issue in the general question of whether every woman should receive an obstetric ultrasound examination. As reviewed above, there is extensive literature documenting the benefits of routine ultrasound screening. However, there is also a decisive role for the exercise of the pregnant woman's autonomy to judge the benefits and harms of routine ultrasound examination and the worth to her of the information yielded by high-quality ultrasound. The authors of the RADIUS trial explicitly oppose routine ultrasound screening, because most pregnant women will accept ultrasound when it is routinely offered. In their view this drives up cost and expectations[31]. In effect, they and those who agree with them propose paternalistic denial of important information to pregnant women without any convincing ethical or scientific justification. Thus, it invites the obstetrician to abandon the ethical obligation to serve as an advocate for the pregnant woman.

References

1. U. S. Department of Health and Human Services (1984). *Diagnostic Ultrasound Imaging in Pregnancy*, Publication no. 84–667. (Bethesda, Maryland: National Institutes of Health)
2. Royal College of Obstetricians and Gynaecologists (1984). *Report of RCOG Working Party on Routine Ultrasound Examination in Pregnancy.* (London: Royal College of Obstetricians and Gynaecologists)
3. Ewigman, B. G., Crane, J. P., Frigoletto, F. D. *et al.* (1993). Effect of prenatal ultrasound screening on perinatal outcome. *N. Engl. J. Med.*, **329**, 821–7
4. LeFevre, M. L., Bain, R. P., Ewigman, B. G. *et al.* (1993). A randomized trial of prenatal ultrasonographic screening: impact on maternal management and outcome. *Am. J. Obstet. Gynecol.*, **169**, 483–9
5. Stark, C., Orleans, M., Haverkamp, A. *et al.* (1984). Short and long-term risks after exposure to diagnostic ultrasound *in utero*. *Obstet. Gynecol.*, **63**, 194
6. Salvensen, K. A., Bakketeig, L. S., Eik-Nes, S. H. *et al.* (1992). Routine ultrasonography *in utero* and school performance at age 8–9 years. *Lancet*, **339**, 85
7. Hobbins, J. (1995). Bioeffect and safety of ultrasound: is it necessary to regulate the use during pregnancy? *Ultrasound Obstet. Gynecol.*, **6** (Suppl. 2), 2
8. American Institute of Ultrasound in Medicine Bioeffects Committee (1988). Bioeffects considerations for the safety of diagnostic ultrasound. *J. Ultrasound Med.*, **7**, 10
9. Rosendahl, H. and Kivinen, S. (1989). Antenatal detection of congenital malformations by routine ultrasonography. *Obstet. Gynecol.*, **73**, 947–51
10. Levi, S., Hyjazi, Y., Schaaps, J. P. *et al.* (1991). Sensitivity and specificity of routine antenatal screening for congenital anomalies by ultrasound: the Belgian multicentric study. *Ultrasound Obstet. Gynecol.*, **1**, 102–10
11. Chitty, L. S., Hunt, G. H., Moore, J. and Lobb, M. O. (1991). Effectiveness of routine ultrasonography in detecting fetal structural abnormalities in a low risk population. *Br. Med. J.*, **303**, 1165–9
12. Luck, C. A. (1992). Value of routine ultrasound scanning at 19 weeks: a four year study of 8849 deliveries. *Br. Med. J.*, **304**, 1474–8
13. Shirley, I. M., Bottomley, F. and Robinson, V. P. (1992). Routine radiographer screening for fetal abnormalities by ultrasound in an un-selected low risk population. *Br. J. Radiol.*, **65**, 564–9
14. Romero, R. (1993). Routine obstetric ultrasound (Editorial). *Ultrasound Obstet. Gynecol.*, **3**, 303–7
15. Saari-Kemppainen, A., Karjalainen, O., Ylöstalo, P. and Heinonen, O. P. (1990). Ultrasound screening and perinatal mortality: controlled trial of systematic one-stage screening in pregnancy. The Helsinki Ultrasound Trial. *Lancet*, **336**, 387–91
16. Bennett, M. J., Little, G., Dewhurst, J. and Chamberlain, G. (1982). Predictive value of ultrasound measurement in early pregnancy: a randomized controlled trial. *Br. J. Obstet. Gynaecol.*, **89**, 338–41
17. Neilson, J. P., Munjanja, S. P. and Whitfield, C. R. (1984). Screening for small for dates fetuses: a controlled trial. *Br. Med. J.*, **289**, 1179–84
18. Bakketeig, L. S., Eik-Nes, S. H., Jacobsen, G. *et al.* (1984). Randomised controlled trial of ultrasonographic screening in pregnancy. *Lancet*, **2**, 207–10
19. Eik-Nes, S. H., Okland, O. and Aure, J. C. (1984). Ultrasound screening in pregnancy: a randomised controlled trial (Letter to the Editor). *Lancet*, **1**, 1347
20. Thacker, S. B. (1985). Quality of controlled clinical trials. The case of imaging ultrasound in obstetrics: a review. *Br. J. Obstet. Gynaecol.*, **92**, 437–44
21. Waldenstrom, U., Axelsson, O., Nilsson, S. *et al.* (1988). Effects of routine one-stage ultrasound screening in pregnancy: a randomised controlled trial. *Lancet*, **2**, 585–8
22. Bucher, H. C. and Schmidt, J. G. (1993). Does routine ultrasound scanning improve outcome in pregnancy? Meta-analysis of various outcome measures. *Br. Med. J.*, **307**, 13–17
23. Ewigman, B., LeFevre, M. and Hesser, J. (1990). A randomized trial of routine prenatal ultrasound. *Obstet. Gynecol.*, **76**, 189–94
24. Goncalves, L. F. and Romero, R. (1993). A critical appraisal of the RADIUS study. *Fetus*, **3.6**, 7–17
25. DeVore, G. (1994). The routine antenatal diagnostic imaging with ultrasound study: another perspective. *Obstet. Gynecol.*, **84**, 622–6
26. Chervenak, F. A. and McCullough, L. B. (1991). Ethics, an emerging subdiscipline of obstetric ultrasound, and its relevance to the routine obstetric scan. *Ultrasound Obstet. Gynecol.*, **1**, 18–20
27. Faden, R. R. and Beauchamp, T. L. (1986). *A History and Theory of Informed Consent.* (New York: Oxford University Press)

28. McCullough, L. B. and Chervenak, F. A. (1994). *Ethics in Obstetrics and Gynecology.* (New York: Oxford University Press)

29. Chervenak, F. A., McCullough, L. B. and Chervenak, J. L. (1989). Prenatal informed consent for sonogram: an indication for obstetric ultrasonography. *Am. J. Obstet. Gynecol.*, **161**, 857–60

30. Chervenak, F. A. and McCullough, L. B. (1996). The threat of the new managed practice of medicine to patient autonomy. *J. Clin. Ethics*, in press

31. Ewigman, B. G., LeFevre, M.L., Bain, R. P. *et al.* (1990). Ethics and routine ultrasonography in pregnancy (Letter). *Am. J. Obstet. Gynecol.*, **163**, 256–7

32. Beauchamp, T. L. and Childress, J. F. (1989). *Principles of Biomedical Ethics*, 3rd edn. (New York: Oxford University Press)

33. Berkowitz, R. A. (1993). Should every pregnant woman undergo ultrasonography? *N. Engl. J. Med.*, **329**, 874–5

Malformations and karyotype

16

G. D'Ottavio, M. A. Rustico, V. Pecile, A. Maieron, G. Conoscenti, R. Natale and G. P. Mandruzzato

INTRODUCTION

The possibility of performing early diagnosis of an increasing number of genetic diseases in the human fetus today represents an important means of preventing those severe diseases for which no satisfactory therapeutic solutions are available. Prenatal diagnosis has substantially modified the very content of genetic advice for many of these incurable illnesses, so that a couple at risk can now face pregnancy with the prospect of discovering if the fetus does in fact suffer from any of these diseases at an early stage. In which case, selective abortion is an available option.

The development of obstetric techniques for visualization of the fetus, as well as for sampling cells, blood and tissues from the fetus, has turned fetal diagnostic into a widely-applied procedure.

Chromosomal anomalies represent a large proportion of genetic diseases. The aim of cytogenetic analysis is to study the chromosomal constitution of the cells as a factor organizing their genome, and, as such, constituting the karyotype, i.e. that set of chromosomes which – based on their number, morphology and structure – is characteristic of the species to which the genome belongs. Subsequent to karyotype mutations, the number and morphology of the chromosomes can change. Constitutional chromosomal anomalies can be found in 50% of the cases of spontaneous abortions; 10–40% of fetuses with malformations and/or growth retardation; 5–10% of stillbirths or perinatal deaths; 0.8% of newborns; 4–8% of newborns with severe congenital defects; 12–33% of subjects with mental retardation; 5% of infertile males (15% of males with azoospermia); and 9% of primary amenorrheas (in 55% of those as-sociated with a short stature and 73% of those with Turner phenotypes).

In mature gametes, chromosomal anomalies are present in 10% of spermatozoa and up to 25% of oocytes. Such abnormalities originate during gametogenesis in subjects with normal karyotypes, even though in a few rare cases, they may be confined to germinal stem cells. This situation of germinal mosaicism entails a higher risk of recurrence of unbalanced gametes[1–3].

Amniocentesis in the second trimester, and, more recently, the sampling of chorionic villi in the first trimester of pregnancy allow prenatal detection of chromosomal aberrations. Despite the widespread adoption of these techniques, the reduction in the incidence of chromosomal anomalies at birth has been only minimal. The main reasons for this are as follows:

(1) Less than 3% of pregnancies with chromosomal anomalies have a risk factor that can be identified before conception (e.g. a translocation of a parental origin, or a previous child with chromosomal anomalies);

(2) Screening based on the mother's advanced age would enable detection of about 30% of autosomal trisomies, but only 50% of the women at risk because of their age undergo a prenatal diagnosis examination.

In recent years, among the risk factors for aneuploidies, and, in particular, for Down syndrome, besides maternal age, the presence of some particular markers in the mother's serum has been shown to be indicative. In fact, it has been demonstrated that between the 15th and 18th week of gestation, the level of α-fetoprotein and non-conjugated estriol is lower, whereas the content of chorionic gonadotropin is higher, in the serum of pregnant women with Down fetuses, compared to pregnancies with normal fetuses[4-6]. Wald and colleagues[7] proposed a statistical method which, starting from multiples of the median values of individual markers and the risk associated to the mother's age, enables an 'individualized' assessment to be made of the risk of Down syndrome. The combination between a mother's advanced age and a biochemical test showing a risk threshold of 1 in 250 (being equal to that of women who are 37 at the time of childbirth) should enable detection of more than 50% of pregnancies with trisomy 21 syndrome.

Yet another complementary method for screening chromosomal anomalies is ultrasonography, as many fetuses with chromosomal rearrangements have malformations that can be detected echographically.

In evaluating a fetus with congenital anomalies, it is important to determine whether one single anomaly (isolated) or multiple anomalies (multiplex) are present. Common single malformations are usually included in the group of multifactorial disorders, whereas multiplex malformations represent a syndrome and could be due to one single gene defect, to a chromosomal abnormality, or to a teratogen.

In the case of ultrasonically-diagnosed prenatal malformations it would be more correct to define a single anomaly as an 'apparently' isolated one because we are not always able to rule out either some subtle anomalies (i.e. intestinal malrotation, anomalous lung lobation, facial dismorphic features, etc.) or some microscopic parenchymal changes, as pathologists are.

While there are no doubts about the need to check fetal karyotype when multiple malformations are associated, controversy still exists over the advisability of offering the patient a genetic amniocentesis when an 'isolated' defect is discovered during ultrasound evaluation. At the present, the decision is often left to the discretion of the individual obstetrician. In an attempt to clarify this important management issue we have reviewed the recent literature dealing with this problem, also reporting our own experience.

OUR EXPERIENCE

In a series of 606 ultrasonically-diagnosed malformed fetuses, we selected 442 cases useful for evaluation either because of karyotype availability (390 cases) or because normality was clinically stated in a follow-up lasting more than 2 years (52 cases, mainly of unilateral renal pathology). In this sample the overall chromosomal abnormality rate was 21.5%.

The chromosomal aberration rate was 62.3% (38 out of 61 cases) in the case of multiple anomaly and 15.2% (58 out of 381 cases) in the case of an isolated malformation (Table 1). The most common strongly indicative isolated malformation was cystic hygroma (76.5%), followed by cardiovascular defects (with an incidence of

Table 1 *Distribution of abnormal karyotypes in fetuses affected by isolated or multiple malformations*

	Total (n)	Karyotypes performed	Abnormal karyotype	
			n	%
Isolated malformations				
Central nervous system	160	120	11	9.1
Cardiovascular	77	55	12	21.8
Urinary tract	121	92	2	2.2
Gastrointestinal	41	38	7	18.4
Lymphatic	42	34	26	76.5
Skeleton	78	36	0	0
Pulmonary	14	6	0	0
Total	533	381	58	15.2
Multiple malformations	73	61	38	62.3

aneuploidy of 21.8%), gastrointestinal and abdominal wall defects (18.4%) and central nervous system abnormalities (9.1%).

In the following paragraphs we will discuss each pathology in detail, grouping them by system, and making reference to the experiences of other authors as well as our own.

CENTRAL NERVOUS SYSTEM MALFORMATIONS

In a large series of children and fetuses with chromosomal anomalies, two-thirds of brains showed no pathological changes[8]. The brains of the infants may have been small and they may have shown a variety of minor morphological abnormalities, but there was no unique or specific anomaly associated with a chromosomal aberration, except for agyria-pachygiria with the deletion of the short arm of chromosome 17 in Miller–Dieker syndrome[8]. Similarly, in other series of perinatal and pediatric autopsies, an incidence of chromosomal abnormality ranging between 5.4 and 6.5% was reported in newborns with multiple abnormalities, whereas no cytogenetic abnormalities were observed in infants with isolated central nervous system (CNS) defects[9,10].

Nevertheless, in pre-viable fetuses, some malformations are quite often associated with chromosomal abnormalities. They represent an indication for chromosome analysis in the affected fetus even when no other anomaly can be recognized outside the central nervous system. The most common aberrations associated with CNS defects in embryos are triploidy, 45,X and trisomies 13 and 15. In contrast, no CNS anomalies were found in 45,X cases, which later spontaneously aborted (or were terminated)[11].

There is a strong but not invariable association of *holoprosencephaly* with trisomy 13 (or its variants) and about one-third of fetuses with trisomy 13 show holoprosencephaly[12]. An abnormal growth and differentiation of the prosencephalon walls results in the wide spectrum of cerebral anomalies found in holoprosencephalic disorders. They range from absence of olfactory bulbs to a small brain with single ventricle and no cerebral hemispheres, no corpus

callosum or septum pellucidum, although only the most severe features are recognizable at the prenatal ultrasonographic examination[13]. Since the median face is derived from the mesenchyma, ventral to the prosencephalon, facial abnormalities, including cyclopia, presence of proboscis, hypothelorism and medial cleft lip and palate, may be associated with brain malformations. Facial malformations appear to increase the risk of chromosomal aberrations as well as the association with omphalocele or cystic kidneys (including duplications or deletion of chromosome 18, trisomy 21 and triploidy).

In our series of seven cases of isolated holoprosencephaly we found one trisomy 13 out of five cases with facial anomalies and none in the two cases without facial anomalies. Four aneuploidies (all of them trisomy 13 or its variants) were detected out of the six cases with multiplex malformations and facial anomalies (Table 2).

Although the increased amount of intraventricular cerebrospinal fluid, resulting in various degrees of *hydrocephaly*, may be due to overproduction or defective absorption of the fluid, in the pre-viable period the vast majority of cases are due to obstruction. There are several causes of obstruction including malformation of hindbrain (i.e. Arnold–Chiari malformation, commonly seen in myelocele), infections (toxoplasmosis, cytomegalovirus, etc.), or mutant genes[14].

An X-linked recessive aqueductal stenosis occurs in about 2% of cases in which no other anomalies are found. Prenatal series report a frequency of chromosomal abnormalities associated with isolated hydrocephaly ranging between 3 and 8% depending on the presence or absence of spina bifida.

In our series of 39 cases of isolated brain ventricle enlargement with karyotype available, we found five chromosomal abnormalities equal to an incidence of 12.8%. They included one trisomy 21 in a 44-year-old pregnant women, two triploidies in severely growth retarded fetuses and one unbalanced translocation. In the sample there was also a balanced translocation of maternal origin (Table 2). In general, mild ventriculomegaly, either isolated or associated with other malformations, resulted in a greater

Table 2 *Central nervous system malformations and abnormality of karyotype*

Central nervous system malformation	Isolated		Associated	
	Abnormal karyo-type/anomalies observed	Abnormality of karyotype	Abnormal karyo-type/anomalies observed	Abnormality of karyotype

Hydrocephaly	5/39	1 × trisomy 21
		2 × triploidies
		1 × 46,XY,−7 +
		  der(7),t(7;8)
		1 × 46,XX,
		  t(8;9)mat
			6/15	1 × trisomy 21
				1 × triploidy
				1 × 46,XY/47,XY
				1 × 46,XY,iso (18q)
				1 × 47,XX,t(18;21), + 21
				1 × 46,XY,inv(10)

Dandy–Walker malformation	0/8		2/2	1 × trisomy 18 1 × 46,XX,− 18, + idic(18)
Agenesis of corpus callosum	2/9		2/5	2 × trisomy 18
Holoprosencephaly	1/7	1 × trisomy 8 1 × 46,XY,7 q+	4/6	2 × trisomy 13 2 × 46,XX,− 14, + t(13;14)
Anencephaly	0/20	1 × trisomy 13	1/1	1 × trisomy 18
Cephalocele	0/4		0/1	
Spina bifida	3/29		—	
Microcephaly	0/4	2 × trisomy 18 1 × trisomy 21	1/2	1 × 46,XY,der(4),t(4;10)
Total	11/120 (9.1%)		16/32 (50.0%)	

risk of chromosomal aberration, if compared to severe hydrocephaly.

The Dandy–Walker malformation was originally described as a variant of congenital hydrocephalus. In more recent antenatal series, the incidence of ventriculomegaly has been established as being between 50 and 70% and it is responsible for about 12% of congenital hydrocephalus cases. This malformation consists of hypoplastic or absent cerebellar vermis and an enlarged posterior fossa due to the cystic dilatation of the fourth ventricle. In a series of 34 Dandy–Walker malformation cases, Pilu and co-workers[15] reported three anomalous karyotypes out of 29 available ones. In all cases a partial defect was found with normal or borderline lateral ventricles. Similarly, in a larger but more heterogeneous series, generically including all cases of enlarged cysterna magna, Nyberg and colleagues[16] found that the absence of ventricular dilatation correlated most strongly with a chromosome abnormality. In both series the fetuses had other associated malformations, all detected at ultrasonography.

In 10 cases of our series, all karyotypes were found to be normal in the fetuses of eight women below 35 years of age in which the Dandy–Walker malformation was isolated. In the other two cases in which the CNS disorder was associated with a congenital heart defect, a trisomy 18 and an isodicentric chromosome 18 (idic 18) were detected, despite the very young maternal age (Table 2).

As far as neural tube defects are concerned, it is well known that they have a multifactorial etiology, which is expressed when a genetically predisposed individual is exposed to one or more environmental insults (i.e. folic acid deficiency)[17]. According to Kalousek and colleagues[18], 16% of fetuses with triploidy had lumbosacral defects, 11% of fetuses with trisomy 13 had encephalocele and 4% of fetuses with trisomy 18 had meningomyelocele. It has not been reported whether the fetuses also had extra CNS anomalies.

In a recently published paper[19], seven chromosomal anomalies were detected in 43 cases of isolated spina bifida (16.3%) even though in this sample the theoretical risk of chromosomal abnormalities was no greater than 0.3%. The difference is statistically significant ($p = 0.012$). Previous papers report a frequency as high as 50%, but in only very small series[19].

In 29 cases of isolated myelomeningocele, we found three chromosomal disorders (10.3%): one trisomy 21 in a 44-year-old woman and two cases of trisomy 18 in women younger than 35 (Table 2).

Non-syndromal anencephaly is usually multifactorial or, in some rare cases, may be caused by such chromosomal abnormalities as triploidy. Furthermore, anencephaly may occur with or without rachischisis; in the former case, associated abnormalities are more frequent and more severe.

Cephalocele occurs in many syndromes, and occasionally in some chromosomal disorders, mainly in cases of triploidy, trisomy 14, trisomy 15 and monosomy X. In four cases of isolated cephalocele and 21 cases of anencephaly no chromosomal abnormalities were found except for one trisomy 18 associated with advanced maternal age and complete rachischisis (Table 2).

The diagnosis of apparently isolated fetal agenesis of corpus callosus appears to carry an excellent prognosis[20]. However, fetal karyotyping may be indicated for all cases of agenesis of the corpus callosus since three of the four fetuses with trisomy 8 reported in the literature had agenesis of the corpus callosus as the only sonographic finding, representing a one in 10 risk of aneuploidy[21]. In 14 cases referred to our institution we found four chromosomal anomalies including a trisomy 8, in an otherwise normal fetus, and a duplication of long arm of chromosome 7 (46XY,7q+) associated with bilateral pleural effusion. Trisomy 18 was found in the two other fetuses showing multiple anomalies (Table 2).

CARDIOVASCULAR MALFORMATIONS

Heart malformations are amongst the most frequent abnormalities found at birth. They alone account for about one-third of all malformations and are thought to be responsible for 30% of perinatal deaths[22]. They represent a heterogeneous group of diseases, whose origin is often due to chromosomal aberrations, Mendelian disorders, or teratogenic agents. In particular, a well-known association is the one with karyotype abnormalities, which has been documented in 13% of the cases observed after birth[23].

The experience of centers with large numbers of case histories of sonographic diagnosis of fetal heart disease has shown that a much higher percentage of chromosomal anomalies is associated with heart diseases detected *in utero* than in live-born infants. Berg and associates[24] estimated, for example, that the diagnosis of heart malformation during the second trimester of pregnancy is associated with a risk of aneuploidy which is three times as high as that found in postnatal life. The frequency with which cardiac malformations are associated with karyotype abnormalities ranges from 16 to 65%, based on the authors or the selection criteria used. The frequency is also high in the pilot studies performed during the early stages of pregnancy by transvaginal sonography[25].

Cardiovascular malformations are found in over 90% of fetuses with trisomy 18 and 13, in about 50% of fetuses with trisomy 21, and in 15–20% of those with monosomy X. Therefore, the presence of cardiac anomaly increases the risk of aneuploidy. We have observed 135 cases of cardiac anomaly. The heart diseases most frequently observed were: conotruncal anomalies (41 cases, 30.3%), complete atrioventricular canal (23 cases, 17%), isolated ventricular septal defect (17 cases, 12.5%), coarctation and/or hypoplasia of the aortic arch (12 cases, 8.8%). The karyotype – available in 108 cases – was altered in 41.7% of the subjects. In 77 fetuses, heart disease was an isolated malformation. In this group, the karyotype was performed in 55 cases. In 12 cases, it was shown to be altered (21.8%) (Table 3). The most common form of aneuploidy was trisomy 21 (5 cases out of 12). In the forms associated with other malformations (58 cases), karyotype abnormalities were present in 60.4% of the cases (32 cases out of 53 karyotypes performed). The chromosome anomaly most frequently observed in this group

Table 3 *Congenital heart malformations and abnormality of karyotype*

Congenital heart malformation	Isolated		Associated	
	Abnormal karyo-type/anomalies observed	Abnormality of karyotype	Abnormal karyo-type/anomalies observed	Abnormality of karyotype
Atrioventricular defect	7/15	5 × trisomy 21 1 × trisomy 18 1 × 46,XX,del (8) (p23.1)	5/6	2 × trisomy 21 3 × trisomy 18
Tetralogy of Fallot	0/6		3/6	1 × trisomy 18 1 × trisomy 13 1 × 46,XY,del(9) (q22)
Truncus arteriosus	1/1	1 × trisomy 18	3/4	2 × trisomy 18 1 × trisomy 13
Double outlet right ventricle	1/4	1 × trisomy 18	3/4	2 × trisomy 18 1 × 46,XY/47,XY + 16
Pulmonary valve atresia	0/3		1/2	1 × trisomy 13
Transposition great arteries	0/2		0/1	
Ventricular septal defect	1/1	1 × trisomy 18	7/12	7 × trisomy 18
Atrial septal defect	0/1		2/2	1 × trisomy 13 1 × 46,XX,del(18) (q21q23)
Hypoplastic left ventricle	0/5		—	
Tricuspid valve atresia	0/4		0/2	
Coarctation/hypoplastic aorta	1/3	1 × 46,XY,del(18) (q21q23)	6/8	6 × 45,X
Pulmonary valve stenosis	1/2	1 × 46,XY,t(2;17) (q11.2;p11.2)mat	1/1	1 × trisomy 18
Aortic stenosis	0/5		1/1	1 × 46,XX,del(11) (q22q23)
Univentricular heart	0/2		0/2	
Other*	0/1		0/2	
Total	12/55 (21.8%)		32/53 (60.4%)	

*Other, 1 × mitral valve + tricuspid valve stenosis and 2 × myocardiopathy

was trisomy 18 (16 cases out of 32) (Table 3). In six fetuses with cystic hygromas, aortic coarctation was associated with an X-monosomy. Trisomy 13 and other chromosome anomalies (deletions, translocations, mosaicisms) were less frequent.

In agreement with the data reported in the pediatric literature, trisomy 21 was consistently observed in the presence of a complete atrioventricular canal (in two of these fetuses extracardiac anomalies were also observed). Studies on heart morphogenesis have explained the process leading to the formation of atrioventricular valves, and have demonstrated that in trisomy 21 there is an increased cell adhesiveness preventing fusion of endocardial cush-

ions[26]. In cases of aortic coarctation, tetralogy of Fallot and tricuspid valve dysplasia, which are unusual in postnatal life, were also reported.

In trisomy 18, the most frequent heart defect was ventricular septal defect, with misalignment of the anteroposterior conal septum (eight cases). Less frequent anomalies were double outlet right ventricle and truncus arteriosus, complete atrioventricular canal and stenosis of the pulmonary valve associated with tricuspid valve dysplasia. The most common associations with extracardial anomalies were multiple-malformation syndromes and brain abnormalities. In two cases, the only association observed was between cysts of the chorioid plexus and ventricular septal defect, which was observed in two women who were over 38 years of age. In the only case of isolated ventricular septal defect associated with trisomy 18, the mother was 38.

Trisomy 13 was found in three conotruncal anomalies and in one atrial septal defect of secundum type, always in conjunction with severe diseases affecting the central nervous system or the urinary tract.

The cases of aortic coarctation, as well as aortic and pulmonary stenosis associated with deletions, translocations or mosaicisms are unusual and unexpected if compared to the data on postnatal life.

All X-monosomies were associated – as has already been described in the literature[27] – with cystic hygromas of the neck and aortic coarctation. In order to explain this typical association, Clark[27] suggested that the increased pressure exerted by the dilated lymphatic system might compress the ascending aorta and increase flow resistance in the left part of the heart. Intracavitary flow redistribution is then supposed to be responsible for coarctation and also for the other defects of the left heart described in this disease, such as the aortic bicuspid valve or aortic atresia. Thus, the proportion of chromosomal anomalies varies within individual heart diseases. For example, among all cases of complete atrioventricular canal with an abnormal karyotype (12 cases), trisomy 21 was found to be the most common disorder (seven cases). In the group of conotruncal defects – which are thought to be due to anomalies in mesenchymal tissue migration – there is a whole range of possibilities, from the frequent association of truncus or double outlet right ventricle with trisomy 18, to the absence of any association for transposition of great arteries.

In our series, hypoplastic left ventricle was not diagnosed in association with aneuploidies or extracardiac malformations. This is unlike the series of Respondek and co-workers[28] who reported four cases of hypoplastic left ventricle with trisomy 13, two of which were associated with other abnormalities.

Furthermore, atrial isomerism present in three cases) was not found in conjunction with karyotype anomalies.

URINARY TRACT MALFORMATIONS

Postnatal and postmortem studies have established that urinary tract defects are commonly found in many chromosomal abnormalities. The most frequently reported associations are between horseshoe kidney and trisomy 18, microscopic renal cortical cysts and trisomy 13, and renal hypoplasia and triploidy. Furthermore, bilateral or unilateral renal agenesis occurs in some chromosomal abnormalities such as 22q- or 4p-[18].

The largest prenatal study in the literature refers to 682 fetuses with renal defects diagnosed by ultrasonography with available karyotypes. The authors demonstrated that the maternal age-related risk for fetal aneuploidy increased three-fold when the renal malformation was isolated and 30-fold when there were other associated anomalies.

In this series no differences were found relating to the unilateral or bilateral nature of the lesions to the presence of oligohydramnios or the type of malformation. In mild hydronephrosis the most frequent abnormality found was trisomy 21, whereas in moderate/severe hydronephrosis, multicystic kidneys, or renal agenesis the commonest abnormalities were trisomies 18 and 13. Moreover the pattern of associated malformations varied according to the type of chromosomal abnormality. In trisomy 13 the commonest associated findings were holoprosencephaly, facial cleft, cardiac defects and upper limb deformities. In trisomy 18, choroid plexus cysts, omphalocele, cardiac malformations and overlapping fingers were the most frequent associations. In trisomy 21 minor anomalies were associated, including nuchal thickening, macroglossia and clinodactily[29].

In a total of 92 cases of prenatally diagnosed isolated renal pathology we found two chromosomal aberrations, equal to a frequency of 2.2%, whereas in 20 cases associated with extrarenal malformations, the rate rose to 40.0% (Table 4). In particular we had one aneuploidy out of 38 cases of isolated obstructive uropathy. It was a trisomy 21 in a 40-year-old pregnant woman, whose fetus, at ultrasonographic examination, showed a megacystis due to congenital urethral

Table 4 *Urinary tract malformation and abnormality of karyotype*

Urinary tract malformation	Isolated		Associated	
	Abnormal karyo-type/anomalies observed	Abnormality of karyotype	Abnormal karyo-type/anomalies observed	Abnormality of karyotype
Megacystis	1/9	1 × trisomy 21	5/7	1 × trisomy 13 4 × trisomy 18
Obstructive megaureter	0/15			
Uretero pelvic junction stenosis	0/14		1/3	1 × 46,XX,20 q+
Uretero vesical reflux	0/2			
Cystic dysplasia (Potter type I and II)	0/22			
Cystic cortical dysplasia	1/2	1 × 46,XX/46,XX, t(7;13)	1/1	1 × 46,X, + mar
Single cyst	0/3			
Bilateral renal agenesis	0/7		1/9	1 × 45,XX,t(14;21)
Unilateral renal agenesis, ectopia, duplicity	0/18			
Total	2/92 (2.2%)		8/20 (40.0%)	

stenosis. Four cases of trisomy 18 and one of trisomy 13 were detected in fetuses showing a multiple anomaly associated with megacystis, and one 1 20 q+ was found in a fetus with unilateral hydronephrosis, hypertelorism and clinodactily. We also found a fetus affected by Morris syndrome associated with megacystis and horseshoe kidney, in a woman with a previously affected infant. Among 27 cases of cystic kidneys, two aneuploidies were found: a translocation 7;13 associated with isolated bilateral multicystic kidneys and a 46,X + mar associated with renal cortical cysts, non-septated cystic hygroma and skeletal deformities.

None of the 18 cases of isolated unilateral agenesis or ectopia had anomalous karyotypes. The same was true for seven cases in which bilateral renal agenesis was the only malformation detected. Among nine cases of bilateral agenesis associated with other anomalies, a balanced Robertsonian translocation (14;21) was found in a fetus showing also a complete rachischisis and bilateral talipes (Table 4).

GASTROINTESTINAL AND ABDOMINAL WALL DEFECTS

The finding of a digestive anomaly is a good indication for performing fetal karyotyping even when an isolated malformation is found especially in case of duodenal stenosis or esophageal atresia. It has been reported that the most frequent malformations found associated with *esophageal atresia* are gastrointestinal defects (about one-half consisting in imperforate anus)[38]. The second most common associated defects are cardiovascular malformations, while urogenital defects, including renal agenesis and hydronephrosis, are the third most common association.

When detection was dependent solely on associated malformations, chromosomal anomalies, including trisomy 18 and 21, were detected in 4% of newborns and 14% of fetuses when esophageal atresia was diagnosed[30].

Duodenal atresia is an isolated anomaly in only 30–52% of cases being frequently associated with other gastrointestinal anomalies (26%), vertebral anomalies and cardiac defects (20%). Approximately one-third of cases of duodenal atresia are related to trisomy 21. The lesion also occurs in association with interstitial deletion of the long arm of the chromosome 9. The strong association with chromosomal abnormalities and other structural anomalies supports the view that the lesion is due to an early embryonic insult, as opposed to lower atresias which arise after organogenesis has already taken place, and in which ischemia appears to be the major pathogenetic mechanism. The critical period is likely to be identified between the 30th and 40th day of gestation as shown in affected fetuses exposed to thalidomide[31].

In our series of six fetuses affected by isolated duodenal stenosis or atresia, we found four cases of trisomy 21, as against a normal karyotype in our nine cases of isolated atresia of small intestine.

About 50% of fetuses with prenatally diagnosed *omphalocele* have an abnormal karyotype: while trisomy 18 is common, triploidy, trisomy 13, trisomy 21, 45,X and 47,XXY have also been reported[32].

Dott[33] divided omphalocele into two types. Small omphaloceles usually contain only intestine, while the umbilical cord arises from the apex of the sac and it probably results from the failure of mid-gut in returning into the abdominal cavity. In larger omphalocele, the abdominal wall superior to the cord insertion is absent and the sac may contain liver and other abdominal organs, while the umbilical cord stems from the inferior part of the sac.

The frequency of chromosomal abnormalities associated to omphalocele differs according to the type of omphalocele, the smaller one being the most affected one, and the difference is statistically significant. The association with extraintestinal anomalies increases the risk of chromosomal aberrations as well[34]. In our group one of the seven fetuses with isolated exomphalos had an abnormal karyotype, in contrast four of the six cases with additional malfor-

mations were found to be chromosomally abnormal (Table 5).

None of the eight cases of *gastroschisis* either as single or multiple malformation, showed any abnormality in karyotype. There are only a few reports of diaphragmatic hernia associated with trisomies 13, 18 or 21, and 45,X. Benacerraf and Azdick[35] found chromosomal abnormalities in 21% of 19 fetuses with a diaphragmatic defect. In our study, we found two chromosomal aberrations (a mosaic trisomy 8 and a trisomy 21) out of 11 isolated diaphragmatic hernias and two aneuploidies (two trisomies 18) out of four cases associated with other malformations (Table 5).

About 50% of infants with diaphragmatic abnormalities have associated defects including, in order of frequency: CNS anomalies (especially myelocele), gastrointestinal malformations, genitourinary and cardiovascular defects. Adjunctive abnormalities increase the risk of associated chromosomal aberrations, and should be carefully investigated, even in cases of normal karyotype.

CYSTIC HYGROMA

Cystic hygroma of the neck is a congenital malformation characterized by lymph accumulation in the cervical region, caused by impaired communication between the lymphatic and the venous systems, this problem is normally already present on the 40th day of gestation.

The dilatation of the jugular lymphatic sacs along the sides of the neck is accompanied, in

Table 5 *Gastrointestinal malformations, abdominal wall defects and abnormality of karyotype*

Gastrointestinal malformations and abdominal wall defects	Isolated		Associated	
	Abnormal karyotype/anomalies observed	Abnormality of karyotype	Abnormal karyotype/anomalies observed	Abnormality of karyotype
Duodenal stenosis	4/6	4 × trisomy 21	1/3	1 × trisomy 21
Atresia of small intestine	0/9			
Omphalocele	1/7	1 × trisomy 18	4/6	4 × trisomy 18
Gastroschisis	0/5		0/3	
Diaphragmatic hernia	2/11	1 × trisomy 21 1 × 46,XY/47,XY,+ 8	2/4	2 × trisomy 18
Total	7/38 (18.4%)		7/16 (43.7%)	

most cases, by generalized lymph stasis, which may cause hydrops and fetal death[36,37]. This abnormality is frequently associated with karyotype anomalies, in varying – according to the different authors – but consistently extremely high percentages (60–70% of the cases)[36,38]. Turner syndrome 45,X accounts for 40–80% of chromosomal abnormalities in the different case histories[38].

Some phenotypic characteristics of this syndrome (pterygium colli, edema of the extremities due to peripheral lymphatic hypoplasia) suggest the presence of lymphatic impairment in the embryo, which was spontaneously resolved during intrauterine life. The lack of lymphatic drainage might in turn influence the genesis of cardiovascular anomalies, and aortic coarctation in particular, which are frequently associated with cystic hygromas in fetuses with monosomy X[27].

Other aneuploidies described in association with cystic hygromas are Turner mosaic (46,XX/45,X), trisomy 21 and trisomy 18, the 13 q- and 18 p- syndromes, partial 11q/22q trisomy, the mosaic-type trisomy 22 and Klinefelter's syndrome[36,38,39]. Bronshtein and coworkers[39,40] distinguished two types of cystic hygromas, i.e. septated and non-septated lesions. The former type of hygroma is frequently associated with aneuploidies (72%) and structural anomalies (52%), and is apparently characterized by an unfavorable prognosis, with a low percentage of liveborn infants (12%). Non-septated forms, probably due to transient lymphatic obstruction or retarded lymphatic-venous communication, seem to be associated with an abnormal karyotype only in 5.7% of the cases, and with other malformations in 15%. Furthermore, they appear to be transient in 98% of the cases, with 94% liveborn infants. According to Shulman and associates[41], however, non-septated forms are also associated with karyotype anomalies in a fairly significant percentage of cases (12.5%). So the karyotype needs to be performed in both cases.

Our case series included 58 fetuses with cystic hygroma. We found 42 cases of isolated cystic hygroma and 16 cases of hygroma associated with other structural abnormalities. The karyotype, obtained by amniocentesis or cordocentesis, or by means of cell culture after spontaneous or induced abortion, was available in 34 and 14 cases, respectively (Table 6). It was aneuploid – in agreement with the data reported in the literature – in 76.5% of the cases (Table 1). In cases with isolated cystic hygroma, 17 were monosomy X, six were cases of trisomy 21 (all in women who were 35 years of age or older), one was a case of trisomy 13 and two were cases of trisomy 18. In one case, the postmortem examination showed that the normal female karyotype 46,XX was accompanied by a male phenotype.

In hygromas combined with other malformations, associated chromosomal abnormalities accounted for 78.5% of the cases; in six cases aortic coarctation was found. All hygromas associated with aortic coarctation showed a monosomy X, of which one was a monosomy X mosaicism. In another case, the monosomy X was associated with renal defects (horseshoe kidney). Three cases of trisomy 18 were found: one case of hygroma was associated with clenched hands and talipes, one with an atrioventricular canal, and a third case was associated with gastroschisis and an atrioventricular canal. There was only one case of trisomy 21. Here, the hygroma was accompanied by cerebral ventriculomegaly. Six out of 58 cases of cystic hygroma were non-septated forms. Three cases were associated with chromosomal anomalies (two cases of trisomy 21, in women of 35 and 36 years of age, and one case of trisomy 18). No other associated malformations were found.

Table 6 *Cystic hygroma and abnormality of karyotype*

	Number of cases (%)	Abnormality of karyotype
Isolated	26/34 (76.5%)	17 × 45,X 6 × trisomy 21 2 × trisomy 18 1 × trisomy 13
Associated	11/14 (78.5%)	6 × 45,X 1 × 46,XX/45,X 1 × trisomy 21 3 × trisomy 18

SKELETAL MALFORMATIONS

Skeletal abnormalities represent a heterogeneous group of diseases, including different clinical entities where ossification disorders are associated with defects in other organs or tissues. These illnesses are so complex as to prevent their definitive classification. In fact, the cases described vary widely in numbers and characteristics, presenting as they do signs that are typical of other forms, or failing to exhibit other signs that are considered specific to the disease in question. Based on the International Classification of skeletal malformation reported in reference 18, we can distinguish:

(1) Osteochondrodysplasias, including a series of syndromes where cartilage anomalies are associated with abnormal bone development;

(2) Dysostoses, including all abnormalities involving limb shortening and congenital bending of long bones;

(3) Idiopathic osteolysis;

(4) Primary metabolic abnormalities;

(5) Miscellaneous disorders with osseous involvement;

(6) Chromosomal anomalies.

Some skeletal abnormalities exhibit an almost constant association with chromosomal aberrations, with particular regard to trisomies.

In trisomy 18, frequent findings include clenched hands with overlapping fingers, most frequently with the index finger overlapping the middle finger, with the fifth finger curved inward. Other skeletal problems include rocker-bottom feet, talipes and arthrogryposis. Cleft lip and/or palate is less common in trisomy 18 than in trisomy 13. In addition, a variety of different anomalies involving virtually every system have been described in conjunction with trisomy 18: cardiovascular malformations, omphalocele, urinary tract anomalies and central nervous system malformations[42,43].

The characteristic findings of trisomy 13 include microcephaly, anophthalmia or microphthalmia, cleft lip and palate, flexed and overlapping fingers, polydactyly and clubfoot. Of internal anomalies, malformations of the central nervous system, (like holoprosencephaly), cardiovascular anomalies (also of minor entity) and anomalies of genitourinary tract are common.

The ultrasonographic markers of trisomy 21 related to the skeletal system are the relative shortening of the femur and humerus, clinodactily and sandal gap. In triploidies, together with the characteristic ultrasonographic findings, such as early growth retardation and placental anomalies, syndactyly of the third and fourth fingers and talipes equinovarus are commonly found[44]. Limb abnormalities are therefore characteristic of various chromosomal anomalies, and ultrasonographic detection of hand and foot alterations should stimulate the search for associated defects.

In our series of 78 isolated skeletal abnormalities (including 16 cases of osteochondrodysplasias, seven cases of focal limb loss, three cases of clubfoot, eight cases of cleft lip and palate and three cases of miscellanea) the karyotype was shown to be normal in all the 37 karyotypes performed.

In 22 cases, skeletal defects were associated with other malformations. Of the 20 karyotypes performed, 17 were shown to be pathological. The sonographic findings – in various associations – most frequently associated with chromosomal aberrations were: the overlapping fingers in trisomy 18, cleft lip/palate in trisomy 13 and syndactyly in triploidy[45] (Table 7). While an isolated picture is not associated with aneuploidy, skeletal abnormalities found in conjunction with multiple malformations can thus play a role as of sonographic markers of karyotype anomaly[46].

RESPIRATORY SYSTEM MALFORMATIONS

In accordance with the data reported in the literature, our experience also showed that respiratory system abnormalities were not associated with karyotype anomalies.

Table 7 *Minor skeletal malformations and abnormality of karyotype*

Malformation	Trisomy 18	Trisomy 13	Other	Triploidy
Overlapping fingers	6	2	1 × 46,XY,+ inv(10)	—
			1 × 46,XX,10 q+	
Clubfoot	3	1	—	—
Flexed hands	2	1	1 × 46,XY/47,XY,+ 18	—
Cleft lip/palate	2	3	—	1
Upper limb reduction	1	—	—	—
Syndactyly	—	—	—	1
Micrognathia	1	—	—	—

Other possible markers of fetal chromosomal anomalies

Identification through non-invasive techniques of fetuses with potential karyotype anomalies is one of the objectives pursued by ultrasound prenatal diagnostics in recent years.

With few exceptions, performance of fetal karyotype after sonographic detection of major – isolated or multiple – malformations is a routine practice. This approach does not allow diagnosis of all fetuses with chromosome anomalies. Many of these, in fact, have a perfectly normal appearance even under the closest examination by an experienced operator, or indeed show the alterations characteristic of chromosomal anomalies only at a later stage in pregnancy. Sometimes they do exhibit, however, subtle variations of biometric or morphological parameters, and many authors have focused on these aspects. A wide range of sonographic pictures have been described, which can be helpful in order to identify fetuses with aneuploidy with varying degrees of reproducibility and sensitivity: from a thickened nuchal fold, to relative limb shortness, hypoplasia of the middle phalanx of the fifth finger and a dilated cisterna magna, which are all discussed in detail in a different section of this book. Here we will only consider borderline ventriculomegaly.

The lateral ventricles are visualized and measured during routine sonography, so deviations from what are considered normal values can be detected. Deviations from the normal range of values frequently represent a reason for referral in order to define the risk of aneuploidy.

Borderline ventriculomegaly

Ever since it became known that the width of the atrium of the lateral ventricle is a parameter which is independent of gestational age, it has been accepted that borderline deviations from these values (generally between 10 and 15 mm) are characteristic of a group of subjects with mild ventriculomegaly who deserve attention[47]. Some studies also referring to postnatal life do report, in fact, their association with karyotype anomalies, and with trisomy 21 in particular. Even though the cause for ventricular dilatation in Down syndrome and in other aneuploidies is uncertain, it is thought to be due to non-obstructive phenomena related to cerebral mass reduction or atrophy.

The studies published so far, providing homogeneous definitions of borderline ventriculomegaly, are summarized in Table 8. They refer to cases of ventriculomegaly that were diagnosed at different stages of pregnancy in populations at high risk, with the exception of a perspective study on low-risk pregnancies in the second trimester. Mahoney and associates[48] studied a series of 20 fetuses with isolated ventriculomegaly. They observed one case of trisomy 21 that was diagnosed after birth and was associated with other malformations, out of a total of 11 karyotypes performed.

In the 55 fetuses studied by Goldstein and colleagues[49], ventriculomegaly was isolated in 13 cases. In the five karyotypes performed in this group, chromosomes were found to be normal. In 42 fetuses, ventriculomegaly was found in conjunction with other malformations: in this condition the karyotype was altered in eight out of 25 karyotypes performed[49]. In the series

Table 8 *Mild ventriculomegaly and abnormal karyotype*

Study	Isolated karyotypes performed/anomalies observed	Associated karyotypes performed/anomalies observed	Abnormality of karyotype
Mahoney *et al.*, 1988[48]	11/20	—	1 × trisomy 21*
Goldstein *et al.*, 1990[49]	5/13	—	0
Bromley *et al.*, 1991[50]	—	25/42	8 not specified
	—	12/44	3 × trisomy 21
			1 × trisomy 18
			1 × del 7 p
D'Ottavio *et al.*, 1995 (our data)	11/15	—	1 × trisomy 21
			1 × triploidy
			1 × 46,XY,− 7,+
			der (7)t(7;8)pat
Achiron *et al.*, 1993[51]	—	1/1	1 × trisomy 21
	2/4	—	1 × trisomy 21
	—	4/4	1 × trisomy 18

*Additional anomalies and karyotype detected after birth

of Bromley and co-workers[50] (44 fetuses with associated ventriculomegaly), the group of 12 karyotypes performed showed five cases of chromosome aberration.

We have observed 15 cases of isolated ventriculomegaly. The karyotype, available for 11 fetuses, was altered in three cases: one trisomy 21 and one triploidy in women above 35 years of age; one unbalanced translocation 7/8 of a paternal origin. One fetus with ventriculomegaly associated with nuchal edema had trisomy 21. In this case the mother's age was above 35. A perspective study by Achiron and associates[51], conducted on a low-risk population in the second trimester of pregnancy, highlighted eight cases of ventriculomegaly. Out of the six karyotypes performed (two in isolated forms, four in conjunction with other pathological findings) two aneuploidies were diagnosed.

CONCLUSIONS

Although chromosomal abnormalities are not amenable to treatment, if the diagnosis is made before viability, a termination of pregnancy can be offered to the parents or unnecessary interventions (i.e. Cesarean section in case of fetal distress) can be avoided, later in pregnancy.

As previously mentioned, antenatal diagnosis of chromosomal defects, in a low-risk population, is based not only on biochemical screening, but, mainly on ultrasonographic detection of certain malformations, especially in multiple association. Nicolaides and colleagues[45] have shown an increasing correlation between the number of anomalies and the risk of chromosomal aberrations. For example, when two abnormalities were associated, the risk of chromosomal abnormality amounted to 29%, whereas, when five major or minor anomalies were associated, the risk increased up to 70%. Similarly, other authors have demonstrated an increased risk of chromosomal anomaly in cases of malformations associated with intrauterine growth retardation or with polyhydramnios[52]. Nevertheless, even single specific anomalies carry a relatively high risk of chromosomal aberration. Fetal karyotyping is therefore advisable any time such malformations are detected, even when no other defects can be recognized[53].

Malformations, albeit isolated, indicating possible association with chromosomal abnormalities include facial cleft, esophageal atresia, duodenal stenosis, omphalocele, diaphragmatic hernia, major and minor cardiac defects, distal urinary tract obstruction and cystic kidneys, holoprosencephaly and agenesis of corpus callosum, neural tube defect, cystic hygroma and polidactily[46,54]. In contrast, gastroschisis and atresia of small intestine, unilateral hydronephrosis, skeletal dysplasia and transposition of the great arteries, if isolated, do not seem to represent an increased risk of chromosomal anomaly.

Given a malformation, it is important to point out that the risk of chromosomal abnormality is inversely related to the severity of the defect. Indeed, a fetus with a small omphalocele has a much higher risk of chromosomal aberration than one with a large omphalocele (containing either bowel or liver). The same applies to fetuses with mild ventriculomegaly or bilateral pyelectasis, as compared to those with clearly defined hydrocephaly or hydronephrosis.

Ultrasonographic markers of chromosomal abnormalities are a controversial issue in prenatal diagnosis. Indeed, the number of such markers is continually increasing and they may even be found in some normal fetuses. This makes it difficult to decide whether or not to perform an invasive diagnostic procedure. Nevertheless many authors agree that when at least some of these sonographic markers (e.g. ventriculomegaly or nuchal thickening) are present, the risk of aneuploidy is such as to justify an invasive test.

When carrying out a sonographic examination, the real problem consists of not detecting, or underestimating those slight changes in anatomy or in biometry which actually put the fetus at risk of a chromosomal aberration. It is commonly accepted that the likelihood of having a fetus with chromosomal abnormalities increases with increasing maternal age, and decreases with the growing of gestational age (because of the greater rate of spontaneous abortions of fetuses with abnormal karyotype). Therefore in each individual case one should carefully evaluate the risk of losing a pregnancy, entailed in the use of invasive techniques, as against the risk of giving birth to a child with karyotype abnormalities.

Another point to be considered is a possible association of abnormal sonographic findings with genetic syndromes, metabolic errors or anatomical abnormalities, which cannot be definitely ruled out, even when a karyotype is normal. Despite this limitation, fetal karyotype plays an essential role in prenatal diagnosis, especially considering the great impact that a child with a chromosomal anomaly has on the family and on the community at large.

References

1. Milunsky, A. (ed.) (1992). *Genetic Disorders and The Fetus*, 3rd edn. (Baltimore, London: The Johns Hopkins University Press)
2. Brock, K. J. H., Rodeck, Ch. H. and Ferguson-Smith, M. A. (eds.) (1992). *Prenatal Diagnosis and Screening*. (London: Churchill Livingstone)
3. Hook, E. B. and Porter, I. H. (eds.) (1977). *Population Cytogenetics*. (New York, San Francisco, London: Academic Press)
4. Bogart, M. H., Pandian, M. R. and Jones, O. W. (1987). Abnormal maternal serum chorionic gonadotropin levels in pregnancies with fetal chromosome abnormalities. *Prenat. Diagn.*, **7**, 623–30
5. Bogart, M. H., Golbus, M. S., Sorg, N. D. and Jones, O. W. (1989). Human chorionic gonadotropin levels in pregnancies with aneuploid fetuses. *Prenat. Diagn.*, **9**, 379–84
6. Canick, J. A., Knight, G. J., Palomaki, G. E., Haddow, J. E., Cuckle, H. S. and Wald, N. J. (1988). Low second trimester maternal serum unconjugated oestriol in pregnancies with Down's syndrome. *Br. J. Obstet. Gynaecol.*, **95**, 330–33
7. Wald, N. J., Cuckle, H. S., Densem, J. W., Nanchahal, K., Canick, J. A., Haddow, J. E., Knight, G. J. and Palomaki, G. E. (1988). Maternal serum screening for Down's syndrome in early pregnancy. *Br. J. Obstet. Gynaecol.*, **95**, 334–41
8. Gulotta, F., Rehder, H. and Gropp, A. (1981). Descriptive neuropathology of chromosomal disorders in man. *Hum. Genet.*, **57**, 337–51
9. Machin, G. A. and Crolla, J. A. (1974). Chromosome constitution of 500 infants dying during the perinatal period. *Humangenetik*, **23**, 183–7
10. Sutherland, G. R., Carter, R. F., Bauld, R., Smith, I. I. and Bain, A. D. (1978). Chromosome studies at the paediatric necropsy. *Ann. Hum. Genet.*, **42**, 173–6
11. McFadden, D. and Kalousek, D. (1989). Survey of neural tube defects in spontaneously aborted embryos. *Am. J. Med. Genet.*, **32**, 356–8

12. Demyer, W. (1977). Holoprosencephaly. In Vinknen, P. and Bruyn, G. (eds.) *Congenital Malformations of the Brain and Skull, Handbook of Clinical Neurology*, Vol. 30, pp. 431–9. (Amsterdam: Elsevier North Holland Publishing Co.)

13. Cohen, M. (1982). An update on the holoprosencephalic disorders. *J. Pediatr.*, **101**, 865–9

14. Laurence, K. (1987). Hydrocephalus and malformations of the central nervous system. In Keeling, J. W. (ed.) *Fetal and Neonatal Pathology*, pp. 463–5. (Berlin, Heidelberg, New York: Springer-Verlag)

15. Pilu, G., Goldstein, I., Reece, E. A., Perolo, A., Foschini, M. P., Hobbins, J. C. and Bovicelli, L. (1992). Sonography of fetal Dandy–Walker malformation: a reappraisal. *Ultrasound Obstet. Gynecol.*, **2**, 151–7

16. Nyberg, D. A., Mahony, B. S., Hegge, F. N., Hickok, D., Luthy, D. A. and Kapur, R. (1991). Enlarged cisterna magna and the Dandy–Walker malformation: factors associated with chromosome abnormalities. *Obstet. Gynecol.*, **77**, 436–42

17. Campbell, L., Dayton, D. and Sohal, G. (1986). Neural tube defects: a review of human and animal studies of the etiology of neural tube defects. *Teratology*, **34**, 171–87

18. Kalousek, D. K., Fitch, N. and Paradice, B. A. (1990). *Pathology of the Human Embryo and Previable Fetus*, pp. 128–39. (New York, Berlin, Heidelberg: Springer-Verlag)

19. Harmon, J. P., Hiett, A. K., Palmer, C. G. and Golichowski, A. M. (1995). Prenatal ultrasound detection of isolated neural tube defects: is cytogenetic evaluation warranted? *Obstet. Gynecol.*, **86**, 595–9

20. Vergani, P., Ghidini, A., Strobelt, N., Locatelli, A., Mariani, S., Bertalero, C. and Cavallone, M. (1994). Prognostic indicators in the prenatal diagnosis of agenesis of corpus callosum. *Am. J. Obstet. Gynecol.*, **170**, 753–8

21. Gupta, J. K. and Lilford, R. J. (1995). Assessment and management of fetal agenesis of the corpus callosum. *Prenat. Diagn.*, **15**, 301–12

22. Šamànek, M., Goetzova, J. and Benesova, D. (1986). Causes of death in neonates born with a heart malformation. *Int. J. Cardiol.*, **11**, 63–74

23. Ferencz, C., Neill, C. A., Boughman, J. A., Rubin, J. D., Brenner, J. I. and Perry, L. W. (1989). Congenital cardiovascular malformations associated with chromosome abnormalities: an epidemiologic study. *J. Pediatr.*, **114**, 79–86

24. Berg, K. A., Clark, E. B., Astemborski, J. A. and Boughman, J. A. (1988). Prenatal detection of cardiovascular malformations by echocardiography: an indication for cytogenetic evaluation. *Am. J. Obstet. Gynecol.*, **159**, 477–81

25. Bronshtein, M., Zimmer, E. Z., Milo, S., Ho, S. Y., Lorber, A. and Gerlis, L. M. (1991). Fetal cardiac abnormalities detected by transvaginal sonography at 12–16 weeks' gestation. *Obstet. Gynecol.*, **78**, 374

26. Kurnit, D. M., Aldridge, J. F., Matsuoka, R. and Matthysse, S. (1985). Increased adhesiveness of trisomy 21 cells and atrioventricular canal malformations in Down's syndrome: a stochastic model. *Am. J. Med. Genet.*, **20**, 385–99

27. Clark, E. B. (1984). Neck web and congenital heart defects: a pathogenic association in 45 X-O Turner syndrome? *Teratology*, **29**, 355–61

28. Respondek, M. L., Binotto, C. N., Smith, S., Donnenfeld, A., Weil, S. R. and Huhta, J. C. (1994). Extracardiac anomalies, aneuploidy and growth retardation in 100 consecutive fetal congenital heart defects. *Ultrasound Obstet. Gynecol.*, **4**, 272–8

29. Nicolaides, K. H., Cheng, H., Snijders, R. J. M. and Gosden, C. M. (1992). Fetal renal defects: associated malformations and chromosomal defects. *Fetal Diagn. Ther.*, **7**, 1–11

30. German, J. C., Mahour, G. H. and Wooley, M. M. (1976). Esophageal atresia and associated anomalies. *J. Pediatr. Surg.*, **11**, 299–306

31. Tibboel, D., van Nie, C. J. and Molenavar, J. C. (1980). The effect of temporary general hypoxia and local ischemia on the development of the intestine: an experimental study. *J. Pediatr. Surg.*, **15**, 57–64

32. Hughes, M. D., Nyberg, D. A., Mack, L. A. and Pretorius, D. H. (1989). Fetal omphalocele: prenatal US detection of concurrent anomalies and other predictors of outcome. *Radiology*, **173**, 371–6

33. Dott, N. (1932). Clinical record of case of exomphalos, illustrating embryonic type and its surgical treatment. *Trans. Edinburgh Obstet. Soc.*, **52**, 105–8

34. Getachew, M. M., Goldstein, R. B., Edge, V., Goldberg, J. D. and Filly, R. A. (1991). Correlation between omphalocele contents and karyotypic abnormalities: sonographic study in 37 cases. *Am. J. Roentgenol.*, **158**, 133–6

35. Benacerraf, B. and Adzick, N. (1987). Fetal diaphragmatic hernia: ultrasound diagnosis and clinical outcome in 19 cases. *Am. J. Obstet. Gynecol.*, **156**, 573–6

36. Chervenak, F. A., Isaacson, G., Blakemore, K. J., Breg, W. R., Hobbins, J. C., Berkowitz, R. L., Tortora, M., Mayden, K. and Mahoney, M. J. (1983). Fetal cystic hygroma. Cause and natural history. *N. Engl. J. Med.*, **309**, 822–5

37. Cullen, M. T., Gabrielli, S., Green, J. J., Rizzo, N., Mahoney, M. J., Salafia, C., Bovicelli, L. and Hobbins, J. C. (1990). Diagnosis and significance

of cystic hygroma in the first trimester. *Prenat. Diagn.*, **10**, 643–51

38. Abramowicz, J. S., Warsof, S. L., Lochner Doyle, D., Smith, D. and Levy, D. L. (1989). Congenital cystic hygroma of the neck diagnosed prenatally: outcome with normal and abnormal karyotype. *Prenat. Diagn.*, **9**, 321–27

39. Bronshtein, M., Bar-Hava, I., Blumenfeld, I., Bejar, J., Toder, V. and Blumenfeld, Z. (1993). The difference between septated and non septated nuchal cystic hygroma in the early second trimester. *Obstet. Gynecol.*, **81**, 683–7

40. Bronshtein, M., Rottem, S., Yoffe, N. and Blumenfeld, Z. (1989). First-trimester and early second-trimester diagnosis of nuchal cystic hygroma by transvaginal sonography: diverse prognosis of the septated from the non septated lesion. *Am. J. Obstet. Gynecol.*, **161**, 78–82

41. Shulman, L. P., Raafat, N. A., Mace, P. C., Emerson, D. S., Felker, R. E., Simpson, J. L. and Elias, S. (1994). Significance of septations in isolated fetal cystic hygroma detected in the first trimester. *Prenat. Diagn.*, **14**, 223–6

42. Nicolaides, K. H. and Campbell, S. (1992). Ultrasound diagnosis congenital abnormalities. In Milunsky, A. (ed.) *Genetic Disorders and Fetus*, pp. 593–648. (Baltimore, London: The Johns Hopkins, University Press)

43. Sepulveda, W., Treadwell, M. C. and Fisk, N. M. (1995). Prenatal detection of preaxial upper limb reduction in trisomy 18. *Obstet. Gynecol.*, **85**, 847–50

44. Sanders, R. C. (1993). Ultrasonic clues to the detection of chromosomal anomalies. *Obstet. Gynecol. Clin. North Am.*, **20**, 455–83

45. Nicolaides, K. H., Snijders, R. J. M., Gosdan, C. M., Berry, C. and Campbell, S. (1992). Ultrasonographically detectable markers of fetal chromosomal abnormalities. *Lancet*, **340**, 704–7

46. Eydoux, P., Choiset, A., Le Porrier, N., Thepot, F., Szpiro-Tapia, S., Alliet, J., Ramond, S., Viel, J. F., Gautier, E., Morichon, N. and Girard-Orgeolet, S. (1989). Chromosomal prenatal diagnosis: study of 936 cases of intrauterine abnormalities after ultrasound assessment. *Prenat. Diagn.*, **9**, 255–68

47. Cardoza, J. D., Goldstein, R. B. and Filly, R. A. (1988). Exclusion of fetal ventriculomegaly with a single measurement: the width of the lateral ventricular atrium. *Radiology*, **169**, 711–14

48. Mahony, B. S., Nyberg, D. A., Hirsch, J. H., Petty, C. N., Hendricks, S. K. and Mack, L. A. (1988). Mild idiopathic lateral cerebral ventricular dilatation *in utero*: sonographic evaluation. *Radiology*, **169**, 715–21

49. Goldstein, R. B., La Pidus, A. S., Filly, R. A. and Cardoza, J. (1990). Mild lateral cerebral ventricular dilatation *in utero*: clinical significance and prognosis. *Radiology*, **176**, 237–42

50. Bromley, B., Frigoletto, Jr, F. D. and Benacerraf, B. R. (1991). Mild fetal lateral cerebral ventriculomegaly: clinical course and outcome. *Am. J. Obstet. Gynecol.*, **164**, 863–7

51. Achiron, R., Schimmel, M., Achiron, A. and Mashiach, S. (1993). Fetal mild idiopathic lateral ventriculomegaly: is there a correlation with fetal trisomy? *Ultrasound Obstet. Gynecol.*, **3**, 89–92

52. Gagnon, S., Fraser, W., Fouquette, B., Bastide, A., Bureau, M., Fontaine, J. Y. and Huot, C. (1992). Nature and frequency of chromosomal abnormalities in pregnancies with abnormal ultrasound findings: an analysis of 117 cases with review of the literature. *Prenat. Diagn.*, **12**, 9–18

53. Rizzo, N., Pittalis, M. C., Pilu, G. L., Orsini, L. F., Perolo, A. and Bovicelli, L. (1990). Prenatal karyotyping in malformed fetuses. *Prenat. Diagn.*, **10**, 17–23

54. Nicolaides, K., Shawwa, L., Brizot, M. and Snijders, R. (1993). Ultrasonographically detectable markers of fetal chromosomal defects. *Ultrasound Obstet. Gynecol.*, **3**, 56–69

Nuchal translucency screening for chromosomal abnormalities in the first trimester

17

N. J. Sebire, R. J. M. Snijders, A. Kalogeropoulos, N. Psara and K. H. Nicolaides

INTRODUCTION

Increased nuchal translucency at 10–14 weeks of gestation is a common phenotypic expression of trisomies, Turner syndrome and triploidy. This chapter examines the development of a new method of screening for chromosomal defects based on the combination of fetal nuchal translucency thickness, maternal age and maternal serum biochemistry during the first trimester of pregnancy.

METHODS OF SCREENING FOR CHROMOSOMAL DEFECTS

The first method of selecting pregnancies for invasive testing was based on the observation, made at the beginning of this century, that the incidence of fetal chromosomal abnormalities is associated with maternal age[1]. Since the early 1970s, when amniocentesis for fetal karyotyping was introduced, the procedure has been offered to women on the basis of advanced maternal age, 37 years or over; this 'high-risk' group constitute approximately 5% of the pregnant population. Twenty-five years later we now know that the high-risk group contributes only about 30% of trisomy 21 babies and that screening on the basis of maternal age has not resulted in a substantial fall in the proportion of infants born with this condition[2].

In the late 1980s a new method of screening was introduced that takes into account not only maternal age but also the concentration of various fetoplacental products in the maternal circulation. At 16 weeks of gestation the median maternal serum concentrations of α-fetoprotein, estriol and chorionic gonadotropin (total, free α- and free β-hCG) in trisomy 21 pregnancies are sufficiently different from the median in normal pregnancies to allow the use of combinations of some or all of these substances to select a 'high-risk' group. This method of screening is proving to be more effective than maternal age alone and for the same rate of invasive testing (about 5%) it can identify about 60% of the fetuses with trisomy 21[3–5].

An alternative method of screening is ultrasound examination in the first trimester of pregnancy[6]. Increased fetal nuchal translucency thickness at 10–14 weeks of gestation is a common phenotypic expression of trisomies 21, 18 and 13, Turner syndrome and triploidy. This method has now been proven to identify more than 80% of affected fetuses for a false positive rate of about 5%[7]. When fetal heart rate and maternal serum free β-hCG are also taken into account the detection rate of chromosomal defects is about 90%[8,9].

ABNORMAL NUCHAL FLUID

During the second and third trimesters of pregnancy, abnormal accumulation of fluid behind the fetal neck can be classified as nuchal cystic hygromas and nuchal edema, in the first trimester the term translucency is used.

Nuchal cystic hygromas

Nuchal cystic hygromas are developmental abnormalities of the lymphatic system. Prenatal diagnosis by ultrasonography is based on the demonstration of a bilateral, septated, cystic structure, located in the occipitocervical region. Reports on antenatally diagnosed cystic hygromas have established an association with hydrops fetalis (40–100% of cases), congenital heart defects (0–90% of cases) and chromosomal defects (45–90% of fetuses); the commonest being Turner syndrome[10]. The wide range in the reported incidence of hydrops fetalis, cardiac defects and both the presence and types of chromosomal defects may be a consequence of differences in the diagnostic criteria for cystic hygromas used in the various reports. Azar and colleagues[10] examined only fetuses with septated, cervical, dorsal hygromata and 75% had chromosomal defects; Turner syndrome accounted for about 95% of the chromosomal defects.

Nuchal edema

Nuchal edema is due to subcutaneous accumulation of fluid that produces a characteristic tremor on ballotment of the fetal heart[11]. It may be considered as an early sign of hydrops fetalis, which has a diverse etiology including trisomies, cardiovascular and pulmonary defects, skeletal dysplasias, congenital infection and metabolic and hematological disorders. Benacerraf and co-workers[12,13] noted the association between increased soft tissue thickening on the posterior aspect of the neck and trisomy 21. In a series of 1704 consecutive amniocenteses at 15–20 weeks of gestation in which there were 11 fetuses with trisomy 21, 45% of the trisomic and 0.06% of the normal fetuses had nuchal thickness > 5 mm. Nicolaides and associates[11] considered nuchal edema to be present if in the mid-sagittal plane of the neck there was subcutaneous edema > 7 mm. This was distinguished from nuchal cystic hygromata and hydrops fetalis (accompanying generalized edema). In a series of 144 fetuses with nuchal edema, 37% had chromosomal defects, mainly trisomy 21, but also other trisomies, deletions or translocations, triploidy and Turner syndrome[11]. Furthermore, the chromosomally normal fetuses had a very poor prognosis because in many cases there was an underlying skeletal dysplasia, genetic syndrome or cardiac defect[11].

Nuchal translucency

In the first trimester abnormal accumulation of nuchal fluid is referred to as nuchal translucency[6]. Although in some studies the condition was defined as multiseptated thin-walled cystic mass similar to that seen in the second trimester, in others the term was used loosely to include nuchal thickening or edema. We prefer the use of the term translucency, as opposed to cystic hygroma or nuchal edema, because this is the ultrasonographic feature that is observed; during the second trimester the translucency usually resolves and in a few cases it persists as nuchal edema or evolves into generalized hydrops.

ASSESSMENT OF NUCHAL TRANSLUCENCY THICKNESS

Measurement

Transabdominal ultrasound examination is performed to obtain a sagittal section of the fetus for measurement of fetal crown–rump length. The maximum thickness of the subcutaneous translucency between the skin and the soft tissue overlying the cervical spine is measured[6]. Care is taken to distinguish between fetal skin and amnion because at this gestation both structures appear as thin membranes (Figure 1). This is

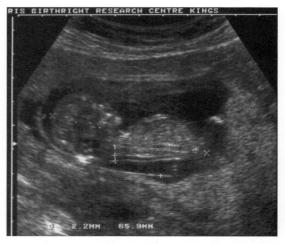

Figure 1 *An ultrasound image showing the measurement of the fetal nuchal translucency. The amnion can be seen as a separate membrane from the fetal skin*

achieved by waiting for spontaneous fetal movement away from the amniotic membrane; alternatively the fetus is bounced off the amnion by asking the mother to cough and/or by tapping the maternal abdomen. All sonographers performing fetal scans should be capable of measuring reliably the crown–rump length and obtaining a proper sagittal view of the fetal spine. For such sonographers it is easy to acquire, within a few hours, the skill to measure accurately nuchal translucency thickness.

Repeatability

A potential criticism of screening by ultrasound is that scanning requires not only highly-skilled operators but it is also prone to operator variability. This issue was addressed by a prospective study at 10–14 weeks of gestation in which the translucency was measured by two of four operators in 200 pregnant women[14]. To assess repeatability of different components of variability six measurements of nuchal translucency were made on each fetus. The first operator generated the appropriate image and measured the translucency and then generated a new image and repeated the measurement (intra-observer repeatability). This second image was frozen on the screen but the calipers were removed and the second operator reset the calipers and made a measurement (caliper placement repeatability). The process was then repeated with the operators reversed (inter-observer repeatability). This study demonstrated that when the nuchal translucency thickness is measured by well-trained operators the measurement is highly reproducible. The repeatability was unrelated to the size of the nuchal translucency and when the mean of two measurements was used 95% of the time the intra- and interobserver repeatability was 0.54 and 0.62 mm, respectively. Additionally, the study demonstrated that the caliper placement repeatability was similar to the intra- and interobserver repeatability, suggesting that a large part of the variation in measurements can be accounted for by the placement of the calipers rather than the generation of the image.

Increase with gestational age

In a multicenter study involving more than 20 000 pregnancies, the fetal nuchal translucency thickness increased with crown–rump length (Figure 2)[7]. Therefore in determining whether a given nuchal translucency thickness is increased it is essential to take gestation into account.

NUCHAL TRANSLUCENCY AND CHROMOSOMAL DEFECTS

In the early 1990s several reports of small series in high-risk pregnancies demonstrated a possible association between abnormal nuchal fluid and chromosomal defects in the first trimester of pregnancy. Subsequently, a series of screening studies in high-risk pregnancies were carried out; these involved measurement of nuchal translucency thickness immediately before fetal karyotyping, mainly for advanced maternal age. These studies reported that the prevalence of chromosomal defects is dependent on both the

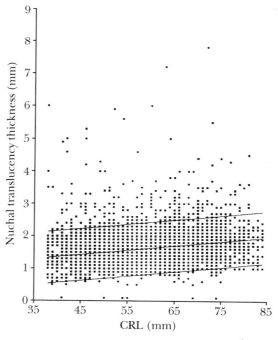

Figure 2 *Fetal nuchal translucency thickness plotted against crown–rump length (CRL) in 20 217 chromosomally normal fetuses (median, 5th and 95th centiles)*

fetal nuchal translucency thickness and maternal age. More recently, screening studies of unselected populations were carried out. These studies established the distribution of nuchal translucency thickness with crown–rump length in chromosomally normal and abnormal fetuses and from the overlapping distributions it was possible to calculate risks for chromosomal defects with any given nuchal translucency thickness. Such studies also established that the risks for trisomies can be derived by combining data from maternal age, fetal nuchal translucency thickness, fetal heart rate and maternal serum concentrations of placental products.

Observational studies

Several studies documented a strong association between abnormal nuchal translucency and chromosomal defects (Table 1)[6,15–33].

Although the mean prevalence of chromosomal defects in 20 series involving a total of 1698 patients was 29%, there were large differences between the studies with the prevalence ranging from 19 to 88%. This variation in results was presumably the consequence of both the failure to take into account the maternal age distribution of the populations examined, and differences in the definition of minimum thickness of the abnormal translucency, ranging from 2 to 10 mm.

Screening in high-risk populations

In a prospective study of 827 women with singleton pregnancies undergoing first-trimester fetal karyotyping because of advanced maternal age, parental anxiety, or a family history of a chromosomal abnormality in the absence of balanced parental translocation, the translucency thickness was measured[6]. This study suggested that invasive testing for patients with translucency of > 2.5 mm would identify 77% of the fetuses with trisomy 21 with a false positive rate of 4.1%. In

Table 1 *Summary of reported series on first-trimester fetal nuchal translucency providing data on gestational age, criteria for diagnosis and the presence of associated chromosomal defects*

Author	Gestation (weeks)	Translucency thickness (mm)	n	Total n	Total %	Tr21	Tr18	Tr13	45,X	Other
Johnson *et al.* 1993[15]	10–14	≥ 2.0	68	41	60	16	9	2	9	5
Hewitt *et al.* 1993[16]	10–14	≥ 2.0	29	12	41	5	3	1	2	1
Shulman *et al.* 1992[17]	10–13	≥ 2.5	32	15	47	4	4	3	4	—
Nicolaides *et al.* 1992[6,18]	10–13	≥ 3.0	88	33	38	21	8	2	—	2
Pandya *et al.* 1994[19,20]	10–13	≥ 3.0	1015	194	19	101	51	13	14	15
Szabo and Gellen, 1990[21]	11–12	≥ 3.0	8	7	88	7	—	—	—	—
Wilson *et al.* 1992[22]	8–11	≥ 3.0	14	3	21	—	—	—	1	2
Ville *et al.* 1992[23]	9–14	≥ 3.0	29	8	28	4	3	1	—	—
Trauffer *et al.* 1994[24]	10–14	≥ 3.0	43	21	49	9	4	1	4	3
Brambati *et al.* 1995[25]	8–15	≥ 3.0	70	13	19	?	?	?	?	?
Comas *et al.* 1995[26]	9–13	≥ 3.0	51	9	18	4	4	—	—	1
Szabo *et al.* 1995[27]	9–12	≥ 3.0	96	43	45	28	10	—	2	3
Nadel *et al.* 1993[28]	10–15	≥ 4.0	63	43	68	15	15	1	10	2
Savoldelli *et al.* 1993[29]	9–12	≥ 4.0	24	19	79	15	2	1	1	—
Shulte-Vallentin and Schindler, 1992[30]	10–14	≥ 4.0	8	7	88	7	—	—	—	—
van Zalen-Sprock *et al.* 1992[31]	10–14	≥ 4.0	18	6	33	3	1	—	1	1
Cullen *et al.* 1990[32]	11–13	≥ 6.0	29	15	52	6	2	—	4	3
Suchet *et al.* 1992[33]	8–14	≥ 10.0	13	8	62	—	—	—	7	1
Total	8–15		1698	497	29	245	116	25	59	39

Tr21, trisomy 21; Tr18, trisomy 18; Tr13, trisomy 13; 45,X, Turner syndrome

an expanded series of 1273 women the translucency thickness was > 2.5 mm in 84% of the fetuses with trisomy 21 and in 4.5% of the chromosomally normal fetuses; the corresponding values for translucencies of > 3.5 mm were 60 and 1% respectively[18].

Similar findings were obtained in an additional four studies of pregnancies undergoing first-trimester fetal karyotyping (Table 2)[26,27,29,30]. However, in another study involving 1819 pregnancies, nuchal translucency thickness of > 3 mm identified only 30% of the chromosomally abnormal fetuses (no data were provided specifically for trisomy 21) and the false positive rate was 3.2%[25].

Pandya and colleagues[19] in a study of 560 pregnancies with increased fetal nuchal translucency thickness (2.5–9 mm) at 10–14 weeks of gestation, reported that the incidence of chromosomal defects increased with both maternal age and translucency thickness. In an expanded series of 1015 pregnancies with increased nuchal translucency the observed number of trisomies 21, 18 and 13 fetuses with translucencies of

3, 4, 5 and > 6 mm was approximately three-, 18-, 28- and 36-times higher than the respective number expected on the basis of maternal age (Table 3, Figure 3); the incidence of Turner syndrome and triploidy was nine- and eight-times higher, respectively, but the incidence of other sex chromosome aneuploidies was similar to that expected[20].

Screening in unselected populations

The Frimley Park and St Peter's study

Frimley Park and St Peter's are general hospitals within the NHS with a combined annual number of deliveries of approximately 6000. Prior to the introduction of nuchal translucency scanning, the policy of these hospitals was to offer amniocentesis to women aged 35 years or older. During 1993 there were 11 fetuses with Down syndrome and only two of these were detected prenatally[34].

Subsequently, nuchal translucency screening was introduced and the implementation of this

Table 2 *The sensitivity and false positive rate of screening with fetal nuchal translucency ≥ 3 and ≥ 4 mm in five screening studies*

Author	Gestation (weeks)	n	Trisomy 21	Nuchal translucency ≥ 3 mm		Nuchal translucency ≥ 4 mm	
				Sensitivity (%)	False positive (%)	Sensitivity (%)	False positive (%)
Shulte-Vallentin et al. 1992[30]	10–14	632	7	—	—	100	0.2
Savoldelli et al. 1993[29]	9–12	1400	28	—	—	53.6	0.4
Nicolaides et al. 1994[18]	10–14	1273	25	84.0	4.5	60.0	1.0
Comas et al. 1995[26]	9–13	481	7	57.1	9.5	57.1	0.7
Szabo et al. 1995[27]	9–12	3380	31	90.0	1.6	67.7	0.4
Total		7166	98	84.1	3.0	63.3	0.5

Table 3 *Observed number of trisomies 21, 18 and 13 in relation to fetal nuchal translucency thickness and the expected number on the basis of maternal age*[20]

Nuchal thickness (mm)	n	Observed		Expected		Observed : expected ratio	
		21	18 and 13	21	18 and 13	21	18 and 13
3	696	24	10	7.47	3.23	3.2	3.1
4	139	26	8	1.31	0.56	19.8	14.3
5	66	24	10	0.84	0.36	28.6	27.8
≥ 6	114	26	36	1.20	0.52	21.7	69.2
Total	1015	100	64	10.82	4.67	9.2	13.7

policy was achieved without the need for increasing the number of staff or the equipment. Women with fetal translucency of 2.5 mm or more were offered fetal karyotyping. In addition, women aged 35 years or older were offered amniocentesis at 16 weeks' gestation.

The data of the first 5 months after the introduction of the new policy were analyzed following completion of the pregnancies[34]. During this period 74% of women delivering in the two hospitals attended for first-trimester scanning and the nuchal translucency was successfully measured in all pregnancies. The translucency was raised in 3.6% of cases and the total percentage of invasive procedures was 5.1%. All four cases of Down syndrome that occurred in this period were diagnosed prenatally.

The Austrian study

In a prospective screening study of 1972 low-risk women with singleton pregnancies attending for routine antenatal care, transabdominal measurement of fetal nuchal translucency thickness was performed in all cases[35]. The nuchal translucency thickness was ≥ 2.5 mm in 1.3% of the cases and this group included 73% of those with chromosomal abnormalities.

The multicenter screening study

In an ongoing multicenter study, co-ordinated by the Fetal Medicine Foundation, nuchal translucency screening has been carried out in more than 50 000 pregnancies at the Harris Birthright Research Centre for Fetal Medicine and 18 district general hospitals.

The data from the first 20 804 completed pregnancies[7] have demonstrated that:

(1) In normal pregnancies nuchal translucency thickness increases with gestation;

(2) In chromosomally abnormal pregnancies nuchal translucency thickness is increased (Figure 4);

(3) The risk for trisomies can be derived by multiplying the background maternal age and gestation-related risk by a likelihood

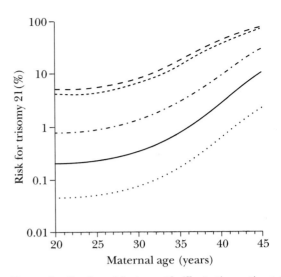

Figure 3 *Semilogarithmic graph illustrating estimated risks for fetal trisomy 21 at 10–14 weeks of gestation on the basis of maternal age alone (background) and maternal age with fetal nuchal translucency thickness of < 3, 3, 4 and > 4 mm[20]*

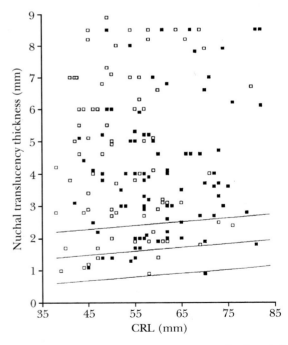

Figure 4 *The multicenter screening study. Fetal nuchal translucency (NT) in 86 fetuses with trisomy 21 (■) and in 78 fetuses with other chromosomal abnormalities (□) plotted on the reference range (median, 5th and 95th centiles) with crown–rump length (CRL)*

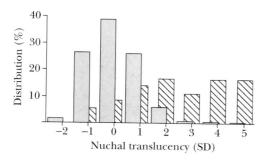

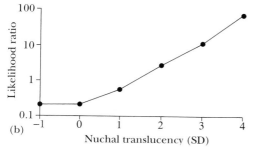

Figure 5 *The multicenter screening study. Graph (a) shows the distribution of fetal nuchal translucency expressed as number of standard deviations (SD) from the normal mean in chromosomally normal fetuses (stippled bars) and 86 with trisomy 21 (hatched bars). Graph (b) shows likelihood ratios derived from the incidences in the two groups*

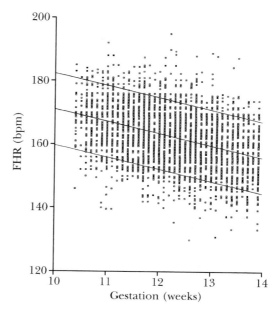

Figure 6 *Fetal heart rate (FHR) plotted against gestation calculated from the crown–rump length in normal pregnancies. The lines indicate the normal median, 5th and 95th centiles*

ratio, which depends on the degree of deviation in nuchal translucency from the normal mean for gestation (Figure 5);

(4) In about 5% of pregnancies the estimated risk for trisomy 21 was at least 1 in 100 and this group included 80% of fetuses with trisomy 21 and 77% of those with other chromosomal abnormalities.

This study has now proven that combining maternal age with fetal nuchal translucency thickness is currently the most sensitive method of screening for chromosomal abnormalities.

More widespread introduction of this method of screening, as with any new technology in medicine, requires appropriate training and continuous audit. One of the aims of the Fetal Medicine Foundation is to ensure that such high standards are maintained and the Foundation will provide the necessary computer program for calculation of risks only to those

sonographers that receive the appropriate certificate of competence and participate in continuing audit of results.

NUCHAL TRANSLUCENCY AND FETAL HEART RATE

In an ultrasound screening study of fetal nuchal translucency thickness at 10–14 weeks of gestation the fetal heart rate was also measured[8]. In 6903 normal singleton pregnancies fetal heart rate decreased from a mean of 171 bpm at 10 weeks of gestation to 156 bpm at 14 weeks (Figure 6). In 85 trisomy 21 pregnancies, the mean fetal heart rate was significantly higher than in the normal group (Figure 7). Similarly, the heart rate was increased in 16 fetuses with trisomy 13 and 19 with Turner syndrome. In contrast, the heart rate was decreased in 34 fetuses with trisomy 18 and 8 with triploidy (Figure 7).

In both the trisomy 21 and the normal pregnancies there was no significant association between the nuchal translucency thickness and fetal heart rate. Therefore, fetal nuchal translucency and heart rate can be combined in calculating the risk for trisomies. In a study of 6961 pregnancies at 10–14 weeks of gestation it was estimated that inclusion of fetal heart rate can improve the sensitivity of screening for trisomy 21 by a combination of maternal age and fetal nuchal translucency thickness from 80% to about 85%[8].

NUCHAL TRANSLUCENCY AND MATERNAL SERUM BIOCHEMISTRY

In trisomy 21 during the first trimester of pregnancy the maternal serum concentration of free β-human chorionic gonadotropin (free β-hCG) is higher and pregnancy associated plasma protein-A (PAPP-A) is lower than in chromosomally normal pregnancies (Table 4)[36–46]. Pregnancy-specific β1-glycoprotien (SP1) and α-fetoprotein do not provide useful distinction between affected and normal pregnancies[40,47].

Studies examining the relationship between maternal serum PAPP-A or free β-hCG concentrations and fetal nuchal translucency thickness have demonstrated no significant association between biochemistry and ultrasound findings in either the chromosomally normal or the trisomy 21 pregnancies[9,41,46]. Therefore, maternal serumal PAPP-A and free β-hCG and fetal nuchal translucency can be combined in calculating risks for fetal trisomies. In a study of 2529 pregnancies at 10–14 weeks of gestation it was estimated that inclusion of maternal serum free β-hCG can improve the sensitivity of screening for trisomy 21 by a combination of maternal age and fetal nuchal translucency thickness from 80% to about 85%[9].

PATHOLOGICAL FINDINGS IN TRISOMIC FETUSES WITH INCREASED TRANSLUCENCY

Hyett and colleagues[48–50] reported on the pathological examination of the fetal heart and great arteries in chromosomally abnormal fetuses with increased nuchal translucency at 10–14 weeks of gestation. After suction termination of pregnancy the heart and great arteries were identified, fixed with paraformaldehyde

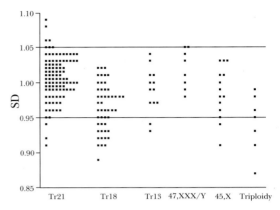

Figure 7 *Distribution of fetal heart rate (FHR) measurements expressed as number of standard deviations (SD) from the normal mean for gestation in fetuses with trisomy 21 (Tr21), trisomy 18 (Tr18), trisomy 13 (Tr13), sex chromosome aneuploidies (47,XXX/Y), Turner syndrome (45,X) and triploidy*

Table 4 *Maternal serum PAPP-A and free β-hCG in pregnancies with fetal trisomy 21 during the first trimester of pregnancy*

		Trisomy 21	
	Gestation (weeks)	n	Median (MoM)
PAPP-A			
Wald *et al.* 1992[36]	9–12	19	0.23
Brambati *et al.* 1993[37]	6–11	14	0.30
Hurley *et al.* 1993[38]	8–12	7	0.33
Muller *et al.* 1993[39]	9–14	17	0.42
Bersinger *et al.* 1994[40]	10–13	29	0.53
Brizot *et al.* 1994[41]	10–13	45	0.50
Free β-hCG			
Ozturk *et al.* 1990[42]	8–12	9	1.60
Aitken *et al.* 1993[43]	7–13	14	2.00
Macri *et al.* 1993[44]	10–13	29	2.20
Macintosh *et al.* 1994[45]	8–12	14	2.10
Brizot *et al.* 1995[46]	10–13	41	2.00

and examined using a step-wise microdissection method and scanning electron microscopy.

The commonest cardiac lesions seen in fetuses affected by trisomy 21 were atrioventricular or ventricular septal defect. Trisomy 18 was associated with ventricular septal defects and/or polyvalvular abnormalities; in trisomy 13, there were atrioventricular or ventricular

236

septal defects, valvular abnormalities and either narrowing of the isthmus or truncus arteriosus, and Turner syndrome was associated with severe narrowing of the whole aortic arch.

The aortic isthmus was significantly narrower than in normal fetuses in all four groups of chromosomally abnormal fetuses and the degree of narrowing of the isthmus was significantly greater in fetuses with high nuchal translucency thickness. It could therefore be postulated that narrowing of the aortic isthmus, the common pathological feature in all four groups of chromosomally abnormal fetuses, is the basis of increased nuchal translucency thickness.

LETHALITY OF TRISOMY 21 FETUSES WITH INCREASED TRANSLUCENCY

Screening for chromosomal defects in the first rather than the second trimester has the advantage of earlier prenatal diagnosis and consequently less traumatic termination of pregnancy for those couples that chose this option. A potential disadvantage is that earlier screening preferentially identifies those chromosomally abnormal pregnancies that are destined to miscarry. Snijders and co-workers[51] compared the prevalence of trisomy 21 at 12 weeks with that in live births and estimated that approximately 40% of affected fetuses die *in utero*. This issue of

preferential intrauterine lethality of chromosomal defects is of course a potential criticism of all methods of antenatal screening, including second-trimester maternal serum biochemistry; the estimated rate of intrauterine lethality between 16 weeks and term is about 30%[51]. This section examines the interrelation between increased nuchal translucency in trisomy 21 and fetal lethality.

Decision to continue with the pregnancy after the diagnosis of trisomy 21

In a study of 108 fetuses with trisomy 21 diagnosed in the first trimester because of increased nuchal translucency thickness, in five cases the parents chose to continue with the pregnancy whereas in 103 they had termination; trisomy 21 was also diagnosed in one of the fetuses in a twin pregnancy where the parents elected to avoid invasive prenatal diagnosis or selective fetocide[52]. The maternal age, ultrasound findings and outcome of the six trisomy 21 fetuses are shown in Table 5.

In five of the six fetuses the nuchal translucency resolved and at the second trimester scan the nuchal fold thickness was normal (less than 7 mm)[52]. At the second-trimester scan, one fetus had nuchal edema, three had septal defects, two had echogenic bowel and one had mild hydronephrosis or pyelectasia. All six trisomy 21

Table 5 *Maternal age, gestational age, ultrasound findings and outcome including sex, anomalies, gestation at delivery and birth weight in six trisomy 21 fetuses with increased nuchal translucency thickness[52]*

Case	Maternal age (years)	Gestational age (weeks)	Ultrasound findings	Outcome
1	22	13	NT 10	healthy male
		20	NF 6	37 weeks, 2458 g
2	40	11	NT 7	healthy male
		18	NF 4	37 weeks, 3260 g
3	26	11	NT 5	female, small VSD
		21	NF 5, echogenic bowel, septal defect	39 weeks, 3934 g
4	27	12	NT 5	male, small VSD
		20	NF 5, echogenic bowel, pylectasia, septal defect	39 weeks, 3771 g
5	41	12	NT 4	female, large VSD*
		18	NF 4, septal defect	32 weeks, 1640 g
6	40	12	NT 8	healthy female
		20	NF 8	36 weeks, 1510 g

NT, nuchal translucency thickness (mm); NF, nuchal fold thickness (mm); VSD, ventricular septal defect; *, baby died at age 6 months

babies were born alive and five are healthy. One had a major atrioventricular septal defect and died at the age of 6 months. Another two of the babies had small ventricular septal defects and these are being managed conservatively awaiting spontaneous closure. These data suggest that increased nuchal translucency does not necessarily identify those trisomic fetuses that are destined to die *in utero*.

Decision to terminate the pregnancy after the diagnosis of trisomy 21

In a study of 70 pregnancies where trisomy 21 was diagnosed at 12 (range 11–14) weeks of gestation and the parents opted for elective termination which was carried out at 14 (12–20) weeks, ultrasound examination to establish viability was carried out at the time of chorionic villus sampling (CVS) and just before termination[53]. Eight fetuses died in the interval between CVS and termination and the rate of lethality increased with translucency thickness from 5.3% for those with translucency of 1–3 mm to 23.5% for translucency of > 7 mm.

On the extreme assumption that the relative rate of intrauterine lethality of trisomy 21 fetuses according to translucency thickness stays the same throughout pregnancy, it was estimated that a policy of screening by maternal age and fetal nuchal translucency followed by selective termination of affected fetuses would be associated with a more than 70% reduction in the live birth incidence of trisomy 21[53].

NUCHAL TRANSLUCENCY IN MULTIPLE PREGNANCIES

During the last 20 years, both the average maternal age and the use of assisted reproduction techniques have increased with a consequent increase in the number of multiple pregnancies at high risk of chromosomal defects. In multiple pregnancies compared to singletons, prenatal diagnosis is complicated because first, effective methods of screening, such as maternal serum biochemistry, are not applicable, second, the techniques of invasive testing may provide uncertain results or may be associated with higher risks of miscarriage, and, third, the fetuses may be discordant for an abnormality in which case one of the options for the subsequent management of the pregnancy is selective fetocide.

In singleton pregnancies the method of choice for fetal karyotyping may be CVS because of the advantages of early diagnosis, whilst in twin pregnancies, the method of choice for fetal karyotyping is amniocentesis. However, cytogenetic results from amniocentesis are not usually available until around 18–20 weeks of gestation; if one fetus is chromosomally abnormal and the parents choose selective fetocide the risk of miscarriage is three times higher than with fetocide before 16 weeks[54]. Therefore, there is a need for selection of the appropriate diagnostic technique depending on the likelihood for selective fetocide; if the risk is high (more than 1 in 50) then CVS should be the technique of choice, otherwise amniocentesis is preferable[55].

Pandya and co-workers[56] examined nuchal translucency thickness of each fetus in eight twin pregnancies where karyotyping at 10–14 weeks of gestation demonstrated that at least one of the fetuses was chromosomally abnormal. Eight fetuses had trisomy 21 and two had trisomy 18. The nuchal translucency thickness was more than 2.5 mm in nine (90%) of the trisomic fetuses and in one of the chromosomally normal ones. In the Harris Birthright screening study at 10–14 weeks there were 20 543 singleton pregnancies and 392 twin pregnancies. This study demonstrated that in twin pregnancies screening for trisomy 21 by measurement of fetal nuchal translucency thickness and maternal age had a similar sensitivity to that found in singletons. However, the false positive rate of the test is higher in twin compared to singleton pregnancies, due to a higher prevalence of increased translucency in chromosomally normal fetuses from monochorionic pregnancies (about 9%, compared to about 6% in singletons). The most likely explanation for this high false positive rate is that increased nuchal translucency in one of the fetuses in monochorionic twins is an early manifestation of heart failure due to twin–twin transfusion syndrome.

INCREASED TRANSLUCENCY IN CHROMOSOMALLY NORMAL FETUSES

In two studies examining a total of 32 chromosomally normal fetuses with increased nuchal translucency (≥ 2 mm) there were four terminations of pregnancy (three because of progressive hydrops and one because of amnion disruption sequence), one intrauterine death in a fetus with obstructive uropathy, one spontaneous abortion and 26 live births[15,24]. The 26 live births, included 23 healthy ones, two with non-specific dysmorphic features and one with Noonan syndrome.

Shulman and associates[57] reported on 32 chromosomally normal fetuses with increased nuchal translucency (≥ 2.5 mm). In one case there were persistent hygromas that were successfully repaired at birth and in the other 31 cases the translucency resolved by 20 weeks and all babies were healthy at birth; follow-up examination at 12 months demonstrated normal growth and development in all infants.

Pandya and co-workers[20] reported on the outcome of 565 chromosomally normal fetuses with nuchal translucency 3–9 mm. The incidence of structural defects, mainly cardiac, diaphragmatic, renal and abdominal wall, was approximately 4%, which is higher than would be expected in an unselected population. Additionally, fetuses with increased translucency, as with nuchal edema in later pregnancy, may be at increased risk of rare genetic syndromes such as Stickler syndrome, Smith–Lemli–Opitz syndrome, Jarco Lavine syndrome or arthrogryposis[58]. The overall survival, taking into account perinatal deaths and terminations of pregnancy for fetal defects, decreased with nuchal translucency thickness from 97% for 3 mm to 53% for ≥ 5 mm[20].

Hyett and colleagues[58] performed pathological studies in fetuses with increased translucency and reported a high prevalence of cardiac abnormalities and genetic syndromes. In this respect, measurement of nuchal translucency thickness may prove to be a useful method of screening for cardiac and other abnormalities in addition to its role in screening for chromosomal defects. It is therefore recommended that in all cases with increased nuchal translucency at 10–14 weeks detailed ultrasound scans are subsequently performed to diagnose fetal abnormalities and markers of possible genetic syndromes.

References

1. Shuttleworth (1909). Mongoloid imbecility. *Br. Med. J.*, **2**, 661–65
2. Cuckle, H., Nanchahal, K. and Wald, N. (1991). Birth prevalence of Down's syndrome in England and Wales. *Prenat. Diagn.*, **11**, 29–34
3. Phillips, O. P., Elias, S., Shulman, L. P., Andersen, R. N., Morgan, C. D. and Simpson, J. L. (1992). Maternal serum screening for fetal Down syndrome in women less than 35 years of age using α-fetoprotein, hCG and unconjugated estriol: a prospective 2-year study. *Obstet. Gynecol.*, **80**, 353–8
4. Wald, N. J., Kennard, A., Densem, J. W., Cuckle, H. S., Chard, T. and Butler, L. (1992). Antenatal maternal serum screening for Down's syndrome: results of a demonstration project. *Br. Med. J.*, **305**, 391–4
5. Haddow, J. E., Palomaki, G. E., Knight, G. J., Williams, J., Pulkinen, A., Canick, J. A., Saller, D. N. and Bowers, G. B. (1992). Prenatal screening for Down's syndrome with use of maternal serum markers. *N. Engl. J. Med.*, **327**, 588–93
6. Nicolaides, K. H., Azar, G., Byrne, D., Mansur, C. and Marks, K. (1992). Fetal nuchal translucency: ultrasound screening for chromosomal defects in first trimester of pregnancy. *Br. Med. J.*, **304**, 867–9
7. Pandya, P. P., Snijders, R. J. M., Johnson, S. J., Brizot, M. and Nicolaides, K. H. (1995). Screening for fetal trisomies by maternal age and fetal nuchal translucency thickness at 10 to 14 weeks of gestation. *Br. J. Obstet. Gynaecol.*, **102**, 957–62
8. Noble, P. L., Abraham, H. D., Snijders, R. J. M., Sherwood, R. and Nicolaides, K. H. (1996).

Screening for fetal trisomy 21 in the first trimester of pregnancy: maternal serum free β-hCG and fetal nuchal translucency thickness. *Ultrasound Obstet. Gynecol.*, **6**, 390–5

9. Hyett, J. A., Noble, P. L., Snijders, R. J. M., Montenegro, N. and Nicolaides, K. H. (1996). Fetal heart rate in trisomy 21 and other chromosomal abnormalities at 10–14 weeks of gestation. *Ultrasound Obstet. Gynecol.*, **7**, in press

10. Azar, G. B., Snijders, R. J. M., Gosden, C. and Nicolaides, K. H. (1991). Fetal nuchal cystic hygromata: associated malformations and chromosomal defects. *Fetal Diagn. Ther.*, **6**, 46–57

11. Nicolaides, K. H., Azar, G., Snijders, R. J. M. and Gosden, C. M. (1992). Fetal nuchal oedema: associated malformations and chromosomal defects. *Fetal Diagn. Ther.*, **7**, 123–31

12. Benacerraf, B. R. and Frigoletto, F. D. (1987). Soft tissue nuchal fold in the second-trimester fetus: standards for normal measurements compared with those in Down syndrome. *Am. J. Obstet. Gynecol.*, **157**, 1146–9

13. Nadel, A., Bromley, B. and Benacerraf, B. R. (1993). Nuchal thickening or cystic hygromas in first- and early second-trimester fetuses: prognosis and outcome. *Obstet. Gynecol.*, **82**, 43–8

14. Pandya, P. P., Altman, D., Brizot, M. L., Pettersen, H. and Nicolaides, K. H. (1995). Repeatability of measurement of fetal nuchal translucency thickness. *Ultrasound Obstet. Gynecol.*, **5**, 334–7

15. Johnson, M. P., Johnson, A., Holzgreve, W., Isada, N. B., Wapner, R. J., Treadwell, M. C., Heeger, S. and Evans, M. (1993). First-trimester simple hygroma: cause and outcome. *Am. J. Obstet. Gynecol.*, **168**, 156–61

16. Hewitt, B. (1993). Nuchal translucency in the first trimester. *Aust. NZ J. Obstet. Gynaecol.*, **33**, 389–91

17. Shulman, L. P., Emerson, D., Felker, R., Phillips, O., Simpson, J. and Elias, S. (1992). High frequency of cytogenetic abnormalities with cystic hygroma diagnosed in the first trimester. *Obstet. Gynecol.*, **80**, 80–2

18. Nicolaides, K. H., Brizot, M. L. and Snijders, R. J. M. (1994). Fetal nuchal translucency: ultrasound screening for fetal trisomy in the first trimester of pregnancy. *Br. J. Obstet. Gynaecol.*, **101**, 782–6

19. Pandya, P. P., Brizot, M. L., Kuhn, P., Snijders, R. J. M. and Nicolaides, K. H. (1994). First trimester fetal nuchal translucency thickness and risk for trisomies. *Obstet. Gynecol.*, **84**, 420–3

20. Pandya, P. P., Kondylios, A., Hilbert, L., Snijders, R. J. M. and Nicolaides, K. H. (1995). Chromosomal defects and outcome in 1015 fetuses with increased nuchal translucency. *Ultrasound Obstet. Gynecol.*, **5**, 15–19

21. Szabo, J. and Gellen, J. (1990). Nuchal fluid accumulation in trisomy-21 detected by vaginal sonography in first trimester. *Lancet*, **336**, 1133

22. Wilson, R. D., Venir, N. and Farquharson, D. F. (1992). Fetal nuchal fluid – physiological or pathological? – in pregnancies less than 17 menstrual weeks. *Prenat. Diagn.*, **12**, 755–63

23. Ville, Y., Lalondrelle, C., Doumerc, S., Daffos, F., Frydman, R., Oury, J. F. and Dumez, Y. (1992). First-trimester diagnosis of nuchal anomalies: significance and fetal outcome. *Ultrasound Obstet. Gynecol.*, **2**, 314–16

24. Trauffer, M. L., Anderson, C. E., Johnson, A., Heeger, S., Morgan, P. and Wapner, R. J. (1994). The natural history of euploid pregnancies with first-trimester cystic hygromas. *Am. J. Obstet. Gynecol.*, **170**, 1279–84

25. Brambati, B., Cislaghi, C., Tului, L., Alberti, E., Amidani, M., Colombo, U. and Zuliani, G. (1995). First-trimester Down's syndrome screening using nuchal translucency: a prospective study. *Ultrasound Obstet. Gynecol.*, **5**, 9–14

26. Comas, C., Martinez, J. M., Ojuel, J., Casals, E., Puerto, B., Borrell, A. and Fortuny, A. (1995). First-trimester nuchal edema as a marker of aneuploidy. *Ultrasound Obstet. Gynecol.*, **5**, 26–9

27. Szabo, J., Gellen, J. and Szemere, G. (1995). First-trimester ultrasound screening for fetal aneuploidies in women over 35 and under 35 years of age. *Ultrasound Obstet. Gynecol.*, **5**, 161–3

28. Nadel, A., Bromley, B. and Benacerraf, B. R. (1993). Nuchal thickening or cystic hygromas in first- and early second-trimester fetuses: prognosis and outcome. *Obstet. Gynecol.*, **82**, 43–8

29. Savoldelli, G., Binkert, F., Achermann, J. and Schmid, W. (1993). Ultrasound screening for chromosomal anomalies in the first trimester of pregnancy. *Prenat. Diagn.*, **13**, 513–18

30. Schulte-Vallentin, M. and Schindler, H. (1992). Non-echogenic nuchal oedema as a marker in trisomy 21 screening. *Lancet*, **339**, 1053

31. Van Zalen-Sprock, M. M., van Vugt, J. M. G. and van Geijn, H. P. (1992). First-trimester diagnosis of cystic hygroma – course and outcome. *Am. J. Obstet. Gynecol.*, **167**, 94–8

32. Cullen, M. T., Gabrielli, S., Green, J. J., Rizzo, N., Mahoney, M. J., Salafia, C., Bovicelli, L. and Hobbins, J. C. (1990). Diagnosis and significance of cystic hygroma in the first trimester. *Prenat. Diagn.*, **10**, 643–51

33. Suchet, I. B., van der Westhuizen, N. G. and Labatte, M. F. (1992). Fetal cystic hygromas: further insights into their natural history. *Can. Assoc. Radiol. J.*, **6**, 420–4

34. Pandya, P. P., Goldberg, H., Walton, B., Riddle, A., Shelley, S., Snijders, R. J. M. and Nicolaides, K. H. (1995). The implementation of first

trimester scanning at 10–13 weeks' gestation and the measurement of fetal nuchal translucency thickness in two maternity units. *Ultrasound Obstet. Gynecol.*, **5**, 20–5

35. Hafner, E., Schuchter, K. and Philipp, K. (1995). Screening for chromosomal abnormalities in an unselected population by fetal nuchal translucency. *Ultrasound Obstet. Gynecol.*, **6**, 330–3

36. Wald, N., Stone, R., Cuckle, H. S., Grudzinskas, J. G., Barkai, G., Brambati, B., Teisner, B. and Fuhrmann, W. (1992). First trimester concentrations of pregnancy associated plasma protein A and placental protein 14 in Down's syndrome. *Br. Med. J.*, **305**, 28

37. Brambati, B., Macintosh, M. C. M., Teisner, B., Maguiness, S., Shrimanker, K., Lanzani, A., Bonacchi, I., Tului, L., Chard, T. and Grudzinskas, T. J. (1993). Low maternal serum level of pregnancy associated plasma protein (PAPP-A) in the first trimester in association with abnormal fetal karyotype. *Br. J. Obstet. Gynaecol.*, **100**, 324–6

38. Hurley, P. A., Ward, R. H. T., Teisner, B., Iles, R. K., Lucas, M. and Grudzinskas, J. G. (1993). Serum PAPP-A measurements in first-trimester screening for Down syndrome. *Prenat. Diagn.*, **13**, 903–8

39. Muller, F., Cuckle, H., Teisner, B. and Grudzinskas, J. G. (1993). Serum PAPP-A levels are depressed in women with fetal Down syndrome in early pregnancy. *Prenat. Diagn.*, **13**, 633–6

40. Bersinger, N. A., Brizot, M. L., Johnson, A., Snijders, R. J. M., Abbott, J., Schneider, H. and Nicolaides, K. H. (1994). First trimester maternal serum pregnancy-associated plasma protein A and pregnancy-specific β1-glycoprotein in fetal trisomies. *Br. J. Obstet. Gynaecol.*, **101**, 970–4

41. Brizot, M. L., Snijders, R. J. M., Bersinger, N. A., Kuhn, P. and Nicolaides, K. H. (1994). Maternal serum pregnancy associated placental protein A and fetal nuchal translucency thickness for the prediction of fetal trisomies in early pregnancy. *Obstet. Gynecol.*, **84**, 918–22

42. Ozturk, M., Milunsky, A., Brambati, B., Sachs, E. S., Miller, S. and Wands, J. R. (1990). Abnormal maternal serum levels of human chorionic gonadotropin free subunits in trisomy 18. *Am. J. Med. Genet.*, **36**, 480–3

43. Aitken, D. A., McCaw, G., Crossley, J. A., Berry, C., Connor, J. M., Spencer, K. and Macri, J. N. (1993). First-trimester biochemical screening for fetal chromosome abnormalities and neural tube defects. *Prenat. Diagn.*, **13**, 681–9

44. Macri, J. N., Kasturi, R. V., Krantz, D. A., Cook, E. J., Moore, N. D., Young, J. A., Romero, K. and Larsen, J. W. (1993). Maternal serum Down syndrome screening: free beta protein is a more effective marker than human

chorionic gonadotrophin. *Am. J. Obstet. Gynecol.*, **163**, 1248–53

45. Macintosh, M. C., Iles, R., Teisner, B., Sharma, V., Chard, T. and Grudzinskas, J. G. (1994). Maternal serum human chorionic gonadotrophin and pregnancy associated plasma protein A, markers for fetal Down syndrome at 8–14 weeks. *Prenat. Diagn.*, **14**, 203–8

46. Brizot, M. L., Snijders, R. J. M., Butler, J., Bersinger, N. A. and Nicolaides, K. H. (1995). Maternal serum hCG and fetal nuchal translucency thickness for the prediction of fetal trisomies in the first trimester of pregnancy. *Br. J. Obstet. Gynaecol.*, **102**, 127–32

47. Brizot, M. L., Kuhn, P., Bersinger, N. A., Snijders, R. J. M. and Nicolaides, K. H. (1995). First trimester maternal serum alpha-fetoprotein in fetal trisomies. *Br. J. Obstet. Gynaecol.*, **102**, 31–4

48. Hyett, J. A., Moscoso, G. and Nicolaides, K. H. (1995). First trimester nuchal translucency and cardiac septal defects in fetuses with trisomy 21. *Am. J. Obstet. Gynecol.*, **172**, 1411–13

49. Hyett, J. A., Moscoso, G. and Nicolaides, K. H. (1995). Cardiac defects in trisomy 18 fetuses affected by increased first trimester nuchal translucency. *Fetal Diagn. Ther.*, **10**, 381–6

50. Hyett, J. A., Moscoso, G. and Nicolaides, K. H. (1995). Increased nuchal translucency in trisomy 21 fetuses: relation to narrowing of the aortic isthmus. *Hum. Reprod.*, **10**, 3049–51

51. Snijders, R. J. M., Sebire, N. J. and Nicolaides, K. H. (1995). Maternal age and gestational age specific risk for chromosomal defects. *Fetal Diagn. Ther.*, **10**, 356–67

52. Pandya, P. P., Snijders, R. J. M., Johnson, S. and Nicolaides, K. H. (1995). Natural history of trisomy 21 fetuses with fetal nuchal translucency. *Ultrasound Obstet. Gynecol.*, **5**, 381–3

53. Hyett, J. A., Sebire, N. J., Snijders, R. J. M. and Nicolaides, K. H. (1996). Intrauterine lethality of trisomy 21 fetuses with increased nuchal translucency thickness. *Ultrasound Obstet. Gynecol.*, in press

54. Evans, M. I., Goldberg, J. D., Dommergues, M., Wapner, R. J., Lynch, L., Dock, B. S., Horenstein, J., Golbus, M. S., Rodeck, C. H., Dumez, Y., Holzgreve, W., Timor-Tritsch, I., Johnson, M. P., Isada, N. B., Monteagudo, A. and Berkowitz, R. L. (1994). Efficacy of second-trimester selective termination for fetal abnormalities: international collaborative experience among the world's largest centers. *Am. J. Obstet. Gynecol.*, **171**, 90–4

55. Sebire, N. J., Noble, P. L., Psarra, A., Papapanagiotou, G. and Nicolaides, K. H. (1996). Fetal karyotyping in twin pregnancies: selection of technique by measurement of fetal nuchal

translucency thickness. *Br. J. Obstet. Gynaecol.*, in press

56. Pandya, P. P., Hilbert, F., Snijders, R. J. M. and Nicolaides, K. H. (1995). Nuchal translucency thickness and crown–rump length in twin pregnancies with chromosomally abnormal fetuses. *J. Ultrasound Med.*, **14**, 565–8

57. Shulman, L. P., Emerson, D. S., Grevengood, C., Felker, R. E., Gross, S. J., Phillips, O. P. and Elias, S. (1994). Clinical course and outcome of fetuses with isolated cystic nuchal lesions and normal karyotypes detected in the first trimester. *Am. J. Obstet. Gynecol.*, **171**, 1278–81

58. Hyett, J. A., Moscoso, G., Papapanagiotou, G., Perdu, M. and Nicolaides, K. H. (1996). Abnormalities of the heart and great vessels in chromosomally normal fetuses with increased nuchal translucency thickness at 10–13 weeks of gestation. *Ultrasound Obstet. Gynecol.*, **7**, in press

The role of second-trimester ultrasound examination in the detection of fetal aneuploidy

18

A. M. Vintzileos, J. C. Smulian and D. L. Day-Salvatore

INTRODUCTION

Until a few years ago the prenatal diagnosis of trisomy 21 in the second trimester was confined to offering genetic amniocentesis to women 35 years of age or older. This approach resulted in identification of approximately 20–30% of fetuses with trisomy 21, with a false-positive rate of 5–7%[1,2]. The average risk for pregnancy loss of normal fetuses associated with genetic amniocentesis is approximately 1 in 270. Experience has shown that using advanced maternal age alone as an indication for genetic amniocentesis requires approximately 140 amniocenteses to identify one fetus with trisomy 21. Therefore, one normal fetus may be lost as a result of the procedure for every two fetuses identified with trisomy 21. In the mid-1980s, maternal serum biochemical screening was added to the armamentarium of prenatal diagnosis of fetal aneuploidy. This approach was introduced to increase the detection rate of fetuses with aneuploidy born from women younger than 35 years old. Recently, the combination of maternal age and multiple serum biochemical markers (maternal serum α-fetoprotein, estriol, human chorionic gonadotropin) has increased the prenatal detection rate to 60–65% for trisomy 21[3]. However, even with the use of the most current practices, 35–40% of fetuses with trisomy 21 remain undetected, whereas 5–10% of pregnant women are subjected to genetic amniocentesis. Most importantly, by using a combination of maternal age and multiple serum biochemical markers, 60–80 amniocenteses are still required to identify one fetus with trisomy 21. This implies that a normal fetus may be lost due to genetic amniocentesis for every 3–4 fetuses identified with trisomy 21. In summary, the prenatal diagnosis of fetal aneuploidy in the second trimester of pregnancy relying on current practices has been less than ideal.

Since the mid-1980s several studies have been published on the use of first- and second-trimester ultrasonography in the prenatal detection of fetal aneuploidy[4–34]. First-trimester ultrasonography for the detection of fetal aneuploidy has been the subject of numerous investigations in Europe, where it has been shown to hold promise as a screening tool. The use of first-trimester ultrasound in the detection of fetal aneuploidy is discussed in another chapter of this book. In the United States routine ultrasonography is not standard care and therefore has not been used to screen for fetal aneuploidy. However, research and experience have shown that second-trimester ultrasonography may assist in the prenatal detection of fetuses with chromosome abnormalities and modify the counselling and therefore the need for amniocentesis by adjusting the *a priori* risk for trisomy 21[35]. The usefulness of second-trimester ultrasonography rests on the identification of structural anomalies, abnormal fetal biometry or other ultrasound 'markers' for aneuploidy.

FETAL STRUCTURAL ANOMALIES

In general, the presence of one fetal structural anomaly characterizes disorders of multifactorial origin, whereas multiple anomalies strongly suggest the presence of a chromosome abnormality. Table 1 lists the most common fetal structural malformations typically

Table 1 *Structural anomalies associated with fetal aneuploidy*

Central nervous system lesions
Facial malformations
Neck anomalies
Non-immune hydrops
Cardiac lesions
Duodenal atresia
Omphalocele
Hydrothorax
Diaphragmatic hernia
Genitourinary anomalies
Limb malformations

associated with fetal aneuploidy[36]. All these malformations are diagnosable by experienced sonographers during the second trimester of pregnancy, except duodenal atresia, which may not be detectable until after 24 weeks of pregnancy. Of these malformations, non-immune hydrops, duodenal atresia and hydrothorax are often associated with trisomy 21, whereas all the others are mainly associated with trisomy 18 or 13. Fetal central nervous system (CNS) anomalies are typically associated with trisomies 18 and 13. More specifically, approximately 3–8% of fetuses with prenatally diagnosed ventriculomegaly are chromosomally abnormal, with trisomies 13, 18, 21 or triploidy being the most frequent[36]. Dandy–Walker anomaly is associated with trisomies 18 or 13 in 29–50% of the prenatally diagnosed cases, holoprosencephaly (alobar/semilobar) with trisomies 13, 18 or triploidy in 43–59% of the cases, and agenesis of the corpus callosum with trisomies 13, 18 or triploidy in 14–20% of the cases[36]. An enlarged cisterna magna (> 10 mm) may be seen in association with trisomies 18 or 13 and is associated with chromosome abnormalities in 55% of cases. If ventriculomegaly is present in addition to an enlarged cisterna magna, the risk for a fetal chromosome abnormality is 9%, whereas the absence of ventriculomegaly increases the risk to approximately 77%. Although choroid plexus cysts are not structural anomalies, they have been associated with increased frequency of fetal aneuploidy, especially trisomy 18. However, most trisomy 18 fetuses have early growth restric-

tion and also other ultrasonically demonstrable structural malformations. The literature is controversial about whether or not genetic amniocentesis should be offered to women carrying fetuses with choroid plexus cysts in the second trimester of pregnancy. Without regard to associated anomalies, the overall risk for trisomy 18 in the presence of choroid plexus cysts is approximately 6.2%, which seems high enough to justify amniocentesis[37]. However, an analysis of 13 prospective studies showed that isolated choroid plexus cysts (without associated fetal anomalies) carry a risk for aneuploidy of 1 : 374[37]. Although this risk for fetal aneuploidy is higher than that of the general population, it may not be high enough to justify amniocentesis. Also, it should be emphasized that approximately 60% of fetuses with trisomy 18 are already growth restricted by the second trimester of pregnancy[38]. Therefore, documentation of normal fetal growth in addition to exclusion of associated structural malformations is mandatory before genetic counselling is given. Fetal facial abnormalities may also be associated with fetal aneuploidy. Cleft lip or palate when associated with other structural anomalies carries a risk for trisomies 13 or 18 of approximately 40–75%; however, in the absence of other ultrasonically demonstrable anomalies, there is no increased risk for fetal chromosome abnormalities[36]. Ocular abnormalities, such as those seen with holoprosencephaly, are associated with trisomies 13 or 18 in over 50% of cases[36]. Micrognathia or small ears are also associated with fetal chromosome abnormalities, mainly trisomies 13, 18 or 21.

The frequency of fetal chromosome abnormalities among prenatally diagnosed cases of cystic hygroma is approximately 75%. The most common aneuploidy is 45,X, which is seen in 66% of chromosomally abnormal fetuses. When a nuchal cystic hygroma is associated with non-immune hydrops, the risk for fetal chromosome abnormality is extremely high (80–90%). In this setting the most frequent chromosome abnormalities are 45,X, trisomy 21 or trisomy 18[36]. If non-immune hydrops is not associated with cystic hygroma, the risk for trisomy 21 is approximately 14–18%.

Congenital heart disease carries a significant risk for fetal aneuploidy, especially in the prenatally diagnosed cases. When fetal cardiac disease is diagnosed prenatally, the risk for fetal aneuploidy is approximately 60–70% in the presence of other structural malformations, whereas in the absence of other anomalies the risk is approximately 15–20%. In the prenatally diagnosed cases of fetal cardiac disease the main trisomies (13, 18 and 21) have a similar frequency. In contrast, the most frequent chromosome abnormality seen in newborns with congenital heart disease is trisomy 21. Approximately 50% of fetuses with trisomy 21, 99% of fetuses with trisomy 18 and 90% of fetuses with trisomy 13 have congenital heart disease. This implies that expert fetal echocardiography, if normal, has the theoretical potential to decrease the *a priori* risk for trisomy 21 by approximately 50% and almost eliminate the risk for trisomies 18 or 13. Expert fetal echocardiography in the second trimester of pregnancy has been reported to detect 60% of fetuses with trisomy 21[39].

The prenatal diagnosis of duodenal atresia is associated with a risk for trisomy 21 of approximately 20–30%. However, only 5–8% of fetuses with trisomy 21 have duodenal atresia[36]. The 'double bubble' sign, which suggests the presence of duodenal atresia, may not be manifested until the late second trimester or third trimester of pregnancy.

The presence of a fetal omphalocele should strongly increase the suspicion for trisomy 18. Approximately 30–40% of prenatally diagnosed cases of omphalocele have been associated with fetal chromosome abnormalities, the most common of which are trisomies 18, 13 or 21[36]. The risk for a chromosome abnormality depends on the presence of other anomalies, the contents of the sac (small bowel vs. liver) as well as the size of the omphalocele.

Trisomy 21 and 45,X are the most common chromosome abnormalities associated with fetal hydrothorax. In the presence of hydrothorax the risk for these chromosome abnormalities is 9–12%. The most frequent chromosome abnormalities associated with diaphragmatic hernia are trisomies 18 and 21, which are seen in 4–25% of the prenatally diagnosed cases[36]. Of the genitourinary abnormalities, isolated ureteropelvic junction obstruction or multicystic/dysplastic kidney are not associated with increased risk for aneuploidy. However, if ureteropelvic junction obstruction is associated with other fetal anomalies, the risk for trisomy 18 is approximately 4%. In the presence of multicystic/dysplastic kidney associated with other anomalies, the risk for trisomy 13 is approximately 12.5%. Bladder outlet obstruction carries a risk for fetal aneuploidy of approximately 23%, with trisomies 18 or 13 being the most common[36].

The strength of the association between fetal extremity malformations and aneuploidy has not been adequately investigated in prenatally diagnosed cases. Extremity malformations such as limb reduction anomalies, radial thumb aplasia, overlapping fingers, flexion deformities and polydactyly are associated with trisomy 18 or 13. Malformations such as hypoplasia of the middle phalanx of the fifth digit and a wide space between the first and second toe are associated with trisomy 21. In chromosomally abnormal fetuses, extremity malformations are usually found in association with other structural anomalies or 'markers' of fetal aneuploidy.

The aforementioned fetal structural anomalies, when multiple, are associated mainly with trisomy 18 or 13. Expert ultrasonography should identify over 80% of fetuses with trisomy 18 or 13, because these fetuses exhibit one or more structural anomalies. However, only 28% of fetuses with trisomy 21 exhibit one or more structural malformations[35]. Since most fetuses with trisomy 21 do not exhibit any ultrasonically demonstrable anomalies during the second trimester of pregnancy, research efforts have been focused on the role of fetal biometry or other ultrasound 'markers'[4–34].

FETAL BIOMETRY AND OTHER ANEUPLOIDY MARKERS

Since the mid-1980s, numerous ultrasound markers for fetal aneuploidy have been investigated (Table 2). Intrauterine growth restriction in the second or early third trimester may be associated with fetal chromosome abnormalities in approximately 13% of cases, with the most common being trisomy 18 or triploidy. However, most of these fetuses have associated structural malformations in addition to intrauterine growth restriction. There are several conflicting reports regarding the usefulness of the ultrasound markers shown in Table 2. A literature review[35] to establish the usefulness of these markers revealed that biparietal diameter, occipitofrontal diameter, cephalic index, transverse cerebellar diameter and neck circumference (if used alone) were not useful in the prenatal detection of fetal aneuploidy. On the other hand, some of the ultrasound markers, such as frontal lobe dimensions, femur/foot length ratio, humerus/foot length ratio, iliac bone length and length of the middle phalanx of the fifth digit have not been studied extensively[40–46]. We recently undertook a MEDLINE computer search (years 1983–94) of all studies that examined the usefulness of ultrasound markers in the prenatal detection of fetal trisomy 21[35]. In that review only studies from

Table 2 *Fetal biometry markers for aneuploidy*

Intrauterine growth restriction (early onset)
Biparietal diameter
Occipitofrontal diameter
Cephalic index
Transverse cerebellar diameter
Frontal lobe dimensions
Neck circumference
Femur length
Femur/foot length ratio
Humerus length
Humerus/foot length ratio
Pyelectasis
Ear length
Iliac bone length
Length of middle phalanx of the fifth digit

Table 3 *Studies using femur length measurements to detect trisomy 21 in the second trimester*

Authors	'Abnormal' test	Number of fetuses with trisomy 21	Sensitivity n	Sensitivity %	False-positive rate n	False-positive rate %
Benacerraf et al. (1987)[6]	O/E (xBPD) ≤ 0.91	28	19	68	4/192	2
Lockwood et al. (1987)[7]	BPD/FL > 1.5 SD					
New Haven group		35	18	51	26/349	7
Boston group		20	14	70	9/195	5
Perrella et al. (1988)[8]	O/E (xBPD) ≤ 0.91	19	5	26	29/128	23
Brumfield et al. (1989)[9]	BPD/FL ≥ 1.80	15	6	40	1/45	2.2
LaFollette et al. (1989)[10]	O/E (xBPD) ≤ 0.91	30	4	13	27/229	12
Lynch et al. (1989)[11]	O/E (xBPD) ≤ 0.91	9	5	55	5/9	56
	BPD/FL > 1.5 SD	9	2	22	1/9	11
Dicke et al. (1989)[12]	O/E (xGA) < 0.91	33	5	15	18/177	10
	BPD/FL > 1.5 SD	33	6	18	7/177	4
Cuckle et al (1989)[13]	O/E (xBPD) < 0.91	83	20	24	84/1340	6.3
Hill et al (1989)[14]	O/E (xBPD) ≤ 0.91	22	11	50	43/286	15
	BPD/FL > 1.5 SD	22	8	36	20/286	7
Benacerraf et al. (1989)[15]	O/E (xBPD) ≤ 0.91	20	8	40	35/709	5
Shah et al. (1990)[16]	BPD/FL (xGA) > 90th centile	17	3	18	1/17	6
Ginsberg et al. (1990)[17]	BPD/FL > 1.5 SD	11	5	46	14/212	6.6
Rodis et al. (1991)[18]	BPD/FL > 95th centile for GA	11	2	18	95/1890	5
	FL < 5th centile for GA	11	2	18	95/1890	5
Rotmensch et al. (1992)[19]	O/E (xBPD) < 0.91	43	8	19	18/204	9
Nyberg et al. (1993)[20]	O/E (xBPD) ≤ 0.91	45	11	24	44/942	4.7
Lockwood et al. (1993)[21]	O–E (xBPD) < –3.4 mm	42	6	15	163/4949	3.3
Total*		483	151	31	616/11 873	5

BPD, biparietal diameter; FL, femur length; O, observed; E, expected (mean); GA, gestational age; xBPD, for a given BPD measurement; xGA, for a given gestational age
*If the study reports two different methods, only the numbers of the first method were added into the total
Reprinted with permission from the *American Journal of Obstetrics and Gynecology*[35]

which sensitivities and specificities could be calculated were included. Table 3 summarizes the studies that used femur length measurements to detect trisomy 21 in the second trimester of pregnancy. Although a variety of methodologies were used to define 'shortness' of the femur, the overall sensitivity was 31%. However, the range of sensitivities was between 13 and 70%. The overall false-positive rate was 5%. Since different methodologies were used in many of these studies, the results were also analyzed according to the specific methodologies used. Eight studies used the biparietal diameter/femur length ratio[7,9,11,12,14,16–18] and ten used the observed/expected femur length ratio according to the measured biparietal diameter[6,8,10–15,19,20] (Table 4). The biparietal diameter/femur length ratio had better overall sensitivity (37% vs. 29%), which was not statistically significant, and a significantly lower overall false-positive rate (5.6% vs. 7.3%). Table 5 summarizes studies that used

humerus length measurement to detect trisomy 21. The overall sensitivity by using short humerus was 33% and the overall false-positive rate 4.5%. Studies using the combination of short femur and short humerus (by observed/expected length ratios) showed an overall sensitivity of 32% and specificity 98%[5,20]. Table 6 summarizes studies that used nuchal fold thickening (≥ 6 mm) to detect trisomy 21. With the use of nuchal fold thickening of ≥ 6 mm, the overall sensitivity was 34% and the specificity was 99.5%. There were three studies that examined fetal pyelectasis (anteroposterior diameter of renal pelvis ≥ 4 mm) as a possible marker for trisomy 21[5,23,24]. Although the overall sensitivity of pyelectasis in these three studies was 21%, in the overwhelming majority of trisomy 21 cases pyelectasis was associated with other abnormal ultrasound findings (e.g. cardiac defects, short femur or short humerus). Review of the literature supports the conclusion

Table 4 *Comparison of efficacy for predicting trisomy 21 between the biparietal diameter/femur length ratio (BPD/FL) (eight studies) and the observed/expected femur length ratio (O/E (FL)) (ten studies)*

	BPD/FL References 7, 9, 11, 12, 14, 16–18	O/E (FL) References 6, 8, 10, 11, 12–15, 19, 20	P-value
Number of fetuses with trisomy 21	173	332	
Sensitivity (average)	64/173 (37%)	96/332 (29%)	$p = 0.14$
Range of sensitivities	18–70%	13–68%	
False-positive rate (average)	129/2290 (5.6%)	307/4216 (7.3%)	$p = 0.02$
Range of false-positive rates	2.2–11%	2–56%	

Reprinted with permission from the *American Journal of Obstetrics and Gynecology*[35]

Table 5 *Studies using humerus length (HL) measurements to detect trisomy 21 in the second trimester*

Authors	'Abnormal' test	Number of fetuses with trisomy 21	Sensitivity n	Sensitivity %	False-positive rate n	False-positive rate %
Rodis *et al.* (1991)[18]	< 5th centile for GA	11	7	64	95/1890	5
	BPD/HL > 95th centile for GA	11	7	64	95/1890	5
Benacerraf *et al.* (1991)[22]	O/E (xBPD) < 0.90	24	12	50	25/400	6.2
Rotmensch *et al.* (1992)[29]	O/E (xBPD) < 0.90	43	12	28	18/204	9
Nyberg *et al.* (1993)[20]	O/E (xBPD) $\leq$ 0.89	45	11	24	42/942	4.5
Lockwood *et al.* (1993)[21]	O–E (xBPD) < –3.6 mm	42	12	29	198/4949	4
Total		165	54	33	378/8385	4.5

GA, gestational age; BPD, biparietal diameter; O, observed; E, expected (mean); xBPD, for a given BPD measurement
Reprinted with permission from the *American Journal of Obstetrics and Gynecology*[35]

Table 6 *Studies using nuchal fold thickening (≥ 6 mm) to detect trisomy 21 in the second trimester*

Authors	Number of fetuses with trisomy 21	Sensitivity		False-positive rate	
		n	%	n	%
Benacerraf and Frigoletto (1987)[25]	28	12	43	4/3825	0.1
Toi *et al.* (1987)[26]	11	2	18	1/1693	0.05
Perrella *et al.* (1988)[8]	14	3	21	12/128	9
Lynch *et al.* (1989)[11]	9	5	56	0/9	0
Hill *et al.* (1989)[14]	22	2	9	—	0
Benacerraf *et al.* (1989)[15]	20	8	40	—	0
Ginsberg *et al.* (1990)[17]	12	5	41	0/212	0
Nyberg *et al.* (1990)[4]	25	4	16	10/3500	0.3
Crane and Gray (1991)[27]	16	12	75	47/3338	1.4
Benacerraf *et al.* (1991)[22]	24	12	50	0/400	0
Lockwood *et al.* (1993)[21]	42	6	14	30/4949	0.6
Kirk *et al.* (1992)[28]	19	9	47	21/7087	0.3
De Vore and Alfi (1993)[29]	35	7	20	14/2752	0.5
Watson *et al.* (1994)[30]	14	7	50	27/1381	2
Total	291	94	33	170/29 274	0.5

Reprinted with permission from the *American Journal of Obstetrics and Gynecology*[35]

Table 7 *Efficacy of sonographic markers for trisomy 21*

Marker	Sensitivity	Specificity
Short femur (by BPD/FL)	0.37	0.94
Short femur (by O/E)	0.29	0.92
Short humerus (by O/E)	0.31	0.95
Short femur and humerus (both by O/E)	0.32	0.98
Pyelectasis + (i.e. short femur or humerus by O/E)	0.21	0.97
Nuchal fold thickening (≥ 6 mm)	0.33	0.99
Echogenic bowel	0.09	0.99
Short ear length (< 10th centile for GA)	0.71	0.92

BPD, biparietal diameter; FL, femur length; O, observed; E, expected; GA, gestational age
Reprinted with permission from the *American Journal of Obstetrics and Gynecology*[35]

that isolated pyelectasis without any other abnormal ultrasound findings does not increase the risk for fetal aneuploidy to a degree justifying genetic amniocentesis[35]. Studies examining the value of fetal ear length measurements in detecting trisomy 21 suggest an overall sensitivity of 71% and specificity 92%[33,34]. Echogenic bowel is not a fetal biometric parameter, but it has been proposed as a possible marker for fetal aneuploidy in the second trimester of pregnancy[4,31,32]. Our review showed that the overall sensitivity and specificity of echogenic bowel in detecting fetal trisomy 21 in the second trimester were 9.5% and 99.6%, respectively[4]. The efficacy of ultrasonographic markers for detecting trisomy 21 in terms of sensitivity and specificity is summarized in Table 7.

ADJUSTING THE RISK FOR TRISOMY 21 ON THE BASIS OF SECOND-TRIMESTER ULTRASOUND EXAMINATION

The overwhelming majority of the aforementioned studies on the usefulness of various ultrasound markers for the prenatal detection of fetal aneuploidy have been performed in high-risk patients, i.e. women ≥ 35 years old or women with abnormal serum biochemistry results. The results of these studies, therefore, cannot be directly applied to low-risk women, women ≤ 35 years old or women with normal serum biochemistry results, without appropriate mathematical manipulation. Bayes' theorem allows the calculation of positive and negative predictive values of a test if the sensitivity, specificity and prevalence of the disease are

Table 8 *Mid-trimester risk, as modified by ultrasound findings, for trisomy 21, based on maternal age in a structurally normal fetus. (All risks are expressed as 1/x)*

Maternal age (years)	Age alone*	Normal by ultrasound	Short femur by BPD/FL	Short femur by O/E	Short humerus by O/E	Short femur and humerus by O/E	Pyelectasis with short femur or humerus	Nuchal fold	Echogenic bowel	Short ear
20	1231	18 871	260	463	301	108	194	29	91	194
21	1145	17 553	242	431	280	100	181	27	85	180
22	1065	16 326	225	401	261	93	168	26	79	168
23	1000	15 330	212	376	245	88	158	24	74	157
24	942	14 441	199	354	231	83	149	23	70	148
25	887	14 598	188	334	217	78	140	21	66	140
26	842	12 908	178	317	206	74	133	20	63	133
27	798	12 233	169	300	196	70	126	19	59	126
28	755	11 574	160	284	185	66	120	18	56	119
29	721	11 053	153	271	177	64	114	18	54	114
30	685	10 501	145	258	168	60	109	17	51	108
31	650	9964	138	245	159	57	103	16	49	103
32	563	8631	120	212	138	50	89	14	42	89
33	452	6929	96	170	111	40	72	11	34	72
34	352	5396	75	133	87	31	56	9	27	56
35	274	4200	59	104	68	25	44	7	21	44
36	213	3265	46	81	53	19	34	6	17	34
37	166	2545	36	63	41	15	27	5	13	27
38	129	1978	28	49	32	12	21	4	10	21
39	100	1533	22	38	25	10	17	3	8	17
40	78	1196	17	30	20	8	13	3	7	13
41	61	935	14	24	16	6	10	2	5	10
42	47	721	11	18	12	5	8	2	4	8
43	37	567	9	15	10	4	7	2	4	7
44	29	445	7	12	8	3	5	2	3	5
45	22	337	5	9	6	3	4	1	3	4
46	17	261	4	7	5	2	4	1	2	4
47	13	199	4	6	4	2	3	1	2	3
48	10	153	3	4	3	2	2	1	2	2
49	8	123	3	4	3	2	2	1	2	2

BPD, biparietal diameter; FL, femur length; O, observed; E, expected (mean)
*Adapted from reference 1
Reprinted with permission from the *American Journal of Obstetrics and Gynecology*[35]

known[47,48]. The sensitivities and specificities of the various ultrasound markers as established by literature review are shown in Table 7. Using the *a priori* risk for trisomy 21 as 'prevalence' of the disease, tables have been generated to adjust the risk for trisomy 21 on the basis of ultrasound findings and maternal age (Table 8) or maternal serum biochemistry results (Table 9). The ultrasound-adjusted risks assume that the fetus (or fetuses) are free of ultrasonically demonstrable structural anomalies. The ultrasound-adjusted risk for trisomy 21 with normal ultrasonography was based on a sensitivity of 91% when a combination of ultrasound markers was used[5,49]. Normal ultrasonography is considered as the absence of any aneuploidy markers, e.g. major anomaly (including cardiac), nuchal fold ≥ 6 mm, short femur, short humerus, pyelectasis and choroid plexus cysts. During the last 3 years we have used a combination of aneuploidy markers to manage patients at increased risk for fetal trisomy 21. In addition to the aforementioned markers we have included echogenic bowel, hypoplastic middle phalanx of the fifth digit, wide space between the first and second toe and a two-vessel

Table 9 *Mid-trimester risk, as modified by ultrasound findings, for trisomy 21, based on triple screen in a structurally normal fetus. (All risks are expressed as 1/x)*

Triple screen risk	Normal by ultrasound	Short femur by BPD/FL	Short femur by O/E	Short humerus by O/E	Short femur and humerus by O/E	Pyelectasis with short femur or humerus	Nuchal fold	Echogenic bowel	Short ear
15 000	160 000	3163	5631	3661	1303	2359	347	1100	2348
14 500	154 667	3057	5444	3539	1260	2281	335	1063	2270
14 000	149 333	2952	5256	3417	1216	2202	324	1026	2192
13 500	144 000	2846	5068	3295	1173	2124	312	990	2114
13 000	138 667	2741	4881	3173	1129	2045	300	953	2035
12 500	133 333	2636	4693	3051	1086	1966	289	917	1957
12 000	128 000	2530	4505	2929	1043	1888	277	880	1879
11 500	122 667	2425	4318	2807	999	1809	266	843	1801
11 000	117 333	2319	4130	2685	956	1730	254	807	1722
10 500	112 000	2214	3942	2563	912	1652	243	770	1644
10 000	106 667	2109	3754	2441	869	1573	231	733	1566
9500	101 333	2003	3567	2319	826	1495	220	697	1488
9000	96 000	1898	3379	2197	782	1416	208	660	1409
8500	90 667	1792	3191	2075	739	1337	197	624	1331
8000	85 333	1687	3004	1953	695	1259	185	587	1253
7500	80 000	1582	2816	1831	652	1180	174	550	1175
7000	74 667	1476	2628	1709	609	1102	162	514	1096
6500	69 333	1371	2441	1587	565	1023	151	477	1018
6000	64 000	1266	2253	1465	522	944	139	440	940
5500	58 667	1160	2065	1343	478	866	128	404	862
5000	53 333	1055	1878	1221	435	787	116	367	783
4500	48 000	949	1690	1099	392	708	135	331	705
4000	42 667	844	1502	977	348	630	93	294	627
3500	37 333	739	1315	855	305	551	82	257	549
3000	32 000	633	1127	733	261	473	70	221	470
2500	26 667	528	939	611	218	394	59	184	392
2000	21 333	422	751	489	175	315	47	147	314
1500	16 000	317	564	367	131	237	36	111	236

BPD, biparietal diameter; FL, femur length; O, observed; E, expected (mean)
Reprinted with permission from the *American Journal of Obstetrics and Gynecology*[35]

umbilical cord. At the time of this writing we have evaluated over 500 patients between 15 and 23 weeks' gestation who either had declined genetic amniocentesis or chose to have a sonogram prior to deciding whether to undergo amniocentesis. We have encountered 14 fetuses with trisomy 21, one fetus with trisomy 13 and one fetus with triploidy. Twelve of the 14 fetuses with trisomy 21, the one fetus with trisomy 13 and the one fetus with triploidy had two or more abnormal ultrasound markers present; one fetus with trisomy 21 had one abnormal marker and one had a completely normal ultrasound examination. The most important aneuploidy markers were: abnormal nuchal fold thickening (present in nine trisomy 21 fetuses) short humerus (present in seven trisomy 21 fetuses) and cardiac defects (present in five trisomy 21 fetuses). When one or more abnormal ultrasound markers were present the sensitivity, specificity and positive and negative predictive values for trisomy 21 were 93%, 87%, 18% and 99.7%, respectively. When two or more abnormal ultrasound markers were present, the sensitivity, specificity, positive and negative predictive values for trisomy 21 were 86%, 97%, 48% and 99.5%, respectively. In our view, a second-trimester genetic sonogram may be a reasonable alternative for patients at increased risk for fetal trisomy 21 who wish to avoid amniocentesis. In this group of patients the detection rate of trisomy 21 was very high (93%) with an amniocentesis rate less than 20%.

The prerequisites for a 'genetic' sonogram are obviously skill and experience in diagnosing fetal structural anomalies, especially congenital heart disease. Another problem may be the accuracy of fetal measurements and the applicability of the published ratios between different populations and different ultrasound units. Therefore, extreme caution should be exercised before ultrasound-adjusted risks are used clinically. The data from which the ultrasound-adjusted risks were generated have been produced by experienced units and sonographers and may not apply to general practices. On the other hand, the use of ultrasound-adjusted risk for fetal trisomy 21 has the potential dramatically to decrease the number of genetic amniocenteses in high-risk patients when targeted 'genetic' sonography by experienced personnel reveals no abnormal ultrasound markers. As a matter of fact, genetic amniocentesis may not be indicated in the presence of normal ultrasono-

graphy for women 45 years of age or younger (see Table 8). In contrast, the presence of short femur (by biparietal diameter/femur length ratio), combination of short femur and short humerus, pyelectasis associated with other abnormal ultrasound findings, increased nuchal fold thickening, echogenic bowel or short fetal ear may indicate the need for offering amniocentesis to women < 35 years old[35]. Since the birth of a child with trisomy 21 does not carry the same significance as the loss of a normal fetus (due to genetic amniocentesis) for all patients, the use of individual ultrasound-adjusted risks is very attractive. Other compelling arguments for the use of ultrasound-adjusted risks are respect for maternal autonomy and better selection of candidates for genetic amniocentesis, thus minimizing the procedure-related losses of normal fetuses. However, there is no doubt that more studies are needed to define the role of ultrasound in the prenatal detection of fetal aneuploidy in both individual populations and in general practice.

References

1. Palomaki, G. E. and Haddow, J. E. (1987). Maternal serum alpha-fetoprotein, age, and Down syndrome risk. *Am. J. Obstet. Gynecol.*, **156**, 460–3
2. Adams, M., Erickson, J., Leyde, P. and Oakley, G. (1981). Down's syndrome: recent trend in the United States. *J. Am. Med. Assoc.*, **246**, 758–60
3. Wald, N. J., Cuckle, H. S., Densem, J. W. *et al.* (1988). Maternal serum screening for Down's syndrome in early pregnancy. *Br. Med. J.*, **297**, 883–7
4. Nyberg, D. A., Resta, R. G., Luthy, D. A., Hickok, D. E., Mahony, B. S. and Hirsch, J. H. (1990). Prenatal sonographic findings of Down syndrome: review of 94 cases. *Obstet. Gynecol.*, **76**, 370–7
5. Benacerraf, B. R., Neuberg, D., Bromley, B. and Frigoletto, F. D. (1992). Sonographic scoring index for prenatal detection of chromosomal abnormalities. *J. Ultrasound Med.*, **11**, 449–58
6. Benacerraf, B. R., Gelman, R. and Frigoletto, F. D. (1987). Sonographic identification of second-trimester fetuses with Down's syndrome. *N. Engl. J. Med.*, **317**, 1371–6
7. Lockwood, C., Benacerraf, B., Krinsky, A. *et al.* (1987). A sonographic screening method for Down syndrome. *Am. J. Obstet. Gynecol.*, **157**, 803–8
8. Perrella, R., Duerinck, A. J., Grant, E. G., Tessler, F., Tabsh, K. and Crandall, B. F. (1988). Second-trimester sonographic diagnosis of Down syndrome: role of femur-length shortening and nuchal-fold thickening. *Am. J. Roentgenol.*, **151**, 981–5
9. Brumfield, C. G., Hauth, J. C., Cloud, G. A., Davis, R. O., Henson, B. V. and Cosper, P. (1989). Sonographic measurements and ratios in fetuses with Down syndrome. *Obstet. Gynecol.*, **73**, 644–6
10. LaFollette, L., Filly, R. A., Anderson, R. *et al.* (1989). Fetal femur length to detect trisomy 21. *J. Ultrasound Med.*, **8**, 657–60
11. Lynch, L., Berkowitz, G. S., Chitkara, U., Wilkins, I. A., Mehalek, K. E. and Berkowitz, R. L. (1989). Ultrasound detection of Down syndrome: is it really possible? *Obstet. Gynecol.*, **73**, 267–70

12. Dicke, J. M., Gray, D. L., Songster, G. S. and Crane, J. P. (1989). Fetal biometry as a screening tool for the detection of chromosomally abnormal pregnancies. *Obstet. Gynecol.*, **74**, 726–9

13. Cuckle, H., Wald, N., Quinn, J., Royston, P. and Butler, L. (1989). Ultrasound fetal femur length measurement in the screening for Down's syndrome. *Br. J. Obstet. Gynaecol.*, **96**, 1373–8

14. Hill, L. M., Guzick, D., Belfar, H. L., Hixson, J., Rivello, D. and Rusnak, J. (1989). The current role of sonography in the detection of Down syndrome. *Obstet. Gynecol.*, **74**, 620–3

15. Benacerraf, B. R., Cnann, A., Gelman, R., Laboda, L. A. and Frigoletto, F. D. (1989). Can sonographers reliably identify anatomic features associated with Down syndrome in fetuses? *Radiology*, **173**, 377–80

16. Shah, Y. G., Eckl, C. J., Stinson, S. K. and Woods, J. R. (1990). Biparietal diameter/femur length ratio, cephalic index, and femur length measurements: not reliable screening techniques for Down syndrome. *Obstet. Gynecol.*, **75**, 186–8

17. Ginsberg, N., Cadkin, A., Pergament, E. and Verlinsky, Y. (1990). Ultrasonographic detection of the second-trimester fetus with trisomy 18 and trisomy 21. *Am. J. Obstet. Gynecol.*, **163**, 1186–90

18. Rodis, J. F., Vintzileos, A. M., Fleming, A. D. *et al.* (1991). Comparison of humerus length versus femur length in fetuses with Down syndrome. *Am. J. Obstet. Gynecol.*, **165**, 1051–6

19. Rotmensch, S., Luo, J. S., Liberati, M., Belanger, K., Mahoney, M. J. and Hobbins, J. C. (1992). Fetal humeral length to detect Down syndrome. *Am. J. Obstet. Gynecol.*, **166**, 1330–4

20. Nyberg, D. A., Resta, R. G., Luthy, D. A., Hickok, D. E. and Williams, M. A. (1993). Humerus and femur length shortening in the detection of Down's syndrome. *Am. J. Obstet. Gynecol.*, **168**, 534–8

21. Lockwood, C. J., Lynch, L., Ghidini, A., Lapinski, R., Berkowitz, G., Thayer, B. and Miller, W. A. (1993). The effect of fetal gender on the prediction of Down syndrome by means of maternal serum α-fetoprotein and ultrasonographic parameters. *Am. J. Obstet. Gynecol.*, **169**, 1190–7

22. Benacerraf, B. R., Neuberg, D. and Frigoletto, F. D. (1991). Humeral shortening in second-trimester fetuses with Down syndrome. *Obstet. Gynecol.*, **77**, 223–7

23. Benacerraf, B. R., Mandell, J., Estroff, J. A., Harlow, B. L. and Frigoletto, F. D. (1990). Fetal pyelectasis: a possible association with Down syndrome. *Obstet. Gynecol.*, **76**, 58–60

24. Corteville, J. E., Dicke, J. M. and Crane, J. P. (1992). Fetal pyelectasis and Down syndrome: is genetic amniocentesis warranted? *Obstet. Gynecol.*, **79**, 770–2

25. Benacerraf, B. R. and Frigoletto, F. D. (1987). Soft tissue nuchal fold in the second-trimester fetus: standards for normal measurements compared with those in Down syndrome. *Am. J. Obstet. Gynecol.*, **157**, 1146–9

26. Toi, A., Simpson, G. F. and Filly, R. A. (1987). Ultrasonically evident fetal nuchal skin thickening: is it specific for Down syndrome? *Am. J. Obstet. Gynecol.*, **156**, 150–3

27. Crane, J. P. and Gray, D. L. (1991). Sonographically measured nuchal skinfold thickness as a screening tool for Down syndrome: results of a prospective clinical trial. *Obstet. Gynecol.*, **77**, 533–6

28. Kirk, J. S., Cornstock, C. H., Fassnacht, M. A., Yang, S. S. and Lee, W. (1992). Routine measurement of nuchal thickness in the second trimester. *J. Matern. Fetal Med.*, **1**, 82–6

29. DeVore, G. R. and Alfi, O. (1993). The association between an abnormal nuchal skin fold, trisomy 21, and ultrasound abnormalities identified during the second trimester of pregnancy. *Ultrasound Obstet. Gynecol.*, **3**, 387–94

30. Watson, W. J., Miller, R. C., Menard, M. R. *et al.* (1994). Ultrasonographic measurement of fetal nuchal skin to screen for chromosomal abnormalities. *Am. J. Obstet. Gynecol.*, **170**, 583–6

31. Scioscia, A. L., Pretorius, D. H., Budorick, N. E., Cahill, T. C., Axelrod, F. T. and Leopold, G. R. (1992). Second trimester echogenic bowel and chromosomal abnormalities. *Am. J. Obstet. Gynecol.*, **167**, 889–94

32. Dicke, J. M. and Crane, J. P. (1992). Sonographically detected hyperechoic fetal bowel: significance and implications for pregnancy management. *Obstet. Gynecol.*, **80**, 778–82

33. Birnholz, J. C. and Farrell, E. E. (1988). Fetal ear lengths. *Pediatrics*, **81**, 555–8

34. Lettieri, L., Rodis, J. F., Vintzileos, A. M., Feeney, L., Ciarleglio, L. and Craffey, A. (1993). Ear length in second trimester aneuploid fetuses. *Obstet. Gynecol.*, **81**, 57–60

35. Vintzileos, A. M. and Egan, J. F. X. (1995). Adjusting the risk for trisomy 21 on the basis of second trimester ultrasonography. *Am. J. Obstet. Gynecol.*, **172**, 837–44

36. Nyberg, D. A. and Crane, J. P. (1990). Chromosome abnormalities. In Nyberg, D. A., Mahony, B. S. and Pretorius, D. H. (eds.) *Diagnostic Ultrasound of Fetal Anomalies – Text and Atlas*, pp. 676–724. (Chicago: Year Book Medical Publishers)

37. Gross, S. J., Shulman, L. P., Tollery, E. A., Emerson, D. S., Felker, R. E. Simpson, J. L. and Elias, S. (1995). Isolated fetal choroid plexus cysts and

trisomy 18. A review and meta-analysis. *Am. J. Obstet. Gynecol.*, **172**, 83–7

38. Gray, S. E., Tsapanos, V., McLean, D. A., Nardi, D. A. and Vintzileos, A. M. (1995). Ultrasound detection of trisomy 18 and 21 by second trimester growth curves. *J. Matern. Fetal Invest.*, **5**, 135–9

39. DeVore, G. R. and Alfi, O. (1995). The use of color Doppler ultrasound to identify fetuses at increased risk for trisomy 21: an alternative for high-risk patients who decline amniocentesis. *Obstet. Gynecol.*, **85**, 378–86

40. Perry, T. B., Benzie, R. J., Cassar, N. *et al.* (1984). Fetal cephalometry by ultrasound as a screening procedure for the prenatal detection of Down's syndrome. *Br. J. Obstet. Gynaecol.*, **91**, 138–43

41. Hill, L. M., Rivello, D., Peterson, C. and Marchese, S. (1991). The transverse cerebellar diameter in the second trimester is unaffected by Down's syndrome. *Am. J. Obstet. Gynecol.*, **164**, 101–3

42. Turner, G. W., Vintzileos, A. M., Nardi, D. A., Feeney, L., Campbell, W. A. and Rodis, J. F. (1992). Neck circumference measurements in second trimester fetuses with Down syndrome. *J. Matern. Fetal Med.*, **1**, 65–9

43. Bahado-Singh, R. O., Wyse, L., Dor, M. A., Copel, J. A., O'Connor, T. and Hobbins, J. C. (1992). Fetuses with Down syndrome have disproportionately shortened frontal lobe dimensions on ultrasonographic examination. *Am. J. Obstet. Gynecol.*, **167**, 1009–14

44. Johnson, M. P., Barr, M., Treadwell, M. C. *et al.* (1993). Fetal leg and femur/foot length ratio: a marker for trisomy 21. *Am. J. Obstet. Gynecol.*, **169**, 557–63

45. Johnson, M. P., Michaelson, J. E., Barr, M. *et al.* (1994). Sonographic screening for trisomy 21: femur humerus : foot length ratio, a useful marker. *Fetal Diagn. Ther.*, **9**, 130–8

46. Benacerraf, B. R., Harlow, B. L. and Frigoletto, F. D. (1990). Hypoplasia of the middle phalanx of the fifth digit. *J. Ultrasound Med.*, **9**, 389–94

47. Peipert, J. F. and Sweeney, P. J. (1993). Diagnostic testing in obstetrics and gynecology: a clinician's guide. *Obstet. Gynecol.*, **82**, 619–23

48. Kramer, M. S. (1988) *Clinical Epidemiology and Biostatistics*, pp. 201–19. (New York: Springer-Verlag)

49. Nadel, A. S., Bromley, B., Frigoletto, F. D. and Benacerraf, B. R. (1995). Can the presumed risk of autosomal trisomy be decreased in fetuses of older women following a normal sonogram? *J. Ultrasound Med.*, **14**, 297–302

Section 3

Challenges in fetal therapy

Fetal surgery

19

K. J. VanderWall and M. R. Harrison

INTRODUCTION

Until recently, the womb shielded the fetus from observation. Powerful new imaging and sampling techniques have unveiled the mystery of the fetus, improved our understanding of fetal physiology and defined the natural history of several congenital anomalies. Fetal therapy has emerged as we continue to push the limits of fetal diagnosis. In other words, the fetus is now a patient[1].

The fetus as a patient involves the maternal–fetal unit. Whatever intervention is performed in the fetus also directly affects the mother. Although most prenatal malformations are best managed by appropriate medical and surgical therapy after maternal transport to a tertiary medical center for planned delivery, a few simple anatomic abnormalities with predictable developmental consequences may require treatment before birth.

Tremendous progress has been made in solving the technical aspects of fetal surgery and the intraoperative and postoperative care and monitoring of the maternal–fetal unit. However, the general application of fetal surgery still remains hampered by preterm labor and ineffective tocolysis after fetal interventions. Preterm labor has limited success in fetal surgery, much as rejection has limited success in transplantation. An intensive effort to solve the vexing problem of preterm labor after hysterotomy for fetal surgery continues and has yielded new insight into the role of nitric oxide in myometrial contractions and the use of nitric oxide donors for the treatment of preterm labor[2,3]. More recently, the advancement of fetal surgery through small puncture sites in the uterus, or fetoscopic surgery, may obviate the morbidity of preterm labor and reduce the maternal–fetal risk.

RISKS AND BENEFITS OF FETAL SURGERY

The risks and benefits for the mother are difficult to assess. Clearly, the healthy mother accepts some risk to help her unborn child. She may choose to accept the risk in exchange for alleviating her own burden in raising a child with a severe malformation. For the fetus, the risk of the procedure is weighed against the benefit of correcting a fatal or debilitating defect.

Because maternal safety is the primary concern in fetal surgery, the best perioperative management of the maternal–fetal unit requires continuous monitoring of mother and fetus in an intensive care setting. Only a few open fetal surgery cases have been treated at other institutions, so the 50 cases performed at our center provide the best data on maternal outcome. There have been no maternal deaths and few postoperative maternal complications, but all mothers had uterine contractions after fetal surgery, accounting for some morbidity from the treatment regimen. In our early experience, seven patients developed amniotic fluid leaks; two from the hysterotomy site, requiring repair, and five from the vagina. Four patients developed pulmonary edema while receiving high doses of tocolytic drugs. Although this frightening complication was reversible, it emphasized the need for close, continuous monitoring in an intensive care unit the first few days following surgery. Experimental studies have not revealed what causes the pulmonary edema, but most probably the etiology is multifactorial and related to the stress of surgery, pregnancy, and the use of tocolytic drugs (J. F. Bealer and colleagues, and M. R. Harrison and associates, unpublished data).

Because the hysterotomy site is usually in the upper segment of the uterine corpus, and thus comparable to a classic Cesarean section, all future deliveries should be by Cesarean section. In our series, uterine disruptions occurred in two subsequent pregnancies; maternal and neonatal outcome were excellent in both cases. Finally, future reproductive potential does not appear to be jeopardized by fetal surgery; 19 mothers have had subsequent pregnancies without complication.

MANAGEMENT OF MOTHER AND FETUS

Figure 1 summarizes the technical aspects of open fetal surgery that have evolved over 15 years of experimental and clinical work. Intraoperatively, mothers are monitored with a central venous pressure catheter and a radial arterial line. Postoperative care in the first 48 h is provided in a fetal intensive care unit by a trained cadre of physicians and nurses with a specially designed fetal monitor that continuously records fetal electrocardiogram, temperature and intra-amniotic pressure[4]. Maternal arterial pressure, central venous pressure, urine output and oxygen saturation are continuously monitored. Patient-controlled analgesia and/or epidural analgesics ease maternal stress and aid tocolysis. A second generation cephalosporin is given prophylactically for 48 h. Obstetric ultrasound examinations and fetal echocardiography are performed daily to assess amniotic fluid volume, fetal well being and cardiac function. Maternal–fetal monitoring continues on the obstetric ward for 5–7 days postoperatively, followed by outpatient examinations, sonograms and tocolysis, with subcutaneous terbutaline via a portable pump. Cesarean section is performed when either the membranes rupture or labor cannot be controlled, usually before 36 weeks' gestation.

Breeching the uterus, whether by puncture or by incision, incites uterine contractions. In spite of technical advances, preterm labor remains the nemesis of fetal surgery, and the tocolytic regimen that was successful in non-human primate experiments is fraught with potential clinical difficulties. In humans, aggressive treatment of postoperative labor with maximal doses of indomethacin, magnesium sulfate and β-mimetics has had adverse effects on the mother and the fetus/neonate[5–7]. Indomethacin constricts the fetal ductus arteriosus and may lead to tricuspid regurgitation, significant right-heart failure and pulmonary hypertension[8]. Although halogenated inhalation agents provide satisfactory anesthesia for mother and fetus, this regimen can depress fetal and maternal myocardial function and decrease placental perfusion[9]. Maternal pulmonary edema is a known side effect of the magnesium sulfate and the β-mimetics used for tocolysis, and fluid restriction to avoid this complication may compromise maternal–placental–fetal circulation and exacerbate preterm labor[10]. The search for a more effective and less toxic tocolytic regimen led to the demonstration in monkeys that exogenous nitric oxide ablates preterm labor induced by hysterotomy[3]. For the last 2 years, we have used intravenous nitroglycerin intraoperatively and postoperatively with successful ablation of hysterotomy-induced preterm labor, but its safety and efficacy for mother and fetus remain unclear (M. R. Harrison and co-workers, unpublished data).

FETAL PROBLEMS AMENABLE TO SURGICAL CORRECTION BEFORE BIRTH

A few simple anatomic abnormalities with predictable life-threatening consequences may benefit from surgical correction before birth (Table 1). At present, only a small number of malformations have been successfully corrected. Others (e.g. complete heart block, aqueductal stenosis, pulmonary or aortic valve obstruction and tracheal atresia) may be appropriate for fetal surgery, once their pathophysiology and natural history are better understood. Finally, if the risk of the procedure could be reduced to that of postnatal repair, particularly if the *in utero* intervention is minimally invasive, a few non-lethal anomalies (e.g. myelomeningocele, cleft lip and palate,

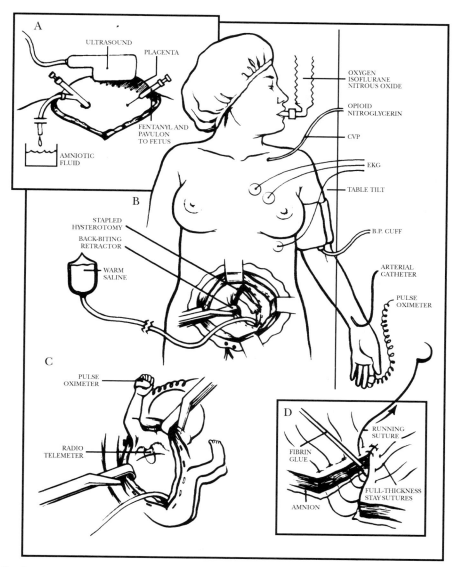

Figure 1 *Fetal surgery techniques. A. The uterus is exposed through a low, transverse, abdominal incision. Ultrasound is used to localize the placenta, inject the fetus with narcotic and muscle relaxant and aspirate amniotic fluid. B. The uterus is opened with staples that provide homeostasis and seal the membranes. Warm saline is continuously infused around the fetus. Maternal anesthesia, tocolysis and monitoring are shown. C. Absorbable staples and back-biting clamps facilitate hysterotomy exposure of the pertinent fetal part. A miniaturized pulse oximeter records pulse rate and oxygen saturation intraoperatively. A radiotelemeter monitors fetal electrocardiogram (EKG) and amniotic pressure during and after operation. D. After fetal repair, the uterine incision is closed with absorbable sutures and fibrin glue. Amniotic fluid is restored with warm Ringer's lactate. (A videotape of fetal surgery techniques is available)*

craniosynostosis) might be better repaired *in utero*.

As minimally invasive techniques become developed and refined, the way we treat life-threatening malformations may change. In addition, with the advance of gene therapy, fetal stem cell transplantation and chronic fetal vascular access, the treatment of debilitating but non-lethal anomalies may soon become a clinical reality.

Table 1 *Malformations potentially amenable to fetal surgery. From reference 63 with permission*

Fetal defect	Effect on development/rationale for treatment		Treatment
	Effect	*Likely result*	*Treatment*
Life threatening			
Diaphragmatic hernia	lung hypoplasia	respiratory failure	open repair, temporary tracheal occlusion
Cystic adenomatoid malformation	lung hypoplasia hydrops	hydrops and death	open pulmonary lobectomy
Posterior urethral valves	lung hypoplasia renal dysplasia	respiratory failure/renal failure	percutaneous catheter placement, open vesicostomy
Sacrococcygeal teratoma	high output failure	hydrops and death	open tumor resection
Aqueductal stenosis	hydrocephalus	neurological damage	ventriculoamniotic shunt, open ventriculoperitoneal shunt*
Complete heart block	low output failure	hydrops and death	percutaneous pacemaker, open pacemaker
Pulmonary artery or aortic obstruction	ventricular hypertrophy	heart failure	percutaneous valvuloplasty, open valvuloplasty*
Tracheal atresia or stenosis	overdistension by lung fluid	hydrops and death	open tracheostomy*
Not life threatening			
Myelomeningocele	spinal cord damage	paralysis, neurogenic bowel/bladder	fetoscopic coverage, open repair*
Cleft lip/palate	facial defect	persistent deformity	fetoscopic or open repair*

*Not yet attempted in human fetuses

Congenital diaphragmatic hernia

Congenital diaphragmatic hernia results when the diaphragm fails to close in the first trimester. The abdominal viscera herniate into the chest and cause lung underdevelopment in both size and maturity[11–13]. Despite advances in prenatal care, maternal transport for planned delivery, neonatal resuscitation and extracorporeal membrane oxygenation, the mortality for babies with isolated congenital diaphragmatic hernia diagnosed before 25 weeks' gestation remains 60%[14]. Babies who die *in utero* and soon after birth account for a substantial 'hidden mortality'.

Although there are no 100% accurate prognostic criteria for predicting survival for babies with congenital diaphragmatic hernia, we have developed an algorithm for managing this condition in the fetus (Figure 2). We have shown experimentally that repair before birth, allowing the lungs time to grow while the fetus remains on placental support, is physiologically sound and technically feasible[15]. Repair *in utero*

has proven to be a formidable challenge, particularly when the left lobe of the liver is incarcerated in the chest (approximately 50% of the cases). Reduction of the liver in these cases compromises umbilical venous flow and leads to fetal demise[16].

To evaluate the extent of liver incarcerated into the chest in fetuses with congenital diaphragmatic hernia, color Doppler imaging has been used for careful definition of the anatomy of the umbilical vein or ductus venosus. When the umbilical vein is deviated far to the left, the liver is usually up in the chest. If the course of the sinus venosus appears well up in the chest, the liver cannot be reduced without compromising umbilical flow. Thus, fetuses with either of these two vessels above the level of the diaphragm cannot be treated with the current complete repair.

For fetuses deemed 'unfixable' by virtue of liver herniation, we have developed experimentally and now tested clinically a new approach to improving fetal lung development.

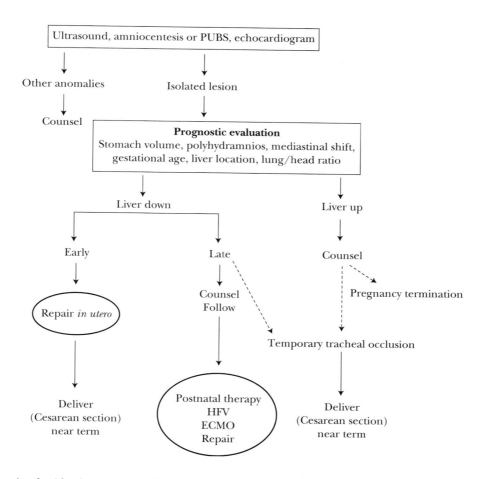

Figure 2 *An algorithm for managing a fetus with diaphragmatic hernia. PUBS, percutaneous umbilical blood sampling; HFV, high-frequency ventilation; ECMO, extracorporeal membrane oxygenation. From reference 63, with permission*

Experimental work in our laboratory and others has shown that fetal tracheal obstruction can correct the pulmonary hypoplasia associated with congenital diaphragmatic hernia[17–21]. Normally, the fetal lung produces a continuous flow of lung fluid that exits through the trachea into the amniotic fluid. Experimentally, external drainage of fetal lung fluid retards lung growth, resulting in pulmonary hypoplasia[22,23], whereas tracheal obstruction markedly accelerates lung growth, resulting in pulmonary hyperplasia[18,19,23–26]. In fetal lambs with surgically created diaphragmatic hernias, tracheal obstruction expands the fetal lung, which not only pushes the viscera back into the abdomen but

also produces lungs that at birth are larger and functionally better than those of untreated controls. Thus, fetal trachea obstruction does more than passively distend the fetal lung; it accelerates growth and improves function.

Using the technology developed for laparoscopic surgery and for temporary tracheal occlusion, we have now developed a fetal endoscopic technique for tracheal occlusion in fetal sheep[27,28]. This fetal endoscopic ('Fetendo') technique offers significant advantages over open fetal surgery. Fetendo is minimally invasive, may decrease maternal and fetal risks, and hopefully decreases preterm labor, because of decreased uterine manipulation

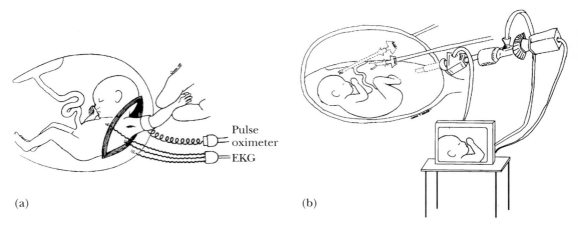

(a)   (b)

Figure 3   *Comparison of open fetal surgery vs. fetoscopic surgery (Fetendo). Drawings demonstrate the basics of open fetal surgery (a) and fetoscopic surgery (b)*

(Figure 3). Continuing to explore minimally invasive techniques is critical for the future of fetal therapy.

Congenital cystic adenomatoid malformation

Congenital cystic adenomatoid malformation (CCAM) is a benign pulmonary mass that is almost always unilateral and is usually confined to one pulmonary lobe. When it is diagnosed *in utero*, the overall prognosis depends on the size of the lung mass and the secondary physiological effects. A large mass can cause mediastinal shift, pulmonary hypoplasia and cardiovascular compromise, leading to hydrops and eventually fetal demise.

Our experience with more than 80 cases of CCAM confirms that the development of fetal hydrops rapidly leads to fetal demise. Fetal hydrops appears to result from vena caval obstruction or cardiac compression by the huge chest mass[29]. Although most lesions can be successfully treated after birth and some even resolve before birth, for the severe cases (less than 10%) that develop hydrops before 26 weeks, *in utero* lobectomy has been successful[30].

After demonstrating in a fetal lamb model that *in utero* pulmonary resection is feasible and compensatory growth of the opposite lung occurs, we then developed an algorithm for management of the fetus with a CCAM[31,32]

(Figure 4). Initial evaluation should include an ultrasound examination to confirm the diagnosis, amniocentesis or percutaneous umbilical blood sampling to rule out any chromosomal abnormalities, and a fetal echocardiogram to detect congenital heart disease and to evaluate cardiac function. Careful serial sonographic surveillance of large lesions is necessary to detect the first signs of hydrops.

Nine fetuses have undergone open fetal surgery for resection of a CCAM tumor; five of these had rapid resolution of hydrops, impressive lung growth *in utero*, and normal postnatal growth and development with a follow-up of 12–45 months[30]. In most cases, fetal lobectomy will be necessary, but for a lesion with a single large cyst, thoracoamniotic shunting has also been successful[33].

Sacrococcygeal teratoma

Sacrococcygeal teratoma, the most common tumor of the newborn, is rarely malignant and is usually amenable to simple resection[34]. However, sacrococcygeal teratoma diagnosed early in fetal life may follow a dramatically different course. A large tumor can steal distal aortic blood flow and shunt blood away from the placenta and toward the tumor (vascular steal phenomenon). Serial sonograms of prenatally diagnosed sacrococcygeal teratoma have revealed that large tumors found early in gestation

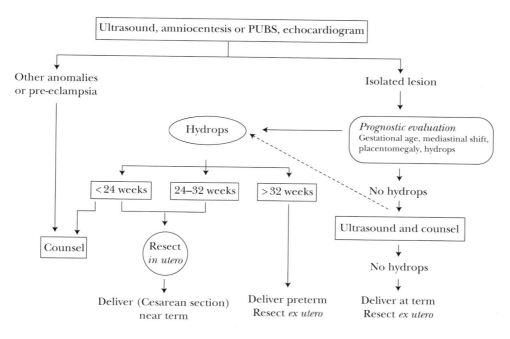

Figure 4 *An algorithm for managing a fetus with a congenital cystic adenomatoid malformation. PUBS, percutaneous umbilical blood sampling. From reference 64, with permission*

are frequently associated with rapid fetal demise[35]. Signs of impending fetal demise include fetal hydrops (pleural or pericardial effusion, cardiomegaly, ascites and skin edema), placentomegaly, or polyhydramnios. The development of placentomegaly and polyhydramnios can lead to the potentially devastating 'mirror syndrome', in which the maternal condition begins to mirror that of the fetus. The mother can develop progressive symptoms of pre-eclampsia, including vomiting, hypertension, proteinuria and peripheral edema. Endothelial toxins or vasoactive factors released from the edematous placenta are thought to be the etiology of this syndrome[36].

Our current recommendations for management of sacrococcygeal teratoma are detailed in Figure 5. Briefly, all fetuses diagnosed with this condition should have a detailed sonographic examination to confirm the diagnosis and rule out any other associated anomalies. An assessment should be made of placental size, type of sacrococcygeal teratoma and presence of hydrops. Color flow Doppler ultrasonography

and echocardiography should be performed to document the presence of high output failure secondary to the vascular steal phenomenon[37]. Although most sacrococcygeal teratomas can be managed postnatally, the immature fetus with a large sacrococcygeal teratoma who develops high output failure will initiate maternal pre-eclampsia, preterm labor and possibly fetal death. In this desperate situation, the only hope for fetal survival may be fetal surgical resection of the tumor or fetoscopic interruption of the vascular supply to the tumor vessels.

Urinary tract obstruction

The natural history of untreated fetal urinary tract obstruction is well documented, and selection criteria based on fetal urine electrolyte and β_2-microglobulin levels and the sonographic appearance of the fetal kidneys have proven reliable[38,39]. Renal dysplasia secondary to early complete obstruction affects tubular and glomerular development. Renal dysplasia, however,

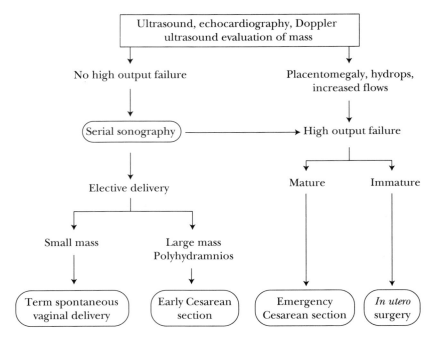

Figure 5 *An algorithm for managing a fetus with sacrococcygeal teratoma. From reference 65, with permission*

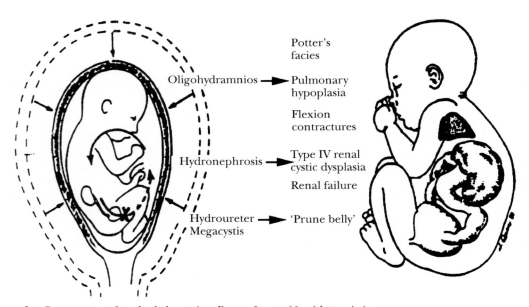

Figure 6 *Consequences of urethral obstruction. From reference 66, with permission*

is not the immediate cause of death in neonates with high-grade urethral obstruction. Markedly decreased urinary output leads to oligohydramnios and pulmonary hypoplasia (Figure 6).

Ninety per cent of fetuses with urinary tract obstruction do not require *in utero* intervention. Fetuses with bilateral hydronephrosis due to urethral obstruction and oligohydramnios

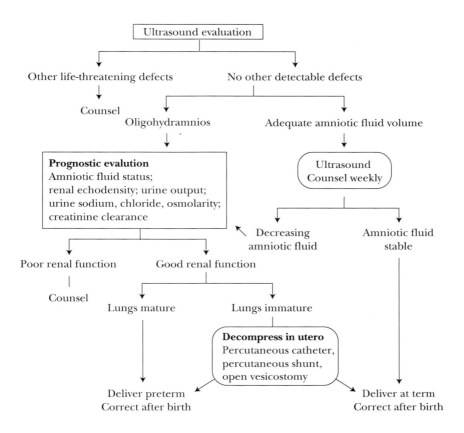

Figure 7 *An algorithm for managing a fetus with bilateral hydronephrosis. From reference 67, with permission*

should have a prompt evaluation of fetal renal function by ultrasound examination and urinalysis.

From our cumulative clinical and experimental studies, we have derived general guidelines for management of the fetus with hydronephrosis (Figure 7). The maturity of the lungs is critical for survival. If the lungs are mature, the fetus can be delivered early for postnatal decompression. If the lungs are immature, choices for fetal intervention include ultrasound-guided percutaneous vesicoamniotic shunt (catheter or wire mesh stent), fetoscopic vesicostomy or open fetal vesicostomy[40–42]. *In utero* decompression with restoration of amniotic fluid can prevent the development of fatal pulmonary hypoplasia. It is not clear if decompression can arrest or reverse renal dysplastic changes that compromise renal function.

Inherited defects as candidates for fetal stem cell transplantation

A wide variety of inherited defects that can now be diagnosed early in gestation, such as hemoglobinopathies and immunodeficiencies, are currently treated after birth by bone marrow transplantation. However, postnatal treatment is limited by donor availability, graft rejection, graft-versus-host disease (GVHD), and patient deterioration prior to transplantation[43,44]. In contrast, *in utero* transplantation of normal fetal hematopoietic stem cells in the preimmune fetus maintains stable long-term chimerism. A fetus early in gestation (less than 16 weeks) is an ideal recipient, because it will not reject the transplanted cells, obviating the need for immunosuppression. In addition, the bone marrow is primed to receive stem cells migrating from the fetal liver, obviating the need for marrow ablation. We have confirmed these hypotheses by transplanting fetal hematopoietic stem cells into early-gestation sheep and monkeys and demonstrated long-term hematopoietic chimerism of all cell lines without rejection, GVHD, or the need for immunosuppression[45,46].

Clinical experience with fetal stem cell transplantation may be limited, in part by an insufficient degree of engraftment or chimerism to cure or palliate some diseases. In the few cases attempted, donor cell engraftment levels have been low and have had limited clinical efficacy[47]. Low levels of donor engraftment may be sufficient in diseases such as chronic granulomatous disease and severe combined immunodeficiency, but a higher degree of expression in the periphery might be necessary to change the course of diseases such as β-thalassemia or sickle cell disease. In those diseases that may require a high percentage of donor cell engraftment, it might be necessary to induce tolerance *in utero* and then deliver 'booster' injections from a living relative postnatally. After a decade of preparation in experimental animal models, we have opened a trial to transplant hematopoietic stem cells obtained from fetal liver or prepared from a parent's bone marrow into fetuses of less than 15 weeks' gestation diagnosed with chronic granulomatous disease or severe combined immune deficiency disease.

Another application for fetal hematopoietic stem cell transplantation is the fetus that is diagnosed prenatally with predictable neonatal organ failure. The induction of specific immune tolerance by transplanting hematopoietic stem cells *in utero* may allow organ replacement after birth, without rejection or the need for immunosuppression[48]. For a fetus that needs a kidney, lung or heart, T cell-depleted hematopoietic stem cells from a relative could be used to induce tolerance for a living-related transplant after birth. Although this is promising, a great deal of experimental work is necessary before clinical application is attempted.

Twin–twin transfusion syndrome

In some twin pregnancies, abnormal placental chorionic vessels connect the circulation of the two fetuses, leading to an imbalance of blood flow. Both twins can be in jeopardy because of marked changes in amniotic fluid volume, growth retardation, or hydrops. In many cases, serial amniocenteses of the polyhydramniotic sac has restored the imbalance and allowed the pregnancy to continue. For severe cases, recent therapy has focused on interrupting the abnormal placental vascular connections, by ligating the umbilical circulation (of an acardiac–acephalus twin), dividing the abnormal placental vessels fetoscopically, or by removing the abnormal fetus by hysterotomy[49–51]. Future interventions will most probably continue to be less invasive, using sonographically guided or fetoscopic techniques.

Myelomeningocele

Myelomeningocele, a devastating congenital malformation, can lead to varying degrees of sensorimotor paraplegia, hydrocephalus and skeletal deformities. Previously, the defect was thought to result from failure of the embryological neural elements to form a normal spinal cord; however, recent studies suggest that neurological impairment after birth may be due to exposure of the spinal cord *in utero*[52]. We have shown in fetal lambs that exposure of the spinal cord to the intrauterine environment causes neurological damage resembling human myelomeningocele that can be prevented by repairing the anatomic defect *in utero*[53]. Before attempting *in utero* repair, we must determine at what point in gestation the neurological damage occurs.

Craniofacial anomalies

During fetal animal studies, we learned that the fetus heals surgical incisions without scar formation. This unique repair process does not depend on the sterile, aqueous intrauterine environment[54]. The differences between fetal and adult skin healing reflect processes intrinsic to fetal tissue such as an extracellular wound matrix rich in hyaluronic acid and a substantially reduced inflammatory infiltrate, and cytokine profile[55,56]. Scarless fetal wound healing has prompted therapeutic strategies for *in utero* correction of cleft lip and palate, midfacial growth restriction and secondary nasal deformities[57,58]. We are continuing to develop less invasive fetoscopic techniques for repair before justifying the risks of intervention.

Cardiac anomalies

A few simple structural cardiac defects that interfere with development may benefit from prenatal correction. For example, balloon valvuloplasty across a stenotic valve may allow normal development of the ventricles. While the physiology remains to be proven experimentally, aortic stenosis has been dilated by a balloon catheter placed percutaneously[59]. Other exciting experimental techniques include pacemaker placement for complete heart block (unpublished data) and fetal cardiac bypass[60].

THE FUTURE OF FETAL SURGERY

Research on fetal surgery has expanded fetal biology with implications beyond fetal surgery. The observation that a fetus heals surgical incisions without scarring has provided new insights into the natural history of wound healing and stimulated efforts to mimic the fetal process postnatally[55,61]. Fetal tissue appears to be biologically and immunologically superior for transplantation and for gene therapy, and fetal immune tolerance may allow a wide variety of inherited non-surgical diseases to be cured by fetal hematopoietic stem cell transplantation[45].

The future of fetal surgery depends on scientific and technical progress, primarily in two areas. Advancing our scientific knowledge of the normal regulation of parturition and of the pathophysiological induction of preterm labor should result in new and more effective pharmacological therapies that will induce uterine relaxation, provide effective tocolysis after fetal intervention, and be safe both to mother and fetus.

The future of fetal surgery also depends on adapting minimally invasive surgery for repairing fetal defects *in utero*[28,62]. The era of minimally invasive surgery has arrived and must be translated to the womb. If improvements in these two areas are achieved, the promise to fetal surgery, i.e. that for some diseases the earliest possible intervention will produce the best result, may become a reality. However, the promise of cost-effective, preventive fetal therapy can be subverted by misguided clinical applications, such as an *in utero* procedure that 'saves' an otherwise doomed fetus for prolonged neonatal or lifelong intensive care. Enthusiasm for fetal therapy must be tempered by respect for the interests of the mother and the family, by the careful study of disease in animal models and untreated human fetuses, and by a willingness to abandon the therapy that does not prove to be both effective and cost effective in properly controlled trials.

References

1. Harrison, M. R., Golbus, M. S. and Filly, R. A. (1990). *The Unborn Patient: Prenatal Diagnosis and Treatment*. (Philadelphia: W. B. Saunders)
2. Natuzzi, E. S., Ursell, P. C., Harrison, M. R. and Reimer, K. (1993). Nitric oxide synthase activity in the pregnant uterus decreases at parturition. *Biochem. Biophys. Res. Commun.*, **179**, 1–8
3. Jennings, R. W., MacGillivray, T. E. and Harrison, M. R. (1993). Nitric oxide inhibits preterm labor in the Rhesus monkey. *J. Matern. Fetal Med.*, **2**, 170–5
4. Jennings, R. W., Adzick, N. S. and Longaker, M. T. (1993). Radio-telemetric fetal monitoring during and after open fetal surgery. *Surg. Obstet. Gynecol.*, **176**, 59–64
5. Groome, L. J., Goldenberg, R. L., Cliver, S. P., Davis, R. O. and Copper, R. L. (1992). Neonatal periventricular–intraventricular hemorrhage after maternal β-sympathomimetic tocolysis. *Am. J. Obstet. Gynecol.*, **167**, 873–9
6. Morales, W. J. and Madhav, H. (1993). Efficacy and safety of indomethacin compared with magnesium sulfate in the management of

preterm labor: a randomized study. *Am. J. Obstet. Gynecol.*, **169**, 97–102

7. Norton, M. E., Merrill, J., Cooper, B., Kuller, J. A. and Clyman, R. (1993). Neonatal complications after the administration of indomethacin for preterm labor. *N. Engl. J. Med.*, **329**, 1602–7

8. Manchester, D., Margolis, H. S. and Sheldon, R. E. (1976). Possible association between maternal indomethacin therapy and primary pulmonary hypertension of the newborn. *Am. J. Obstet. Gynecol.*, **126**, 467–9

9. Sabik, J. F., Assad, R. S. and Hanley, F. L. (1993). Halothane as an anesthetic for fetal surgery. *J. Pediatr. Surg.*, **28**, 542–7

10. Besinger, R. E. and Niebyl, J. R. (1990). The safety and efficacy of tocolytic agents for treatment of preterm labor. *Obstet. Gynecol. Surg.*, **45**, 415–40

11. Reid, L. (1977). The lung: its growth and remodeling in health and disease. *Am. J. Roentgenol.*, **129**, 777–88

12. Naeye, R. L., Shochat, S. J., Whitman, V. and Maisels, M. J. (1976). Unsuspected pulmonary vascular abnormalities associated with diaphragmatic hernia. *Pediatrics*, **58**, 902–6

13. Glick, P. L., Stannard, V. A., Leach, C. L., Rossman, J., Hosada, Y., Morin, F. C., Cooney, D. R., Allen, J. E. and Holm, B. (1992). Pathophysiology of congenital diaphragmatic hernia. II: The fetal lamb CDH model is surfactant deficient. *J. Pediatr. Surg.*, **27**, 382–8

14. Harrison, M. R., Adzick, N. S., Flake, A. W., Jennings, R. W., Estes, J. M., MacGillivray, T. E., Chueh, J. T., Goldberg, J. D., Filly, R. A., Goldstein, R. B., Rosen, M. A., Cauldwell, C., Levine, A. H. and Howell, L. J. (1993). Correction of congenital diaphragmatic hernia *in utero*. VI. Hard-earned lessons. *J. Pediatr. Surg.*, **28**, 1411–18

15. Adzick, N. S., Outwater, K. M., Harrison, M. R. and Reid, L. M. (1985). Correction of congenital diaphragmatic hernia *in utero*. IV. An early gestational model for pulmonary vascular morphometric analysis. *J. Pediatr. Surg.*, **20**, 673–90

16. Harrison, M. R., Adzick, N. S., Flake, A. W. and Jennings, R. W. (1993). The CDH two-step: a dance of necessity. *J. Pediatr. Surg.*, **28**, 813–16

17. Wilson, J. M., DeFiore, J. W. and Peters, C. A. (1993). Experimental fetal tracheal ligation prevents the pulmonary hypoplasia associated with fetal nephrectomy: possible application for congenital diaphragmatic hernia. *J. Pediatr. Surg.*, **28**, 1433–40

18. Hedrick, M. H., Estes, J. M., Sullivan, K. M., Bealer, J. F., Kitterman, J. A., Flake, A. W., Adzick, N. S. and Harrison, M. R. (1994). Plug the lung until it grows (PLUG): a new method to treat congenital diaphragmatic hernia *in utero*. *J. Pediatr. Surg.*, **29**, 612–17

19. DiFiore, J. W., Fauza, D. O., Slavin, R., Peters, C. A., Fackler, J. C. and Wilson, J. M. (1994). Experimental fetal tracheal ligation reverses the structural and physiological effects of pulmonary hypoplasia in congenital diaphragmatic hernia. *J. Pediatr. Surg.*, **29**, 248–57

20. Bealer, J. F., Skarsgard, E. D., Hedrick, M. H., Meuli, M., VanderWall, K. J., Flake, A. W., Adzick, N. S. and Harrison, M. R. (1995). The 'PLUG' odyssey: adventures in experimental fetal tracheal occlusion. *J. Pediatr. Surg.*, **30**, 361–5

21. Beierle, E. A., Langham, M. R. and Cassin, S. (1996). *In utero* lung growth in fetal sheep with diaphragmatic hernia and tracheal stenosis. *J. Pediatr. Surg.*, in press

22. Carmel, J., Freidman, F. and Adams, F. (1965). Fetal tracheal ligation and tracheal development. *Am. J. Dis. Child.*, **109**, 452–6

23. Alcorn, D., Adamson, T. and Lambert, T. (1976). Morphologic effects of chronic tracheal ligation and drainage in the fetal lamb lung. *J. Anat.*, **22**, 649–60

24. Moessinger, A. C., Harding, R., Adamson, T. M., Singh, M. and Kin, G. T. (1990). Role of lung fluid in growth and maturation of the fetal sheep lung. *J. Clin. Invest.*, **86**, 1270–7

25. Hooper, S. B., Man, V. K. M. and Harding, K. (1993). Changes in lung expansion after pulmonary DNA synthesis and IGFII gene expression in fetal sheep. *Am. J. Phys.*, **265**, L403–9

26. Hooper, S. B. and Harding, R. (1995). Fetal lung liquid: a major determinant of the growth and functional development of the fetal lung. *Clin. Exp. Pharmacol. Physiol.*, **22**, 235–47

27. Skarsgard, E. D., Meuli, M., VanderWall, K. J., Bealer, J. F., Adzick, N. S. and Harrison, M. R. (1996). Fetal endoscopic tracheal occlusion ('Fetendo-Plug') for congenital diaphragmatic hernia. *J. Pediatr. Surg.*, in press

28. VanderWall, K. J., Bruch, S. W., Meuli, M., Kohl, T., Szabo, Z., Adzick, N. S. and Harrison, M. R. (1996). Fetal endoscopic ('Fetendo') tracheal clip. *J. Pediatr. Surg.*, in press

29. Rice, H. E., Estes, J. M., Hedrick, M. H., Bealer, J. F., Harrison, M. R. and Adzick, N. S. (1994). Congenital cystic adenomatoid malformation: a sheep model of fetal hydrops. *J. Pediatr. Surg.*, **29**, 692–6

30. Adzick, N. S. (1994). Fetal cystic adenomatoid malformation of the lung: diagnosis, perinatal management, and outcome. *Semin. Thorac. Cardiovasc. Surg.*, **6**, 247–52

31. Adzick, N. S., Hu, L. M., Davies, P., Flake, A. W., Reid, L. M. and Harrison, M. (1986).

Compensatory lung growth after pneumon-ectomy in the fetus. *Surg. Forum*, **37**, 648

32. Adzick, N. S. (1993). Fetal thoracic lesions. *Semin. Pediatr. Surg.*, **2**, 103–8

33. Nicolaides, K. H., Blott, A. J. and Greenough, A. (1987). Chronic drainage of fetal pulmonary cyst. *Lancet*, **2**, 618

34. Bale, P. M. (1984). Sacrococcygeal developmental abnormalities and tumors in children. *Perspect. Pediatr. Pathol.*, **1**, 9–56

35. Flake, A. W., Harrison, M. R., Adzick, N. S., Laberge, J. M. and Warsof, S. L. (1986). Fetal sacrococcygeal teratoma. *J. Pediatr. Surg.*, **21**, 563–6

36. Nisula, B. C. and Taliadouros, G. S. (1980). Thyroid function in gestational trophoblastic neoplasia: evidence that thyrotropic activity of chorionic gonadotropin mediates the thyrotoxicosis of choriocarcinoma. *Am. J. Obstet. Gynecol.*, **138**, 77–85

37. Langer, J. C., Harrison, M. R., Schmidt, K. G., Silverman, N. H., Anderson, R. L., Goldberg, J. D., Filly, R. A., Crombleholme, T. M., Longaker, M. T. and Golbus, M. S. (1989). Fetal hydrops and death from sacrococcygeal teratoma: rationale for fetal surgery. *Am. J. Obstet. Gynecol.*, **160**, 1145–50

38. Nicolaides, K. H., Cheng, H. H., Snijders, R. J. M. and Moniz, C. F. (1992). Fetal urine biochemistry in the assessment of obstructive uropathy. *Am. J. Obstet. Gynecol.*, **166**, 932–7

39. Johnson, M. P., Bukowski, T. P., Reitleman, C., Isada, N. B., Pryde, P. G. and Eraus, M. I. (1994). *In utero* surgical treatment of fetal obstructive uropathy: a new comprehensive approach to identify appropriate candidates for vesicoamniotic shunt therapy. *Am. J. Obstet. Gynecol.*, **170**, 1770–9

40. Manning, F. A., Harrison, M. R. and Rodeck, C. H. (1986). Special report: catheter shunts for fetal hydronephrosis and hydrocephalus. *N. Engl. J. Med.*, **315**, 336–40

41. MacMahan, R. A., Renou, P. M., Shekelton, P. A. and Paterson, R. J. (1991). *In utero* cystostomy. *Lancet*, **340**, 1234

42. Crombleholme, T. M., Harrison, M. R., Langer, J. C. and Adzick, N. S. (1988). Early experience with open fetal surgery for congenital hydronephrosis. *J. Pediatr. Surg.*, **23**, 1114–21

43. Clark, J. (1990). The challenge of bone marrow transplantation. *Mayo Clin. Proc.*, **65**, 111–14

44. Parkman, R. (1986). The application of bone marrow transplantation to the treatment of genetic diseases. *Science*, **232**, 1373–8

45. Flake, A. W., Harrison, M. R., Adzick, M. S. and Zanjani, E. D. (1986). Transplantation of fetal hematopoietic stem cells *in utero*: the creation of hematopoietic chimeras. *Science*, **233**, 776–8

46. Harrison, M. R., Slotnick, R. N., Crombleholme, T. M., Golbus, M. S., Tarantal, A. F. and Zanjani, E. D. (1989). *In utero* transplantation of fetal liver hematopoietic stem cells in monkeys. *Lancet*, **2**, 1425–7

47. Cowan, M. J. and Golbus, M. S. (1994). *In utero* hematopoietic stem cell transplants for inherited diseases. *Am. J. Pediatr. Hem. Oncol.*, **16**, 35–42

48. Hedrick, M. H., Rice, H. E., Sacks, D. H., Zanjani, E. D. and Flake, A. W. (1993). Creation of pig–sheep xenogeneic hematopoietic stem cells. *Transplant Sci.*, **3**, 23–6

49. Porreco, R. P., Barton, S. M. and Havercamp, A. D. (1991). Occlusion of umbilical artery in acardiac, acephalic twin. *Lancet*, **337**, 326–7

50. DeLia, J. E., Cruikshank, D. P. and Keye, W. R. (1990). YAG laser occlusion of placental vessels in severe twin–twin transfusion syndrome. *Obstet. Gynecol.*, **75**, 1046–53

51. Fries, M. H., Goldberg, J. D. and Golbus, M. S. (1991). Treatment of acardius–acephalus twin gestations by hysterotomy and selective delivery. *Obstet. Gynecol.*, **79**, 601–4

52. Meuli, M., Meuli-Simmen, C., Yingling, C. D., Hoffman, K. B., Harrison, M. R. and Adzick, N. S. (1995). A new model of myelomeningocele: studies in fetal lambs. *J. Pediatr. Surg.*, **30**, 1034–7

53. Meuli, M., Meuli-Simmen, C., Hutchins, G. M., Yingling, C. D., McBiles-Hoffman, K., Harrison, M. R. and Adzick, N. S. (1995). *In utero* surgery rescues neurological function at birth in sheep with spina bifida. *Nature Med.*, **1**, 342–7

54. Ferguson, M. W. and Howarth, G. F. (1992). Marsupial models of scarless fetal wound healing. In Adzick, N. S. and Longaker, M. T. (eds.) *Fetal Wound Healing*, pp. 95–124. (New York: Elsevier)

55. Whitby, D. J. and Ferguson, M. W. J. (1992). Immunohistochemical studies of the extracellular matrix and soluble growth factors in fetal and adult wound healing. In Adzick, N. S. and Longaker, M. T. (eds.) *Fetal Wound Healing*, pp. 161–75. (New York: Elsevier)

56. Stern, M. G., Longaker, M. T. and Stern, R. (1992). Hyaluronic acid and its modulation in fetal and adult wounds. In Adzick, N. S. and Longaker, M. T. (eds.) *Fetal Wound Healing*, pp. 189–98. (New York: Elsevier)

57. Duncan, B. W., Adzick, N. S., Bradley, S. M., Longaker, M. T., Crombleholme, T. M., Levinsohn, D. G., Moelleken, B. R., Chua, J., Harrison, M. R. and Kaban, L. B. (1989). An *in utero* model of craniosynostosis. *Surg. Forum*, **40**, 608–9

58. Longaker, M. T, Stern, M., Lorenz, H. P., Whitby, D. J., Harrison, M. R., Adzick, N. S. and

Kaban, L. B. (1992). A model for fetal cleft lip repair in lambs. *Plast. Reconstr. Surg.*, **90**, 950–4

59. Allan, L. D., Maxwell, D. and Tynan, M. (1991). Progressive obstructive lesions of the heart – an opportunity for fetal therapy. *Fetal Ther.*, **6**, 173–7

60. Hanley, F. L. (1994). Fetal cardiac surgery. *Adv. Cardiac. Surg.*, **5**, 47–74

61. Lorenz, H. P., Longaker, M. T. and Perchoka, L. A. (1992). Scarless wound repair: a human fetal skin model. *Development*, **114**, 253–9

62. Estes, J. M., Adzick, N. S. and Harrison, M. R. (1994). *Fetoscopic surgery*. In Holcomb, G. W. (ed.) *Pediatric Endoscopic Surgery*, pp. 155–62. (Norwalk, CT: Appleton & Lange)

63. Flake, A. W. and Harrison, M. R. (1995). Fetal Surgery. *Annu. Rev.*, **46**, 67–78

64. Adzick, N. S., Harrison, M. R. and Flake, A. W. (1993). Fetal surgery for cystic adenomatoid malformation of the lung. *J. Pediatr. Surg.*, **28**, 806–12

65. Flake, A. W. (1993). Fetal sacrococcygeal teratoma. *Semin. Pediatr. Surg.*, **2**, 113–20

66. Crombleholme, T. M., Harrison, M. R., Longaker, M. T. and Langer, J. C. (1988). Prenatal diagnosis and management of bilateral hydronephrosis. *Pediatr. Nephr.*, **2**, 334–42

67. Glick, P. L., Harrison, M. R., Golbus, M. S., Adzick, N. S., Filly, R. A. and Callen, P. W. (1985). Management of the fetus with congenital hydronephrosis. II. Prognostic criteria and selection for treatment. *J. Pediatr. Surg.*, **20**, 376–87

Endoscopic laser coagulation in the management of severe twin–twin transfusion syndrome

20

N. J. Sebire, J. Hyett, Y. Ville and K. H. Nicolaides

INTRODUCTION

In monozygotic twin pregnancies embryonic splitting within 3 days of fertilization, which occurs in approximately one-third of cases, results in two separate fetuses with independent placental circulations[1,2]. Splitting after the third day of fertilization is associated with vascular communications between the placentas; when cleavage is delayed beyond day 12 the fetuses are conjoint. In some monochorionic twin pregnancies imbalance in the net flow of blood across the placental vascular communications from one fetus, the donor, to the other, the recipient, results in twin–twin transfusion syndrome (TTTS).

PATHOPHYSIOLOGY OF TWIN–TWIN TRANSFUSION SYNDROME

The phenomenon of a shared circulation between monochorionic twins was first described by Schatz[3] in 1875. Although anastomoses of arteries and veins are present in almost all monochorionic placentas, it is the arteriovenous anastomoses which are responsible for TTTS. The anatomical studies of Bernischke and Kim[1] demonstrated that arteriovenous anastomoses are deep in the placenta but almost always proceed through the cotyledonary capillary bed. Schatz[3] showed that this third circulation was usually accompanied by another arteriovenous anastomosis in the opposite direction, which tended to balance the flow and minimize hemodynamic shifts. Mild, moderate or severe TTTS may develop depending on the net flow between these anastomoses which are common, variable in size, number and direction[1].

The precise underlying mechanisms by which a select population of those monochorionic pregnancies with vascular communications go on to develop TTTS is not fully understood. However, it has been hypothesized that primary maldevelopment of the placenta of the donor twin may cause increased peripheral resistance in the placental circulation which promotes shunting of blood to the recipient; the donor therefore suffers from both hypovolemia due to blood loss and hypoxia due to placental insufficiency[4,5]. The recipient fetus compensates for its expanded blood volume with polyuria[6] but since protein and cellular components remain in its circulation the consequent increase in colloid oncotic pressure draws water from the maternal compartment across the placenta. A vicious cycle of hypervolemia, polyuria, hyperosmolality is established leading to high-output heart failure and polyhydramnios.

Studies examining fetal blood obtained by cordocentesis in pregnancies with severe TTTS have reported large intertwin differences in plasma albumin and total protein concentrations[7,8] but no consistent differences in hemoglobin concentration between donor and recipient fetuses[5,7–9].

Fries and colleagues[10] have noted that in monochorionic diamniotic twins the prevalence of velamentous cord insertion was much higher in those with than without TTTS (64% and 19%, respectively); they suggested that the membranously inserted cord can be easily compressed reducing blood flow to one twin and this may also contribute to the pathogenesis of the syndrome.

DIAGNOSIS OF TWIN–TWIN TRANSFUSION SYNDROME

Traditionally, the diagnosis of TTTS was made retrospectively, in the neonatal period, on the basis of an intertwin difference in birth weight of 20% or more and hemoglobin concentration of 5 g/dl or more[11–13]. These observations were made in live births and therefore the criteria may only apply to relatively mild TTTS, since severe cases result in miscarriage or stillbirth. Additionally, large intertwin differences, in hemoglobin and birth weight are found in some dichorionic twin pregnancies and are not pathognomonic of TTTS[14].

Severe disease often becomes apparent in the early second trimester of pregnancy, with the mother complaining of a sudden increase in abdominal girth associated with extreme discomfort, and occasionally respiratory distress. On examination, there is tense polyhydramnios, which is pathognomonic of TTTS when observed at this early gestation. In such cases ultrasound examination will reveal a twin pregnancy with the polyhydramnios/anhydramnios sequence. There may be discordance in the size of the fetuses. However, the pathognomonic features of severe TTTS are the presence of a large bladder in the polyuric recipient fetus in the polyhydramniotic sac and 'absent' bladder in the anuric donor that is found 'stuck' and immobile at an edge of the placenta or the uterine wall where it is held fixed by the collapsed membranes of the anhydramniotic sac (Figure 1).

These features can occasionally lead to the mistaken diagnosis of bilateral renal agenesis or obstructive uropathy in a twin pregnancy where one of the fetuses is abnormal. Another relatively common mistake is that the pregnancy is monoamniotic because the collapsed intertwin membrane is not visualized, being closely wrapped around the donor fetus.

Other sonographic findings that may prove to be of prognostic significance include the presence of a hypertrophic, dilated and dyskinetic

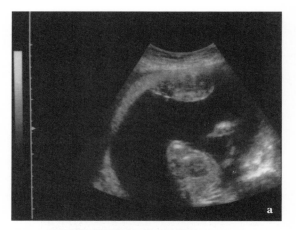

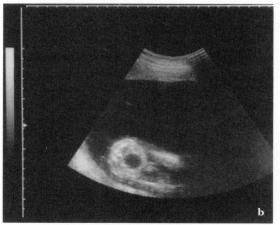

Figure 1 *Ultrasound images demonstrating the features of twin–twin transfusion syndrome. (a) Is the 'stuck' donor fetus in its anhydramniotic sac with no visible bladder, whilst (b) is the recipient fetus, with polyhydramnios and a large bladder visible*

heart in the recipient fetus, whilst in the donor, the heart may be dilated and the bowel hyperechogenic; these fetuses are manifestations of hypoxia and are commonly seen in hypoxemic fetuses from pregnancies complicated by severe uteroplacental insufficiency. The donor fetus may also demonstrate ventriculomegaly and/or microcephaly.

Color Doppler studies in severe TTTS presenting with acute polyhydramnios during the second trimester of pregnancy have demonstrated the presence of several superficial vessels connecting the two circulations[15]. Additionally, the umbilical artery pulsatility index (PI) has been reported to be increased in both donor and recipient fetuses; the former may be the consequence of abnormal placental development and the latter may be the result of polyhydramnios-related compression[16].

Doppler findings in the circulation of the donor fetus (decreased blood flow velocity in both the thoracic aorta and middle cerebral artery) suggest that this fetus is compromised by severe uteroplacental insufficiency but with the additional disadvantage imposed by chronic hemorrhage and hypovolemia[16]. In the recipient fetus, there may be decreased PI in the middle cerebral artery and decreased velocity in the aorta, which may be the consequence of hypervolemia-related congestive heart failure, which worsens with advancing gestation.

Although Doppler abnormalities have been described in TTTS, at present the use of these investigations is generally limited, because they are neither useful in the diagnosis of TTTS nor do they appear to provide useful prediction of prognosis.

LASER COAGULATION OF THE COMMUNICATING PLACENTAL VESSELS

Technique

The method of choice for treating severe TTTS is endoscopic Nd : YAG laser coagulation of the placental blood vessels that connect the circulations of the two fetuses. De Lia and co-workers[17] described a technique involving general or regional anesthesia and the endoscope was introduced into the uterus after laparotomy, hysterotomy and the insertion of a purse-string suture to control bleeding and amniotic fluid leakage. This was attempted in 30 twin pregnancies and successful laser coagulation was achieved in 26; 18 of the pregnancies resulted in delivery of at least one live baby[18]. However, despite the advantages of this approach the technique has not gained widespread application, presumably because of its invasive nature.

Recently, Ville and associates[19,20] reported a sonoendoscopic technique performed under local anesthesia for successful separation of

chorioangiopagus twins. Detailed ultrasound examination, including color flow mapping, is first performed to localize the placenta, the intertwin amniotic membrane, the placental insertion of the umbilical cords and the communicating blood vessels on the chorionic plate[19]. The appropriate site of entry on the maternal abdomen is chosen to avoid injury to the placenta or fetuses and to allow access to the suspected area of vascular communications.

Under continuous ultrasound visualization, a rigid 2-mm diameter fetoscope (field of vision 75°) housed in a 2.7-mm diameter cannula (KeyMed, Southend, UK) is introduced transabdominally into the amniotic cavity of the recipient twin. A 400-μm diameter Nd : YAG laser fiber (MBB, Munich, Germany) is then passed down the side-arm of the cannula to 1 cm beyond the tip of the fetoscope. A combination of ultrasonographic and direct vision is used to examine systematically the chorionic plate along the whole length of the intertwin membrane and identify the crossing vessels, which are coagulated by the administration of a total of 1000–4500 J delivered by 3-second shots using an output of 30–50 W at a distance of 1 cm[19]. Subsequently, amniotic fluid is drained through the fetoscope cannula over a period of 10–15 min to obtain subjective normalization of the amniotic fluid volume on ultrasonographic examination. The total procedure usually takes 30–45 min to complete.

Rationale/advantages

The aim of systematic coagulation of all superficial placental vessels that cross or are adjacent to the intertwin membrane is to interrupt the vascular communications between the circulations of the two fetuses. Arteriovenous anastomoses (which are thought to play the major role in the hemodynamic disturbance underlying fetofetal transfusion) are found deep in common cotyledons but their afferent and efferent branches are superficial[1]. Although the intertwin membrane does not necessarily overlie these common cotyledons[21], coagulation of all crossing vessels will inevitably include the afferent and efferent branches of these anastomoses.

Laser coagulation of communicating vessels potentially avoids many of the complications associated with severe TTTS treated by other means. Cerebral palsy with periventricular leukomalacia is a well-recognised complication of monochorionic twin pregnancies and is usually attributed to vascular accidents following the intrauterine death of one of the fetuses[22-25]. This complication is commonly seen in survivors after amniodrainage or other methods of treatment. Suggested mechanisms include a severe hypotensive episode due to hemorrhage from the survivor into the placenta of the dead fetus or disseminated intravascular coagulation after the release of thromboplastin from the dead twin. Laser coagulation of communicating vessels should potentially avoid these complications. However, brain damage observed in association with TTTS does not occur only when one of the fetuses dies and in some cases it may be the consequence of intrauterine ischemic-hypoxic brain injury; in the donor fetus hypoxia may be the consequence of hypovolemia and uteroplacental insufficiency, whereas in the recipient hypoxia may be due to increased blood viscosity and hypervolemia-related congestive heart failure.

Results from the Harris Birthright Centre

Endoscopic laser coagulation was performed at the Harris Birthright Centre on a total of 96 pregnancies; 74 are now completed and 22 are continuing. Good visualization of the intertwin membrane and coagulation of the crossing vessels was achieved in all cases at the first procedure but more difficulty was experienced with those cases where the placentas were anterior. In one case laser coagulation was performed at 17 weeks but this was repeated at 22 weeks because there was recurrence of TTTS.

In the 74 completed pregnancies, there were 53 (72%) with at least one survivor and the total number of babies that survived was 80 of 148 (54%). In 27 pregnancies both babies were born alive, in 26 one baby was born alive and in 21 there were no survivors. The gestation at laser coagulation and at delivery of each case are illustrated in Figure 2. There was no significant difference between the three outcome groups in gestation at presentation, intertwin

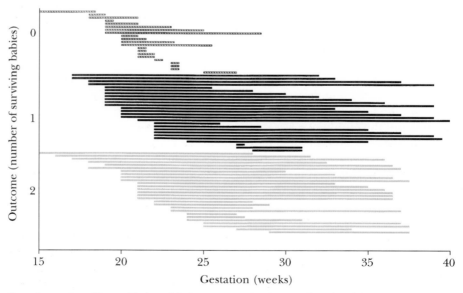

Figure 2 *Gestation at time of laser ablation of the intercommunicating vessels and at delivery in pregnancies complicated by twin–twin transfusion syndrome at the Harris Birthright Centre. The three shades of bar represent the outcome groups; cases where both babies died (top), where one baby survived (middle) and where both babies survived (bottom)*

difference in estimated fetal weight, or degree of polyhydramnios both in terms of deepest vertical pool of amniotic fluid and the volume of amniotic fluid that was drained at fetoscopy, or the incidence of anterior placentas.

In three cases the donor fetus had ventriculomegaly at presentation and selective fetocide was performed after laser coagulation at 20, 21 and 23 weeks, respectively; in the first two cases there was spontaneous abortion one week later but in the third a normal baby was delivered at 40 weeks. There were another 19 pregnancies with no survivors. In 11 pregnancies both fetuses died *in utero*; in six death occurred within 24 h of laser coagulation and in five cases 2–5 weeks after an apparently successful procedure. In eight other cases the patients presented with vaginal bleeding and contractions; in five there was spontaneous miscarriage of both twins whilst in three the donor fetus had died within 24 h of laser coagulation and although the recipient was alive spontaneous abortion occurred 1–6 weeks later. In two of these cases the amniotic fluid at the time of fetoscopy was black from a previous intra-amniotic hemorrhage and exchange with Hartmans solution was performed before the communicating placental vessels could be visualized for coagulation.

In one of the pregnancies where both babies survived, the donor fetus was noted to have progressive microcephaly and the parents were offered the option of selective fetocide but declined; this child now at 9 months of age has cerebral palsy. All other survivors are developing normally. In the group with one survivor, death of the donor (20 of the 26 pregnancies) usually occurred either within 24 h of the procedure or a few weeks later due to progressive intrauterine growth retardation (IUGR). In the cases where the recipient died (six of the 26 pregnancies) the fetuses were hydropic at presentation. In this group, one of the donor fetuses was noted to have ventriculomegaly, and after delivery at 34 weeks obstructive hydrocephalus was diagnosed. This was successfully treated by ventriculoperitoneal shunting and the child who is now 21 months old is developing normally.

In TTTS the donor fetus may not only be subjected to chronic hemorrhage and hypovolemia but also to severe placental insufficiency[4,5]. In monochorionic twin pregnancies there are many vascular communications between the circulations of the two fetuses and although the donor suffers an overall loss of blood this fetus might be dependent for oxygenation on blood from the recipient. It could be postulated that laser coagulation of all communicating vessels deprived the donor from this source of oxygen and hastened its death. Alternatively, coagulation of all placental vessels that cross the intertwin membrane may have interrupted the vascular supply to more than the common cotyledons destroying whatever little reserve previously existed in an already compromised placenta. The extent to which we will be able to restrict coagulation to the common cotyledons and the potential increase in survival without increasing handicap remains to be determined.

ALTERNATIVE METHODS OF MANAGING SEVERE TWIN–TWIN TRANSFUSION

Expectant management

In twin pregnancies with presumed TTTS development of acute polyhydramnios at less than 28 weeks of gestation is associated with a high perinatal mortality rate, primarily because of spontaneous abortion or very preterm delivery of growth-retarded babies or babies with hydrops. Saunders and colleagues[5] reviewed 53 such pregnancies in the literature before 1992 and the fetal survival rate was only 5%.

In the few babies that survive with expectant management there is a high incidence of morbidity. Brain damage may occur due to a combination of factors including intrauterine hypoxia and preterm delivery[5,26]. In addition, death of one fetus, usually the donor, may be associated with subsequent death or hypoxic/ischemic sequelae in the co-twin[22–25,27,28].

Medical therapy

Indomethacin has been used in an attempt to prevent the onset of preterm delivery both through its tocolytic properties and by its action in reducing fetal urine production and therefore polyhydramnios. In a study reporting the administration of indomethacin in three pregnancies with TTTS presenting with polyhydramnios at 20–25 weeks of gestation one patient delivered at 25 weeks and both babies died[29]. In each of the other two pregnancies one fetus died within 4 days of the onset of treatment; the pregnancies continued to 30 and 36 weeks, respectively, and the two babies survived but one of the neonates had multicystic encephalomalacia.

Selective fetocide

The poor prognosis of untreated TTTS, particularly when one of the fetuses is severely compromised, has led various groups to consider selective fetocide as a method of treatment. The rationale behind this approach is to interrupt TTTS and maximize the chances of survival of one of the fetuses mainly by potentially reducing the chance of severe preterm delivery.

Several techniques have been described including surgical removal of one fetus by hysterotomy[30], ultrasound-guided pericardial injection of saline to achieve cardiac tamponade or the intracardiac injection of potassium chloride[7,25,31–34], ultrasound-guided insertion of thrombogenic coils or fibrin into the heart or the umbilical vein of one of the fetuses[35,36], and ultrasound-guided ligation of one umbilical cord[37].

In 15 pregnancies that were managed by selective fetocide at 20–26 weeks of gestation there were eight survivors (27% of the total).

Serial amniodrainage

An 18-gauge needle is introduced into the uterus under ultrasound guidance. The amniotic fluid is allowed to drain freely into a sterile bag through a plastic tube attached to the hub of the needle over a period of 40–120 min until there is subjective normalization of amniotic fluid volume on ultrasonographic examination. Patients are assessed every week and further amniodrainage is indicated with recurrence of polyhydramnios.

This treatment presumably prevents the polyhydramnios-mediated risk of spontaneous abortion or very premature delivery[5,38–40]. It is also possible that with advancing gestation and increasing fetoplacental blood volume the relative significance of the hemodynamic effects of placental anastomoses is reduced. In this respect repeated amniocenteses may, at least in some cases allow the fetal cardiovascular system to outgrow the deleterious effect of placental anastomoses[5,6]. In addition, amniodrainage reduces amniotic fluid pressure and may relieve the compression of the membranously inserted cord or superficial vessels which could improve blood flow in the donor fetus[10].

In studies published before 1992 amniodrainage was associated with survival in 30–40% of the cases[5]. However, five recent papers from three centers have reported survivals of 72–83% of fetuses and the number of pregnancies with at least one survivor was 81–100%[38–42]. One of these series examined 37 pregnancies with the stuck-twin syndrome, including dichorionic pregnancies where the discordancy in amniotic fluid volume could be attributed to fetal or placental abnormalities rather than TTTS[42]. Five pregnancies were terminated, five were managed conservatively with 40% fetal survival, and 27 were treated with serial amniocenteses with 72% fetal survival; 36% of survivors had cerebral palsy. In the second series of nine pregnancies that were managed with serial amniocenteses the fetal survival was 83%, but 53% had neonatal morbidity; another four pregnancies were managed conservatively because the disease was apparently milder and in this group fetal survival was 75%[40]. In the third series the survival rate in five pregnancies managed conservatively was 0%, and in the 17 pregnancies treated with amniocenteses fetal survival was 79%; no data were provided on follow up[38,41].

The marked improvement in survival with serial amniodrainage, or even with conservative management in two of the series, compared to

Table 1 *Comparison of features at presentation and delivery of pregnancies with twin–twin transfusion syndrome which had antenatal intervention, either by serial amniodrainage or by laser coagulation of the communicating placental circulation*

Feature	Amniodrainage ($n = 25$)	Laser coagulation ($n = 74$)
Gestation at presentation (weeks)	2 (17–26)	21 (15–29)
Intertwin weight difference (% of recipient)	32 (15–56)	30 (5–71)
Amniotic fluid depth (cm)	13 (10–16)	13 (8–20)
Initial amniodrainage (ml)	2850 (600–6700)	2500 (400–6500)
Babies surviving* (%)	32%	52%
Interval to delivery* (weeks)	6 (0–18)	13 (0–21)
Gestation at delivery in livebirths (weeks)*	31 (26–37)	34 (25–40)
Birthweight in livebirths (g)*	1550 (700–2900)	1960 (550–4250)
Prevalence of cerebral palsy*	4 (25%)	1 (1.3%)

*Statistical difference demonstrated by Mann–Whitney test, $p < 0.05$

previous studies that apparently used the same treatment protocols, presumably reflect differences in the severity of the disease. Nevertheless, it is universally acknowledged that a very high proportion of survivors suffer chronic handicap and presumably a high proportion of parents that are counselled as to this risk may choose to have their pregnancies terminated rather than treated with amniocenteses.

COMPARISON OF LASER COAGULATION AND SERIAL AMNIOCENTESES

Comparison of survival and handicap following these techniques may ultimately require a randomized study. In the meantime it is possible to draw some conclusions from the data in our center because the same entry criteria were used.

Serial amniocenteses was the treatment of choice during 1988–1992. We used this treatment in 25 monochorionic twin pregnancies with acute polyhydramnios at less than 28 weeks of gestation. The total number of babies that survived was 16 of 50 (32%) and the number of pregnancies with at least one survivor was 11 of 25 (44%). Four (25%) of the survivors had cerebral palsy and brain scans demonstrated lesions compatible with intrauterine hypoxia/ischemia. Although this survival rate was higher than that reported in the literature with expectant management, the very high level of handicap in survivors prompted us to seek alternative therapeutic option and since 1992 endoscopic laser coagulation has been used.

The amniodrainage and laser coagulation groups are compared in Table 1. At presentation there were no significant differences between the groups in gestation, intertwin differences in estimated fetal weight or degree of polyhydramnios both in terms of the deepest vertical pool of amniotic fluid and the volume of amniotic fluid that was drained at the first procedure.

The data suggest that laser coagulation is associated with higher survival, with increased interval between presentation and delivery, later gestation at delivery and higher birth weight. Furthermore, there is a substantially lower risk of cerebral palsy than that seen following treatment with serial amniodrainage.

References

1. Benirschke, K. and Kim, C. K. (1973). Multiple pregnancy. *N. Engl. J. Med.*, **228**, 1276–84

2. Hrubec, Z. and Robinette, D. (1984). The study of human twins in medical research. *N. Engl. J. Med.*, **310**, 435–41

3. Schatz, F. (1882). Eine besondere Art von einseitiger Polyhydramnie mit anderseitiger Oligohydramnie bei eineiigen Zwillingen. *Arch. Gynakol.*, **19**, 329

4. Saunders, N. J., Snijders, R. J. M. and Nicolaides, K. H. (1991). Twin–twin transfusion syndrome in the second trimester is associated with small inter-twin hemoglobin differences. *Fetal Diagn. Ther.*, **6**, 34–6

5. Saunders, N. J., Snijders, R. J. M. and Nicolaides, K. H. (1992). Therapeutic amniocentesis in twin–twin transfusion syndrome appearing in the second trimester of pregnancy. *Am. J. Obstet. Gynecol.*, **166**, 820–24

6. Rosen, D., Rabinowitz, R., Beyth, Y., Feijgin, M. D. and Nicolaides, K. H. (1990). Fetal urine production in normal twins and in twins with acute polyhydramnios. *Fetal Diagn. Ther.*, **5**, 57–60

7. Weiner, C. P. and Ludomirski, A. (1994). Diagnosis, pathophysiology, and treatment of chronic twin to twin transfusion syndrome. *Fetal Diagn. Ther.*, **9**, 283–90

8. Berry, S. M., Puder, K. S., Bottoms, S. F., Uckele, J. E., Romero, R. and Cotton, D. B. (1995). Comparison of intrauterine hematologic and biochemical values between twin pairs with and without stuck twin syndrome. *Am. J. Obstet. Gynecol.*, **172**, 1403–10

9. Fisk, N. M., Borrell, A., Hubinont, C., Tannirandorn, Y., Nicolini, U. and Rodeck, C. H. (1990). Fetofetal transfusion syndrome: do the neonatal criteria apply *in utero*? *Arch. Dis. Child.*, **65**, 657–61

10. Fries, M. H., Goldstein, R. B., Kilpatrick, S. J., Golbus, M. S., Callen, P. W. and Filly, R. A. (1993). The role of velamentous cord insertion in the etiology of twin–twin transfusion syndrome. *Obstet. Gynecol.*, **81**, 569–74

11. Rausen, A. R., Seki, M. and Strauss, L. (1965). Twin transfusion syndrome. *J. Pediatr.*, **66**, 613–28

12. Abraham, J. M. (1969). Character of placentation in twins, as related to hemoglobin levels. *Clin. Pediatr. Phila.*, **8**, 526–30

13. Tan, K. L., Tan, R., Tan, S. H. and Tan, A. M. (1979). The twin transfusion syndrome. Clinical observations on 35 affected pairs. *Clin. Pediatr. Phila.*, **18**, 111–14

14. Danskin, F. H. and Neilson, J. P. (1989). Twin-to-twin transfusion syndrome: what are appropriate diagnostic criteria? *Am. J. Obstet. Gynecol.*, **161**, 365–9

15. Hecher, K., Ville, Y. and Nicolaides, K. H. (1995). Doppler studies of the fetal circulation in twin–twin transfusion syndrome. *Ultrasound Obstet. Gynecol.*, **5**, 318–24

16. Hecher, K., Ville, Y. and Nicolaides, K. H. (1995). Color Doppler ultrasound in the identification of communicating vessels in twin to twin transfusion syndrome and acardiac twins. *J. Ultrasound Med.*, **14**, 37–40

17. De Lia, J. E., Cruikshank, D. P. and Keye, W. R. (1990). Fetoscopic neodymium : YAG laser occlusion of placental vessels in severe twin–twin transfusion syndrome. *Obstet. Gynecol.*, **75**, 1046–53

18. De Lia, J. E., Kuhlmann, R. S., Harstad, T. W. and Cruikshank, D. P. (1995). Fetoscopic laser ablation of placental vessels in severe previable twin–twin transfusion syndrome. *Am. J. Obstet. Gynecol.*, **172**, 1202–11

19. Ville, Y., Hecher, K., Ogg, D., Warren, R. and Nicolaides, K. (1992). Successful outcome after Nd : YAG laser separation of chorioangiopagus-twins under sonoendoscopic control. *Ultrasound Obstet. Gynecol.*, **2**, 429–31

20. Ville, Y., Hyett, J., Hecher, K. and Nicolaides, K. (1995). Preliminary experience with endoscopic laser surgery for severe twin twin transfusion syndrome. *N. Engl. J. Med.*, **332**, 224–27

21. De Lia, J. E., Kuhlmaa, R. S., Cruikshank, D. P. and O'Bee, L. R. (1993). Placental surgery: a new frontier. *Placenta*, **14**, 477–85

22. Bendon, R. W. and Siddiqi, T. (1989). Acute twin to twin *in utero* transfusion. *Pediatr. Pathol.*, **9**, 951–58

23. Bejar, R., Vigliocco, G., Gramajo, H., Solana, C., Benirschke, K., Berry, C., Coen, R. and Resnick, R. (1990). Antenatal origin of neurologic damage in newborn infants. II. Multiple gestations. *Am. J. Obstet. Gynecol.*, **162**, 1230–36

24. Fusi, L., MacOharland, P., Fisk, N., Nicolini, U. and Wigglesworth, J. (1991). Acute twin–twin transfusion: a possible mechanism for brain damaged survivors after intrauterine death of a monozygotic twin. *Obstet. Gynecol.*, **78**, 517–22

25. Mahone, P. R., Sherer, D. M., Abramowicz, J. S. and Woods, J. R. (1993). Twin–twin transfusion syndrome: rapid development of severe hydrops of the donor following selective feticide of the hydropic recipient. *Am. J. Obstet. Gynecol.*, **169**, 166–68

26. Larroche, J. C., Droulle, P., Delezoide, A. L., Narcy, F. and Nessmann, C. (1990). Brain damage in monozygous twins. *Biol. Neonate*, **57**, 261–78

27. Sherer, D. M., Abramowicz, J. S., Jaffe, R., Smith, S. A., Metlay, L. A. and Woods, J. R. (1993). Twin–twin transfusion with abrupt onset of microcephaly in the surviving recipient following spontaneous death of the donor twin. *Am. J. Obstet. Gynecol.*, **169**, 85–8

28. Margono, F., Feinkind, L. and Minkoff, H. L. (1992). Foot necrosis in a surviving fetus associated with twin–twin transfusion syndrome and monochorionic placenta. *Obstet. Gynecol.*, **79**, 867–69

29. Jones, J. M., Sbarra, A. J., Dililklo, L., Cetrulo, C. L. and D'Altan, M. E. (1993). Indomethacin in severe twin to twin transfusion syndrome. *Am. J. Perinatol.*, **10**, 24–6

30. Urig, M. A., Simpson, G. F., Elliott, J. P. and Clewell, W. H. (1988). Twin twin transfusion syndrome: the surgical removal of one twin as a treatment option. *Fetal Ther.*, **3**, 185–8

31. Wittmann, B. K., Farquharson, D. F., Thomas, W. D. S., Baldwin, V. J. and Wadsworth, L. D. (1986). The role of feticide in the management of severe twin transfusion syndrome. *Am. J. Obstet. Gynecol.*, **155**, 1023–26

32. Weiner, C. P. (1987). Diagnosis and treatment of twin to twin transfusion in the mid- second trimester of pregnancy. *Fetal Ther.*, **2**, 71–4

33. Chescheir, N. C. and Seeds, J. W. (1988). Polyhydramnios and oligohydramnios in twin gestations. *Obstet. Gynecol.*, **71**, 882–86

34. Donnenfield, A. E., Glazerman, L. R., Cutillo, D. M., Librizzi, R. J. and Weiner, S. (1989). Fetal exsanguination following intrauterine angiographic assessment and selective termination of a hydrocephalic, monozygotic co-twin. *Prenat. Diagn.*, **9**, 301–9

35. Bebbington, M. W., Wilson, R. D., Machan, L. and Wittmann, B. K. (1995). Selective fetocide in twin transfusion syndrome using ultrasound guided insertion of thrombogenic coils. *Fetal Diagn. Ther.*, **10**, 32–6

36. Dommergues, M., Mandelbrot, L., Delezoide, A. L., Aubry, M. C., Fermont, L., Caputo-Manko, D. and Dumez, Y. (1995). Twin-to-twin transfusion syndrome: selective fetocide by embolisation of the hydropic fetus. *Fetal Diagn. Ther.*, **10**, 26–31

37. Lemery, D. J., Vanilieferinghen, P., Gasq, M., Finkeltin, F., Beaufrere, A. M. and Beytout, M. (1994). Fetal umbilical cord ligation under ultrasound guidance. *Ultrasound Obstet. Gynecol.*, **4**, 339–401

38. Elliott, J. P., Urig, M. A. and Clewell, W. H. (1991). Aggressive therapeutic amniocentesis for treatment of twin–twin transfusion syndrome. *Obstet. Gynecol.*, **77**, 537–40

39. Reisner, D. P., Mahony, B. S., Petty, C. N., Nyberg, D. A., Porter, T. F., Zingheim, R. W., Williams, M. A. and Lutuy, D. A. (1993). Stuck twin syndrome: outcome in thirty-seven consecutive cases. *Am. J. Obstet. Gynecol.*, **169**, 991–95

40. Pinette, M. G., Pan, Y., Pinette, S. G. and Stubblefield, P. G. (1993). Treatment of twin–twin transfusion syndrome. *Obstet. Gynecol.*, **82**, 841–46

41. Urig, M. A., Clewell, W. H. and Elliott, J. P. (1990). Twin twin transfusion syndrome. *Am. J. Obstet. Gynecol.*, **163**, 1522–26

42. Mahony, B. S., Petty, C. N., Nyberg, D. A., Luthy, D. A., Hickok, D. E. and Hirsch, J. H. (1990). The stuck twin phenomenon: ultrasonographic findings, pregnancy outcome and management with serial amniocentesis. *Am. J. Obstet. Gynecol.*, **163**, 1513–22

Prenatal diagnosis and management of fetal tumors

21

V. D'Addario and V. De Salvia

Fetal tumors are rare congenital anomalies that can be located in different parts of the fetal body. As in the adults, fetal tumors may arise from any tissue and are consequently characterized by a variety of pathophysiological findings. The prenatal diagnosis of a fetal tumor has important implications for the fetal and neonatal, as well as the maternal, outcome. Such a diagnosis, however, can sometimes be difficult or incomplete, due to limitations in identifying the type and/or the site of the tumor, thus precluding optimal perinatal management. The most common types and sites of fetal tumors are listed in Tables 1 and 2.

This chapter summarizes the current knowledge on the prenatal diagnosis, natural history and perinatal management of the most common fetal tumors.

SACROCOCCYGEAL TERATOMA

Sacrococcygeal teratoma is one of the most common tumors in newborns, with a reported incidence of 1 in 35 000 to 1 in 40 000 live births[1]. It is thought to develop from totipotential cells in Hensen's node or in reproductive tract anlage[2]. A 'twinning accident', with incomplete separation during embryogenesis and abnormal development of one fetus, has also been suggested as a possible etiology of sacrococcygeal teratoma[3]. This hypothesis is supported by the fact that organoid elements are occasionally found in the tumor and by the family history of twinning in many of the patients affected.

The size of these tumors is extremely variable and an unpredictable growth can occur *in utero*. Tumors as large as 25 cm have been reported to obstruct labor[4]. As regards their location, sacro-

coccygeal teratoma may be entirely external, may have a partial intrapelvic extension or may be completely intrapelvic. According to their site, they have been divided by the American Academy of Pediatrics Surgical Section (AAPSS) into four types[5]:

(1) Type 1 tumors, predominantly exophytic;

(2) Type II tumors, mainly external but with a significant intrapelvic retroperitoneal extension;

(3) Type III tumors, apparently external but with the main part of the mass extending into the abdomen and displacing the abdominal structures; and

(4) Type IV tumors, presacral with no external presentation.

In the AAPSS survey of 405 cases, 46% were of type I, 36% of type II, 9% of type III and 10% of type IV.

Most sacrococcygeal teratomas are solid or mixed solid and cystic. Purely cystic forms are

Table 1 *Most common types of fetal tumor*

Cyst	Hamartoma
Teratoma	Neuroblastoma
Lymphangioma	Sarcoma
Hemangioma	Other

Table 2 *Most common sites of fetal tumors*

Sacrococcygeal
Cervical
Intracranial
Chest (lung, heart, mediastinum)
Abdominal (liver, kidneys, adrenals, spleen, mesentery, omentum, ovaries, uterus, retroperitoneal space)
Skin

rare. In about 80% of the cases they are histologically benign[6]. Malignancy is more common in males, in the solid and in the type III tumors. The malignant potential seems to increase with advancing delay in diagnosis. In the AAPSS survey the mortality rate was 7% in the cases diagnosed on the first day of life, and rose to 38% in the patients who underwent surgery at the age of 2 years and after[5]. Other important factors influencing the prognosis are the size and the morphological type of the tumor: large and mainly solid tumors carry a higher mortality rate, due to difficulty in resection and tumor hemorrhage[7,8]. These considerations emphasize the importance of the ultrasonographic prenatal diagnosis, which reveals the internal structure as well as the size and the intra-abdominal extension of the tumor.

The first report of prenatal ultrasound diagnosis of sacrococcygeal teratoma was published in 1979[9]. Since then several cases have been reported, all confirming the high accuracy of ultrasound in diagnosis of tumors[10–15]. The most common ultrasonic finding of a fetal sacrococcygeal teratoma is that of a mixed or predominantly solid mass located near the caudal spine of the fetus[10] (Figures 1 and 2). A mainly cystic appearance is rare[12]. Calcifications may be present. Color Doppler study can demonstrate their rich vascularization. Polyhydramnios is present in most cases of prenatally diagnosed sacrococcygeal teratomas, although the mechanism is not clear[10]. Fetal hydrops can be a further complication associated with large tumors; it is secondary to fetal heart failure, which can be due to two possible mechanisms: either severe fetal anemia secondary to tumor hemorrhage[16] or high cardiac output from arteriovenous shunting within the tumor[17]. Fetal hydrops is always an ominous finding.

The differential diagnosis of sacrococcygeal teratoma mainly includes meningomyeloceles: however, these anomalies are virtually never solid, do not contain calcifications and demonstrate the typical spinal defect. Other anomalies that can simulate a sacrococcygeal teratoma are lymphomas, retrorectal hamartomas, intracanalicular epidermoid tumors, neuroblastomas, hemangiomas, gliomas and many other

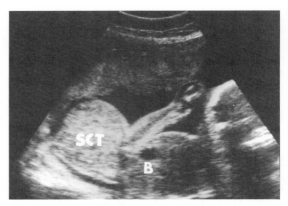

Figure 1 *Type I sacrococcygeal teratoma (SCT). The tumor is predominantly exophytic and solid*

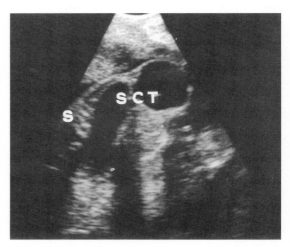

Figure 2 *Type II mainly cystic sacrococcygeal teratoma (SCT). The tumor is mainly external, but with a significant intrapelvic extension. S, Sacrum*

rare conditions (more than 50) that can occur with skin-covered lesions in the sacrococcygeal region[18].

Associated anomalies are reported in 11–38% of the cases[11,19,20]. Some of the local abnormalities, such as rectovaginal fistula and imperforate anus, are thought to be directly related to the tumor growth during fetal development[21]. Association with aneuploidies is extremely rare[19,22]. Biochemical markers such as α-fetoprotein and acetylcholinesterase are not useful in differential diagnosis of sacrococcygeal teratoma from other fetal caudal abnormalities.

The prognosis of sacrococcygeal teratoma is usually good after neonatal surgery; the only exceptions are represented by the rare cases of malignant teratomas and by the type III lesions, due to the cranial displacement of abdominal organs, sometimes even resulting in lung hypoplasia. The main complications that can occur in fetal sacrococcygeal teratomas are prematurity, fetal hydrops and tumor hemorrhage *in utero* or during delivery. Once the prenatal diagnosis is made, serial ultrasound examinations should be performed, in order to assess tumor growth, amniotic fluid volume and early evidence of fetal hydrops. Fetal renal and gastrointestinal functions should also be evaluated, since the tumor can cause compression of the urethra as well as of the bowel, causing hydronephrosis or intestinal tract obstruction[23].

The mode of delivery depends on the size of the tumor. Vaginal delivery may be possible with small tumors. However, since the main complication is represented by rupture or hemorrhage during delivery, Cesarean section is recommended to avoid hemorrhage or dystocia, especially in large tumors[10,24]. Prenatal ultrasonically guided aspiration of cystic sacrococcygeal teratomas can be performed in order to facilitate delivery[15,25,26]. Prenatal treatment may also include fetal digitalization in cases of hydrops developing before lung maturity has been achieved.

Fetal surgery has also been attempted. Langer and colleagues[27] operated on a 21-week hydropic fetus and found that the resection of the tumor resulted in the reversal of hydrops, but preterm labor, unfortunately, occurred after operation, with the delivery of a non-viable fetus. Flake[13] operated on a 26-week hydropic fetus, with subsequent resolution of the hydrops; preterm delivery resulted in a healthy neonate, who unfortunately died during a subsequent surgical procedure. *In utero* ligation of the main artery leading to the tumor has also been considered, to prevent tumor growth and subsequent development of hydrops before extrauterine viability of the child is possible[27]. The potential benefit of such prenatal surgery, however, must be balanced against the potential risks for the mother and the fetus.

Table 3 *Tumors of the neck*

Teratoma	Branchial cyst
Lymphangioma	Thyroglossal cyst
Hemangioma	Other

Delivery should be performed in a tertiary center, with neonatologists present and pediatric surgeons available for prompt surgical resection.

TUMORS OF THE NECK

Tumors of the fetal neck are mainly represented by cervical teratomas and other differentiated soft tissue masses, such as lymphangiomas and hemangiomas (Table 3).

Cervical teratomas are very rare tumors, composed of tissues foreign to a particular anatomic site, with all three germ layers represented. Sonographically, they appear as unilateral, asymmetric masses located in the lateral and anterior regions of the fetal neck. They usually extend to the mastoid process and to the mandible, displacing the ear. Extension into the oral vault and the mediastinum has also been reported. Their structure is usually that of a complex mass, with solid and cystic components (Figure 3); color Doppler can visualize their rich vascularization. Their size can be extremely variable: tumor masses greater than the fetal head have been reported[28-30]. Polyhydramnios is associated with 20–40% of cases, and is due to esophageal obstruction by the large cervical mass.

The differential diagnosis mainly includes cystic hygroma. This is the cervical mass most commonly diagnosed in the prenatal period. It is not a true tumor, but a developmental abnormality of the lymphatic system characterized by the lack of jugular lymph sac drainage into the jugular vein with consequent formation of a cystic structure located in the posterior aspect of the fetal neck; the cyst is typically flaccid and presents thin borders with thin septa. Cystic hygroma can be recognized early in the first trimester by using transvaginal sonography; association with hydrops, cardiac defects and chromosomal abnormalities (mainly Turner

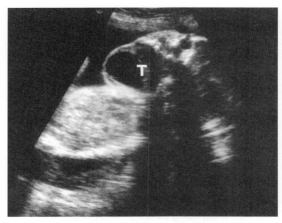

Figure 3 *Cervical teratoma (T), anterior mainly cystic*

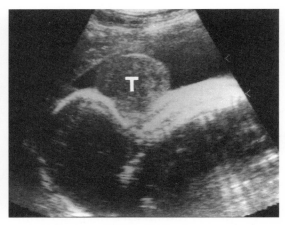

Figure 5 *Solid mass (T) on the posterior aspect of the fetal neck, proving to be a fibroid tumor*

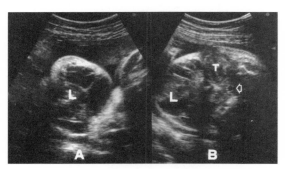

Figure 4 *Lateral cervical lymphangioma. A, parasagittal scan of the fetal neck, showing a huge complex mass with solid and cystic components; B, axial scan at the level of the fetal mouth; L, lymphangioma; T, tongue; arrow, pharynx*

Table 4 *Intracranial tumors*

Teratomas	Vascular tumors
Glial tumors	Cysts (intra/extra-axial)
Neuroblastic tumors	

cal teratoma represents an indication for Cesarean section to avoid malpresentation and dystocia caused by hyperextension of the neck and large tumor size. Since the tumor can obstruct the airway, the delivery should be planned in a tertiary care unit, where pediatric surgeons are ready for tracheal intubation and prompt intervention[34].

INTRACRANIAL TUMORS

Brain tumors are extremely rare congenital abnormalities, represented, in approximately 50% of the cases, by teratomas; glial tumors (glioblastomas, astroblastomas and spongioblastomas) are second in frequency (Table 4). Independently from their benign or malignant attitude, these tumors tend to have dramatic consequences for the developing fetal brain. Although such lesions may be small and potentially resectable at delivery, to date only large lesions have been detected prenatally[35–38].

Teratomas appear as irregularly shaped, mixed solid and cystic masses distorting the brain anatomy (Figure 6). When the cystic component is prevalent, the differential diagnosis

syndrome) has been reported in up to 90% of the cases[31].

Other conditions mimicking a cervical teratoma, whose differential diagnosis is not always possible, are sarcomas, hemangiomas, lymphangiomas (Figure 4), congenital goiter and, less frequently, branchial cysts, laryngoceles, thyroglossal cysts and other very rare conditions (Figure 5). Cervical teratomas should also be differentiated from epignathus, a teratoma arising from the oral cavity or pharynx, which is recognizable by its anterior location in respect to the fetal neck.

Although rare cases of malignancies have been reported[32,33], most cases of cervical teratomas in fetuses, infants and children are benign. The prenatal diagnosis of a large cervi-

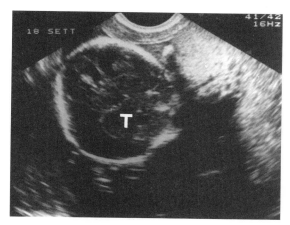

Figure 6 *Intracranial teratoma. The tumor (T) appears as a complex mass, displacing the cerebral hemispheres upward*

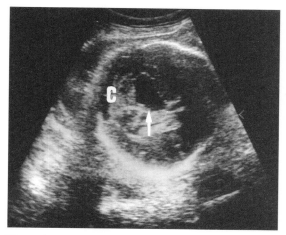

Figure 7 *Supratentorial arachnoid cyst (arrow). C, cerebellum*

The prognosis of the prenatally detected fetal brain tumor is ominous; in each of the reported cases, the baby has been stillborn or has died in the neonatal period.

Other cystic tumors that can be ultrasonically detected *in utero* are the arachnoid cysts. They may be supratentorial or retrocerebellar. The former may present a more variable appearance, due to the larger supratentorial compartment. They appear as cystic structures of variable size that do not cause brain maldevelopment (Figure 7), but cause pressure and a mass effect that may result in hydrocephalus[39]. For this reason the prognosis of arachnoid cysts is better than that of teratomas and glial tumors, if treated before irreversible brain damage occurs.

The differential diagnosis of arachnoid cysts includes porencephalic cysts, mainly cystic teratomas, interhemispheric cysts associated with agenesis of the corpus callosum, cysts of the corpus callosum and Galen vein aneurysm. Differently from arachnoid cysts, porencephalic cysts usually communicate with the lateral ventricle. Cystic teratomas usually present some amount of solid tissue associated with the cystic components. Interhemispheric cysts associated with agenesis of the corpus callosum usually communicate with the third ventricle, due to the absence of the callosal fibers. Corpus callosum cysts show the typical C-shaped appearance in sagittal section (Figure 8). Finally, Galen vein aneurysm is easily recognizable for the typical turbulent Doppler signal generated by the 'cystic' lesion.

Among the intracranial tumors, those arising from the choroid plexuses must also be considered. Choroid plexus papilloma is an extremely rare intracranial neoplasm, accounting for only 3% of all brain tumors found in children. It is generally a benign tumor arising mainly from the choroid plexuses located in the lateral ventricles. The tumor is usually associated with hydrocephalus, due to either an overproduction of cerebrospinal fluid, or to an obstruction to its flow. The prenatal diagnosis can be suspected when ultrasound demonstrates an echogenic mass located at the level of the atrium of one lateral ventricle in an hydrocephalic fetus[40]. The main postnatal complication of this benign

from an arachnoid cyst can be difficult. The only case of fetal glioblastoma reported in the literature presented as a diffusely hyperechoic mass with an appearance similar to that of a large hemorrhage[36]. The tumors are more commonly supratentorial, although a precise location is not possible in cases of huge masses. Hydrocephalus is commonly associated as a consequence of the ventricular obstruction by the mass. Macrocephaly can develop, due both to the size of the tumor mass and to the increasing ventriculomegaly, and can make vaginal delivery impossible even after cephalocentesis.

lesion is hemorrhage; for this reason, the choice of a Cesarean section may be offered in order to reduce the risk of birth trauma and consequent tumor bleeding.

Choroid plexus cysts are thought to originate from neuroepithelial folds within the choroid plexus that become filled with fluid and cellular debris. They cannot be considered true tumors, since they are found in approximately 1% of the fetuses at 16–24 weeks of gestation and, in more than 90% of the cases, they resolve by 26–28 weeks and are of no pathological significance. Their clinical relevance is due to the fact that several reports have documented an association between choroid plexus cysts and chromosomal defects, particularly trisomy 18. An analysis of all published data shows a mean prevalence of chromosomal defects of 8% with a 1% prevalence for apparently isolated lesions and 46% for those with additional abnormalities[41]. However, it is possible that the wide range in the reported prevalence of chromosomal defects is the mere consequence of differences in the maternal age distribution of the populations examined in the various studies. For this reason, if the choroid plexus cysts are apparently isolated, then the maternal age-related risk for trisomy 18 is only marginally increased[42].

CHEST TUMORS

Chest tumors are rare congenital anomalies arising from the lung, the mediastinal space or the heart (Table 5).

Lung tumors

The most common congenital lung tumor is represented by cystic adenomatoid malformations. This is a hamartoma characterized by overgrowth of terminal bronchioles. A classification into three types of cystic adenomatoid malformation has been proposed by Stocker and colleagues[43]: type I has large cysts; type II has multiple small cysts; type III is the microcystic variety and involves the entire lobe with regularly spaced bronchiole-like structures, causing mediastinal shift. Other authors separate these malformations into two groups, based on the

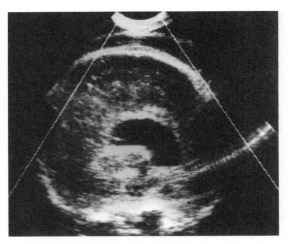

Figure 8 *Cyst of the corpus callosum. Sagittal section of the fetal brain, showing the C-shaped appearance of the cyst*

Table 5 *Chest tumors*

Lung
Cystic adenomatoid malformation
Bronchogenic cyst

Heart
Rhabdomyoma
Myxoma
Teratoma

Mediastinal space
Teratoma
Neurogenic tumor
Thymus neoplasm

predominant component of the lesion (cystic or solid)[44]. Adzick[45] has proposed two categories (macro- and microcystic tumors) based on gross anatomy, ultrasound findings and prognosis; the former contain single or multiple cysts of 5 mm or more in diameter (Figure 9); the latter appear as a solid mass, since the cysts are too small to be visualized by ultrasound, but produce an echo enhancement due to the innumerable interfaces (Figure 10). The macrocystic type is more common and has a more favorable prognosis, whereas the microcystic (solid) type is almost invariably fatal, because of the development of fetal hydrops and hypoplasia of the normal lung tissue, secondary to vena cava or cardiac compression.

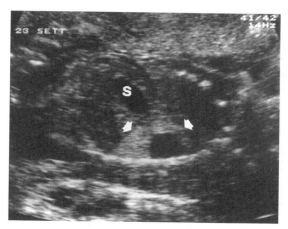

Figure 9 *Cystic adenomatoid malformation of the lung (macrocystic type). A large cyst surrounded by a hyperechoic area is located in the lower lobe of the left fetal lung (arrow). S, stomach*

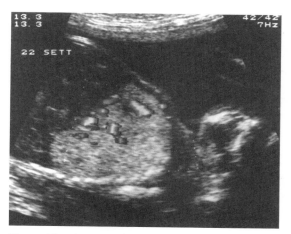

Figure 10 *Cystic adenomatoid malformation (microcystic type). The mass shows a solid appearance, since the cysts are too small to be visualized by ultrasound, but produce echo enhancement, due to the innumerable interfaces*

The differential diagnosis includes bronchogenic cysts, pulmonary sequestration and some very rare mediastinal masses, such as teratomas, pericardial cysts, thymus neoplasms and neurogenic tumors. A bronchogenic cyst appears as an isolated regular hypoechoic area in the lung[46]. Pulmonary sequestration is a mass of pulmonary parenchyma separated from the normal lung, usually not communicating with an airway and receiving its blood supply from the systemic circulation. It appears as a triangularly shaped hyperechogenic mass within the fetal chest, whose differentiation from the microcystic variety of cystic adenomatoid malformation remains difficult. The most characteristic sign of pulmonary sequestration is the visualization of its anomalous arterial supply arising from the aorta[47]. This demonstration, however, remains difficult, despite the use of color Doppler, due to the small size of the vessel and its proximity to the heart, and prevertebral vessels. In addition, other authors have demonstrated that even cystic adenomatoid malformation can present an atypical vascularization of aortic and pulmonary origin[48]. Finally, cases have been reported in which the two malformations coexist[49].

The prognosis of cystic adenomatoid malformation depends on the type and severity of the disease. Depending on the size, it can produce a mass effect on the developing lungs, with subsequent pulmonary hypoplasia. Usually the prognosis is worse in the microcystic type, frequently complicated by mediastinal shift, hydrops and polyhydramnios. Hydrops is the most important sign predictive of an unfavorable outcome. It is probably secondary to vena cava obstruction or cardiac compression from the mediastinal shift caused by the lesion. The absence of hydrops till the end of pregnancy carries a good prognosis for the neonate. The delivery, however, should be planned in a tertiary care center, where immediate resuscitation and thoracic surgery can be planned. Prenatal treatment, consisting of intrauterine shunting of the lung cysts, resulted in a successful outcome in two cases[50,51]. Intrauterine surgery is still an optional experimental treatment[52].

Recently, attention has been focused on the possible spontaneous resolution *in utero* of hyperechogenic lung lesions diagnosed during the second trimester[53,54]. These hyperechoic lesions probably do not represent true lung anomalies, such as cystic adenomatoid malformation or lung sequestration, but only transient airway obstruction by mucous plug[55]. However, these observations invite caution in counselling the parents and indicate follow-up.

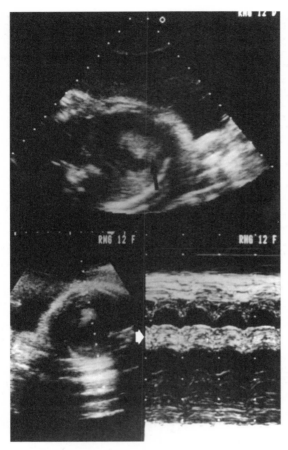

Figure 11 *Large rhabdomyoma of the heart. The hyper-echoic mass is located on the interventricular septum (black arrow). The M-mode shows the thickness of the tumor and its movements with the septum (white arrow)*

Tumors of the heart

Congenital cardiac tumors are extremely rare lesions, mainly represented by rhabdomyomas. Teratomas, fibromas and myxomas are less common. In most cases the tumors are benign. Rhabdomyomas are typically associated in up to 85% of the cases with tuberous sclerosis[56]. However, despite the development of modern imaging, the typical brain and skin lesions of tuberous sclerosis cannot be detected in the fetal stage. Rhabdomyomas, on the other hand, as well as other cardiac tumors, are easily detectable, in the prenatal period; they appear as hyperechoic masses occupying the cardiac area (Figure 11). They can be isolated or, more

Table 6 *Abdominal tumors*

Liver
Hemangioma
Hamartoma
Adenoma
Hepatoblastoma
Isolated cyst

Kidney
Mesoblastic nephroma
Wilms' tumor
Teratoma

Adrenals
Neuroblastoma

Intra-abdominal cysts
Choledochal
Ovarian
Splenic
Mesenteric
Omental
Retroperitoneal

frequently, multiple and can be located on any structure of the heart, including the septum[57]. They can also present as diffuse myocardial thickening[58].

The prognosis depends on the number, size and location of the tumors and on the association with tuberous sclerosis. The presence of hydrops is a severe complication, indicating heart failure. This carries a very poor prognosis. Since a surgical resection of the tumors may be possible, the prenatal diagnosis allows planning of the delivery in a tertiary care center, where pediatric cardiologists and cardiac surgeons are available[59].

ABDOMINAL TUMORS

Abdominal tumors include both solid and cystic lesions arising from different intra-abdominal organs (liver, kidneys, adrenal glands, spleen, mesentery, omentum, ovaries, uterus, retroperitoneal space) (Table 6). The correct prenatal diagnosis of these abnormalities is not always possible by ultrasound, because of the difficulties in defining the organ from which the tumor originates. However, the location of the mass, its relation with other structures and the normality of other organs may be helpful in suggesting a reliable diagnosis.

Hepatic tumors

Primary liver tumors are very rare conditions, which can occasionally be seen in the prenatal period. They include hemangioma, mesenchymal hamartoma, adenoma, hepatoblastoma, metastatic neuroblastoma and isolated cysts.

The sonographic appearance of hepatic hemangioma varies, depending on the degree of fibrosis and stage of involution of the tumor[60–63]: it can be hypoechogenic, hyperechogenic or mixed in appearance. The size can vary from a few millimeters to some centimeters (Figure 12). The vascular nature of hemangioma can be confirmed by pulsed Doppler with color flow only in cases with large vessels and turbulent flow[63] (Figure 13). Polyhydramnios can be associated[64]. A possible reduction in size, or even disappearance *in utero* of the small lesions is possible, as a consequence of the progressive fibrosis and involution of the tumor[61].

Mesenchymal hamartomas ultrasonically appear as irregular cysts, which can also reach huge size[65,66]; however, a case with a solid appearance has been reported[67].

The solid appearance of the mass is common also to hepatoblastoma[64] and adenoma[68]. For this reason a prenatal differential diagnosis among the above different pathological conditions is not possible.

Isolated hepatic cysts appear as well defined anechoic lesions in the liver area[69]; their differential diagnosis from a choledochal cyst could be difficult. This can be suspected when tubular structures referred to dilated hepatic ducts can be seen, adjacent or leading to the cyst[70] (Figure 14).

The management of a fetus affected by a hepatic tumor is expectant, with monitoring of the size and evolution of the tumor. Huge hemangiomas associated with arteriovenous shunting can be the cause of fetal heart failure; small hemangiomas, on the other hand, may undergo no change or even spontaneous reso-

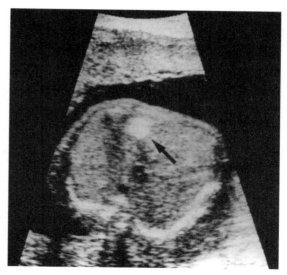

Figure 12 *Small hepatic hemangioma appearing as a hyperechoic mass (arrow) in the liver*

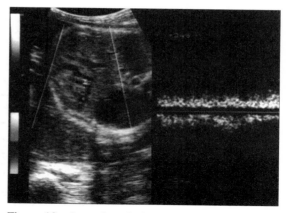

Figure 13 *Large hepatic hemangioma appearing as a complex mass in the left lobe of the liver. Pulsed Doppler with color flow shows large vessels and turbulent flow at the periphery of the mass*

lution[71]. Very large tumors may represent an indication for Cesarean section, to avoid rupture or dystocia during vaginal delivery. After delivery, once the diagnosis is confirmed by computed tomography or magnetic resonance imaging, surgical resection is indicated in cases of large tumors; if the tumor is small and the neonate is asymptomatic, no treatment is indicated.

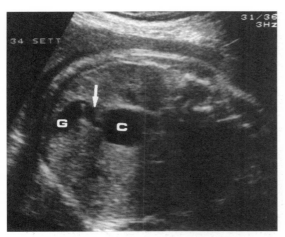

Figure 14 *Choledochal cyst (C). The gallbladder (G) and the dilated cystic duct (arrow) can also be recognized*

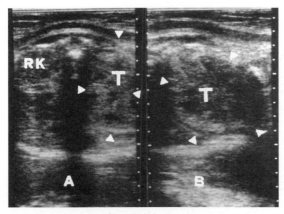

Figure 15 *Transverse (A) and longitudinal (B) sections of the fetal abdomen, showing a tumor of the left kidney, postnatally proved to be a mesoblastic nephroma. T, tumor; RK, right kidney*

Renal tumors

The most common renal mass ultrasonically identified during prenatal life is multicystic kidney[72]; however, this space-occupying lesion cannot be considered as a true tumor, but as a cystic dysplasia resulting from arrest of the complex embryogenetic process, which, starting from the serial dichotomous branching of the ureteric bud, leads to formation of the tubules and consequent induction of nephron development.

The most common renal tumor developing during prenatal life is mesoblastic nephroma, also known as mesenchymal hamartoma. Although the tumor is not encapsulated, it is a benign neoplasm, which in very rare instances may show a malignant pattern. The sonographic appearance of the mesoblastic nephroma is that of a solid mass in one of the upper quadrants of the fetus, compressing the kidney; cystic areas may occasionally be seen in case of hemorrhage and consequent cystic degeneration[73–75] (Figure 15). The tumor may also appear as a diffuse enlargement of the kidney. Polyhydramnios is frequently associated[76]. Possible explanations of the mechanism of polyhydramnios are compression of the tumor on the gastrointestinal tract, and an increase in renal blood flow or impaired renal concentrating ability.

The differential diagnosis should include Wilms' tumor and other congenital tumors such as teratomas, as well as multicystic kidney. Although Wilms' tumor tends to have a well defined capsule, it may be indistinguishable from mesoblastic nephroma. Multicystic kidney can be differentiated by its typical cystic appearance. Focal dysplasia should also be considered in the differential diagnosis[77]. One must also exclude tumors from adjacent organs such as adrenal glands. The most common tumor of adrenal glands is neuroblastoma, whose sonographic appearance is not dissimilar to mesoblastic nephroma. However, a careful examination can allow the recognition of the kidney compressed and displaced caudally by the adrenal mass, which can also present a rich vascularization on color Doppler examination[78].

The diagnosis of a renal tumor requires only serial sonography to monitor the tumor growth. The surgical treatment can be planned in the neonatal period.

Ovarian cysts

Fetal ovarian cysts are the most common intra-abdominal cysts detected in the prenatal period. This is not surprising if one considers that ovarian follicular cysts are found in about one-third of newborns at autopsy, although they are usually small and asymptomatic[79]. Most fetal ovarian cysts are of follicular origin. Granulosa cell tumors, teratomas and mesonephromas have been reported in the neonatal period, but are extremely rare in comparison to the cysts of Graafian origin. Fetal ovarian cysts are hormone sensitive and usually develop in the late second and third trimesters of pregnancy, following the completion of functional maturity of the fetal gonads[80].

The sonographic diagnosis of a fetal ovarian cyst should be suspected when a well defined cystic mass is detected in the lower abdomen of a female fetus with normally structured and functioning intra-abdominal organs[81] (Figure 16). Their size can be extremely variable, with the largest reported cyst measuring 11 cm in diameter[82]. They can be unilateral or, less frequently, bilateral; thin septa may occasionally be seen inside the cystic structure[83]. Sometimes the cysts contain irregular echoes and debris (Figure 17). These are signs of complications in the cyst, such as torsion and hemorrhage[81,84], as confirmed by the occurrence of such findings during the monitoring with serial sonography of cysts that originally were transonic. Association with polyhydramnios can be possible, perhaps as a consequence of intestinal compression by the mass.

The sonographic differential diagnosis includes urachal cysts, enteric duplication, duodenal atresia, bowel obstruction, hydrometrocolpos, mesenteric and omental cysts. Urachal cysts are tubular in shape and extend from the bladder to the umbilicus. Enteric duplication tends to present a tubular more than a round shape. Duodenal atresia shows the typical double bubble appearance with the 'cysts' located in the upper abdomen. Bowel obstruction shows multiple dilated loops and increased peristalsis. In hydrometrocolpos the cyst is located on the middle pelvis between the bladder and the sacrum, and may present low-level echoes inside[85]. Mesenteric and omental cysts may be indistinguishable from those of ovarian origin.

The prognosis of fetal ovarian cysts is usually good. The simple uncomplicated cysts frequently undergo spontaneous resolution by the end of pregnancy or in the first few months of life, thus confirming their functional origin[86]. The complicated cysts will need surgery after

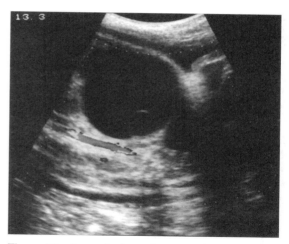

Figure 16 *Large fetal ovarian cyst, showing a small daughter cyst inside*

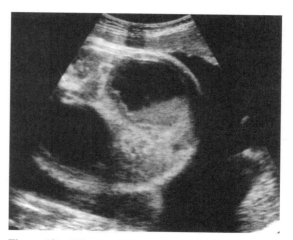

Figure 17 *Bilateral ovarian cysts. The cyst on the left is completely echo-free; the cyst on the right contains debris that is a sign of intracystic hemorrhage*

delivery, although a spontaneous resolution *in utero* has been reported even in these cases[81]. Very large cysts may cause dystocia; to prevent this complication a Cesarean section can be planned. An alternative approach is the ultrasound-guided needle aspiration of the cysts[82]. This procedure may avoid the need for a Cesarean section and diminish the risk of intrauterine torsion, but the puncture of the cyst may carry the risk of rupture of the cyst wall, with intraperitoneal bleeding.

Other intra-abdominal cysts

Other abdominal cysts that can be prenatally detected with ultrasound may be located in the bowel mesentery, in the omentum, in the spleen and in the retroperitoneal space. Among these cases, the only one that can be diagnosed with good reliability is the cyst of the spleen, thanks to the peculiar location of the cyst in the upper left quadrant of the abdomen, above the stomach. Congenital true cysts of the spleen are in most cases epidermoid cysts that are thought to arise from mesothelial inclusion of the visceral peritoneum during fetal spleen development or from an 'in utero trauma' (vascular accident). Neoplastic cysts (hemangioma, lymphangioma, sarcoma) are extremely rare. Small cysts of the spleen should not be operated upon, since their spontaneous resolution is possible in the first years of life[86].

Mesenteric, omental and retroperitoneal cysts may represent obstructed lymphatic drainage or lymphatic hamartomas[87,88]. Ultrasonically, they appear as multiseptated or unilocular cystic masses of variable size. A solid appearance may be due to intracystic hemorrhage. Their location is usually on the middle part of the fetal abdomen (Figure 18); however, their differentiation from ovarian or even choledochal cysts may not be possible. Postnatally the treatment is conservative, but surgery may be required for symptomatic cases.

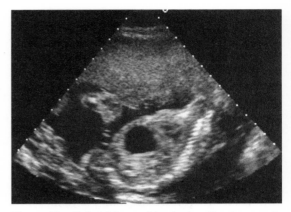

Figure 18 *Isolated intra-abdominal unilocular cyst, located in the middle part of the fetal abdomen. Postnatally it proved to be a mesenteric cyst*

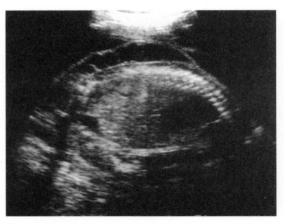

Figure 19 *Large cutaneous hemangioma, appearing as a septated cystic structure on the surface of the fetal chest*

TUMORS OF THE SKIN

Tumors of the skin that can be prenatally detected by ultrasound are hemangiomas and related angiomatous malformations. These lesions may occur as isolated tumors, frequently located on the scalp, ear, eyelid or extremities, or may be part of more complex syndromes, such as Klippel–Trenaunay–Weber syndrome (large cutaneous hemangiomas and hypertrophy of the related bones and soft tissues)[89]; Sturge–Weber syndrome (nevus flammeus of the face and angiomas of the meninges); and von Hippel–Lindau syndrome (angiomas of the retina and cerebellum). Sonographically they appear as septated cystic areas on the fetal surface (Figure 19), which may occasionally be so large that vaginal delivery can be precluded[90].

References

1. Schiffer, M. A. and Greenberg, E. (1956). Sacrococcygeal teratoma in labor and the newborn. *Am. J. Obstet. Gynecol.*, **72**, 1054–62

2. Bale, P. M. (1984). Sacrococcygeal developmental abnormalities and tumors in children. *Perspect. Pediatr. Pathol.*, **1**, 9–18

3. Ashley, D. J. B. (1973). Origin of teratomas. *Cancer*, **32**, 390–4

4. Litwiller, M. R. (1969). Dystocia caused by sacrococcygeal teratoma. *Obstet. Gynecol.*, **34**, 783–6

5. Altmann, R. P., Randolph, J. G. and Lilly, J. R. (1974). Sacrococcygeal teratoma: an American Academy of Pediatrics Surgical Section survey. *J. Pediatr. Surg.*, **9**, 389–95

6. Donnellan, W. A. and Swenson, O. (1988). Benign and malignant sacrococcygeal teratomas. *Pediatr. Surg.*, **64**, 834–46

7. Grisoni, E. R., Gauderer, M. W. L. and Wolfson, R. N. (1988). Antenatal diagnosis of sacrococcygeal teratomas: prognostic features. *Pediatr. Surg. Int.*, **3**, 173–5

8. Flake, A. W., Harrison, M. R. and Adzick, N. S. (1986). Fetal sacrococcygeal teratoma. *J. Pediatr. Surg.*, **21**, 563–6

9. Horger, E. and McCarter, L. M. (1979). Prenatal diagnosis of sacrococcygeal teratoma. *Am. J. Obstet. Gynecol.*, **134**, 228–9

10. Chervenak, F. A., Isaacson, G. and Touloukian, R. (1985). Diagnosis and management of fetal teratomas. *Obstet. Gynecol.*, **66**, 666–71

11. Holzgreve, W., Mahony, B. S. and Glick, P. L. (1985). Sonographic demonstration of fetal sacrococcygeal teratoma. *Prenat. Diagn*, **5**, 545–57

12. Hogge, W. A., Thiagarajah, S. and Barber, V. G. (1987). Cystic sacrococcygeal teratoma: ultrasound diagnosis and perinatal management. *J. Ultrasound. Med.*, **6**, 707–10

13. Flake, A. W. (1993). Fetal sacrococcygeal teratoma. *Semin. Pediatr. Surg.*, **2**, 113–20

14. Garmel, S. H., Crombleholme, T. M. and Semple, J. P. (1994). Prenatal diagnosis and management of fetal tumors. *Semin. Perinatol.*, **18**, 350–65

15. Kurjak, A., Zalud, I., Jurkovic, D., Alfirevic, Z. and Tomic, K. (1989). Ultrasound diagnosis and evaluation of fetal tumors. *J. Perinat. Med.*, **17**, 173–93

16. Alter, D. N., Reed, K. L. and Marx, G. R. (1988). Prenatal diagnosis of congestive heart failure in a fetus with sacrococcygeal teratoma. *Obstet. Gynecol.*, **71**, 978–81

17. Schmidt, K. G., Silverman, N. H., Harrison, M. R. and Callen, P. W. (1989). High-output cardiac failure in fetuses with large SCT: diagnosis by echocardiography and Doppler ultrasound. *J. Pediatr.*, **114**, 1023–8

18. Lemire, R. J. and Beckwith, J. B. (1982). Pathogenesis of congenital tumors and malformations of the sacrococcygeal region. *Teratology*, **25**, 201–11

19. Kuhlman, R. S., Warsof, S. L. and Levy, D. L. (1987). Fetal sacrococcygeal teratoma. *Fetal Ther.*, **2**, 95–100

20. Werb, P., Scurry, J. and Ostor, A. (1992). Survey of congenital tumors in perinatal necroscopies. *Pathology*, **24**, 247–53

21. Berry, C. L., Keeling, J. and Hilton, C. (1970). Coincidence of congenital malformation and embryonic tumors of childhood. *Arch. Dis. Child.*, **45**, 229–31

22. Holzgreve, W., Miny, P., Anderson, R. and Golbus, M. S. (1987). Experience with 8 cases of prenatally diagnosed sacrococcygeal teratomas. *Fetal. Ther.*, **2**, 88–94

23. Holzgreve, W. and Willital, G. H. (1993). Fetal tumors. In Chervenak, F., Isaacson, G. C. and Campbell, S. (eds.) *Ultrasound in Obstetrics and Gynecology*, vol. II, pp. 1009–206. (Boston: Little, Brown and Co.)

24. El-Qarmalui, M. A., Saddik, M. and El Abdel Hadi, F. (1990). Diagnosis and management of sacrococcygeal teratoma. *Int. J. Gynecol. Obstet.*, **31**, 275–81

25. Mintz, M. C., Mennuti, M. and Fishman, M. (1983). Prenatal aspiration of sacrococcygeal teratoma. *Am. J. Roentgenol.*, **141**, 367–8

26. Jurkovic, D. and Kurjak, A. (1988). Prenatal diagnosis and management of fetal tumors. In Cagnazzo, G. and D'Addario, V. (eds.) *The Fetus as a Patient '88*. pp. 49–62. (Amsterdam: Elsevier Science)

27. Langer, J. C., Harrison, M. R. and Schmidt, K. G. (1989). Fetal hydrops and death from sacrococcygeal teratoma: rationale for fetal surgery. *Am. J. Obstet. Gynecol.*, **160**, 1145–50

28. Patel, R. B., Gibson, J. Y., De Cruz, C. A. and Burkhalter, J. L. (1982). Sonographic diagnosis of cervical teratoma *in utero*. *Am. J. Roentgenol.*, **139**, 1220–2

29. Trecet, J. C., Claramunt, V. and Larraz, J. (1984). Prenatal ultrasound diagnosis of fetal teratoma of the neck. *J. Clin. Ultrasound*, **12**, 509–11

30. Roodhooft, A. M., Delbeke, L. and Vaneerdeweg, W. (1987). Cervical teratoma: prenatal detection and management in the neonate. *Pediatr. Surg. Int.*, **2**, 181–4

31. Azar, G., Snijders, R. J. M., Gosden, C. M. and Nicolaides, K. H. (1991). Fetal nuchal cystic hygromata : associated malformations

and chromosomal defects. *Fetal Diagn. Ther.*, **6**, 46–57

32. Baumann, F. R. and Nerlich, A. (1993). Metastasizing cervical teratoma of the fetus. *Pediatr. Pathol.*, **13**, 21–7

33. Thurkow, A. L., Visser, G. H. A., Oosterhuis, J. W. and de Vries, J. A. (1983). Ultrasound observations of a malignant cervical teratoma of the fetus in a case of polyhydramnios. Case history and review. *Eur. J. Obstet. Gynecol. Reprod. Biol.*, **14**, 375–84

34. Zerella, J. T. and Finberg, F. J. (1990). Obstruction of the neonatal airway from teratomas. *Surg. Gynecol. Obstet.*, **170**, 126–31

35. Lipman, S. P., Pretorius, D. H., Rumack, C. M. and Manco-Johnson, M. L. (1985). Fetal intracranial teratomas: US diagnosis of three cases and review of the literature. *Radiology*, **157**, 491–6

36. Riboni, G., De Simoni, L., Leonardi, O. and Molla, R. (1985). Ultrasound appearance of a glioblastoma in a 33 week fetus *in utero*. *J. Clin. Ultrasound*, **13**, 345–7

37. Hoff, N. R. and Mackay, I. M. (1980). Prenatal ultrasound diagnosis of intracranial teratoma. *J. Clin. Ultrasound*, **8**, 247–50

38. Shawker, T. H. and Schwartz, R. M. (1983). Ultrasound appearance of a malignant fetal brain tumor. *J. Clin. Ultrasound*, **11**, 35–7

39. Diakoumakis, E. E., Weinberg, B. and Mollin, J. (1986). Prenatal sonographic diagnosis of a suprasellar arachnoid cyst. *J. Ultrasound Med.*, **5**, 529–30

40. Pilu, G., De Palma, L. and Romero, R. (1986). The fetal subarachnoid cysterns: an ultrasound study with report of a case of congenital communicating hydrocephalus. *J. Ultrasound Med.*, **5**, 365–71

41. Snijders, R. J. M., Farrias, C., von Kaisenberg, C. and Nicolaides, K. H. (1996). Fetal abnormalities (choroid plexus cysts). In Snijders, R. J. M. and Nicolaides, K. H. (eds.) *Ultrasound Markers for Fetal Chromosomal Defects*, pp. 12–14. (Casterton, UK: Parthenon Publishing)

42. Snijders, R. J. M., Shawwa, L. and Nicolaides, K. H. (1994). Fetal choroid plexus cysts and trisomy 18: assessment of the risk based on ultrasound findings and maternal age. *Prenat. Diagn.*, **14**, 1119–27

43. Stocker, T., Madewell, J. and Drake, R. (1975). Congenital cystic adenomatoid malformation of the lung: classification and morphological spectrum. *Hum. Pathol.*, **8**, 155–66

44. Bale, P. M. (1979). Congenital cystic malformation of the lung. *Am. J. Clin. Pathol.*, **71**, 411–21

45. Adzick, N. S. (1990). The fetus with a cystic adenomatoid malformation. In Harrison, M. R., Golbus, M. S. and Filly, R. A. (eds.) *The Unborn Patient*, pp. 320–9. (Philadelphia: Saunders)

46. Mayden, K. L., Tortora, M. and Chervenak, F. A. (1984). The antenatal sonographic detection of lung masses. *Am. J. Obstet. Gynecol.*, **148**, 349–62

47. Sauerbrei, E. (1991). Lung sequestration. *J. Ultrasound Med.*, **10**, 101–6

48. Ellis, K. (1991). Developmental abnormalities in the systemic blood supply to the lungs. *Am. J. Roentgenol.*, **156**, 669–74

49. Zangwill, B. C. and Stocker, J. T. (1993). Congenital cyst adenomatoid malformation within an extralobar pulmonary sequestration. *Pediatr. Pathol.*, **13**, 309–12

50. Clark, S. L., Vitale, D. J. and Minton, S. D. (1987). Successful fetal therapy for cystic adenomatoid malformation associated with second trimester hydrops. *Am. J. Obstet. Gynecol.*, **157**, 294–7

51. Nicolaides, K. H., Blott, M. and Greenough, A. (1987). Chronic drainage of fetal pulmonary cyst. *Lancet*, **1**, 618

52. Harrison, M. R., Adzick, N. S. and Jenning, R. W. (1990). Antenatal intervention for congenital cystic adenomatoid malformation. *Lancet*, **336**, 965–6

53. Budorick, N. E., Pretorius, D. H., Leopold, G. R. and Stamm, E. R. (1992). Spontaneous improvement of intrathoracic masses diagnosed *in utero*. *J. Ultrasound Med.*, **11**, 653–5

54. MacGillivray, T. E., Harrison, M. R., Goldstein, R. B. and Adzick, N. S. (1993). Disappearing fetal lung lesions. *J. Pediatr. Surg.*, **28**, 1321–4

55. Sepulveda, W. and Fisk, N. M. (1995). Resolving fetal hyperechogenic lung lesions: an unresolved issue. *Ultrasound Obstet. Gynecol.*, **6**, 4

56. Bordarier, C., Lellouch-Tubiana, A. and Robain, O. (1994). Cardiac rhabdomioma and tuberous sclerosis in three fetuses: a neuropathological study. *Brain. Dev.*, **16**, 467–71

57. DeVore, G. R., Hakim, S. and Kleinman, C. (1982). The *in utero* diagnosis of an interventricular septal cardiac rhabdyoma by means of real-time directed M-mode echocardiography. *Am. J. Obstet. Gynecol.*, **143**, 967–9

58. Coates, T. L. and McGahan, J. P. (1994). Fetal cardiac rhabdyomas presenting as diffuse myocardial thickening. *J. Ultrasound Med.*, **13**, 813–16

59. Hwa, J., Ward, C., Nunn, G., Cooper, S., Lau, K. C. and Scholler, G. (1994). Primary intraventricular cardiac tumors in children: contemporary diagnostic and management options. *Pediatr. Cardiol.*, **15**, 233–7

60. Nakamoto, S. K., Dreilinger, A. and Dattel, B. (1983). The sonographic appearance of hepatic hemangioma *in utero*. *J. Ultrasound Med.*, **2**, 239–41

61. Sepulveda, W. H., Donetch, G. and Giuliano, A. (1993). Prenatal sonographic diagnosis of fetal

hepatic hemangioma. *Eur. J. Obstet. Gynecol. Reprod. Biol.*, **48**, 73–6

62. Petrovic, O., Haller, H. and Rukavina, B. (1992). Prenatal diagnosis of a large liver cavernous hemangioma associated with polyhydramnios. *Prenat. Diagn.*, **12**, 70–1

63. Gonen, R., Fong, K. and Chiasson, D. A. (1989). Prenatal sonographic diagnosis of hepatic hemangioendothelioma with secondary nonimmune hydrops fetalis. *Obstet. Gynecol.*, **73**, 485–7

64. Van der Bor, M., Verwey, R. A. and Van Pel, R. (1985). Acute polyhydramnios associated with fetal hepatoblastoma. *Eur. J. Obstet. Gynecol. Reprod. Biol.*, **20**, 65–9

65. Foucar, E., Williamson, R. A. and Yiu-Chiu, V. (1983). Mesenchymal hamartoma of the liver identified by fetal sonography. *Am. J. Roentgenol.*, **140**, 970–2

66. Hirata, G. I., Matsunaga, M. L. and Medearis, A. L. (1990). Ultrasonographic diagnosis of a fetal abdominal mass: a case of a mesenchymal liver hamartoma and a review of the literature. *Prenat. Diagn.*, **10**, 507–12

67. Mason, B. A., Hodges, W. and Goodman, J. R. (1992). Antenatal sonographic detection of a rare solid hepatic mesenchymal hamartoma. *J. Matern. Fetal Med.*, **1**, 134–6

68. Marks, F., Thomas, P. and Lustig, I. (1990). *In utero* sonographic description of a fetal adenoma. *J. Ultrasound Med.*, **9**, 119–22

69. Chung, W. M. (1986). Antenatal detection of hepatic cyst. *J. Clin. Ultrasound*, **14**, 217–20

70. Elrad, H., Mayden, K. L. and Ahart, S. (1985). Prenatal ultrasound diagnosis of choledocal cyst. *J. Ultrasound Med.*, **4**, 553–5

71. Porter, K. B. and Plottner, M. S. (1992). Fetal abdominal hyperechoic mass: diagnosis and management. *Fetal Diagn. Ther.*, **7**, 116–21

72. Kurjak, A., Latin, V., Mandruzzato, G. P., D'Addario, V. and Rajhvain, B. (1984). Ultrasound diagnosis and perinatal management of fetal genito-urinary abnormalities. *J. Perinat. Med.*, **12**, 291–312

73. Giulian, B. B. (1984). Prenatal ultrasonographic diagnosis of fetal renal tumors. *Radiology*, **152**, 69–70

74. Rempen, A., Kirchner, T., Frauendienst-Egger, G. and Hocht, B. (1992). Congenital mesoblastic nephroma. *Fetus*, **2**, 1–5

75. Apuzzio, J. J., Unwin, W., Adhate, A. and Nichols, R. (1986). Prenatal diagnosis of fetal renal mesoblastic nephroma. *Am. J. Obstet. Gynecol.*, **154**, 636–9

76. Geirsson, R. T., Ricketts, N. E. M., Taylor, D. J. and Coghill, S. (1985). Prenatal appearance of a mesoblastic nephroma associated with polyhydramnios. *J. Clin Ultrasound*, **13**, 488–90

77. Gordillo, R., Vilaro, M. and Sherman, N. H. (1987). Circumscribed renal mass in dysplastic kidney. *J. Ultrasound Med.*, **6**, 613–17

78. Goldstein, I., Gomez, K. and Copel, J. A. (1994). The real time and color Doppler appearance of adrenal neuroblastoma in a third trimester fetus. *Obstet. Gynecol.*, **83**, 854–6

79. De Sa, D. J. (1975). Follicular ovarian cysts in the stillbirth and neonates. *Arch. Dis. Child.*, **50**, 45–52

80. Di Zerega, G. S. and Ross, G. Y. (1980). Clinical relevance of fetal gonadal structure and function. *Clin. Obstet. Gynecol.*, **23**, 849–56

81. D'Addario, V., Volpe, G., Kurjak, A., Lituania, M. and Zmijanac, J. (1990). Ultrasonic diagnosis and perinatal management of uncomplicated and complicated fetal ovarian cysts: a collaborative study. *J. Perinat. Med.*, **18**, 375–81

82. Landrum, B., Ogburn, P. Jr and Feinberg, S. (1986). Intrauterine aspiration of a large ovarian cyst. *Obstet. Gynecol.*, **68**, 118–19

83. Sandler, R. M. A., Smith, S. J., Pope, S. G. and Madrazo, B. L. (1985). Prenatal diagnosis of septated ovarian cysts. *J. Clin. Ultrasound*, **13**, 55–7

84. Preziosi, P., Fariello, G., Maiorana, A., Malena, S. and Ferro, F. (1986). Antenatal sonographic diagnosis of complicated ovarian cysts. *J. Clin. Ultrasound*, **14**, 196–8

85. Davis, G. H., Wapner, R. J. and Kurtz, A. B. (1984). Antenatal diagnosis of hydrometrocolpos by ultrasound examination. *J. Ultrasound Med.*, **3**, 371–2

86. Musy, P. A., Roche, B., Belli, D., Bugman, P., Nussle, D. and Le Coultre, C. (1992). Splenic cysts in pediatric patients. A report of 8 cases and review of the literature. *Eur. J. Pediatr. Surg.*, **2**, 137–40

87. Helin, I. and Persson, P. H. (1985). Intra-abdominal cysts detected at prenatal ultrasound screening. *Helv. Pediatr. Acta*, **40**, 55–60

88. Kurtz, R. J., Heinmann, T. M. and Beck, A. R. (1986). Mesenteric and retroperitoneal cysts. *Ann. Surg.*, **203**, 109–16

89. Douglas Lewis, B., Doubilet, P. M., Heller, V., Bierre, A. and Bieber, F. R. (1986). Cutaneous and visceral haemangiomata in the Klippel–Trenaunay–Weber syndrome: antenatal sonographic detection. *Am. J. Roentgenol.*, **147**, 598–600

90. Suma, V., Marini, A., Gamba, P. and Luzzatto, C. (1990). Giant hemangioma of the thigh: prenatal sonographic diagnosis. *J. Clin. Ultrasound*, **18**, 421–2

Fetal cardiac intervention in congenital heart disease

22

T. Kohl

INTRODUCTION

Fetal cardiac intervention in congenital heart disease is a very recent subspeciality in prenatal medicine. The experience with procedures for fetal cardiac intervention is, therefore, limited and criteria to select fetuses for cardiac intervention merely exist. Scientific evidence to justify fetal cardiac interventions can presently only be derived from careful interpretation of case reports and retrospective echocardiographic studies focusing on specific lesions[1–12]. Case reports, as well as retrospective studies, have allowed inferences on the natural history and *in utero* progression of fetal heart disease. It became clear that although most cardiac malformations develop during embryonic life, some lesions continue to evolve during gestation and result in severe secondary damage to dependent cardiovascular structures. Although this secondary damage is in most cases compatible with normal fetal development, it significantly increases mortality and reduces treatment options after birth. In addition, functional anomalies can result in life-threatening fetal cardiac failure if left untreated. The frustration at not being able to influence the prenatal progression of anatomical lesions or functional anomalies has prompted the interest in exploring the feasibility of fetal cardiac interventions[13–22].

Based on general criteria developed to select lesions for fetal intervention in non-cardiac anomalies[23], similar criteria can be proposed to select congenital heart lesions for fetal cardiac intervention (Table 1). With these criteria in mind, fetal cardiac intervention seems most desirable for severe obstructions of the fetal aortic and pulmonary valves[24] (Table 2). In addition, fetal cardiac intervention may be beneficial in the fetus with congenital complete heart block and normal cardiac anatomy resulting in heart failure refractory to medical therapy[17,20,22]. Prenatal cardiac intervention has also been suggested for prenatal closure of the foramen ovale and ductus arteriosus as well as for tetralogy of Fallot with absent pulmonary valve[17,24]. The purpose of this chapter is to describe the treatment rationale and current experience with fetal cardiac intervention in human fetuses with severe aortic and pulmonary valvar obstructions, and congenital complete heart block. It also suggests specific selection criteria for some of these lesions and provides a preview of potential future therapeutic approaches.

Table 1   *General selection criteria for fetal cardiac intervention*

The primary cardiac abnormality results from a simple anatomical or functional defect
The cardiac abnormality is isolated. Chromosomal and other abnormalities have been ruled out
The cardiac abnormality is life-threatening either *in utero* or after birth
The intervention must either be life saving *in utero* or possess the potential to improve significantly postnatal surgical options and results
The intervention has the potential to abolish, arrest or even reverse the progression of pathological secondary changes caused by the primary cardiac abnormality
The intervention can be performed with minimal or acceptable maternal morbidity
Competence in performing the planned intervention with a high degree of success has been successfully achieved in animal models

Table 2 *Cardiac lesions amenable to fetal cardiac intervention*

Cardiac lesion	Effect	Result	Treatment options
Semilunar valvar obstructions	ventricular outflow obstruction	ventricular dilatation, or more common ventricular hypertrophy and hypoplasia, loss of ventricular function, hypoplasia of atrioventricular valves and great vessels, endocardial fibroelastosis	ultrasound-guided balloon valvuloplasty, *fetoscopic cardiac catheterization and balloonvalvuloplasty, *fetal cardiac surgery and valvotomy
Premature closure of foramen ovale 'primary form'	reduced flow to left heart	right ventricular dilatation, cardiac failure, hypoplasia of left heart structures	ultrasound or *fetoscopic cardiac catheterization and balloon dilatation, *fetal cardiac surgery and opening of foramen ovale
Premature closure of ductus arteriosus	right ventricular and pulmonary hypertension	right ventricular dilatation, hypertrophy, cardiac failure, pulmonary hypertension	*fetal cardiac surgery and insertion of aortopulmonary shunt
Complete heart block	low cardiac output	low-output cardiac failure	*fetoscopic cardiac intervention or open *fetal cardiac surgery for pacemaker placement
Tetralogy of Fallot with absent pulmonary valve	pulmonary regurgitation	aneurysmal dilatation of main and branch pulmonary arteries. Compression of airways and esophagus, polyhydramnios, cardiac failure. Postnatal respiratory failure	*fetal cardiac surgery for creation of pulmonary atresia and aortopulmonary shunt

*Experimental or potential procedures that have not yet been performed in human fetuses

SEMILUNAR VALVAR OBSTRUCTIONS

Treatment rationale

Severe obstructions of the pulmonary and aortic valve, including fetuses with hypoplastic left and right heart syndrome account for more than 7.5% of all newborns with congenital heart disease, and for more than 25% of neonatal cardiac death within the first week of life[25]. In a prospective series of 1006 consecutive fetuses with fetal congenital heart disease, these lesions were observed in about 25% of the fetuses[26]. Although pulmonary and aortic valve obstructions start as simple anatomical defects early in embryonic or later in fetal life, both can result in extensive secondary damage to the obstructed ventricle and dependent cardiovascular structures over the remainder of gestation[3,4,7,9,12,27,28]. Postnatal surgical options and overall prognosis depend to a large extent on the severity of this secondary damage. Unrepaired, almost all infants will die soon after birth, at the time the ductus arteriosus closes, and for survival an in-series circulation with two functioning ventricles is required. However, postnatal surgical options are often limited to palliative one-ventricle repairs by staged modified Fontan procedures and carry a high mortality rate[29–31]. Alternatively, neonatal cardiac transplantation had early and intermediate results superior to those of palliative one-ventricle repairs[32–35]. However, difficulties with the selection and supply of donor organs, graft rejection and the occurrence of post-transplant coronary artery disease remain major obstacles to this therapeutic approach[32,36,37].

Because of the poor postnatal outcome and limited long-term prognosis of severe fetal semilunar valvar obstructions, termination of gestation in previable fetuses is now frequently considered[26–28,38,39]. If the gestation is continued, *in utero* transport to a specialized center where cardiac procedures are routinely performed has been advised to improve perinatal management[40]. Scheduled premature delivery for early catheter-based cardiac intervention or surgical valvotomy has been chosen in individual fetuses to prevent further *in utero* deterioration of cardiac function over the last weeks of gestation[41–43]. This approach, however, may introduce additional postnatal complicating factors related to prematurity[40] and must be decided on an individual basis.

The goal of fetal cardiac intervention in severe pulmonary and aortic valvar obstructions is to prevent, arrest, or reverse secondary cardiovascular damage so that after birth, survival with two functioning ventricles is possible. Although further interventions can be anticipated after birth, the prenatal procedure should change the natural disease course such that catheter interventions or reconstructive instead of palliative surgical procedures can be performed. The fetal circulation and fetal cardiovascular tissue as well as the intrauterine environment may offer several advantages for fetal cardiac intervention. The parallel arrangement of the fetal circulation[44] may allow for slow recovery of the unloaded ventricle over the remainder of gestation[16,38]. The ability for ongoing myocyte hyperplasia and continued formation of capillaries in fetal cardiac tissue may allow for catch-up growth of hypoplastic cardiovascular structures[16]. In addition, the occurrence or progression of endocardial fibroelastosis may be prevented. Furthermore, the *in utero* milieu obviates the need for postinterventional intensive care management[24].

Pathophysiology

Fetal pulmonary and aortic valvar obstructions result in pressure overload of the obstructed ventricle. With little or absent flow across the obstructed valve, sufficient cardiac output for fetal survival can be maintained only by rerouting of blood flow via the foramen ovale and the ductus arteriosus[45]. The degree of blood flow across these fetal shunt connections is determined by the severity of the valvar stenosis and by atrioventricular compliance on the obstructed and non-obstructed sides of the heart[45]. Over the course of gestation, different degrees

of ventricular hypertrophy and hypoplasia as well as growth failure of associated cardiovascular structures develop (i.e. atrioventricular valve, great artery). The degree of these changes depends on the severity of the obstruction and when it occurs in gestation. Ventricular hypertrophy and hypoplasia as well as growth failure of associated cardiovascular structures may be explained by altered flow and pressure patterns in the developing heart[45] and have been induced in experimental studies. In fetal sheep, short-term survivors of ascending aorta banding showed left ventricular hypertrophy, decrease in left ventricular volume and partially fused aortic valve commissures with normal annulus size[46]. These changes resembled those seen in moderately severe aortic stenosis. In long-term survivors of the same surgery, the disease progressed to massive left ventricular hypertrophy, diminutive left ventricular volume, thickened aortic valve leaflets and hypoplastic valve annulus. These changes resembled those seen in severe aortic stenosis.

Natural history

The prenatal histories of severe pulmonary or aortic valvar obstructions in human fetuses share many similarities and are described together. Serial echocardiographic studies suggest that initial dilatation of the obstructed ventricle occurs, which is followed by either further dilatation with or without cardiac decompensation, or is compensated by adaptive cardiovascular changes involving the obstructed and non-obstructed sides of the heart[3,9,28,47].

Progressive ventricular dilatation and fetal hydrops reflect the inability of the fetal heart to accommodate to the required circulatory changes[28]. Cardiac enlargement can be so pronounced that secondary lung hypoplasia develops as the heart and lungs compete for space in the fetal chest[3] (Color plate 26a–e). Ventricular dilatation without hydrops is common in late-gestation fetuses with critical aortic stenosis. After birth, the left ventricle is dilated and functions poorly, but no signs of cardiac failure are encountered if right heart function is normal. The absence of cardiac failure in these older fetuses suggests that both ventricular response and hemodynamic effects may vary with the gestational age at which the obstruction becomes effective. Fetal and neonatal survival have been poor in cases of ventricular dilatation whether it is left or right ventricular outflow obstruction[3,48].

Conversely, a slow gradual progression or a milder degree of semilunar valvar obstruction may provide the time needed for cardiovascular adaptation[45]. In this situation, the obstructed ventricle hypertrophies and thus may stop or retard growth[4,9,12,28,48] (Color plates 27 and 28). Ventricular growth failure is accompanied by various degrees of atrioventricular valvar and great vessel hypoplasia. This hypertrophic-hypoplastic response of the obstructed ventricle is seen more often than ventricular dilatation. The extreme disease forms are classified among the hypoplastic left and right heart syndromes. Endocardial fibroelastosis is common in fetuses with severe semilunar valvar obstruction and has been associated with poor prognosis in post-natal life[28,49].

Medical therapy

No pharmacological treatment regimen for fetal pulmonary or aortic valvar obstructions has yet been defined. Anecdotal evidence indicates that inotropic support and anticongestive therapy may benefit fetuses with these lesions who are in cardiac failure[39].

Since the ductus arteriosus provides the main conduit for systemic or pulmonary blood flow in these lesions, administration of cyclooxygenase inhibitors to the mothers should be avoided because of the potential for ductal constriction. For the same reason, tocolysis with indomethacin and attempts to induce fetal lung maturation with steroids need to be monitored closely in fetuses with ductus-dependent heart disease[50,51].

Fetal balloon valvuloplasty

To date, balloon valvuloplasty has been attempted in ten fetuses to alleviate severe obstructions of the aortic or pulmonary valve. Six of these fetuses had aortic valvar stenoses, one had aortic valvar atresia, two had pulmonary valvar atresia and one had pulmonary valvar atresia associated with critical aortic valvar stenosis[13–15,18,19,38] (Allan, L. D., Huhta, J. C., Chaoui, R. and Lopes, L. – personal communications). Fetal balloon valvuloplasty in these initial catheter-based interventions was performed under ultrasound guidance (Figure 1 and Color plate 29). A needle is inserted through the maternal abdomen into the uterus. The needle is then advanced through the fetal chest into the obstructed ventricle. Then a small guide wire and balloon valvuloplasty catheter are delivered through the needle across the obstructed valve. The balloon is inflated within the valve ring and then all interventional devices are withdrawn. This procedure was completed in six human fetuses. In two fetuses with aortic and pulmonary valvar atresia, the imperforate valves could not be passed with interventional devices. In one fetus with pulmonary valve atresia, only a small opening in the imperforate valve was created using a radio frequency catheter[19]. In one fetus with pulmonary atresia and intact septum associated with critical aortic stenosis, a 4-French catheter sheath was placed into the left ventricle and a guide wire could be positioned across the stenotic aortic valve. Persistent fetal bradycardia and displacement of the catheter sheath required abandonment of this procedure before valvuloplasty could be performed.

There has been one long-term survivor after fetal balloon valvuloplasty in a fetus with aortic valve stenosis[38]. In this child, comparison of prenatal with postnatal echocardiographic studies showed recovery of left ventricular function. All other fetuses but two survived attempted or completed fetal balloon valvuloplasty for several weeks but then died either *in utero* or after delivery. It seems likely that these late fetal or neonatal deaths were not related to the intervention but rather to 'worst case' selection. There were only two early deaths, observed within 24 h after the procedure. In the first of these cases, bilateral hematothorax was found at autopsy[14]. In the second case, intracardiac positioning of

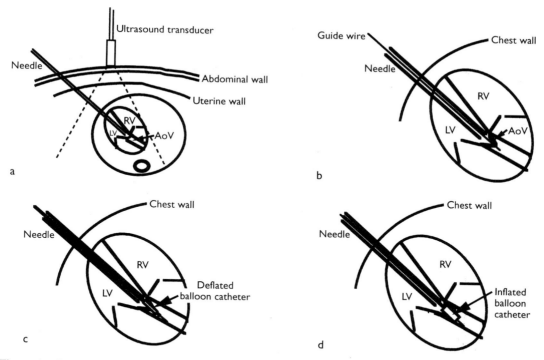

Figure 1 *Line drawing of ultrasound-guided fetal balloon valvuloplasty in fetal aortic stenosis. (a) A 16–18-gauge needle is inserted through the maternal abdomen into the uterus. The needle is then advanced through the fetal chest into the left ventricle (LV) as coaxial as possible to the left ventricular outflow tract. (b) A guide wire (GW) is advanced across the stenotic aortic valve (AoV) into the ascending aorta. (c) A balloon catheter is positioned over the wire across the valve annulus. (d) The balloon is inflated in order to dilate the stenotic valve. After valvuloplasty, all interventional material is removed. RV, right ventricle*

interventional devices resulted in persistent fetal bradycardia.

These initial results of fetal balloon valvuloplasty, namely ventricular recovery in the survivor as well as the low rate of acute fetal mortality in these patients (20%) are encouraging. Further investigation, however, would be welcomed to improve catheter-based fetal cardiac intervention and to define specific criteria to select fetuses who would most benefit from the procedure[38].

Selection for fetal cardiac intervention in fetuses with aortic or pulmonary valvar obstructions

It is likely that initially most fetal cardiac interventions will be performed after 24 weeks of gestation for two reasons. First, many parents would choose termination of pregnancy if severe fetal heart disease is diagnosed earlier in fetal life[26–28,38,39]. Second, because the small heart size of younger fetuses poses technical limits to surgical or catheter-based procedures for fetal cardiac intervention. Despite the small heart size and technical difficulties, it would be desirable to perform fetal cardiac interventions even earlier in gestation. The deleterious effects of fetal semilunar valvar obstructions could then be abolished sooner and cardiac recovery during the postinterventional course would allow re-evaluation of whether termination of pregnancy should still be considered.

Specific selection criteria may help to differentiate the subgroup of fetuses which is most likely to benefit from prenatal cardiac intervention from two subgroups which seem less likely to benefit from this approach. The group that may benefit consists of fetuses with a moderate to severe degree of semilunar valvar obstruction, decreased ventricular function and growth failure of cardiovascular structures. In this group, prenatal intervention may prevent, arrest, or reverse secondary cardiovascular damage and preserve ventricular function. The two groups that seem less likely to benefit from prenatal cardiac intervention consist of, first, fetuses with less severe semilunar valvar obstruction, sufficient ventricular function and near-normal growth of cardiovascular structures, and, second, fetuses with severe semilunar valvar obstruction, loss of ventricular function and severe hypoplasia of cardiovascular structures. In these two groups, prenatal intervention may not be indicated because of either too mild or too advanced a stage of fetal cardiac disease.

Specific selection criteria for assigning fetuses to these groups could be determined by extrapolation and inference from postnatal risk factors necessitating palliative surgical one-ventricle repair. These postnatal risk factors are in aortic valvar obstructions, ventricular hypoplasia in concert with small ventricular inflow or outflow dimensions and endocardial fibroelastosis[49,52]; in pulmonary valvar obstructions, ventricular hypoplasia in concert with a small tricuspid valve[31]. Since postnatal survival with two functioning ventricles is the goal of fetal cardiac intervention, the *in utero* development of these risk factors needs to be prevented.

Recently available data in human fetuses with left heart obstructive lesions suggest that serial measurements of left heart growth and assessment of flow direction across the foramen ovale and distal aortic arch may predict postnatal left heart size[9]. In this study, fetuses that required postnatal surgical one-ventricle repair showed decreased growth of the left ventricle, mitral valve and ascending aorta. Mitral valve, ascending aortic growth and the ratio of ascending aortic to main pulmonary artery diameter were found to correlate best with postnatal left ventricular volume. In addition, left to right shunting across the foramen ovale and retrograde flow in the distal aortic arch were observed in this group. Based on these findings, fetuses at risk for left heart hypoplasia can be identified, and fetal cardiac intervention can be justified if the mitral valve or ascending aorta do not grow sufficiently, reversed flow across the foramen ovale and the ductus arteriosus are encountered, and ventricular function is sufficient.

Less information is available to establish selection criteria for fetal cardiac intervention in the fetus with pulmonary valve obstruction. Data from prenatal studies indicate that the severity of pulmonary valve obstructions may be assessed *in utero* by the direction of ductal flow, the presence of pulmonary insufficiency, the degree of tricuspid insufficiency and the size of the pulmonary valve and arteries[53]. In postnatal individuals with pulmonary atresia and intact septum, a simple echocardiographic measurement of the tricuspid valve diameter has been useful to predict the necessity of surgical one-ventricle repair in this lesion[31]. It remains to be seen if serial studies of *in utero* tricuspid valve growth in fetal pulmonary valve obstructions allow inference of the degree of postnatal right heart hypoplasia.

Assessment of ventricular function in severe fetal pulmonary or aortic valvar stenoses could be performed by measuring the maximum velocity of a pulsed Doppler mitral or tricuspid valvar regurgitation signal. In fetuses with aortic valve obstructions, deterioration of ventricular function was identified by a progressive decrease in regurgitant velocity across the mitral valve[48]. Using the modified Bernoulli equation, the regurgitant velocity allows estimation of the amount of pressure that is generated by the obstructed ventricle[54]. If the velocity of the atrioventricular regurgitant jet is high, sufficient ventricular function may be assumed to justify fetal cardiac intervention (Color plate 27c). However, if the velocity of the atrioventricular regurgitant jet is low, lack of sufficient ventricular function can be assumed and fetal cardiac intervention may no longer be beneficial (Color plate 26c).

Summary

In conclusion, obstructions of the fetal aortic and pulmonary valves are encountered in a significant number of fetuses and can result in extensive secondary damage to dependent cardiovascular structures. Postnatal treatment options are often limited to palliative surgical one-ventricular repairs. Cardiac intervention in fetuses with these lesions aims to preserve the function and growth of the obstructed ventricle and dependent structures such that survival with two ventricles is possible after birth. Fetal cardiac intervention by ultrasound-guided balloon valvuloplasty has been performed with limited success in a small number of fetuses. Outcome in future cases may be improved by further developments in surgical and catheter-based procedures and improved fetal selection.

CONGENITAL COMPLETE HEART BLOCK

Treatment rationale

Congenital complete heart block (CCHB) is a rare cardiac condition; its incidence is about 1 in 20 000 live births[55]. CCHB needs to be differentiated from non-sustained and other sustained bradycardias in fetal life[56]. This differentiation can be readily performed by fetal echocardiography[57-59].

CCHB in the fetus can be divided into two types: fetuses with CCHB associated with structural heart defects and fetuses with isolated CCHB. CCHB associated with structural heart defects can be seen in left atrial isomerism, atrioventricular discordance and atrioventricular septal defects[60-62]. Isolated fetal CCHB with normal cardiac anatomy occurs most commonly in mothers with clinical or subclinical maternal connective tissue disease. In association with maternal connective tissue disease, fetal CCHB develops secondary to transplacental passage of maternal immunoglobulin class G autoantibodies to soluble ribonucleoproteins SSA (Ro) and SSB (La)[60,63-70]. These antibodies bind to fetal cardiac and other tissues between the 18th and 24th weeks of gestation and can induce irreversible fibrotic destruction of the fetal atrioventricular node as well as fetal myocarditis and general inflammation of fetal tissues[63,67,71-73]. In one study, the risk for mothers with lupus erythematodes and anti-Ro antibodies to deliver a first child with CCHB has been reported to be about 1 in 20 pregnancies[70]. In the same study, the recurrence risk for CCHB in second pregnancy increased to 1 in 3–4 pregnancies if a previous child with CCHB was born to a mother with SSA antibodies. In another study, the risk of having a third child affected among three pregnancies was estimated as high as 60%[74].

The prognosis of fetal CCHB depends on the ventricular escape rate as well as on the presence of fetal hydrops and additional cardiac malformations[60]. Most fetuses with CCHB and normal cardiac anatomy will survive until term and throughout the neonatal period if their ventricular escape rate is higher than 55 beats per minute (bpm). If the ventricular escape rate falls below 55 bpm, fetal hydrops may occur and the prognosis is guarded. Almost all fetuses with CCHB and hydrops will die *in utero*, regardless of normal or abnormal cardiac anatomy[60-62,75].

Pathophysiology

The normal fetal heart operates near the peak of the Starling curve that relates atrial filling pressure and ventricular stroke volume[76]. Therefore, cardiac output cannot be increased by increases in preload but depends on changes in heart rate, ventricular size, cardiac contractility and afterload. In the presence of CCHB, however, since heart rate is decreased and cannot be manipulated, fetal cardiac output can only be maintained by changes in ventricular size, cardiac contractility and afterload. Compensatory increases in ventricular size and cardiac contractility have been described in human fetuses with CCHB[77,78]. Increased arteriovenous oxygen extraction and afterload control by preferred perfusion of individual vascular beds may provide additional compensatory mechanisms. It may be important for the disease course whether CCHB occurs acutely or after a period of progressive deterioration of atrioventricular conduction. Like fetal lambs[79], human fetuses may not tolerate the acute onset of CCHB. A slow and gradual decrease in heart rate, however, would provide the time required for cardiovascular adaptation.

Medical therapy

No optimal treatment regimen for CCHB has yet been defined. Sympathomimetic or anti-cholinergic drugs have been used to increase fetal heart rate[60]. For this purpose, isoprenaline, terbutaline, ritodrine and atropine have been administered to the mother[22,60,80–82]. In many cases, however, these drugs will not raise the ventricular escape rhythm sufficiently. Nevertheless, since β-receptors are present in the fetal myocardium[83], sympathomimetic drugs may still benefit the fetus by increasing cardiac contractility and stroke volume. In addition, transplacental anticongestive therapy with digoxin and lasix may be effective[80]. Fetal delivery is indicated when the fetal condition is deteriorating despite pharmacological therapy and if the fetus is mature enough to survive. Fetal cardiac intervention by cardiac pacing will be a treatment option for the immature fetus in heart failure refractory to medical therapy.

CCHB caused by transplacental passage of antibodies may benefit from anti-inflammatory therapy because further damage to cardiac and non-cardiac structures may be prevented or alleviated. Dexamethasone administration may improve the degree of heart block in some fetuses and has the potential to prevent progression of incomplete to complete block[84]. In addition, inflammational changes of the atrioventricular valves resulting in severe valvar insufficiency as well as cardiomyopathy have been ascribed to antibody antigen reactivity in fetal cardiac tissues[82]. Since fetal hydrops in antibody-mediated CCHB may occur as a result of general tissue inflammation rather than low cardiac output, administration of corticosteroids, immunoglobulins, plasmapheresis or plasma exchange may be useful to treat or prevent additional cardiac lesions and to suppress inflammation in other fetal tissues[63,66,71,72,82,84]. Dexamethasone and betamethasone are superior to prednisolone for the treatment of CCHB because both are barely metabolized by the placenta[85]. Conversely, prednisolone undergoes extensive transformation to relatively inactive prednisone when crossing the placenta[85,86].

Fetal cardiac pacing

Fetal cardiac pacing in CCHB will be reserved for those few fetuses with CCHB and normal cardiac anatomy that develop heart failure refractory to medical therapy and are too young to be delivered. To date, fetal cardiac pacing has only been attempted in three human fetuses. In one of these fetuses, open fetal surgery at 22 weeks of gestation for placement of epicardial pacing leads failed[17]. In the two other fetuses, at 24 and 26 weeks of gestation, ultrasound-guided positioning of pacing wires into the right ventricle via the inferior caval vein or by direct transthoracic ventricular puncture was successfully performed[20,22]. The capture time, however, in these two cases ranged only between 4 and 8 h. After this period, in one fetus the pacing wire was displaced from the right ventricle; the second fetus died with the wire still in place. Both cases illustrate that fetal cardiac pacing is feasible in the human fetus. However, future attempts to pace the fetal heart in CCHB ultimately depend on a reliable and safe method to secure the pacing leads to the fetus.

Long-term pacing of the fetal left ventricle between 5 and 26 days was performed in fetal lambs after lead and pacemaker implantation by open fetal surgery[87]. Although this experimental study shows that ventricular pacing alone has the potential to maintain sufficient cardiac output, atrioventricular sequential pacing may be more desirable because of the important contribution of atrial contraction to ventricular filling in the fetus. The advantages of atrioventricular sequential pacing on cardiac filling were studied in fetal lambs. In those lambs, ventricular pacing consistently resulted in significantly lower cardiac outputs than atrioventricular sequential pacing and sinus rhythm[79]. During only ventricular pacing, the loss of atrial contraction resulted in a 50% decrease in right and a 29% decrease in left ventricular stroke volume.

Prevention

The transplacental passage of maternal class G antibodies is dependent on active transport mechanisms that mature around the 20th week of gestation. Since Ro- and La-antigens are expressed in fetal tissues at the same time, reduction of maternal antibodies before transplacental passage occurs or antigens are expressed may offer the best protection[88,89]. Prophylactic treatment in mothers who are for the first time pregnant is difficult because most cases of fetal CCHB associated with maternal autoimmune disease occur in women with subclinical symptoms[69,90]. Prophylactic treatment, however, was attempted in three high-risk groups[68]. These groups included first, mothers with previously known connective tissue disease with anti-Ro and anti-La antibodies, second, mothers who had a previous child with CCHB associated with these antibodies. The third group included mothers with anti-Ro antibody titer higher than $1 : 16$[70]. To lower maternal anti-Ro antibody levels, prophylactic therapy with corticosteroids, azathioprine and immunoglobulin therapy as well as plasmapheresis or plasma exchange was attempted[74,91–93]. Since these prophylactic therapies were followed by delivery of healthy newborns, they may have suppressed the development of CCHB.

If prophylactic therapy is attempted, it should be instituted before 18–20 weeks of gestation to lower maternal antibody levels before significant transplacental passage can occur and before Ro- and La-antigens are expressed in the fetal heart. However, prophylactic therapy should not be instituted during the first trimester, when major organogenesis occurs.

Summary

In summary, CCHB is a rare cardiac lesion with an incidence of about 1 in 20 000 live births. It can be divided into two groups: fetuses with CCHB associated with structural heart defects and fetuses with isolated CCHB. Isolated CCHB is usually associated with transplacental passage of maternal autoantibodies. The prognosis of fetal CCHB depends most importantly on ventricular escape rate, the presence of fetal hydrops and additional cardiac malformations. Treatment with sympathomimetic drugs can increase ventricular escape rate and improve cardiac contractility. In maternal autoantibody-associated CCHB, therapeutic lowering of antibodies has the potential to prevent the progression of heart block, and can improve fetal hydrops. In addition, prophylactic lowering of antibodies may be beneficial to prevent recurrence of fetal CCHB in some high-risk groups. Fetal cardiac pacing should be reserved for the rare fetus with CCHB and normal cardiac anatomy in cardiac failure refractory to medical therapy.

OTHER LESIONS

Premature closure of foramen ovale

The foramen ovale allows preferential streaming of umbilical venous return to the left heart during fetal life. Thus, oxygen-enriched blood is supplied to the coronary arteries and the developing brain[94]. Since the foramen ovale is traversed by about 40% of the blood returning via the ductus venosus and inferior caval vein, it provides the main source of blood flow to the left side of the fetal heart[45]. Premature closure or obstruction of the foramen ovale requires rerouting of blood flow through the right ventricle. The additional volume load on the right ventricle may result in right heart dilatation, cardiac failure and hydrops fetalis[6]. However, prenatal closure of the foramen ovale without fetal hydrops has also been described[95].

Premature closure of the foramen ovale may occur as a primary or secondary lesion, the latter in association with other cardiovascular anomalies. Primary closure of the foramen ovale early in gestation has been implicated in the development of the hypoplastic left heart syndrome[96,97]. This implication is supported by experimental studies in fetal lambs, in which hypoplasia of the left heart was induced by surgical closure of the foramen ovale in mid-gestation[46]. Secondary closure of the foramen ovale may occur in the presence of left ventricular inflow obstructions, mitral regurgitation and left atrial tachycardias[98–100]. These lesions may result in increased left atrial pressure, which keeps the septum primum in a closed position. This closure may be only functional; however, anatomical closure by secondary formation of adhesions can occur.

Differentiation between primary and secondary closure of the foramen ovale can be inferred from the location of the septum primum. In the case of primary closure, bulging of the septum primum through the foramen ovale into the left atrium has been described[101]. Conversely, in the case of secondary closure associated with increased left atrial pressures, bulging into the right atrium has been observed[98,102].

Prenatal intervention in premature closure of the foramen ovale has not yet been performed but could be achieved by either open surgical procedures or by fetal cardiac catheterization. Differentiation between primary and secondary forms of closure bears important implications for the success of these procedures. In the case of primary closure of the foramen ovale and hypoplasia of the left heart, prenatal opening of the foramen ovale has the potential to increase left heart blood flow and this may promote catch-up growth of left heart structures. In the case of secondary closure of the foramen ovale related to left ventricular inflow or outflow obstructions, prenatal opening of all obstructed structures seems necessary and opening the foramen ovale as the only procedure may not be useful.

Premature closure of ductus arteriosus

Premature closure of the ductus arteriosus is rare. It is usually related to tocolysis or treatment of polyhydramnios with indomethacin, and maternal administration of non-steroidal analgesics[103–105]. It has also been described after betamethasone treatment to induce fetal lung maturity[50]. With cessation of the responsible drug, ductal patency can usually be restored within 1–3 days and no invasive fetal therapy is needed[13]. In some fetuses, premature closure of the ductus arteriosus occurs unrelated to fetal or maternal therapy[106]. Hemodynamically, ductal closure results in right ventricular and pulmonary hypertension[107]. Right ventricular dilatation, tricuspid insufficiency and severe cardiac failure threatening fetal survival may ensue[50,108,109]. Fetal cardiac intervention in

these cases could be performed by open fetal cardiac surgery and aortopulmonary shunting.

Tetralogy of Fallot with absent pulmonary valve

Tetralogy of Fallot with absent pulmonary valve is a rare cardiac defect which may result in right ventricular dilatation, fetal cardiac failure and hydrops[110]. The to-and-fro flow pattern from the right ventricle into the pulmonary arteries leads to aneurysmal dilatation of the main and branch pulmonary arteries during fetal life (Figure 2). Pulmonary artery dilatation may be so severe that it interferes with normal development of fetal airways resulting in life-threatening respiratory failure after birth[111,112]. As an additional complicating factor, persistence of the ductus arteriosus, which is usually absent in this syndrome, may be encountered in some fetuses and has been associated with poor postnatal survival[113]. Prenatal intervention in severe cases by open fetal cardiac surgery may prevent or reverse aneurysmal dilatation of main and branch pulmonary arteries as well as compression of fetal airways. To prevent to-and-fro flow from the right ventricle into the pulmonary arteries, surgical creation of pulmonary atresia would be required. If a patent ductus arteriosus is found, it should be ligated. Pulmonary blood flow after surgery would be maintained by placement of a small-caliber aortopulmonary shunt. Over the remainder of gestation, reduction in pulmonary blood flow may allow normalization of pulmonary artery size as well as decompression and growth of adjacent airway structures.

FUTURE THERAPEUTIC APPROACHES

Fetal cardiac surgery

Although intracardiac surgical procedures have not yet been performed in human fetuses, many of the necessary techniques have been defined in animal experiments[16,21]. Cardiac bypass in fetal lambs (Figure 3) can now be performed with survival to term[114,115]. Fetal demise in

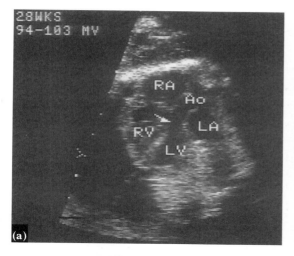

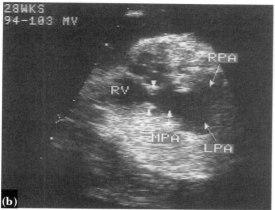

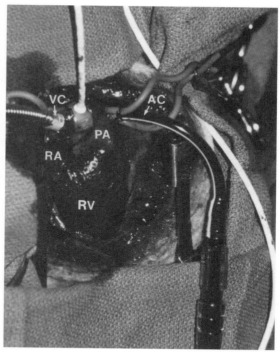

Figure 3 *Cardiac bypass in a late-gestation fetal lamb. A single venous cannula (VC) drains the venous blood from the right atrium (RA) to the pump circuit. The oxygenated blood returns to the heart via an arterial cannula (AC) that extends into the ductus arteriosus. Alternatively, peripheral cannulation of the carotid artery and jugular vein can be performed. RV, right ventricle; PA, pulmonary artery. (Courtesy of V. M. Reddy and F. L. Hanley)*

Figure 2 *Tetralogy of Fallot with absent pulmonary valve in cardiac failure at 28 weeks of gestation. (a) The aorta (Ao) is overriding the large ventricular septal defect (arrow). Note the significant amount of ascites. (b) In this lesion, massive aneurysmal dilatation of the main (MPA) as well as branch pulmonary arteries (RPA, LPA) interferes with the normal development of fetal airways which can result in life-threatening respiratory failure after birth. Rudimentary pulmonary valve tissue (arrow heads) is usually present. Fetal cardiac intervention in tetralogy of Fallot with absent pulmonary valve is directed towards normalization of pulmonary artery and airway development and requires open fetal surgery for creation of pulmonary atresia and aortopulmonary shunting. RA, right atrium; LA, left atrium; RV, right ventricle; LV, left ventricle. (Courtesy of N. H. Silverman)*

earlier experiments was related to placental dysfunction and fetal metabolic acidosis after bypass and has been overcome by several advances[16]. Among these advances are the inhibition of prostaglandin synthesis with indomethacin and corticosteroids, suppression of fetal stress response by total spinal anesthesia with tetracine, and removal of the placenta from the bypass circuit[114,116–121]. Utilizing a novel fetal bypass-circuit requiring no priming volume, eight of nine fetal lambs progressed to term and were delivered normally[115]. Placental function and fetal hemodynamics were preserved significantly better by this new circuit than with previous ones, and even pharmacological blunting of fetal stress response or inhibition of prostaglandin synthesis were not required. Actual techniques for fetal cardiac surgery (e.g. valvotomy, pacemaker-implantation) are technically straightforward procedures and resemble the postnatal approach to the respective lesions[16]. Cardiac monitoring during repair can be achieved by fetal transesophageal echocardiography[122].

Despite these remarkable advances in the development of surgical fetal cardiac intervention, it is important to keep in mind that most animal experiments to train and assess the feasibility of these procedures have been performed in fetal sheep. The sheep uterus, however, does not at all reflect the strong tendency of the human uterus for pharmacologically uncontrollable uterine contractions after hysterotomy for fetal repair. To date, the suppression of these contractions remains the Achilles' heel of current fetal surgical attempts in human fetuses[17] and will affect the safety of open fetal cardiac surgery.

Fetoscopic fetal cardiac catheterization

The effort to perform fetal cardiac catheterization and balloon valvuloplasty in fetal semilunar valvar obstructions is supported by the experience that postnatally this technique can be performed with similar results to surgical valvotomy[123]. Fetal cardiac catheterization is less invasive than open fetal cardiac surgery for both mother and fetus because fetal cardiovascular access can be achieved percutaneously by small punctures[13–15,18,38] and does not require maternal laparotomy, hysterotomy, fetal thoracotomy or cardiac bypass.

However, the experience gained from the initial fetal balloon valvuloplasties also illustrates that fetal cardiac catheterization may be improved by special equipment and a safer and more reliable method for fetal cardiovascular access. For example during fetal balloon valvuloplasty, parts of the balloon catheters impacted on the edge of the needle used for cardiac access and were cut off from the main body of the catheter[14,18,38]. In addition, repeated punctures of the heart were necessary to optimize positioning of interventional devices[14]. This strategy, however, increases the risk of bleeding complications and injury to healthy myocardium as well as other cardiovascular and intrathoracic structures. Although the acute mortality of the reported balloon valvuloplasties in human fetuses has been low (20%), direct

needle punctures of the fetal heart have accounted for severe bradycardia, asystole, hemopericardium, hematothorax, cardiac laceration and fetal death in these and other fetuses[14,124].

Alternatively, fetoscopic techniques under direct visualization may offer a safer means for fetal cardiac catheterization than ultrasound-guided direct punctures of the heart. Fetoscopic techniques to access the uterus and perform minor fetal surgical procedures have recently been described in human fetuses and in animal models[125–129]. These techniques may also be valuable to obtain access to the fetal circulation. Fetal cardiac catheterization for balloon valvuloplasty by itself will then resemble the postnatal approach.

The development of open and fetoscopic procedures for fetal cardiac intervention may require imaging capabilities not attended by conventional fetal echocardiography[122]. Conventional fetal echocardiography may interfere with the positioning of trocars and interventional devices or may be limited by unfavorable imaging windows or quality. Therefore, fetal intracardiac and transesophageal imaging utilizing an intravascular ultrasound catheter for cardiac monitoring have been developed in fetal lambs[122,130]. Both approaches permit real-time imaging of fetal cardiac anatomy, function and positioning of intravascular devices (Figure 4). Because it is less invasive, fetal transesophageal echocardiography seems at present to be more practicable than intracardiac echocardiography. Intraesophageal placement of the ultrasound catheter can be achieved by fetoscopy (Figure 5).

Fetoscopic cardiac catheterization for balloon valvuloplasty may also reduce the incidence of premature fetal delivery generally observed after open fetal surgery[131]. In addition, fetoscopic techniques may not require Cesarean section for fetal delivery since the uterus is accessed through minimal openings. Cesarean section, however, is obligatory after open fetal surgery for the treated as well as for any future child because of the risk of uterine rupture during normal delivery[131].

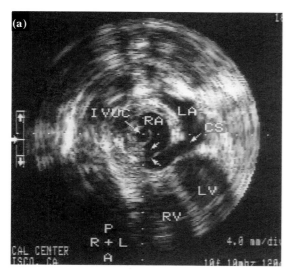

Figure 4 *Fetal intracardiac and transesophageal echocardiography utilizing an intravascular ultrasound catheter (IVUC) in fetal lambs. Basal four-chamber view of the fetal heart obtained by (a) intracardiac echocardiography at 132 days of gestation and (b) transesophageal echocardiography at 90 days of gestation. The basal imaging plane was chosen to delineate the course of the coronary sinus (CS). Both imaging positions permit detailed definition of fetal cardiac anatomy and positioning of interventional devices. (c) Shows intracardiac imaging of a deflated balloon valvuloplasty catheter in the ascending aorta (AoA) in a late-gestation fetus. RV, right ventricle; LV, left ventricle; RA, right atrium; LA, left atrium; LPA, left pulmonary artery; RPA, right pulmonary artery; T, trachea; A, anterior; P, posterior; L, left; R, right. Distance between markers is 4 mm*

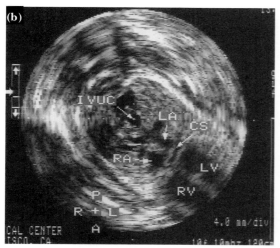

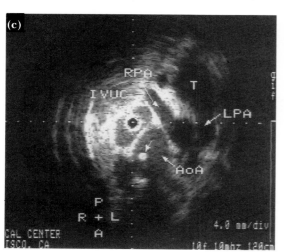

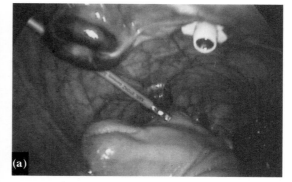

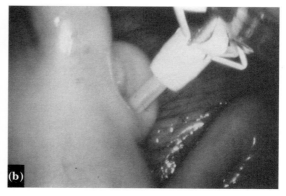

Figure 5 *Fetoscopic set-up for fetal transesophageal echocardiography in a fetal lamb at 95 days of gestation. Some amniotic fluid has been evacuated and a low pressure (3–5 mmHg) gaseous inflation of the uterus has been carried out to facilitate fetal visualization. A trocar has been placed above the fetal head (a) and a laparoscopic forceps is used for fetal head manipulation and imaging catheter insertion. (b) shows the inserted imaging catheter*

SUMMARY

Fetal cardiac intervention in congenital heart disease is a very recent subspecialty in prenatal medicine. Despite its invasive nature, fetal cardiac intervention may be beneficial for severe obstructions of the fetal semilunar valves, congenital complete heart block with normal cardiac anatomy resulting in heart failure refractory to medical therapy, and some other lesions. The goal of fetal cardiac intervention is to prevent, arrest, or reverse secondary cardiovascular damage or treat life-threatening fetal cardiac failure that can result from these lesions. To date, only a few, mostly ultrasound-guided interventions in severe obstructions of the fetal semilunar valves and in congenital complete heart block have been performed. The experience gained from these initial interventions demonstrates that the success of fetal cardiac intervention will ultimately depend on safer methods for fetal cardiovascular access and specific criteria for fetal selection. Remarkable advances in the development of procedures for fetal cardiac intervention have been made over the last few years. Cardiac bypass in fetal lambs can now be performed with survival to term and may soon be applicable in the human fetus. Alternatively, fetoscopic techniques for fetal cardiac catheterization seem possible to perform fetal balloon valvuloplasties or other interventional procedures. Based on the increasing amount of information about the prenatal history of fetal congenital heart disease and by extrapolating and inferring from known postnatal risk factors, the group of fetuses that is most likely to benefit from fetal cardiac intervention may be defined. Both technical advances and a rising awareness of the necessity to improve fetal selection offer great promise for fetal cardiac intervention in the near future.

ACKNOWLEDGEMENTS

I gratefully acknowledge the collaborative support of Drs Lindsey D. Allan and Rabih Chaoui as well as the editorial assistance of Ms Mimi Zeiger in preparing this manuscript. This work was supported by a research grant (Ko 1484/2-1) from the German Research Society (DFG).

References

1. Hornberger, L. K., Sahn, D. J., Kleinman, C. S., Copel, J. and Silverman, N. H. (1994). Antenatal diagnosis of coarctation of the aorta: a multicenter experience. *J. Am. Coll. Cardiol.*, **23**, 417–23

2. Allan, L. D., Crawford, D. C. and Tynan, M. J. (1984). Evolution of coarctation of the aorta in intrauterine life. *Br. Heart J.*, **52**, 471–3

3. Allan, L. D., Crawford, D. C. and Tynan, M. J. (1986). Pulmonary atresia in prenatal life. *J. Am. Coll. Cardiol.*, **8**, 1131–6

4. Allan, L. D., Sharland, G. K. and Tynan, M. J. (1989). The natural history of the hypoplastic left heart syndrome. *Int. J. Cardiol.*, **25**, 341–3

5. Allan, L. D. and Sharland, G. K. (1992). Prognosis in fetal tetralogy of Fallot. *Pediatr. Cardiol.*, **13**, 1–4

6. Chobot, V., Hornberger, L. K., Hagen-Ansert, S. and Sahn, D. J. (1990). Prenatal detection of restrictive foramen ovale. *J. Am. Soc. Echocardiogr.*, **3**, 15–19

7. Danford, D. A. and Cronican, P. (1992). Hypoplastic left heart syndrome: progression of left ventricular dilation and dysfunction to left ventricular hypoplasia *in utero*. *Am. Heart J.*, **123**, 1712–13

8. Holley, D. G., Martin, G. R., Brenner, J. I., Fyfe, D. A., Huhta, J. C., Kleinman, C. S., Ritter, S. B. and Silverman, N. H. (1995). Diagnosis and management of fetal cardiac tumors: a multicenter experience and review of published reports. *J. Am. Coll. Cardiol.*, **26**, 516–20

9. Hornberger, L. K., Sanders, S. P., Rein, A. J., Spevak, P. J., Parness, I. A. and Colan, S. D. (1995). Left heart obstructive lesions and left ventricular growth in the midtrimester fetus. A longitudinal study. *Circulation*, **92**, 1531–8

10. Hornberger, L. K., Sanders, S. P., Sahn, D. J., Rice, M. J., Spevak, P. J., Benacerraf, B. R., McDonald, R. W. and Colan, S. D. (1995). *In utero* pulmonary artery and aortic growth and potential for progression of pulmonary outflow

tract obstruction in tetralogy of Fallot. *J. Am. Coll. Cardiol.*, **25**, 739–45

11. Rice, M. J., McDonald, R. W. and Reller, M. D. (1993). Progressive pulmonary stenosis in the fetus: two case reports. *Am. J. Perinatol.*, **10**, 424–7

12. Todros, T., Presbitero, P., Gaglioti, P. and Demarie, P. (1988). Pulmonary stenosis with intact ventricular septum: documentation of development of the lesion echocardiographically during fetal life. *Int. J. Cardiol.*, **8**, 1131–6

13. Huhta, J. C. (1996). Fetal echocardiography in the detection and management of fetal heart disease. In Spitzer, A. R. (ed.) *Intensive Care of the Fetus and Neonate*, pp. 772–86. (St Louis, Baltimore, Boston: Mosby)

14. Maxwell, D., Allan, L. and Tynan, M. J. (1991). Balloon dilatation of the aortic valve in the fetus: a report of two cases. *Br. Heart J.*, **65**, 256–8

15. Chaoui, R., Bollmann, R., Goeldner, B. and Rogalski, V. (1994). Aortic balloon valvuloplasty in the human fetus under ultrasound guidance: a report of two cases. *Ultrasound Obstet. Gynecol.*, **4** (Suppl.), 162A

16. Hanley, F. L. (1994). Fetal cardiac surgery. *Adv. Card. Surg.*, **5**, 47–74

17. Harrison, M. R. (1993). Fetal surgery. *West. J. Med.*, **159**, 341–9

18. Lopes, L. M., Cha, S. C., Kajita, L. J., Aiello, V. D., Jatene, A. and Zugaib, M. (1995). Balloon dilatation of the aortic valve in the fetus – a case report. *Fetal Diagn. Ther.*, in press

19. Wright, J. G. C., Skinner, J. R. and Stumper, O. (1994). Radiofrequency assisted pulmonary valvotomy in a fetus with pulmonary atresia and intact ventricular septum. Presented at the *13th Meeting of The International Fetal Medicine and Surgery Society*, Antwerp, Belgium, May

20. Walkinshaw, S. A., Welch, C. R., McCormack, J. and Walsh, K. (1994). *In utero* pacing for fetal congenital heart block. *Fetal Diagn. Ther.*, **9**, 183–5

21. Turley, K., Vlahakes, G. J., Harrison, M. R., Messina, L., Hanley, F., Uhlig, P. N. and Ebert, P. A. (1982). Intrauterine cardiothoracic surgery: the fetal lamb model. *Ann. Thorac. Surg.*, **34**, 422–6

22. Carpenter, R. Jr, Strasburger, J. F., Garson, A. Jr, Smith, R. T., Deter, R. L. and Engelhardt, H. Jr (1986). Fetal ventricular pacing for hydrops secondary to complete atrioventricular block. *J. Am. Coll. Cardiol.*, **8**, 1434–6

23. Adzick, N. S. and Harrison, M. R. (1994). The unborn surgical patient. *Curr. Probl. Surg.*, **31**, 1–76

24. Dunn, J. M., Weil, S. R. and Russo, P. (1993). Management of fetal cardiac anomalies. In Hanson, M. A., Spencer, J. A. D. and Rodeck, C. H. (eds.) *Fetus and Neonate. Physiology and Clinical Applications – The Circulation*, pp 377–95. (Cambridge: Cambridge University Press)

25. Fyler, D. C., Buckley, L. P., Hellenbrand, W. E. and Cohn, H. E. (1980). Report of the New England Regional Infant Care Program. *Pediatrics*, **65**, 375–461

26. Allan, L. D., Sharland, G. K., Milburn, A., Lockhart, S. M., Groves, A. M., Anderson, R. H., Cook, A. C. and Fagg, N. L. (1994). Prospective diagnosis of 1006 consecutive cases of congenital heart disease in the fetus. *J. Am. Coll. Cardiol.*, **23**, 1452–8

27. Hornberger, L. K., Benacerraf, B. R., Bromley, B. S., Spevak, P. J. and Sanders, S. P. (1994). Prenatal detection of severe right ventricular outflow tract obstruction: pulmonary stenosis and pulmonary atresia. *J. Ultrasound Med.*, **13**, 743–50

28. Sharland, G. K., Chita, S. K., Fagg, N. L., Anderson, R. H., Tynan, M. J., Cook, A. C. and Allan, L. D. (1991). Left ventricular dysfunction in the fetus: relation to aortic valve anomalies and endocardial fibroelastosis. *Br. Heart J.*, **66**, 419–24

29. Forbess, J. M., Cook, N., Roth, S. J., Serraf, A., Mayer, J. E. and Jonas, R. A. (1995). Ten-year institutional experience with palliative surgery for hypoplastic left heart syndrome. *Circulation*, **92** (Suppl. II), 262–6

30. Norwood, W. I., Lang, P. and Hansen, D. D. (1983). Physiologic repair of aortic atresia-hypoplastic left heart syndrome. *N. Engl. J. Med.*, **308**, 23–6

31. Hanley, F. L., Sade, R. M., Blackstone, E. H., Kirklin, J. W., Freedom, R. M. and Nanda, N. C. (1993). Outcomes in neonatal pulmonary atresia with intact ventricular septum. A multi-institutional study. *J. Thorac. Cardiovasc. Surg.*, **105**, 406–27

32. Chinnock, R. E., Larsen, R. L., Emery, J. R. and Bailey, L. L. (1995). Pretransplant risk factors and causes of death or graft loss after heart transplantation during early infancy. *Circulation*, **92** (Suppl. II), 206–9

33. Bailey, L. L., Nehlsen-Cannarella, S. L., Doroshow, R. W., Jacobson, J. G., Martin, R. D., Allard, M. W., Hyde, M. R., Dang Bui, R. H. and Petry, E. L. (1986). Cardiac allotransplantation in newborns as therapy for hypoplastic left heart syndrome. *N. Engl. J. Med.*, **315**, 949–51

34. Bailey, L. L., Gundry, S. R., Razzouk, A. J., Wang, N., Sciolaro, C. M. and Chiavarelli, M. (1993). Bless the babies: one hundred and fifteen late survivors of heart transplantation during the first year of life. The Loma Linda

University Pediatric Heart Transplant Group. *J. Thorac. Cardiovasc. Surg.*, **105**, 805–15

35. Chiavarelli, M., Gundry, S. R., Razzouk, A. J. and Bailey, L. L. (1993). Cardiac transplantation for infants with hypoplastic left heart syndrome. *J. Am. Med. Assoc.*, **270**, 2944–7

36. Doroshow, R. W., Ashwal, S. and Saukel, G. W. (1995). Availability and selection of donors for pediatric heart transplantation. *J. Heart Lung Transplant.*, **14**, 52–8

37. Pahl, E., Zales, V. R., Fricker, F. J. and Addonizio, L. J. (1994). Post-transplant coronary artery disease in children. A multicenter national survey. *Circulation*, **90** (Suppl. II), 56–60

38. Allan, L. D., Maxwell, D. J., Carminati, M. and Tynan, M. J. (1995). Survival after fetal aortic balloon valvoplasty. *Ultrasound Obstet. Gynecol.*, **5**, 90–1

39. Blake, D. M., Copel, J. A. and Kleinman, C. S. (1991). Hypoplastic left heart syndrome: prenatal diagnosis, clinical profile, and management. *Am. J. Obstet. Gynecol.*, **165**, 529–34

40. Chang, A. C., Huhta, J. C., Yoon, G. Y., Wood, D. C., Tulzer, G., Cohen, A., Mennuti, M. and Norwood, W. I. (1991). Diagnosis, transport, and outcome in fetuses with left ventricular outflow tract obstruction. *J. Thorac. Cardiovasc. Surg.*, **102**, 841–8

41. Yasukochi, S., Satomi, G. and Harada, Y. (1995). Successful neonatal balloon aortic valvuloplasty following prenatal diagnosis of critical aortic stenosis. *Cardiol. Young*, **5**, 363–6

42. Robertson, M. A., Byrne, P. J. and Penkoske, P. A. (1989). Perinatal management of critical aortic valve stenosis diagnosed by fetal echocardiography. *Br. Heart J.*, **61**, 365–7

43. Huhta, J. C., Carpenter, R. Jr, Moise, K. Jr, Deter, R. L., Ott, D. A. and McNamara, D. G. (1987). Prenatal diagnosis and postnatal management of critical aortic stenosis. *Circulation*, **75**, 573–6

44. Rudolph, A. M. (1974). The fetal circulation. In *Congenital Heart Disease*, pp. 1–16. (Chicago: Year Book Medical Publishers)

45. Rudolph, A. M. (1974). *Congenital Diseases of the Heart*. (Chicago: Year Book Medical Publishers)

46. Fishman, N. H., Hof, R. B., Rudolph, A. M. and Heymann, M. A. (1978). Models of congenital heart disease in fetal lambs. *Circulation*, **58**, 354–64

47. Vincent, R N., Menticoglou, S., Chanas, D., Manning, F., Collins, G. F. and Smallhorn, J. (1987). Prenatal diagnosis of an unusual form of hypoplastic left heart syndrome. *J. Ultrasound Med.*, **6**, 261–4

48. McCaffrey, F. M. and Sherman, F. S. (1994). Prenatal diagnosis of severe aortic stenosis. *Pediatr. Cardiol.*, **15**, 255A

49. Mocellin, R., Sauer, U., Simon, B., Comazzi, M., Sebening, F. and Buhlmeyer, K. (1983). Reduced left ventricular size and endocardial fibroelastosis as correlates of mortality in newborns and young infants with severe aortic valve stenosis. *Pediatr. Cardiol.*, **4**, 265–72

50. Azancot-Benisty, A., Benifla, J. L., Matias, A., De Crepy, A. and Madelenat, P. (1995). Constriction of the fetal ductus arteriosus during prenatal betamethasone therapy. *Obstet. Gynecol.*, **85**, 874–6

51. Saenger, J. S., Mayer, D. C., D'Angelo, L. J. and Manci, E. A. (1992). Ductus-dependent fetal cardiac defects contraindicate indomethacin tocolysis. *J. Perinatol.*, **12**, 41–7

52. Rhodes, L. A., Colan, S. D., Perry, S. B., Jonas, R. A. and Sanders, S. P. (1991). Predictors of survival in neonates with critical aortic stenosis. *Circulation*, **84**, 2325–35

53. Hornberger, L. K., Spevak, P. J., McDonald, R. W., Rice, M. J., Martin, G. R., Sanders, S. P., Colan, S. D. and Sahn, D. J. (1995). *In utero* pulmonary outflow obstruction: natural history and predictors of postnatal severity. *J. Am. Coll. Cardiol.*, **25**, 349A

54. Yock, P. G. and Popp, R. L. (1984). Noninvasive estimation of right ventricular systolic pressure by Doppler ultrasound in patients with tricuspid regurgitation. *Circulation*, **70**, 657–62

55. Michaelsson, M. and Engle, M. A. (1972). Congenital complete heart block: an international study of the natural history. *Cardiovasc. Clin.*, **4**, 85–101

56. Wladimiroff, J. W., Stewart, P. A. and Tonge, H. M. (1988). Fetal bradyarrhythmia: diagnosis and outcome. *Prenat. Diagn.*, **8**, 53–7

57. Allan, L. D., Anderson, R. H., Sullivan, I. D., Campbell, S., Holt, D. W. and Tynan, M. J. (1983). Evaluation of fetal arrhythmias by echocardiography. *Br. Heart J.*, **50**, 240–5

58. Kleinman, C. S., Donnerstein, R. L., Jaffe, C. C., DeVore, G. R., Weinstein, E. M., Lynch, D. C., Talner, N. S., Berkowitz, R. L. and Hobbins, J. C. (1983). Fetal echocardiography. A tool for evaluation of *in utero* cardiac arrhythmias and monitoring of *in utero* therapy: analysis of 71 patients. *Am. J. Cardiol.*, **51**, 237–43

59. Silverman, N. H., Enderlein, M. A., Stanger, P., Teitel, D. F., Heymann, M. A. and Golbus, M. S. (1985). Recognition of fetal arrhythmias by echocardiography. *J. Clin. Ultrasound*, **13**, 255–63

60. Schmidt, K. G., Ulmer, H. E., Silverman, N. H., Kleinman, C. S. and Copel, J. A. (1991). Perinatal outcome of fetal complete

atrioventricular block: a multicenter experience. *J. Am. Coll. Cardiol.*, **17**, 1360–6

61. Shenker, L., Reed, K. L., Anderson, C. F., Marx, G. R., Sobonya, R. E. and Graham, A. R. (1987). Congenital heart block and cardiac anomalies in the absence of maternal connective tissue disease. *Am. J. Obstet. Gynecol.*, **157**, 248–53

62. Garcia, O. L., Metha, A. V., Pickoff, A S., Tamer, D. F., Ferrer, P. L., Wolff, G. S. and Gelband, H. (1981). Left isomerism and complete atrioventricular block: a report of six cases. *Am. J. Cardiol.*, **48**, 1103–7

63. Buyon, J. P., Swersky, S. H., Fox, H. E., Bierman, F. Z. and Winchester, R. J. (1987). Intrauterine therapy for presumptive fetal myocarditis with acquired heart block due to systemic lupus erythematosus. Experience in a mother with a predominance of SSB (La) antibodies. *Arthritis Rheum.*, **30**, 44–9

64. Buyon, J. P. (1989). Neonatal lupus and congenital complete heart block: manifestations of passively acquired autoimmunity. *Clin. Exp. Rheumatol.*, **7**, S199–203

65. Buyon, J. P., Ben-Chetrit, E., Karp, S., Roubey, R. A., Pompeo, L., Reeves, W. H., Tan, E. M. and Winchester, R. J. (1989). Acquired congenital heart block. Pattern of maternal antibody response to biochemically defined antigens of the SSA/Ro-SSB/La system in neonatal lupus. *J. Clin. Invest.*, **84**, 627–34

66. Carreira, P. E., Gutierrez-Larraya, F. and Gomez-Reino, J. J. (1993). Successful intrauterine therapy with dexamethasone for fetal myocarditis and heart block in a woman with systemic lupus erythematosus. *J. Rheumatol.*, **20**, 1204–7

67. Knolle, P., Mayet, W., Lohse, A. W., Treichel, U., Meyer zum Buschenfelde, K. H. and Gerken, G. (1994). Complete congenital heart block in autoimmune hepatitis (SLA-positive). *J. Hepatol.*, **21**, 224–6

68. Olah, K. S. and Gee, H. (1991). Fetal heart block associated with maternal anti-Ro (SSA) antibody – current management. A review. *Br. J. Obstet. Gynaecol.*, **98**, 751–5

69. Petri, M., Watson, R. and Hochberg, M. C. (1989). Anti-Ro antibodies and neonatal lupus. *Rheum. Dis. Clin. North Am.*, **15**, 335–60

70. Ramsey-Goldman, R., Hom, D., Deng, J. S., Ziegler, G. C., Kahl, L. E., Steen, V. D., LaPorte, R. E. and Medsger, T. Jr (1986). Anti-SSA antibodies and fetal outcome in maternal systemic lupus erythematosus. *Arthritis Rheum.*, **29**, 1269–73

71. Watson, W. J. and Katz, V. L. (1991). Steroid therapy for hydrops associated with antibody-mediated congenital heart block. *Am. J. Obstet. Gynecol.*, **165**, 553–4

72. Richards, D. S., Wagman, A. J. and Cabaniss, M. L. (1990). Ascites not due to congestive heart failure in a fetus with lupus-induced heart block. *Obstet. Gynecol.*, **76**, 957–9

73. Arroyave, C. M., Puente Ledezma, F., Montiel Amoroso, G. and Martinez Garcia, A. C. (1995). Myocardiopathy diagnosed *in utero* in a mother with SSA antibodies treated with plasmapheresis. *Ginecol. Obstet. Mex.*, **63**, 134–7

74. Buyon, J., Roubey, R., Swersky, S., Pompeo, L., Parke, A., Baxi, L. and Winchester, R. J. (1988). Complete congenital heart block: risk of occurrence and therapeutic approach to prevention. *J. Rheumatol.*, **15**, 1104–8

75. Machado, M. V., Tynan, M. J., Curry, P. V. and Allan, L. D. (1988). Fetal complete heart block. *Br. Heart J.*, **60**, 512–15

76. Reller, M. D., Morton, M. J., Reid, D. L. and Thornburg, K. L. (1987). Fetal lamb ventricles respond differently to filling and arterial pressures and to *in utero* ventilation. *Pediatr. Res.*, **22**, 621–6

77. Koyanagi, T., Hara, K., Satoh, S., Yoshizato, T. and Nakano, H. (1990). Relationship between heart rate and rhythm, and cardiac performance assessed in the human fetus *in utero*. *Int. J. Cardiol.*, **28**, 163–71

78. Veille, J. C. and Covitz, W. (1994). Fetal cardiovascular hemodynamics in the presence of complete atrioventricular block. *Am. J. Obstet. Gynecol.*, **170**, 1258–62

79. Crombleholme, T. M., Harrison, M. R., Longaker, M. T., Langer, J. C., Adzick, N. S., Bradley, S., Duncan, B. and Verrier, E. D. (1990). Complete heart block in fetal lambs. I. Technique and acute physiological response. *J. Pediatr. Surg.*, **25**, 587–93

80. Harris, J. P., Alexson, C. G., Manning, J. A. and Thompson, H. O. (1993). Medical therapy for the hydropic fetus with congenital complete atrioventricular block. *Am. J. Perinatol.*, **10**, 217–19

81. Sokol, R. J., Hutchison, P., Krouskop, R. W., Brown, E. G., Reed, G. and Vasquez, H. (1974). Congenital complete heart block diagnosed during intrauterine fetal monitoring. *Am. J. Obstet. Gynecol.*, **120**, 1115–17

82. Weber, H. S. and Myers, J. L. (1994). Maternal collagen vascular disease associated with fetal heart block and degenerative changes of the atrioventricular valves. *Pediatr. Cardiol.*, **15**, 204–6

83. Whitsett, J. A., Pollinger, J. and Matz, S. (1982). Beta-adrenergic receptors and catecholamine sensitive adenylate cyclase in developing rat ventricular myocardium: effect of thyroid status. *Pediatr. Res.*, **16**, 463–9

84. Copel, J. A., Buyon, J. P. and Kleinman, C. S. (1995). Successful *in utero* therapy of fetal heart block. *Am. J. Obstet. Gynecol.*, **173**, 1384–90

85. Blanford, A. T. and Murphy, B. E. (1977). *In vitro* metabolism of prednisolone, dexamethasone, betamethasone, and cortisol by the human placenta. *Am. J. Obstet. Gynecol.*, **127**, 264–7

86. Beitins, I. Z., Bayard, F., Ances, I. G., Kowarski, A. and Migeon, C. J. (1972). The transplacental passage of prednisone and prednisolone in pregnancy near term. *J. Pediatr.*, **81**, 936–45

87. Scagliotti, D., Shimokochi, D. D. and Pringle, K. C. (1987). Permanent cardiac pacemaker implant in the fetal lamb. *Pace. Pacing Clin. Electrophysiol.*, **10**, 1253–61

88. Rote, N. (1985). Maternal fetal immunology. In Scott, J. and Rote, N. (eds.) *Immunology in Obstetrics and Gynecology*, pp. 55–76. (Norwalk, CT: Appleton-Century-Crofts)

89. Stiehm, E. R. (1975). Fetal defense mechanisms. *Am. J. Dis. Child.*, **129**, 438–43

90. Reichlin, M., Friday, K. and Harley, J. B. (1988). Complete congenital heart block followed by anti-Ro/SSA in adult life. Studies of an informative family. *Am. J. Med.*, **84**, 339–44

91. Barclay, C. S., French, M. A., Ross, L. D. and Sokol, R. J. (1987). Successful pregnancy following steroid therapy and plasma exchange in a woman with anti-Ro (SSA) antibodies. Case report. *Br. J. Obstet. Gynaecol.*, **94**, 369–71

92. Kaaja, R., Julkunen, H., Ammala, P., Teppo, A. M. and Kurki, P. (1991). Congenital heart block: successful prophylactic treatment with intravenous gamma globulin and corticosteroid therapy. *Am. J. Obstet. Gynecol.*, **165**, 1333–4

93. van der Leij, J. N., Visser, G. H., Bink-Boelkens, M. T., Meilof, J. F. and Kallenberg, C. G. (1994). Successful outcome of pregnancy after treatment of maternal anti-Ro (SSA) antibodies with immunosuppressive therapy and plasmapheresis. *Prenat. Diagn.*, **14**, 1003–7

94. Edelstone, D. I. and Rudolph, A. M. (1979). Preferential streaming of ductus venosus blood to the brain and heart in fetal lambs. *Am. J. Physiol.*, **237**, H724–9

95. Phillipos, E. Z., Robertson, M. A. and Still, D. K. (1990). Prenatal detection of foramen ovale obstruction without hydrops fetalis. *J. Am. Soc. Echocardiogr.*, **3**, 495–8

96. Lev, M., Arcilla, R., Rimoldi, H. J., Licata, R. M. and Gasul, B. M. (1963). Premature narrowing of the foramen ovale. *Am. Heart J.*, **65**, 638–47

97. Raghib, G., Bloemendahl, R. D., Kanjuh, V. I. and Edwards, J. E. (1965). Aortic atresia and premature closure of the foramen ovale. *Am. Heart J.*, **70**, 476–80

98. Bharati, S., Patel, A. G., Varga, P., Husain, A. N. and Lev, M. (1991). *In utero* echocardiographic diagnosis of premature closure of the foramen ovale with mitral regurgitation and large left atrium. *Am. Heart J.*, **122**, 597–600

99. Kleinman, C. S., Dubin, A. M., Nehgme, R. A., Rosenfeld, L. E. and Copel, J. A. (1996). Left atrial tachycardia in the human fetus: identifying the fetus at greatest risk for developing nonimmune hydrops fetalis. *Ultrasound Obstet. Gynecol.*, in press

100. Buis-Liem, T. N., Ottenkamp, J., Meerman, R. H. and Verwey, R. (1987). The concurrence of fetal supraventricular tachycardia and obstruction of the foramen ovale. *Prenat. Diagn.*, **7**, 425–31

101. de Groot, R., Essed, C. E., Gaillard, J. L., Mettau, J. W. and Villeneuve, V. H. (1984). Primary restrictive foramen ovale. *Eur. J. Pediatr.*, **141**, 248–9

102. Pesonen, E., Haavisto, H., Ammala, P. and Teramo, K. (1983). Intrauterine hydrops caused by premature closure of the foramen ovale. *Arch. Dis. Child.*, **58**, 1015–16

103. Respondek, M., Weil, S. R. and Huhta, J. C. (1995). Fetal echocardiography during indomethacin treatment. *Ultrasound Obstet. Gynecol.*, **5**, 86–9

104. Rasanen, J. and Jouppila, P. (1995). Fetal cardiac function and ductus arteriosus during indomethacin and sulindac therapy for threatened preterm labor: a randomized study. *Am. J. Obstet. Gynecol.*, **173**, 20–5

105. Carmona, F., Martinez-Roman, S., Mortera, C., Puerto, B., Cararach, V. and Iglesias, X. (1993). Efficacy and safety of indomethacin therapy for polyhydramnios. *Eur. J. Obstet. Gynecol. Reprod. Biol.*, **52**, 175–80

106. Chao, R. C., Ho, E. S. and Hsieh, K. S. (1993). Doppler echocardiographic diagnosis of intrauterine closure of the ductus arteriosus. *Prenat. Diagn.*, **13**, 989–94

107. Huhta, J. C., Cohen, A. W. and Wood, D. C. (1990). Premature constriction of the ductus arteriosus. *J. Am. Soc. Echocardiogr.*, **3**, 30–4

108. Arcilla, R. A., Thilenius, O. G. and Ranniger, K. (1969). Congestive heart failure from suspected ductal closure *in utero*. *J. Pediatr.*, **75**, 74–8

109. Becker, A. E., Becker, M. J. and Wagenvoort, C. A. (1977). Premature contraction of the ductus arteriosus: a cause of foetal death. *J. Pathol.*, **121**, 187–91

110. Sameshima, H., Nishibatake, M., Ninomiya, Y. and Tokudome, T. (1993). Antenatal diagnosis of tetralogy of Fallot with absent pulmonary valve accompanied by hydrops fetalis and polyhydramnios. *Fetal Diagn. Ther.*, **8**, 305–8

111. Watterson, K. G., Malm, T. K., Karl, T. R. and Mee, R. B. (1992). Absent pulmonary valve syndrome: operation in infants with airway obstruction. *Ann. Thorac. Surg.*, **54**, 1116–19

112. Heinemann, M. K. and Hanley, F. L. (1993). Preoperative management of neonatal tetralogy of Fallot with absent pulmonary valve syndrome. *Ann. Thorac. Surg.*, **55**, 172–4

113. Ettedgui, J. A., Sharland, G. K., Chita, S. K., Cook, A., Fagg, N. and Allan, L. D. (1990). Absent pulmonary valve syndrome with ventricular septal defect: role of the arterial duct. *Am. J. Cardiol.*, **66**, 233–4

114. Fenton, K. N., Zinn, H. E., Heinemann, M. K., Liddicoat, J. R. and Hanley, F. L. (1994). Longterm survivors of fetal cardiac bypass in lambs. *J. Thorac. Cardiovasc. Surg.*, **107**, 1423–7

115. Reddy, V. M., Liddicoat, J. R., Klein, J. R., Wangler, R. K. and Hanley, F. L. (1996). Longterm fetal outcome after fetal cardiac bypass: fetal survival to full term and organ pathology. *J. Thorac. Cardiovasc. Surg.*, **111**, 536–44

116. Fenton, K. N., Heinemann, M. K., Hickey, P. R., Klautz, R. J., Liddicoat, J. R., Hanley, F. L. (1994). Inhibition of the fetal stress response improves cardiac output and gas exchange after fetal cardiac bypass. *J. Thorac. Cardiovasc. Surg.*, **107**, 1416–22

117. Fenton, K. N., Heinemann, M. K. and Hanley, F. L. (1993). Exclusion of the placenta during fetal cardiac bypass augments systemic flow and provides important information about the mechanism of placental injury. *J. Thorac. Cardiovasc. Surg.*, **105**, 502–10

118. Bradley, S. M., Hanley, F. L., Duncan, B. W., Jennings, R. W., Jester, J. A., Harrison, M. R. and Verrier, E. D. (1992). Fetal cardiac bypass alters regional blood flows, arterial blood gases, and hemodynamics in sheep. *Am. J. Physiol.*, **263**, H919–28

119. Hawkins, J. A., Clark, S. M., Shaddy, R. E. and Gay, W. Jr (1994). Fetal cardiac bypass: improved placental function with moderately high flow rates. *Ann. Thorac. Surg.*, **57**, 293–7

120. Sabik, J. F., Assad, R. S. and Hanley, F. L. (1992). Prostaglandin synthesis inhibition prevents placental dysfunction after fetal cardiac bypass. *J. Thorac. Cardiovasc. Surg.*, **103**, 733–42

121. Sabik, J. F., Heinemann, M. K., Assad, R. S. and Hanley, F. L. (1994). High-dose steroids prevent placental dysfunction after fetal cardiac bypass. *J. Thorac. Cardiovasc. Surg.*, **107**, 116–24

122. Kohl, T., Szabo, Z., VanderWall, K. J., Hutchison, S. J., Stelnicki, E. J., Meuli, M., Harrison, M. R., Silverman, N. H. and Chou, T. M. (1996). Experimental fetal transesophageal and intracardiac echocardiography utilizing an intravascular ultrasound catheter. *Am. J. Cardiol.*, **77**, 899–903

123. Zeevi, B., Keane, J. F., Castaneda, A. R., Perry, S. B. and Lock, J. E. (1989). Neonatal critical valvar aortic stenosis. A comparison of surgical and balloon dilation therapy. *Circulation*, **80**, 831–9

124. Westgren, M., Selbing, A. and Stangenberg, M. (1988). Fetal intracardiac transfusions in patients with severe rhesus isoimmunisation. *Br. Med. J.*, **296**, 885–6

125. Estes, J. M., Szabo, Z. and Harrison, M. R. (1992). Techniques for *in utero* endoscopic surgery. A new approach for fetal intervention. *Surg. Endosc.*, **6**, 215–18

126. Estes, J. M., MacGillivray, T. E., Hedrick, M. H., Adzick, N. S. and Harrison, M. R. (1992). Fetoscopic surgery for the treatment of congenital anomalies. *J. Pediatr. Surg.*, **27**, 950–4

127. Quintero, R. A., Reich, H., Puder, K. S., Bardicef, M., Evans, M. I., Cotton, D. B. and Romero, R. (1994). Brief report: umbilical-cord ligation of an acardiac twin by fetoscopy at 19 weeks of gestation. *N. Engl. J. Med.*, **330**, 469–71

128. Quintero, R. A., Hume, R., Smith, C., Johnson, M. P., Cotton, D. B., Romero, R. and Evans, M. I. (1995). Percutaneous fetal cytoscopy and endoscopic fulguration of posterior urethral valves. *Am. J. Obstet. Gynecol.*, **172**, 206–9

129. VanderWall, K. J., Meuli, M., Szabo, Z., Bruch, S. W., Kohl, T., Hoffman, W. Y., Adzick, N. S. and Harrison, M. R. (1996). Percutaneous access to the uterus for fetal surgery. *J. Laparoendosc. Surg.*, in press

130. Kohl, T., Stelnicki, E. J., VanderWall, K. J., Szabo, Z., Ko, E., Bruch, S. W., Harrison, M. R., Silverman, N. H., Hanley, F. L. and Chou, T. M. (1996). Transesophageal echocardiography in fetal sheep – a new monitoring tool for open and fetoscopic cardiac procedures. *Surg. Endosc.*, in press

131. Longaker, M. T., Golbus, M. S., Filly, R. A., Rosen, M. A., Chang, S. W. and Harrison, M. R. (1991). Maternal outcome after open fetal surgery. A review of the first 17 human cases. *J. Am. Med. Assoc.*, **265**, 737–41

Thoracoamniotic shunting for fetal pleural effusions

23

N. J. Sebire and K. H. Nicolaides

INTRODUCTION

Prolonged intrathoracic compression of the fetal lung, by conditions such as pleural effusions, is associated with pulmonary hypoplasia and neonatal death. Additionally, in some cases mediastinal compression leads to the development of fetal hydrops with a high risk of perinatal death. The extent to which these complications can be prevented by intrauterine decompression is being investigated in both animal and human studies.

PLEURAL EFFUSIONS

Hydrops fetalis, with an incidence of about one per 1000 pregnancies, is characterized by generalized skin edema and pericardial, pleural, or ascitic effusions. This is a non-specific finding in a wide variety of fetal[1] and maternal disorders, including hematological, chromosomal, cardiovascular, pulmonary, gastrointestinal, hepatic and metabolic abnormalities, congenital infection, neoplasms and malformations of the placenta or umbilical cord. While in many cases the cause may be determined, frequently the abnormality remains unexplained even after fetal blood sampling or expert postmortem examination.

Fetal pleural effusions may be an isolated finding or they may occur in association with generalized edema and ascites. Irrespective of the underlying cause, infants affected by pleural effusions usually present in the neonatal period with severe, and often fatal, respiratory insufficiency. This is either a direct result of pulmonary compression caused by the effusions, or due to pulmonary hypoplasia secondary to chronic intrathoracic compression. The overall mortality of neonates with pleural effusions is 25%, with a range from 15% in infants with isolated pleural effusions to 95% in those with gross hydrops[1]. Chromosomal abnormalities, mainly trisomy 21, are found in about 6% of fetuses with apparently isolated pleural effusions.

PULMONARY DEVELOPMENT

In the human, the bronchial tree is fully developed by the 16th week of gestation at which time the full adult number of airways is established. The aveoli continue to develop even after birth, increasing in number and size until the growth of the chest wall is completed in adulthood. The growth of blood vessels supplying the acinus (intra-acinar vessels) parallels alveolar development, while the growth of pre-acinar vessels follows the development of the airways[2].

Animal studies

Studies in the sheep have shown that the inflation of a balloon in the fetal thorax from day 100 of development to term results in respiratory insufficiency at birth which is not improved by postnatal decompression[3]. Lambs with inflated intrathoracic balloons, although vigorous at delivery, developed progressive hypoxemia, hypercapnia and acidemia and died of respiratory insufficiency despite maximal resuscitation and ventilatory support. Deflation of the intrathoracic balloon in the neonatal period did not improve survival, because the lungs were already hypoplastic with decreased compliance and decreased cross-sectional area of pulmonary vessels. In contrast, prenatal decompression, on day 120 of gestation, was associated with improved postnatal survival, and a significant increase in lung weight, air capacity, compliance and area of the pulmonary vascular bed[3].

CONSERVATIVE MANAGEMENT

A series of case reports have described the spontaneous antenatal resolution of pleural effusions within 2–12 weeks of diagnosis at 16–32 weeks of gestation (Table 1). In addition, spontaneous resolution occurred in a total of five (15%) of 33 fetuses in two series examining the natural history of antenatally-diagnosed pleural effusions[7,9] (Table 1).

There are also several cases of antenatally-diagnosed pleural effusions that were managed conservatively and, although the effusions did not resolve, the babies survived after appropriate postnatal treatment (Table 2).

In contrast, there are many reported cases of fetal pleural effusions that were managed con-servatively where the outcome was poor, either intrauterine or early neonatal death mainly due to pulmonary hypoplasia (Table 3).

Intrapartum thoracocentesis

Thoracocentesis involves the aspiration of fluid from the pleural cavity of the fetus. When thoracocentesis is performed antenatally the effusion usually reaccumulates within 48 h and the babies die either antenatally or in the neonatal period; however, there are reports of antenatal resolution following one or more thoraco-centesis (Table 4).

Intrapartum thoracocentesis has been carried out to facilitate neonatal resuscitation, and this may be useful particularly in those units without constant availability of highly-trained neonatal staff and the appropriate equipment to perform drainage within seconds of delivery. Petres and colleagues[33] drained the right

Table 1 Reports documenting spontaneous antenatal resolution of isolated fetal pleural effusions. Site of the effusion indicated as right (R) or left (L)

Author	Cases	Site	GA at diagnosis (weeks)	GA at resolution (weeks)	GA at delivery (weeks)	Outcome
Lien et al. 1990[4]	1	L	16	19	41	alive
Adams et al. 1988[5]	1	L	16	28	40	alive
Sherer et al. 1992[6]	1	R + L	30	34	36	alive
Pijpers et al. 1989[7]	2	R + L	> 24	33–37	33–41	alive
Jaffe et al. 1986[8]	1	R + L	32	37	40	alive
Longaker et al. 1989[9]	3	R + L	26	—	37	alive
		R + L	29	—	38	alive
		R + L	30	—	40	alive

GA, gestational age

Table 2 Reports on antenatally-diagnosed pleural effusions managed conservatively in which the babies survived after postnatal treatment. Site of the effusion indicated as right (R) or left (L)

Author	Cases	Site	Hydrops	GA at diagnosis (weeks)	GA at delivery (weeks)	Outcome
Lange and Manning, 1981[10]	2	R + L	no	39	39	alive
		R + L	yes	32	32	alive
Meizner et al., 1986[11]	1	R	no	38	38	alive
Booth et al., 1987[12]	1	R + L	yes	34	34	alive
Bruno et al., 1988[13]	1	R + L	yes	35	35	alive
Adams et al., 1988[5]	1	R + L	no	36	38	alive
Longaker et al., 1989[9]	10	*	—	34 (28–38)	36 (34–38)	alive
Carmant and Guennec, 1989[14]	1	R + L	no	32	33	alive
Pijpers et al., 1989[7]	6	R + L	no	25-39	33-41	alive
Petrikovsky et al., 1991[15]	1	R + L	no	34	34	alive

GA, gestational age; *seven cases bilateral and three unilateral

Table 3 *Reports on antenatally diagnosed pleural effusions managed conservatively in which the babies died either in utero (IUD) or in the neonatal period (NND). Site of the effusion indicated as right (R) or left (L)*

Author	Cases	Site	Hydrops	GA at diagnosis (weeks)	GA at delivery (weeks)	Outcome
Carrol, 1977[16]	1	R + L	yes	36	36	IUD
Thomas and Anderson, 1979[17]	1	R + L	no	32	35	NND
Bovicelli *et al.*, 1981[18]	1	R + L	no	35	38	NND
Jouppila *et al.*, 1983[19]	2	R + L	no	33	40	NND
		R	yes	26	28	IUD
Peleg *et al.*, 1985[20]	3	R + L	yes	34	35	NND
		R + L	yes	33	33	NND
		R + L	no	34	34	NND
Castillo *et al.*, 1987[21]	6	R + L	yes	26	32	NND
			yes	26	40	NND
			no	30	38	NND
			yes	26	27	NND
			yes	25	28	IUD
			yes	18	19	NND
Adams *et al.*, 1988[5]	1	L	no	25	39	NND
Longaker *et al.*, 1989[9]	10	R + L	—	29 (18–35)	32 (22–37)	NND
Saltzmans *et al.*, 1989[22]	9	R + L	yes	28	—	NND
		R + L	yes	24	—	IUD
		R + L	yes	24	—	IUD
		R + L	yes	31	—	NND
		R + L	yes	34	—	NND
		R + L	yes	30	—	NND
		R + L	yes	26	—	NND
		R + L	yes	25	—	IUD
		R + L	yes	27	—	NND
Moerman *et al.*, 1993[23]	5	R + L	yes	29	29	NND
		R + L	yes	40	40	IUD
		R + L	yes	35	35	NND
		R + L	yes	32	32	IUD
		R + L	yes	30	30	NND

GA, gestational age

pleural effusion of a fetus at 36 weeks' gestation, but this reaccumulated within 24 h. At 37 weeks, when the mother was in labor, the effusion was again drained and the infant was born in good condition. Similarly, Schmidt and co-workers[34] reported the successful intrapartum thoracocentesis and paracentesis in a fetus at 35 weeks of gestation; the infant required assisted ventilation until the 20th day after birth and survived.

PLEUROAMNIOTIC SHUNTING

Technique of pleuroamniotic shunting

Pleural effusions or pulmonary cysts can be drained into the amniotic cavity through a double pigtail silastic catheter (Rocket, London). The catheter, with external and internal diameters of 0.21 and 0.15 mm, has radio-opaque stainless-steel inserts at each end and lateral holes around the coil.

In our center pleuroamniotic shunting is performed as an outpatient procedure, without maternal sedation or fetal paralysis[35]. Ultrasound scanning, with a curvilinear transducer, is used to obtain a transverse section of the fetal thorax. With the transducer in one hand, held parallel to the intended course of the cannula, the chosen site of entry on the maternal abdomen is cleaned with antiseptic solution and local anesthetic

Table 4 *Reports on antenatal thoracocentesis for drainage of fetal pleural effusions. In seven cases the babies survived and in ten they died either in utero (IUD) or in the neonatal period (NND). Site of the effusion indicated as right (R) or left (L)*

Author	Cases	Site	Hydrops	GA at thoracocentesis (weeks)	GA at delivery (weeks)	Outcome
Benacerraf and Frigoletto, 1985[24]	1	L	no	19 +21 + 22 resolved at 24 weeks	40	alive
Benacerraf et al., 1986[25]	1	L	no	20 + 21 + 22 + 23 + 24 resolved at 26 weeks	40	alive
Murayama et al., 1987[26]	1	L	no	30	33	alive
Philippe et al., 1990[27]	1	R + L	yes	33	37	alive
King et al., 1991[28]	1	R + L	yes	34	35	alive
Eddleman et al., 1991[29]	2	R + L	no	32 resolved at 33 weeks	33	alive
		R + L	yes	30	36	NND
Mandelbrot et al., 1992[30]	2	R + L	yes	35	35	alive
		R + L	yes	34 + 35	35	IUD
Meizner, 1989[31]	1	L	no	29	33	NND
Longaker et al., 1989[9]	4	L	yes	28	28	IUD
		R + L	yes	28	30	NND
		L	no	34 + 34	34	NND
		R	no	28 + 29 + 31 + 32	32	NND
Landy et al., 1990[32]	1	L	no	30 + 31 + 31 + 32 + 32	32	NND
Moerman et al., 1993[23]	2	R + L	yes	30	30	NND
		R + L	yes	35	35	NND

GA, gestational age

is infiltrated down to the myometrium. Under ultrasound guidance, a metal cannula with a trochar (external diameter 3 mm, length 15 cm; RMS surgical developments) is introduced transabdominally into the amniotic cavity and inserted through the fetal chest wall, in the mid-thoracic region, into the effusion or cyst. The trochar is removed and the catheter inserted into the cannula. A short introducer rod is then used to deposit half of the catheter into the effusion or cyst. Subsequently, the cannula is gradually removed into the amniotic cavity where the other half of the catheter is pushed by a long introducer. If drainage of the contralateral lung is also needed the appropriate fetal position is achieved by rotation of the fetal body using the tip of the cannula.

After insertion of the shunt serial ultrasound scans are performed at weekly intervals to determine if the effusions reaccumulate, in which case another shunt may be inserted. After delivery the chest drains are immediately clamped and removed to avoid development of pneumothorax.

Pregnancy outcome after pleuroamniotic shunting

Data are available from 16 published series from other centers, as well as from 74 cases from the Harris Birthright Research Centre for Fetal Medicine.

Roberts and associates[36] inserted one end of an epidural catheter into the unilateral pleural effusion of a fetus at 25 weeks' gestation; the other end of the catheter was placed in a bag on the mother's abdomen. During the first 24 h, 70 ml of bright-yellow fluid was drained, but only 30 ml drained over the next 5 days and subsequently the catheter was removed. The effusion did not reaccumulate and a healthy infant was delivered at term. Seeds and Bowes[37] inserted pleuroamniotic catheters in a fetus with large pleural effusions at 30 weeks' gestation. Postproceduraly, fetal activity increased, polyhydramnios decreased and there was cessation of the uterine contractions that were present before shunting. However, after 3 days the effusions reaccumulated because one of the catheters had migrated out of the fetal chest, and the other catheter had been drawn under the fetal skin surface. Polyhydramnios increased and the infant, delivered 48 h later, made a good recovery after drainage and ventilatory support.

Weiner and colleagues[38] performed pleuroamniotic shunting at 25 weeks in a hydropic fetus with extralobar sequestration. Although there was resolution of the edema and ascites, the infant born at 29 weeks died in the neonatal period.

Rodeck and co-workers[39] reported eight cases with pleural effusions, including five with hydrops, that were shunted at 25–35 weeks' gestation. The infants were delivered at 32–39 weeks' gestation; six infants survived with good respiratory function and two died in the neonatal period due to pulmonary hypoplasia. In the latter two cases the lungs did not expand after pleuroamniotic shunting (Table 5).

Results from the Harris Birthright Centre

During a 10-year period (1985–1994), pleuroamniotic shunting was performed in 74 singleton pregnancies. The data of the first 47 cases were reported previously[35,42]. Pleuroamniotic shunting was considered if there was associated fetal hydrops, polyhydramnios or major, progressive pulmonary compression and/or mediastinal shift. Fetal karyotyping was performed at the time of shunting and if abnormal or hydrops worsened, the option of termination was discussed with the parents. If intrathoracic fluid reaccumulated, further shunting was considered.

In five cases the pregnancies were terminated at the request of the parents because the fetuses were found to have Down syndrome ($n = 3$), Turner syndrome ($n = 1$), or progressive hydrops despite successful drainage of the effusions ($n = 1$). In the 69 cases where the pregnancies continued, the effusions were bilateral in 38 (55%) and unilateral with associated mediastinal shift in 31. Fetal ascites and/or generalized skin edema was present in seven (23%) of the 31 with unilateral effusions and in 34 (89%) of the 38 with bilateral effusions. All of this group had normal karyotypes, except for one fetus with trisomy 21.

Insertion of pleuroamniotic shunts resulted in rapid expansion of the lungs in all but one fetus which was subsequently found to have

Table 5 *Reported cases of pleuroamniotic shunting in centers other than the Harris Birthright Research Centre. Site of the effusion indicated as right (R) or left (L)*

Author	Cases	Site	Hydrops	GA at shunting (weeks)	GA at delivery (weeks)	Outcome	Comments
Seeds and Bowes, 1986[37]	1	R + L	yes	30	31	alive	
Weiner et al., 1986[38]	1	L	yes	25 + 27 + 27	29	NND	extralobar sequestration
Rodeck et al., 1988[39]	8	L	no	27	39	alive	
		R + L	yes	28	32	alive	
		R	no	32	34	alive	trisomy 21
		R	no	25	39	alive	
		R + L	yes	35 + 36	39	alive	
		R + L	yes	31 + 32	34	alive	
		R + L	yes	31	32	NND	
		R + L	yes	29	32	NND	
Longaker et al., 1989[9]	1	R + L	yes	30 + 31	32	alive	
King et al., 1991[28]	1	R + L	yes	34	38	IUD	
Mandelbrot et al., 1992[30]	2	R + L	yes	31	32	NND	Opitz trigonocephaly
		R + L	yes	31	34	alive	
Ronderos-Dumit et al., 1991[40]	1	R + L	yes	33	37	alive	
Becker et al., 1993[41]	1	L	yes	23 + 27	36	alive	

GA, gestational age; NND, neonatal death; IUD, intrauterine death

arthrogryposis. In cases with unilateral effusions, there was a simultaneous shift of the heart to its normal position within the thorax. In eight cases (12%) the effusions reaccumulated 1–3 weeks after shunting, presumably because the shunts blocked or the fetus pulled out the shunt; in these cases further shunts were inserted. Polyhydramnios was present in 43 (62%) of the 69 cases and this resolved within 1–3 weeks after shunting in 28 (65%). Similarly, hydrops resolved in 19 (46%) of the 41 affected pregnancies.

All 28 non-hydropic fetuses survived (Table 6) but in the hydropic group 19 (46%) of the 41 babies survived and 22 (54%) died *in utero* or in the neonatal period (Table 7). The six intrauterine deaths occurred 1–8 weeks after

shunting which was effective in draining the pleural effusions but did not prevent progressive increase in skin edema. In the group of neonatal deaths, there were two cases of diaphragmatic hernia and one case each of major cardiac defect, arthrogryposis, pseudomonas septicemia and disseminated intravascular coagulation; in 10 cases death was due to a combination of respiratory, cardiovascular and renal failure. In the 47 surviving infants, seven (15%) required surgery for atrioventricular septal defect, coarctation of the aorta, thyroid teratoma, congenital portocaval shunt, congenital diaphragmatic hernia, pulmonary extralobar sequestration, or cystic hygroma.

Booth and colleagues[12] examined the neonatal course of two babies with hydrops

Table 6 *Results of pleuroamniotic shunting at the Harris Birthright Research Centre in fetuses with pleural effusions in the absence of hydrops. Site of effusion indicated as right (R) or left (L)*

Case	Site	AFV	GA at shunt (weeks)	GA at delivery (weeks)	Outcome	Comments
1	L	N	20	32	alive	
2	L	N	20	36	alive	
3	L	N	20	39	alive	
4	L	N	20	41	alive	
5	R + L	N	21	37	alive	
6	L	N	21	41	alive	
7	R	N	22	38	alive	diaphragmatic hernia
8	L	N	22	39	alive	
9	R	P*	24	39	alive	
10	L	P*	24 + 26	39	alive	
11	L	P	27	32	alive	
12	R + L	N	27	37	alive	
13	L	N	27	39	alive	
14	L	N	28	39	alive	
15	R	N	29	31	alive	
16	R	N	29	41	alive	
17	L	P	30	30	alive	
18	L	P*	30	34	alive	
19	R	P*	30	34	alive	
20	L	N	31	36	alive	extralobar sequestration
21	R	N	31	38	alive	
22	R	P*	31	38	alive	
23	R	P*	32	35	alive	atrioventricular septal defect, trisomy 21
24	R	P	32 + 34	35	alive	
25	R	P	33	35	alive	cystic hygroma
26	L	P*	33	39	alive	
27	R + L	P*	34	37	alive	
28	R + L	P*	35	39	alive	

GA, gestational age; N, normal, P; polyhydramnios; AVP, amniotic fluid volume; *resolution of polyhydramnios after shunting

Table 7 *Pleuroamniotic shunting at the Harris Birthright Research Centre in hydropic fetuses with pleural effusions. Site of the effusion indicated as right (R) or left (L)*

Case	Site	Ascetes	Edema	AFV	GA at shunt (weeks)	GA at delivery (weeks)	Outcome	Comments
1	R + L	++	++	N	20	33	alive	congenital porto-caval shunt
2	R + L	++	+	N	21	37	alive[R]	
3	R + L	+	+	P*	22	38	alive[R]	
4	R + L	+	+	N	24 + 26 + 29	39	alive[R]	
5	R + L	++	−	N	25	38	alive[R]	
6	R	+	+	P*	26	37	alive[R]	
7	R + L	+	++	P*	30	36	alive[R]	
8	R + L	+	+	P*	30 + 32	38	alive[R]	
9	R + L	++	+	P*	31	37	alive[R]	
10	R + L	+	+	N	32	33	alive[R]	
11	R + L	+	+	P	32	33	alive	
12	R + L	++	+	P*	32	35	alive[R]	
13	R + L	++	−	P*	32	39	alive[R]	
14	L	+	++	P*	32	40	alive[R]	
15	R	−	++	P	33	34	alive	thyroid teratoma
16	R + L	++	++	P*	33	37	alive[R]	
17	R	++	++	P*	33	38	alive[R]	supraventricular tachycardia
18	R	+	++	P*	33	38	alive[R]	coarctation of the aorta
19	L	++	+	P	34	36	alive	
20	R + L	++	+	N	22	23	IUD	mucopolysac-charroidosis VII
21	R + L	++	++	N	22	30	IUD	
22	R + L	+	++	N	23	25	IUD	recurrent hydrops
23	R + L	++	++	P*	24	26	IUD	
24	R + L	+	++	P	26	27	IUD	
25	R + L	+	++	P	35	36	IUD	
26	R + L	++	++	N	20	29	NND	
27	R + L	+	++	P*	25	32	NND[R]	recurrent hydrops
28	R + L	++	++	O	26	35	NND	
29	R + L	−	++	P*	28	32	NND	
30	R + L	+	++	P*	28 + 31	33	NND[R]	
31	R + L	++	+	P*	29 + 30	31	NND	
32	R + L	++	++	P*	29	32	NND	disseminated intravascular coagulation
33	R + L	++	++	P*	29 + 32	35	NND	Pseudomonas septicemia
34	R + L	+	++	P	30	31	NND	
35	R + L	++	++	P*	30	31	NND[R]	
36	R + L	++	+	N	30	35	NND[R]	diaphragmatic hernia
37	R + L	+	+	P	31	32	NND	
38	R + L	+	++	P	31 + 32	35	NND	arthrogryposis
39	R + L	−	++	P	33	34	NND	univentricular heart
40	R + L	+	++	P	35	36	NND	
41	R	+	++	P	35	37	NND	diaphragmatic hernia

GA, gestational age; −, none detected; +, mild/moderate; ++, severe; N, normal; P, polyhydramnios; O, oligohydramnios; *resolution of polyhydramnios after shunting; [R], resolution of hydrops after shunting; IUD, intrauterine death; NND, neonatal death; AFV, amniotic fluid volume

Table 8 *Overall outcome in non-hydropic and hydropic fetuses with pleural effusions treated by antenatal thoracocentesis or pleuroamniotic shunting*

| | Non-hydrops | | Hydrops | |
Management	Total	Alive	Total	Alive
Thoracocentesis	8	4 (50%)	9	3 (33%)
Pleuroamniotic shunting	31	31 (100%)	54	27 (50%)

fetalis associated with pleural effusions. One baby who was treated by pleuroamniotic shunting had no effusion at birth and required less resuscitation than the baby with no antenatal intervention.

Infant follow-up

Thompson and co-workers[43] examined the respiratory status at 3–60 months of age in 17 of the infants who had undergone pleuroamniotic shunting. Although six (35%) suffered from recurrent respiratory symptoms, this frequency is similar to that found in healthy infants[44]. The mean functional residual capacity of these infants was normal, suggesting that pleuroamniotic shunting may also have permitted normal lung growth[43]; infants with impaired lung growth tend to have small-volume lungs[45].

Maternal morbidity

Ronderos-Dumit and associates[40] described a case of bilateral pleural effusions, hydrops and polyhydramnios in which pleuroamniotic shunting was complicated by the development of massive maternal ascites and oligohydramnios. This was presumably the result of amniotic fluid leakage through the uterine wall. After 24 h there was resolution of maternal ascites and reaccumulation of amniotic fluid. Subsequently the pregnancy progressed uneventfully and a healthy infant was delivered at 37 weeks' gestation, 4 weeks after shunting.

Becker and colleagues[41] performed pleuroamniotic shunting in a hydropic fetus at 23 weeks' gestation. However, the shunt got stuck in the uterine wall. A further shunt was introduced a few days later. Serial scans demonstrated effective drainage of the effusions and resolution of the hydrops. However, ultrasound examination at 36 weeks, after spontaneous onset of labor, failed to demonstrate any of the shunts. Abdominal X-ray was performed which identified one of the catheters in the uterine wall and the other in the upper maternal abdomen. After delivery one of the catheters was found in the amniotic membranes and the second was removed by laparoscopy. The infant was well.

Summary of results

Table 8 summarizes the results of outcome after antenatal thoracocentesis or pleuroamniotic shunting in fetuses with pleural effusions. In the non-hydropic group treated by thoracocentesis 50% survived compared to 100% for those that had pleuroamniotic shunting. Survival in the hyropic group was lower after thoracocentesis (33%) than after pleuroamniotic shunting (50%). Polyhydramnios independent of the presence or absence of hydrops does not appear to influence the chance of survival.

CONCLUSIONS

Isolated fetal pleural effusions may either resolve spontaneously or be treated after birth. Nevertheless, in some cases severe and chronic compression of the fetal lungs can result in pulmonary hypoplasia and neonatal death. In others, mediastinal compression leads to the development of fetal hydrops and polyhydramnios which are associated with a high risk of premature delivery and subsequent perinatal death.

The data from fetuses with isolated pleural effusions suggest that certainly in some cases short-term decompression by thoracocentesis or temporary drainage may disrupt the underlying pathology. However, in the majority of cases the fluid reaccumulates within 24 h requiring repeated procedures which are likely to be more traumatic than chronic pleuroamniotic shunting.

The data on pleuroamniotic shunting demonstrate the value of this technique both for diagnosis and therapy. First, the diagnosis of an underlying cardiac abnormality or other intrathoracic lesion may become apparent only after effective decompression and return of the mediastinum to its normal position. Second, it may help distinguish between hydrops due to primary accumulation of pleural effusions, in which case the ascites and skin edema may resolve after shunting, and other causes of hydrops such as infection, in which drainage of the effusions does not prevent worsening of the hydrops. This technique is also an effective and safe method of chronic drainage of fetal pleural effusions to reverse fetal hydrops, resolve polyhydramnios and potentially prevent the development of pulmonary hypoplasia. Nevertheless, in half of the hydropic fetuses pleuroamniotic shunting does not prevent their ultimate death, which is the consequence of the underlying disease.

References

1. Beischer, N. A., Fortune, D. W. and Macafee, J. (1971). Nonimmunologic hydrops fetalis and congenital abnormalities. *Obstet. Gynecol.*, **38**, 86–95

2. Hislop, A. (1996). Fetal and postnatal anatomical development. In Greenough, A., Robertson, N. R. C. and Milner, A. D. (eds.) *Neonatal Respiratory Disorders*, pp. 3–12. (London: Oxford University Press)

3. Harrison, M. R., Bressack, M. A., Churg, A. M. and Lorimier, A. A. (1980). Correction of congenital diaphragmatic hernia *in utero*. II. Simulated correction permits fetal lung growth with survival at birth. *Surgery*, **88**, 260–8

4. Lien, J. M., Colmorgen, G. H. C., Gehret, J. F. and Evantash, A. B. (1990). Spontaneous resolution of fetal effusion diagnosed during the second trimester. *J. Clin. Ultrasound*, **18**, 54–6

5. Adams, H., Jones, A. and Hayward, C. (1988). The sonographic features and implications of fetal pleural effusions. *Clin. Radiol.*, **39**, 398–401

6. Sherer, D. M., Abramowicz, J. S., Eggers, P. C. and Woods, J. R. Jr (1992). Transient severe unilateral and subsequent bilateral primary fetal hydrothorax with spontaneous resolution at 34 weeks' gestation associated with normal neonatal outcome. *Am. J. Obstet. Gynecol.*, **166**, 169–70

7. Pijpers, L., Reuss, A., Stewart, P. A. and Wladimiroff, J. W. (1989). Noninvasive management of isolated bilateral fetal hydrothorax. *Am. J. Obstet. Gynecol.*, **161**, 330–2

8. Jaffe, R., Segni, E. D., Altaras, M., Loebel, R. and Aderet, N. B. (1986). Ultrasonic real-time diagnosis of transitory fetal pleural and pericardial effusion. *Diagnostic Imaging Clin. Med.*, **55**, 373–5

9. Longaker, M. T., Laberge, J. M., Dansereau, J., Langer, J. C., Crombleholme, T. M., Callen, P. W., Golbus, M. S. and Harrison, M. R. (1989). Primary fetal hydrothorax: natural history and management. *J. Ped. Surg*, **24**, 573–6

10. Lange, I. R. and Manning, F. A. (1981). Antenatal diagnosis of congenital pleural effusions. *Am. J. Obstet. Gynecol.*, **140**, 839–40

11. Meizner, I., Carmi, R. and Bar-Siv, J. (1986) Congenital chylothorax – prenatal ultrasonic diagnosis and successful post partum management. *Prenat. Diagn.*, **6**, 217–21

12. Booth, P., Nicolaides, K. H., Greenough, A. and Gamsu, H. R. (1987). Pleuro-amniotic shunting for fetal chylothorax. *Early Hum. Dev.*, **15**, 365–7

13. Bruno, M., Iskra, L., Dolfin, G. and Farina, D. (1988). Congenital pleural effusion: prenatal ultrasonic diagnosis and therapeutic management. *Prenat. Diagn.*, **8**, 157–9

14. Carmant, L. and Guennec, J. C. (1989). Congenital chylothorax and persistent pulmonary hypertension of the neonate. *Acta Paediatr. Scand.*, **78**, 789–92

15. Petrikovsky, B. M., Shmoys, S. M., Baker, D. A. and Monheit, A. G. (1991). Pleural effusion in aneuploidy. *Am. J. Perinatol.*, **91**, 214–6

16. Carrol, B. (1977). Pulmonary hypoplasia and pleural effusions associated with fetal death *in utero*: ultrasonic findings. *Am. J. Roentgenol*, **129**, 749–50

17. Thomas, D. B. and Anderson, J. C. (1979). Antenatal detection of fetal pleural effusion and neonatal management. *Med. J. Aust.*, **2**, 435–6

18. Bovicelli, L., Rizzo, N., Orsini, L. F. and Calderoni, P. (1981). Ultrasonic real-time diagnosis of

fetal hydrothorax and lung hypoplasia. *J. Clin. Ultrasound*, **9**, 253–4

19. Jouppila, P., Kirkinen, P., Herva, R. and Koivisto, M. (1983). Prenatal diagnosis of pleural effusions by ultrasound. *J. Clin. Ultrasound*, **11**, 516–9

20. Peleg, D., Golichowski, A. M. and Ragan, W. D. (1985). Fetal hydrothorax and bilateral pulmonary hypoplasia. *Acta Obstet. Gynecol. Scand.*, **64**, 451–3

21. Castillo, R. A., Devoe, L. D., Falls, G., Holzman, G. B., Hadi, H. A. and Fadel, H. E. (1987). Pleural effusion and pulmonary hypoplasia. *Am. J. Obstet. Gynecol.*, **157**, 1252–5

22. Saltzman, D. H., Frigoletto, F. D., Harlow, B. L., Barss, V. A. and Benacerraf, B. R. (1989). Sonographic evaluation of hydrops fetalis. *Obstet. Gynecol.*, **74**, 106–11

23. Moerman, P., Vandenberghe, K., Devlieger, H., Hole, C. V., Fryns, J. P. and Lauweryns, J. M. (1993). Congenital pulmonary lymphangiectasis with chylothorax: a heterogeneous lymphatic vessel abnormality. *Am. J. Med. Genet.*, **47**, 54–8

24. Benacerraf, B. R. and Frigoletto, F. D. Jr (1985). Mid-trimester fetal thoracentesis. *J. Clin. Ultrasound*, **13**, 202–4

25. Benacerraf, B. R., Frigoletto, F. D. Jr and Wilson, M. (1986). Successful midtrimester thoracentesis with analysis of the lymphocyte population in the pleural effusion. *Am. J. Obstet. Gynecol.*, **155**, 398–9

26. Murayama, K., Jimbo, T., Matsumoto, Y., Mitsuishi, C. and Nishida, H. (1987). Fetal pulmonary hypoplasia with hydrothorax. *Am. J. Obstet. Gynecol.*, **157**, 119–20

27. Philippe, H. J., Paupe, A., DoÚípeyre, P., Jacquemard, F., Lenclen, R., Muller, F., Blanc, P., Olivier-Martin, M. and Lewin, D. (1990). Diagnostic antenatal et prise en charge du chylothorax congenital. *Arch. Fr. Ped.*, **47**, 737–40

28. King, P. A., Ghosh, A., Tang, M. H. Y. and Lam, S. K. (1991). Recurrent congenital chylothorax. *Prenat Diagn.*, **11**, 809–11

29. Eddleman, K. A., Levine, A. B., Chitkara, U. and Berkowitz, R. L. (1991). Reliability of pleural fluid lymphocyte counts in the antenatal diagnosis of congenital chylothorax. *Obstet. Gynecol.*, **78**, 530–2

30. Mandelbrot, L., Aubry, M. C., Mussat, P., Dumez, Y. and Dommergues (1992). Reversal of fetal distress by emergency *in utero* decompression of hydrothorax. *Am. J. Obstet. Gynecol.*, **167**, 1278–83

31. Meizner, I. (1989). Pleuroamniotic shunting for decompression of fetal pleural effusions. *Obstet. Gynecol.*, **73**, 298–9

32. Landy, H. J., Daly, V., Heyl, P. S. and Khoury, A. N. (1990). Fetal thoracocentesis with

unsuccessful outcome. *J. Clin. Ultrasound*, **18**, 50–3

33. Petres, R. E., Redwine, F. O. and Cruikshank, D. P. (1982). Congenital bilateral chylothorax. Antepartum diagnosis and successful intrauterine surgical management. *J. Am. Med. Assoc.*, **248**, 1360–1

34. Schmidt, W., Harms, E. and Wolf, D. (1985). Successful prenatal treatment of non-immune hydrops fetalis due to congenital chylothorax. Case report. *Br. J. Obstet. Gynaecol.*, **92**, 685–7

35. Blott, M., Nicolaides, K. H. and Greenough, A. (1988). Pleuroamniotic shunting for decompression of fetal pleural effusions. *Obstet. Gynecol.*, **71**, 798–800

36. Roberts, A. B., Clarkson, P. M., Pattison, N. S., Jamieson, M. G. and Mok, P. M. (1986). Fetal hydrothorax in the second trimester of pregnancy: successful intra-uterine treatment at 24 weeks gestation. *Fetal Ther.*, **1**, 203–9

37. Seeds, J. W. and Bowes, W. A. Jr (1986). Results of treatment of severe fetal hydrothorax with bilateral pleuroamniotic catheters. *Obstet. Gynecol.*, **68**, 577–9

38. Weiner, C. P., Varner, M., Pringle, K., Hein, H., Williamson, R. and Smith, W. L. (1986). Antenatal diagnosis and palliative treatment of nonimmune hydrops fetalis secondary to pulmonary extralobar sequestration. *Obstet. Gynecol.*, **68**, 275–80

39. Rodeck, C. H., Fisk, N. M., Fraser, D. I. and Nicolini, U. (1988). Long-term *in utero* drainage of fetal pleural effusion. *N. Engl. J. Med.*, **319**, 1135–8

40. Ronderos-Dumit, D., Nicolini, U., Vaughan, J., Fisk, N. M., Chamberlain, P. F. and Rodeck, C. H. (1991). Uterine-peritoneal amniotic fluid leakage: an unusual complication of intrauterine shunting. *Obstet. Gynecol.*, **78**, 913–5

41. Becker, R., Arabin, B., Novak, A., Entezami, M. and Weitzel, H. K. (1993). Successful treatment of primary fetal hydrothorax by long-time drainage from week 23. *Fetal Diagn. Ther.*, **8**, 331–7

42. Nicolaides, K. H. and Azar, G. B. (1990). Thoraco-amniotic shunting. *Fetal Diagn. Ther.*, **5**, 153–64

43. Thompson, P. J., Greenough, A. and Nicolaides, K. H. (1993). Respiratory function in infancy following pleuro-amniotic shunting. *Fetal Diagn. Ther.*, **8**, 79–83

44. Greenough, A., Maconochie, I. and Yuksel, B. (1990). Recurrent respiratory symptoms in the first year of life following preterm delivery. *J. Perinat. Med.*, **8**, 489–94

45. Helms, P. (1982). Lung function in infants with congenital pulmonary hypoplasia. *J. Pediatr.*, **101**, 918–22

Techniques for pediatric and fetal surgery

Z. Szabo, A. Cuschieri and G. Berci

24

INTRODUCTION

Laparoscopic surgery has become an important modality in pediatric surgery in numerous applications including thoracic, abdominal, genitourinary, and other applications. Fetal surgery has shown similar promise by using the endoscopic approach in treatment of debilitating or life-threatening congenital defects. Fetoscopic surgery obviated the need for maternal hysterotomy which was an important development, since uterine irritation resulted in spontaneous abortion. A percutaneous approach, that is without hysterotomy and laparotomy, has been developed to minimize other ill effects associated with current fetoscopic techniques.

An equally important development in laparoscopic surgery, which has affected pediatric and fetal surgeons, has been the development of intracorporeal suturing and knotting techniques. Although in laparoscopic surgery there are easier mechanical means of approximating tissue edges and aids for knotting, manually executed instrument-suturing and knotting is still an essential and fundamental skill. Laparoscopic suturing and knotting can be applied to vastly different types of tissues, operative sites, and degrees of access, and can be a contributing factor to improve health-care economy.

The skills required efficiently to approximate tissues demand focused attention, considerable dexterity, and creativity. They enable the surgeon to repair iatrogenic injuries expediently, and, moreover, to expand application to other procedures that may have been daunting otherwise. The development of proficiency in laparoscopic suturing and internal knotting requires the surgeon to commit adequate time to partake in formal training and further hone his skills through regular practice. As laparoscopic surgery is a form of magnified surgery, those trained or at least exposed to microsurgery may experience a less arduous path to technique development. In laparoscopic surgery, these skills have freed the surgeon from dependence on mechanical devices and are therefore more economical.

Fetoscopic surgery differs from laparoscopic surgery in a number of different aspects, from the smaller size and greater friability of tissues involved, to the instruments, port sizes and locations, the overall strategy, and other factors. Nonetheless, the fundamental principles are the same, although they must be observed to a more critical degree. In the following sections, these overall principles and techniques of intracorporeal suturing and knotting are described in detail. When the surgeon, or any member of his or her team, understands what is involved and that consistently successful technique is the result of careful planning and purpose, he or she will be able to meet the challenges successfully and with confidence.

CHALLENGES

The minimal access approach represents an evolutionary advancement in surgery, especially with regard to improvement in patient recovery (from reducing access trauma) and health-care costs. However, this benefit is gained at the expense of the surgeon who has to work proportionately harder. He or she must contend with a more restrictive position to accomplish the surgical task, and this position is more physically and mentally stressful for the surgeon. If we compare the difficulty level of the traditional open technique to laparoscopic suturing, there is a distinct difference[1] (Figure 1). The consequent challenges center mainly around four areas: visual perception, eye–hand coordination, set-up and the mental framework.

The *visual perception* challenge is caused by indirect viewing of the operative field from an altered perspective through a closed-circuit video system. Using current technology, a flat, two-dimensional image on a 14–19 inch monitor is provided that is sometimes inadequate in illumination and clarity. While an image thus obtained is marginal, it is adequate to carry out most suturing needs. Keeping the optical components clean and the video system fine-tuned, or 'tweaked', is of great significance, although often a neglected factor. The surgeon would be best served by making certain that an optimal image (including centering the action on the

monitor) is preserved throughout the procedure. With substantial practice and experience, the image becomes more informative to the surgeon, especially with regard to the different spatial relationships, references points, and altered view of anatomy.

The *eye–hand coordination* challenge is produced by two factors, first, the optical magnification from the laparoscope, and second, the long length of the instruments (22–33 cm) and their distant fulcrums. When attempting to suture without formal, systematic training[1–3], this endeavor can be quite intimidating; in fact, only a handful of individuals have learned to suture adequately on their own but not without first investing an inordinate amount of time and effort in the process.

The third challenge is *the set-up*, i.e. how the surgeon is positioned in relation to his or her suturing environment as well as the placement of the view and suturing ports. The two key elements entailed are the coaxial alignment of the visual path, and the triad relationship between the view and two hands (Figure 2). A study comparing the efficiency of the lateral versus the coaxial set-up for suturing clearly demonstrated the lower efficiency of the lateral positioning[4].

The increased challenges associated with laparoscopic suturing can be met by proper training, appropriate equipment and

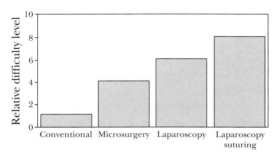

Figure 1 *Relative difficulty levels between open and laparoscopic surgery*

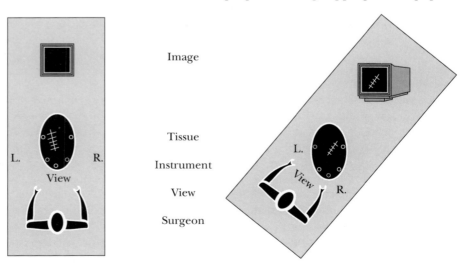

Figure 2 *Coaxial alignment of the visual path*

instrumentation, and the adaptation of a philosophy and lifestyle that enables the surgeon to concentrate and develop the stamina necessary for this work[5].

PRINCIPLES

Reducing movement speed and range of motion (slowing down)

Magnification and the reduction of the operative field size require a proportionate reduction of movement speed and range (path) in order to regain eye–hand coordination and overall control. The use of long-stemmed instruments with distant fulcrums adds to the challenge. The best remedy to any situation that is 'out of control' is to slow down; and slow down in proportion to the degree of magnification and focus one's attention exclusively on the task at hand.

Traditionally, surgeons are in a hurry. In the handicapped laparoscopic suturing setting, a great deal of frustration and fumbling can be seen, particularly in the novice. As tissues are magnified and instruments moved, it is very difficult visually to trace the trajectory of the two instrument tips, particularly when these movements are fast and erratic. Even for experienced surgeons, movements must be slowed down in order to regain control of the movements and restore precision.

The greater the magnification and/or the more difficult the port position set-up, the more one must slow down when suturing tissue edges together or tying an intracorporeal knot. Slowed movement not only permits recognition of impending error and consequential correction of action, it also provides good control which in turn builds confidence. In short, slowed, error-free movements lead to faster finishes.

Choreography of movements

Although slowing down restores the necessary control and movement precision, it also increases operating time. This increase will be in proportion to the magnification and the degree of difficulty of the set-up. Certain components of the suturing technique involve repetitious movements such as needle driving and knot tying. These movements can be analyzed, broken down to their most basic components, then reassembled into the most efficient and intuitive process. Every movement made should flow into the next (hence the term 'choreography'). This choreography, coupled with a reduction in movement speed, will enable precision-controlled movements and a reduction of operating time. When this choreography is memorized, it benefits the surgeon when learning a new procedure. It arms him or her with a technique that is standardized and frees the surgeon to focus on the variable aspects of the procedure. It provides a visual memory that, even under the stress of surgery, can easily be recalled and duplicated.

Economy of motion

A complementary component of movement choreography, application of the economy of motion principle, will further shorten operating time. Random, nervous and uncertain movements need to be eliminated and replaced with deliberate, purposeful maneuvers. Simply by eliminating unnecessary movements, even subtle ones such as regrasping tissue that falls away from the grasp of an instrument, a great deal of time will be saved. These movements have to be planned out in one's mind and slowly executed following this mental image, keeping it as close as possible to the ideal. It does take considerable time and effort to develop smooth choreography, flawless technique and maximum motion economy but the reward is commensurate. An individual style can be developed by incorporating these combined principles which is effective, efficient and elegant. One of the best demonstrations of the economy of motion principle is during the very beginning of suturing when loading the needle; this will be described later.

Ambidextrous technique

When suturing in a handicapped surgical set-up such as the laparoscopic field, the surgeon really cannot afford to be dominantly single-handed.

Even with the most careful preplanning and placement of instrument ports, a situation can easily enough arise that favors a non-dominant (e.g. left-handed) movement for needle driving and knot tying. Although the tissues could be adjusted to a more favorable right-handed execution, or a forced right-handed move can be made, this is done at the expense of tissue damage. Further, a less-than-ideal stitch placement and/or an awkward looking style may result. To achieve maximum potential from laparoscopic surgery, the surgeon is advised to develop an ambidextrous suturing technique.

Set-up

Coaxial line-up

Coaxial alignment means that the position of the surgeon, the view port (laparoscope and camera), the instrument ports, target tissue and the video monitor are arranged along a straight line. The distance between the surgeon and the monitor should be no greater than 180 cm. This alignment maximizes the surgeon's access, and reduces the stress on the human brain when calculating and translating the relationships of instruments and tissues.

Ideally, the video system should include a high-resolution 19-inch monitor and be viewed no further than 150–180 cm away. The laparoscope and instrument ports need to be placed in a fashion that duplicates the natural anatomy of the surgeon; that is, placing the camera in the middle and the suturing ports on either side in advance of the surgeon's frontal plane, just like the human eyes are in the middle and the hands on either side. The distance between the suturing ports should be about 20 cm. Having the ports closer or further apart would still enable the surgeon to suture; however, it would be significantly more difficult.

Use of a *laparoscope holder*, whether mechanical, pneumatic, or robotic, is desirable, preferably with a zooming device for difficult suturing situations. It will provide a rock-solid image that a surgical assistant would be hard pressed to duplicate over a prolonged period of time. The zooming device will allow magnification

changes, i.e. a close-up or panoramic view, as required for varying circumstances.

Triad port positions (Figure 3)

Suturing essentially requires three ports, one for viewing, and one each for the right- and left-hand instruments. The most intuitive arrangement of these ports consists of the view port being in between the right and the left instrument ports in a triangular formation, duplicating human anatomy (i.e. vision or the eyes in the middle, parallel with the axis of the coaxial line-up). When attempting to suture in a different location, these three ports can be shifted in

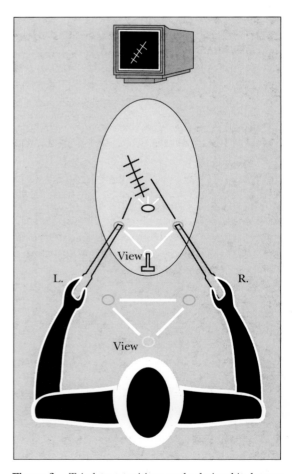

Figure 3 *Triad port positions and relationship between the view and two hands*

unison to the new position. Most target tissues can be accessed from the base position of putting the laparoscope in the umbilicus and having the assistant position tissues in a favorable location.

Ideal directions

The ideal directions for suturing in a magnified surgical field again follow pre-established routines from ordinary activities. For the right-handed surgeon, the suture line should be in the 11 o'clock–5 o'clock position and the stitches placed in the 1 o'clock–7 o'clock direction. Paper positioned at this angle facilitates writing in a straight line, parallel to the top and bottom edges of the paper (or perpendicular to the left and right edges). In a similar manner, this suture line should be positioned in the same angle, so that the stitches would be perpendicular to it. For the left-hander, the suture line should be positioned at a 1 o'clock–7 o'clock position and the stitches placed in the 11 o'clock–5 o'clock direction. Positioning tissues in this manner, as with any aspect of good set-up, facilitates proper techniques and favorable results.

Touch confirmation

In laparoscopic suturing, the locations of various objects in the field are often difficult to judge when relying solely on visual information from a two-dimensional image. A simple technique can be employed to enhance movement accuracy which consists of touching the targeted structure lightly (gentle probing) to verify one's estimation of its correct location. By practicing the 'touch confirmation' technique, the surgeon can gain critical clues to an object's true whereabouts before expending the effort to grasp it. In the process, actual spatial relationships become apparent and should be incorporated in the surgeon's visual memory. With this information, the surgeon is able to transform a two-dimensional image into a 'virtual three-dimensional' image. Touch confirmation is only one component of 'virtual three dimensions'; it also involves experienced visual perception as well as logical reasoning. The touch confirmation technique can result in movements that are remarkably accurate when coupled with the principles of slowed movements, sequential choreography, flawless technique, and the economy of motion.

Instrument rotation

Laparoscopic suturing requires frequent instrument rotation such as the scooping motion of needle driving and rotating sutures during knot tying. Instruments with the traditional pistol or angled ring grip are unsuitable for these techniques since rotation is particularly difficult and awkward. While a highly skilled surgeon could use such instruments, it is an unnecessary burden that leads more quickly to surgeon fatigue.

Instrument fulcrum

The importance of port positioning is not only to provide the proper angle of access but also to provide a fulcrum for the instruments that is exactly halfway between the tip and the handle, in other words 50% of the instrument shaft is inside the body cavity and 50% is outside. This provides a 1 : 1 ratio of movement between the handle and tip.

EQUIPMENT, INSTRUMENTATION AND SUTURE MATERIAL

Although high-quality equipment benefits every aspect of laparoscopic surgery, it is suturing that commands the highest standards. Since laparoscopic suturing is an inherently difficult task, close attention must be paid to selecting, arranging, and optimizing equipment and instrumentation to minimize surgeon fatigue and consequent error.

Optics

The optical component of minimal access surgical equipment is the laparoscope with its built-in illumination channel and a separate source delivering the light via fiberoptic or liquid cables. Laparoscopes vary in their physical

Laparoscope and instrument axis

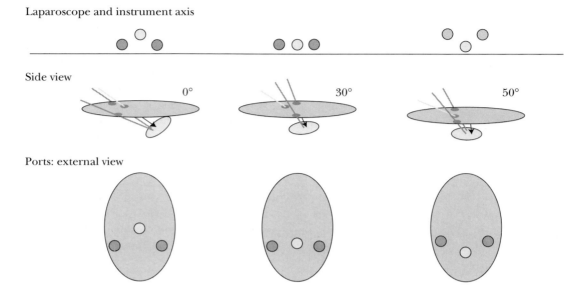

Side view

Ports: external view

Figure 4 *Laparoscopic view angles and suturing port positions for the 0°, 30° and 50° laparoscopes*

dimensions; however, the most practical sizes involve diameters of 2, 4, 5 and 10 mm and lengths of 15–30 cm.

The objective lens of a 0° laparoscope provides a straightforward view; the 30° laparoscope, a forward oblique view, which when rotated provides a broader range of views. In most cases, the 30° laparoscope is preferred for suturing, since it provides more flexible viewing. Although the 0° laparoscope will provide a brighter, sharper image, it has a shallow perspective and therefore is not recommended when an overhead view is needed (Figure 4).

Since the laparoscope's objective lens is in relatively close proximity to the target tissues, fluids and tissue debris can easily adhere to the lens, especially when tissues and instruments are moved about actively. A deterioration of the image clarity is the consequence. The laparoscope's lens should be frequently cleaned, even if the procedure needs to be halted briefly. Cleaning of the objective is accomplished by first removing the laparoscope from the port, then wiping it off (and the laparoscope shaft as well) with a warm wet gauze, followed by a dry gauze, and then applying a solution with antifogging properties or betadine solution. The

entrance of the viewing port should also be cleaned before reintroducing the laparoscope through it. (Also, after surgery and sterilization of the laparoscope, the optical components should be wiped immaculately clean and polished.)

A common but questionable method of cleaning the lens involves touching the lens to tissue in the operative site. While this solves the clarity problem temporarily, it has a potentially detrimental effect. Tissue fluids can dry onto the surface of the lens during the procedure. Since these fluids contain proteins, it is harder to clean them off the objective and, when force is applied, it may result in removing some of the optical coating applied by the manufacturer, thereby permanently reducing optical quality.

The coupler between the laparoscope and the video camera is equipped with a focusing ring and a zooming ring both of which are very useful features and important components. When increasing or decreasing the magnification by twisting the laparoscope's zooming ring, or if the laparoscope is pushed closer to the image or pulled further back, the focus must be adjusted by twisting the focusing ring.

Video systems

Currently, state-of-the-art equipment includes a three-chip color camera and 19-inch monitor, with a maximum resolution of 600 lines, plus a digital image enhancer. Although a properly assembled and tuned laparoscopic system provides a reasonable image, complicated reconstructive and suturing tasks present an increased visual challenge. In order to address the lack of a stereopsis, three-dimensional (3-D) laparoscopes have been designed but they still require viewing through a TV monitor (with 3-D glasses). While usable, the results have been less than ideal because of the compromises built into such systems. Lack of consistent image clarity, illumination, and field size have been the primary problems and, thus 2-D systems are still the equipment of choice. High-definition television (HDTV) may offer the next practical improvement. The first step will most likely be a sharp 2-D HDTV color image, followed by development of the 3-D version of it. In comparing the image available through a stereoscopic surgical microscope, which is the benchmark, further advances are still in the future. This, in fact, is the image quality for which industry should strive.

In the meantime, a high-quality 2-D video system will suffice, especially if the surgeon develops the necessary visual perception and visual memory skills, transforming this information into a 'virtual 3-D' image. In other words, the surgeon 'feels' his way around and augments retinal stimuli with reasoning.

Instrumentation

Suturing instruments are very different from the traditional endoscopic instruments (e.g. graspers) since they need to meet special requirements. Since suturing is a two-handed task, the non-dominant hand holds an assisting grasper and the dominant hand holds the needle driver. Each instrument is designed to perform its specific tasks. The needle driver's role is primarily to handle the needle and suture material (including knotting) while having adequate facility to handle the tissue to the appro-

priate extent. The assisting grasper's main function is to grasp and hold the tissues as well as handle the suture material and assist in knot tying. The assisting grasper should be able to hold the needle for left-handed suturing if the situation mandates it. The suturing process requires both instruments to be rotated frequently and thus the handle of the instrument should be rounded to facilitate this type of movement.

Although one can successfully suture with traditional pistol-gripped instruments (Roman scissor-handles), the coaxial design where the handle, stem, and tips are aligned along a straight line is much easier to work with and promotes a more intuitive eye–hand coordination (Figure 5). A lock mechanism can be built into the handle which allows the surgeon to lock the needle into a preferred position during needle driving. This lock can be useful for experienced suturers but can get in the way during the initial stages of learning. This lock also has

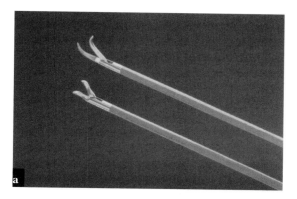

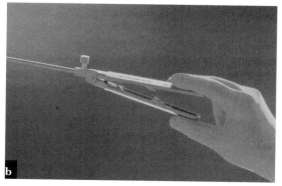

Figure 5 *Coaxial suturing instruments with curved tips. (a) Tips: above, assisting grasper, below, needle driver; (b) handles: coaxial Castroviejo style*

to be intuitive, unobtrusive, and not distractive during suturing. The shaft of the instrument should be at least 33 cm for general purpose use (22 cm for pediatric use), and it should be sealed to prevent loss of insufflation.

Although the handle and stems are identical for both instruments, the jaws differ significantly since they are designed for different functions. The needle driver jaw is configured primarily for needle driving and secondarily for suture and tissue handling. The tips are short and powerfully leveraged, maximizing the grasping power; they have a slight curve with a distinct point to facilitate the suture looping during knot tying, and delicate tissue and suture pick-up from a wet tissue surface. The assisting grasper's narrow jaws are aggressively curved and pointed for maximum grasping capability.

Suture materials

The high level of difficulty that laparoscopic suturing involves requires careful selection of the suture. The selection of the needle and the thread combination can make suturing and knotting either easier or more difficult. There are two other important characteristics in regard to the needle aside from wire strength and sharpness – that is visibility and curvature. The early pioneers in this field used straight needles because of the inability to pass curved needles through the ports. Next came the ski needle, which provided the ease of passing through the port with an added curvature at the tip for tissue pick-up. The preference of experienced surgeons, however, seems to be gravitating back toward curved needles because of the familiar and intuitive scooping motion involved.

With regard to the thread, the important characteristics are visibility, pliability, and knot-holding security. For laparoscopic application, 2-0 silk is used since it has good pliability and is easy to work with. The absorbable polyglactin or lactomer suture material is also easy to handle; however its visibility is significantly reduced because of its pastel violet (lavender) color. Polyester, polyglycolic acid, and polyglyconate sutures have similar visibility disadvantages since they are likely to be stained on contact with blood. The ideal suture material should have vibrant, fluorescent (yellow, green, pink, etc.) colors[6] to provide easy visibility, such as ePTFE which is fluorescent white and resistant to staining.

Monofilament polypropylene, polydiaxanone and nylon are strong, although their stiffness, or excessive memory, can be frustrating to use. Braided materials hold a square knot securely but they are unsuitable for an extracorporeal slip knot. For this purpose, a monofilament material is more suitable because of its slippery surface. If an intracorporeal square knot is tied with these sutures, one must remember to throw three of four hitches to provide adequate knot-holding security.

TRAINING APPROACH

Intracorporeal suturing and knotting provide an excellent focus for training. The choreographed square slip knot, surgeon's knot and Aberdeen knot give the surgeon a tangible, achievable goal to accomplish. Time standards are introduced such as tying a square knot in 30 s, or placing a complete stitch in 1.5 min, or performing an end-to-end or side-to-side anastomosis in under 60 min. These accomplishable tasks build confidence, and should be first practiced on inanimate material, then animal tissue, and finally progressing to the live animal. As the efficacy of this technique has become apparent, it has become the focus of many advanced laparoscopic training programs and workshops. A simulator (trainer box)[7] designed especially for laparoscopic suturing is practical for use with inanimate materials and animal tissues. In the author's opinion, 80 h of formal training and supervised practice time are required to become comfortable with intracorporeal suturing and anastomosis techniques (Figure 6).

Curriculum

The goal of advanced laparoscopic courses is to impart the method of adapting the traditional open techniques to laparoscopic setting. However, this transition is not straightforward but can be facilitated by explaining some of the differences and important technical details. A brief description of the equipment and instruments used during the training sessions should be provided and the use of new or modified instruments also demonstrated.

Training should begin with exercises in a simulator (suturing trainer box) using inanimate material (Figure 7). This provides an opportunity to become familiar with the equipment, instrumentation, and the particulars of intracorporeal suturing and knot tying. Exercises begin with suturing a latex glove that has two rows of dots marked; a cut made through it facilitates the acquisition of the skills of needle handling, precision suturing, and the knot tying sequence. It is particularly important to develop a good technique, such as targeting entrance and exit points, early on in training to avoid the development of bad habits. This is a physically and mentally stressful event, therefore it is rec-

ommended that students should be well rested and avoid caffeine.

The techniques presented during the didactic session should be personally demonstrated by the lecturer to course participants. Ideally, two course participants per trainer set-up allows adequate practice time. First, one surgeon assumes the suturing role while the other provides camera holding and assistance with positioning the target materials, etc. Each participant should work for approximately 3–5 min to accomplish a specific task, then rotate roles. An experienced instructor should be readily on hand to provide guidance if any questions or difficulty arise.

Exercises

In this initial phase, it is important to discuss and practice the vital set-up principles as well as to develop an appreciation for the economy of motion principle, choreographed movements, and flawless technique involved with suturing and knotting techniques. It is also necessary to approach these exercises with relaxed muscles, slowed movements, and tightly focused attention. Furthermore, one needs to recognize that this is a form of precision technique where finesse triumphs over brute force.

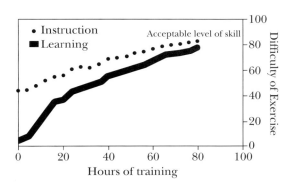

Figure 6 *Skill acquisition in limited access magnified surgical field*

TECHNIQUE

Suture length

After the appropriate suture has been selected for the procedure, the proper length of suture should be carefully considered and calculated prior to its introduction to the operative field. Generally, the length of suture to be inserted into the field should be the minimum length necessary to accomplish the suturing task (usually no more than 17–20 cm). First, introducing a suture longer than this would result in thread tangling and thus require excessive handling. Repeated manipulations and struggles with a long suture can be quite time-consuming and frustrating. Second, inserting the ideal length of suture necessary to accomplish the suturing task eliminates the need for the repeated process of

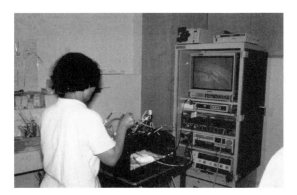

Figure 7 *Trainer set-up*

removal of the used needle and introduction of a new one. By reducing the suture passage traffic through the ports, the likelihood of losing the needle in the port or field is also reduced. Third, a complementary component of this concept is the position of the knot on the thread. The knot should always be tied at the end of the thread. This is a basic principle in magnified surgery (e.g. microsurgery) and is necessary to practice laparoscopically. In contrast, by tying the knot conveniently in the middle of the thread, as is practiced in open surgery, the result will be the uneconomical use of several sutures for a given task. Consequentially, the problems associated with heavy traffic of suture passage through the ports (potential needle loss) is a factor.

Furthermore, the suture line should be kept clear of suture tails and those not used as stay sutures should be snipped reasonably close to the knot to minimize visual clutter and maintain a clean and orderly surgical field.

Needle loading and driving

Straight and ski needles can be inserted through smaller diameter ports but curved needles (especially 1/2 circle needles) may require entry through a larger port, depending on the size of the needle. By grasping the thread 2 cm from the end of the needle with the assisting grasper and positioning it in the proper needle-driving direction, the needle can be introduced and prepared for loading into the jaws of the needle driver instrument without significant extraneous movements. By continuing to hold the thread at this point, the needle can be dangled above the tissue surface and slowly lowered so that the tip of the needle touches the tissue. The instrument can then be moved in such a manner that the needle points in the proper direction for suturing and the needle driver can carefully take hold of the needle and make small adjustments as needed. If the needle is grasped in the proper part but is pointing in the wrong direction, the needle tip can be hooked into the tissue slightly (in an avascular area) and, by pushing the instrument in one direction or another, swiveled into the proper position.

The appropriate grasping point on the needle shaft is approximately two-thirds of its length from the tip of the needle for a 3/8 circle needle, and roughly one-half of the way back for a half circle needle.

Holding the needle perpendicular to its plane by the needle driver provides the most effective grasp for driving through tissues. Furthermore, the needle should also be driven perpendicular through the entrance and exit points, following its curvature to minimize on tissue trauma at these points. In doing so, minimal tissue resistance will be encountered and needle driving will be a straightforward procedure. Slow movements enhance a smooth process.

Deviations from this perpendicular approach lead to a variety of difficulties, frustrations, and wasted time. Needle deflection commonly results from attempting to drive the needle through tissues while the tip has not fully penetrated all tissue layers. To correct needle deflection (when the needle flips out of the proper position), the surgeon can simply reverse the erroneous movement he or she has just made, or the thread can be gently grasped about 1 cm behind the needle end and pulled in a direction to restore the proper position. The surgeon's grip on the needle driver must be loosened somewhat to allow this adjustment, but not excessively or the needle will be dropped altogether.

Suture lines

The appropriate suture line for a given repair can be determined by assessing the type and length of the defect, type of tissues involved, and their function. A continuous suture line can be completed more rapidly because it involves far fewer knots (Table 1), but it is more difficult to accomplish with the same level of precision that can be obtained with an interrupted suture line.

Table 1 *Intracorporeal and extracorporeal knots*

Intracorporeal	*Extracorporeal*
Square-slip	Roeder
Surgeon's	Sliding square
Aberdeen	Pretied

Identification of the tissue edges is necessary as is careful adjustment of the tension on each stitch as the suture line progresses. One method is to use the assisting grasper to lift the suture which provides some degree of countertraction during stitch placement. By using the tail of the first stitch to elevate the tissue, and the thread exteriorized using a suture retrieval device, it is anchored with a hemostat on the surface of the skin. Moderate tension is applied to the suture line and the tissue, then the suture line can be positioned favorably for completion of the repair. Another method is to have the assistant elevate the stitch just completed, or to lock the suture line every few stitches. In the end, if any gaps or loose stitches are found, an interrupted stitch can be added.

An interrupted suture line is more conducive to a precise repair and in some cases, such as a hand-sewn gastrojejunostomy, use of both types of suture lines is recommended at different aspects of the repair.

Intracorporeal knotting

Square knot[8] (Figure 8)

This is the most flexible, practical, and economical way to secure two suture ends approximating tissue edges. The important advantage of this traditional, instrument-tied *square knot* is that, while it is a locking knot, it is forgiving. That is, it can be converted to a *slip knot*[9] and in this slipping configuration the thread can be adjusted to the ideal position and tension, then reconverted to its original locking configura-

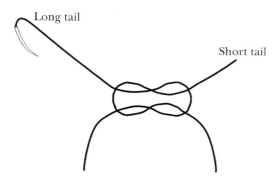

Figure 8 *The square knot*

tion. Therefore, if the knot initially locks outside of the intended position, it does not need to be removed and replaced. Also, if used temporarily to secure a stay suture, the same knot can be converted for use in tissue approximation by making the proper conversions. If stiff monofilament suture is used, a third throw may be placed for additional security.

Although the properly choreographed sequence is initially challenging to learn and requires considerable time and practice to master, the surgeon is manifested the benefit of the increased awareness of the dexterity possible in the laparoscopic approach (Figure 9).

Surgeon's knot

If modest tension exists at the tissue edges to be approximated, the first single throw easily unravels, and therefore a double throw would be more secure. Like the square knot, the surgeon's knot is secured with a single throw in the opposite direction. The disadvantage is that this becomes a permanent knot which cannot be adjusted. One might be convinced that, after placing a surgeon's knot, the tissue is properly approximated, only to discover later that the stitch is loose. As with all permanent knots, if adjustment are needed, the surgeon's knot has to be cut out and replaced. Considering the labor intensiveness of suturing and knotting, the square-slip knot holds a clear advantage.

Granny knot

This is composed of two half-hitches placed in the same direction. This is an unpredictable knot – sometimes it will slip and other times it will jam. It is usually the result of an incorrectly tied square knot.

Twist knot

This knot was promoted because it avoid the complex choreography required by the square knot. The long tail is grasped by the needle driver instrument and rotated three or more times around its axis, then the short tail is pulled through the created loops and pulled tight,

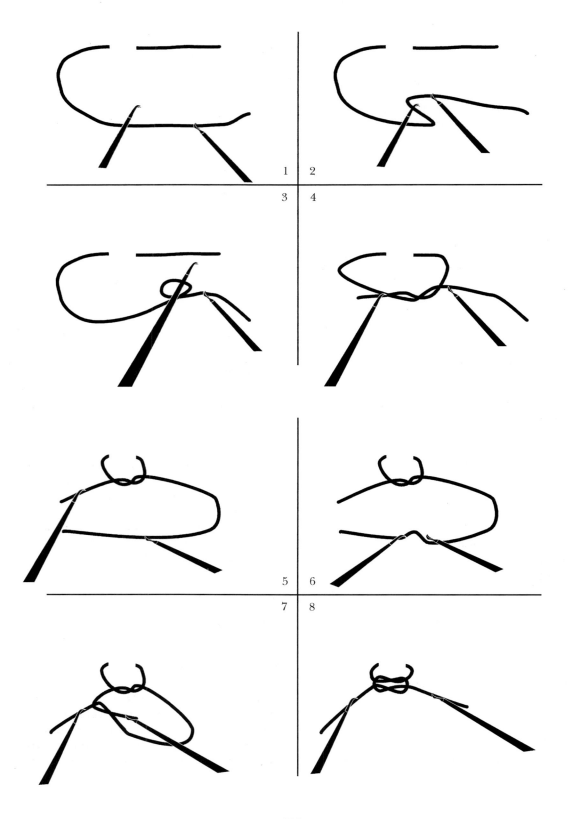

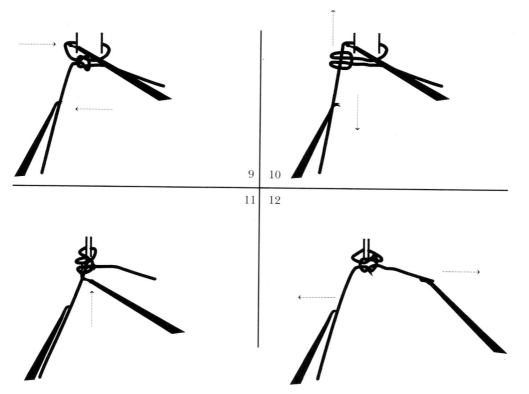

Figure 9 *Choreographed square knot: starting position (steps 1–4), forming the square knot (steps 5–8), conversion to its sliding configuration (steps 9–10); pushing the knot down (step 11), and reconverting to locking configuration (square knot)*

creating a knot. Although it seems simple, it takes considerable skill to accomplish it correctly.

Lasso knot

The end of the suture is doubled up and tied approximately 3–5 mm from the end, creating a loop. This can be either a permanent or slip knot. As the needle is driven through the entrance and exit points, it is brought back and passed through this loop at the end. As the thread is pulled, the tissue edges are brought together. The slip knot version can be tightened to hold and the permanent version will stay loose and its use is preferable for a continuous suture line.

Prelooped suture

The 'prelooped' suture is introduced to the surgical field through a port. The needle is driven through the entrance and exit points, and then threaded through the pretied suture loop, secured by the tip of the applicator. Then the thread is held taut and the applicator handle is pushed, tightening the loop and creating the knot. The threads are then cut. Again, it takes some skill to apply this device.

Aberdeen knot (Figure 10)

Securing a continuous suture line can be accomplished two ways. One possibility is to loosen the last loop and use it as the 'short tail' for the traditional square or surgeon's knot tying of a three-legged tie.

Another method is the Aberdeen knot, which also requires loosening up the last loop. It is also known as the crochet or french knot. Although this knotting technique requires minimal rotation of the instrument, it still requires considerable skill to execute properly.

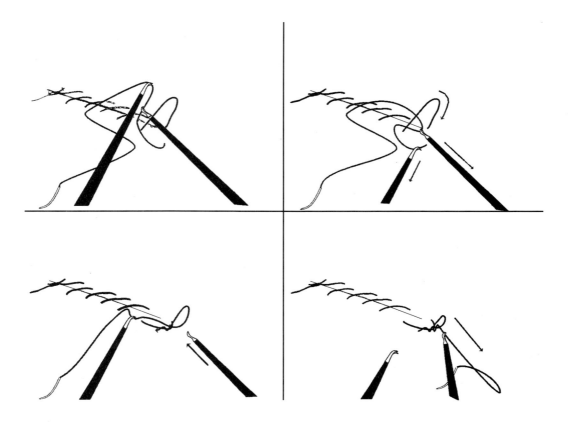

Figure 10   *The Aberdeen knot*

It is recommended that the participants begin with the choreographed square knot, and, once they have gained confidence, they can try the other methods.

Extracorporeal knotting

This type of knot, where the knot is tied outside of the body cavity and reintroduced using an instrument, is useful when the surgeon lacks intracorporeal knotting skills. It can be used on sturdier tissues and, therefore, there is little application for the extracorporeal knot in fetal surgery. It is sometimes used when the operating space is too tight for the instrument tips to maneuver in, although an intracorporeal square knot can be tied away from the stitch in a more spacious area, converted to a slip knot and slid down into place. These knots work best with slippery monofilament suture materials.

Knots tied with braided suture have a tendency to lock prematurely. A common misconception about extracorporeal knots is that they require less skill to perform than the tying of an intracorporeal knot. On the contrary, to tie extracorporeal knots safely, considerable skill and cognizance of the pitfalls, and therefore strategies to avoid potential tissue trauma are required.

SUTURING IN THE FETAL PATIENT

Once good access is established, suturing, knotting and operative techniques are basically the same as for standard laparoscopy – with the exception that greater control is required. The smaller structures and tissues require higher magnification, smaller sutures, and greater precision in stitch placement. The friability of fetal tissue requires a more delicate approach and familiarity with the limits of tissue strength (i.e. when they will tear). Shorter instruments have proven to be easier to control for fetoscopic surgery[10] and therefore are preferred to standard-length laparoscopic instruments.

Needle selection should be focused on those with a special curvature and suture material should be chosen that is strong, pliable, and contrasting in color, ranging from 3-0 to 6-0 in size.

References

1. Szabo, Z. and Henderson, S. R. (1993). Organizing training programs in laparoscopic microsurgery: set-up, curriculum, and standards. In *Endoscopy in Gynecology, AAGL 20th Annual Meeting Proceedings*, pp. 259–65. American Association of Gynecologic Laparoscopists, Santa Fe Springs, CA

2. Wolfe, B. M., Szabo, Z., Moran, M. E. *et al.* (1993). Training for minimally invasive surgery: need for surgical skills. *Surg. Endosc.*, **7**, 93–5

3. Azziz, R. (1992). Operative endoscopy: the pressing need for a structured training and credentialing process. *Fertil. Steril.*, **58**, 1100–2

4. Cuschieri, A. and Szabo, Z. (1995). *Tissue Approximation in Endoscopic Surgery : Suturing & Knotting Techniques.* (Oxford: Isis Medical Media)

5. Szabo, Z. (1993). Laparoscopic suturing and tissue approximation. In Hunter, J. G. and Sackier, J. M. (eds.) *Minimally Invasive Surgery*, pp. 141–55. (New York: McGraw-Hill)

6. Bowyer, D. W., Moran, M. E. and Szabo, Z. (1992). Laparoscopic suturing in urology: a model for vesicourethral anastomosis following radical prostatectomy. *Min. Invas. Ther.*, **4**, 165–70

7. Szabo, Z. Endoscopic suturing and knotting. In Braverman, M. H. and Tawes, R. L. (eds.) *Surgical Technology International*, 2nd edn., pp. 123–8. (San Francisco: Surgical Technology International)

8. Buncke, H. J., Chater, N. L. and Szabo, Z. (1975). *Manual of Microvascular Surgery.* (Danbury: Davis & Geck)

9. Szabo, Z., Stellini, L., Rose, E. H. *et al.* (1992). Slip-knot suspension technique: a fail-safe microanastomosis technique for small caliber vessels. *Microsurgery*, **13**, 100–2

10. Estes, J. M., Szabo, Z. and Harrison, M. R. (1992). Techniques for *in utero* endoscopic surgery: a new approach for fetal intervention. *Surg. Endosc.*, **6**, 215–18

Section 4

Assessment of the fetal condition

The embryo as a patient: early pregnancy loss

25

J. C. Birnholz and F. B. Kent

INTRODUCTION

'Miscarriage' implies misbehavior, mismanagement, mishap, and disaster. From literature through romances and old wives' tales, early pregnancy loss is associated with accusation and irony, which prompts a fear of miscarriage when pregnancy is suspected or anticipated. Women often assume that they have been responsible for a miscarriage themselves or they may be blamed for one by their partner or relatives; they regret their helplessness and they regard miscarriage as a failure of their own bodies. Grief and guilt, shame and depression can be devastating and prolonged.

Until recently, early pregnancy was often unrecognized. Miscarriages were only identified as those occurring after the fact of pregnancy had been established. There was usually no medical or biological explanation for the loss, so that most women would associate the bleeding and passage of conceptual products with some recent, stressful event. We now identify pregnancy soon after conception, we appreciate the frequency of very early pregnancy failure, and we have some understanding of the biological foundations (and necessity) of early pregnancy loss. The ultrasound examiner can provide reassurance when viability is confirmed and an informative and educational perspective (Color plate 30) that can be sustaining and uplifting for patients confronted with an extant or inevitable loss.

We believe that most early pregnancy losses are a normal mechanism for prevention of fetal malformations and of severe developmental disabilities. We believe we can predict which pregnancies will continue into the second trimester and which will terminate spontaneously by the mid-first trimester from findings in the initial ultrasound survey, and we are beginning to extend the potential for anatomic diagnosis into the embryonic phase of development. Our observations began with a predictive analysis of gestational sac features in 1973[1] and our current database consists of 1589 first-trimester examinations utilizing large-aperture, high-frequency endovaginal-array ultrasound equipment with high-performance pulsed Doppler capabilities, technical advances which extend diagnostic capabilities from fetal into embryonic phases of development.

BIOLOGY, DEFINITIONS AND IMAGING

Under most ordinary circumstances, in the absence of overt toxic environmental or occupational exposures, drug use, or chronic illness, we expect that at least half of all conceptions will fail to produce a viable embryo[2,3]. Conception occurs within the tube, with implantation within an hormonally prepared endometrium about a week later. Most early pregnancy losses result from implantation failures, and the occurrence of conception may not have been appreciated. Symptoms may be limited to physical tiredness and a delayed, heavy menstrual flow with some clotted material. Subfertile women bear a double burden of a low conception rate and an early loss rate of the order of 80%[4].

The majority of early pregnancy losses are associated with chromosomal abnormalities[5,6], despite the cellular selection processes associated with ovulation, spermatogenesis, sperm migration, and competition for exclusive ovum penetration. Conversely, the miscarriage rate is increased for all forms of aneuploidy[7].

Fetal survival is possible with minimal genetic disruption, such as an extra one of the smaller chromosomes with sparse genetic information, i.e. trisomies 13, 18, and 21 or monosomy X. Non-disjunctions of the larger chromosomes terminate a cell line. Triploidy is found in about 16% of abortuses[8], but is an extremely rare finding at birth. A sac that appears empty ultrasonically (Figure 1) is referred to as an 'anembryonic' pregnancy, which differs from a pregnancy failure with a visible embryo only in the timing (or number of cell divisions) between conception and growth cessation. Growth arrest may precede and preclude trophoblast development, which is why most of the sacs have thin walls without an obvious decidual rim. The embryo, the membranes, and the decidual/placental components of an early pregnancy each have their individual chromosome components derived from the conceptus. Aneuploidy may occur for all or any of these compartments in complete or mosaic forms. The primary division of embryo and placental lines from the zygote is the formation of the blastocyst within the morula, at about 4 days of age.

Espey and Ben Halin have hypothesized that the physical mechanism of ovulation involves an inflammatory type reaction at the ovarian capsule[9]. Something similar may be presumed to occur as a conceptus burrows within the endometrium and, again, when the trophoblast invades the myometrium. If cell divisions cease soon after conception, genes are not activated for synthesis of substances required for invasion and implantation. The conceptus will be retained for a variable time at the endometrial surface before expulsion occurs (Figure 2). Factors in the endometrial microenvironment affecting cell adhesion and local inflammatory responses may also interfere with implantation. Selenium, cadmium, chromium, lead and, perhaps, alcohol may interfere at multiple sites in the developmental chain, including implantation.

The common clinical correlates of pregnancy, tiredness, breast tenderness, pelvic vascular engorgement, and 'morning' sickness, relate to hormone production from the corpus luteum and the developing placenta. After embryonic

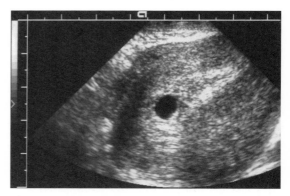

Figure 1 *Anembryonic pregnancy appears as an anechoic void, usually with a thin wall (lack of trophoblast differentiation), which has not penetrated the endometrium*

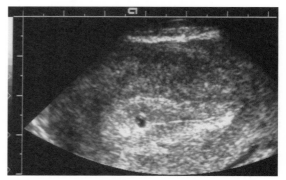

Figure 2 *A (secondary) yolk sac appears within a minute gestational sac, near the border of the endometrium. There has been an embryonic growth arrest, probably around day 7, with arrested implantation. The yolk sac is the first structure to become visible within the gestational sac*

or trophoblast cell divisions cease, the sac separates, the corpus luteum involutes, progesterone levels fall, and coordinated, expulsive, myometrial contractions begin. When hormone production continues, patients will feel pregnant, even though there may be no visible embryo or no embryonic life. This condition is referred to as a 'missed abortion'. Declining progesterone levels signal embryonic demise and impending miscarriage[10]. Giving progesterone exogenously will prevent contractions, but it cannot rescue or retrieve a malformed or maldeveloped embryo.

The myometrial dynamics of a miscarriage seem to be identical to those of menstrual flow[7]. The secretory endometrium separates during the 1st day of menstruation, and emptying depends entirely upon contractions, at first in the longitudinal periendometrial zone and later, during peak flow, involving the transverse, central layer. Contractions become coordinated and have a net force applied sequentially from fundus towards the lower segment. A pacemaker is inferred, although the control of contractile force and periodicity have not been determined. It is likely that progesterone (or its lack) affects the induction of myometrial receptors for prostaglandin, influencing contractile efficiency. The multilevel variability in hormone production, intrauterine circulation, receptor number, and receptor efficiency in early pregnancy explains the marked variation in the timing and thoroughness of spontaneous abortion after embryonic demise. Forceful contractions decrease intrauterine blood flow, first in subendometrial veins and then in radial arteries. Sustained contractions with myometrial anoxia are painful. In terms of early pregnancy loss, hemorrhage at the margin of the sac, sac separation, and myometrial contractions are separate events and not necessarily associated or sequential.

The effectiveness of ultrasound imaging depends upon instrumentation type and use, the skill and experience of the operator, and the habitus of the patient[11]. Instrument features must be selected for optimization of spatial, contrast, and temporal resolutions simultaneously. All early pregnancy viewing is performed with an endovaginal probe, because of the low noise content of these images[12]. Supplemental, transabdominal viewing is only applicable with a grossly myomatous, anteverted uterus with a fundal or cornual implantation site, when intervening tissue compromises endovaginal viewing. The probe should be a linear or area array with large aperture. There should be dynamic beam formation and dynamic display allocation. A linear array is preferred to a tightly curved array, and the field of view should be limited to the region of interest and magnified to maximize the number of display pixels allocated per tissue area. Frame averaging, gray or pseudo color imaging, and dynamic range should be selected for noise reduction. Newer

forms of ultrasound image formation with higher levels of noise (side and grating lobe) reduction will be of particular value in early pregnancy studies. Doppler imaging should be obtained in an energy or power mode at the highest available frequency.

Intrauterine pregnancy can be recognized 2 weeks after conception as a minute, approximately, 1-mm, thin-walled fluid locule with an hypoechoic corona. The corona is reminiscent of the lysozyme-rich boundary of an invasive metastatic tumor. Within a week, the gestational sac will have burrowed through the basal layer of the endometrium and there will be a highly reflective trophoblastic boundary. A small (secondary) yolk sac should be visible by this time, suspended within the gelatinous primary yolk sac substance of the extracoelomic space (Figure 2). Visualization of the yolk sac precedes ultrasonic definition of the embryo which will reach a length of 1 mm just before 6 weeks' gestational age (i.e. idealized menstrual dating equal to conceptual age plus 2 weeks). Cardiac motion will be obvious from this stage at television-frame rates in magnification mode, and intraembryonic blood flow velocity should surpass conventional, pulsed Doppler signal-to-noise threshold by a body length of 2.5 mm (Figure 3). Central circulatory features become defined with energy Doppler imaging near the start of the 7th week (Color plate 31).

The embryo tends to be positioned adjacent to the yolk sac attached by a stalk containing allantoic vessels. The embryo develops within the amnion, which is fused to the cord and so closely applied to the body that it is not resolved as separate at 6 weeks. Amniotic fluid is transuded through the skin with the volume increasing linearly with embryonic surface area in the mid-first trimester[13]. The amnion is visualized from about 7 weeks and afterwards (Figure 4). Fluid volume increases exponentially after about 9½ weeks, when fetal urine production begins. The terms 'conceptus'. 'embryo', and 'fetus' are loosely divided by age, with 'fetus' being applied, conventionally, after about 10 weeks, when organogenesis is established and the risk of subsequent, spontaneous pregnancy loss is presumed to be low.

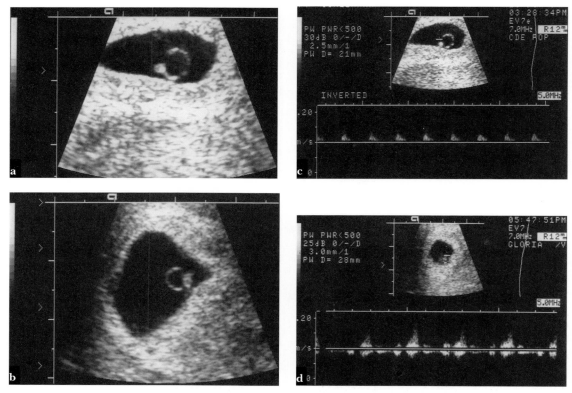

Figure 3 *Embryonic cardiac motion is usually perceptible by the time the yolk sac is about 2 mm in diameter. These are examples at 5.7 and 6.2 weeks' gestation ((a) and (c)) with pulsed Doppler patterns. The earlier pattern has just barely perceptible secondary peaks while the later tracing shows multiple flow events*

ULTRASOUND OBSERVATIONS

Discussion is limited herein to intrauterine pregnancy with a reasonably central implantation site and thick decidual boundary. In practice, this starting point may follow one or more examinations resolving issues of ectopic pregnancy, referral within 10 days of conception, or referral after spontaneous, complete abortion. An embryo should become visible before 6.5 weeks, next to a (spherical) yolk sac between 2 and 3 mm in diameter. Viability is ascertained by the presence or absence of a heart beat. The circulation is the first physiological system to become activated, with cardiac motion beginning when the heart is still in tubular form around day 23 after conception. A heart beat may not be seen with an embryonic plate less than 0.5 mm in length; however, cardiac motion should be obvious with current instrumentation

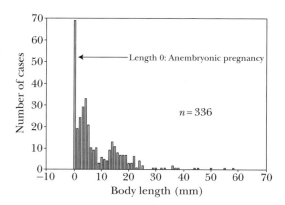

Figure 4 *Histogram distribution of all cases of missed abortion by body length. The most common group consists of those with embryonic growth arrest within the first few days after conception*

by the time the embryonic length reaches 2.0 mm[14]. Restudy can be obtained for either operator or patient certainty of embryonic demise.

The 'blighted twin' phenomenon[15] is now well recognized. Diagnosis requires visualization of a distinct, encapsulated fluid locule, with or without an embryonic remnant. Intraendometrial collections occur with a peridecidual (implantation) hemorrhage. When there is an anembryonic sac, well separated from a viable embryo/gestational sac complex, the remnant may have been retained from an unrecognized conception a month or more earlier. Loss of one or more embryos of a multiple pregnancy is an indication for amniocentesis. Any instance of monochorionic multiples identified in the first trimester requires close serial observation, because of the risk of parabiotic syndrome, which can be treated under some conditions by ablation of communicating vessels. Color flow Doppler (especially Energy mode) will depict the umbilical cords clearly and identify those at highest risk for compromise because of a common or closely spaced cord origin.

Body length (a linear estimator of embryonic volume) is used to determine the timing of conception of a viable embryo with reasonable precision[16–18]. In our series of nearly 1600 first-trimester examinations, there were 1176 viable (scrupulously normal) embryos and 336 missed abortions. Embryonic length distribution with missed abortion is shown in Figure 4. The commonest group were anembryonic (length 0) or length less than 1 mm, representing growth arrest within the first few weeks after conception. Embryonic length (equivalent to age at demise and representing the probability of demise with age) decreases exponentially after 6 weeks gestational age except for a small secondary peak at around 8 weeks' gestation (Figure 5). Some inference is required for timing conception in missed abortion with visible embryo, because of the variable and generally unknown time of sac retention and because growth rate may have been abnormal. However, when we estimate the timing of conception by month for the viable cases and for some cases of embryonic demise and missed abortion (Figure 6), we find a statistically significant seasonal pattern. Peak conception in our population occurs in July, typically

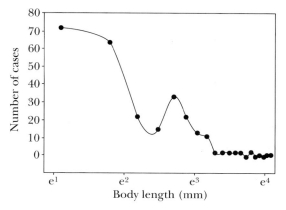

Figure 5 *Smoothed (3 mm bin) distribution of body length for 267 cases of missed abortion. An embryo could be visualized in each of these cases. The x-axis (body length) is scaled to powers of e (2.72). The secondary peak occurs at about 15 mm and there is a minimal shoulder at 20 mm*

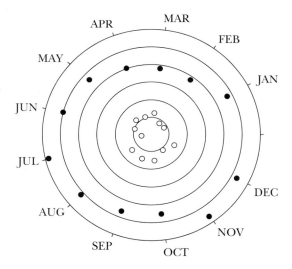

Figure 6 *Polar plot of number of cases by estimated month of conception. The highest number of viable embryos (solid circles) and the lowest number of missed abortions (empty circles) fall along the July radius*

including vacation time, and also the month with lowest missed abortion rate. Additional conception peaks occur in November and December.

The yolk sac is the first structure to become visible within the gestational sac. The yolk sac is an energy source for the developing embryo and generates hematopoietic stem cells. Reece and colleagues[19] proposed that the allantoic circulation is a site of injury for hyperglycemia and may be responsible for early pregnancy loss and some malformation complexes typical of uncontrolled maternal diabetes. A relatively small or flat yolk sac is a common finding with early pregnancy loss, and, in true anembryonic pregnancy, there is no visible yolk sac. The yolk sac expands when there is decreased allantoic venous flow. Preterminal thrombosis of the allantoic stalk may calcify when uterine expulsion is delayed. Allantoic blood flow in larger vessels comprising the stalk is revealed by Energy Doppler.

Motion of the embryonic heart beat becomes visible with electronically scanned images within a few days of the start of contractions. We document and study cardiac activity with a brief pulsed Doppler tracing, usually of about 2 s duration. The smallest sampling window will often encompass the entire embryo. Composite blood flow velocity may not surpass a pulsed Doppler detection threshold when the embryonic length is less than 1 mm; however, recording should be uncomplicated technically by the time an embryo has elongated to 3 mm. The shape of the Doppler tracing will depend upon the relative sizes of the sampling window and of the embryo, insonification bandwidth, transducer focal pattern, and the angle of insonification relative to the torso. The pattern should have two high-velocity peaks corresponding to ventricular filling and ejection. The first-trimester embryonic heart is without external nervous control, so that the pattern should always have an absolute and monotonous regularity (Figure 7). Transient decelerations, representing unbalanced vagal effects, occur in the early second trimester, and sympathetic accelerations do not become possible until the third trimester. The heart rate is closely related to body size and consequently age (Figure 8), increasing to a maximal value at about 9 weeks' gestation[20]. The mechanism for this rate control remains to be clarified, although elegant studies in an embryonic avian model suggest that the rate effect may be related to changes in peripheral vascular resistance during that period of development[21]. The standard deviation of heart rate (HR) ver-

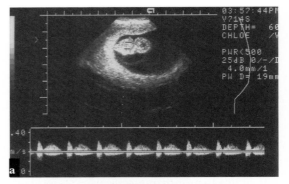

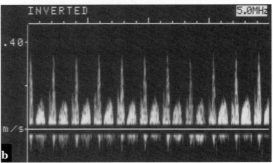

Figure 7 *(a) The short high-velocity peak is ventricular filling, the lower phase is composite ejection and outflow. The filling phase will reveal separate diastolic inflow and atrial systolic components by 10 weeks' gestation (b)*

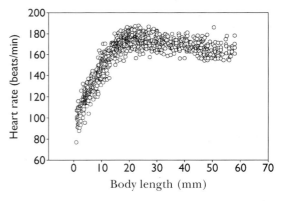

Figure 8 *Graph of heart rate versus body length (a non-interpretive indicator of time) in the first trimester for 900 viable, normal cases with crown–rump length < 50 mm. Rates are calculated from Doppler tracings and have an estimated precision of about a beat per minute*

sus embryo length (which can be related to age) is low, between 1 and 20 mm. The relationship is given by the pair of equations derived from 500 cases (Figure 9):

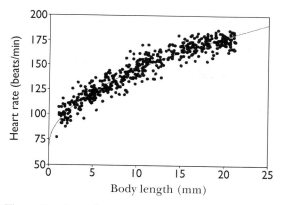

Figure 9 *Curve fit parameters for heart rate versus body length during the near linear initial portion of the first-trimester rate pattern between 4 and 6 weeks' gestation*

$$HR = 66.820307 + 24.872632 \, Length^{\frac{1}{2}}$$

$$Length = -4.214787 + 0.12418928 HR^{\frac{1}{2}} Ln\,(HR)$$

with each relationship having a correlation coefficient of about 0.90. Embryonic heart rates below 80 beats/min after 7 weeks (as observed visually or sampled with M mode) have been reported as conveying a poor prognosis for further survival[22]. Achiron and colleagues have reported that rates above 180 beats/min in the early second trimester are also a negative prognostic sign, which they speculate represents a direct myocardial effect of fetal infection following chorioamnionitis[23].

The Doppler pattern looks something like an electrocardiogram; however, it displays blood flow velocity changes with time and, as such, it is a direct indicator of myocardial mechanics. We score as 'feeble' any visible heart rate that does not trigger the Doppler at or beyond a fetal length of 2.5 mm, as 'single' when only a portion of the pump cycle is depicted by Doppler, and an 'arrhythmia' with any type of intermittent disturbance of a regular two-phase pattern (Figure 10). Eleven of 15 'feebles' had subsequent loss, with three of four survivors less than 1.5 mm in body length. There was loss of 23 of 36 'single' patterns or 23 of 29 singles with body length greater than 2.0 mm. Twenty of 20 irregular patterns had subsequent demise. Twenty-two of 1196 cases with regular heart rate patterns had subsequent demise (including cases of parabiotic syndrome and aneuploidy).

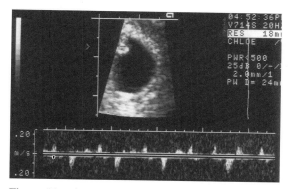

Figure 10 *A complex arrhythmia at 6.5 weeks resembling an A : V dissociation with a variable ventricular rate*

Each of these Doppler categories represents beats that are ineffective mechanically, entirely (feeble), partially (single), or intermittently (the commonest type of arrhythmia resembling a variable A : V block with a dropping out of a portion of some beats). The Doppler pattern demonstrates pump function, and any depression in contractile efficiency represents heart failure. In those cases that have survived a few days, we have observed a marked increase in amniotic fluid volume and usually some slight distention of the yolk sac (Figure 11). Amniotic fluid is transuded through skin in the first trimester, and, with systemic venous hypertension, resorption of fluid into the body is impeded and the amnion becomes distended. As the skin becomes cornified, skin edema becomes possible. Amniotic fluid excess is an analog of pulmonary edema with left heart failure and of peripheral edema with right heart failure later in life. Fetal ventricles pump in parallel (rather than in series), and the amnion is 'insulated' by the coelomic space from fluid exchange through the chorion. Figure 12 compares free amniotic volume for viable embryos with missed abortion. We infer that the majority of cases with amniotic fluid excess sustained congestive heart failure as a terminal episode. Arrhythmias precede heart failure and demise in anoxic embryonic mammalian and avian models[24]. Cases after 8 weeks' gestation with preterminal decline in cardiac output will demonstrate a pericardial effusion (Figure 13), followed sequentially by proximal skin edema, pleural effusions, and ascites if the time course

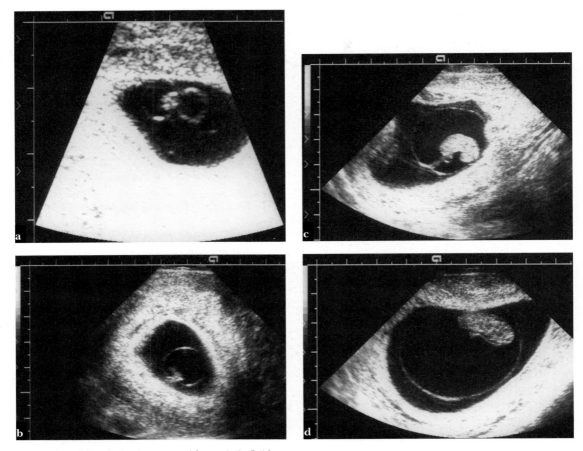

Figure 11 *Missed abortion cases with amniotic fluid excess*

is sufficiently protracted. Arrhythmia cases tend to have ventricular rates below the age-adjusted norm, especially before 7 weeks' gestation, while regular heart rate cases prior to loss tend to be above average, particularly those with intrauterine hematomas with potential for diffusion of vasoactive substances into the fetal circulation.

Ultrasonic demonstration of viability alone decreases the age-adjusted miscarriage risk significantly[25,26]. Our experience is that, once normal pump function is demonstrated with a supra-threshold Doppler pattern with distinct phases, with a regular rate in the normal range, and without any visible dysmorphic features, the likelihood of pregnancy continuation is at least 98%, independent of age or signs of intrauterine bleeding. For the majority of

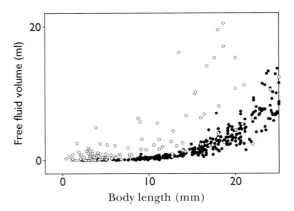

Figure 12 *The open circles are cases of missed abortion. Note the limited data dispersion in normal cases before 20-mm body length and the preponderance of fluid excess with missed abortion*

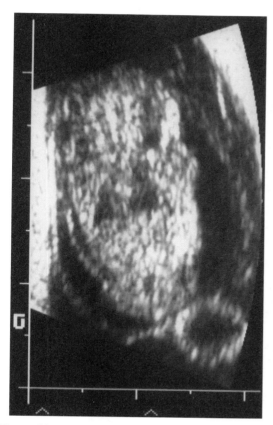

Figure 13 *A large mediastinal fluid collection appears as a central triangle in this 22-mm embryo. There is also elevation of nuchal and torso skin*

first-trimester subjects, ultrasound serves to provide reassurance.

As detail resolution improves, the potential for first-trimester recognition of anomalies is also enhanced[27,28]. Central circulatory features are disclosed by Energy Doppler imaging by 6.5 weeks' gestational age, and a 'four-chamber' view is obtained after the mid-first trimester (Color plate 32). We have identified one example of cardiac exstrophy first seen at about 7 weeks (Color plate 33). Another case of ectopia cordis was found at the end of the first trimester using Doppler color imaging[29]. A rudimentary spine can be perceived as early as 7 weeks and paired choroid glomi, implying mid-line division of a developing brain, is already evident by 8½ weeks, indicating the potential for early detection of anencephaly (Figure 14) and holoprosencephaly (Figure 15) by the mid-first

trimester. Recent studies have suggested an increased prevalence of nuchal, scalp, or torso skin edema in first-trimester examinations, these presumably representing cases with aneuploidy (with lymphedema) who would have succumbed and miscarried before a, conventional, mid-second-trimester examination. Skeletal features, including the hands, are in evidence by the 10th week (Figure 16), and facial features are well defined by the end of the first trimester (Figure 17).

Chronologies of spontaneous movements have been reported as indicators of neuromotor development, especially in the second trimester when the sizes of extremities, hands, lenses, and facial features were more in keeping with performance features of early ultrasound equipment[30,31]. Visual observations of abortuses in the first trimester by Hooker, Humphries, Windle, and others[32-34] have led to foundation theories of behavior as a differentiation and refinement of primitive 'reflexes'. High-speed, high-resolution ultrasound enables observation of motor activity under physiological conditions with the potential for associating regressive activities as indicating hypoxia or other environmental disturbance. Simple, infrequent, extensile twitches of the torso are seen by 30–35 days after conception, and we have observed movements of the forearms and shrug-like movements of the shoulders and upper torso by 20-mm length. Tools now exist for detailed study of first-trimester motoric behavior.

There is little variation in normal embryonic growth patterns. Cell division rates are retarded with aneuploidy[35], resulting in a size discrepancy in the first trimester, the effects being most pronounced for triploidy and mosaic forms of trisomies that do not survive in their full form, such as trisomy 16. Most, but not all, instances of size less than anticipated from last menstrual period dating will represent conception late in a cycle. The issue may be clarified whenever the date of conception is known or when the patient can limit the probable time of conception to a few widely spaced dates. Embryonic length should be estimated from separate, concordant determinations. A substandard growth rate between studies a week or more

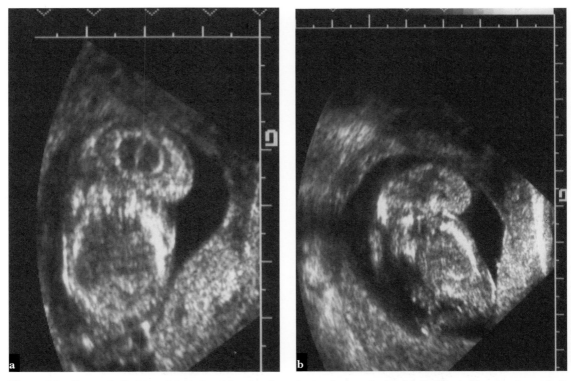

Figure 14 *Exencephalia (acrania) in the mid- to late first trimester has a soft, dumb-bell-shaped, fibrovascular cephalic bundle. When this breaks down, amniotic fluid clouds transiently and the cranial base has a typical truncated appearance*

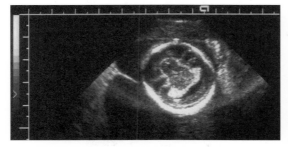

Figure 15 *Alobar holoprosencephaly can be identified before the end of the first trimester. This case had multiple anomalies and was found to have trisomy 13*

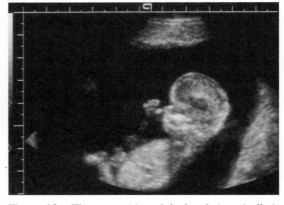

Figure 16 *The rest position of the hands is typically in front of the face in the first and second trimesters*

apart reconfirms the growth deficit and conveys a poor prognosis.

PERSPECTIVE

The common and old term for anembryonic pregnancy is a 'blighted ovum', which seems to imply a deficiency of the female component of the conceptus. This is an example of the sub-liminal or unintentional assignment of blame for early pregnancy loss that contributes to its psychological toll for both partners. The term 'threatened abortion' has been used with vaginal bleeding early in pregnancy, with the presumption that larger and repetitive episodes of

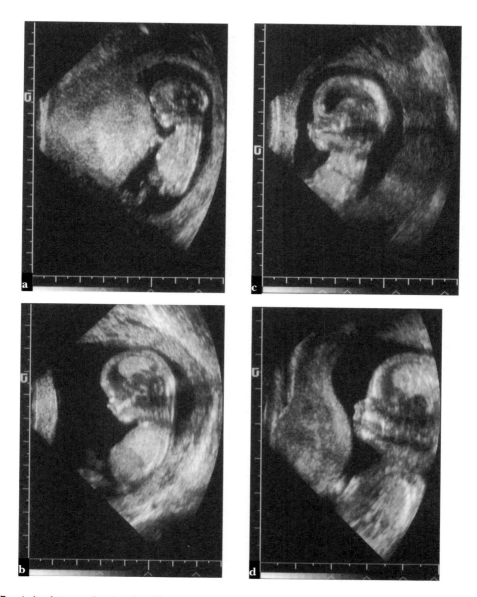

Figure 17 *A developmental series of profiles*

hemorrhage would signal an 'inevitable' abortion, which might be pre-empted by emptying the uterus surgically. The last 20 years of ultrasound use has removed the early gravid uterus as terra incognita. Ultrasonic observations of the uterus and its contents should resolve issues of implantation, embryonic presence, number and viability, and present information for correlation with an emerging arsenal of biochemical,

physiological, cytogenetic, and immunological tools for sampling the uterine environment.

We advocate an ultrasound survey when a woman first believes that she may be pregnant. Standard practice predicates ultrasound usage on indications, such as bleeding, although frequent monitoring has become the norm with assisted reproduction. We have observed a disproportionate incidence of embryonic arrhythmias and subsequent losses in self-referred women without typical indications. The study is performed from an endovaginal viewing portal and can be limited to less than 1 min without loss in information retrieval.

In most instances of an ultrasound examination in early pregnancy, we anticipate confirmation of central, intrauterine implantation with a viable embryo having a two-phase cardiac cycle. When there is a missed abortion, the patient is informed immediately and the information placed in the context of the high incidence of early pregnancy loss as well as her own past history. The association of aneuploidy and early pregnancy loss is reiterated, especially when there is embryonic skin edema. More important for the patient will be an understanding of the lack of effect of daily external life events on the course of embryonic development after implantation has occurred. The fact of conception itself is reinforced, since there is an important prognostic distinction between early loss and infertility. The examiner should convey a level of certainty about the findings for the patient and her physician and repeat the study as necessary until findings are unequivocal.

We emphasize the performance of ultrasound instrumentation in attempting to visualize and evaluate embryos that may be only a few millimeters in length. Clinical practice spans a range of instrumentation performance. Units offering the very best spatial resolution and the least power output should be applied preferentially for early pregnancy studies. Current units just surpass the 1-mm lateral resolution barrier under ordinary scanning conditions. Significant technical advances portending further refinement and sophistication for early pregnancy viewing are now in progress.

The embryonic phase of development is distinct clinically from the remainder of gestation, as are the interactions between the embryo and its immediate environment. New techniques for exploring this microcosm have already provided the capabilities for forming prognoses and making rudimentary diagnoses. There is a potential for therapeutic maneuvers even at this frontier of gestation.

ACKNOWLEDGEMENT

The authors wish to thank Dr Anya Kowalik, New York Hospital for reviewing the manuscript.

References

1. Birnholz, J. C. and Barnes, A. B. (1973). Early diagnosis of hydatidiform mole by ultrasound imaging. *J. Am. Med. Assoc.*, **225**, 1359–60
2. Wilcox, A. J., Weinberg, C. R., O'Connor, J. F. *et al.* (1992). Incidence of early pregnancy loss. *N. Eng. J. Med.*, **319**, 189–94
3. Edwards, R. G. (1986). Causes of early embryonic loss in human pregnancy. *Hum. Reprod.*, **1**, 185–98
4. Hakim, R. B., Gray, R. H. and Zacur, H. (1995). Infertility and early pregnancy loss. *Am. J. Obstet. Gynecol.*, **172**, 1510–17
5. Guerneri, S., Bettio, D., Simoni, G., Brambati, B. *et al.* (1991). Prevalence and distribution of chromosome abnormalities in a sample of first trimester internal abortions. *Hum. Reprod.*, **2**, 736–9
6. Ohno, M., Maeda, T. and Matsunobu, A. (1991). A cystogenetic study of spontaneous abortions with direct analysis of chorionic villi. *Obstet. Gynecol.*, **77**, 394–8
7. Poland, B. J., Miller, J. R., Harris, M. and Livinston, J. (1981). Spontaneous abortion. A study of 1961 women and their conceptuses. *Acta Obstet. Gynecol. Scand. Suppl.*, **102**, 1–32
8. Boue, J., Boue, A. and Lazar, P. (1975). Retrospective and prospective epidemiologic studies of 1500 karyotyped spontaneous human abortions. *Teratology*, **12**, 11–26
9. Espey, L. L. and Ben Halin, A. (1990). Characteristics and control of the normal menstrual cycle. *Obstet. Gynecol. Clin. North Am.*, **17**, 275–98
10. Al-Sebai, M. A. H., Kingsland, C. R., Diver, M., Hipkin, L. and McFadyen, I. R. (1995). The role

of a single progesterone measurement in the diagnosis of early pregnancy failure and the prognosis of fetal viability. *Br. J. Obstet. Gynaecol.*, **102**, 364–9

11. Birnholz, J. C. and Hayes, T. (1987). The effect of instrumentation and examination. In McGahan, J. P. (ed.) *Controversies in Ultrasound*, pp. 143–52. (New York: Churchill Livingstone)

12. Birnholz, J. C. (1992). Smaller parts scanning of the fetus. *Radiol. Clin. North Am.*, **30**, 977–91

13. Birnholz, J. C. and Madanes, A. E. (1995). Amniotic fluid accumulation in the first trimester. *J. Ultrasound Med.*, **14**, 597–602

14. Goldstein, I., Zimmer, E. A., Tamir, A., Peretz, B. A. and Paldi, E. (1991). Evaluation of normal gestational sac growth: appearance of embryonic heartbeat and embryo body movements using the transvaginal technique. *Obstet. Gynecol.*, **77**, 885–8

15. Finberg, H. J. and Birnholz, J. C. (1979). Ultrasound observations in multiple gestation with first trimester bleeding: the blighted twin. *Radiology*, **132**, 137–42

16. Robinson, H. P. and Fleming, J. E. E. (1979). A critical evaluation of sonar 'crown–rump length' measurements. *Br. J. Obstet. Gynaecol.*, **82**, 702–10

17. Daya, S. (1993). Accuracy of gestational age estimation by means of fetal crown–rump length measurement. *Am. J. Obstet. Gynecol.*, **168**, 903–8

18. Hadlock, F. P., Shah, Y. P., Kanon, D. J. *et al.* (1992). Fetal crown–rump length: reevaluation of relation to menstrual age (5–18 weeks) with high resolution real time U.S. *Radiology*, **182**, 501–5

19. Reece, E. A., Pinter, E., Honko, C., Wu, Y.-K. and Naftolin, F. (1994). The yolk sac theory: closing the circle on why diabetes-associated malformations occur. *J. Soc. Gynecol. Invest.*, **1**, 3–13

20. Wisser, J. and Dirschedl, P. (1994). Embryonic heart rate in dated human embryos. *Early Hum. Dev.*, **37**, 107–15

21. Dunnigan, A., Hu, N., Benson, D. W. Jr, and Clark, E. B. (1987). Effect of heart rate increase on dorsal aortic flow in stage 24 chick embryo. *Pediatr. Res.*, **22**, 442–4

22. Laboda, L., Estroff, J. A. and Benacerraf, B. R. (1989). First trimester bradycardia: a sign of impending fetal loss. *J. Ultrasound Med.*, **8**, 561–3

23. Achiron, R., Tadmor, O. and Mashiach, S. (1991). Heart rate as a predictor of first-trimester spontaneous abortion after ultrasound-proven viability. *Obstet. Gynecol.*, **78**, 330–4

24. Senges, J., Brachmann, J., Pelzer, D., Kramer, B. and Kubler, W. (1980). Combined effects of glucose and hypoxia on cardiac automaticity and conduction. *J. Molec. Cell Cardiol.*, **12**, 311–23

25. Frates, M. C., Benson, C. B. and Doubilet, P. M. (1993). Pregnancy outcome after a first trimester sonogram demonstrating fetal cardiac activity. *J. Ultrasound Med.*, **12**, 383–6

26. Simpson, J. L., Mills, J. L., Holmes, L. B. *et al.* (1987). Low fetal loss rates after ultrasound-proved viability in early pregnancy. *J. Am. Med. Assoc.*, **258**, 2555–7

27. Gembruch, U., Knopfle, G., Chatterjee, M., Bald, R. and Hansmann, M. (1990). First-trimester diagnosis of fetal congenital heart disease by transvaginal two-dimensional and Doppler echocardiography. *Obstet. Gynecol.*, **75**, 496–8

28. Nelson, L. H. and King, M. (1992). Early diagnosis of holoprosencephaly. *J. Ultrasound Med.*, **11**, 57–9

29. Bennett, T. L., Burlbaw, J., Drake, C. K. and Finley, B. E. (1991). Diagnosis of ectopia cordis at 12 weeks gestation using transabdominal ultrasonography with color flow Doppler. *J. Ultrasound Med.*, **10**, 695–6

30. Birnholz, J. C., Stephens, J. C. and Faria, M. (1978). A possible means of defining neurologic developmental milestones *in utero*. *Am. J. Roentgenol.*, **138**, 537–40

31. DeVries, J. I. P., Visser, G. H. A. and Prechtl, H. F. R. (1982). The emergence of fetal behavior. I. Quantitative aspects. *Early Hum. Dev.*, **7**, 301–22

32. Humphrey, T. (1964). Some correlations between the appearance of human fetal reflexes and the development of the nervous system. *Prog. Brain Res.*, **4**, 93–135

33. Hooker, D. (1952). *The Prenatal Origin of Behavior*. (Lawrence: University of Kansas Press)

34. Windle, W. F. and Orr, D. W. (1937). The development of behavior in chick embryos: spinal cord structure correlated with early somatic mobility. *Comp. Neurol.*, **60**, 287–307

35. Paton, G. R., Silver, M. F. and Allison, A. C. (1974). Comparison of cell cycle time in normal and trisomic cells. *Hum. Genet.*, **23**, 173–6

357

New advances in understanding fetal hypoxia

26

A. Salihagic, A. Fignon, A. Locatelli, J. Lansac and Ph. Arbeille

INTRODUCTION

Fetal oxygenation, which represents the process of transporting molecular oxygen to the tissues of the fetal body, includes: (1) oxygen transfer across the placenta; (2) reversible binding of oxygen to fetal hemoglobin and fetal blood flow; and (3) oxygen consumption for growth and metabolism[1]. Under physiological condition, about 55% and 45% of cardiac output is distributed to the fetal body and to the placenta, respectively. During normoxemia, relatively small fractions of cardiac output are directed to the fetal brain, heart, kidneys and adrenals[2].

Hypoxia is defined as a decreased concentration of oxygen in the tissues. It leads to a conversion from aerobic to anaerobic metabolism, which produces less energy and more acid. There are three types of fetal hypoxia:

(1) Hypoxemic hypoxia – reduced placental perfusion and consequent decrease in fetal arterial blood oxygen content due to low pO_2.

(2) Anemic hypoxia – reduced arterial blood oxygen content due to low fetal hemoglobin concentration; and

(3) Ischemic hypoxia – reduced blood flow to the fetal tissues.

If the oxygen supply is not restored, prolonged hypoxia from any cause will lead to fetal death[1].

The effects of hypoxia on the fetus are of great interest to clinicians. Hypoxic insult is thought to be a major cause of fetal and neonatal morbidity and mortality[3]. The cardiovascular responses to hypoxia are probably the most important adaptive reactions responsible for maintaining fetal homeostasis[4].

They are co-ordinated to centralize blood flow to organs important for maintenance of life, such as the fetal heart and brain. Decreased pO_2 dilates the cerebral and myocardial vessels to maintain constant delivery of oxygen and other metabolic substrates[5,6]. The circulatory centralization acts in concert with metabolic centralization to ensure intact survival of the fetus during hypoxia. The fetus is able to reduce oxygen consumption by decreasing the oxygen delivery to peripheral organs, to defend delivery and consumption of oxygen to the brain and to the heart, i.e. 'metabolic centralization'[2].

Knowledge on fetal hypoxia is primarily derived from animal experiments. In recent years Doppler ultrasound has enabled studies of the vascular response to hypoxia to be carried out in human fetuses.

HEMODYNAMIC DOPPLER INDICES AND FETAL HYPOXIA

Accessibility to the main fetal hemodynamics by Doppler has led to the development of various hemodynamic indices. The amplitude of the end-diastolic flow in the fetal vessels is directly related to vascular resistance in the area supplied by these vessels[7]. In order to quantify the vascular resistances, various indices (which measure the proportion of systolic flow within the total forward flow (M) during one cardiac cycle, or the relative amplitude of systolic (S) to diastolic (D) flow), have been proposed: pulsatility index (PI) $= (S-D)/M$[8], $R = D/S$[9], resistance index (RI) $= (S-D)/S$[10], $R = S/D$[11]. Most of these parameters change as the resistance to flow into the vascular territory

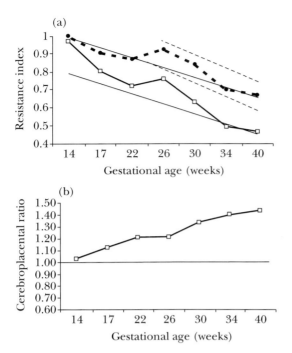

Figure 1 *(a) Evolution of the cerebral resistance index (CRI, circles) and placental vascular resistance (umbilical resistance index, URI, squares) in the same fetus during a normal gestation. The fluctuations in parallel of the two indices are related to the variations of the fetal heart rate. Note that the cerebral resistances are higher than the placental resistances at any gestational age. (b) Evolution of the cerebroplacental ratio during a normal gestation (CRI > URI, therefore CRI/URI always > 1)*

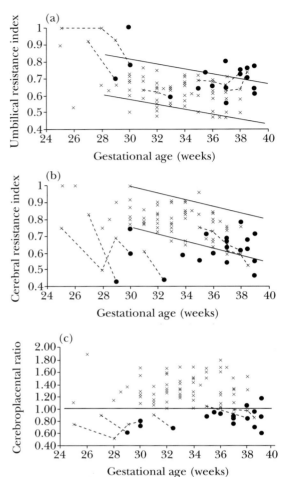

Figure 2 *(a) Evolution of the umbilical (URI) vascular resistance in normal (stars) and growth-retarded fetuses (circles). (b) Evolution of the cerebral vascular resistance (URI) in normal (stars) and growth-retarded fetuses (circles). The sensitivity of these indices for the detection of intrauterine growth retardation (IUGR) is about 60%. (c) Cerebroplacental ratio for normal (stars) and growth-retarded fetuses (circles). The sensitivity of this index for the detection of IUGR is about 85%. The population consisted of 90 hypertensive pregnancies, 17 (19%) with moderate IUGR*

investigated changes $((S-D)/M$, $(S-D)/S$, $S/D))$. Therefore, for these indices, any abnormally increased values are found above the upper limit of the normal range (Figures 1 and 2a). However, the D/S index decreases as the resistance to flow increases. Such an increase in vascular resistance may be due to vascular disease (placental infarction or fibrosis) or to distal arterial vasoconstriction (brain response to increased pO_2 or to drugs). Conversely, abnormally decreased resistance to flow values are displayed below the lower limit of the normal range of the index for $(S-D)/M$, $(S-D)/S$, S/D (Figures 1 and 2b) and above the upper limit for the D/S index. The decrease in flow resistance may be due to the existence of arteriovenous shunts or to an arterial vasodilatation (brain adaptation to hypoxia or to drugs). In

some pathological conditions, such as severe fetal hypoxemia or acidemia, there is absence of frequencies at the end of diastole in some vessels.

In order to assess the vascular resistance when there is no diastolic flow in the artery (umbilical, renal artery), we also use an

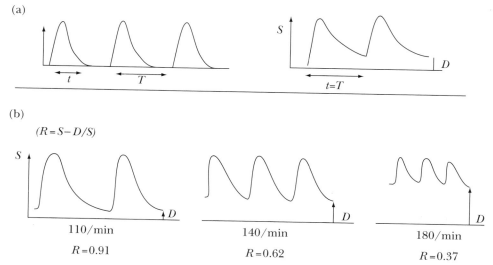

Figure 3 *(a) Modified resistance index (MRI) for the evaluation of the vascular resistances, even in the case of absent end-diastolic flow. MRI = ((S − D)/S) × (T/t). T, cardiac cycle duration; t, time of forward flow; S and D, maximum systolic and end-diastolic amplitude, respectively. (b) Effect of the heart rate on the end-diastolic flow and on the resistance index (R)*

extended resistance index (ERI) that takes into account either the amplitude of the end-diastolic flow or the duration of the forward flow. This index is expressed as follows: $R = (S − D)/S × (T/t)$, where T is the cardiac cycle duration and t the duration of the forward flow (Figure 3). When the forward flow extends to the next systolic peak, the ratio (T/t) is 1 and the index is usually expressed as $R = (S − D)/S$. As the vascular resistance increases, the amplitude of the diastolic component decreases to zero and the index R increases to 1. If the resistance increases more, we observe a reduction in the duration of the diastolic perfusion. The ratio T/t becomes greater than 1, and consequently the resistance index rises. Conversely, when the vascular resistance decreases (placental development), the duration of the diastolic flow (within the umbilical artery) increases progressively until the end-diastolic flow amplitude becomes greater than zero. This ERI has been validated *in vitro* on a hydrodynamic system. The results of this test demonstrate that the extended index changes in proportion to the vascular resistance even if there is no diastolic flow. The extended index as one of the classical indices is virtually angle independent. On the

classical resistance index the systolic as well as the diastolic amplitude are affected to the same extent by the angle variations. On the ERI, we take into consideration the time duration of the forward flow and the time duration of the cardiac cycle, which are not angle dependent.

At about the same time as these indices were formulated, an index of peripheral fetal flow distribution was proposed. This parameter, based on the comparison of the cerebral vascular resistance index (CRI), and the placental resistance index (URI) is expressed as either CRI/URI[12,13] or URI/CRI[14]. By measurement of the flow redistribution between the placenta and the brain, the use of these cerebroplacental ratios (in cases of pathological pregnancies) takes into account the placental disturbances due to the vascular disease at this level, and the cerebral response (vasodilatation) to the hypoxia induced by placental dysfunction. In normal pregnancies the diastolic component in the cerebral arteries is lower than in the umbilical arteries at any gestational age. Therefore, the cerebrovascular resistance remains higher than the placental resistance and the cerebroplacental ratio (CPR = CRI/URI) is greater than 1 (Figures 1 and 2c). The CPR becomes less than

1 if any flow redistribution in favor of the brain occurs. The URI/CRI ratio changes in the opposite direction. The CPR is not heart rate dependent, as are the resistance indices. It is well known that an elevation of the fetal heart rate increases the end-diastolic velocity and therefore decreases the resistance index (Figure 3b). On the other hand, the diminution of the heart rate increases the value of the index. This effect of the heart rate is eliminated by the use of the CPR, because both indices, CRI and URI, are measured on the same fetus with the same heart rate. Figure 1 shows, in a normal pregnancy, the fluctuations of both the placental and the umbilical indices (due to the heart rate variations) and the stability of the CPR. Finally, it was demonstrated that the normal range of the CPR is limited by a single lower cut-off value of 1–1.1, at least for the second half of the pregnancy (Figure 1).

During the past 10 years, the objective has been to check whether a simple relationship exists between these indices, measured as the variations of the diastolic flow in one artery or the fetal flow distribution, and the development of intrauterine growth retardation (IUGR) or hypoxia, and whether one or a combination of these indices could be used as a predictor of fetal outcome.

Cerebroplacental ratio, hypoxia and fetal outcome

The comparison of the cerebral and the placental vascular resistance for the assessment of IUGR was proposed in 1986[12] and the results confirmed in 1987[13,14]. In pathological pregnancies (hypertensive pregnancies, for example) with IUGR we frequently observe a reduction in placental perfusion and an increase in flow towards the brain. This phenomenon, called the brain sparing effect, is supposed to compensate for fetal hypoxia and is associated most of the time with fetal growth retardation. The main advantage of comparing placental and cerebrovascular resistance is that we take into account first, the existence of placental disease which can be responsible for an alteration of the maternal to fetal exchanges and second, the

cerebral hemodynamic consequences of these abnormalities.

Nevertheless, the cerebroplacental ratio may become pathological in various situations:

(1) There is an increase in the placental resistance but no hypoxia and normal cerebral perfusion;

(2) The placental resistance is normal but hypoxia exists and so the cerebral resistance is abnormally decreased;

(3) Both placental and cerebral resistances are abnormal; and

(4) Both indices are within their normal range but the cerebral index is lower than the placental index (Figure 4).

All these combinations describe a fetal flow redistribution and are associated in most cases with IUGR. Several studies based on the same philosophy, using either the ratio between the anterior cerebral artery index and the umbilical

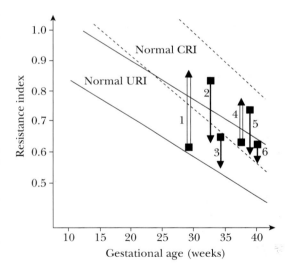

Figure 4 *Cerebral resistance index (CRI, triangles) and umbilical resistance index (URI, squares) associated with either a normal fetus (cerebroplacental ratio, CPR > 1) or a growth-retarded fetus (IUGR, CPR < 1). 1, 4: normal URI and normal CRI (CPR > 1), normal fetus; 2: abnormal CRI and abnormal URI (CPR < 1), IUGR; 3: abnormal CRI and normal URI (CPR < 1), IUGR; 5: normal CRI and abnormal URI (CPR < 1), IUGR; 6: normal CRI and normal URI (CPR < 1), IUGR*

index (CRI/URI), which is pathological when less than 1 (Figures 1 and 2c)[12,13,15–17], or the ratio between the umbilical index and the internal carotid index (URI/CRI), which is pathological when greater than 1[14,18], demonstrated a sensibility of approximately 86% and a specificity of about 98%.

The cerebroplacental ratio has been tested on hypertensive pregnancies with severe IUGR, idiopathic IUGR, or twin gestations[19], and showed the same accuracy in all these cases. At present, this parameter is the most widely used in clinical practice.

Recently, the cerebroplacental ratio was also tested on a population of pregnancy-induced hypertension with only moderate IUGR[20,21]. The objective was to check the sensitivity of this parameter in the detection of fetal flow redistribution at an early stage of development of IUGR, on a population with only moderate IUGR (Figure 2). The population consisted of 90 hypertensive pregnant mothers, aged 26.33 ± 5.3 years. The patients were included in the study when their blood pressure measured more than 140/90. All patients were treated by labetalol and dihydralazine. Of the 90 neonates, 73 (81%) were of normal growth and 17 (19%) were growth retarded. The duration of gestation (mean $\pm$ standard error of mean) was 38.2 ± 1.35 weeks for the normal growth group and 36.4 ± 3.1 for the growth-retarded group. Eighty-two pregnancies (91.1%) were delivered normally, and eight (8.9%) required a Cesarean section; four or 4.4% because of fetal distress and four or 4.4% for other reasons (e.g. placenta previa). Five of the 17 IUGR fetuses showed abnormal fetal heart rate (dip I or II), and eight had an abnormal Apgar score.

Doppler investigation of the fetal cerebral, renal and umbilical arteries was performed 3–4 times during the pregnancy, the last examination being performed approximately a week before delivery (1.7 ± 1.3 weeks). The vascular resistances in the brain (CRI), the kidney (RRI), and the placenta (URI) were evaluated using the resistance index and the cerebroplacental ratio. Eighty-eight per cent of the growth-retarded fetuses had an abnormal cerebroplacental ratio, but only 41% an abnormal

umbilical index and 53% an abnormal cerebral index (Figure 2). In the normal-growth fetuses, 97% had a normal cerebroplacental ratio as well as normal umbilical and cerebral indices.

This high sensitivity and specificity of the cerebroplacental ratio as a predictor of IUGR confirms that, even at the early stage of development of IUGR, the fetal flow redistribution in favor of the brain always exists and is detectable by Doppler. Nevertheless, this adaptation of the fetus may have several origins, such as hypoxia, malnutrition and hypovolemia, and the role of these factors has to be investigated in animals or computerized models.

Kjellmer and colleagues[22] demonstrated in animals that IUGR is generally associated with cerebral metabolism disturbances (monoamines) and delayed development of the brain. Moreover, Fouron and associates[23] showed that in the case of fetal flow redistribution there is a reverse diastolic flow into the aortic arch which confirms the presence, in the flow moving to the brain, of hypoxic blood coming from the right ventricle. This phenomenon probably limits the beneficial activity of the brain sparing effect. Therefore, the cerebroplacental ratio was tested as an indicator of adverse perinatal outcome. Gramellini and co-workers[16] found, in a population of 45 growth-retarded fetuses, a sensitivity of 90% for the cerebroplacental ratio, when it was used as a predictor of poor perinatal outcome, compared with 78% for the middle-cerebral artery and 83% for the umbilical artery indices. In this study, the parameters taken into account to evaluate fetal well-being were fetal heart rate, gestational age, birth weight, Cesarean rate, umbilical vein pH, 5-min Apgar score, incidence of admission to the neonatal intensive care unit, and neonatal complications.

FETAL HEMODYNAMIC CHANGES ASSOCIATED WITH HYPOXIA

Umbilical circulation and hypoxia

To date, most of the clinical applications of the fetal Doppler method have been concerned with the investigation of placental arterial hemodynamics. In normal pregnancy, impedance to flow in the umbilical arteries decreases with advancing gestation, due to progressive maturation of the placenta and increase in the number of tertiary stem villi[1,14,24–26]. Several studies have already demonstrated the possibilities and the limits of using umbilical Doppler for the assessment of fetal growth[25–36]. Most of these studies used the S/D ratio, the RI ($(S-D)/S$), or the PI ($(S-D)/M$), measured on the umbilical arterial Doppler velocity waveform. All these umbilical vascular resistance indices, when greater than the upper limit of the normal range (> 2 SD), are frequently associated with IUGR. The sensitivity of this method in this application is generally about 65–70%. A cross-sectional study in pregnancies with IUGR fetuses has shown that increased impedance to flow in the uterine and umbilical arteries is associated with fetal hypoxemia and acidemia[37]. However, when these indices were used as a predictor of fetal well-being, several authors showed that only strong disturbances of the umbilical arterial flow, such as absent end-diastolic flow, were associated with acute fetal patency, but in this case it is still difficult to evaluate the degree of hypoxia and fetal distress, according to the reduction in placental perfusion[38–41].

There are several reasons for these results, but we have to keep in mind that umbilical Doppler detects only local hemodynamic abnormalities, which are not in all cases associated with a deterioration of placental function. These indices measure the resistance to flow, due to the presence of vascular disease at the placental level, and are not influenced by other central hemodynamic parameters, such as fetal volemia or fetal hypoxia. Therefore, one can accept that placental vascular disease exists (reduction of arteriolar density, limited infarctions, fibrosis) without fetal hypoxia being induced. Conversely, the alteration of the mother-to-fetus oxygen exchange may be disturbed without any placental hemodynamic lesion.

The fetal cerebral circulation was subsequently investigated, the objective being to study the brain response to placental dysfunction and hypoxia and to test the sensitivity of cerebral Doppler as a predictor of fetal outcome.

Cerebral circulation and hypoxia

The main intracerebral arteries, such as the middle and the anterior cerebral arteries[12,13,18] and the internal carotid artery[42], are easy to identify from the well-known intracranial anatomic structures. The reduced diastolic flow in these vessels at the beginning of the second half of the pregnancy (20–25 weeks) develops progressively later on. The increase in the diastolic component as the pregnancy progresses is interpreted as a decrease in the cerebral resistance due to brain development. These findings also suggest that in the later part of pregnancy a proportionally greater fraction of the cardiac output is directed to the fetal brain, presumably to compensate for the progressive fall with gestational age in fetal blood pO_2 and increase in pCO_2[1]. The same Doppler indices for the placenta are used for the evaluation of the cerebrovascular resistance changes (Figures 1 and 2b).

The Doppler indices measured on the spectrum of the main fetal cerebral arteries are sensitive to any vasoconstriction or vasodilatation of the brain vessels. The increase in the diastolic cerebral flow is interpreted as a vasomotor response (vasodilatation) to hypoxia. Even if hypoxia is confirmed in most of the cases, it remains difficult to quantify and to follow up this hypoxia[43,44]. Comparisons between the cerebral Doppler index and the measurement of pO_2, pCO_2, pH and O_2 content by cordocentesis have demonstrated a good correlation between pO_2 and the cerebral Doppler index during the early development of hypoxia (the cerebral index decreases with decreasing pO_2). Nevertheless, when acidosis appeared, an increase in the cerebral vascular resistance index was observed, due to a decrease in the diastolic flow[37,45].

In a first approach, it appears difficult to use the cerebral index to quantify hypoxia, but if in fetuses with abnormally decreased cerebral resistance index this index is measured every 2 days, one can expect to follow up the evolution of hypoxia through the cerebrovascular changes:

(1) The cerebrovascular index decreases progressively, as in normal fetuses, so the hypoxia seems to be compensated by the brain hyperperfusion;

(2) The cerebral index decreases significantly and becomes more and more pathological; hypoxia develops but the fetus is probably not acidemic; and

(3) The cerebral index, which was much lower than the normal limit, increases and enters the normal range again. In this case the capability of the brain vessels to vasodilate has been overloaded, or the vessel(s) cannot expand further, due to the development of cerebral edema. Hypoxia is decompensated for, and the fetus becomes acidemic.

These hypotheses are still under clinical evaluation, but it is now clear that it is hazardous to use only the absolute value of the cerebral Doppler index for the assessment of hypoxia and to make the decision of delivery. Only the evolution of the cerebral index or the cerebroplacental ratio over several days may provide information on the development of fetal hypoxia. Nevertheless, a good correlation has been found between the existence of significantly decreased (< 0.2 SD) cerebral resistance and the development of post-asphyxial encephalopathy in the neonate[46]. In this study, the specificity and the sensitivity of cerebral Doppler, as a predictor of neonatal outcome, were about 75% and 87%, respectively.

Regional cerebral flow

With color Doppler technology it is now possible to investigate the main cerebral arteries and to evaluate vascular resistance in various brain vascular areas supplied by these arteries[47]. In normal fetuses the resistance index was significantly higher in the middle cerebral artery than in the anterior and posterior cerebral arteries. In pathological pregnancies with hypoxia and cerebral vasodilatation (decreased cerebral index), the sensitivity of the cerebral Doppler index was not dependent on the choice of the cerebral artery explored.

Cerebrovascular reactivity

When the cerebral Doppler index is lower than the normal range or when the cerebroplacental ratio points to a fetal flow redistribution, the fetus is considered hypoxic, but it is difficult to evaluate the consequences of this exposure to hypoxia on the brain structures and their development, as well as on cerebral functions[43,46].

The oxygen test (maternal oxygenation administration) has been used to test fetal brain reactivity[48–50]. During oxygen treatment the cerebral index was measured at the level of the internal carotid. In fetuses with brain sparing effect (cerebral resistance below normal), but that did not develop fetal distress, the oxygen treatment induced an increase in cerebral resistance. However, those fetuses with cerebral vasodilatation that did not respond to the oxygen test (no cerebral resistance increase), developed fetal distress (Figure 5). The sensitivity of the oxygen test, when used as a predictor of imminent fetal distress, is about 70%[48]. The positive cerebral response proves a maintained placental transfer; this condition could justify the intrauterine treatment of fetuses with long-term maternal oxygen therapy. Conversely, the absence of a vascular response to the oxygen test means that the placental transfer and/or the cerebral reactivity is impaired.

The cerebrovascular resistance of the fetus is also sensitive to the variation of CO_2 content in the air inspired by the mother. A recent study[51] demonstrated that a mixture with 2% CO_2 induces a decrease in fetal cerebral resistance but does not affect the fetal heart rate or the umbilical flow.

Recent investigation has also shown that the middle cerebral arterial PI decreases week-by-week in hypoxic human fetuses without fetal distress, but remains relatively stable during the same period in acidemic fetuses[52]. This suggests the loss of cerebrovascular reactivity in fetuses with fetal distress.

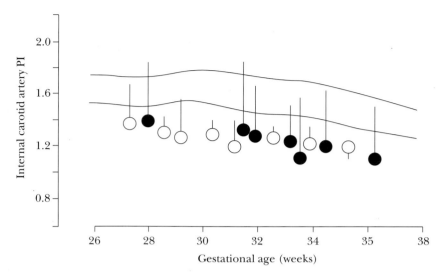

Figure 5 *Pulsatility index (PI) from the internal carotid artery before (circles) and 20 min after (top of vertical lines) maternal administration of 60% humidified oxygen. The open circles indicate those fetuses that developed acute fetal distress. Normal range for gestation is shown as the mean − 1 SD (from reference 48)*

Aortic circulation and hypoxia

In the situation of highly impaired blood flow in a vessel, the diastolic velocities might disappear. This finding in the umbilical artery and/or fetal descending aorta has been shown to correlate well with an unfavorable pregnancy outcome[53,54]. A semiquantitative method of assessing the waveform, 'four blood flow classes (BFC)', has been defined to describe the appearance of the waveform, with emphasis on its diastolic part[55]. These classes are as follows:

BFC 0   (Normal) positive flow throughout the heart cycle and a normal PI;

BFC I   Positive flow throughout the cycle and a PI > mean ± 2 SD of normal;

BFC II Non-detectable end-diastolic velocity;

BFC III Absence of positive flow throughout the major part of diastole and/or reverse flow in diastole.

The BFC was abnormal (BFC I–III) in 57% of the IUGR fetuses and in 93% of those IUGR fetuses that subsequently developed signs of fetal distress requiring operative delivery. The sensitivity in predicting IUGR was 41% for the aortic PI and 57% for the aortic BFC. In predict-

ing delivery for fetal distress, the corresponding values were 76 and 87%, respectively. Another approach to the description of the aortic or umbilical velocity waveform that has also been adopted in a clinical context is a simple qualitative evaluation of the presence or absence of end-diastolic velocity.

The degree of intrauterine and neonatal morbidity was found to be reflected in pathological changes in the fetal aortic blood velocity[55–57]. Furthermore, a relationship has been found to exist between the mean fetal aortic velocity and the degree of fetal hypoxia, hypercapnia, acidosis and hyperlactemia, as diagnosed in blood samples obtained by cordocentesis in growth-retarded fetuses[58].

Renal circulation and hypoxia

The change in pO_2, pH and O_2 content may affect several vascular systems, such as the renal or the splanchnic circulation. In order to make the Doppler method more sensitive in the evaluation of fetal hypoxia, several groups have conducted studies on the fetal renal circulation[59,60]. Some studies concerning severe IUGR and hypoxic fetuses have demonstrated a reduction in

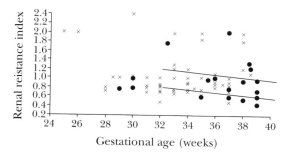

Figure 6 *Renal resistance index, RRI = (S − D)/S × T/t in hypertensive pregnancies: n = 90; 18 IUGR fetuses (circles). In this population of moderately growth-retarded fetuses, we observed three different renal vascular responses: seven with decreased RRI; four with increased RRI; and seven with normal RRI*

renal perfusion, which is expressed as an increase in the PI[60].

Conversely, the study carried out by our group on a population with moderate IUGR, with no sign of severe hypoxia or fetal distress, has shown that the renal response could be a vasoconstriction or a vasodilatation. In the IUGR group (abnormal cerebroplacental ratio in 88% of the cases), the renal index was normal in 33% of the cases, or elevated (27%), or decreased (40%). In the normal group (normal cerebroplacental ratio in 97% of the cases), the renal index was normal (73%), or increased (15.5%), or decreased (11.5%) (Figure 6)[20]. Our recent investigations have also demonstrated that the renal RI correlates very poorly with fetal growth[21,61].

These contradictory findings of renal RI may be explained by the fact that the renal flow is sensitive to many factors other than hypoxia[59]. One can suggest that in the case of severe IUGR, with long-term exposure to hypoxia, the fetal adaptation consists of cerebral vasodilatation along with vasoconstriction of the rest of the vascular bed. Conversely, in the early phase of development of the pathology, the renal vasculature still adapts, like the cerebral, to fetal pO_2 changes. Moreover, in the case of oligohydramnios or polyhydramnios, for instance, the renal resistance increases or decreases and probably the renal flow is also affected by any change in fetal volemia. During ischemic hypoxia in animals and human beings, both polyuria and

oliguria have been reported, depending on the experimental conditions and the degree of the insult[62]. In severe or prolonged hypoxia, renal blood flow and eventually the glomerular filtration rate are reduced, leading to oliguria. Conversely, mild hypoxia, both in the adult and the newborn, leads to a rise in renal blood flow and in urine excretion. Therefore, it seems that at present the renal index needs to be evaluated in larger populations and in several pathologies in order to establish if it is a reliable parameter for the evaluation and the follow-up of fetal hypoxia.

Venous circulation and hypoxia

Changes in venous Doppler waveforms can be induced by an increased afterload, after fetal arterial redistribution is established[63]. Severe hypoxemia combined with acidosis causes redistribution of umbilical vein blood towards the ductus venosus, at the expense of hepatic blood flow[64,65]. It has recently been proposed that changes in the venous circulation indicate failure of the compensatory circulatory mechanisms, implying the development of right failure secondary to an increase in afterload[66]. This considered that arterial redistribution has reached its maximum before alterations on the venous side occur.

FETAL RESPONSE TO THE ACUTE AND CHRONIC TYPE OF HYPOXIA

Induced hypoxia in lamb fetuses has demonstrated a very sensitive and rapid brain vasodilatation. Our data are in agreement with *in vitro* findings that fetal cerebral vessels relax markedly and quickly in response to hypoxia, in contrast to the common carotid artery, which relaxes only very slowly and to a much smaller degree[5]. The fetal cerebral and umbilical flows have been assessed by Doppler sensors implanted in the fetus[67] during fetal hypoxia induced by cord compression, aorta compression and drug injection.

Cord compression ($n = 8$) decreased the venous return and the umbilical arterial flow, which induced hypoxia instantaneously and simulated fetal central hypovolemia. During such a compression of 10-min duration, the cerebrovascular resistances decreased and the cerebral flow was maintained, or only slightly decreased. Simultaneous recordings of the cerebral and umbilical Doppler waveforms together with the pO_2 showed that the cerebroplacental ratio decreased proportionally with the pO_2. The umbilical flow decreased in the same direction but to a greater extent (Figure 7a, b). The pH and heart rate stayed normal. In the case of progressive cord compression (progressive changes of the umbilical resistances), the cerebroplacental ratio followed the changes in fetal pO_2 very closely (Figure 7c).

Maternal aortic compression ($n = 6$) reduced the uterine flow and induced fetal hypoxia after about 30 s. After 1 min of compression, the heart rate dropped, so the compression was interrupted. The heart rate recovered 30 s after the end of the compression, and the pH did not change during the test. The umbilical flow remained stable; however, the umbilical resistances increased and the cerebral resistances decreased. As in the previous case, the cerebroplacental ratio followed the variations of the fetal pO_2, but the amplitude of its variations was weaker than during the cord compression (Figure 8).

As shown in Figure 9, good correlation was found between the absolute values of the cerebroplacental ratio and corresponding pO_2 values in the two hypoxic studies ($r = 0.65$ for the aorta compression test; $r = 0.70$ for cord compression). When comparing the URI and pO_2 absolute values, we found much lower correlations ($r = 0.27$ for aorta compression; $r = 0.54$ for cord compression). When comparing the CRI and pO_2 absolute values, we again found much lower correlations ($r = 0.21$ for aorta compression; $r = 0.39$ for cord compression).

Propranolol ($4\,\mu g/kg$) was injected into pregnant ewes intravenously ($n = 3$). From the first minute after injection, the umbilical resistances increased and the cerebral resistances decreased[67]. In this study, the pO_2 was not measured, but the fetal flow redistribution detected by the cerebroplacental ratio after each injection leads us to suspect that repeated injec-

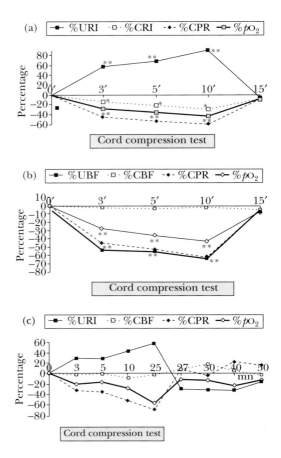

Figure 7 Cord compression test in lamb fetuses. Variations in percentage from the pre-test value of the (a) umbilical vascular resistance (URI), the cerebral resistance (CRI), the cerebroplacental ratio (CPR) and the fetal pO_2. (b) The umbilical flow volume (UBF), the cerebral flow (CBF), the CPR, and the fetal pO_2, on lamb fetuses, during a period of chord compression. The CPR decreases in proportion to the fetal pO_2 and the umbilical flow volume and the cerebral flow remain constant. (c) Variations of the umbilical vascular resistance (URI), and the cerebral flow (CBF), the CPR, and the fetal pO_2. Note that the CPR follows the pO_2 changes very closely. (*$p < 0.01$; **$p < 0.001$)

tions of this drug may induce repeated hypoxic stresses for the fetus, and the question is to evaluate the beneficial effect of any drug (on the mother), and its deleterious effects (hypoxia?) on the fetus.

The fetal cerebral and umbilical flows were monitored during maternal anesthesia of 7-h duration, the objective being to detect any fetal hemodynamic change (hypoxia) in relation to

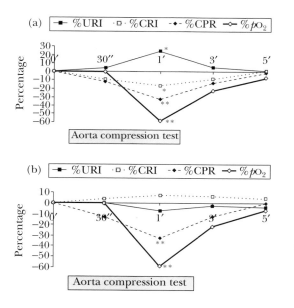

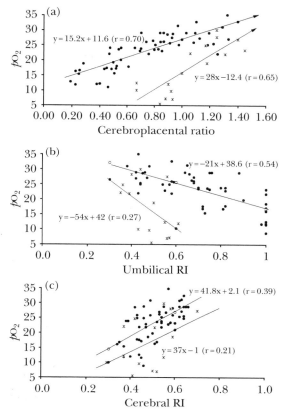

Figure 8 *Maternal aortic compression test. Variations in percentage from the pre-test value of the (a) umbilical vascular resistances (URI), the cerebral resistance (CRI), the cerebroplacental ratio (CPR), and the fetal pO₂. (b) The umbilical flow volume (UBF), the cerebral flow (CBF), the CPR and the fetal pO₂ on lamb fetuses, during a period of maternal aortic compression. The CPR decreases in proportion with the fetal pO₂, as in the cord compression, but the variations of this parameter are of lower amplitude than during the cord compression. In this case the umbilical flow volume does not change, the cerebral flow is slightly increased. (*p < 0.01; **p < 0.001)*

Figure 9 *Comparison between absolute values of (a) fetal pO₂ and cerebroplacental ratio, for the aortic compression test (stars) and the cord compression test (circles); (b) pO₂ and umbilical RI; and (C) pO₂ and cerebral RI, in normal and hypoxic periods, induced either by cord compression or by aortic compression. The closest correlation was seen with the cerebroplacental ratio*

the different drugs used during this period (phenoperidine 7.5 mg, thiopental 500 mg, Gamma-OH 6 g and Forane 0.3–0.5% at +1 h 30 min after the beginning of the anesthesia). The patient was operated on at 21 weeks' gestation for angioma of the posterior cranial fossa. Doppler recordings of the umbilical arteries and the fetal anterior cerebral arteries were obtained before anesthesia, during anesthesia (+ 10 min, +45 min, +1 h, +1 h 30 min, +3 h, +7 h) and after anesthesia (+2 h, +7 days, +5 months). The fetal heart rate decreased progressively +2 h after the beginning of the anesthesia (from 150/min to 110/min at +3 h), and recovered partially at +2 h after the end of the anesthesia. Seven days and 5 months later, the fetal heart rate was normal for the gestational age (145/min). At the same time, the

CRI and the URI decreased together moderately; however, the cerebroplacental ratio oscillated around its basal value. These three parameters stayed within the normal range for the gestational age during the whole period of anesthesia. After the anesthesia, the cerebral and placental indices decreased normally from 22 to 40 weeks, and the cerebroplacental ratio remained stable. The evolution of the fetal vascular parameters showed the effects of the drugs on the fetal heart rate (significant decrease) but also the good stability of the fetal flow distribution (cerebral and placental), despite the strong hemodynamic changes in the mother.

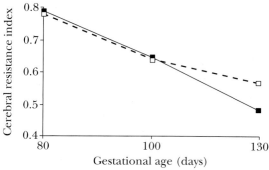

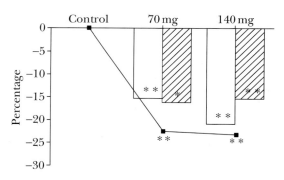

Figure 10 *Variations of the fetal cerebral resistance index in lamb fetuses in a test of the effects of nicotine, during gestation (from days 80 to 130). In the control (placebo) group (unbroken line) the cerebral index decreased progressively until the end of the gestation, but not in the 'nicotine group' (dashed line), submitted to repeated maternal injections of nicotine from gestation day 30 until delivery*

Figure 11 *Effect of long-term cocaine administration in pregnant ewes, on fetal weight (white bars), pO_2 (hatched bars) and cerebroplacental ratio (squares). The mean fetal weight was significantly lower in the two cocaine groups. The cerebroplacental ratio and the fetal pO_2 decreased with a similar amplitude in the two cocaine groups in comparison with the control group (*p < 0.01, **p < 0.001)*

The effect of chronic nicotine treatment on fetal cerebral flow and reactivity has been studied in pregnant ewes receiving a daily dose of nicotine equivalent to 20 cigarettes[68]. The results showed the absence of a decrease in vascular resistance at the end of gestation, as is normally observed (Figure 10). This phenomenon, more evident in the cerebral than in the placental vessels, could be interpreted as a cerebral vasoconstriction or as delayed brain development. In addition to these hemodynamic findings, it was observed that there was a higher percentage of stillborns in the nicotine group (63%) than in the control group (13%). The newborns in the nicotine group showed an abnormal cerebrovascular response when submitted to a CO_2 inhalation test (no cerebral vasodilatation). The conclusion of the study was that repeated administration of nicotine is responsible for abnormal brain vascular development, with loss of cerebral reactivity, and poor fetal outcome. These results lead to the hypothesis that, if fetal hypoxia develops in 'nicotine fetuses', the capability of the brain vessels to adapt by vasodilatation will be reduced because of nicotine's vasoconstrictive effect and because of the deleterious effects of the drug on the growth and the maturation of the brain structures.

The effect of long-term cocaine administration on pO_2 and fetal growth has been investi-gated in pregnant ewes daily treated with 1 or 2 mg/kg cocaine (from day 60 of gestation). All fetuses ($n = 14$, cocaine groups; $n = 7$, control group) were alive at delivery (Cesarean section at 134 days). The mean fetal weight was significantly lower in the cocaine groups. The values of pO_2 in the two cocaine groups confirmed the presence of a moderate but significant hypoxia in these groups compared with the control group (Figure 11). Fetal growth retardation is probably the result of a direct or indirect vasoconstrictor effect of cocaine which reduces placental blood flow[69,70]. Decreased blood flow in the placental bed may lead to a disturbance in the transfer of nutrients and oxygen to the fetus and induce both fetal growth retardation and hypoxia. Moreover, the fetal flow redistribution was present in the two cocaine groups, and the cerebroplacental ratio decreased with the pO_2 in these two groups, as in acute hypoxia (Figure 11).

General remarks

Various studies have already shown relationships between Doppler parameters and fetal hypoxia during human and animal gestations, but no parameter has been found accurately to follow the fetal pO_2 changes[37,45]. These results confirm that the cerebroplacental ratio can detect and follow the development of fetal hypoxia with good accuracy. Nevertheless, the variations of the cerebroplacental ratio are not of the same amplitude in the cord and in the aorta compression tests. This may be explained by the fact that the cord compression induces both, hypoxia and hypovolemia, and that the cerebroplacental ratio is influenced by these two phenomena. Conversely, on the other 'induced hypoxia' tests (aorta compression, drugs) the venous return was not mechanically reduced and volemia remained stable during the test. Recent investigation also suggests that the decrease of the pO_2 and the cerebroplacental ratio occur quite simultaneously and any pO_2 change (even of some per cent) is associated with a cerebroplacental ratio change of similar amplitude. The cerebroplacental ratio appears to be the most suitable parameter for detecting and quantifying the early development of hypoxia, in the case of acute hypoxia[71]. Furthermore, it may also be considered to be a reliable parameter for the follow-up of the fetal pO_2 in case of chronic hypoxia.

Our human and animal data also confirm the existence of physiological compensatory mechanisms that protect the fetal life during the acute as well as the chronic type of hypoxia. Although the fetus is able to adapt to hypoxia, increased cerebral perfusion triggered by hypoxia could induce the formation of brain lesions. A recent epidemiological study has shown that, although the fetus may adapt to undernutrition and thereby survive, permanent changes in the body's physiology and metabolism may lead to cardiovascular disease in adult life[72].

MONITORING OF THE FETAL ADAPTATION TO HYPOXIA – A HUMAN CASE REPORT

In one growth-retarded and hypoxic fetus the cerebral and umbilical hemodynamic changes were assessed (by Doppler), daily during 18 days. The fetal brain was investigated by magnetic resonance imaging (MRI) close to the delivery, and because the fetus died at delivery we performed an anatomical study of the fetal brain. The evolution of the fetal hemodynamics

(day by day) was interpreted according to the clinical, MRI and anatomical findings.

Case report

A 31-year-old pregnant woman, para 1, a smoker (less than 10 cigarettes per day), with history of hypertension, psoriasis and obesity, was admitted to the hospital at 26 weeks of gestation because of hypertension and a growth-retarded fetus. The pregnancy was normal until the 22nd gestational week.

When the patient was admitted to the hospital, the ultrasound examination showed intrauterine growth retardation (IUGR) below the 5th centile of our normal range and oligohydramnios.

Doppler examinations of the umbilical and cerebral arteries were performed every day from week 26 + 4 days (186 days) until 2 days prior to delivery (week 29 + 1 day; 204 days). The umbilical and cerebral resistance index (URI and CRI) and the cerebroplacental ratio (CRI/URI) were calculated. There was no diastolic flow in the umbilical artery at any time during the study (URI = 1) and the time of perfusion (during the cardiac cycle) did not change significantly in this vessel. Therefore, the umbilical vascular resistance was considered as constant during the period of the study. As a consequence, the CRI and the cerebroplacental ratio (CRI/URI) showed the same variations. At the first measurement (26 weeks + 4 days; 186 days) the CRI and the cerebroplacental ratio values (0.74) were abnormal; the lower limit of the normal range being 0.87 for the CRI and 1 for the cerebroplacental ratio. The CRI and cerebroplacental ratio increased and decreased alternately around 0.7 until week 27 + 2 days (191 days) of gestation. Afterwards, the CRI and the cerebroplacental ratio remained stable at 0.67 until week 28 + 3 days (199 days), then increased progressively until 0.7 (week 29; 203 days), and finally reached their highest value, 0.88, at 29 weeks + 2 days (205 days), 2 days prior to delivery (Figure 12).

During the Doppler investigation, the fetal heart rate was between 121 and 139 beats per min (bpm). Several episodes of bradycardia

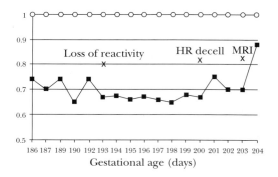

Gestational age (days)

Figure 12 *Doppler monitoring over 18 days. The cerebral resistance index and the cerebroplacental ratio are represented by the same curve (squares), because in this case the umbilical resistance index (circles) remained constant, and equal to 1. At the beginning of the surveillance period the cerebroplacental ratio showed significant variations from one day to the next, and after this period remained constant until the heart rate deceleration (HR decell) occurred (day 199). It then increased significantly until fetal death (at delivery)*

(75 bpm) were noted from week 28 + 3 days (199 days), i.e. 6 days prior to delivery, and became more frequent during the last 3 days. At week 29 (203 days), an MRI examination, focused on the fetal brain, was performed. The transverse incidences in T1 weighted spin-echo and in T2 weighted fast spin-echo acquisitions did not show any abnormal pattern. The contrast between gray and white matter was consistent with gestation plus age, and the white matter signal was homogeneous. There was no asymmetry between the two hemispheres and both ventricles were of normal size.

Because of an abnormal biophysical profile score with abnormal heart rate patterns, development of severe oligohydramnios and persistence of a very high level of the mother's blood pressure (despite anti-hypertensive therapy: Aldomet, Trandate), the pregnancy was interrupted (week 29 + 3 days; 206 days).

Postmortem examination confirmed the presence of IUGR with growth parameters corresponding to approximately 26 weeks' gestation. Gross examination of the brain showed a development compatible with obstetric gestational age, a brain weight under the 10th centile for age and a cerebellar diameter of 30 mm. There was meningeal congestion as-

sociated with periventricular radial congestion. Histological examination showed cerebellar development compatible with gestational age. Staining for immunoreactivity to glial fibrillary acidic protein (GFAP) demonstrated the presence of pathological gliosis in the germinal matrix, centrum semiovale and the cerebellum. Histology also showed a marked vasodilatation of both anterior and middle cerebral arteries. Although the placenta was not examined, its weight, 140 g, was abnormally low for both fetal weight and gestational age.

Discussion

In severe and/or prolonged hypoxia, myocardial blood flow is also increased to defend delivery of oxygen to the fetal myocardium[73]. If placental insufficiency persists and placental resistance increases, this defence will be overloaded, leading to abnormal findings on the biophysical score[63]. An abnormal biophysical profile score, heart rate abnormality and development of severe oligohydramnios are the main reasons for interruption of the pregnancy with severe hypoxia.

In the present case, the cerebroplacental ratio was always significantly lower than 1 and close to 0.7 (– 30% from the normal limit), leading to suspicion of a significantly low level for the fetal pO_2. On the other hand, the CRI reflects the vasomotor response of the brain vessels to hypoxia. Before day 192 (27 weeks + 2 days) the CRI and cerebroplacental ratio decreased, but not uniformly, which may indicate that the cerebrovascular reactivity was still efficient (Figure 12). From day 192 until day 199, these two indices remained unchanged. This pattern is more likely to favor an absence of vascular reactivity. Two hypotheses may support this observation: (1) the cerebral vessels have reached their maximal level of vasodilatation; and (2) the prolonged brain hyperperfusion (brain sparing effect) and the hypoxia have induced the formation of brain edema, which limits the dilatation of the vessels. At the end of week 29 (days 200 to 203) the CRI increased irregularly, and then increased strongly up to 0.88 (+26%), which reduced the brain perfusion. This increase of the CRI may correspond to a vasoconstrictive process (due to the acidemia) and/or to the combination of the vasoconstriction and the development of the perivascular edema. At this stage the breakdown of compensatory mechanisms has occurred and acidosis has developed. Arduini and co-workers[74] have shown that maximal cerebral redistribution of flow is reached approximately 2 weeks before the onset of fetal heart rate decelerations. We found the episodes of bradycardia a week after maximal cerebral redistribution (a few days before fetal death). In two published reports an increase of the PI in the middle cerebral artery, preceding fetal death, have been described in a case of lupus anticoagulant[75] and proteinuric pre-eclampsia with essential hypertension and IUGR[76]. Pre-term brain edema has been proposed as the underlying cause of this phenomenon[77].

The MRI results could seem to be inconsistent with the Doppler findings, but it is well known that discrete processes affecting the brain tissue (such as edema) may not be visible on conventional MRI as used in the present case. Hypoxia induces delayed injuries which are detectable throughout MRI investigations only if significant alteration of relaxation time occurs (ischemic lesions)[78]. Nevertheless, brain edema (not visible on the MRI) may be responsible for the increased CRI and the loss of cerebrovascular reactivity.

It is already established that IUGR can be associated with hypoxic–ischemic brain pathology, including pathological gliosis and periventricular leukomalacia[79]. Nevertheless, it is important to stress the development of brain damage during redistribution. Indeed, recent work has shown that brain damage can develop despite the existence of redistribution (brain sparing effect)[80] (R. N. Laurini, unpublished data). This leads to a question of redistribution as a purely physiological phenomenon[79].

In this context, one must bear in mind the distinctive anatomy of the cerebral macro- and microcirculation and their possible role in autoregulation, as discussed elsewhere[81]. It is suggested that the vasodilatation of cerebral arteries, demonstrated on morphological exami-

nation of the brain, represents a form of 'vessel paralysis', after the initial period, reducing the capacity of arteries for further adaptation[81]. Furthermore, the presence of arterial vasodilatation excludes the possibility of vasoconstriction.

Moreover, it is known that the early stages of hypoxic–ischemic brain pathology, in particular pathological gliosis, are difficult to detect by means of sonography. The lack of correlation between MRI and morphological findings emphasizes once more the importance of a comprehensive neuropathological evaluation of all fetuses.

In conclusion, even though no tissue damage was shown on MRI (3 days prior to fetal death), it is evident that fetal behavior was severely affected during the 2 last weeks of the pregnancy. During this period of sustained hypoxia the fetal deterioration was characterized by: (1) the progressive development of oligohydramnios (190 days); (2) the disappearance of the vascular reactivity (7 successive RIs constant at 194 days); (3) the occurrence of fetal heart rate decelerations (199 days); and finally (4) the increase of cerebral vascular resistances with reduction of brain perfusion (204 days). The chronology of these events shows that the fetal deterioration process extended over approximately 2 weeks. Finally, in addition to single Doppler measurements performed 1 week before delivery (for prediction of fetal outcome), one can suggest use of the 'loss of fluctuation of the cerebral RI' to identify the beginning of the period of very high risk for the fetus[82]. This hypothesis may have to be confirmed on a larger number of pathological pregnancies.

CONCLUSION

The cerebral flow changes in relation to hypoxia and fetal distress remain one of the most interesting areas to be investigated. Even though many studies have already demonstrated good correlations between cerebral Doppler data and fetal hypoxia, or fetal well being, it is too early to draw conclusions about how to use this cerebral Doppler in routine practice for the management of fetal distress

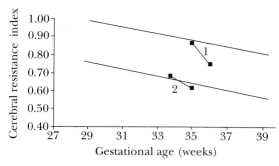

Figure 13 *Example 1: Fetus number 1, with a relatively low heart rate, has the cerebral resistance index in the upper part of the normal range (see Figure 1). One week later, the cerebral index decreases by 25%, but it remains in the normal range. Without the results of previous examinations, the fetus appears to be in a perfectly normal hemodynamic state. Example 2: Fetus number 2, with a relatively high heart rate, has the cerebral resistance index in the low part of the normal range. If this index decreases by 10% 1 week later, it will become pathological. In fact, fetus number 2 has a hemodynamic development more normal than that of fetus number 1, although the absolute value of the cerebral index at the second examination shows the opposite*

and for making the decision to interrupt a gestation.

The umbilical resistance index has been used to confirm the existence of placental hemodynamic disorders in the case of IUGR, but the sensitivity of this parameter for the follow-up of fetal growth remains close to 60%. Nevertheless, the absence of end-diastolic flow on the umbilical or aortic Doppler waveform is an indicator of severe fetal distress and neonatal cerebral complications.

The cerebroplacental index that measures the proportion of flow supplying the brain and the placenta is now the most widely used parameter for the assessment of IUGR and hypoxia. One reason is that it takes into account the causes and the consequences of the placental insufficiency responsible for IUGR and hypoxia. The second reason is that this parameter is not heart rate dependent, and has a single cut-off value (normal if > 1, or 1.1), at least during the second half of pregnancy. On the other hand, because IUGR is usually associated with brain metabolism disturbances and delayed brain development, the cerebroplacental ratio, already an indicator of IUGR and hypoxia, is also

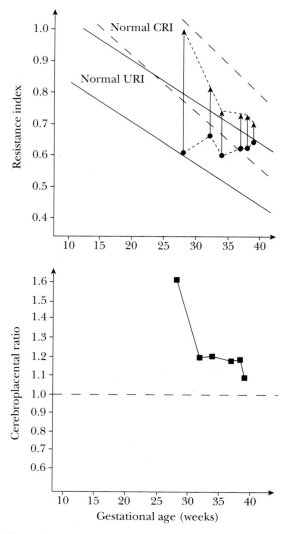

Figure 14 *Evolution of both the umbilical (URI) and the cerebral resistance index (CRI) during the early phase of development of moderate intrauterine growth retardation (normal delivery, fetal weight in the 10th centile), and the corresponding cerebroplacental ratio. These two resistance indices showed large fluctuations, even within their normal range or at its limit; however, the cerebroplacental ratio decreased regularly towards its cut-off line of normality, in agreement with a progressive redistribution of the fetal flows usually induced by the development of a hypoxic process*

an accurate parameter for the prediction of poor perinatal outcome.

It is also clear that, because the resistance indices are heart rate dependent, it is hazardous to draw any conclusions from one absolute value of any of these parameters. As shown in the examples in Figure 13, fetus number 1, with a relatively low heart rate, had the cerebral resistance index in the upper part of the normal range. One week later, the cerebral index decreased by 25%, but it remained in the normal range. Without knowledge of the results of previous examinations, one would consider that the fetus was in a perfectly normal hemodynamic state. If the evolution of the cerebral index was followed, the decrease of the cerebral resistance may lead to suspicion of an increase of the cerebral flow in response to a decrease of the fetal pO_2. Fetus number 2, with a relatively high heart rate, had the cerebral resistance index in the low part of the normal range. If this index had decreased by 10% 1 week later, it would have become pathological. In fact, fetus number 2 had a hemodynamic development more normal than that of fetus number 1, although the absolute value of the index in the second examination showed the opposite.

Only several successive daily measurements of the Doppler indices will lead to a more realistic evaluation of fetal hemodynamics. Moreover, any increase in the umbilical index or decrease in the cerebral or cerebroplacental index, even inside the normal range, will have to be considered as pathological. Conversely, the progressive decrease in the umbilical index, the progressive decrease in the cerebral index or the stability of the cerebroplacental ratio, even out of the normal limits on the diagram, will be considered as normal. Figure 14 shows the fluctuations of both the umbilical and cerebral resistance indices; however, the cerebroplacental ratio decreased regularly during the early phase of development of moderate IUGR (normal delivery, fetal weight in the 10th centile). It was noted that all these indices stayed within or at the limit of their normal range.

Our recent studies[67,71] demonstrated that the cerebroplacental ratio changes followed very closely and significantly the fetal pO_2 changes during the period of acute hypoxia (Figures 7, 8 and 9). If this ratio shows the same accuracy in the monitoring of the pO_2 changes in chronic as in acute hypoxia, it will be of great interest to measure this parameter frequently with the objective of atraumatically quantifying the fetal pO_2 change, especially in the case of moderate IUGR. Our preliminary data confirm that the cerebroplacental ratio is also a good indicator of the fetal pO_2 level in a case of chronic hypoxia (Figure 11). The remaining question to be taken into consideration is: What reduction in the cerebroplacental ratio (i.e. pO_2) remains acceptable for the fetal brain, and for what duration?

ACKNOWLEDGEMENTS

We thank the technicians of the animal station (INRA) for their active contribution to this work. This work was supported by INSERM and Region Centre grants.

References

1. Nicolaides, K. H. and Campbell, S. (1991). Fetal oxygenation and circulation. In Philipp, E. E., Barnes, J. and Newton, M. (eds.) *Scientific Foundations of Obstetrics and Gynaecology*, pp. 304–15. (London: William Heinemann Medical Books)
2. Jensen, A., Roman, C. and Rudolph, A. M. (1991). Effects of reducing uterine blood flow on fetal blood flow distribution and oxygen delivery. *J. Dev. Physiol.*, **15**, 309–23
3. Brace, R. A. (1993). Regulation of blood volume *in utero*. In Hanson, M. A., Spencer, J. A. D. and Rodeck, C. H. (eds.) *Fetus and Neonate. Physiology and Clinical Applications*, vol. 1: *The Circulation*, pp. 73–99. (Cambridge: Cambridge University Press)
4. Wood, C. E. (1993). Local and endocrine factors in the control of the circulation. In Hanson, M. A., Spencer, J. A. D. and Rodeck, C. H. (eds.) *Fetus and Neonate. Physiology and Clinical Applications*, vol. 1: *The Circulation*, pp. 700–15. (Cambridge: Cambridge University Press)
5. Gilbert, R. D., Pearce, W. J., Ashwal, S. *et al.* (1990). Effects of hypoxia on contractility of

isolated fetal lamb cerebral arteries. *J. Dev. Physiol.*, **13**, 199–203

6. Reuss, M. L., Parer, J. T., Harris, J. L. *et al.* (1982). Haemodynamic effects of alpha-adrenergic blockade during hypoxia in fetal sheep. *Am. J. Obstet. Gynecol.*, **142**, 410–15

7. Adamson, S. L., Morrow, R. J., Langille, B. L. *et al.* (1990). Site-dependent effects of increases in placental vascular resistance on the umbilical arterial velocity waveform in fetal sheep. *Ultrasound Med. Biol.*, **16**, 19–27

8. Gosling, R. G. and King, D. H. (1975). Ultrasonic angiology. In Harius, A. W. and Adamson, S. L. (eds.) *Arteries and veins*, pp. 61–98. (Edinburgh: Churchill Livingstone)

9. Maulik, D., Yarlagadda, P., Nathanielsz, P. *et al.* (1989). Hemodynamic validation of Doppler assessment of fetoplacental circulation in a sheep model system. *J. Ultrasound Med.*, **8**, 177–81

10. Pourcelot, L. (1974). Applications cliniques de l'examen doppler transcutané: vélocimétrie ultrasonore doppler. *Sem. INSERM*, **34**, 213–40

11. Stuart, B., Drumm, J., Fitzgerald, D. E. and Duignan, N. M. (1980). Fetal blood velocity waveforms in normal pregnancies. *Br. J. Obstet. Gynaecol.*, **87**, 780–6

12. Arbeille, P., Ttanquart, F., Body, G. *et al.* (1986). Evolution de la circulation artérielle ombilicale et cérébrale du foetus au cours de la grossesse. XVI Journées Nationales de Néonatologie. Progrès en néonatologie. *Karger Edit*, **6**, 30–7

13. Arbeille, P., Roncin, A., Berson, M. *et al.* (1987). Exploration of the fetal cerebral blood flow by Doppler ultrasound in normal and pathological pregnancies. *Ultrasound Med. Biol.*, **13**, 329–37

14. Wladimiroff, J. W., Van de Wijngaard, J. A., Degani, S. *et al.* (1987). Cerebral and umbilical arterial blood flow velocity wave form in normal and growth retarded pregnancies. *Obstet. Gynaecol.*, **69**, 705–9

15. Brar, H. S., Horenstein, J., Medearis, A. L. *et al.* (1989). Cerebral, umbilical and uterine resistance using Doppler velocimetry in postterm pregnancy. *J. Ultrasound Med.*, **8**, 187–91

16. Gramellini, D., Folli, M. C. and Raboni, S. (1992). Cerebral–umbilical Doppler ratio as predictor of adverse outcome. *Obstet. Gynecol.*, **79**, 416–20

17. Arbeille, P., Leguyader, P., Fignon, A. *et al.* (1994). Fetal hemodynamics and flow velocity indices. In Copel, J. and Reeds, K. (eds.) *Doppler in Obstetrics and Gynecology*, pp. 19–29. (New York: Raven Press)

18. Woo, J. S. K., Liang, S. T., Lo, R. L. S. *et al.* (1987). Middle cerebral artery doppler flow velocity waveform. *Obstet. Gynaecol.*, **70**, 613–16

19. Arbeille, P., Henrion, C. H., Paillet, C. H. *et al.* (1988). Hemodynamique cerebrale et placentaire dans les grossesses gemellaires. Progrès en néonatologie. *Karger Edit*, **7**, 223–9

20. Arbeille, P. and Leguyader, P. (1992). Cerebral, renal, and umbilical Doppler in the evaluation of IUGR and fetal well being on hypertensive pregnancies. *J. Ultrasound Med.*, **11**, 31

21. Arbeille, P., Maulik, D., Stree, J. L. *et al.* (1994). Fetal cerebral and renal Doppler in small for gestational age fetuses in hypertensive pregnancies. *Eur. J. Obstet. Gynecol. Reprod. Biol.*, **56**, 111–16

22. Kjellmer, I., Thordstein, M. and Wennergren, M. (1992). Cerebral function in the growth-retarded fetus and neonate. *Biol.Neonate*, **62**, 265–70

23. Fouron, J. C., Teyssier, G., Maroto, E. *et al.* (1991). Diastolic circulatory dynamics in the presence of elevated placental resistance and retrograde diastolic flow in the umbilical artery: Doppler echographic study in lambs. *Am. J. Obstet. Gynecol.*, **164**, 195–203

24. Arbeille, P., Giovangrandi, Y., Pourcelot, D. *et al.* (1984). Les ultrasons dans l'exploration de la circulation foeto-placentaire. *J. Mal. Vasc.*, **9**, 297–300

25. Schulman, H., Fleischer, A. and Stern, W. (1984). Umbilical velocity wave ratios in human pregnancy. *Am. J. Obstet. Gynecol.*, **148**, 985–90

26. Gudmundsson, S. and Marsal, K. (1988). Umbilical artery and uteroplacental blood flow velocity waveforms in normal pregnancy – a cross-sectional study. *Acta Obstet. Gynecol. Scand.*, **67**, 347–54

27. Arbeille, P., Asquier, E., Moxhon, E. *et al.* (1983). Nouvelle technique dans la surveillance de la grossesse: l'étude de la circulation foetale et placentaire par les ultrasons. *J. Gynecol. Obstet. Biol. Reprod.*, **12**, 851–9

28. Cameron, A. D., Nicholson, S. F. and Nimrod, C. A. (1988). Doppler waveforms in the fetal aorta and umbilical artery in patients with hypertension in pregnancy. *Am. J. Obstet. Gynecol.*, **158**, 339–45

29. Eik-Nes, S. H., Marsal, K. and Kristoffersen, K. (1984). Methodology and basic problems related to blood flow studies in the human fetus. *Ultrasound Med. Biol.*, **10**, 329–37

30. Erskine, R. L. A. and Ritchie, J. W. K. (1985). Quantitative measurement of fetal blood flow using doppler ultrasound. *Br. J. Obstet. Gynaecol.*, **92**, 600–4

31. Fleischer, A., Schulman, M., Farmakides, G. *et al.* (1985). Umbilical artery velocity waveform and intrauterine growth retardation. *Am. J. Obstet. Gynecol.*, **151**, 502–5

32. McCallum, W. D., Williams, C. S. and Daigle, R. E. (1978). Fetal blood velocity waveforms. *Am. J. Obstet. Gynecol.*, **132**, 425–9

33. Maulik, D., Arbeille, P. and Kadado, T. (1992). Hemodynamic foundation of umbilical arterial Doppler waveform analysis. *Biol. Neonate*, **62**, 280–9

34. Reuwer, P. J. H. M., Nuyen, W. C., Beijer, H. J. M. *et al.* (1984). Characteristics of flow velocities in the umbilical arteries, assessed by Doppler ultrasound. *Eur. J. Obstet. Gynecol. Reprod. Biol.*, **17**, 397–408

35. Trudinger, B. J., Giles, W. B., Cook, C. M. *et al.* (1985). Fetal umbilical artery flow velocity waveforms and placental resistance: clinical significance. *Br. J. Obstet. Gynaecol.*, **92**, 20–3

36. Trudinger, B. J., Cook, C. M., Giles, W. B. *et al.* (1987). Umbilical artery flow velocity waveforms in high-risk pregnancies. *Lancet*, **1**, 188–90

37. Bilardo, C. M., Nicolaides, K. H. and Campbell, S. (1990). Doppler measurements of fetal and uteroplacental circulations: relationship with umbilical venous blood gases measured at cordocentesis. *Am. J. Obstet. Gynecol.*, **162**, 115–20

38. Brar, H. S. and Platt, L. D. (1988). Reverse end-diastolic flow on umbilical artery velocimetry in high-risk pregnancies: an ominous finding with adverse pregnancy outcome. *Am. J. Obstet. Gynecol.*, **159**, 559–61

39. Divon, M. Y., Girz, B. A., Lieblich, R. *et al.* (1989). Clinical management of the fetus with markedly diminished umbilical artery end-diastolic flow. *Am. J. Obstet. Gynecol.*, **161**, 1523–7

40. Nicolaides, K. H., Bilardo, C. M., Soothill, P. W. *et al.* (1988). Absence of end diastolic frequencies in umbilical artery: a sign of fetal hypoxia and acidosis. *Br. Med. J.*, **297**, 1026–7

41. Rochelson, B., Schulman, H., Farmakides, G. *et al.* (1987). The significance of absent end-diastolic velocity in umbilical artery velocity waveforms. *Am. J. Obstet. Gynecol.*, **156**, 1213–18

42. Wladimiroff, J. W., Tonge, H. M. and Stewart, P. A. (1986). Doppler ultrasound assessment of cerebral blood flow in the human fetus. *Br. J. Obstet. Gynaecol.*, **93**, 471–5

43. Archer, L., Levene, M. I. and Evans, D. H. (1986). Cerebral artery Doppler ultrasonography and prediction of outcome after perinatal asphyxia. *Lancet*, **2**, 1116–18

44. Laurin, J., Marsal, K., Persson, P. *et al.* (1987). Ultrasound measurement of fetal blood flow in predicting fetal outcome. *Br. J. Obstet. Gynaecol.*, **94**, 940

45. Bonnin, P., Guyot, O., Blot, P. *et al.* (1992). Relationship between umbilical and fetal cerebral flow velocity waveforms and umbilical venous blood gases. *Ultrasound Obstet. Gynecol.*, **2**, 18–22

46. Rizzo, G., Arduini, D., Luciano, R. *et al.* (1989). Prenatal cerebral Doppler ultrasonography and neonatal neurologic outcome. *J. Ultrasound Med.*, **8**, 237–40

47. Arbeille, P., Collet, M., Fignon, A. *et al.* (1989). Cerebral flow assessment by conventional and color-coded doppler in human fetuses during pregnancies with hypertension. *Echocardiogr. J.*, **6**, 265–70

48. Arduini, D., Rizzo, G., Romanini, C. *et al.* (1989). Hemodynamic changes in growth retarded fetuses during maternal oxygen administration as predictors of fetal outcome. *J. Ultrasound Med.*, **8**, 193–6

49. Edelstone, D. I., Peticca, B. B. and Goldblum, L. J. (1985). Effects of maternal oxygen administration on fetal oxygenation during reductions in umbilical blood flow in fetal lambs. *Am. J. Obstet. Gynecol.*, **152**, 351–8

50. Nicolaides, K. H., Bradley, R. J., Soothill, P. W. *et al.* (1987). Maternal oxygen therapy for intrauterine growth retardation. *Lancet*, **1**, 942

51. Richardson, B., Potts, P., Connors, G. *et al.* (1990). The effect of carbon dioxide on cerebral flow velocity waveforms in the human fetus. Proceedings of *IIIrd International Perinatal Doppler Society*, Los Angeles, 26–28 September, p.56

52. Mori, A., Iwashita, M., Nakabayashi, M. *et al.* (1992). Effect of maternal oxygen inhalation on fetal hemodynamics in chronic hypoxia with IUGR. *J. Matern. Fetal Invest.*, **2**, 93–9

53. Jouppila, P. and Kirkinen, P. (1984). Increased vascular resistance in the descending aorta of the human fetus in hypoxia. *Br. J. Obstet. Gynaecol.*, **91**, 853–6

54. Lingman, G., Laurin, J. and Marsal, K. (1986). Circulatory changes in fetuses with imminent asphyxia. *Biol. Beonate*, **49**, 66–73

55. Laurin, J., Lingman, G., Marsal, K. *et al.* (1987). Fetal blood flow in pregnancies complicated by intrauterine growth retardation. *Obstet. Gynecol.*, **69**, 895–902

56. Hackett, G. A., Campbell, S., Gamsu, H. *et al.* (1987). Doppler studies in the growth retarded fetus and prediction of neonatal necrotising enterocolitis, haemorrhage, and neonatal morbidity. *Br. Med. J.*, **294**, 13–16

57. Griffin, D., Bilardo, K., Masini, L. *et al.* (1984). Doppler blood flow waveforms in the descending thoracic aorta of the human fetus. *Br. J. Obstet. Gynaecol.*, **91**, 997–1006

58. Soothill, P. W., Nicolaides, K. H., Bilardo, C. M. *et al.* (1986). Relation of fetal hypoxia in growth retardation to mean blood velocity in the fetal aorta. *Lancet*, **2**, 1118–20

59. Moretti, M., Mercer, B., Cartier, M. *et al.* (1990). Pulsatility index of the fetal renal artery in post-dates pregnancies and relation to amniotic fluid. Proceedings *IIIrd International Perinatal Doppler Society*, Los Angeles, 26–28 September, p.48

60. Vyas, S., Nicolaides, K. H. and Campbell, S. (1989). Renal artery flow velocity waveforms in normal and hypoxemic fetuses. *Am. J. Obstet. Gynecol.*, **161**, 168–72

61. Arbeille, P., Salihagic, A., Fignon, A. *et al.* (1995). Hémodynamique ombilicale, cérébrale, aortique et rénale foetale: Retard de croissance-hipoxie. *Reprod. Hum. Horm.*, **8**, 357–71

62. Daniel, S. S., Yeh, M. N., Bowe, E. T. *et al.* (1975). Renal response of the lamb fetus to partial occlusion of the umbilical cord. *J. Pediatr.*, **87**, 788–94

63. Hecher, K., Campbell, S., Doyle, P. *et al.* (1995). Assessment of fetal compromise by Doppler ultrasound investigation of the fetal circulation. Arterial, intracardiac and venous blood flow velocity studies. *Circulation*, **91**, 129–38

64. Reuss, M. L. and Rudolph, A. M. (1980). Distribution and recirculation of umbilical and systemic venous blood flow in fetal lambs during hypoxia. *J. Dev. Physiol.*, **2**, 71–84

65. Behram, R. E., Lees, M. H., Peterson, E. N. *et al.* (1970). Distribution of the circulation in the normal and asphyxiated fetal primate. *Am. J. Obstet. Gynecol.*, **108**, 956–69

66. Campbell, S., Harrington, K. and Lees, C. (1994). The prenatal assessment of fetal hypoxia. In Kurjak, A. and Chervenak, F. (eds.) *The Fetus as a Patient. Advances in Diagnosis and Therapy*, pp. 381–8. (Carnforth, UK: Parthenon Publishing)

67. Arbeille, P., Berson, M., Maulik, D. *et al.* (1992). New implanted Doppler sensors for the assessment of the main fetal hemodynamics. *Ultrasound Med. Biol.*, **18**, 97–103

68. Arbeille, P., Bosc. M., Vaillant, M. *et al.* (1992). Nicotine-induced changes in the cerebral circulation in ovine fetuses. *Am. J. Perinatol.*, **4**, 270–4

69. Moore, T. R., Sorg, J., Miller, L. *et al.* (1986). Hemodynamic effects of intravenous cocaine on the pregnant ewe and fetus. *Am. J. Obstet. Gynecol.*, **155**, 883–8

70. Woods, J. R. Jr, Plessinger, M. A. and Clarc, K. E. (1987). Effect of cocaine on uterine blood flow and fetal oxygenation. *J. Am. Med. Assoc.*, **257**, 957–61

71. Arbeille, P., Maulik, D., Fignon, A. *et al.* (1995). Assessment of the fetal pO_2 changes by cerebral and umbilical Doppler on lamb fetuses during acute hypoxia. *Ultrasound Med. Biol.*, **21**, 861–70

72. Barker, D. J. P., Gluckman, P. D., Godfrej, K. M. *et al.* (1993). Fetal nutrition and cardiovascular disease in adult life. *Lancet*, **341**, 938–41

73. Itskowitz, J., Goetzman, B. W., Roman, C. *et al.* (1984). Effect of fetal–maternal exchange transfusion on fetal oxygenation and blood flow distribution. *Am. J. Physiol.*, **247**, H655–60

74. Arduini, D., Rizzo, G. and Romanini, C. (1992). Changes of pulsatility index from fetal vessels preceding the onset of late deceleration in growth-retarded fetuses. *Obstet. Gynecol.*, **79**, 605–10

75. Mari, G. and Wasserstrum, N. (1991). Flow velocity waveforms of the fetal circulation preceding fetal death in a case of lupus anticoagulant. *Am. J. Obstet. Gynecol.*, **164**, 776–8

76. Chandran, R., Serra, S. V., Sellers, S. M. *et al.* (1991). Fetal middle cerebral artery flow velocity waveforms – a terminal pattern. Case report. *Br. J. Obstet. Gynaecol.*, **98**, 937–8

77. Vyas, S., Nicolaides, K. H., Bower, S. *et al.* (1990). Middle cerebral artery flow velocity waveforms in fetal hypoxaemia. *Br. J. Obstet. Gynaecol.*, **91**, 797–803

78. Helperm, J. A., Dereski, M. O., Knight, P. A. *et al.* (1993). Histopathological correlation of nuclear magnetic resonance imaging parameters in experimental cerebral ischemia. *Magn. Reson. Imaging*, **11**, 241–6

79. Laurini, R. M. (1994). Fetal brain pathology. In Kurjak, A. and Chervenak, F. (eds.) *The Fetus as a Patient. Advances in Diagnosis and Therapy*, pp. 89–106. (Carnforth, UK: Parthenon Publishing)

80. Alkalin-Sel, T., Bewleys, S., Van Geijn, H. P. *et al.* (1993). The significance of MCA Doppler assessment in preterminal decompensation of the severely growth retarded fetus. *2nd World Congress of Perinatal Medicine*, Rome

81. Marsal, K., Gunnarsson, G., Ley, D. *et al.* (1994). Cerebral circulation in the perinatal period. In Kurjak, A. and Chervenak, F. (eds.) *The Fetus as a Patient. Advances in Diagnosis and Therapy*, pp. 477–88. (Carnforth, UK: Parthenon Publishing)

82. Fignon, A., Salihagic, A., Akoka, S. *et al.* (1996). Twenty day-cerebral and umbilical Doppler monitoring on a growth retarded and hypoxic fetus. *Eur. J. Obstet. Gynecol. Reprod. Biol.*, in press

Improved fetal outcome by fetal monitoring: 17 years' experience in Yohka Hospital

27

K. Maeda and T. Tsuzaki

INTRODUCTION

The most common fetal monitoring technique is fetal heart rate (FHR) monitoring, because of its high sensitivity for the detection of fetal hypoxia and the possibility of continuous and easy application during pregnancy and labor. The application of fetal monitoring in our hospital has reduced fetal death, hypoxic damage and cerebral palsy.

REDUCED PERINATAL MORTALITY AFTER FETAL MONITORING

FHR indications of fetal hypoxia and impending fetal death were studied in labor. As acute fetal hypoxia was the main cause of intrapartum fetal death, the detection of fetal distress by FHR was thought to be useful in the prevention of fetal death. After the diagnosis of fetal distress by FHR monitoring, Cesarean section was carried out in the first stage of labor, or forceps, vacuum extraction or Cesarean delivery were carried out in the second stage. Fetal death was prevented by immediate delivery and, therefore, short-term fetal outcome was greatly improved by the decrease of stillbirths, after introduction of FHR monitoring. The use of fetal monitoring was extended to include the detection of fetal distress during the antepartum period.

Perinatal mortality was greatly reduced by the introduction of fetal monitoring. In our early controlled study from 1974 to 1976 (Figure 1)[1], perinatal mortality was decreased in the fetal monitoring group to one-third of the non-monitored group. Improvement was obtained by the prevention of fetal death, and also by the reduc-

tion of neonatal asphyxia and subsequent early neonatal deaths, by rapid delivery in cases of abnormal intrapartum FHR.

STUDIES ON THE DEVELOPMENT OF CEREBRAL PALSY

The decrease in the incidence of infantile cerebral palsy was another expectation of the introduction of fetal monitoring. Some authors[2-4], however, reported no effect of electronic fetal monitoring (EFM) on the reduction of cerebral

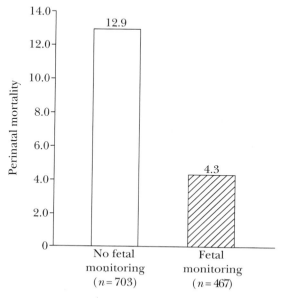

Figure 1 *Perinatal mortality in the groups of no fetal monitoring and fetal monitoring in Tottori University Hospital in 1974–76*

palsy. However, in these studies the EFM was employed after rupture of membranes and therefore there would be less chance to detect abnormal FHR in early labor. Insignificant reduction of the incidence of cerebral palsy after the application of EFM in these studies might be explained by this reason.

External monitoring, however, employs transducers on the maternal abdomen, so that FHR changes can be detected not only in labor after membrane rupture, but also in early labor as well as during the antepartum period. The fetus can be monitored in every pregnant woman because of its non-invasive nature and the absence of medical contraindications. For these reasons, the outcome after external monitoring was studied in our experience of Yohka hospital, separately from the EFM report[4].

Character and history of Yohka Hospital

Perinatal mortality and the development of cerebral palsy were studied in Yohka Hospital, a municipal general hospital located in the Japanese countryside, covering an area of more than five towns in Yabu county. The inhabitants rarely moved from this region. The department of obstetrics and gynecology introduced fetal monitoring in 1977, and fetal heart rate monitoring has been continued to date. The registered number of cerebral palsy sufferers was the subject of this report. Infantile cerebral palsy was diagnosed by pediatric doctors, and recorded in the registry of the Wadayama regional medical center.

The method of fetal monitoring in Yohka Hospital

Fetal monitoring was performed by the external method. The external transducer was attached to the patient immediately after admission, and the cardiotocograph was recorded as continuously as possible in almost all patients in labor[5]. Rapid delivery was carried out by Cesarean section, forceps or vacuum extraction, if the patient was diagnosed with fetal distress due to FHR abnormality by using the standard criteria, including bradycardia, late deceleration, severe variable deceleration, loss of variability and sinusoidal pattern.

Perinatal status after fetal monitoring in Yohka Hospital

Neonatal asphyxia decreased significantly immediately after the introduction of fetal monitoring. The perinatal mortality rate of the hospital, only excluding referred fetal death and referred anencephaly, was low at 6 per 1000 before the introduction of fetal monitoring, but it decreased significantly to 3 per 1000 after the use of the antepartum non-stress test (NST) (Table 1).

The rate of registered cerebral palsy was 2.2 per 1000 before the use of fetal monitoring, and decreased to 0.2–0.3 per 1000 after its introduction. This represents a 90% reduction. The Cesarean section rate was only slightly increased to 9.8% (Table 1)[5]. This low Cesarean section rate might have been obtained by the correct

Table 1 *Outcome and intrapartum monitoring during a 10-year period in Yohka Hospital*[5]

Perinatal status	Period A (1975–76)	Period B (1977–82)	Period C (1983–86)	Statistics		
				A–B	B–C	A–C
Number of births	661	3417	2903			
Non-stress test (%)	0	< 20	> 20			
Perinatal mortality (/1000)	6.1	6.1	3.1	NS	S	S
Neonatal depression (%)	7.3	5.2	4.3	S	NS	S
Registered cerebral palsy (/1000)*	2.2	0.2	0.3	S	NS	S
Very low birth weight infants (%)	0.9	0.6	0.6	NS	NS	NS
Cesarean sections (%)	7.0	11.7	9.8	S	S	S

Period A, no fetal monitoring; period B and C, full intrapartum monitoring. *the registry of regional Wadayama medical center. NS, not statistically significant; S, statistically significant ($p < 0.05$)

Table 2 *Cerebral palsy during the period of fetal monitoring and during the control period in the total live births in Wadayama registry*

| | Total births | | Cerebral palsy | |
		n	Rate (/1000)	Fisher's exact test
Control	1827	4	2.19	p = 0.0249*
Fetal monitoring	13211	6	0.45	

*significant

Table 3 *Cerebral palsy during the period of fetal monitoring and during the control period in term deliveries*

| | Term births | | Cerebral palsy | |
		n	Rate (/1000)	Fisher's exact test
Control	1767	4	2.26	p = 0.0106*
Fetal monitoring	12611	4	0.32	

*significant

Table 4 *Cerebral palsy during the period of fetal monitoring and during the control period in preterm deliveries*

| | Preterm births | | Cerebral palsy | |
		n	Rate (/1000)	Fisher's exact test
Control	60	0	0	p = 0.1737**
Fetal monitoring	600	2	3.33	

**not significant

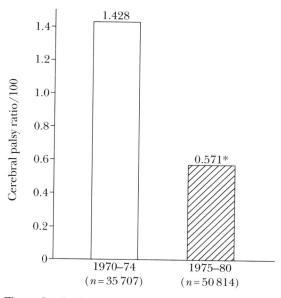

Figure 2 *Cerebral palsy incidences per 1000 livebirths in two connected periods in Tottori area[6]. 1970–74: rare use of fetal monitoring; 1975–80: frequent use of fetal monitoring. *Significant reduction for about 60%*

diagnosis of fetal distress, without unnecessary operation.

The cerebral palsy rate was studied in another independent report among 85 000 deliveries in the Tottori area by pediatric neurologists[6], and they concluded that the incidence of cerebral palsy decreased by 60% after the use of fetal monitoring (Figure 2). This study confirmed our results.

The cerebral palsy rate in term and preterm deliveries during 17 years of fetal monitoring

Cerebral palsy development data were limited to term deliveries in order to exclude the influence of preterm deliveries[7].

Cerebral palsy development was 2.2 per 1000 during the control years before the use of fetal monitoring, and 0.45 per 1000 in 13 211 deliveries during the 17-year period of fetal monitoring. This represented an 80% reduction in cerebral palsy. Fisher's exact test confirmed the statistical significance of the reduction (Table 2).

In term deliveries, cerebral palsy development was 0.32 per 1000 in 12 611 term deliveries during the 17-year period of fetal monitoring in Yohka Hospital (Table 3). This represented an 86% reduction which was significant.

Conversely, there was no reduction of cerebral palsy incidence in preterm deliveries. Cerebral palsy development was 3.33 per 1000 in preterm deliveries during the 17-year period. No significant change was determined with Fisher's test or the χ^2 test (Table 4). It might be suspected that there would be an increasing tendency to cerebral palsy in preterm deliveries, although this trend would be explained by increased survival of very low birth weight infants due to the recent progress in neonatal care. In fact, it has been reported that neurological

Table 5 *Cerebral palsy in the preterm and term deliveries during the monitored period*

| | Number of births | Cerebral palsy | | Fisher's exact test |
		n	Rate (/1000)	
Preterm	600	2	3.33	$p = 0.0274$*
Term	12 611	4	0.32	

*significant

problems were found in about 10% of the infants born with very low birth weight.

Cerebral palsy has a significantly higher incidence in preterm than in term deliveries during the 17-year period of fetal monitoring, and the cerebral palsy ratio was significantly higher (approximately 10 times) in preterm than in term deliveries (Table 5). These results demonstrate the importance of reducing preterm deliveries.

FUTURE ASPECTS AND STRATEGIES

The cerebral palsy rate was reduced by 80–90%, after the introduction of external fetal monitoring during labor. However, cerebral palsy infants still occur. It is our opinion that we must try to find future strategies to reduce further the remaining cases of cerebral palsy.

First, congenital brain anomalies have been reported to be an important cause of cerebral palsy. Congenital anomalies are diagnosed in early pregnancy by ultrasound, particularly with the use of transvaginal sonography. The prevention of congenital brain anomalies needs to be studied further in the future.

Periventricular leukomalacia (PVL) has been reported to be an important and frequent cause of cerebral palsy in preterm neonates. It has been recognized that the appearance of PVL cysts in the neonatal brain suggests the antepartum development of PVL. Therefore, the development of PVL in the fetus should be looked for by sonography. During the antepartum period, PVL is diagnosed not only by characteristic cysts, but also by periventricular echodensity (PVE). We[8] have already found the development of fetal PVE during pregnancy, which evolved into PVL cysts in the neonatal period. High-risk factors for PVL include pre-maturity, maternal hemorrhage, hypoxia and infection. In our experience umbilical cord abnormalities, including excessive twisting, associated with frequent variable FHR decelerations, may be a risk factor. The fetuses who show high-risk factors for PVL should be carefully monitored by sonography and Doppler ultrasound during pregnancy.

Intraventricular hemorrhage (IVH) is an important cause of cerebral palsy, and its antepartum development has been reported in early neonatal life and also during the antepartum period. Fetal IVH requires further study in the future to develop strategies to prevent cerebral palsy.

Although most hypoxic brain damage is prevented by careful fetal monitoring and appropriate intervention, occasional hypoxia will still occur. This rare cause of cerebral palsy occurs as a result of sudden, severe and unavoidable anoxia. The role of delayed neuronal death (DND), which was initially reported in adult cases of the interruption of brain circulation in the 1980s, and recently studied in neonatal brain damage after anoxic insults in pediatric neurology, needs to be studied in the fetus. DND of the fetus may also appear after the persistence of severe anoxia associated with prolonged FHR bradycardia below 60 bpm.

DND was reported to be caused by increased glutamate, Ca ions and free radicals after the anoxia. The brain damage progresses for more than 10 h after the initiation of DND. Reoxygenation and recirculation are ineffective in curing the DND, but it may be treated by blockers of glutamate and Ca ions, and free radical scavengers[9]. Such effective postanoxic therapy should be evaluated for future use in the fetal patient. This would represent a significant advance in the treatment of fetal brain damage after an unavoidable anoxic event before the birth.

SUMMARY

During the 17 years of experience after the introduction of external fetal monitoring, in Yohka Hospital, the outcome was significantly improved in terms of neonatal asphyxia, perinatal mortality and the cerebral palsy rate. An independent report by pediatric neurologists supported the results. The improvement was recognized both in total deliveries and in term deliveries. The cerebral palsy rate in preterm deliveries was not changed significantly during the 17-year period, and had a significantly higher incidence than in term deliveries. Future strategies to reduce cerebral palsy include the reduction of prematurity, detection and prevention of congenital brain anomalies, antepartum PVL, IVH and the possible treatment of DND after the anoxia.

References

1. Maeda, K. (1979). Healthy baby and reduced fetal death by improved obstetric management. In Karim, S. M. M. and Tan, K. L. (eds.) *Problems in Perinatology, Proceedings of 1st Asia Oceania Congress of Perinatology*, pp. 525–9. (Singapore: University of Singapore)
2. Naeye, R. L., Peters, E. C. Bartholomew, M. and Landis, J. R. (1989). Origins of cerebral palsy. *Am. J. Dis. Child.*, **143**, 1154–61
3. Nelson, K. B. and Ellenberg, J. H. (1986). Antecedents of cerebral palsy, multivariate analysis of risk. *N. Engl. J. Med.*, **315**, 81–6
4. MacDonald, D., Grant, A., Sheridan-Perenia, M., Boyland, P. and Chalmers, I. (1985). The Dublin randomized controlled trial of intrapartum fetal heart rate monitoring. *Am. J. Obstet. Gynecol.*, **152**, 524–39
5. Tsuzaki, T., Sekijima, A., Morishita, K., Takeuchi, Y., Mizuta, M., Minagawa, Y., Nakajima, K. and Maeda, K. (1990). The survey on the perinatal variables and the incidence of cerebral palsy for 12 years before and after the application of the fetal monitoring systems. *Acta Obstet. Gynaecol. Jpn.*, **42**, 99–105
6. Takeshita, K., Ando, Y., Ohtani, K. and Takashima, S. (1989). Cerebral palsy in Tottori, Japan. *Neuroepidemiology*, **8**, 184–92
7. Quilligan, E. J. (1994). Personal communication. *5th Japan-Taiwan Conference on Perinatal Ultrasound, Kagoshima.*
8. Utsu, M., Serizawa, M., Yamamoto, N., Yamazaki, T., Oi, H. and Maeda, K. (1995). Blood flow and fetal damages in the excessive umbilical cord twisting. *Ultrasound Obstet. Gynecol.*, **6** (Suppl. 2), Abstr. 41
9. Espinoza, M. I. and Parer, J. T. (1991). Mechanism of asphyxial brain damage, and possible pharmacologic intervention, in the fetus. *Am. J. Obstet. Gynecol.*, **164**, 1582–91

Systematic antenatal functional evaluation $\qquad$ 28

B. Arabin, D. Oepkes and J. van Eyck

INTRODUCTION

The 'fetus as a patient' has become a classical term in perinatal medicine. A major advance in knowledge has been achieved by innovative techniques[1] addressing fetal health as an issue of concern. Subsequent changes in everyday practice dealing with both mother and fetus as possible patients have been reflected by ethical concepts[2], which had otherwise been left to the speculation or intuition of parents, obstetricians and society. Nevertheless, we still emphasize that unborn children being initiative, responsive and even communicative[3] should be protected with care, not solely because late problems can arise. Unless there are inborn errors, intrauterine patients seem only to be the victims of a hostile environment. Primary prevention in order to maintain fetal health throughout pregnancy would be an ideal tool. Assuming that the fetus is a healthy human being who could just be kept *safe* from threatening conditions would imply several criteria:

(1) Knowledge of the origin of pathophysiological processes;

(2) Ability to select pregnancies with possible risks (epidemiology/history);

(3) Ability to select pregnancies with specific risks (screening examinations);

(4) Knowledge of effective preventive interventions.

Only if these criteria were insufficiently fulfilled, would the fetus require further concern. Again there are several possibilities:

(1) The fetus might adapt to possible temporary reduced life quality;

(2) The fetus can cope with intrauterine but not with extrauterine life;

(3) Adaptation or defence against hostile influence *in utero* become insufficient with the risk of later handicap, impairment, disability or even death.

At advanced gestational age early recognition of risk factors may prevent life-long problems by delivery of the infant. If intrauterine problems arise at early gestational age – although evaluated properly – delivery is not an option. In these cases we have to balance *prenatal* vs. *postnatal life quality* with the objective of maintaining a *life-long life quality*. Dependent on the etiology of the disease there are differences in effectiveness and duration of direct or indirect interventions:

(1) Direct causal or symptomatic fetal therapy with a procedure related risk (e.g. laser therapy in twin–twin transfusion syndrome, blood transfusion in fetal anemia);

(2) Treatment to improve postnatal adaptation (e.g. corticosteroids);

(3) Indirect treatment to maintain or improve long-lasting life quality *in utero* (e.g. early strict treatment of maternal diabetes);

(4) Indirect treatment to maintain or improve temporary life quality *in utero* when prevention or direct treatment is not available (e.g. 'active postponement' in pre-eclampsia).

Systematic fetal medicine and preventive pregnancy care virtually did not exist until approximately 30 years ago. New diagnostic tools are still being introduced. This may be one reason that single results of technical approaches are still overestimated instead of being interpreted in a clinical context in relation to the specific environmental processes and fetal risk factors. For some diseases the clinical and diagnostic tools in use are either unable to identify fetuses at risk or are not interpreted in the correct context. However, to provide the most possible safety, epidemiological risk factors, technical expertise and scientific knowledge of various pathophysiological influences on the fetus have to be pragmatically integrated into a systematic antenatal function evaluation (SAFE) of individual mothers and their growing fetuses when fetal well-being is at risk due to a harmful environment.

CLINICAL EXPERIENCE

In fetuses with inborn health impairments therapeutic measures are either not possible, palliative or combined with method-related risks. Many of these infants will have to live with their disease for the rest of their life. 'Environmental' fetal health problems theoretically can be combined with a normal life after birth. The strong linkage between basic research on etiology, epidemiological risk factors, diagnostic steps, prevention and management options should be considered in everyday practice.

In our routine work we have established protocols related to the variety of fetal diseases incorporating semiquantitative evaluation of defined criteria as SAFE. In addition, we have attempted to document available information to elucidate individual disorders with specific data from procedures and individual information that have not previously been evaluated. Table 1 reflects an overview of what we regard as environmental diseases and some diagnostic, preventive and therapeutic measures. Invasive diagnostic procedures are only used if sufficient information is not given by non-invasive tests.

Our approach and final data will not be explained in detail in this chapter. Within a short period of time single parameters will either have been applied or abandoned according to the

analysis of our own data and/or the review of new literature. We have therefore decided to select three diseases to illustrate differences in achievements concerning etiology, preventive, diagnostic and therapeutic tools rather than to place emphasis on single test results. The state of the art of population-based measures and possibilities at specialized centers, with respect to the life-long future of infants has changed tremendously as in progressive fetal anemia due to red blood cell alloimmunization, moderately as in progressive fetal hypoxia possibly combined with iatrogenic prematurity due to early onset pre-eclampsia, or not significantly as in (sub) acute fetal hypoxia possibly combined with anemia due to abruptio placentae. In those diseases where there are still only poor achievements historical considerations might provoke us to solve unsolved problems. Therefore, we unrestrainedly acknowledge the pioneer work that has been undertaken based on imagination, professional courage and persistence. These attitudes will stimulate the continued search for further advances by subjective observations, individual initiatives and team work[4].

Progressive fetal anemia in red blood cell alloimmunization

Fetal anemia as a consequence of red blood cell alloimmunization is considered a stimulating example of what can and already has been achieved in perinatal medicine. It also enables us to witness the relationship between *basic research* (discovery of the rhesus factor[5], first fetomaternal transfusion[6,7]), *diagnostic techniques* (first amniotic punctures[8–10], first cordocentesis[11–13]), *prevention* (prophylaxis, effectiveness, population-based application[14–16]) and *therapeutic options* (intrauterine transfusions[17–20]) for the goal of life-long life quality.

In the past, what was primarily called hemolytic disease of the newborn or erythroblastosis fetalis has in the meantime been recognized to be what is regarded as a typical environmental disease for the fetus. As such, it has changed from a major contributor to perinatal morbidity and mortality of unknown cause to a condition which can be prevented in most cases, or at least successfully diagnosed and treated providing the fetus with intrauterine and future life quality.

Fetal hypoxia and iatrogenic immaturity in early onset pre-eclampsia and HELLP syndrome

It was only in this century that the indirect measurements of blood pressure and proteinuria were introduced into obstetric practice. This made it possible to recognize at least some conditions which threaten the mother. One of the most severe associated complications, the hemolysis, elevated liver enzymes and low platelet count (HELLP) syndrome, was only described in 1982[21]. Epidemiological risk factors and, recently, an increasing number of hemostatic and metabolic abnormalities have been detected in mothers with early-onset pre-eclampsia and HELLP syndrome, which will have an impact on screening, counselling and pharmacological therapy[22]. Multicenter trials, regarded as pioneering work, have shown that preventive treatment in pregnancies with a history of pre-eclampsia can improve outcome[23]. However, specific knowledge about the origin of pre-eclampsia and HELLP syndrome in primigravidas still remains unclear. Maternal clinical symptoms are often the first warning sign. At this stage, the fetus may already show signs of compromise with the risk of intrauterine hypoxia. Caring for the mother may even require the disregard of fetal or neonatal life quality. Improving maternal health by symptomatic therapy considering the environment primarily may not only prolong pregnancy but also improve temporary life quality of the fetus[24].

Although the exact cause of the final pathophysiological pathway, namely endothelial cell dysfunction, is still unknown, nutritional and respiratory placental dysfunction nearly always impair fetal health in utero. Nevertheless, direct biophysical examinations of fetal functions have replaced biochemical placental function tests[25,26] which, in the late 1970s, were still the most important investigative tools in the second half of pregnancy. In the cascade of a harmful environment, reduced uterine flow primarily reduces fetal respiration[27]. Traditional clinical concepts characterizing the health of the neonate immediately after birth[28] can in the meantime be applied to define respiratory, cardiovascular and neurological sequelae in utero when 'translated' into prenatal medicine[29]. Recently, the venous and intracardic circulation have also been incorporated into our protocols to detect signs of cardiac insufficiency as a consequence of hypoxia[30,31].

(Sub-)acute fetal hypoxia and anemia in progressive abruptio placentae

In the majority of pregnancies with premature separation of a normally implanted placenta specific mechanisms remain unknown. The shorter Latin expression abruptio denotes a sudden accident of clinical manifestation but not a primary cause of underlying chronic diseases reflected by the recurrence rate of around 10%. It is discouraging that in more than half of recurrences abruptio proves fatal to the fetus[32]. Considering that little has been found to elucidate the etiology or underlying disorders, it is not surprising that a classification of abruptio from the 1950s[33], e.g. before fetomaternal medicine and preventive pregnancy care had been established, is still used in the literature.

Most risk factors of abruptio, such as chronic hypertension, pre-eclampsia, premature rupture of membranes (PROM), smoking, drug abuse, high parity, unmarried status and age < 25 years, are confounded by the sociodemographic status. An increasing incidence rate of abruptio was described to occur among women likely to be financially and socially disadvantaged[34]. At this stage, when there are no strictly defined medical options, sociodemographic prevention programs and counselling of mothers at risk in response to early symptoms should not be underestimated. This also holds true for a high number of environmental fetal diseases in which an understanding of the etiology allowing easy screening programs is still insufficiently available.

Table 1 *Summary of 'environmental' risk factors affecting fetal health and possible diagnoses and interventions*

Environmental risk	Fetal or neonatal health impairment	Risk factors	First symptoms, screening tools
Alloimmunization, infection, fetomaternal hemorrhage	chronic anemia, hemolytic disease	obstetric history	indirect: antibody screen, ADCC direct: PCR, amniocytes, fetal blood group
Diabetes (pregnancy induced)	macrosomy, cardiomyopathy, metabolic problems	family and obstetric history	glucosuria, stress tests, macrosomia
Placental dysfunction	IUGR/chronic hypoxia (iatrogenic immaturity)	socioeconomic and lifestyle risks, obstetric history, smoking	'small-for-date baby'
Pre-eclampsia and HELLP syndrome	IUGR/chronic hypoxia (iatrogenic immaturity)	family, medical and obstetric history	DBP > 90 mmHg proteinuria > 0.3, 'small-for-date baby'
Prolonged pregnancy	(sub)acute hypoxia	irregular menstrual cycle	age of pregnancy, amnopscopy?
Premature labor	immaturity	obstetric history, sociodemographic and lifestyle factors	clinical findings, e.g. multiple pregnancy
PROM (< 26 weeks)	long hypoplasia immaturity	actual history	verification PROM clinics/ultrasound, biochemically
	infection, immaturity	—	interleukins, cervical culture
Abruptio placentae	(sub)acute hypoxia, possibly anemia, possibly immaturity	obstetric history, smoking	PROM, pre-eclampsia, trauma? vaginal bleeding, contractions/tone

For abbreviations, see notes at foot of page overleaf

(Continued across from opposite page)

Biochemical diagnosis	Biophysical diagnosis	Prevention primary/ secondary	Management options
indirect: change/type, antibody titers/ADCC direct: bilirubin in amniotic fluid (Liley-index), Hb/Hct (FBS)	liver/spleen size, Doppler studies of hyperdynamic circulation, FHR monitoring, search for early signs of hydrops, valve regurgitation, fluid accumulation	well-matched transfusions, immunoprophylaxis quantitative assessment of FMH	direct: transfusions early delivery?
indirect: Hba1c/glucose level direct: fetal lung maturity, fetal insulin AF	echocardiography, Doppler venous and intracardial circulation	diet, insulin	postponement to term under strict control/ labor induction in macrosomia
indirect: hemoconcentration direct: fetal blood gases?	Doppler uterine arteries, AFI, Doppler arterial venous and intracardiac circulation, FHR/FBM/FM/FT	lifestyle, aspirin, heparin	volume expansion? O_2?
indirect: Hb, Hk, platelets, transaminases, bilirubin direct: fetal blood gases?	indirect: BP/CO/SVR/ PCWP/PAP, Doppler uterine arteries direct: Doppler arterial/ venous and intracardial circulation, FHR/FBM/ FM/FT	aspirin, heparin, pyridoxine, folic acid	volume expansion and vasodilatation, $MgSO_4$, sedation, corticosteroids
indirect: hemoconcentration	AFV/FHR pattern, Doppler cerebral artery, right/left heart diameter	induction of labor	delivery, possibly amnioninfusion in cases with meconium stained AF
indirect: cervix and urine culture, fibronectin/ CRP, interleukin direct: bacterial culture AF, lung maturity tests	Cervical structure, cervical length, tocography, Doppler uterine artery	lifestyle, prophylaxis of infection	tocolytics
—	fetal position, AFV, Doppler ductus arteriosus combined with FMB, nose flow during FBM	—	amnioninfusion? tocolytics
indirect: cervix and urine culture, fibronectin/ CRP, interleukin direct: fetal culture	FHR monitoring, tocography	non-invasive measures	antibiotics
indirect: Hb, Hct, platelets, Fg, FDP, ATIII direct: Kleihauer-Bethke Invasive: fetal Hb/Hk	indirect: Doppler uterine artery, placental echolucency, contractions direct: Doppler umbilical artery and cerebral artery, Doppler aorta ascendens, FHR pattern	lifestyle, treatment of underlying disorders, cessation of smoking, folic acid?	acute delivery, at early gestational age 'active postponement' with close monitoring, tocolysis?

Epidemiology including lifestyle trend analysis, basic research of underlying disorders, diagnostic techniques, preventive and therapeutic options have to be specified to improve fetal life quality in combination with this disease.

SUMMARY

Systematic approaches need to be adapted to local possibilities, individual expertise and future visions, as well as to the individual needs of parents and fetuses. Decision making depends on techniques which in practice do not always work with 100% certainty. Multiple variables reduce failure rates. Future observations will improve diagnostic and therapeutic management. Failure rates can be reduced if the examinations fit into classical concepts of underlying mechanisms. Actual life quality, hopes and feelings of parents, although hard to score, should always be integrated in decision making.

Since a large number of fetuses exposed to a small risk continues to contribute to more risk cases than a small number with greater risks, we have to compromise between 'upstream' and 'downstream' attitudes[35] when reducing threatening environmental conditions for the fetus without decreasing efficiency regarding time and costs.

THE FUTURE

The standardization of clinical management protocols is a prerequisite for education, self-control and comparison with different options. Nevertheless, it should be emphasized, that there must always be space for individualization which is as important in the approach of fetal diseases as it is in adult medicine. Medical science and clinical practice do not pursue truth as an absolute value but from what is happening in the individual. In this way our fetuses help us to define future steps. Their disease manifestations, if unusual, challenge dogma and can lead to reflection and change. Years after unusual encounters we can instantly recall particular fetuses who led to reappraisal of their health status, adaptation or maladaptation towards environmental threats. Further steps are still required to be taken in the prevention, diagnosis and therapy of fetuses at risk, if only we have the patience and enthusiasm to care, to be creative, to value new observations, to maintain our curiosity, to learn from systematic antenatal evaluation and to incorporate protocol results in long-term follow-up of infants who have been our patients *in utero*.

Life expectancy of newborns, of 70–80 years in industrialized countries, has led to maintenance of fetal health and a safe continuation from fetal to neonatal life becoming the most important contributors to primary preventive health care.

Footnote to Table 1

HELLP, syndrome of hemolysis, elevated liver enzymes and low platelet count; PROM, premature rupture of membranes; IUGR, intrauterine growth retardation; PCR, polymerase chain reaction; ADCC, antibody dependent cellular cytotoxicity; DBP, diastolic blood pressure; Hb, hemoglobin; Hct, hematocrit; FBS, fetal blood sampling; AFV, amniotic fluid volume; CRP, C-reactive protein; FDP, fibrinogen degradation products; ATIII, antithrombin III; FHR, fetal heart rate; AFI, amniotic fluid index; FBM, fetal breathing movements; FM, fetal movement; FT, fetal tone; BP, blood pressure; CO, cardiac output; SVR, systemic vascular resistance; PCWP, pulmonary capillary wedge pressure; PAP, pulmonary arterial pressure; FMH, fetomaternal hemorrhage

References

1. Saling, E. and Arabin, B. (1988). Historic landmarks of perinatal medicine. *J. Perinat. Med.*, **16**, 5–21

2. McCullough, L. B. and Chervenak, F. A. (1994). *Ethics in Obstetrics and Gynecology.* (New York, Oxford: Oxford University Press)

3. Arabin, B., Bos, R., Rijlaarsdam, R., Mohnhaupt, A. and van Eyck, J. (1996). The phenomenon of inter-human contacts – how does it start? *Ultrasound Obstet. Gynecol.*, submitted

4. Silvers, R. (1995). *The Hidden History of Science.* New York Review of Books (New York)

5. Landsteiner, K. and Wiener, A. S. (1942). An agglutinable factor in human fetal blood recognized by immune sera for rhesus blood. *Proc. Soc. Exp. Biol. Med.*, **43**, 223–34

6. Wiener, A. S. (1948). Diagnosis and treatment of anemia of the newborn caused by occult placental hemorrhage. *Am. J. Obstet. Gynecol.*, **56**, 717–25

7. Kleihauer, E. and Betke, K. (1960). Praktische Anwendung des Nachweises von HbF-haltigen Zellen in fixierten Blutausstrichen. *Internist*, **1**, 292–300

8. Bevis, D. (1952). Antenatal prediction of hemolytic disease of the newborn. *Lancet*, **1**, 395–9

9. Liley, A. W. (1961). Liquor amnii analysis in the management of pregnancy complicated by rhesus sensitisation. *Am. J. Obstet. Gynecol.*, **82**, 1359–70

10. Whitefield, C. R. (1970). A three-year assessment of an action-line method of timing interventions in rhesus immunization. *Am. J. Obstet. Gynecol.*, **108**, 1239–45

11. Daffos, F., Capella-Pavlovsky, M. and Forestier, F. (1985). Fetal blood sampling during pregnancy with use of a needle guided by ultrasound: a study of 606 consecutive cases. *Am. J. Obstet. Gynecol.*, **153**, 655–60

12. Rhodeck, C. H. and Campbell, S. (1979). Umbilical cord insertion as a source of pure fetal blood for prenatal diagnosis. *Lancet*, **1**, 1244–5

13. Wladimiroff, J. W. and Jahoda, M. C. J. (1977). Real time scanning and transabdominal fetal blood sampling. *Lancet*, **1**, 593–7

14. Finn, R. (1960). Erythroblastosis. *Lancet*, **1**, 526–9

15. Clarke, C. A., Donhoe, W. T. A., McConnell, R. B. *et al.* (1963). Further experimental studies on the prevention of Rh haemolytic disease. *Br. Med. J.*, **1**, 979–84

16. Freda, V. J., Gorman, J. G. and Pollak, W. (1964). Successful prevention of experimental Rh sensitization in amn with an anti-Rh gamma2 globulin antibody preparation: a preliminary report. *Transfusion*, **4**, 26–32

17. Liley, A. W. (1963). Intrauterine transfusions of the fetus in haemolytic disease. *Br. Med. J.*, **2**, 1107–12

18. Rhodeck, C. H., Howman, C. A., Karnicki, J., Kem, J. R., Whitmore, M. and Austin, M. A. (1981). Direct intravascular fetal blood transfusion by fetoscopy in severe rhesus immunisation. *Lancet*, **1**, 625–9

19. Hobbins, J. C., Davis, C. D. and Webster, J. (1976). A new technique utilizing ultrasound to aid an intrauterine transfusion. *J. Clin. Ultrasound*, **4**, 135–7

20. Hansmann, M. and Lang, N. (1972). Intrauterine Transfusion unter Ultraschallkontrolle. *Klin. Wochenschr.*, **50**, 930

21. Weinstein, L. (1982). Syndrome of hemolysis, elevated liver enzymes and low platelet count: a severe consequence of hypertension in pregnancy. *Am. J. Obstet. Gynecol.*, **142**, 159–67

22. Dekker, G. A., de Vries, J., Doelitzsch, P. M., Huijgens, P. C. M., von Blomberg, B. M. E., Jakobs, C. and van Geijn, H. P. (1995). Underlying disorders associated with severe early-onset pre-eclampsia. *Am. J. Obstet. Gynecol.*, **173**, 1042–8

23. CLASP Collaborative Group (1994). A randomized trial of low-dose aspirin for the prevention and treatment of pre-eclampsia among 9346 pregnant women. *Lancet*, **343**, 619–29

24. Visser, W. and Wallenburg, H. C. S. (1995). Temporizing management of severe pre-eclampsia with and without the HELLP syndrome. *Br. J. Obstet. Gynaecol.*, **102**, 111–17

25. Chard, T. (1987). What is happening to placental function tests? *Ann. Clin. Biochem.*, **24**, 435–9

26. Arabin, B., Ragosch, V. and Mohnhaupt, A. (1995). From biochemical to biophysical placental function tests in fetal surveillance. *Am. J. Perinat.*, **12**, 168–71

27. Campbell, S., Pearce, J. M. F., Hackett, G. *et al.* (1986). Quantitative assessment of uteroplacental blood flow: early screening test for high risk pregnancies. *Obstet. Gynecol.*, **68**, 649–53

28. Apgar, V. (1953). A proposal for a new method of evaluation of the newborn infant. *Anesth. Analg. Curr. Res.*, **32**, 260–9

29. Arabin, B., Snyders, R., Mohnhaupt, A., Ragosch, V. and Nicolaides, K. H. (1993). Evaluation of the fetal assessment score in pregnancies at risk for intrauterine hypoxia. *Am. J. Obstet. Gynecol.*, **169**, 549–54

30. Kiserud, T., Eik-Nes, S. H., Blaas, K. H. and Hellevik, L. R. (1991). Ultrasonographic velocimetry of the fetal ductus venosus. *Lancet*, **338**, 1412–14

31. Hecher, K., Snijders, R., Campbell, S. and Nicolaides, K. H. (1995). Fetal venous, intra-cardiac, and arterial blood flow measurements in intrauterine growth retardation: relationship with fetal blood gases. *Am. J. Obstet. Gynecol.*, **173**, 10–15

32. Pritchard, J. A., Cunningham, F. G., Pritchard, S. A. and Mason, R. A. (1991). On reducing the frequency of severe abruptio placentae. *Am. J. Obstet. Gynecol.*, **165**, 1345–51

33. Page, E. W., King, E. B. and Merrill, J. A. (1954). Abruptio placentae: dangers of delay in delivery. *Obstet. Gynecol.*, **3**, 385–90

34. Saftlas, A. F., Olson, D. R., Atrash, H. K., Rochat, R. and Rowley, D. (1991). National trends in the incidence of abruptio placentae, 1979–1987. *Obstet. Gynecol.*, **78**, 1081–6

35. Rose, C. (1992). *Strategies of Preventive Medicine.* (New York: Saunders)

Monitoring fetal hypoxemia: Doppler flow measurement and computerized cardiotocography

29

G. P. Mandruzzato, Y. J. Meir and L. Fischer Tamaro

ANTEPARTUM COMPUTERIZED CARDIOTOCOGRAPHY

Antepartum cardiotocography (CTG) is one of the few techniques available today to assess fetal conditions in high-risk pregnancies. Visual interpretation of CTG traces has been shown to be unreliable. In order to eliminate observer variability and to increase the accuracy of CTG, numerical on-line analysis of fetal heart rate patterns was introduced.

Dawes and collaborators started work on the development of a computerized system to analyze human fetal heart rate patterns in 1978. Initially, their motivation derived from animal experiments that demonstrated that the heart rate was modulated by many rhythms of breathing, associated with sleeps states, age and the time of day[1], and because of their expectation that there could be more information gained by an accurate analysis in the human fetus. Subsequently, with the increasing number of studies that recognized the lack of reproducibility of visual evaluation of CTG, a numerical on-line analysis of fetal heart rate patterns was found to be essential, not only for research, but also as a more accurate tool in the assessment of fetal conditions[2–5]. In 1983 a computerized on-line CTG system entered clinical use in Oxford, and since 1986 this has been used in the Department of Obstetrics and Gynaecology of the Istituto per l'Infanzia of Trieste. In this chapter, the principles of computerized CTG are illustrated and clinical experience with the system is described.

CHARACTERISTICS OF COMPUTERIZED CARDIOTOCOGRAPHY

In a computerized CTG system, results of analysis are given continuously on-line, both in graphic and in written form, on a monitor. Warnings are usually displayed or heard when the signal loss is too high, when fetal movements are deficient or when the trace is abnormally flat or decelerative. A printout of the record with the results of analysis is available. As far as the program is concerned, we will refer mainly to 'System 8000' developed by Dawes and co-workers at the Nuffield Institute in Oxford for Sonicaid[6–8]. The system acquires data continuously for up to 60 min. The fetal monitor is interrogated to acquire the autocorrelation function and tocodynamometer reading, and for fetal movements. The measurement of the fetal pulse interval is controlled by error algorithms. Valid pulse intervals are averaged over an 'epoch' of $1/16$ min (3.75 s) and then stored. The first analysis is performed after 10 min and every 2 min thereafter. The principal parameters calculated are fetal movements, the basal fetal heart rate, the number of accelerations and decelerations, the variation and the episodes of high and low fetal heart rate variation.

Fetal movements

During the monitoring the mother signals all fetal movements with a hand-held event marker.

Each epoch containing one or more perceived movements is identified.

Fetal heart rate baseline and basal heart rate

The baseline has been defined as a running average of heart rate in the absence of accelerations and decelerations. The best technical procedure is still debated. Leaving the technical details to the original descriptions[7,9,10], the baseline is derived using a digital filter (autoregressive to avoid phase changes) and from the frequency distribution of pulse intervals. The basal fetal heart rate is recorded in beats per min (bpm), averaged from episodes of low fetal heart rate variation, or otherwise from the frequency distribution of pulse intervals.

Accelerations and decelerations

Accelerations and decelerations are occasional deviations from the baseline with a certain amplitude and duration. In the Oxford system there are two principal types of deceleration: type I, amplitude > 10 bpm and duration > 1 min; type II, amplitude > 20 bpm and duration > 30 s (other types are specified when the fetal heart rate record is very flat, and a third analysis is performed to identify shallow decelerations associated with contractions). Large decelerations are defined by area, greater than 20 beats below the baseline. Accelerations are identified when the fetal heart rate deviates above the baseline by more than 10 bpm for more than 15 s.

Variation and episodes of high and low variation

With the present instruments there is no point in measuring very short-term beat-to-beat variation, because it is normally so low (about 2 ms), too near to the limit of accuracy. It is underestimated if autocorrelation is used, and overestimated by conventional Doppler detector systems[11,12]. Moreover, the amount of data to be stored and the time required for analysis would be 8–10 times greater. The Oxford system considers two types of variations: long-term and short-term, both excluding decelerations. Long- (or medium-) term variation is expressed as the mean 1-min range of pulse intervals. Short-term variation is calculated as the mean of successive epochal (1/16 min) pulse interval differences. Short- and long-term variations are highly correlated ($R = 0.90$) (Figure 1). Short-term variation is more useful when low-frequency sinusoidal rhythms are present. Episodes of high or low variation are identified when, during consecutive minutes of a trace, the long-term variation exceeds or falls below a certain threshold, defined as the first centile of measurements at 30–33 weeks, to minimize the effects of gestational age.

Over the past 10 years, more than 40 000 clinical records have been collected, from different centers (Oxford, Luton, Southampton and Trieste). The first records were obtained in normal pregnancies, to establish the limits of normality of the different parameters calculated by the system. Later they were made for clinical purposes, predominantly for monitoring fetal conditions in pregnancies complicated by fetal growth retardation or known maternal disease.

Interpretation of computerized analysis

It took several years and thousands of records to elaborate normal tables for the different patterns of the CTG. It must be stressed that for most of the parameters there is a wide range of normality within the same gestational age. The reason for this is that the fetal heart

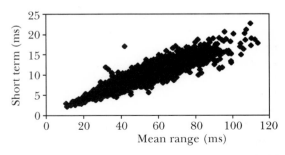

Figure 1 *Correlation between long-term (mean range) and short-term variation of fetal heart rate in 3984 traces ($R = 0.90$)*

Table 1 *Changes in long-term fetal heart rate variation (mean range) at different gestational ages in normal pregnancies*

Gestational age (weeks)	Number of traces	Mean range (ms)				
		Average	Median	SEM	SD	Lower 3rd centile
28–29	293	42.3	40.9	0.6	10.9	25.5
30–31	405	44.5	42.6	0.7	14.1	24.2
32–33	466	46.5	44.0	0.7	14.8	24.6
34–35	491	48.6	46.2	0.7	15.3	25.9
36–37	572	49.5	47.4	0.6	14.8	27.9
38–39	568	50.6	48.4	0.7	16.5	26.8
40	434	50.1	48.2	0.8	16.5	25.3
41	1014	48.5	46.4	0.5	16.2	25.1
42	380	46.4	44.2	0.8	16.3	21.9
43	108	44.7	42.4	1.4	14.4	22.6

rate varies greatly with fetal behavioral states after 28 weeks' gestation, and with gestational age.

The fetal basal heart rate decreases with gestational age; the normal range is 120–160 bpm. The number of accelerations increases with gestational age from 28 to 40 weeks more than three fold, but fetal heart rate accelerations may be absent in many traces of normal fetuses. However, at least one episode of high fetal heart rate variation is always (> 99%) present from 28 weeks on in normal fetuses if the duration of the CTG is sufficient. Episodes of low variation may last up to 50 min in normal fetuses near term. This is why there is no constant length of recording recommended; the length should depend on the fulfilment of certain criteria, i.e. the presence of an episode of high variation of sufficient amplitude, and no evidence of large decelerations or a sinusoidal rhythm. Decelerations are present in some normal fetuses near term, and even when these are associated with low fetal heart rate variation, they are a poor guide to outcome. The diagnostic importance of both accelerations and decelerations has been overstated, probably because exact measurements were difficult without computers. Even though variation demonstrates a wide band of values in the normal fetus, it seems that this is the best measure to evaluate fetal conditions. Long-term variation ('mean minute range' in the Oxford system) tends to increase from 28 weeks to term. Values above 30 ms are considered normal, those between 20 and 30 ms are questionable and those below 20 ms are considered abnormal (Table 1).

Short-term variation is highly correlated with long-term variation. In the presence of low-frequency (1 in 2–5/min) sinusoidal rhythms, short-term variation, in the absence of an episode of high fetal heart rate variation, is a better guide to outcome (Table 2).

Fetal monitoring by computerized CTG: features and clinical considerations

One of the major issues in obstetrics, today as in the past, consists in the evaluation of relative risks. On one side of the scale we find the risk of fetal death or severe damage *in utero*; on the other, neonatal death or severe morbidity as a result of prematurity. Improvements in neonatal care have lowered neonatal mortality and morbidity, but for the obstetrician the problem remains, with the difference that it must be resolved at earlier gestational ages. The introduction of computerized CTG offers a new relative-risk weighing tool. As for all the other means used for the evaluation of the fetal condition, it must be stressed that computerized CTG should be used in conjunction with other biological measurements.

Before the experience with computerized CTG is described, some concepts should be kept in mind.

(1) Antepartum CTG is used as an intermittent examination. The identification of acute

Table 2 *Changes in short-term fetal heart rate variation at different gestational ages in normal pregnancies*

Gestational age (weeks)	Number of traces	Short-term variation (ms)				
		Average	Median	SEM	SD	Lower 3rd centile
< 28	46	7.54	6.85	0.4	2.7	5.1
28–29	60	7.96	7.65	0.3	2.2	4.7
30–31	92	8.13	7.95	0.2	2.1	5.0
32–33	114	8.68	8.20	0.2	2.4	5.3
34–35	148	8.95	8.60	0.2	2.4	4.8
36–37	187	9.27	9.00	0.2	2.8	4.5
38–39	326	9.18	8.90	0.2	2.8	5.0
40–41	697	8.99	8.60	0.1	2.7	5.1
42–43	86	9.03	8.60	0.3	2.9	4.4

events, such as sudden fetal death not preceded by progressive deterioration (e.g. abruption or placental infarction), are excluded;

(2) CTG is not useful for the detection of growth retardation in itself, but it is useful in detecting hypoxemia and alterations of metabolic status, whether or not these are associated with placental vascular disease or growth retardation;

(3) Gross changes in fetal heart rate are late signs of fetal hypoxemia;

(4) In a distressed fetus it is necessary to have reliable means to detect small progressive changes in metabolic status; and

(5) All instrumental and biochemical parameters used today to monitor fetal conditions give a numerical measurement. The only one based on an opinion is 'eye-ball' evaluation of CTG, which is highly unreliable.

Clinical and experimental experience with antepartum CTG has shown that the most reliable single parameter of fetal conditions is variation. Absence of accelerations, the presence of decelerations, reduction of movements and changes in basal fetal heart rate are all likely to occur occasionally in a normal fetus. On the other hand, they may be absent in hypoxemic or anemic fetuses. Some authors[13] have shown that repetitive late decelerations are almost constantly present in advanced stages of fetal deterioration, but the problem is that they may not be present or be so small that they are overlooked by visual assessment. As far as terminal traces are concerned, computerized CTG improves reproducibility by supplying numerical thresholds. Numerical analysis of the CTG detects fetal deterioration at an early stage and enables the obstetrician longitudinally to follow fetuses at risk[14–17]. A constant, progressive reduction in variation has been shown to be associated with progressive deterioration of fetal oxygenation. We emphasize 'progressive', because there is a small proportion of fetuses that persistently exhibit low heart rate variation and neither their outcome, nor their postnatal heart rate features, differ from those of controls with a higher heart rate variation before birth[18]. This gives further evidence that the 'unreactive' trace is not a reliable indication of fetal compromise.

The best way to demonstrate a relationship between fetal heart rate patterns and fetal biochemical status is to find a significant correlation between numerical CTG measurements and numerical values of fetal blood gas analysis[19,20]. While it is easy and non-invasive to perform fetal electronic monitoring, if necessary more than once or twice a day, it is too invasive and too risky to perform fetal blood sampling (cordocentesis) in the same way. However, a sample of blood may be acquired after a Cesarean section in the absence of labor. Smith and colleagues[21] studied the correlation between fetal heart rate patterns and biochemical measurements in cord samples, obtained in three groups of patients delivered by Cesarean section: group 1, for fetal compromise between 28 and 36 weeks' gestation; group 2, for urgent maternal reasons between 28 and 36 weeks' gestation; group 3, electively at 38–40 weeks. The comparison between groups 1 and 2 in this study was not between abnormal and normal, but between compromised fetuses with and without marked fetal heart rate abnormalities.

The authors showed that fetuses with abnormal heart rate patterns (group 1) exhibited lower umbilical arterial PO_2 values than those at a corresponding gestational age but with normal or suboptimal traces (group 2). When groups 1 and 2 were combined there was a significant correlation between the mean minute range of fetal heart rate variation and umbilical artery PO_2. The results demonstrated that measurement of fetal heart rate variation can help identify fetuses that are becoming hypoxemic, without acidemia. They suggested that a mean range of < 20 ms is abnormal, and > 20–30 ms is probably abnormal, especially if associated with decelerations.

The next step was to investigate the clinical implications of very low fetal heart rate variation. Street and co-workers[22] studied retrospectively the outcome of pregnancies in which at least one computerized CTG record displayed a long-term variation (mean range) below 20 ms. They found a mean range below 20 ms in 78 women (961 traces) out of 2582 (7396 traces) who had computerized CTG between 1983 and 1987. They considered as the index trace the first trace with a mean range below 20 ms. Most of the pregnancies were complicated by proteinuric hypertension (73%) or by intrauterine growth retardation (IUGR; 19%). There were five intrauterine deaths and four neonatal deaths for a total perinatal mortality rate of 11.5%. Of the liveborn, eight were acidemic at delivery and 30 had hyaline membrane disease. All deaths occurred when the index trace was taken before 32 weeks. One of the most interesting features is that 27 fetuses were below 30 weeks' gestation when the index trace was taken; nevertheless, pregnancy was safely prolonged in 17 (63%) by an average of 17 days. This fact outlines the utility of having measures, in order to quantify longitudinally the state of fetal compromise, even when ominous signs are already present. While processing their data the authors found that the long-term variation in a sinusoidal fetal heart rate pattern superimposed on an otherwise flat trace is normal or high. Moreover, one out of nine terminal traces is sinusoidal. This led the authors to examine measurements of short-term variation. As mentioned above, beat-to-beat variation cannot be measured accurately with present Doppler-based instruments. Therefore, they defined a new measure of short-term variation as that of successive epochs (3.75 s), during which valid fetal heart rate values are averaged. Of the 78 fetuses in the study, 44 had a short-term variation below 3 ms in at least one record. Four of these fetuses died *in utero*. All four had short-term variation between 0.9 and 2.5 ms in the last trace within 24 h of death. Of the remaining 40 liveborn babies, those who showed short-term variation below 2.6 ms had decreased arterial pH and increased base deficit, suggesting that they were becoming acidotic and that the trace might have been preterminal.

In our series from 1986 to 1994 in pregnancies complicated by pregnancy-induced hypertension and/or severe IUGR, in which intervention was excluded because of extreme prematurity, very low fetal weight estimate or because the consent for intervention was not given by the patient, we had 11 intrauterine deaths (excluding malformed fetuses) that had at least one computerized CTG. Considering as the index trace the first trace with a mean range below 20 ms, in one case it took 60 days from index trace to death, in one it took 41 days, in two cases 17 and 14 days, respectively, and in the other seven it took less than 8 days. No constant was found as far as the time-interval between the day of the lowest mean range and the day of intrauterine death was concerned (Figure 2).

Another important study about short-term variation and its relationship to decelerations and umbilical flow velocity waveforms was published in 1992[23]. The authors studied 89 patients demonstrating at least one record with short-term variation equal to or below 3 ms. If the fetus did not die *in utero*, umbilical artery blood gases were sampled at Cesarean section in the absence of labor. When short-term variation fell

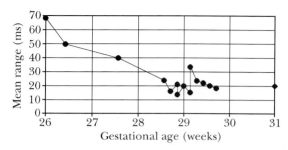

Figure 2 *Mean range in a case of intrauterine death at 31 weeks of a male, 480-g fetus. Pregnancy complicated by severe intrauterine growth retardation and oligohydramnios*

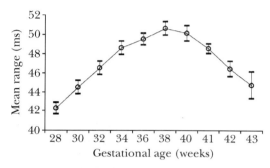

Figure 3 *Mean range in normal pregnancies (average ± SE)*

below 2.6 ms there was a high incidence of metabolic acidemia and intrauterine death (34% combined). On the other hand, there were also eight fetuses in which short-term variation fell transiently below 2.6 ms and within 24 h was above 3 ms, all without acidemia at delivery. In our opinion, the main feature of this study is the relationship between low variation, decelerations and outcome. The authors showed that the presence of decelerations did not predict metabolic acidemia or loss of other vital signs. As for the temporal relationship, decelerations usually appeared late, compared with the fall in fetal heart rate variation below the lower limit of normality (5.7 ms).

Computerized CTG is an essential method to monitor post-term pregnancies when expectant management is adopted. Recently, we have studied the features of computerized CTG in prolonged pregnancies in order to measure changes in fetal heart rate long-term variation

patterns in fetuses with increasing gestational age after term. Computerized measurement of fetal heart rate patterns with the Sonicaid System 8000 was performed in 567 singleton pregnancies at 41–43 weeks between 1987 and 1993, obtaining 1502 valid measurements. Our results show that after 41 weeks long-term fetal heart rate variation decreased progressively from an average value of 48.5 ms at 41 weeks to 46.4 ms and 44.7 ms at 42 and 43 or more weeks, respectively. Whereas long-term fetal pulse interval variation has been shown to rise progressively with increasing gestational age from 28–29 weeks, it reaches a peak at 39–40 weeks in normal patients. Thereafter, not only is there no further rise, but values decrease progressively (Figure 3).

Conclusions

Computerized CTG analysis offers new perspectives for a more reliable assessment of fetuses at risk and for the interpretation of fetal heart rate patterns. The advantages of computerized CTG may be summarized as follows.

(1) Predefined criteria to be satisfied are always interpreted in the same way, obtaining an objective reading of the fetal heart rate trace which eliminates the observer variability;

(2) Numerical measurements of fetal heart rate patterns are available and can be stored in large databases. This allows statistical evaluation of the different parameters of the fetal heart rate, introducing a better scientific approach for the definition of normality and abnormality;

(3) The quality of the record is improved;

(4) The time required for the test is reduced;

(5) Computerized systems can be programmed to be interactive and give warning signals when necessary;

(6) With sufficient data accumulated, it is possible to extrapolate the measure of the fetal heart rate that gives the best estimate of fetal well-being. To date the best single

measure to be taken into consideration seems to be variation (long-term or short-term);

(7) A more accurate comparison between fetal heart rate patterns and other biological measurements is possible; and

(8) Computerized CTG enables the detection of small changes in fetal heart rate occurring in time, so that, when initial deterioration signs arise, the single fetus can be followed up longitudinally.

In conclusion, computerized analysis of CTG, as offered by System 8000 and other systems, greatly improves the reliability of fetal heart rate evaluation in clinical practice. It is, in fact, possible to distinguish, with good accuracy, fetuses that are truly jeopardized because of hypoxemia or acidemia, from those that are not.

DOPPLER FLOWMETRY

Characteristics

This non-invasive method, used to assess the patterns of blood flow in a vessel, is based on the fact that the frequency of the ultrasound beam emitted by the probe is altered when it reaches a moving target. The reflected frequency is increased when the target is moving toward the probe and reduced when it is moving away. The alteration of the frequency is proportional to the target speed. In our case the targets are the blood cells reflecting the ultrasound beam. By using this technology it is possible to obtain a sonogram that is the graphic display of the different blood velocities that are present in the vessel during the cardiac cycle. In order to have a numerical identification of the sonogram, different formulas have been proposed, mainly based on the principle of comparing the maximum systolic with the minimum diastolic velocities. As the latter is particularly influenced by the resistance to flow downstream in the vessel's explored segment, it is possible to obtain information regarding the level of the peripheral resistance. Assuming that the possible error in

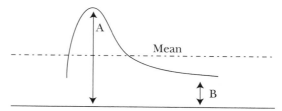

Figure 4 *Sonogram and angle-independent parameters (A, maximum systolic velocity; B, minimum diastolic velocity):* $\frac{A}{B}$ = A/B *ratio (reference 24);* $\frac{A-B}{A}$ = *resistance index (reference 25);* $\frac{A-B}{Mean}$ = *pulsatility index (reference 26)*

the absolute estimation of the velocity, due to the angle of insonation, is the same for both phases of the cycle, so-called 'angle-independent' parameters have been proposed. The most commonly used are represented in Figure 4. It can be observed that only the pulsatility index (PI) takes into consideration the value of the mean velocity, offering perhaps more information regarding the shape of the sonogram.

A sonogram can be obtained by using continuous wave or pulsed wave Doppler. As compared to the continuous wave technique, the pulsed wave technique offers an axial resolution that allows selective investigation of a single vessel after visualization on the screen. By adding color flow imaging, it is possible also to identify very tiny vessels and to study their flow, putting the sample volume of the pulsed wave exactly where it is required.

Patterns in normal pregnancies

It is possible to study the hemodynamic patterns of most fetal vessels (somatic, splanchnic and cerebral) and umbilical vessels. A clear diastolic flow is present in the fetal aorta (Figure 5) and is more prominent in the umbilical artery (Figure 6). It has been shown that in normally evolving pregnancies the peripheral resistance progressively decreases in umbilical arteries and to a lesser extent in fetal vessels. Therefore, in order to draw correct clinical conclusions, it is necessary to compare the obtained values with charts describing the range of normality for each gestational age.

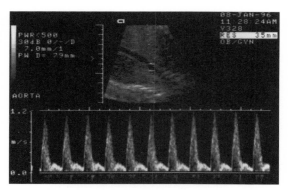

Figure 5 *Normal Doppler waveform in the fetal descending aorta*

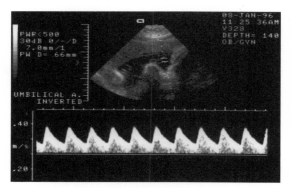

Figure 6 *Normal Doppler waveform in the umbilical artery*

Patterns in complicated pregnancies

In the presence of fetal hypoxemia the situation is different. As a consequence of blood flow redistribution, somatic and splanchnic vessels undergo vasoconstriction that is represented by increased peripheral resistance, as shown by a reduction of diastolic flow velocity that in some cases may be absent (Color plate 34) or reversed (Color plate 35). On the other hand, cerebral vessels depict a reduction of peripheral resistance with increased diastolic blood flow. Increased resistance in somatic vessels together with reduced resistance in cerebral vessels is defined as the 'brain-sparing effect' and represents the phenomenon of fetal adaptation to hypoxemia.

In case of hypoxemia, peripheral resistance can also be increased at the level of the umbilical arteries, representing alterations of fetal–maternal exchanges. It has been shown that the peripheral resistance observable in umbilical arteries is proportional to the obliteration of the vascular bed of the placenta, but this obliteration must involve at least 60% before the sonogram is altered[27,28]. Absent or reversed end-diastolic flow velocity, collected under the acronym ARED, can also be observed in umbilical arteries. Alterations of diastolic flow in umbilical arteries, reflecting reduction of maternal–fetal changes, indicate the cause of fetal hypoxemia, while alterations of flow in all fetal vessels first represent the fetal adaptation to hypoxemia and in worsening cases the inability of the fetus to sustain the adverse condition, losing the capacity to adapt. This condition is also shown by an increase of peripheral resistance in cerebral vessels after the first observed reduction.

A schematic representation of hemodynamic patterns in fetal and umbilical arteries is represented in Figure 7.

Interpretation and clinical use

As far as clinical use of Doppler flowmetry is concerned, according to our experience (Table 3) and to the medical literature[29], this technique seems not to be recommended as a mass screening procedure for the prediction of IUGR or hypoxemia. In fact, although its specificity for hypoxemia is good, particularly in the umbilical artery, its sensitivity is too low, considering what is believed to be acceptable for a mass screening test.

However, Doppler flowmetry on fetal and umbilical arteries has shown to be a suitable second-level test in pregnancies carrying an increased risk of fetal hypoxemia[30–32]. A good human fetal model to check the accuracy of this test is represented by IUGR cases. In the presence of reduced fetal growth, the risk that hypoxemia is present or will develop is high, about 30% of the cases, as a consequence of reduced fetal–maternal exchange of nutrients and gases. On the other hand, about 60% of fetuses showing a growth defect at ultrasound biometry have normal oxygenation and do not require

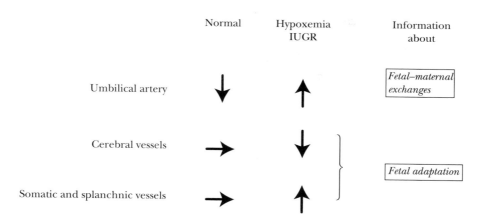

	Normal	Hypoxemia IUGR	Information about
Umbilical artery	↓	↑	Fetal–maternal exchanges
Cerebral vessels	→	↓	Fetal adaptation
Somatic and splanchnic vessels	→	↑	

Figure 7 *Peripheral resistance in normal and complicated pregnancies – those with hypoxemia or intrauterine growth retardation (IUGR)*

Table 3 *Accuracy of Doppler flowmetry (pulsatility index > 2 SD) for predicting intrauterine growth retardation (IUGR) and hypoxemia in 291 unselected pregnancies submitted to ultrasound biometry and Doppler investigation at a 15-day interval from the 28th week of pregnancy*

	IUGR		Fetal hypoxemia	
	UA	FDAo	UA	FDAo
Sensitivity (%)	13.8	51.7	15.4	60.0
Specificity (%)	100.0	99.2	99.3	97.1
Positive predictive value (%)	100.0	88.2	50.0	52.9
Negative predictive value (%)	91.3	94.9	96.2	97.8
True positives (*n*)	4	15	2	9
True negatives (*n*)	25	14	11	6
False positives (*n*)	0	2	2	8
False negatives (*n*)	262	260	276	268

FDAo, fetal descending aorta; UA, umbilical artery

interventions; only an intermediate control can be recommended.

It is therefore necessary to identify the two groups of IUGR fetuses (hypoxemic or not), in order that their management be properly modulated. Doppler flowmetry seems to be able to provide the answer. Our experience is presented in Table 4. A group of 470 IUGR fetuses underwent Doppler flowmetry on the fetal thoracic descending aorta and the umbilical artery during periods of apnea and absence of movements, and the PI was calculated. Accord-

ing to the results of Doppler flowmetry, the fetuses were divided into four groups. The first group was represented by cases in which ARED flow had been observed. In the second group, cases with PI values over 2 SD in both vessels were collected. In the third group abnormal PI values were encountered only in the aorta. In the fourth group, both vessels depicted values within the normal range. The prevalence of hypoxemia was calculated and compared in the four groups. The difference appeared to be statistically significant. Hypoxemia is always en-

Table 4 *Prevalence of fetal hypoxemia according to Doppler flowmetry in 470 cases of intrauterine growth retardation. The perinatal mortality rate was 4.2%; 20 cases all presented absent or reversed end-diastolic flow*

	ARED		> 2 SD, FDAo + UA		> 2 SD, FDAo		< 2 SD, Normal		Total	
	n	%	n	%	n	%	n	%	n	%
Fetal distress*	58	100.0	38	79.2	30	41.1	40	13.7	166	35.3
No fetal distress	—		10	20.9	43	58.9	251	86.3	304	64.7
Total	58	12.3	48	10.2	73	15.5	291	61.9	470	100.0

FDAo, fetal descending aorta; UA, umbilical artery; *$p = 0.001$

Table 5 *Accuracy of Doppler flowmetry for predicting fetal hypoxemia in the umbilical artery or fetal aorta, in the same group of fetuses with intrauterine growth retardation, after the exclusion of absent or reversed end-diastolic flow*

	Umbilical artery	Descending aorta
Sensitivity (%)	35.2	62.7
Specificity (%)	96.7	82.6
Positive predictive value (%)	79.2	56.2
Negative predictive value (%)	80.8	86.3
True positives (n)	38	68
True negatives (n)	294	251
False positives (n)	10	53
False negatives (n)	70	40

countered in cases presenting ARED flow and was very frequent in the second group. In the third group, it was still present in about 40% of the cases, but became much lower in the last group.

Comparing the accuracy of Doppler flowmetry in predicting fetal hypoxemia, there is a clear difference in sensitivity and also in specificity between the aorta and the umbilical artery (Table 5). As already mentioned, the pathophysiological background of the hemodynamic response is different in the fetal vessels and in the umbilical arteries. By using and correctly interpreting Doppler flowmetry information, it is possible to modulate the intensity of control and management.

It has also been advocated that Doppler flowmetry information from cerebral vessels should be used as a guide to management. More recently, its utility has been discussed[33].

The clinical implication of ARED flow must be discussed separately. This hemodynamic condition is always associated with severe hypoxemia, as shown also by studies on fetal blood gases in this situation. Usually in the medical literature ARED cases are presented and discussed together. This is not completely correct, and makes it difficult to compare the clinical results[34]. As shown in Table 6, both conditions (absent and reversed end-diastolic flow) are associated with IUGR, low birth weight, low gestational age at delivery, fetal malformations and/or karyotype aberrations and high perinatal mortality and morbidity. However, there is a significant difference in mean birth weight and particularly in perinatal mortality rate.

When a longitudinal observation is possible, after the observation of absent end-diastolic flow, sooner or later reverse flow will become evident. From a practical point of view, absent end-diastolic flow observation does not always mean the necessity of an immediate delivery. Conversely, in cases of reverse flow, intrauterine death must be expected in a few days. As a consequence, if no other contraindications are present, the delivery should be immediate. In our experience the survivors have all been extracted by Cesarean section at the first appearance of reverse flow. However, also among survivors, the rate of later observed handicaps is high, therefore an exhaustive counselling with the family is mandatory before applying active management.

Conclusions

Doppler flowmetry offers the possibility of investigation by a non-invasive technique of the

Table 6 *Prevalence of abnormalities (structural and/or karyotypic), mean birth weight and perinatal mortality rate in absent end-diastolic flow (EDFA) and reverse flow, or these two considered together (ARED)*

	ARED (n = 78)	EDFA (n = 40)	Reverse flow (n = 38)
Fetal abnormalities	13 (16.7%)	6 (15.0%)	7 (18.4%)
Mean birth weight	1312 (530–3150)	1577 (700–3150)	1048 (530–1800)
Perinatal mortality	33 (423/1000)	7 (175/1000)	26 (684/1000)
Intrauterine death	30	5	25
Neonatal death	3	2	1

hemodynamic patterns of fetal adaptation to hypoxemia and/or the presence of a severe reduction of oxygen supply to fetal blood and organs.

By using this as a second-level test in complicated pregnancies it is possible to modulate the characteristics of control and management, according to the Doppler findings. Due to the fact that this technique is easy to perform, is not time-consuming and can be repeated, accurate monitoring is possible of the level of fetal oxygenation, and a progressively worsening condition can be detected in good time.

CONCLUDING REMARKS

Fetal hypoxemia is a condition of high risk and should be recognized and monitored in an objective way in order to optimize clinical management, avoiding unnecessary intervention or not delaying it too much when it is necessary.

For this purpose, the clinician should rely on objective evaluations offering numerical results that can easily be compared. In such a way each fetus can become its own control, and the choice of the treatment may be more rational. Evaluation of computerized cardiotocography and Doppler flowmetry of fetal and umbilical arteries is likely to fulfil these criteria.

References

1. Dalton, K. J., Dawes, G. S. and Patrick, J. E. (1977). Diurnal, respiratory and other rhythms of fetal heart rate in lambs. *Am. J. Obstet. Gynecol.*, **89**, 276–84

2. Dawes, G. S., Redman, C. W. G. and Smith, J. (1985). Improvements in the registration and analysis of fetal heart rate records at the bedside. *Br. J. Obstet. Gynaecol.*, **92**, 317–25

3. Lawson, G. W., Dawes, G. S. and Redman, C. W. G. (1984). Analysis of fetal heart rate on-line at 32 weeks gestation. *Br. J. Obstet. Gynaecol.*, **91**, 542–50

4. Visser, G. H. A., Dawes, G. S. and Redman, C. W. G. (1981). Numerical analysis of the normal human antenatal fetal heart rate. *Br. J. Obstet. Gynaecol.*, **88**, 792–802

5. Visser, G. H. A., Goodman, J. D. S., Levine, D. H. and Dawes, G. S. (1982). Diurnal and other cyclic variations in human fetal heart near term. *Am. J. Obstet. Gynecol.*, **142**, 535–44

6. Dawes, G. S., Moulden, M. and Redman, C. W. G. (1991). System 8000: computerized antenatal FHR analysis. *J. Perinat. Med.*, **19**, 47–51

7. Dawes, G. S., Moulden, M. and Redman, C. W. G. (1990). Criteria for the design of fetal heart rate systems. *Int. J. Biomed. Comput.*, **25**, 287–94

8. Mantel, R., Van Geijn, H. P., Ververs, I. A. P. and Copray, F. J. A. (1991). Automated analysis of near term antepartum fetal heart rate in relation to fetal behavioural states: The Sonicaid System 8000*. *Am. J. Obstet. Gynecol.*, **165**, 57–65

9. Arduini, D. and Rizzo, G. (1990). Quantitative analysis of fetal heart rate: its application in antepartum clinical monitoring and behavioural pattern recognition. *Int. J. Biomed. Comput.*, **25**, 247–52

10. Mantel, R., Van Geijn, H. P., Caron, F. J. M. *et al.* (1990). Computer analysis of antepartum fetal heart rate. I. Baseline determination. *Int. J. Biomed. Comput.*, **25**, 261–72

11. Lawson, G. W., Dawes, G. S. and Redman, C. W. G. (1982). A comparison of two fetal heart rate ultrasound detector systems. *Am. J. Obstet. Gynecol.*, **143**, 840–2

12. Lawson, G. W., Belcher, R., Dawes, G. S. and Redman, C. W. G. (1983). A comparison of ultrasound (with autocorrelation) and direct electrocardiogram fetal heart rate detector systems. *Am. J. Obstet. Gynecol.*, **147**, 721–2

13. Beckedam, D. J., Visser, G. H. A., Mulder, E. J. H. *et al.* (1987). Heart rate variation and movement incidence in growth retarded fetuses: the significance of antenatal late heart rate decelerations. *Am. J. Obstet. Gynecol.*, **157**, 126–33

14. Mandruzzato, G. P., Conoscenti, G. C., Casaccia, R., Fischer Tamaro, L. and Gigli, C. (1991). Clinical validity of doppler fluximetry and computerized CTG in the assessment of fetal wellbeing. *Perspect. Gynaecol. Obstet.*, **8**, 5–11

15. Ribbert, L. S. M., Fidler, V. and Visser, G. H. A. (1991). Computer-assisted analysis of normal second trimester fetal heart rate patterns. *J. Perinat. Med.*, **19**, 53–9

16. Schneider, E. P., Schulman, H., Farmakides, G. and Chan, L. (1992). Clinical experience with antepartum computerized fetal heart monitoring. *J. Matern. Fetal Invest.*, **2**, 41–4

17. Searle, J. R., Devoe, L. D., Phillips, M. C. and Searle, N. S. (1988). Computerized analysis of resting fetal heart rate tracings. *Obstet. Gynecol.*, **71**, 407–11

18. Smith, J. H., Dawes, G. S. and Redman, C. W. G. (1987). Low human fetal heart rate variation in normal pregnancy. *Br. J. Obstet. Gynaecol.*, **94**, 656–64

19. Henson, G. L., Dawes, G. S. and Redman, C. W. G. (1983). Antenatal fetal heart rate variability in relation to fetal acid–base status at cesarean section. *Br. J. Obstet. Gynaecol.*, **90**, 516–21

20. Ribbert, L. S. M., Snijders, R. J. M., Nicolaides, K. H. and Visser, G. H. (1991). Relation of fetal blood gases and data from computer-assisted fetal heart patterns in small for gestational age fetuses. *Br. J. Obstet. Gynaecol.*, **98**, 820–3

21. Smith, J. H., Anand, K. J. S., Cotes, P. M. *et al.* (1988). Antenatal fetal heart rate variation in relation to the respiratory and metabolic status of the compromised human fetus. *Br. J. Obstet. Gynaecol.*, **95**, 980–9

22. Street, P., Dawes, G. S., Moulden, M. and Redman, C. W. G. (1991). Short term variation in abnormal antenatal fetal heart rate records. *Am. J. Obstet. Gynecol.*, **165**, 515–23

23. Dawes, G. S., Moulden, M. and Redman, C. W. G. (1992). Short term fetal heart rate variation, decelerations, and umbilical flow velocity waveforms before labor. *Obstet. Gynecol.*, **80**, 673–80

24. Stuart, B., Drumm, J., FitzGerald, D. E. and Duigman, N. M. (1980). Fetal blood velocity waveforms in normal pregnancy. *Br. J. Obstet. Gynaecol.*, **87**, 780–5

25. Pourcelot, L. (1974). Aplications clinique de l'examen Doppler transcutane. In Peronneau, P. (ed.) *Velocimetric ultrasonore Doppler*, pp. 213–40. (Paris: Inserm)

26. Gosling, R. G. and King, D. H. (1975). Ultrasonic angiology. In Harcus, A. W. and Adamson, L. (eds.) *Arteries and Veins*, pp. 61–98. (Edinburgh: Churchill Livingstone)

27. Trudinger, B. and Cook, C. M. (1990). Doppler umbilical and uterine flow waveforms in severe pregnancy hypertension. *Br. J. Obstet. Gynaecol.*, **97**, 142

28. Giles, W., Trudinger, B. and Baird, P. (1985). Fetal umbilical artery flow velocity waveforms and placental resistance: pathological correlations. *Br. J. Obstet Gynaecol.*, **92**, 31

29. Newnham, J. P., Patterson, L. L., James, I. R., Diepeveen, D. A. and Reid, S. E. (1990). An evaluation of the efficacy of Doppler flow velocity waveform analysis as a screening test in pregnancy. *Am. J. Obstet. Gynecol.*, **162**, 403–10

30. Marsal, K. and Persson, P. H. (1988). Ultrasonic measurement of fetal blood velocity wave form as a secondary diagnostic test in screening for intrauterine growth retardation. *J. Clin. Ultrasound*, **16**, 239–44

31. Bogatti, P., Veglio, P. C., Rustja, D. and Mandruzzato, G. P. (1989). Feto-placental haemodynamics in growth retardation: a pulsed Doppler study. *Eur. J. Obstet. Gynaecol. Reprod. Biol.*, **31**, 213–19

32. Mandruzzato, G. P., Bogatti, P., Veglio, P. C., Gigli, C., Rustja, D., Casaccia, R. and Fischer, L. (1990). Human fetal haemodynamic adaptation of intrauterine growth retardation. In Dawes, G. S., Borruto, F., Zacutti, A. and Zacutti A. Jr (eds.) *Fetal Autonomy and Adaptation*, pp. 165–74. (Chichester, UK: John Wiley & Sons)

33. Scherjon, S. A., Smolders-DeHaas, H., Kok, J. H. and Zondervan, H. A. (1993). The 'brain-sparing' effect: antenatal cerebral Doppler findings in relation to neurologic outcome in very preterm infants. *Am. J. Obstet. Gynecol.*, **169**, 175

34. Mandruzzato, G. P., Bogatti, P., Fischer, L. and Gigli, C. (1991). The clinical significance of absent or reverse end-diastolic flow in the fetal aorta and umbilical artery. *Ultrasound Obstet. Gynecol.*, **1**, 192–6

Uterine Doppler waveform: prediction and management of pregnancy complications

30

B. Haddad and S. Uzan

INTRODUCTION

Pre-eclampsia and intrauterine growth retardation are still the main causes of maternal and perinatal morbidity and mortality[1]. Pre-eclampsia and many cases of intrauterine growth retardation seem to be related to a failure of trophoblastic invasion into the uterine spiral arteries during the first 20 weeks of pregnancy, leading to a uteroplacental insufficiency[2,3]. These phenomena occur much earlier in pregnancy than do hypertensive complications.

Although the treatment of hypertension during pregnancy reduces maternal risks, it seems not to have any influence on the development of the hypertensive disease or on the frequency of fetal complications. Therefore the aim of last year's research in hypertensive disease has been to find early markers of pre-eclampsia or intrauterine growth retardation, to evaluate their usefulness and to study the effect, in the prevention of pre-eclampsia and intrauterine growth retardation, of low-dose aspirin therapy introduced early in pregnancy.

A poor previous obstetric history, particularly pre-eclampsia or intrauterine growth retardation, is predictive of a high risk of recurrence of vascular complications in the next pregnancy[4,5]. In the EPREDA trial[5], the rates of recurrence of poor outcome, hypertension and proteinuria in patients taking a placebo were 34, 11 and 33%, respectively. However, recurrence can only be used in multiparous patients.

Roll-over test or mid-trimester blood pressure examination can be used to select patients at high risk of hypertensive disease, however, these tests are effective at about 28–32 weeks of pregnancy, a time when prophylaxis for intrauterine

growth retardation seems to be too late[6]. Other tests such as blood platelet count, plasma uric acid, hematocrit and microalbuminuria become abnormal just prior to or at the onset of hypertensive disease, certainly too late to introduce a preventive therapy[4]. Recently, α-fetoprotein[7], fibronectin[8,9] and human chorionic gonadotropin[10,11] have been proposed as early markers, but further studies are needed to ascertain that these tests could be used to predict hypertensive disease. The usefulness of early uterine Doppler examination in the detection of patients at high risk of hypertensive disease has been studied by several authors leading, in some studies, to evaluation of low-dose aspirin treatment in these selected patients in order to reduce hypertensive disease.

DOPPLER ULTRASOUND IN THE PREDICTION OF HYPERTENSIVE DISEASE

The spiral arteries of non-pregnant women, which nourish the endometrium and intervillous space during pregnancy, require 'physiological changes' to permit an increase of blood flow that is necessary to the fetus and placenta[12]. These changes, transforming spiral arteries to uteroplacental arteries, from the decidua to the inner myometrium, are the result of two waves of endovascular trophoblast migration in the first and second trimester[13]. In pre-eclampsia and in a proportion of pregnancies with small-for-gestational age infants the physiological changes of spiral arteries are restricted to the decidual segments alone[3]. The reason for defective trophoblastic invasion of spiral arteries remains unknown. However, the result is an impaired blood supply to the placenta. Since 1983, it has been possible to assess this phenomenon by using Doppler ultrasound on uterine arteries[14].

Initially, several studies[14-17] used uterine Doppler to assess uterine blood flow in patients having fetal growth retardation or severe hypertensive disease. Trudinger and colleagues[15] found a low diastolic uterine artery flow velocity waveform in 60% of pregnancies with growth-retarded infants and in 75% of pregnancies with severe hypertensive disease. Fleischer and associates[16] studied uterine artery Doppler waveforms in 71 women with hypertensive disease. These pregnancies were complicated by stillbirth, premature birth, intrauterine growth retardation and maternal pre-eclampsia when uterine Doppler index S/D ratio was found to be higher than 2.6 and associated to a notch. In order to distinguish evolution of hypertensive disorders in pregnancy Ducey and colleagues[17] examined, in 136 pregnant women with hypertensive disease, pregnancy outcome as a function of both uterine and umbilical artery Doppler velocimetry. Uterine S/D ratio and umbilical S/D ratio were considered abnormal when they were higher than 2.6 from 26 weeks onward and higher than 3 after 30 weeks, respectively. These patients were divided into four groups. The most important group concerning patients having normal uterine and umbilical Doppler velocity (45%), most women had chronic or pregnancy-induced hypertension; deliveries and newborns were usually normal. The three other groups had either isolated abnormal uterine or umbilical Doppler velocity or both. The two-thirds of patients (24%) with both abnormal uterine and umbilical Doppler velocity had pre-eclampsia. Gestational age and perinatal outcome were found to be worst in this group when compared to other groups. Therefore, a normal uterine and umbilical Doppler velocimetry in patients with chronic hypertension or pregnancy-induced hypertension should lead clinicians to be less aggressive in the management of these pregnancies, compared to that of those patients having pre-eclampsia.

Most studies concerning uterine Doppler velocity in pregnant patients with hypertensive disease show a difference between normal and complicated pregnancies. However, the increasing knowledge of the pathophysiology of uterine arteries in normal and hypertensive pregnancies has directed clinicians to study the usefulness of early uterine Doppler in screening patients at risk of developing hypertensive disease.

Trophoblastic invasion is complete at 20 weeks in nearly all patients, however, the persistence of a diastolic notch can be observed until 26 weeks in some women with normal pregnancies[18], suggesting that the physiological process can be delayed. Therefore, screening studies before 20 weeks[19] can induce a high rate of false positives and a lower specificity. Screening too late, after 26 weeks[20], may not be useful as pathological processes will have developed and preventive treatment is less effective. For these reasons, most screening studies were performed between 20 and 24 weeks gestation. These screening trials were considerably different in the choice of impedance to flow indices, cut-off limits to consider abnormal Doppler, insonation sites, definition of small-for-gestational-age infants and study populations.

The impedance to flow indices usually used were the resistance index (RI)[21], or the A/B (or S/D) ratio[22]. Some authors[14,16] also included the presence of an early diastolic notch as an indicator of impaired uteroplacental blood flow. Cut-off limits generally used were the 90th or 95th centile of normal curves previously obtained for local populations, a fixed cut-off was rarely used. Insonation sites were various, S/D ratio and RI were found to be lower from placental than non-placental sites[23,24] and from arcuate than uterine sites[24]. Moreover, screening studies concerned unselected or selected patients at risk for developing pre-eclampsia or intrauterine growth retardation.

Although the diagnostic criteria and endpoints differ in all these studies, uterine Doppler ultrasound remains a simple non-invasive technique with the potential strength to detect pre-eclampsia and intrauterine growth retardation.

Several authors studied the effectiveness of uterine Doppler ultrasound obtained at 20–24 weeks' gestation in the prediction of fetal and maternal complications of hypertensive disease (intrauterine growth retardation, pre-eclampsia). Screening studies concerned selected or unselected populations.

Three large trials concerned selected women. Steel and colleagues[25] studied the efficiency of continuous-wave Doppler ultrasound examination of uterine arteries in the prediction of hypertensive disease in nulliparous women. Of the 1198 nulliparous women screened initially at 18 weeks' gestation, 12% had a persistent abnormal high resistance index (above 0.58) at 24 weeks' gestation; prevalence of proteinuric hypertension was found in 2%. Among women with abnormal uterine Doppler the authors found a significant increase in the rates of hypertension (25 vs. 5%, $p < 0.001$), proteinuric hypertension (10 vs. 0.8%, $p < 0.001$) and severe intrauterine growth retardation (18 vs. 3%, $p < 0.001$) when compared to women with a normal Doppler waveform. In this study population abnormal uterine resistance index had good sensitivity, specificity and negative predictive value for pre-eclampsia, 63%, 89% and 99%, respectively. However, positive predictive value was poor, at 10%. Sensitivity and specificity for the prediction of both hypertension and intrauterine growth retardation were higher (100% and 90%), but positive predictive value remained low (13%).

North and associates[26] studied a screening test for pre-eclampsia and fetal growth retardation, performed on 458 healthy nulliparous women; uterine Doppler waveform was obtained by means of color-pulsed Doppler ultrasound. This test was based on the placental side of the uterine artery resistance index or the A/C ratio (where A is the peak systolic and C the early diastolic velocity) obtained at 19–24 weeks' gestation. Prevalence of pre-eclampsia in the study population was 3.3%. The authors found an increase of pre-eclampsia and fetal growth retardation when the placental-side uterine index (RI or A/C ratio) was above 90th centile. Predic-

tive tests for pre-eclampsia showed a higher sensitivity when using A/C ratio than resistance index (53 vs. 27%, respectively), with an equal specificity (88 vs. 89%, respectively) and negative predictive value (98 vs. 97%, respectively), however, positive predictive values were poor (14 vs. 8%, respectively).

Chan and colleagues[27] studied 358 patients at medium risk for the development of pre-eclampsia and fetal growth retardation, using several uterine Doppler criteria, obtained at 20, 28 and 36 weeks' gestation by a continuous-wave Doppler ultrasound. They found that the best criterion to predict proteinuric hypertension and intrauterine growth retardation was the existence of a high RI (above the 90th centile) associated with diastolic notches in both uterine arteries at 20 weeks. Sensitivity, specificity, positive predictive values and negative predictive values for clinically significant pregnancy-induced hypertension (including proteinuric pregnancy-induced hypertension or pregnancy-induced hypertension occurring before 37 weeks) were found to be 22, 97, 36 and 94%, respectively.

Other large trials involving unselected women have been published. The aim of these studies was to evaluate the effectiveness of uterine Doppler screening between 20 and 26 weeks' gestation for pre-eclampsia or intrauterine growth retardation in the general population. Harrington and colleagues[28] studied 2437 unselected women to detect the best time-dependent screening test based on an abnormal uterine Doppler (a RI higher than the 95th centile and/or the presence of an early diastolic notch) obtained at 20, 24 and 26 weeks' gestation for the prediction of proteinuric pregnancy-induced hypertension or intrauterine growth retardation. They found that 16% of women had an abnormal uterine Doppler obtained with a continuous-wave Doppler at 20 weeks, this rate decreased to 5.4% at 24 weeks and 4.6% at 26 weeks' gestation when measured with a color-pulsed Doppler. Analysis of predictive tests for proteinuric pregnancy-induced hypertension showed high sensitivity (76%) and negative predictive value (99%) of uterine Doppler at 20, 24 and 26 weeks. The improved specificity (86% at 20 weeks to 96% at 24 weeks) and positive predictive value (13% at 20 weeks to 35% at 24 weeks and 44% at 26 weeks) are related to the disappearance of notches.

Bewley and associates[29] studied the ability of second-trimester uterine continuous-wave Doppler ultrasound to predict pre-eclampsia and small-for-gestational-age infants in unselected women. The authors used the averaged RI (AVRI) from four fixed uteroplacental sites, uterine and arcuate sites. Uterine Doppler was considered to be abnormal when AVRI was found to be higher than 95th centile of normality curve. Prevalence of proteinuric pregnancy-induced hypertension and severe intrauterine growth retardation in this study were found at 4.6 and 3.3%, respectively. Predictive tests showed sensitivity and specificity at 24 and 95%, respectively, for proteinuric pregnancy-induced hypertension and 20 and 95%, respectively, for severe intrauterine growth retardation. Positive predictive values were poor for these two complications at 20 and 12%, respectively.

Bower and colleagues[30] studied the value of the early diastolic notch of the uterine arteries at 24 weeks' gestation in a two-stage screening test for pre-eclampsia, in unselected women. In 2026 screened patients, they found that persistence at 24 weeks' gestation of a diastolic notch in the flow velocity waveform (5.1%) was a better predictor for pre-eclampsia than a high RI. The predictive tests in their study population at 24 weeks' gestation, where the prevalence for the development of pre-eclampsia reached 1.8%, showed a sensitivity, a specificity, a positive pre-

dictive value and a negative predictive value at 78, 96, 28 and 99.5%, respectively. The risk of developing significant pre-eclampsia was increased 68-fold when a notch was observed at 24 weeks' gestation.

Sensitivity, specificity, positive predictive values and negative predictive values of abnormal uterine Doppler for pre-eclampsia in selected and unselected patients fluctuate from 22 to 78%, 89 to 97%, 8 to 35% and 94 to 99%, respectively. These results show an important discrepancy between studies, however, it seems that the use of the persistence of diastolic notch alone or associated with an abnormal resistance index improve predictive value for pre-eclampsia (Table 1).

A new approach to the screening of women using uterine Doppler has been proposed to improve the prediction of pre-eclampsia in women with raised maternal serum α-feto-protein[31]. However, many studies using these selection criteria are needed to ascertain the usefulness of this approach.

EARLY MANAGEMENT OF SELECTED HIGH-RISK PATIENTS

The usefulness of uterine Doppler screening to improve pregnancy outcome in unselected patients has given rise to some controversy. Davies and colleagues[32] studied the usefulness of routine uterine Doppler screening of a general obstetric population. In their trial, all patients had a routine standard care. After randomization, 1246 patients had a uterine Doppler and 1229 were considered as controls. The

Table 1 *Uterine Doppler predictivity for pre-eclampsia at 24 weeks' gestation*

	Population	Doppler criteria	Sensitivity (%)	Specificity (%)	PPV (%)	NPV (%)
Steel *et al.*, 1990[25]	nulliparous	RI	63	89	10	99
North *et al.*, 1994[26]	nulliparous	RI	27	89	8	97
Chan *et al.*, 1995[27]	nulliparous	RI + notch	22	97	36	94
Harrington *et al.*, 1991[28]	unselected	RI + notch	76	96	35	99
Bewley *et al.*, 1991[29]	unselected	AVRI	24	95	20	96
Bower *et al.*, 1993[30]	unselected	notch	78	96	28	99

PPV, positive predictive value; NPV, negative predictive value; RI, resistance index; AVRI, average resistance index obtained from left and right arcuate and uterine arteries authors failed to demonstrate any improvement in pregnancy outcome by routine uterine Doppler. This may be due to the fact that nearly 50% of women in this study were multiparous, and that a finding of an abnormal uterine Doppler was not followed by any specific management, for instance by the prescription of aspirin.

Previous obstetric histories and uterine Doppler waveform identify populations at high risk of developing pre-eclampsia and intrauterine growth retardation. These tests can have a favorable effect if they lead to better management (follow-up of blood pressure and fetal growth by means of ultrasound examinations). Moreover, the recognition of a high-risk population can modify the management and the pregnancy outcome by performing third-trimester umbilical ultrasound. This point has been studied by Giles and Bisits[33] using a meta-analysis of six randomized trials studying the usefulness of umbilical Doppler waveform in improving perinatal outcome in high-risk patients[34–39]. The statistical technique of meta-analysis showed that in patients having an umbilical Doppler ultrasound as a part of obstetric management a significant reduction of perinatal mortality (odds ratio, 0.5; 95% CI (0.34–0.73)), and more specifically a reduction of intrauterine fetal death in otherwise normally-formed fetuses (odds ratio, 0.54; 95% CI (0.32–0.89)) when compared to women having a standard management without Doppler.

Another aspect concerning uterine Doppler in the early management of patients at high-risk selected by previous obstetric history was studied by our team[40]. Fifty-one women were treated with low-dose aspirin (100 mg) from 15 weeks' gestation for severe previous obstetric history. A continuous-wave uterine Doppler ultrasound was performed at 24 weeks' gestation. Three women were lost to follow-up. Uterine Doppler was considered abnormal when diastole/systole index was found lower than 10th centile or when a diastolic notch was persistent at 26 weeks. Twenty-six women had an abnormal uterine Doppler. The rate of hypertensive complications (pre-eclampsia and intrauterine growth retardation) was significantly higher in the group of patients with abnormal

uterine Doppler when compared to the group of women with normal uterine Doppler (8/26 vs. 1/22, $p < 0.05$). Mean birth weight was found to be lower in patients with abnormal uterine Doppler (2419 (SD 679) vs. 2841 g, (SD 482) $p < 0.05$) when compared to patients with normal Doppler. Even though the number of patients was small, it would appear that an abnormal uterine Doppler can predict failures of treatment with aspirin, with a sensitivity of 88%, a specificity of 53%, a positive predictive value of 30% and a negative predictive value of 95%.

LOW-DOSE ASPIRIN IN PREGNANCY

During the last decade, several authors studied the effect of early treatment with low-dose aspirin in the prevention of pre-eclampsia and intrauterine growth retardation in high-risk selected patients. The pharmacology of salicylates has recently been elucidated, leading to their use in certain diseases where the alteration of prostaglandin production seems to be involved in the pathophysiology. Several studies have shown that the adaptation of the utero-placental circulation depends largely on the regulation of the synthesis of prostaglandins during pregnancy, and specifically, on prostacyclin and thromboxane A2[41] which are metabolites of the arachidonic acid cyclo-oxygenase pathway[42]. In normal pregnancy, prostacyclin synthesis seems to be increased[41], leading to a dominance of its effect over thromboxane A2[43]. This results in vasodilatation and a reduction of systemic vascular resistance, which is characteristic of normal pregnancy. An alteration of the regulation of prostaglandin synthesis seems to interfere with pregnancy-induced hypertensive diseases, with a dominance of the effect of thromboxane A2 over prostacyclin. The recognition of this imbalance in pregnancy-induced hypertensive diseases led to the use of aspirin which is a cyclo-oxygenase inhibitor[44]. Aspirin may produce a reversal of the pathological process, by interacting with prostaglandin synthesis. It decreases the synthesis of thromboxane A2 relatively more than that of prostacyclin. This relative decrease of thromboxane A2 synthesis suppresses the dominance of thromboxane A2 over prostacyclin in pregnancy-induced hypertensive diseases and may then restore the physiological balance of prostacyclin and thromboxane A2. This concept constitutes the rationale of clinical attempts in the use of the acetylsalicylic acid (aspirin), in the prevention of hypertensive diseases in women at high risk[41].

Several prospective randomized studies[4-6,45-47] published suggest that low-dose aspirin therapy is effective in reducing the incidence of pre-eclampsia and intrauterine growth retardation in women at high risk. The first[4] was an open prospective randomized trial including 102 patients with a poor previous pregnancy outcome or with known hypertension ($\geq 160/95$ mmHg). Patients enrolled were allocated to take aspirin (150 mg) and dipyridamol (300 mg) daily from the third month of pregnancy until delivery ($n = 52$) or no treatment ($n = 50$). Pre-eclampsia and intrauterine growth retardation were significantly decreased in the aspirin group when compared to the group with no treatment (0 vs. 6, $p < 0.01$ for pre-eclampsia and 0 vs. 4, $p < 0.05$ for intrauterine growth retardation). Another more recent randomized placebo-controlled double-blind trial including 229 patients at 15–18 weeks' gestation with at least two poor previous pregnancy outcomes was published by the same team[5]. Women were allocated to receive either a placebo ($n = 73$), aspirin 150 mg daily ($n = 81$), or aspirin 150 mg plus dipyridamol 225 mg daily ($n = 75$). Aspirin therapy ($n = 156$) resulted in a significant decrease in the recurrence of fetal growth retardation (20/156 (13%) vs. 19/73 (26%), $p < 0.02$) and a significantly higher birth weight (2751 (SD 670) vs. 2526 g SD 848; difference 225 g, 95% CI (129–321 g), $p = 0.029$) when compared to the placebo group. A meta-analysis of these six trials[48] showed that low-dose aspirin treatment significantly decreases the rate of pre-eclampsia (2.1 vs. 16.25%, respectively; odds ratio = 0.16; 95% CI (0.09–0.3)) and intrauterine growth retardation (12 vs. 23.7%, respectively; odds ratio, 0.43; 95% CI (0.27–0.67)) when compared to placebo. However, low-dose aspirin does not seem to be effective in reducing the rate of pre-eclampsia or intrauterine growth retardation in patients at medium or low risk[49].

The results of the CLASP (Collaborative Low-dose Aspirin in Pregnancy) trial[49], a multicenter study (involving 9364 women randomly assigned 60 mg aspirin daily or matching placebo) show that overall the use of aspirin was associated with a non-significant reduction of only 12% of proteinuric pre-eclampsia. Aspirin did, however, significantly reduce the likelihood of preterm delivery, with a significant trend towards progressively greater reductions in proteinuric pre-eclampsia the more preterm the delivery. This trial supports our opinion that routine prophylactic use of aspirin is not recommended and that aspirin (given early in the second trimester) can be useful in high risk pregnancies identified on their past obstetric history.

ASPIRIN TREATMENT IN UTERINE DOPPLER SELECTED PATIENTS

Few trials concerning the effectiveness of low-dose aspirin in women with abnormal uterine Doppler waveform have been published (Table 2). McParland and associates[46] carried out a prospective randomized double-blind placebo-controlled trial in uterine Doppler selected patients. After screening 1226 nulliparous women by means of uterine Doppler flow velocity, 148 patients were selected to be at high risk of pregnancy-induced hypertension at 24 weeks' gestation as uterine Doppler examination was abnormal (defined by an index higher than 90th centile). After exclusions and refusals, 100 nulliparous patients were randomly allocated to take 75 mg of aspirin ($n = 48$) or a placebo ($n = 52$) after the assessment of uterine Doppler. Frequency of pre-eclampsia was found to be significantly decreased in the aspirin group when compared to the placebo group (1/48 (2%) vs. 10/52 (19%), $p < 0.02$). No difference was found between the two groups in the occurrence of intrauterine growth retardation (14 vs. 14%) and pregnancy-induced hypertension (13 vs. 25%). However, the incidence of hypertension occurring before 37 weeks was significantly lower in the aspirin-treated group when compared to the placebo group (0 vs. 17%, $p < 0.01$).

Table 2 *Prospective randomized trials of low-dose aspirin in the prevention of hypertensive diseases in patients with abnormal uterine Doppler*

	Placebo (n)	Aspirin (n)	Dose (mg/day)	Placebo vs. aspirin (%)		
				IUGR	PE	PIH
McParland et al., 1990[46]	52	48	75	14/14	19/2*	25/13
Campbell, 1993[50]	16	15	75	25/13	50/13**	50/80

PIH, pregnancy-induced hypertension; PE, pre-eclampsia; IUGR, intrauterine growth retardation; *$p < 0.01$;**$p = 0.05$

Campbell[50] reported preliminary results of a randomized placebo-controlled trial in progress. In this study, 36 patients at high risk, selected by an abnormal uterine Doppler examination (defined as a notch and/or RI > 95th centile) at 24–26 weeks' gestation, were recruited. They were randomly allocated to take 75 mg of aspirin ($n = 15$, three dropped out) or a placebo ($n = 16$, two dropped out). Although the numbers are small, the results show a slightly significant decrease in the incidence of pre-eclampsia in aspirin-treated group when compared to placebo group (2/15 vs. 8/16, $p = 0.05$).

These two studies differ in patient recruitment (abnormal early uterine Doppler index alone or associated with the persistence of a diastolic notch) and in main outcome measures. However, aspirin treatment seems to be effective in reduction of the incidence of pre-eclampsia. In contrast, aspirin therapy has no beneficial effect on the incidence of intrauterine growth retardation.

In view of the double-blind placebo-controlled studies, it seems that low-dose aspirin is effective in the prevention of pregnancy-induced hypertensive diseases, especially pre-eclampsia and intrauterine growth retardation, in women at high risk. High-risk pregnant women can be defined as patients having either poor past obstetric history (intrauterine growth retardation, pre-eclampsia, eclampsia, and for some authors abruptio placentae), or an impaired uterine circulation detected by an early pathological uterine Doppler waveform. In fact, to be effective, aspirin must be started early in pregnancy. Moreover, the history of poor previous pregnancies constitutes the most common practical indication for the use of low-dose aspirin. In contrast, the use of aspirin treatment after an abnormal uterine Doppler at 20–24 weeks' gestation needs to be re-evaluated.

The optimal dose of aspirin has not yet been established. However, a daily single dose of 60–100mg can be an opportune dosage. Low-dose aspirin can be started between 15 and 18 weeks when the indication is a poor previous history[5]. Before starting the therapy, the platelet count must be normal, as must the primary hemostasis Ivy test (under 10 min). Most authors will stop this therapy around 35–36 weeks and Ivy test will be controlled 10 days later to ensure normal primary hemostasis when entering labor.

CONCLUSION

The purpose of screening patients with uterine Doppler at 20–24 weeks' gestation is to identify women at high risk for the development of hypertensive diseases, and especially pre-eclampsia. Results of uterine Doppler predictive tests show an important discrepancy between studies, however, it seems that the use of the persistence of diastolic notch alone or in association with an abnormal RI improves the predictive value for pre-eclampsia. This early selection may allow close observation and monitoring, and for some authors, the introduction of aspirin therapy. A few studies concerning low-dose aspirin use in pregnant women with early abnormal uterine Doppler examination have been published. Although involving relatively small populations, these studies show a trend towards a decrease of pre-eclampsia in aspirin-treated groups. Larger trials are certainly needed to confirm published studies.

References

1. Sibai, B. M., Spinnato, I. A., Watson, D. L. and Anderson, G. D. (1984). Pregnancy outcome in 303 cases with severe preeclampsia. *Obstet Gynecol.*, **64**, 319–24
2. Sheppard, B. L. and Bonnar, J. (1981). An ultrastructural study of uteroplacental spiral arteries in hypertensive and normotensive pregnancy and fetal growth retardation. *Br. J. Obstet. Gynaecol.*, **88**, 695–705
3. Khong, T. Y., De Wolf, F., Robertson, W. B. and Brossen, I. (1986). Inadequate maternal vascular response to placentation in pregnancies complicated by pre-eclampsia and by small-for-gestational age infants. *Br. J. Obstet. Gynaecol.*, **93**, 1049–59
4. Beaufils, M., Uzan, S., Donsimoni, R. and Colau, J. C. (1985). Prevention of pre-eclampsia by antiplatelet therapy. *Lancet*, **1**, 840–2
5. Uzan, S., Beaufils, M., Bréart, G., Bazin, B., Capitant, C. and Paris, J. (1991). Prevention of fetal growth retardation with low-dose aspirin: findings of the Epreda trial. *Lancet*, **337**, 1427–31
6. Schiff, E., Peleg, E., Goldenberg, M., Rosenthal, T., Ruppin, E., Tamarkin, M., Barkaï, G., Ben Baruk, G., Yahal, I., Blankstein, J., Goldman, B. and Marshiach, S. (1989). The use of aspirin to prevent pregnancy-induced hypertension and lower the ratio of thromboxane A2 to prostacyclin in relatively high risk pregnancies. *N. Engl. J. Med.*, **321**, 351–6
7. Salafia, C. M., Silberman, L., Herrara, N. E. and Mahoney, M. J. (1988). Placental pathology at term associated with elevated midtrimester MSAFP concentration. *Am. J. Obstet. Gynecol.*, **158**, 1064–6
8. Ballegeer, V., Spitz, B., Kieckens, L., Moreau, H., Van Assche, A. and Collen, D. (1989). Predictive value of increased plasma levels of fibronectin in gestational hypertension. *Am. J. Obstet. Gynecol.*, **161**, 432–6
9. Uzan, M., Van Bogaert, R., Heim, N., Haddad, B., Sultan, Y. and Grunfeld, L. (1993). Valeur prédictive du Doppler utérin et du dosage de la fibronectine pour le retard de croissance et la pré-éclampsie. Presented at *IXé Journée de Vélocimétrie Sanguine Foetale et Maternelle*, March, Paris
10. Gonen, R., Perez, R., David, M., Dar, H., Merksamer, R. and Sharf, M. (1992). The association between unexplained second-trimester maternal serum hCG elevation and pregnancy complications. *Obstet. Gynecol.*, **80**, 83–6
11. Sorensen, T. K., Williams, M. A., Zingheim, R. W., Clement, S. J. and Hickok, D. E. (1993). Elevated second trimester human chorionic gonadotropin and subsequent pregnancy-induced hypertension. *Am. J. Obstet. Gynecol.*, **169**, 834–8
12. Brossen, I., Robertson, W. B. and Dixon, H. G. (1967). The physiological response of the vessels of the placental bed to normal pregnancy. *J. Pathol. Bacteriol.*, **93**, 569–79
13. Pijnenborg, R., Bland, J. M., Robertson, W. B. and Brosens, I. (1983). Uteroplacental arterial changes related to interstitial trophoblast migration in early human pregnancy. *Placenta*, **4**, 387–414
14. Campbell, S., Diaz-Recasens, J., Griffin, D. R. *et al.* (1983). New Doppler technique for assessing uteroplacental blood flow. *Lancet*, **1**, 675–7
15. Trudinger, B. J., Giles, W. B. and Cook, C. M. (1985). Uteroplacental blood flow velocity-time waveforms in normal and complicated pregnancy. *Br. J. Obstet. Gynaecol.*, **92**, 39–45
16. Fleischer, A., Schulman, H., Farmakides, G., Bracero, L., Grunfeld, L., Rochelson, B. and Koenigsberg, M. (1986). Uterine artery Doppler velocimetry in pregnant women with hypertension. *Am. J. Obstet. Gynecol.*, **154**, 806–13
17. Ducey, J., Schulman, H., Farmakides, G., Rochelson, B., Bracero, L., Fleischer, A., Guzman, E., Winter, D. and Penny, B. (1987). A classification of hypertension in pregnancy based on Doppler velocimetry. *Am. J. Obstet. Gynecol.*, **157**, 680–5
18. Schulman, H., Fleisher, A., Farmakides, G., Bracero, L., Rochelson, B. and Grunfeld, L. (1986). The development of uterine artery compliance as detected by Doppler ultrasound. *Am. J. Obstet. Gynecol.*, **155**, 1031–6
19. Campbell, S., Pearce, J. M. F., Hackett, G., Cohen-Overbeek, T. and Hernandez, C. (1986). Qualitative assessment of utero-placental blood flow: early screening test for high risk pregnancies. *Obstet. Gynecol.*, **68**, 649–53
20. Hanretty, K. P., Primrose, M. H., Neilson, J. P. and Whittle, M. J. (1989). Pregnancy screening by Doppler uteroplacental and umbilical artery waveforms. *Br. J. Obstet. Gynaecol.*, **96**, 1163–67
21. Pourcelot, L. (1974). Applications cliniques de l'examen Doppler transcutané. In Perroneau, P. (ed.) *Vélocimétrie ultrasonore Doppler*, Vol. 34, pp. 213–40. (Paris: INSERM)
22. Stuart, B., Drumm, J., Fitzgerald, D. E. and Duignan, N. M. (1980). Fetal blood velocity waveforms in normal pregnancy. *Br. J. Obstet. Gynaecol.*, **87**, 780–5
23. Kofinas, A. D., Penry, M., Greiss, F. C., Meiss, P. J. and Nelson, L. H. (1988). The effect of placental

location on uterine artery flow velocity waveforms. *Am. J. Obstet. Gynecol.*, **159**, 1504–8

24. Bewley, S., Campbell, S. and Cooper, D. (1989). Utero-placental Doppler flow velocity waveforms in the second trimester. A complex circulation. *Br. J. Obstet. Gynaecol.*, **96**, 1040–6

25. Steel, S. A., Pearce, J. M., McParland, P. and Chamberlain, G. V. P. (1990). Early Doppler ultrasound screening in prediction of hypertensive disorders of pregnancy. *Lancet*, **335**, 1548–51

26. North, R. A., Ferrier, C., Long, D., Townend, K. and Kincaid-Smith, P. (1994). Uterine artery Doppler flow velocity waveforms in the second trimester for the prediction of preeclampsia and fetal growth retardation. *Obstet. Gynecol.*, **83**, 378–86

27. Chan, F. Y., Pun, T. C., Lam, C., Khoo, J., Lee, C. P. and Lam, Y. H. (1995). Pregnancy screening by uterine artery Doppler velocimetry – which criterion performs best? *Obstet Gynecol.*, **85**, 596–602

28. Harrington, K. F., Campbell, S., Bewley, S. and Bower, S. (1991). Doppler velocimetry studies of the uterine artery in the early prediction of pre-eclampsia and intra-uterine growth retardation. *Eur. J. Obstet. Gynecol. Reprod. Biol.*, **42**, S14–S20

29. Bewley, S., Campbell, S. and Cooper, D. (1991). Doppler investigation of uteroplacental blood flow in the second trimester: a screening study for pre-eclampsia and intra-uterine growth retardation. *Br. J. Obstet. Gynaecol.*, **98**, 871–9

30. Bower, S., Bewley, S. and Campbell, S. (1993). Improved prediction of pre-eclampsia by two stage screening of uterine arteries, using the early diastolic notch and color Doppler imaging. *Obstet. Gynecol.*, **82**, 78–83

31. Aristidou, A., Van Den Hof, F. C., Campbell, C. and Nicolaides, K. (1990). Uterine artery Doppler in the investigation of pregnancies with raised maternal serum alpha-fetoprotein. *Br. J. Obstet. Gynaecol.*, **97**, 431–5

32. Davies, J. A., Gallivan, S. and Spencer, J. A. D. (1992). Randomised controlled trial of Doppler ultrasound screening of placental perfusion during pregnancy. *Lancet*, **340**, 1299–303

33. Giles, W. and Bisits, A. (1993). Clinical use of Doppler ultrasound in pregnancy: information of six randomised trial. *Fetal Diagn. Ther.*, **8**, 247–55

34. Trudinger, B. J., Cook, C. M., Giles, W. B., Connelly, A. and Thompson, R. S. (1987). Umbilical artery flow velocity waveforms in high risk pregnancy. A randomised control trial. *Lancet*, **1**, 188–90

35. McParland, P. and Pearce, J. M. (1988). Review article: Doppler blood flow in pregnancy. *Placenta*, **9**, 427–50

36. Omtzigt, A. W. J. (1990). Clinical value of umbilical Doppler velocimetry – a randomised controlled trial. In (Thesis). (Utrecht: University)

37. Newham, J. P., O'Dea, M. R. A., Reid, K. P. and Diepeveen, D. A. (1991). Doppler flow velocity waveform analysis in high risk pregnancies: a randomised controlled trial. *Br. J. Obstet. Gynaecol.*, **98**, 956–63

38. Almstrom, H., Axelsson, O., Cnattinguis, S., Ekman, G., Maesel, A., Ulmsten, U., Armstrom, K. and Marsal, K. (1991). Comparison of umbilical artery velocimetry and cardiotocography for surveillance of small-for-gestational-age fetuses. A multicenter randomised controlled trial (abstr.). *J. Matern. Fetal. Invest.*, **1**, 127

39. Hofmyer, G. J., Pattinsin, R., Buckley, D., Jennings, J. and Redman, C. W. G. (1991). Umbilical artery resistance index as a screening test for fetal well-being. II. Randomised feasability study. *Obstet. Gynecol.*, **78**, 359–62

40. Haddad, B., Uzan, M., Bréart, G. and Uzan, S. (1995). Uterine Doppler wave form and the prediction of the recurrence of pre-eclampsia and intra-uterine growth retardation in patients treated with low-dose aspirin. *Eur. J. Obstet. Gynecol. Reprod. Biol.*, in press

41. Friedman, S. A. (1988). Preeclampsia: a review of the role of prostaglandins. *Obstet. Gynecol.*, **71**, 122–37

42. Oates, J. A., FitzGerald, G. A., Brand, R. A., Jackson, E. K., Knapp, H. R. and Roberts, L. J. (1988). Clinical implications of prostaglandin and thromboxane A2 formation. *N. Engl. J. Med.*, **319**, 689–98

43. Ylikorkala, O. and Makilà, U. M. (1985). Prostacyclin and thromboxane in gynecology and pregnancy. *Am. J. Obstet. Gynecol.*, **152**, 318–29

44. Vayne, J. R. (1971). Inhibition of prostaglandin synthesis as a mechanism of action of aspirin-like drugs. *Nature (London)*, **231**, 232–5

45. Wallenburg, H. C. S., Dekker, G. A., Makowitz, J. W. and Rotmans, P. (1986). Low-dose aspirin prevents pregnancy induced hypertension and pre-eclampsia in angiotensin-sensitive primigravidae. *Lancet*, **1**, 1–3

46. McParland, P., Pearce, J. M. and Chamberlain, G. V. P. (1990). Doppler ultrasound and aspirin in recognition and prevention of pregnancy-induced hypertension. *Lancet*, **335**, 1552–5

47. Benigni, A., Gregorini, G., Frusca, T., Chiabrando, C., Ballerini, S., Valcamonico, A., Orisio, S., Piccinelli, A., Pinciroli, V., Fanelli, R., Gastaldi, A. and Remuzzi, G. (1989). Effect of low-dose aspirin on fetal and maternal generation of thromboxane by platelets in women at risk for pregnancy-induced hypertension. *N. Engl. J. Med.*, **321**, 357–62

48. Uzan, S. and Haddad, B. (1994). Aspirin in pregnancy. In Kurjak, A. and Chervenak, F. A. (eds.) *The Fetus as a patient*, p. 491–504 (Carnforth, UK: Parthenon Publishing)

49. CLASP: a randomised trial of low dose aspirin for the prevention and treatment of pre-eclampsia among 9364 pregnant women. *Lancet*, **343**, 619–29

50. Campbell, S. (1993). Uterine artery Doppler Presented at *IXé Journée de vélocimétrie*, Paris

Actocardiographic assessment of the fetus

31

K. Maeda

INTRODUCTION

The fetus moves in the maternal womb from early pregnancy onwards. A pregnant woman is aware of fetal well-being when she perceives normal fetal movement. Real-time ultrasound has made it possible to observe fetal movement on the screen. However there has been difficulty in the scientific study of fetal movement, because maternal perception was totally subjective and ultrasonic detection relied on the observer's opinion. In addition, the sensitivity in objective methods including mechanical, electromagnetic and piezoelectric techniques was low. Therefore a more sensitive and simple method was required. In 1983, the idea was developed of transforming the noisy tones of fetal movements, which disturbed fetal heart rate tracing, into meaningful signals of fetal movement[1].

THE PRINCIPLE OF THE ACTOCARDIOGRAM

Fetal movement was detected by the ultrasonic Doppler method. The Doppler shift of fetal movement was 40–60 Hz, when the ultrasound frequency was 2 MHz. The Doppler shift was detected by using a 20–80-Hz band-pass filter. Another high-pass filter separated the signal produced by the fetal heart. The fetal movement signal was further changed into a spike-like deflection, recorded by the cardiotocograph (CTG) recorder in the channel of uterine contraction. This was the fetal actogram. The machine was tested by moving a steel ball in water, and we found that the recorded deflection amplitude increased linearly with the magnitude of movement up to 6 mm. Therefore, fetal movement intensity was estimated by the

recorded deflection. The fetal heart rate curve was recorded by the high-frequency Doppler shift of the fetal heart, at the same time as fetal movement, using a single ultrasonic transducer, and the record was the 'actocardiogram'[1]. The markers of fetal movements were automatically recorded on the chart between fetal heart rate (FHR) and actogram when the fetal movement signal was higher than the preset threshold level. An automatic marker system is utilized also in the Kinetokardiogram.

The actocardiogram is an objective, sensitive and continuous recording of fetal movement and heart rate. It enables precise studies of fetal heart rate changes. The actocardiograms of twins are recorded in a single chart in order to monitor the twins simultaneously using a single device[2].

FETAL BEHAVIORAL STATES

Fetal behavioral states can be classified by the actogram in the second and third trimesters. Actographic deflections formed multiple clusters the duration of which was 10–20 s, and there was no uniformity in the intervals of the clusters. These clusters of fetal movements frequently appeared in the active fetal state, but almost none were recorded in the resting state. The actogram transducer was placed on the maternal abdomen corresponding to the fetal chest. Therefore, most signals originated from the rotating motion of the fetal trunk, and this gross fetal movement was recorded in the actogram[1]. Fetal breathing showed continuous signals of regular interval and low amplitude[2]. Computerized automated detection of fetal behavioral states was successful, in cases who

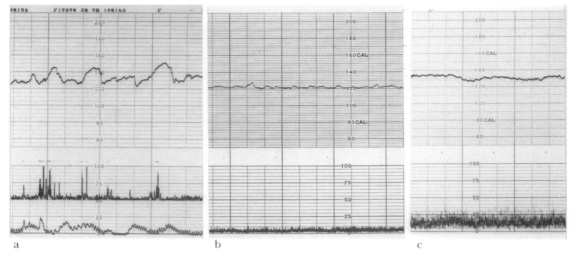

a   b   c

Figure 1   *Three fetal states recorded by actocardiogram in late pregnancy. The upper tracing is fetal heart rate (FHR) and the lower is fetal movement (3 cm/min). (a) Active fetal state, FHR accelerations were accompanied by the clusters of fetal movements. The bottom line is the uterine contraction pattern. (b) Resting fetal state, no fetal movement or FHR acceleration was recorded. FHR baseline variability was within normal range. Active fetal states appeared before and after the resting state. (c) The actocardiogram recorded during fetal breathing movement. Regular low amplitude signals were recorded in the actogram. No acceleration was recorded. FHR baseline was higher than that of the resting state*

showed typical behavioral changes, by processing the actographic output signals[3].

The FHR pattern was characteristic in each of the behavioral states. FHR accelerations were associated with fetal movements in the active fetal state. No FHR accelerations and low FHR baseline were recorded in the resting state[1]. A false-positive non-reactive non-stress test (NST) was frequently reported by the simple CTG in the resting state, but no error occurred with the actocardiogram. No acceleration was recorded in the continuous fetal breathing, but the FHR baseline was slightly higher than that of the resting state[2] (Figure 1). The duration of the active fetal state was 24–150 min, and the resting state 10–36 min, during the daytime in the third trimester[4].

FETAL HICCUPPING MOVEMENTS

Fetal hiccups were recorded by the actogram; they were regular large deflections (Figure 2). Diaphragmatic motion was confirmed by real-time sonography. Chest movement was also confirmed by ultrasonic M-mode. Intervals between hiccupping were 2–3 s, and the duration of hic-

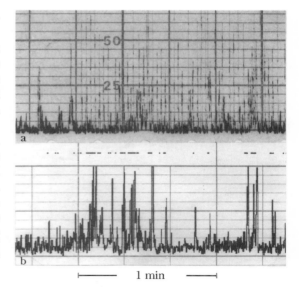

⊢——— 1 min ———⊣

Figure 2   *Fetal hiccupping movements (a) and common fetal movements in the active state (b) of late pregnancy*

cupping was 10–20 min[3]. Fetal hiccups were recorded in many actograms, twice in a day in some cases. The outcome was normal in all cases, therefore, fetal hiccups are physiological and harmless[4].

No FHR acceleration was observed during pure hiccups in the resting state[1]. However, the mother feels fetal hiccupping motion, therefore, this may result in a false-positive non-reactive NST in a simple CTG, if the mother presses the marker switch because of her perception of fetal hiccups. Actographic recognition of the hiccups would resolve any uncertainty.

PSEUDOSINUSOIDAL FETAL HEART RATE PATTERN DETECTED BY THE ACTOCARDIOGRAM

The sinusoidal FHR pattern is a sine wave-like oscillation of the FHR baseline; the pattern is usually ominous when it is associated with fetal anemia or hypoxia. However, we found five cases of physiological sinusoidal FHR pattern, followed by normal outcome, using the actocardiogram in 1000 NSTs. A typical case showed sinusoidal FHR pattern synchronized with cyclic fetal movements of 10-s duration and 10-s interval. The total duration of the change was 10–20 min and normal reactive FHR immediately preceded and followed the pseudosinusoidal pattern[3] (Figure 3). The pattern appeared in the resting fetal state, and the outcome was normal in all cases. The actocardiogram is, therefore, useful for the diagnosis of the pseudosinusoidal pattern, discriminating it from a truly ominous one, and thereby avoiding unnecessary Cesarean sections.

The cyclic movement represents cyclic fetal breathing, because the deflection interval was similar to fetal breathing movements, and sonographically fetal breathing was confirmed with cyclic movements.

ACTOCARDIOGRAM IN FETAL DISTRESS

Decreased fetal movements were observed in a case of mild fetal distress who showed decelerations and the loss of acceleration. Bradycardia was recorded at a later stage in this case. It has been suggested that fetal movements would decrease in the early stage of fetal distress. A case of established fetal distress, diagnosed by the loss of variability, showed no fetal movement[5]. Another case of fetal distress showed a large sinusoidal pattern and the loss of fetal movement. Therefore, the loss of movement would appear to be a late sign in fetal distress caused by fetal hypoxia.

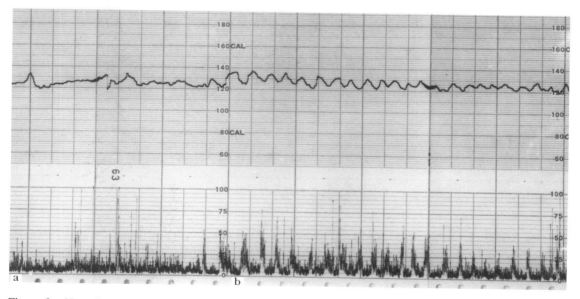

Figure 3 *Normal reactive fetal heart rate (FHR) in the active state (a) and pseudosinusoidal FHR pattern (b) in a normal fetus. Sinusoidal FHR changes synchronized with cyclic fetal movements represent cyclic fetal breathing. The sinusoidal FHR reverted back to a normal pattern after about 10 min*

PREDICTION OF FETAL DISTRESS BY ACTOCARDIOGRAM

The accurate detection of fetal distress is important because early delivery may avoid fetal damage. The simple CTG is insufficient for the detection of impending fetal distress due to the presence of many false-positive non-reactive cases.

The actocardiogram is useful for this purpose. The FHR acceleration associated with fetal movement clusters disappeared in cases which

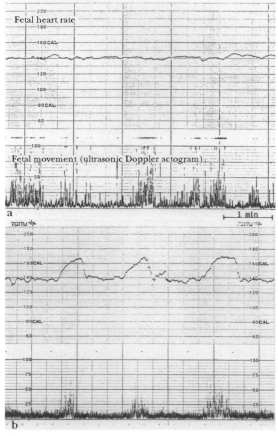

Figure 4 *Non-reactive (a) and reactive (b) actocardiograms. (a) non-reactive pattern, no fetal heart rate (FHR) acceleration was recorded at 35 weeks of gestation in a case of pre-eclampsia and IUGR, in spite of the presence of active fetal movements in the actogram. Two days later, fetal distress was diagnosed due to severe variable decelerations, and a Cesarean section was performed. (b) Normal reactive actocardiogram in normal pregnancy, clear FHR accelerations were accompanied by fetal movement clusters*

showed fetal distress at a later stage. The baseline level and variability were normal; no deceleration or sinusoidal pattern was recorded in these cases. Signs of fetal distress were detected by continuous CTG monitoring a few days after the loss of FHR accelerations, and immediate Cesarean section was performed[3] (Figure 4).

Twenty-five cases of non-reactive actocardiograms were analyzed by Teshima[6], including 20 intrauterine growth retardation (IUGR) cases. They were carefully monitored and fetal distress was present in 19 cases (76%), after non-reactive actocardiograms (Table 1).

Twenty cases of IUGR with non-reactive actocardiograms were compared to 20 cases of IUGR who exhibited normal reactive actocardiograms. Fetal distress appeared in 17 truly non-reactive IUGR fetuses, whereas only four control cases developed fetal distress. This was a significant difference. The sensitivity to predict fetal distress was 81.0%, and the specificity was 84.2%. The sensitivity increased to 94% if it was limited to antepartum fetal distress. Fifteen cases of fetal distress had non-reactive actocardiograms compared to only one of the control cases (Table 2). Fetal distress was detected by intensive CTG monitoring between 0 and 15 days after the detection on a non-reactive actocardiogram (Table 1).

Table 1 *Clinical conditions associated with non-reactive actocardiograms (n = 25)[6]*

Complications
IUGR (n = 20)
Pre-eclampsia
Oligohydramnios
Fetal anomaly
Maternal disease

Subsequent fetal distress
Interval to fetal distress
 0–15 days (n = 19)
 ≤ 7 days (n = 14)
Fetal heart rate change
 loss of variability
 late deceleration
 severe variable deceleration

Cesarean section (n = 22)
1-min Apgar score < 7 (n = 4)

IUGR, intrauterine growth retardation

Table 2 *Outcome of intrauterine growth retarded (IUGR) fetuses with non-reactive actocardiograms. The control cases were IUGR fetuses with a reactive actocardiogram (mean ± SD)*[6]

	IUGR cases	
	Non-reactive actocardiogram	Normal reactive actocardiogram
Number of cases	20	20
Weeks of gestation		
actocardiogram	36.5 ± 2.2	37.0 ± 1.5
birth	36.8 ± 2.2*	39.1 ± 1.7
Fetal distress		
ante- and intra-partum	17/20*	4/20
antepartum	15/18*	1/17
Birth weight (g)	1728 ± 375*	2254 ± 293
1-min Apgar < 7 (cases)	4	0
Number of Cesarean sections	20*	6
Neonatal deaths	2	0

*Significant difference. Prediction of fetal distress by non-reactive actocardiogram: ante- and intra-partum fetal distress; sensitivity, 81.0%; specificity, 84.2%; sensitivity of prediction of antepartum fetal distress, 93.8%

Gestational age at delivery was lower, birth weight was smaller, the rate of fetal distress was higher, the Cesarean section rate was higher, Apgar scores were lower, and neonatal deaths were more common in the cases of IUGR with non-reactive actocardiograms than in the control cases of IUGR. It was concluded that the actocardiogram was valuable for the evaluation of fetal well-being, and very useful in the prediction of fetal distress and unexpected fetal death[6].

After the appearance of fetal distress, immediate Cesarean section should be performed. However, non-invasive treatments, including hospitalization, medication, oxygen inhalation, may be useful. These methods may delay fetal distress and prolong the duration of pregnancy. An immediate Cesarean section may be indicated when there is a non-reactive actocardiogram in a complicated pregnancy, such as IUGR, because the ability to predict fetal distress during pregnancy is high in these cases[6].

CROSS-CORRELATION ANALYSIS OF FETAL HEART RATE AND MOVEMENT

Close correlation of FHR and movement was observed in normal actocardiograms. Loss of this correlation suggested impending fetal distress. More quantitative results were obtained by cross-correlation analysis of fetal movement and FHR. Fetal movement data were delayed for various intervals in order to obtain the highest correlation. The coefficient at 5 min was as high as 0.7 in the active fetal state, when the movement was delayed for 7 s, i.e. fetal movement preceded the acceleration. No correlation was found in the resting fetal state, fetal breathing, or with fetal hiccups[7]. This method will further quantify the correlation of fetal movement and FHR, clearly diagnose the progress of hypoxia, and evaluate the effect of hypoxia treatment, i.e. oxygen inhalation therapy.

FETAL RESPONSE TO SOUND STIMULATION

The use of a vibroacoustic test (VAST), to stimulate a fetus in the resting state, is common. The usual fetal response to VAST is sudden tachycardia. This is a clear response, the sound is intense and the frequency low at 60–70 Hz. The fetus would be surprised by the intense 60-Hz tone.

We intended to test the auditory function of the fetus with varying frequency and tone. The sound was 250–1000 Hz of pure sound and the intensity was controlled by an adult auditory stimulator. The intensity was measured by a noise meter in a silent room. Fetal response was detected by the changes of fetal heart rate and movement. There was FHR acceleration and/or fetal movements on the actocardiogram, when the fetus responded to the stimulation. We attempted to test fetal auditory function by this method, and found that it changed in late pregnancy.

The changes obtained due to 1000-Hz pure sound were significant. The sound intensity necessary to evoke FHR acceleration and/or movement averaged 80 dB at 28 weeks of normal pregnacy, however, the significantly lower intensity of 60 dB was needed to stimulate the fetus at 40 weeks. These results demonstrated that the fetus at 40 weeks of gestation was stimulated by a weaker intensity, by 10 times, than at 28 weeks. In other words, fetal auditory function was 10 times higher at 40 weeks than at 28 weeks of gestation. These data demonstrated that fetal auditory function develops in late pregnancy[8].

FETAL RESPONSE TO STIMULATION WITH LIGHT

The fetus was stimulated by a photographic flash light placed on the maternal abdomen. Fetal response to photic stimulation was detected by FHR acceleration and/or fetal movement. The earliest response to light stimulation appeared at 23 weeks of gestation, and the positive response increased late in pregnancy when 70% of term fetuses responded to the light. Therefore, fetal ability to sense light increases in late pregnancy[8]. It may be possible to perform a fetal audiogram and vision test with fetal actocardiographic responses in the future.

THE AUGMENTED ACTOGRAM

Although the actogram was useful in the analysis of fetal movement, the chart speed was slow at 3 cm/min, and the signal was too small to study greater details of fetal movement. Augmentation of the actogram was needed, and it was possible simply to connect another high-speed pen-writing recorder to the analog output of the actocardiograph (Figure 5). The fetal movement signal was enlarged to about 10 times that of the conventional actogram, and the chart speed was 30 cm/s; these were 10 times faster than the usual actogram.

Fetal hiccupping movements

Fetal hiccupping motion was more clear in the augmented actogram than the conventional one, and the intervals were correctly measured in a case at 32 weeks of gestation. The intervals were about 2 s, and the variation was small (Figure 6).

Assessment of fetal hiccupping motion in early pregnancy

Recently, by motion analysis of the real-time sonographic image, we observed regular movements at 13 weeks of gestation similar to hiccupping movements, i.e. the fetal chin moved upwards, the chest became narrower, the back space widened and the legs stretched, within 0.1 s. The sudden and quick action appeared repeatedly during 3½ min, and was very regular in 30 s. The action interval was measured in the 30-s period and compared to those of hiccupping movements recorded by augmented actogram at 32 weeks of gestation. Intervals of the sudden and regular movements at 13 and 32 weeks were about 2 s and there was no difference between the two fetuses (Table 3).

These results suggest that the quick and regular movements of the fetus may be the initiation of fetal hiccupping at 13 weeks of pregnancy, because we found no regular abrupt motion, only irregular appearances of sudden

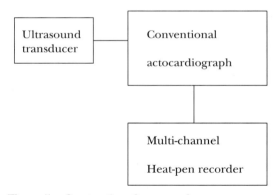

Figure 5 *Construction of augmented actogram system*

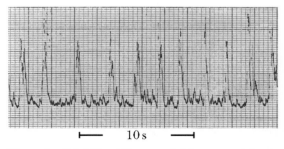

Figure 6 *Fetal hiccupping recorded by augmented actogram*

420

Table 3 *Intervals of quick motion of the fetus at 13 weeks of gestation compared to those of fetal hiccups at 32 weeks*

| | | *Motion intervals* | | |
	n	*Mean ± SD* (s)	*Coefficient of variation* (%)	*Difference*
Quick motion at 13 weeks				
Regular intervals	15	2.01 ± 0.43	21	
All intervals	51	3.27 ± 1.56	48	NS
Hiccups at 32 weeks	67	2.06 ± 0.66	32	S

NS, not significant; S, significant

fetal action, before 13 weeks. As fetal hiccupping is harmless in late pregnancy, early stage hiccupping may also be physiological, and therefore, the sudden movement is harmless in spite of its convulsive appearance.

Fetal breathing movement

Fetal breathing movements were confirmed by sonography and recorded with conventional and augmented actograms. Low-voltage regular signals were recorded, but these were still vague when compared to the conventional actogram. Regular deflections were recorded by the augmented actogram. An active filter was incorporated into the actograph, and connected to the output to improve clarity. The cut-off frequency was 2 or 4 Hz. High frequency was sharply cut off by the filter. A common pen-recorder was connected to the external output of the actograph, the augmented and filtered actogram was then recorded (Figure 7).

The augmented record clearly showed regular changes at 35 weeks of gestation, particularly in the record that used the 2-Hz filter. The regular change continued for 50 s in the fetal resting state. The regular vibration was sporadic after the appearance of gross fetal movements, and completely disappeared in the fetal active state (Figure 8). No regular change was recorded in active fetal state by the augmented and filtered actogram.

The regular fetal movements were compared to other fetal respiratory curves in our previous studies. Breathing detected by computer processing of electrical impedance changes of the maternal abdomen showed cyclic and regular changes[9]. The frequency histogram was studied

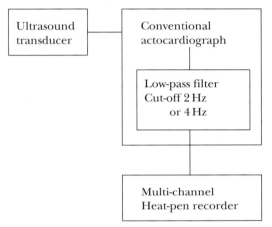

Figure 7 *Block diagram of augmented and filtered actogram*

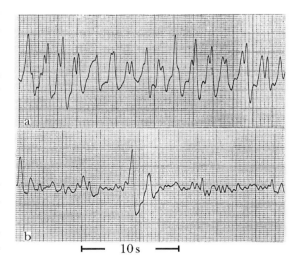

Figure 8 *Fetal breathing movements recorded by the augmented actogram using a 2-Hz low-pass filter. (a) Appearance of regular signals with a frequency of 1-Hz. (b) Disappearance of the regular signals in the active fetal state*

421

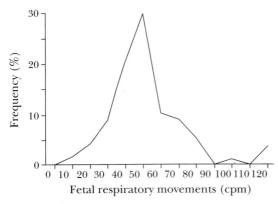

Figure 9 *Distribution of the frequency of fetal respiratory movements. The most frequent fetal respiration was 60 cpm in the fetus in this figure; this pattern was similar to those found in other fetuses. Fetal respiration was measured by electrical impedance[9] of maternal abdomen. cpm, cycles per minute*

Table 4 *The duration of suspected fetal breathing movements recorded with the augmented actogram*

Filter	Duration (s)	
	Mean ± SD	n
No filter	1.00 ± 0.21	38*
2 Hz low-pass	1.08 ± 0.25	43*

*The difference was not significant

in order to analyze the intervals between regular signals. The frequency of fetal respiration was 20–100 times/min, and was most frequently at 60 times/min (Figure 9).

Utsu and colleagues[10] studied fetal tracheal fluid flow by ultrasonic Doppler flow velocimetry, and established the cycle of respiration, the duration of which was about 1 s. The interval of respirations showed various changes, but the

duration remained unchanged in every respiratory cycle.

The durations of the signal cycles in filtered and unfiltered records were about 1 s, i.e. the frequency was about 60/min (Table 4). Therefore, the signals recorded by augmented and filtered actograms were similar to the breathing movements reported in previous studies.

In summary, this chapter shows that regular signals recorded in the augmented actogram represent fetal breathing movements, as confirmed by real-time B-mode sonography. The frequency was 60/min, similar to that of previous studies, and the changes were interrupted by the fetal active state. The augmented actogram will, therefore, be more useful in the study of fetal behavior and in the estimation of fetal well-being than the conventional actogram.

References

1. Maeda, K. (1984). Studies on new ultrasonic Doppler fetal actograph and continuous recording of fetal movement. *Acta Obstet. Gynaecol. Jpn.*, **36**, 280–8
2. Maeda, K. (1990). Recent technical progress in obstetrics and gynecology in Japan. *Front. Med. Biol. Engng.*, **2**, 81–7
3. Maeda, K., Tatsumura, M. and Nakajima, K. (1991). Objective and quantitative evaluation of fetal movement with ultrasonic Doppler actocardiogram. *Biol. Neonate*, **60** (Suppl.), 41–51
4. Ohta, M. (1985). Evaluation of fetal movements with ultrasonic Doppler fetal actograph. *Acta Obstet. Gynaecol. Jpn.*, **37**, 73–82
5. Maeda, K. (1989). Abnormal fetal movement. *Sanfujinkano-Jissai*, **38**, 949–54
6. Teshima, N. (1993). Non-reactive pattern diagnosed by ultrasonic Doppler fetal actocardio-gram and outcome of the fetuses with non-reactive pattern. *Acta Obstet. Gynaecol. Jpn.*, **45**, 423–30
7. Takahashi, H. (1990). Studies on cross-correlation coefficient between fetal heart rate and fetal movement signals detected by ultrasonic Doppler fetal actocardiogram. *Acta Obstet. Gynaecol. Jpn.*, **42**, 443–9
8. Maeda, K. and Tatsumura, M. (1993). Antepartum development of fetal behavior and fetal sensitivity to acoustic and photic stimuli: actocardiographic studies. *Asia Med. J.*, **36**, 277–88
9. Utsu, M. (1981). Studies on the measurement of fetal breathing movement by the impedance method. *Acta Obstet. Gynaecol. Jpn.*, **33**, 87–96
10. Utsu, M., Sakakibara, S., Ishida, T. and Chiba, Y. (1983). Dynamics of tracheal fluid flow in the human fetus, studied with pulsed Doppler ultrasound. *Acta Obstet. Gynaecol. Jpn.*, **35**, 2017–18

Systematic antenatal functional evaluation in pregnancies at risk of progressive fetal anemia

32

D. Oepkes, H. Kanhai and B. Arabin

INTRODUCTION

Fetal anemia may be the consequence of a variety of diseases, such as red blood cell (RBC) alloimmunization, infection, or of complications leading to chronic or acute fetal bleeding. Few data are available about the development and course of non-immune fetal anemia. Due to its sporadic occurrence in women without any detectable risk factors, fetal anemia in these pregnancies is usually only diagnosed at late stages. However, most causes of chronic hemolysis or chronic blood loss leading to progressive fetal anemia are likely to result in pathophysiological changes in the fetus similar to those described in RBC alloimmunization. Fetal hemolytic anemia due to maternal alloantibodies against fetal red cells, represents a distinct example of an environmental hazard to the essentially healthy fetus.

After the introduction of screening and prevention programs, the incidence of RBC alloimmunization, specifically of rhesus (Rh) disease has decreased tremendously. Before the introduction of immune prophylaxis in the late 1960s, Rh-disease occurred in around 1% of births, with 15% of women being Rh-D-negative, this means that 7% of these women gave birth to babies with some degree of hemolytic disease. In the last decade, the incidence has been reduced to around 0.1%. The pregnancies with hemolytic disease which still occur mostly represent failures of the prophylaxis program, such as failure to administer anti-D IgG after abortions, or insufficient amounts of anti-D being given in cases with excessive fetomaternal hemorrhage. Other failures of general preventive health policy occur in those women im-munized by incompatible blood transfusions (especially Kell- and c-antibodies). In those countries, including the Netherlands, where antenatal administration of anti-D IgG is not (yet) routine, early and severe immunization during pregnancy is also a significant contributor to the incidence of new immunizations.

The time of onset and the severity of hemolysis varies, and is in part related to the placental passage of the antibodies, type and subclass of the antibodies and the maturity of the reticuloendothelial system. Furthermore, the development of fetal anemia also depends on the compensatory abilities of the fetus regarding chronically progressive anemia, and, in part, on the gestational age. There is still a lack of insight into the reasons why some fetuses show a surprisingly slow progression of anemia, while others very rapidly deteriorate and die of extreme anemia.

The initial adaptation of the fetus to the increased destruction of red cells is the increase of extramedullary erythropoiesis, occurring primarily in the liver and spleen. When the increased production matches the destruction rate, the only symptom is hepatosplenomegaly. Progressive hemolysis may lead to failure of this adaptation, with actual anemia as a consequence. The reduced oxygen carrying capacity of the blood forces the fetus to increase its blood flow to maintain tissue oxygenation. Cardiac output increases, and, together with the reduced viscosity of the blood, hyperdynamic circulation develops. Further reduction of the hemoglobin level may induce high-output cardiac failure, increased venous pressure,

423

acidemia and capillary leakage due to endothelial cell damage and hypoalbuminemia. These events result in fetal hydrops, and finally death.

When the fetus survives, another risk occurs in the neonatal period, that of hemolysis. Hemolysis may continue for weeks after birth and result in increased bilirubin levels which can no longer be filtered through the placenta and that accumulate in the neonate, particularly in the brain tissues. Cerebral damage (kernicterus) due to hemolytic disease of the newborn used to be a major contributor to the causes of severe mental disability.

Timely recognition of the hazards that threaten the fetus and neonate is necessary to initiate specialized care, which, at present, should lead to the prevention of irreversible damage to the fetus or the neonate. With the application of a variety of diagnostic and therapeutic tools, the great majority of pregnancies complicated by even severe RBC alloimmunization will lead to the birth of a healthy child. Advances in neonatal care have practically resulted in the eradication of kernicterus as a cause of mental disability. Although RBC alloimmunization, when untreated, may have severe consequences for the short- and long-term life quality of the affected child, most children will be completely healthy when effective perinatal care can be provided.

CLINICAL EXPERIENCE

Our center, the University Hospital Leiden, is the national referral center for the treatment of all pregnancies at risk of severe fetal anemia. This means that all the fetal blood transfusions in the country, with a population of 15 million people, are performed at our center. With the introduction of intravascular blood transfusions in 1987 there was an incidence of approximately 200 pregnancies/year with a positive antibody screen. Out of these, around 20/year required fetal blood sampling (FBS) and intravascular blood transfusion. On average, treatment had to be started at 27 weeks, with a mean of three transfusions/fetus.

Until recently, the management of red cell alloimmunized pregnancies was based on repeated use of amniocentesis to measure amniotic fluid bilirubin concentrations (Liley-index). However, this test has disadvantages in detecting the degree of fetal anemia, because fetal compensatory capabilities cannot be taken into account. Also before 27 weeks the Liley-index cannot be used[1]. In addition, a single measurement of amniotic fluid bilirubin is usually insufficient to identify appropriate management options. Serial amniocenteses performed for trend analysis, result in a cumulation of the procedure-related risks including the risk of boosting the antibody levels of the mother by transplacental puncturing[2]. Finally, the relative rarity of the disease has led to a situation where only a few laboratories are able to maintain the necessary expertise in the assessment of the Liley-index.

Prospective study of the clinical value of non-invasive diagnostic tests in the management of severe red cell alloimmunization

To avoid unnecessary hazards due to further 'environmental' risks related to invasive procedures, we decided to develop a systematic non-invasive approach following the classical concept of pathophysiological processes of fetal adaptation. By this means we primarily included only pregnancies with high antibody levels in which fetal blood sampling was performed as a diagnostic tool serving as the gold standard for all our prospectively evaluated non-invasive procedures (Table 1). To determine the fetal response to various degrees of anemia the following tests were performed integrating functional parameters:

(1) Size of liver and spleen reflecting extramedullary erythropoiesis;

(2) Venous and arterial Doppler measurements reflecting hyperdynamic circulation, with classical pictures of fetal anemia;

(3) Placental thickness, amount of amniotic fluid and extent of fetal hydrops.

Table 1 *Primary study group including pregnancies with high antibody levels with or without hydrops. In all patients a non-invasive systematic functional evaluation was performed before cordocentesis*

Subgroup	n	Gestational age at 1st FBS (weeks)	Hb/Ht at 1st FBS (g/dl)	%	Gestational age at delivery (weeks)	Perinatal mortality
Without hydrops	31	26 + 4 (19–34)	5.4 (1.9–10.5)	16 (6–35)	35 + 1 (32–37)	0
With hydrops	7	26 + 2 (18–35)	2.6 (0.3–4.0)	9 (1–16)	33 + 4 (28–37)	4
Total	38	26 + 3	5.1	16	34 + 4	4

FBS, fetal blood sampling; Hb, hemoglobin concentration; Ht, hematocrit. Ranges in parentheses

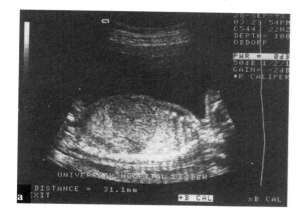

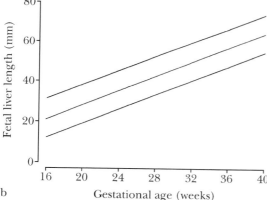

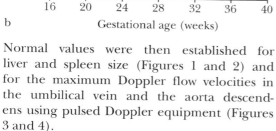

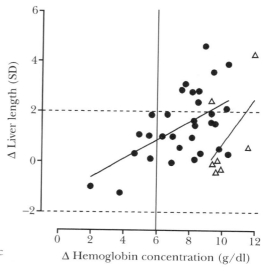

Figure 1 *Parasagittal view (a) through the fetal abdomen at the level of the right liver lobe. Measurement of the liver length is indicated. Reference ranges (b) for fetal liver length in normal pregnancies (y = −7.34 + 1.79x, residuals SD = 4.79). Correlation (c) of Δ fetal liver length with hematocrit deficit at the time of first fetal blood sampling. Circles, non-hydropic fetuses, with regression line (r = 0.55); triangles, hydropic fetuses, with regression line (r = 0.61)*

Normal values were then established for liver and spleen size (Figures 1 and 2) and for the maximum Doppler flow velocities in the umbilical vein and the aorta descendens using pulsed Doppler equipment (Figures 3 and 4).

Liver length was measured in a parasagittal plane, from the diaphragm to the tip of the right liver lobe[3], spleen perimeter was estimated by measuring the transverse (T) and longitudinal (L) diameters in a cross-section of the fetal abdomen, calculating the perimeter using the formula[4] for the ellipsoid: $(T + L) \times 1.57$. Umbilical venous flow velocities were measured by placing the pulsed Doppler sample volume over the proximal intrahepatic part of the vein and correcting for the angle of insonation, ensuring an angle $< 30°$[5]. Aorta descendens time-averaged maximum velocities were measured by placing the sample volume just above the diaphragm, correcting for the angle which was $< 45°$[5].

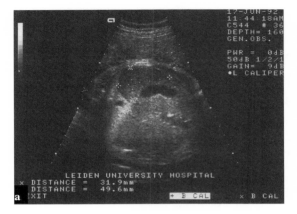

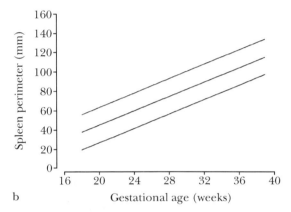

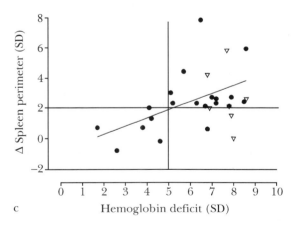

Figure 2 *Transverse view (a) through the fetal abdomen with calipers indicating transverse and longitudinal diameters of the spleen. Reference ranges (b) for fetal spleen perimeter in normal pregnancies (y = −28.33 + 3.66x, residuals SD = 9.14). Correlation (c) of Δ fetal spleen perimeter with hematocrit deficit at the time of first fetal blood sampling. Circles, non-hydropic fetuses, with regression line (r = 0.53); triangles, hydropic fetuses*

The results were then plotted with our own reference ranges, obtained in normal pregnancies. To study the correlation between the ultrasonographic and Doppler measurements with the degree of fetal anemia, the results were plotted against the hematocrit-deficit (difference between actual hematocrit and normal mean for the corresponding gestational age) (Figures 1–4).

The sensitivity, specificity, positive and negative predictive values were calculated using two-by-two tables, classifying the measurements as normal or abnormal, with the cut-off point at 2 standard deviations (SD) above the normal mean. The cut-off level used to define severe anemia was set at a hematocrit level of 5 SD below the normal mean (Table 2).

In clinical practice, decisions are usually made after integrating information from all available test results. We therefore hypothesized that the combined use of ultrasonographic and Doppler parameters based on different adaptation processes in the fetus, might increase their clinical value. Our measurements were used to build a logistic regression model for the prediction of severe anemia, using stepwise forward selection. The most significant contributors to the model were the Doppler results (Table 2).

A recent development in non-invasive assessment of the fetus at risk for hemodynamic compromise is Doppler measurement of the ductus venosus waveform. Apart from the maximum velocity measurement which may be used to detect a hyperdynamic state, the changes in the pulsatile flow pattern, especially a reduced minimal velocity during atrial contraction, have been shown to be associated with increased central venous pressure or right ventricular preload. We studied the ductus venosus waveform changes in 21 RBC alloimmunized pregnancies, at the time of fetal blood sampling. Apart from the expected increased maximum velocities related to anemia, the ratio between peak velocity and minimal velocity was found to be increased, indicating the existence of increased preload in fetal anemia[6].

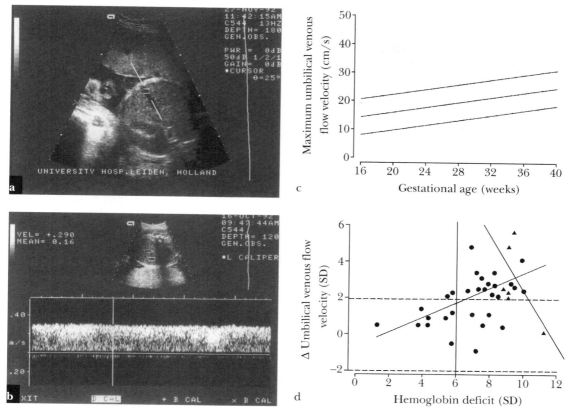

Figure 3 *Longitudinal view (a) through fetal abdomen with pulsed Doppler sample volume in the umbilical vein. Doppler blood flow velocity waveform (b) of umbilical venous blood flow with measurement of maximum velocity. Reference ranges (c) for umbilical venous maximum blood flow velocity in normal pregnancies (y = 7.30 + 0.437x, residuals SD = 3.14). Correlation (d) of Δ umbilical venous maximum velocity with hematocrit deficit at the time of first fetal blood sampling. Circles, non-hydropic fetuses, with regression line (r = 0.48); triangles, hydropic fetuses, with regression line (r = −0.56)*

Current management options using a minimally invasive approach

RBC alloimmunization is an example of a pregnancy complication where the fetus is healthy, but is subject to life-threatening hostile influences as long as she or he is attached to the placenta and the mother. The fetal patient can be saved provided that the disease is recognized and that symptomatic treatment in the form of blood transfusions is given in time. It should be emphasized, however, that the fetus is not only at risk of dying from severe anemia, but also from a number of risks inherent to the invasive nature of the diagnostic and therapeutic interventions. The basic assumption on which our

management protocol is based, is that optimal survival rates can only be achieved by combining timely interventions with a minimum number of invasive diagnostic procedures.

Advanced ultrasound and Doppler technology is used to evaluate fetal biophysical parameters in order to describe signs of the progression of disease and the actual fetal condition. The specific challenge of a non-invasive approach to red cell alloimmunization is motivated not only by the acute risks of amniocentesis or cordocentesis, but also by the increasing awareness of the usually underestimated risk of increased sensitization, which has to be considered together with the procedure-specific risks[7–11].

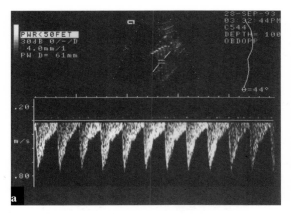

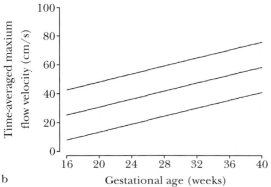

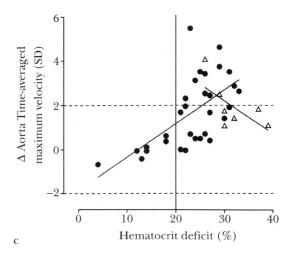

Figure 4 *Doppler waveforms (a) of blood flow velocities in the descending aorta. Reference ranges (b) for time averaged maximum flow velocities in the descending aorta* $(y = -45.63 + 4.989x - 0.064x^2)$. *Correlation (c) of* Δ *aorta descendens time-averaged maximum velocity with hematocrit deficit at the time of first fetal blood sampling. Circles, non-hydropic fetuses, with regression line (r = 0.60); triangles, hydropic fetuses, with regression line (r = -0.59)*

Results from our investigations suggest that Doppler flow velocity measurements, as well as liver and spleen size assessments, can be used to detect fetal changes related to hemolysis and anemia. To derive a complete picture of the fetal health in RBC alloimmunized pregnancies, the classical non-invasive approach to fetal evaluation by searching for early signs of hydrops, should be extended to include the investigation for signs of increased erythropoiesis and hyperdynamic circulation.

Fetal hydrops is known only to develop in a near-terminal stage of the disease, significantly worsening the prognosis for healthy outcome. It can no longer be justified to wait for this sign of severe fetal disease when other parameters associated with developing fetal anemia are available.

The clinical value of amniocentesis is increasingly regarded as limited, not only because it is not reliable before 27 weeks, but also because the data provided by the non-invasive measurements have a more direct correlation with fetal-health status. During the last 5 years we have greatly reduced the number of diagnostic amniocenteses in RBC alloimmunized pregnancies, relying on non-invasive methods for fetal evaluation.

The indications for diagnostic cordocentesis in RBC alloimmunized pregnancies have now changed from only considering the obstetric history and antibody titer to the individualized use of a combination of tests actually describing changes in the fetus. With this approach, we now detect at least moderate anemia in most of our first fetal blood sampling procedures, enabling us immediately to continue the procedure with the transfusion of a significant amount of donor blood. Fetuses exhibiting hydrops at the time of the first transfusion were referred to our center because hydrops was detected unexpectedly in pregnancies that were not considered to be at risk for fetal anemia.

New and promising non-invasive methods for fetal evaluation, such as ductus venosus waveform analyses, are currently being prospectively studied to assess their clinical usefulness.

Table 2 *Diagnostic value of non-invasive techniques in predicting the presence of severe fetal anemia, defined as a hematocrit of < 5 SD of the mean*

Parameter	Sensitivity (%)	Specificity (%)	Positive predictive value (%)	Negative predictive value (%)
Liver length	38	100	100	32
Spleen size	93	100	100	86
Umbilical vein V_{max}	77	80	91	57
Aorta TA V_{max}	50	100	100	37

Logistic regression model (odds = $e^{-23.7 + 0.745\ UV\ V_{max} + 0.157\ AoTA\ V_{max}}$) 100%, 57%, 89% and 100%, respectively. UVV_{max}, umbilical venous maximum velocity; $AoTAV_{max}$, aorta time-averaged maximum velocity

DISCUSSION

During the past 10 years, several investigators have studied the clinical usefulness of ultrasonographic and Doppler parameters in predicting the degree of hemolytic anemia in non-hydropic fetuses. Most studies were designed to assess the predictive values of a single parameter by comparing the measurements with the gold standard, fetal blood sampling. A high positive predictive value was found for fetal liver[12,13] and spleen[4] measurements, reflecting the increased extramedullary hematopoiesis.

Quantitative Doppler studies showed that in fetuses with hemolytic anemia, increased blood flow velocities are present, a situation described as a hyperdynamic circulation. These blood flow changes can be observed by measuring almost any fetal vessel. In clinical practice, the reliability of the measurement depends largely on its reproducibility. The vessel should be easy to visualize in most fetal positions, and allow for a minimal angle between the Doppler sample volume and the direction of flow. The most suitable Doppler parameters for the prediction of fetal anemia are blood flow velocity measurements in the descending aorta, intrahepatic umbilical vein and the middle cerebral artery[5,14–19].

A recent development in the use of Doppler to study the fetal circulation is the measurement of ductus venosus flow velocity waveforms. Fetuses with an increased right ventricular preload have a significantly changed ductus venosus index, which is an angle-independent parameter. In contrast to the other Doppler measurements, this parameter is not used to assess increased flow velocities but is thought to reflect

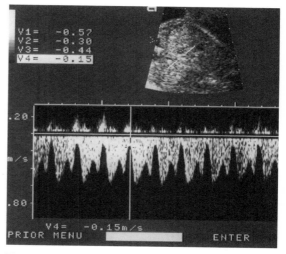

Figure 5 *Doppler flow velocity waveforms in the ductus venosus, with assessment of the minimal velocity during atrial contraction indicated by the caliper*

the degree of cardiac compromise[6,20,21]. Highly abnormal ductus venosus waveforms, with a reverse flow component during atrial systole, can be observed in the presence of hydrops and thus may be regarded as a marker for cardiac failure[19,22,23].

Cardiotocography has been shown to be of limited value, not applicable before about 28 weeks, and not demonstrating any changes until an advanced state of disease is reached. Possibly, the use of computerized measurement of fetal heart rate variations may be of more value in the future[24].

Most of the non-invasive parameters discussed above have positive predictive values as high as 90–100%. Their clinical value is restricted by the number of false negative results in most studies. This has led some investigators to state that diagnostic cordocentesis is the only reliable tool in the management of pregnancies at risk of fetal anemia[16,25]. However, most investigators have focused on the predictive value of a single measurement at a single time, while in practice, clinicians are used to assessing the risk of fetal anemia and the need for an invasive procedure by looking at a series of data, including the obstetric history, antibody titers, gestational age and various repeated ultrasound and Doppler measurements. Our study, using multivariate analysis of a number of ultrasonographic and Doppler parameters to predict the presence or absence of severe anemia showed better results than those using a single parameter[5]. There is no substitute for the clinical experience of the management team with this disease. Decisions whether to perform or postpone invasive diagnostic procedures also depend on factors such as technical difficulties due to placental position, fetal presentation, obesity of the mother etc. Other possible pregnancy complications must be taken into account, as well as logistic problems such as the availability of donor blood. Complications in previous pregnancies can influence patients' and doctors' perspectives on the risks of invasive methods, and lead to them opting for alternative approaches. In conclusion, the above mentioned methods for fetal surveillance are general guidelines, which need to be adapted to the individual patient by experienced clinicians.

SUMMARY

In severely affected pregnancies, the use of a variety of non-invasive tests will at most only postpone the first fetal blood sampling. However, of more importance is the application of the full range of non-invasive methods of fetal evaluation in mild-to-moderate alloimmunized women, who may not require prenatal therapy at all, but are at high risk of having their antibody-levels increased unnecessarily by reassuring invasive tests. In addition, the wide availability and the increasing experience with the use of high-quality ultrasound and Doppler equip-

ment may give physicians not specialized in the treatment of these pregnancies the opportunity to better select the patients and the time for referral, using information from the described ultrasonographic and Doppler evaluation by communicating with the referral center. This is an important advantage particularly in countries or regions where patients need to travel long distances when referred to tertiary care centers.

The methods described herein may be applied to other pregnancy complications associated with chronic fetal anemia, such as parvovirus B19 infection or fetomaternal hemorrhage.

THE FUTURE

Red cell alloimmunization will remain a pregnancy complication, requiring highly-specialized management. Before the effects of the antibodies can be blocked effectively by immunotherapy, we need to attempt to identify all women carrying antibodies against fetal red cells early in pregnancy, to monitor the fetus closely for signs of anemia, and to select those that require invasive diagnosis and therapy. Increasing knowledge of the pathophysiology, including better insight into the development of cardiac failure and hydrops, will undoubtedly result in the development of even more reliable non-invasive tests for fetal evaluation. Apart from ductus venosus studies, new subjects for research include the use of splenic blood flow, and more reliable non-Doppler techniques for volume flow estimation, sophisticated cardiac performance tests and tissue characterization.

In conclusion, RBC alloimmunization remains an important model in fetal medicine. Not only do we almost completely understand its etiology, we also know how to diagnose and treat the most severe cases and, even more important, we have population-based prevention programs. This may serve as an inspiration for investigators and clinicians to find solutions to other major problems in perinatal medicine with the aim of safeguarding the highest possible long-life quality.

References

1. Nicolaides, K. H., Rodeck, C. H., Mibashan, R. S. and Kemp, J. R. (1986). Have Liley-charts outlived their usefulness? *Am. J. Obstet. Gynecol.*, **155**, 90–4

2. Bowman, J. M. and Pollock, J. M. (1985). Transplacental fetal hemorrhage after amniocentesis. *Obstet. Gynecol.*, **66**, 749–54

3. Weiner, S., Bolognese, R. J. and Librizzi, R. J. (1981). Ultrasound in the evaluation and management of the isoimmunized pregnancy. *J. Clin. Ultrasound*, **9**, 315–23

4. Oepkes, D., Meerman, R. H., Vandenbussche, F. P. H. A., van Kamp, I. L., Kok, F. G. and Kanhai, H. H. H. (1993). Ultrasonographic fetal spleen measurements in red cell alloimmunized pregnancies. *Am. J. Obstet. Gynecol.*, **169**, 121–8

5. Oepkes, D., Brand, R., Vandenbussche, F. P. H. A., Meerman, R. H. and Kanhai, H. H. H. (1994). The use of ultrasonography and Doppler in the prediction of fetal haemolytic anaemia: a multivariate analysis. *Br. J. Obstet. Gynaecol.*, **101**, 680–4

6. Oepkes, D., Vandenbussche, F. P., van Bel, F. and Kanhai, H. H. H. (1993). Fetal ductus venosus blood flow velocities before and after transfusion in red-cell alloimmunized pregnancies. *Obstet. Gynecol.*, **82**, 237–41

7. Daffos, F., Capella-Pavlovsky, M. and Forestier, F. (1985). Fetal blood sampling during pregnancy with use of a needle guided by ultrasound: a study of 606 consecutive cases. *Am. J. Obstet. Gynecol.*, **153**, 655–60

8. Pielet, B. W., Socol, M. L., MacGregor, S. N., Ney, J. A. and Dooley, S. L. (1988). Cordocentesis: an appraisal of risks. *Am. J. Obstet. Gynecol.*, **159**, 1497–1500

9. Weiner, C. P., Wenstrom, K. D., Sipes, S. L. and Williamson, R. A. (1991). Risk factors for cordocentesis and fetal intravascular transfusion. *Am. J. Obstet. Gynecol.*, **165**, 1020–5

10. MacGregor, S. N., Silver, R. K. and Sholl, J. S. (1991). Enhanced sensitization after cordocentesis in a rhesus-isoimmunized pregnancy. *Am. J. Obstet. Gynecol.*, **165**, 382–3

11. Bowman, J. M., Pollock, J. M., Peterson, L. E., Harman, C. R., Manning, F. A. and Menticoglou, S. M. (1994). Fetomaternal hemorrhage following funipuncture: increase in severity of maternal red-cell alloimmunization. *Obstet. Gynecol.*, **84**, 839–43

12. Vintzileos, A. M., Neckles, S., Campbell, W. A., Andreoli, J. W. Jr, Kaplan, B. M. and Nochimson, D. J. (1985). Fetal liver ultrasound measurements during normal pregnancy. *Obstet. Gynecol.*, **66**, 477–80

13. Roberts, A. B., Mitchell, J. M. and Pattison, N. S. (1989). Fetal liver length in normal and isoimmunized pregnancies. *Am. J. Obstet. Gynecol.*, **161**, 42–6

14. Rightmire, D. A., Nicolaides, K. H., Rodeck, C. H. and Campbell, S. (1986). Fetal blood velocities in Rh isoimmunization: relationship to gestational age and to fetal hematocrit. *Obstet. Gynecol.*, **68**, 233–6

15. Bilardo, C. M., Nicolaides, K. H. and Campbell, S. (1989). Doppler studies in red cell isoimmunization. *Clin. Obstet. Gynecol.*, **32**, 719–27

16. Nicolaides, K. H., Bilardo, C. M. and Campbell, S. (1990). Prediction of fetal anemia by measurement of the mean blood velocity in the fetal aorta. *Am. J. Obstet. Gynecol.*, **162**, 209–12

17. Vyas, S., Nicolaides, K. H. and Campbell, S. (1990). Doppler examination of the middle cerebral artery in anemic fetuses. *Am. J. Obstet. Gynecol.*, **162**, 1066–8

18. Mari, G., Adrignolo, A., Ahuhamad, A. Z., Pirhonen, J., Jones, D. C., Ludomirsky, A. and Copel, J. A. (1995). Diagnosis of fetal anemia with Doppler ultrasound in the pregnancy complicated by maternal blood group immunization. *Ultrasound Obstet. Gynecol.*, **5**, 400–5

19. Hecher, K., Snijders, R., Campbell, S. and Nicolaides, K. (1995). Fetal venous, arterial and intracardiac blood flows in red blood cell isoimmunization. *Obstet. Gynecol.*, **85**, 122–8

20. Kiserud, T., Eik-Nes, S. H., Blaas, H. G. K. and Hellevik, L. R. (1991). Ultrasonographic velocimetry of the fetal ductus venosus. *Lancet*, **338**, 1412–14

21. DeVore, G. R. and Horenstein, J. (1993). Ductus venosus index: a method for evaluating right ventricular preload in the second-trimester fetus. *Ultrasound Obstet. Gynecol.*, **3**, 338–42

22. Kiserud, T., Eik-Nes, S. H., Hellevik, L. R. and Blaas, H. G. (1993). Ductus venosus blood velocity changes in fetal cardiac diseases. *J. Matern. Fetal Invest.*, **3**, 15–20

23. Oepkes, D., Helbig, A., Meerman, R. H. and Kanhai, H. H. H. (1994). Ductus venosus reversed flow: a sign of fetal cardiac failure. *J. Matern. Fetal Invest.*, **4** (Suppl.), 513 (abstract)

24. Economides, D. L., Selinger, M., Ferguson, J., Bowell, P. J., Dawes, G. S. and MacKenzie, I. Z.

(1992). Computerized measurement of heart rate variation in fetal anemia caused by rhesus alloimmunization. *Am. J. Obstet. Gynecol.*, **167**, 689–93

25. Nicolaides, K. H., Fontanarosa, M., Gabbe, S. G. and Rodeck, C. H. (1988). Failure of ultrasonographic parameters to predict the severity of fetal anemia in rhesus isoimmunization. *Am. J. Obstet. Gynecol.*, **158**, 920–6

Abruptio placentae: from early pregnancy to term

33

R. N. Laurini

INTRODUCTION

Abruptio placentae denotes a detachment of the placenta from its decidual bed. This premature separation of a normally situated placenta can be complete or partial. Furthermore, the hematoma can be central (retroplacental) or marginal.

The rate of placental abruption in an unselected patient population can be variable and only reflects the ability to make the clinical diagnosis. In fact a partial abruptio can go clinically undiagnosed and the pathologist cannot always reliably recognize the presence of an abruptio placentae. Moreover, sonographic examination has significant limitations[1] and there is only some promising but preliminary experience with magnetic resonance imaging in patients with third-trimester bleeding[2]. Notwithstanding, Benirschke and Gille[3] reported an incidence of 3.75% of some degree of abruptio placentae in a series of consecutive placentas past the 20th week of pregnancy.

The correlates of placental abruption are multiple and include hypertensive disease[4], smoking and intrauterine growth retardation[5], and congenital anomalies[6]; however, clinically uncomplicated pregnancies predominate, as demonstrated by Benirschke and Gille[3].

Despite advances in reproductive medicine the etiology and even the origin of the uteroplacental bleeding remain largely unknown. Acute placental separation is currently believed to be related to the pathology of the uteroplacental arterial circulation, or, which is less likely, to that of the pathology of the venous uteroplacental circulation[7]. Independent of its etiology and pathogenesis, abruptio placentae has been traditionally considered as an acute event unlikely to be altered by antepartum surveillance.

Although abruptio placentae remains a poorly understood disorder, it continues to represent an important complication of pregnancy. In effect, abruptio placentae represents a significant contributor to perinatal mortality, mainly as a cause of both preterm delivery and antepartum fetal death[8,9]. Therefore there is a definite need to understand better the natural history of abruptio placentae in order to develop better management of this condition that will result in improved perinatal outcome. In fact, it remains a problem that can benefit from a correlation between the clinical, sonographic and morphological aspects of the condition.

With this in mind, the main aim of this chapter is to define the morphological profile of this disorder and relate it to the clinical, sonographic and hemodynamic findings in this condition. Moreover, and on the basis of this correlation, the author will attempt a brief discussion on the pathophysiology and clinical significance of abruptio placentae developing at different stages in pregnancy.

ABRUPTIO PLACENTAE IN THE FIRST AND SECOND TRIMESTERS

It has been reported that first-trimester vaginal bleeding represents an important predictor of adverse fetal outcome[10]. Furthermore, the work of Eriksen and colleagues[11] has demonstrated that vaginal bleeding in the first and second trimester is associated with an increased risk of placental abruption later in pregnancy.

433

A systematic approach to the morphological assessment of 486 specimens of first-trimester abortion resulted in a classification into six groups to be used for the routine examination of these specimens[12]. Group 2 included hemorrhagic lesions defined as an extensive retroplacental and decidual hemorrhage with or without extension into the intervillous space. These lesions were commonly seen in the presence of normal embryos/fetuses and, on histological examination, the extension of the hemorrhage into the intervillous space represented a common finding. The find of a placental hemorrhage associated with normal embryos or fetuses was considered as an indication that events reminiscent of abruptio placentae also take place in early pregnancy.

A more systematic use of modern ultrasonography has resulted in the recognition of a greater number of pathological conditions in early pregnancy, including the subchorionic hematoma (SCH)[13]. SCH is defined as a sonolucent area located between the chorion and the uterine wall[13,14]. Although different localizations have been described, the most common was subchorionic significantly related to the placental margin[1,14–16].

Table 1 summarizes this author's experience with regard to the morphological findings in specimens from the first and second trimester. Gross examination usually shows the presence of one or more marginal and/or retroplacental blood clots (Figure 1).

In the view of this author it is important to use a terminology that avoids confusion between subchorionic hematoma representing a collection of blood between the chorion and decidua and subchorionic hematoma repre-

senting a subchorionic intervillous thrombus, which is also called a Breus mole. Therefore this author will use the terms marginal placental hematoma (the most common form of subchorionic hematoma) and retroplacental hematoma.

Figures 2 and 3 illustrate the most common macroscopic presentation. In agreement with the sonographic findings, gross examination shows a marginal location of the hematoma in the vast majority of cases. Moreover, these marginally localized hematomas frequently dissect into the intervillous space, predominantly under the chorionic plate.

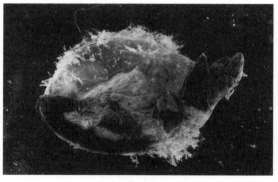

Figure 1 *Spontaneous abortion at 10 weeks' gestation showing an intact gestational sac with an extensive retroplacental hematoma. The fetus was normally developed and showed lesions of acute asphyxia*

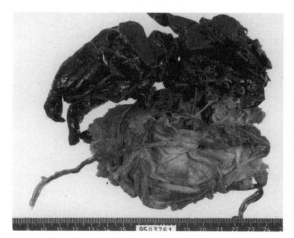

Figure 2 *Twin placenta from a spontaneous abortion at 14 weeks' gestation showing a large marginal hematoma. The patient presented a vaginal bleeding at 12 weeks of gestation*

Table 1 *Morphological findings in the first and second trimester*

Marginal hematoma
Intervillous hemorrhage
Venous sinus congestion and thrombosis
Focal decidual necrosis
Focal decidual hemorrhage
Ischemic villitis
Intravillous hemorrhages
Hemosiderin in chorionic plate

Histological examination of the marginal zones showed lesions mainly affecting the venous circulation. The earliest findings are those of venous sinus congestion as illustrated in Figure 4. Depending on the seriousness of the lesion there can be venous thrombosis associated with focal decidual necrosis and dissecting hemorrhage that often extends into the intervillous space. These morphological findings are in agreement with the view that most placental separations are secondary to events occurring in the venous drainage of the organ[7].

It is probably of diagnostic value to underline the frequent extension of the marginal hematoma into the placenta (Figures 2 and 3). The extension deep into the placenta was occasionally seen by sonography and helped differentiate a subchorionic hemorrhage from a more benign condition called chorioamniotic separation[16]. In the view of the author this finding plays a role in defining the possible clinical significance of this lesion. In fact, the volume of the hematoma is not the main variable to consider.

In addition, histology also shows that chorionic villi are not only affected by the intervillous hemorrhage but also show changes of ischemia in the form of ischemic villitis that represents an early form of infarction. Really these ischemic changes are identical to the placental infarction regularly seen overlying a retroplacental hematoma later in pregnancy.

Finally, histological examination occasionally shows two other morphological changes that have been previously described in abruptio placentae; intravillous hemorrhage and deposits of hemosiderin in the chorionic plate.

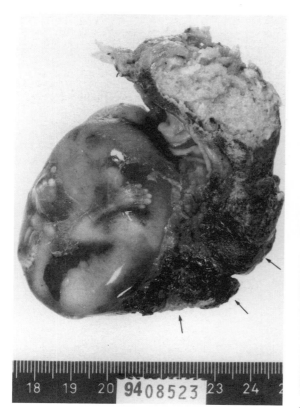

Figure 3 *Amniotic sac with fetus and placenta showing a large marginal hematoma (arrows). Psychosocial termination of pregnancy at 14 weeks' gestation by means of prostaglandin E₂*

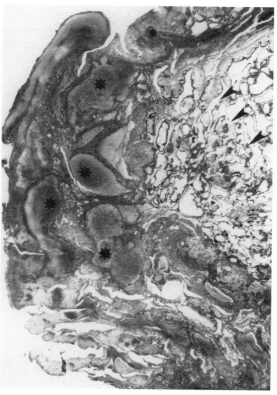

Figure 4 *Gestational sac from a spontaneous abortion at 8 weeks' gestation showing marked congestion of venous sinuses (star) and early marginal hemorrhage (arrows). Hematoxylin–eosin, × 2.5*

In the view of the author, the use of prosta-glandins for termination of pregnancy repre-sents a human model of fetoplacental hypoxic-ischemic pathology in normal pregnancies. A review of 158 placentas from pregnancies termi-nation with prostaglandin E$_2$ for psychosocial reasons demonstrated that it can be considered as a human model of abruptio placentae in the fetal period[17]. The main placental changes were marginal abruptio 75%, early infarction 47%, 'advanced maturation' 53%, villous edema 42%, intravillous hemorrhage 31% and ischemic villi-tis 33%. These findings were compared to those of 22 placentas from cases with abruptio placentae where no prostaglandins were used. In the latter group, the placental findings were identical to those observed in the prostaglandin E$_2$ group. Interestingly, the abruptio placentae group also showed chorioamnionitis and infarc-tion in 64 and 14% of cases, respectively. In the presence of sufficient decidual basalis, both groups showed a normal trophoblastic invasion of spiral arteries associated with a marked con-gestion and focal thrombosis of veins with frequent focal decidual necrosis and hemor-rhage dissecting into the intervillous space. Indeed the morphological appearance in cases of interruption of pregnancies by prostaglandin E$_2$ was identical to that seen in abruptio placentae. Moreover, it is important to under-line that the marginal placental hematoma and associated lesions developed in the presence of normal arterial uteroplacental circulation.

Figures 3, 5, 6 and 7 illustrate both the macro-scopic and histological aspects of the abruptio placentae that develops in the context of psy-chosocial termination of pregnancy by means of prostaglandins.

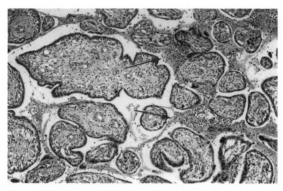

Figure 6 *Placental histology (Figure 3) shows the presence of an ischemic intervillitis (arrows). Hematoxylin–eosin, × 47.9*

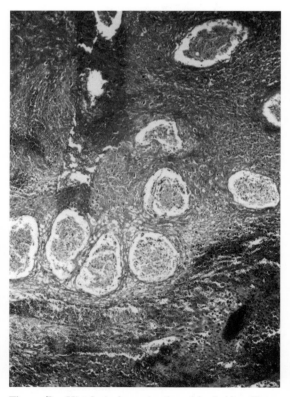

Figure 7 *Histological examination of the decidua (Figure 3) shows multiple foci decidual necrosis including the decidual portion of the spiral arteries. Hematoxylin–eosin, × 44.9*

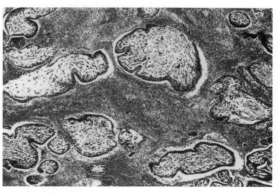

Figure 5 *Histological examination (Figure 3) shows the extension of the marginal hematoma into the intervillous space. Hematoxylin–eosin, × 38.9*

In our experience chorioamnionitis represents the most common cause of placental abruption during fetal life, in particular for the mid-trimester, as illustrated in Figures 8 and 9. Chorioamnionitis was present in 14 out of the 22 cases of placental abruption (gestational age ranged from 13 weeks) used as a control group in our study of placental changes following the use of prostaglandin E_2[17]. Others have also reported a significant association between placental abruption and histological chorioamnionitis[18,19].

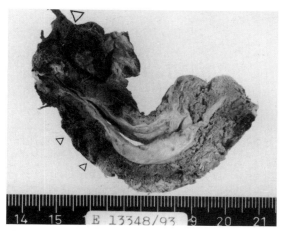

Figure 8 *Placenta from a spontaneous abortion at 13 weeks' gestation showing a marginal hematoma (large arrow) dissecting into the intervillous space (small arrows). Histology demonstrated the presence of a chorioamnionitis*

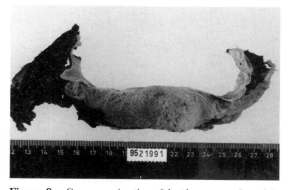

Figure 9 *Gross examination of the placenta confirmed the presence of a large marginal hematoma. Histology showed a severe chorioamnionitis. Patient presented at 21 weeks' gestation with vaginal bleeding, elevated α-fetoprotein, severe oligohydramnios and sonographic findings compatible with a retroplacental hematoma*

A review of the brain pathology in 116 consecutive psychosocial terminations of pregnancy by using prostaglandin E_2 (gestational age ranged from 12 to 23 weeks) showed the following brain lesions: germinal matrix hemorrhage 21%, intraventricular hemorrhage 9%, periventricular congestion 4%, periventricular hemorrhage 9%, pontine hemorrhage 16%, choroid plexus hemorrhage 11% and subarachnoidal hemorrhage 25%. Histology showed that periventricular congestion with or without hemorrhage was associated with a dilatation of thin veins suggesting an important role for the venous lesion[20].

In 1981, Bejar and associates[21] reported that some pathogenic bacteria have phospholipase activity that increases the availability of arachidonate for eicosanoid synthesis. Furthermore, Lamont and co-workers[22] demonstrated that bacterial products increase the production of prostaglandin E by human amnion cells. In view of this and of the similarities between the pathology present with the use of prostaglandin and that associated to chorioamnionitis, in particular abruptio placentae and brain hemorrhage, this author suggested that prostaglandins played a major role in the development of an abruptio placentae in chorioamnionitis[12]. In fact, the increased production of prostaglandin E by the fetal membranes and choriodecidua in unexplained preterm labor associated with chorioamnionitis has been reported in the literature[19].

The possible association between the use of prostaglandin E_2 and placental abruption with or without brain damage merits further studies since prostaglandin E_2 is currently used as a means of induction of labor. In this context one finds several reports in the literature that associate induction of labor by prostaglandin E_2 with both placental abruption and sudden fetal death[23–25].

In this context it is of interest to comment further on the fetal findings from the case illustrated in Figure 9. At postmortem there was a congenital pneumonia associated with important fetal lesions of acute and sustained asphyxia including pathological gliosis. These findings underline the importance of fetal distress that can accompany abruptio placentae and/or chorioamnionitis[26]. In effect, infants born after abruptio placentae should be considered at risk for subsequent neurodevelopmental impairment[27,28].

Nevertheless, as illustrated in Figures 10 and 11, there exists a limited number of abruptio placentae in mid-trimester that fail to show any relationship with either microbiological or morphological findings of infection and/or inflammation. Although rare, some of these cases do show a decidual vasculopathy secondary to a poor trophoblastic invasion of spiral arteries[29]. Moreover, three of the 22 cases of abruptio placentae previously discussed showed the presence of infarctions. Indeed, the placental

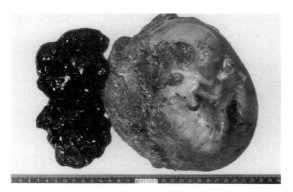

Figure 10 *Amniotic sac and placenta from an abruptio placentae at 20 weeks of gestation showing large (131 g) retroplacental hematoma. Microbiological examination of the placenta and fetal lungs was sterile. The fetus showed lesions of acute asphyxia*

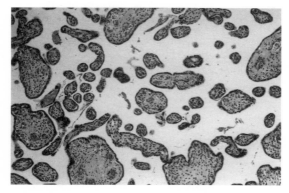

Figure 11 *Histological examination of the placenta (Figure 10) showed the presence of advanced maturation, a sign of placental ischemia. Hematoxylin–eosin, × 47.9*

pathology in Figure 11 is considered as a sign of placental ischemia.

These findings suggest that abruptio placentae developing in the first and second trimester can be represented by two different types; one in which the marginal placental hematoma presentation predominates, associated with a pathology of the venous circulation and the frequent presence of an infected amniotic fluid syndrome; the other in which retroplacental hematomas predominate, associated with an arterial decidual vasculopathy secondary to poor trophoblast invasion in the absence of any infectious and/or inflammatory process. Recent work by Arias and colleagues[30] supports this approach. These authors demonstrated the presence of two distinct subgroups among patients with preterm labor and preterm rupture of membranes; one with infection of the products of conception and another with maternal placental vasculopathy. Interestingly, the incidence of cases with mixed infection and vascular lesions was rare and not significant when compared to the control group. Moreover, abruptio placentae was only present among the group with preterm labor and premature rupture of the membranes.

Color Doppler ultrasound has been used to differentiate the more common finding of subchorionic fluid from that of subchorionic bleeding[14]. Recent work by Kurjak and associates[31] demonstrated the presence of abnormal blood flow patterns in the spiral arteries in the presence of a subchorionic hematoma. These flow abnormalities disappeared with the continuation of pregnancy and were considered as probably secondary to a mechanical effect (compression) from the hematoma.

As previously mentioned, a detailed morphological examination of the decidua shows lesions of the venous circulation associated with foci of decidual necrosis and dissecting hemorrhage. Nevertheless, the trophoblast invasion of spiral arteries in both first and second trimester specimens was normal. In fact marginal or retroplacental hematomas may affect uteroplacental circulation not only by compression but also by destruction of spiral arteries[32]. Independent of the cause of placental abruption, histology shows multiple foci of decidual necrosis that frequently include the decidual portion of spiral arteries (Figure 7). This morphological finding suggests that flow disturbances, as depicted by color Doppler, can also be the result of spiral artery necrosis. In cases where pregnancy progresses, the color Doppler will only read the spiral arteries that are permeable, which can explain the return to normal values reported by Kurjak and co-workers[31]. Nevertheless, this destruction (necrosis) of spiral arteries can play a role in the development of fetal growth retardation in pregnancies that progress into the third trimester. In effect, this destruction of transformed spiral arteries can reduce the total number of spiral arteries available for the perfusion of the feto-placental unit later in gestation.

Moreover, decidual necrosis and associated inflammatory response, whether or not in the presence of chorioamnionitis, may play a major role in activating the prostaglandin cascade or, more importantly, as a source of decidual interleukin-1[33,34]. These chemical mediators, in particular prostaglandins, have been shown to have profound effects on uterine circulation in early pregnancy[35].

ABRUPTIO PLACENTAE IN THE THIRD TRIMESTER

Abruptio placentae in the third trimester is very much related to the risk factors associated with preterm deliveries. Among the most common are hypertension and hypertensive disorders of pregnancy, smoking, drug abuse, abdominal trauma and premature rupture of membranes[36]. In addition one must bear in mind the frequent association with small for gestational age status[5]. Indeed it is during this period of gestation that one can more easily classify the case as that associated with a maternal placental vasculopathy or an infection[30].

In this context the morphological findings in the third trimester are variable (Table 2). In a significant number of cases there are no significant changes and the diagnosis of abruptio placentae remains a clinical one. Notwithstanding, the pathologist must carefully examine the placenta for any signs of an acute or old margi-

nal hematoma (Figure 12). Retroplacental hematomas as illustrated in Figure 13 are readily seen. The latter are commonly associated with an infarction of the overlying placenta.

Histological examination of the hematoma, whether marginal or central, shows the

Table 2 *Morphological findings in the third trimester*

No significant changes
Marginal hematoma
Retroplacental hematoma
Infarction
Intravillous hemorrhages
Hemosiderin in chorionic plate
Abnormal arterial uteroplacental circulation

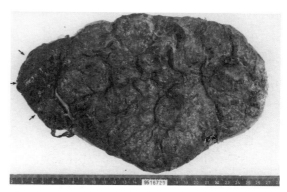

Figure 12 *Macroscopic examination of the placenta showed a marginal hematoma (arrows). Histology demonstrated the presence of a chorioamnionitis. The patient presented with a premature rupture of membranes at 34 weeks of gestation*

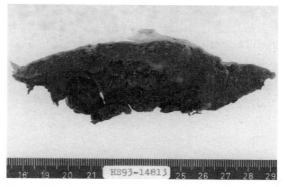

Figure 13 *Placenta showing a massive retroplacental hematoma. Cesarean section was performed at 34 weeks' gestation for abruptio placentae without knowledge of previous vaginal bleeding. Microbiology of placenta was sterile and histology failed to show iron deposition*

presence of congested venous sinuses with focal thrombosis associated with focal decidual necrosis and dissecting hemorrhage (Figure 14). These morphological findings are identical to those previously described for placental hematomas in the first and second trimesters. Such findings are observed independently of the presence or absence of an infection (Figure 13).

In the absence of macroscopic signs of placental abruption, a detailed histological examination can show the presence of focal intravillous hemorrhages (Figure 15). Intervillous hemorrhage consists of rupture of the vessels of chorionic villi resulting in a villous hemorrhage. This lesion was observed in relation to abruptio placentae by Perrin and Sanders[37] and ourselves[38]. Recent work by Mooney and colleagues[39] confirms the relationship between chorionic villous hemorrhage and retroplacental hemorrhage. Nevertheless, in our experience, these intravillous hemorrhages are not specific for placental abruption but can be observed in all conditions with severe fetal distress. These lesions can explain the occurrence of significant fetomaternal hemorrhage with abruptio[40].

Careful examination of the chorionic plate using special stains frequently demonstrates the presence of hemosiderin (iron depositions) (Figure 16). This can represent an isolated finding or, more commonly, be associated with the presence of an acute and/or old marginal placental hematoma. Other authors have also observed histological evidence of old intrauterine bleeding and its frequent association to prematurity[41]. Although this finding is more frequently seen in the third trimester, it is also present in the first and second trimesters as mentioned in Table 1. Such a morphological findings lends support to the concept that premature separation of the placenta, in particular marginal placental hematoma, may occur as a single or repeated event.

In addition, placental abruption in the third trimester frequently showed the presence of a uteroplacental circulation pathology in absence of physiological change (Figure 17).

Except for occasional case reports, few studies have been published using Doppler

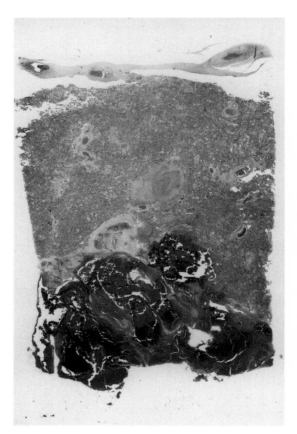

Figure 14 *Histological examination (Figure 13) demonstrated the presence of dilatation of venous sinuses associated with dissecting hemorrhage of the decidua. Hematoxylin–eosin, × 2.4*

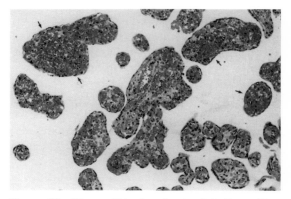

Figure 15 *Placental histology showing foci of intravillous hemorrhages (arrows). Twin pregnancy delivered by Cesarean section after unsuccessful tocolysis at 28 weeks' gestation. Gross examination showed a marginal hematoma and histology demonstrated the presence of a bilateral chorioamnionitis. Hematoxylin–eosin, × 76.6*

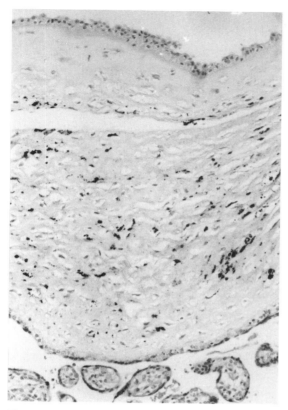

Figure 16 *Histology of chorionic plate shows extensive iron deposition. Gross examination of the placenta showed a sub-acute marginal hematoma. Patient delivered by Cesarean section at 26 weeks of gestation for oligohydramnios and pathological cardiotocogram. Prussian blue, × 71.0*

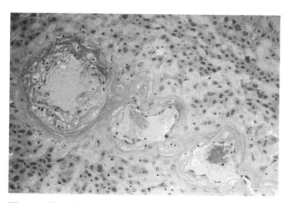

Figure 17 *Histology of decidual samples shows an acute atherosis affecting the decidual portion of the spiral arteries. Gross examination of the placenta revealed a retroplacental hematoma. Patient delivered by Cesarean section at 28 weeks' gestation for decompensated pre-eclampsia. Hematoxylin–eosin, × 76.6*

velocimetry in the surveillance of late pregnancies with clinical suspicion of placental abruption. Malcus and colleagues[38] reported an increased risk for placental abruption if the arcuate and/or umbilical artery flow velocity waveforms were abnormal in patients with third-trimester hemorrhage. A correlation between Doppler velocimetry and morphological examination of the placenta showed that patients with placental centrocotyledon hemorrhages and infarction had more often abnormal umbilical artery flow velocity waveforms at the onset of symptoms. Furthermore, more frequent abnormal arcuate artery flow velocity waveforms were found among those with placental infarction alone. These relationships, however, had disappeared at the final examination before delivery. Similarly to in the first trimester, a possible explanation of these findings is that vessels are read by Doppler velocimetry as pathological as long as there is a flow. If the pathology affecting the fetoplacental and uteroplacental circulation progresses and is severe enough to completely obstruct the lumen, these vessels cease to be read by Doppler velocimetry.

Finally, small for gestational age fetuses were significantly more common when placental morphology showed ischemia, centrocotyledon hemorrhages and infarction or infarction alone.

PHYSIOPATHOLOGY AND CLINICAL SIGNIFICANCE

Independent of its clinical presentation, and whether partial or complete, abruptio placentae or premature separation presents as a detachment of the placenta from its decidual bed. This process can be accompanied by the classical clinical presentation or remain clinically silent.

Table 3 summarizes the main morphological conclusions based on the correlation between the clinical, sonographic and morphological findings in abruptio placentae. However the etiology and pathogenesis of this disorder remains a matter of controversy.

Notwithstanding, there is growing evidence that a significant number of placental abruptions can result from a pathology of the venous

441

Table 3 *Main morphological conclusions*

Marginal or retroplacental hematoma with dissection into intervillous space and/or villous ischemia/infarction

Venous sinuses congestion and thrombosis
Focal decidual necrosis with inflammatory reaction
Focal decidual dissecting hemorrhage

Single or repeated event (hemosiderin and/or organization of hematoma)

UPC pathology (arteries) probably related to associated pathology (PIH, IUGR)

Blood flow changes can be secondary to compression of spiral arteries by the SCH, spiral artery necrosis (decidual necrosis) or secondary to associated pathology (PIH, IUGR)

UPC, uteroplacental circulation; PIH, pregnancy induced hypertension; IUGR, intrauterine growth retardation; SCH, subchorionic hematoma

uteroplacental circulation[7,17]. Increases in venous pressure, predominantly caused by obstruction of the venous drainage, probably play a major role in the development of this hemorrhagic pathology. However, the precise trigger for the rupture of venous structures remains unknown and local anatomical variations in configuration may be implicated[7]. In this context, there remains to be elucidated the role played by the decidual necrosis and inflammation as a source of vasoactive chemical mediators[19,34].

There is no doubt that an abnormal arterial uteroplacental circulation is associated with placental abruption in cases combined with other risk factors such as hypertension, pregnancy induced hypertension, intrauterine growth retardation, smoking and drug abuse. Nevertheless there are no conclusive data to demonstrate that poor trophoblastic invasion of spiral arteries is present in abruptio placentae from clinically uncomplicated pregnancies.

Both published data and that discussed in this chapter clearly show that premature separation of the normally-situated gestational sac and placenta can occur at any time during gestation. A correlation between sonographic and morphological findings has clearly defined the

pathology of marginal/retroplacental hematoma (subchorionic hematoma of the literature). The clinical experience in the literature[6,10,14] as well as our own indicates that significant placental abruption in the first trimester is frequently accompanied by clinical bleeding. This further confirms the reported poor outcome associated with first-trimester vaginal bleeding[10]. The same applies to mid-trimester bleeding which shows the highest perinatal mortality rate when associated with placental abruption[42]. Nevertheless, a significant number of embryonic deaths can occur in the presence of occult subchorionic bleeding. In fact, a careful morphological examination reveals more such cases than expected by clinical findings alone (Laurini, unpublished work).

Moreover, the morphological findings suggest that poor pregnancy outcome is related to the presence of marginal hematomas with extension into the placenta. This underlines the importance of sonographic findings that can allow for a differential diagnosis between this type of subchorionic hemorrhage and similar sonographic images from more benign conditions[14,16].

The occasional presence of hemosiderin in the first-trimester specimens also indicates repeated episodes of bleeding. Furthermore, both first-trimester vaginal bleeding and/or hemosiderin in the chorionic plate can be seen in cases of abruptio placentae occurring in mid- or third trimester. This suggests that abruptio placentae can represent a continuous process showing multiple episodes of bleeding that can already have started in early pregnancy.

Finally, it is also important to underline, once again, the existence of two types of abruptio placentae: that associated with an infection and that associated with a decidual vasculopathy. One can go even further and propose a group that is primarily chemically mediated and the other that is primarily mediated by a decidual vasculopathy. After all there is supporting evidence that placental abruption seen with infections is chemically mediated[19,21,22,33,34]. Moreover decidual necrosis and related inflammatory response can play a major role, even in the absence of infection[34].

The findings discussed in this chapter further demonstrate the clinical significance of the infected amniotic fluid syndrome and of chorioamnionitis as its morphological expression. This is particularly so for the midtrimester but also applies for the third trimester (Figures 12 and 15). Moreover, the relationship between the use of prostaglandins for induction of labor and a possible development of an abruptio placentae and sudden unexpected fetal death merits further studies.

References

1. Nyberg, D. A., Cyr, D. R., Mack, L. A., Wilson, D. A. and Shuman, W. P. (1987). Sonographic spectrum of placental abruption. *Am. J. Roentgenol.*, **148**, 161–4
2. Kay, H. H. and Spritzer, C. E. (1991). Preliminary experience with magnetic resonance imaging in patients with third-trimester bleeding. *Obstet. Gynecol.*, **78**, 424–9
3. Benirschke, K. and Gille, J. (1977). Placental pathology and asphyxia. In Gluck, L. (ed.) *Intrauterine Asphyxia and the Developing Fetal Brain*, (Chicago: Year Book Medical Publishers)
4. Abdella, T. N., Sibai, B. M., Hays, J. M. Jr and Anderson, G. D. (1984). Relationship of hypertensive disease to abruptio placentae. *Obstet. Gynecol.*, **63**, 365–70
5. Voigt, L. F., Hollenbach, K. A., Krohn, M. A., Daling, J. R. and Hickok, D. E. (1990). The relationship of abruptio placentae with maternal smoking and small for gestational age infants. *Obstet. Gynecol.*, **75**, 771–4
6. Krohn, M., Voigt, L., McKnight, B., Daling, J. R., Starzyk, P. and Benedetti, T. J. (1987). Correlates of placental abruption. *Br. J. Obstet. Gynaecol.*, **94**, 333–40
7. Harris, B. A. (1988). Peripheral placental separation: a review. *Obstet. Gynecol. Surv.*, **43**, 577–81
8. McLlewaine, G. M., Hawat, R. C. L., Dunne, F. and McNaughton, M. C. (1979). The Scottish perinatal mortality survey. *Br. Med. J.*, **2**, 1103–6
9. Buckell, E. W. C. and Wood, B. S. B. (1985). Wessex perinatal mortality survey 1982. *Br. J. Obstet. Gynaecol.*, **92**, 550–8
10. Williams, M. A., Mittendorf, R., Leiberman, E. and Monson, R. R. (1991). Adverse infant outcomes associated with first-trimester vaginal bleeding. *Obstet. Gynecol.*, **78**, 14–18
11. Eriksen, G., Wohlert, M., Ersbak, V., Hvidman, L., Hedegaard, M. and Skajaa, K. (1991). Placental abruption. A case-control investigation. *Br. J. Obstet. Gynaecol.*, **98**, 448–52
12. Laurini, R. N. (1986). *Aspects in Developmental Pathology*, pp. 11–33. (Groningen: Drukkerij van denderen BV)
13. Pearlstone, M. and Baxi, I. (1993). Subchorionic hematoma: a review. *Obstet. Gynecol. Surv.*, **48**, 65–8
14. Dickey, R. P., Olar, T. T., Curole, D. N., Taylor, S. N. and Matulich, E. M. (1992). Relationship of first-trimester subchorionic bleeding detected by color Doppler ultrasound to subchorionic fluid, clinical bleeding, and pregnancy outcome. *Obstet. Gynecol.*, **80**, 415–20
15. Sauerbrei, E. E. and Pham, D. H. (1986). Placental abruption and subchorionic hemorrhage in the first half of pregnancy: US appearance and clinical outcome. *Radiology*, **160**, 109–12
16. Abu-Yousef, M. M., Bleicher, J. J., Williamson, R. A. and Weiner, C. P. (1987). Subchorionic hemorrhage: sonographic diagnosis and clinical significance. *Am. J. Roentgenol.*, **149**, 737–40
17. Laurini, R. N. and Akalin-Sel, T. (1993). Placental changes and prostaglandins. *J. Matern. Fetal Invest.*, **3**, 177
18. Darby, M. J., Caritis, S. N. and Shen-Schwarz, S. (1989). Placental abruption in the preterm gestation: an association with chorioamnionitis. *Obstet. Gynecol.*, **74**, 88–92
19. Lopez Bernal, A., Hansell, D. J., Khong, T. Y., Keeling, J. W. and Turnbull, A. C. (1989). Prostaglandin E production by the fetal membranes in unexplained preterm labour and preterm labour associated with chorioamnionitis. *Br. J. Obstet. Gynaecol.*, **96**, 1133–9
20. Laurini, R. N. and Akalin-Sel, T. (1993). Brain lesions and prostaglandins. *J. Matern. Fetal Invest.*, **3**, 176
21. Bejar, R., Curbelo, V., Davis, C. and Gluck, L. (1981). Premature labor. II. Bacterial sources of phospholipase. *Obstet. Gynecol.*, **57**, 479–82
22. Lamont, R. F., Rose, M. and Elder, M. G. (1985). Effect of bacterial products on prostaglandin E production by amnion cells. *Lancet*, **2**, 1331–3
23. Quinn, M. A. and Murphy, A. J. (1981). Fetal death following extra-amniotic prostaglandin gel: report of two cases. *Br. J. Obstet. Gynaecol.*, **88**, 650–1

24. Stewart, P. and Calder, A. A. (1981). Cervical ripening (letter). *Br. J. Obstet. Gynaecol.*, **88**, 1071–2

25. Leung, A., Kwok, P. and Chang, A. (1987). Association between prostaglandin E2 and placental abruption. *Br. J. Obstet. Gynaecol.*, **94**, 1001–2

26. Laurini, R. N. (1994). Fetal brain pathology. In Kurjak, A. and Chervenak, F. A. (eds.) *The Fetus as a Patient*, pp. 89–106. (Carnforth, UK: Parthenon Publishing)

27. Spinillo, A., Fazzi, E., Stronati, M., Ometto, A., Capuzzo, E. and Guaschino, S. (1994). Early morbidity and neurodevelopmental outcome in low-birthweight infants born after third trimester bleeding. *Am. J. Perinatol.*, **11**, 85–90

28. Gibbs, J. M. and Weindling, A. M. (1994). Neonatal intracranial lesions following placental abruption. *Eur. J. Ped.*, **153**, 195–7

29. Laurini, R. N. (1990). Abortion from a morphological viewpoint. In Huisjes, H. J. and Lind, T. (eds.) *Early Pregnancy Failure*, pp. 79–113. (Edinburgh: Churchill Livingstone)

30. Arias, F., Rodriques, L., Rayne, S. C. and Kraus, F. T. (1993). Maternal placental vasculopathy and infection: two distinct subgroups among patients with preterm labor and preterm ruptured membranes. *Am. J. Obstet. Gynecol.*, **168**, 585–91

31. Kurjak, A., Zudenigo, D. and Kupesic, S. Subchorionic hematomas in early pregnancy: clinical outcome and blood flow patterns.

32. Laurini, R. (1995). Abruptio placenta: from early pregnancy to term. *Ultrasound Obstet. Gynecol.*, **6** (suppl. 2), 37

33. Romero, R., Sirtori, M., Oyarzun, E., Avila, C., Mazor, M., Callahan, R., Sabo, V., Athanassiadis, A. P. and Hobbins, J. C. (1989). Infection and labor. V. Prevalence, microbiology, and clinical significance of intraamniotic infection in women with preterm labor and intact membranes. *Am. J Obstet. Gynecol.*, **161**, 817–24

34. Romero, R., Wu, Y. K., Brody, D. T., Oyarzun, E., Duff, G. W. and Durum, S. K. (1989). Human decidua; a source of interleukin-1. *Obstet. Gynecol.*, **73**, 31–4

35. Valentin, L., Sladkevicius, P., Laurini, R., Söderberg, H., Olofsson, P. and Marsal, K. (1995). Effect of a prostaglandin E1 analogue (gemeprost) on uterine and luteal circulation in normal first trimester pregnancies. A Doppler velocimetry study. *Eur. J. Obstet. Gynecol. Reprod. Biol.*, **59**, 25–34

36. Spinillo, A., Capuzzo, E., Colonna, L., Solerte, L, Nicila, S. and Guaschino, S. (1994). Factors associated with abruptio placentae in preterm deliveries. *Acta Obstet. Gynecol. Scand.*, **73**, 307–12

37. Perrin, E. D. V. K. and Sanders, C. H. (1984). Introduction: how to examine the placenta and why. In Perrin, E. D. V. K. (ed.) *Pathology of the Placenta*, pp. 1–36. (New York: Churchill Livingstone)

38. Malcus, P., Laurini, R. and Marsal, K. (1992). Doppler blood flow changes and placental morphology in pregnancies with third trimester hemorrhage. *Acta Obstet. Gynecol. Scand.*, **71**, 39–45

39. Mooney, E. E., Al Shunnar, A., O'Regan, M. and Gillan, J. E. (1994). Chorionic villous haemorrhage is associated with retroplacental haemorrhage. *Br. J. Obstet. Gynaecol.*, **101**, 965–9

40. Cardwell, M. S. (1987). Ultrasound diagnosis of abruptio placentae with fetomaternal hemorrhage. *Am. J. Obstet. Gynecol.*, **157**, 358–9

41. Salafia, C. M., Lopez-Zeno, J. A., Sherer, D. M., Whittington, S. S., Minior, V. K. and Vintzileos, A. M. (1995). Histological evidence of old intrauterine bleeding is more frequent in prematurity. *Am. J. Obstet. Gynecol.*, **173**, 1065–70

42. Nielson, E. C., Varner, M. W. and Scott, J. R. (1991). The outcome of pregnancies complicated by bleeding during the second trimester. *Surg. Gynecol. Obstet.*, **173**, 371–4

Systematic antenatal functional evaluation in pregnancies at risk of progressive abruptio placentae

34

B. Arabin, R. Aardenburg and J. van Eyck

INTRODUCTION

Abruptio placentae is a disease with an incidence of around 0.1–2%, but it is responsible for approximately 15–25% of perinatal deaths[1]. This variation in incidence reflects differences in hospital populations relating not only to sociodemographic factors and longitudinal lifestyle variations[2], but also to difficulties with either the prenatal diagnosis or the postnatal 'gold standard'.

Evidence of abruptio was detected in approximately 4–5% of all placentas suggesting that small episodes may occur more often than expected[3]. However, there have been few attempts to correlate pre- and postnatal morphological findings, such as placental findings or neonatal and maternal morbidity.

Abruptio placentae may be the result of hemorrhage into the decidua basalis leading to separation and possibly to maternal disseminated intravascular coagulation or shock. In subchorionic hematomas in the first and second trimesters, invasion into the villous chorion, ischemic intervillitis and iron depositions in the membranous chorion are found. Abruptio of the third-trimester placenta can manifest itself in a wide variety of ways including: no significant changes, focal intervillous hemorrhage, marginal or retroplacental hematoma and lesions in the decidua suggesting that the venous circulation may play a role in the pathogenesis[4].

Chorionic villous hemorrhage is regarded as a disturbance of fetal vascular dynamics preceding retroplacental hemorrhage and possibly triggering abruptio[5].

Abruptio placentae is one of the most severe environmental threats to the fetus reflected by high rates of perinatal mortality and morbidity because

(1) The general and individual etiology remains unknown in most cases;

(2) There are almost no possibilities of general or specific prevention;

(3) The onset may be concealed, with misinterpreted early symptoms;

(4) It may be combined with fetal anemia, fetal hypoxia and prematurity of the newborn;

(5) The possibly acute onset does not allow fetal adaptation;

(6) Even if suspected there are no real options for causal or symptomatic therapy;

(7) Expectant monitoring to improve fetal maturity in selected cases, requires intensive monitoring ('active postponement') but is still combined with maternal and fetal risks.

Retroplacental hemorrhage provokes early symptoms which may be confused with preterm labor, however, bleeding is suspicious. The classification of abruptio placentae of grade 0–3[6], which is still used in the literature today, was the state of the art already in 1954. It reflects the inadequate approach to clinical consequences and early typical symptoms.

(1) Grade 0, asymptomatic;

(2) Grade 1, vaginal bleeding, uterine tenderness may be present without signs of maternal shock or fetal distress;

(3) Grade 2–3, external bleeding may or may not be present, without maternal shock, but signs of fetal distress (grade 2) or persistent abdominal pain and shock, possible maternal coagulopathy and fetal demise (grade 3).

At stages 2–3 the fetus may be in such a poor condition that the main concerns are directed towards treatment of severe maternal complications.

Due to late onset of acute symptoms, careful evaluation with time-consuming methods is often not appropriate. In fact, every minute shortening the time lag from hospital admission to final delivery might improve long-term prospects for the infant[1]. This has resulted in the concentration on emergency measures rather than on differential diagnosis for the selection of management options. Early diagnosis might help to prevent emergency conditions. At an early gestational age it may be possible to make decisions which may give the very premature fetus a chance to stay or even recover *in utero* and thus maintain her or his life quality.

CLINICAL EXPERIENCE

Overall study group

Since abruptio placentae frequently is an unexpected event, there have been only a few prospective studies. During our observation period the incidence of severe abruptio was 41/4166 deliveries. In all cases there was an adherent macroscopic clot covering more than 10% of the maternal placental surface area based on the maximum surface area of the clot/crater. Nearly half of the pregnancies ($n = 20$) were transferred from home or smaller hospitals where some had been admitted for the following reasons: premature rupture of membranes (PROM), vaginal bleeding and/or uterine tetany at a final stage. They presented as 'emergency cases' at admission (grade 2–3). In eight of the transferred pregnancies maternal symptoms were less severe with varying signs of fetal demise (grade 1–2). In those cases Doppler, real-time ultrasound, actocardiotocography and laboratory values were evaluated and Cesarean

section was indicated on the same or on the following day.

In ten pregnancies abruptio occurred during hospital admission. These patients had all been followed by longitudinal laboratory and biophysical monitoring. Twenty-four pregnancies served as controls presenting with similar symptoms at admission. In three cases delivery was postponed for more than 6 weeks even though there were large echolucent placental areas combined with clinical and laboratory signs of abruptio. The total study group is summarized in Table 1.

Emergency transfer with abruptio placentae grade 2–3

In cases with grade 2–3 ($n = 20$), the mean gestational age at admission was 30 weeks + 2 days ranging between 23 weeks + 5 days and 39 weeks.

In four cases the fetuses had died antenatally and labor was induced immediately. Four mothers delivered vaginally due to progressive dilatation. In 12 cases an emergency Cesarean section was performed, which revealed eight mothers to have a Couvelaire uterus. The mean pH value in the umbilical artery of the live-born infants was 7.1 (6.6–7.3), mean Apgar values after 1 and 5 min were 4 (0–8) and 6 (0–9) respectively, and the mean birth weight was 1450 g (450–3400 g). The perinatal mortality was 6/20. Intracranial hemorrhage grade 2–3 and bronchopulmonary dysplasia were diagnosed in three and two of the infants, respectively.

Primary observation

Not only the poor prognosis for affected fetuses but also the following incidental observation challenged us to follow patients at risk more systematically with combined biophysical and biochemical examinations.

One mother was transferred to our center with intrauterine growth retardation (IUGR) and PROM. Gestational age was 26 weeks and 4 days. Following our protocols for threatening hypoxia we detected: poor uteroplacental blood

SAFE IN PROGRESSIVE ABRUPTIO PLACENTAE

Table 1 Subgroups of the study population with abruptio placentae. Ranges in parentheses

Study group	Supervision	n	Gestational age at admission (weeks + days)	Gestational age at delivery (weeks + days)	Interval between admission and delivery (days)	Birth weight (g)	pH of umbilical artery	1-min Apgar score	5-min Apgar score	Perinatal death
Emergency transfers	no evaluation	20	30 + 2 (23 + 5–39)	30 + 2 (23 + 5 – 39)	0 (0–1)	1450 (450–3400)	7.1 (6.6–7.3)	4 (0–8)	6 (0–9)	6/20
Severe risk of progressive abruptio	only one evaluation	8	31 + 1 (25 + 3–36 + 2)	31 + 2 (25 + 4–36 + 2)	1 (0–2)	1486 (760–2410)	7.15 (6.90–7.40)	5 (2–9)	8 (6–10)	1/8
Moderate risk of progressive abruptio	longitudinal evaluation	10	29 + 5 (26 + 1–36 + 3)	30 + 4 (26 + 5–37)	7 (1–20)	1358 (640–2630)	7.13 (6.75–7.31)	6 (1–8)	8 (4–10)	2/10
Moderate risk (controls)	longitudinal evaluation	24	29 + 4 (24–37 + 3)	33 + 3 (27 + 2–39 + 5)	20 (1–61)	2132 (650–4140)	7.29 (7.17–7.43)	8 (3–10)	9 (6–10)	1/24
Severe risk, expectant monitoring	longitudinal evaluation	3	26 (25 + 4–26 + 4)	33 + 6 (33 + 5–34 + 1)	55 (50–60)	1985 (1830–2140)	7.23 (7.21–7.24)	6 (5–7)	10 (9–10)	0/3

447

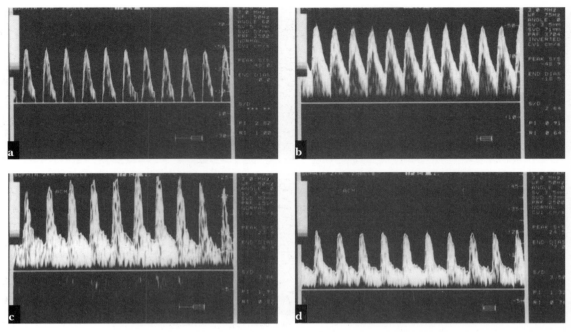

Figure 1 *Doppler velocity waveforms of the umbilical artery at admission (a) and day 2 (b), and the middle cerebral artery at admission (c) and day 2 (d), in a pregnancy with progressive abruptio placentae.*

Table 2 *Semiquantitative biophysical evaluation in progressive abruptio placentae (systematic antenatal functional evaluation (SAFE) score)*

Variables	2 points	1 point	0 point
Doppler uterine arteries	normal	1 × notch	2 × notches
Contractions	none	irregular	regular
Doppler cerebral arteries	PI > 10th centile, ΔPI < 15%	PI > 5th centile and < 10th centile, ΔPI > 15% and < 25%	PI < 5th centile, ΔPI > 25%
Doppler umbilical arteries	PI > 50th centile with brain sparing, ΔPI < 15%	PI > 25th centile and < 50th centile with brain sparing, ΔPI > 15% and < 25%	PI < 25th centile with brain sparing, ΔPI > 25%
FHR pattern	normal	suspicious	pathological
Sonography	normal	echolucent < 4 cm	echolucent > 4 cm

FHR, fetal heart rate; PI, pulsatility index

flow (notches in both uterine arteries), poor umbilical blood flow (zero flow in both umbilical arteries), high cerebral blood flow (pulsatility index (PI) < 10th centile in the internal carotid artery (ICA) and the middle cerebral artery (MCA)) (Figure 1), however, we also detected the presence of fetal reflexes and movements and an uneventful actocardiotocogram.

The following day, contractions increased, which was primarily interpreted as a consequence of PROM. Doppler velocimetry revealed an increase of end diastolic blood flow in the cerebral and umbilical arteries (Figure 1). Simultaneously echolucency was recognized. Due to deterioration of fetal heart rate (FHR) tracing a Cesarean section was indicated. Postnatal investigation revealed retroplacental hematoma. The infant, weighing 720 g, developed normally after an uneventful stay at the neonatal intensive care unit.

Protocol

We observed an increase of end diastolic blood flow in the umbilical artery reflected by a decrease of the PI simultaneously with an increase of end diastolic blood flow velocities in cerebral arteries. This phenomenon was called 'paradoxical fetal blood flow pattern'. The definition of paradoxical blood flow was also applied to cases when the first measurement of high end-diastolic velocities in the cerebral arteries, indicating fetal hypoxia, was combined with normal or high end-diastolic velocity in the umbilical artery in patients with signs of abruptio when delivery was indicated too soon to perform further examinations.

For semiquantitative analysis, the phenomenon of paradoxical blood flow has been integrated with classical biophysical examinations into a scoring system (Table 2). In detail, the cerebral circulation is measured by color Doppler velocimetry of the internal carotid and middle cerebral arteries (*normal*, PI > 10th centile or ΔPI of longitudinal measurements < 15%; *suspicious*, PI < 10th > 5th centile or ΔPI > 15 < 25%; *pathological*, PI < 5th centile or ΔPI > 25%), blood flow in the umbilical arteries is analyzed by color Doppler velocimetry of the mean of both arteries (*normal*, PI > 50th centile combined with brain sparing or ΔPI < 15%; *suspicious*, PI > 25th < 50th centile combined with brain sparing or ΔPI > 15% < 25%; *pathological*, PI < 25th centile combined with brain sparing, ΔPI > 25%). *Uterine blood flow* is detected by color Doppler velocimetry of uterine arteries (*normal*, no diastolic notch; *suspicious*, notch in one uterine artery; *pathological*, notch in both uterine arteries), *contractions* are documented by external tocography (*normal*, no contractions; *suspicious*, irregular contractions; *pathological*, regular contractions or tetany), the *FHR pattern* registered by actocardiography is analyzed according to variability and reactivity, although an improvement could be achieved by using computerized FHR analysis; *the structure of the placenta is* determined by ultrasound (*normal*, no obvious hematoma; *suspicious*, echolucent area > 2 cm < 4 cm; *pathological*, echolucent area > 4 cm).

If time permits, in cases with signs of abruptio placentae, Doppler measurements of the maximal velocity in the aorta ascendens to detect the degree of anemia and ratios of the ductus venosus to determine the degree of hypoxia are also performed. However, these measurements are not integrated in the 'SAFE-score' for abruptio placentae since they are supposed to individualize specific patterns of the disease.

Biochemical results to detect blood loss and the degree of disseminated intravascular coagulation including hemoglobin count, platelets, fibrinogen, fibrinogen degradation products or antithrombin III can also be classified according to standard definitions of absolute values and significant changes during subsequent measurements. Monoclonal anti-bodies specific for cross-linked fibrin degradation and fibrin degradation may be more specific in the prediction of abruptio placentae[7], although we do not yet have data.

Vaginal bleeding, contractions and/or tetany with progressive fetal distress

The case described was a stimulus to investigate fetal blood flow redistribution in combination with standard measurements in pregnancies with clinically suspected abruptio, using the definition of a high end-diastolic blood flow in cerebral arteries (PI < 10th centile) combined with normal or high end-diastolic blood flow velocities in the umbilical arteries (PI < 50th centile). In all eight patients with acute signs of abruptio when delivery was indicated before longitudinal examinations could be performed, we confirmed this phenomenon (Figure 2).

In all eight cases there were pathological blood flow patterns in the uterine arteries, increased frequency of contractions and an impairment of the FHR pattern. In five of eight cases there was even echolucency of > 2 cm. The average score value before delivery was 5.

Vague symptoms without fetal distress at admission

Biophysical examinations and biochemical tests were performed at regular intervals in patients

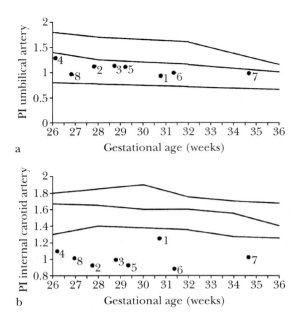

Figure 2 *Pulsatility index (PI) values of the umbilical artery (a) and the internal cerebral artery (b) in pregnancies with abruptio before delivery (n = 8). Top line, 90th centile; middle line, 50th centile; bottom line, 10th centile*

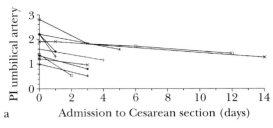

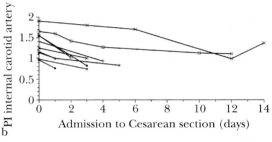

Figure 3 *Course of pulsatility index (PI) of the umbilical artery (a) and of the internal carotid artery (b) in pregnancies with progressive abruptio from admission to delivery (n = 10)*

with warning signs of abruptio. In this group with vaginal bleeding, contractions and/or PROM and/or severe pre-eclampsia and hemolysis, elevated liver enzymes and low platelet count (HELLP) syndrome we have followed ten pregnancies which finally developed abruptio placentae.

The course of umbilical and internal carotid artery blood flow measurements is demonstrated in Figure 3. In all ten patients with consecutive examinations the mean decrease of the PI in the umbilical and internal carotid arteries between admission and delivery were 35% and 30%, respectively, with a mean time interval of 4 days. All ten patients had pathological blood flow values of the uterine arteries. Echolucency was not diagnosed at admission, however, it was detected in seven of the ten cases before delivery.

This group was matched with a control group of, to date, 24 pregnancies of mothers who were also admitted due to vaginal bleeding in combination with contractions and/or PROM and/or severe pre-eclampsia and HELLP syndrome.

Sensitivity and specificity for several cut-off levels were calculated. Receiver operator statistics demonstrated that biophysical evaluation of the combined results of the environment and the fetal response was superior to indirect laboratory tests not only before delivery, but also at admission when clinical symptoms were still vague (Figure 4).

Early onset abruptio placentae, active prolongation and stabilization

To date three pregnancies have been transferred at an early gestational age of around 26 weeks with signs of abruptio in which delivery was postponed for more than 6 weeks. The predominant symptoms were vaginal bleeding and uterine tenderness.

At admission large subchorionic hypo-echogenic areas were detected (Figure 5a). Laboratory findings indicated various degrees of disseminated coagulative disturbances with positive fibrinogen degradation products (0.5–18 mg/l) in all cases, low fibrinogen (1–2.5 g/l) and low platelets (111–140 × 10^9/l). Pathological blood flow in the uterine arteries was present in all cases, there was even negative

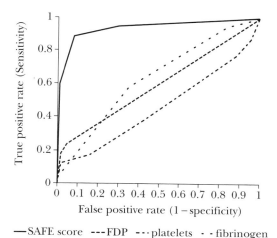

—SAFE score ---FDP ···platelets · ·fibrinogen

Figure 4 *Receiver operator characteristics (ROC) of the biophysical score combined with biochemical parameters to detect fetal abruptio (values at admission, n = 42, 18 cases with abruptio placentae and 24 controls). SAFE, systematic antenatal fetal evaluation; FDP, fibrinogen degradation products*

uterine flow in one case associated with increased tone (Figure 5c). In the same pregnancy maternal and fetal signs of anemia (high maximum velocity in the fetal aorta ascendens) were detected and blood transfusions to the mother were administered. Doppler velocimetry further revealed high maximum end diastolic velocities (PI < 10th centile) in the cerebral arteries and normal end diastolic velocities in the umbilical arteries in all fetuses. After informed consent the parents accepted expectant monitoring due to prematurity of an average of 25 weeks (range: 24 weeks + 5 days–26 weeks + 3 days). Corticoids and nifedipine were administered and the mothers had strict bed rest. Close hand-on monitoring during the first hours and days revealed increasing movements, increasing FHR variability and reversal of the paradoxal blood flow pattern parallel to normalization of laboratory values within the first 2 weeks. The maximal blood flow velocity in the aorta ascendens also decreased in one case within

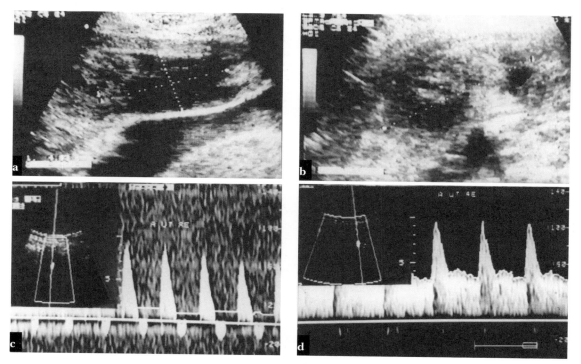

Figure 5 *Course of placental echolucency, at admission at 26 weeks (a) and at 32 weeks after stabilization (b), and uterine blood flow at admission at 26 weeks (c) and after stabilization at 32 weeks (d), in one of the three cases with expectant monitoring and severe subchorionic hematoma*

the first few days. Subchorionic hematomas remained or changed from echolucent to echogenic areas (Figure 5b), even the uterine Doppler velocity waveforms normalized with decreasing tenderness (Figure 5d). All three mothers were sent back to their referral hospital at 34 weeks with normalized laboratory and Doppler values. There they delivered uneventfully. Mean gestational age at delivery was 35 (34 weeks + 4 days–36 weeks + 1 day) weeks.

DISCUSSION

Primarily we have studied severely threatened pregnancies to be able to more readily respond to conditions when the fetus is still at moderate risk or expectant management may be possible. Only clinical experience may leave us alone finding better options for the fetus. Therefore, we have integrated biophysical functional observations with the advantage of results reflecting actual threat and fetal adaptation in the course of abruptio.

Laboratory values indicating local or general coagulation disorders are investigated in patients with suspected abruptio placentae. As abruptio progresses and placental site hemorrhage increases, local consumption of coagulation factors is responsible for clot formation, stabilization and lysis. Fibrinogen, in the presence of platelets or tissue phospholipids, is converted to fibrin which may occlude defects in vessels or tissue. Raised fibrinogen degradation products and increased soluble fibrin complexes may be found[7]. At advanced stages fibrinogen and platelet levels decrease. Although the degree of placental separation and of placental bleeding is somehow related to consumption of coagulation factors, the uncertainty as to how fast the process proceeds and the time lag between etiology, determination and result reduces the diagnostic value for the fetus.

Static ultrasonic imaging detects echolucent areas. The sensitivity depends to a large degree on the site of the bleeding. Marginal attachments have been correctly diagnosed in approximately 60% of symptomatic pregnancies with vaginal bleeding. Nevertheless correct diagnosis has been difficult in cases with retro-placental hematoma, when its echogenic image may be similar to that of a normal placenta and the presentation varies[8]. In large studies visualization of retroplacental hematoma only had a sensitivity of 29%. Anatomically small echolucent areas functionally can lead to severe threats for the fetus and, vice versa, placentas with large echolucent areas may still allow the fetus to cope. Thus, not to react because no echolucency is detected or, vice versa, to panic when large echolucent areas are observed can both be wrong decisions for the long-term future of the fetus.

Pathological blood flow waveforms in the uterine arteries have been described as being associated with abruptio placentae as with pre-eclampsia. Indeed it was diagnosed in all our cases with abruptio indicating chronic hypoxia in the placental bed and later increased tenderness and compression[9]. In addition to primary functional or morphological changes in uteroplacental vessels, which may be an etiological cause of abruptio, uterine compensatory mechanisms, as a response to small insults of decidual hemorrhage, impair uterine blood flow and thus tissue hypoxia and placental infarction. Nevertheless, only a small number of all patients demonstrating pathological uterine blood flow will later develop abruptio placentae. Therefore this parameter may be regarded more as an early risk factor than a specific warning sign. However, it might have high diagnostic value for excluding risks that may lead to the development of abruptio.

Tocography is an immediate direct tool used to diagnose contractions and even tetany. Certain uterine contraction patterns, such as low amplitude, high frequency and high frequency high amplitude contractions (irritable uterus) or increased tone, have been characterized in pregnancies with abruptio. However, none of these patterns has developed to be specific for abruptio to differentiate between threatening premature or prodromal term labor.

FHR monitoring is widely used to detect signs of fetal demise. Frequent FHR monitoring can assist in the detection of placental abruptio even before clinical signs become apparent[10]. Using the computerized sonic aid system in a group of women with pre-eclampsia the course of fetal heart rate variability was detected to be specific for abruptio if there were tracings with a mean minute range of < 20 ms shortly before delivery or if there was an intermediate increase to a mean minute range of > 20 ms within 12–6 h prior to delivery with a terminal drop immediately before delivery. Decelerations were extremely rare in the abruptio group occurring in only two of 30 cases in women with deteriorating minute range[10].

The relatively high variation in the abruptio subgroup may result from increased levels of catecholamines which gradually overcome the vagus stimulation[11].

Doppler velocimetry of the fetal circulation has been widely used to specify fetal risks in IUGR or uninterpretable FHR tracings. In pregnancies with increasing fetal hypoxia we would have expected increasing end diastolic velocities in the cerebral arteries and simultaneously decreasing end diastolic velocities in the umbilical arteries reflecting centralization of the fetal circulation[12]. Fetal blood flow centralization with high end diastolic velocities in cerebral arteries and low, 'zero' or reverse flow in the umbilical arteries is specific for fetal hypoxia and acidemia[13]. Umbilical velocity waveforms are believed to reflect changes in vascular resistance[14]. Conversely, the increased end diastolic umbilical blood flow in pregnancies with progressive abruptio might reflect a decreased downstream impedance caused by mechanical or humoral factors. Simultaneous increase of the maximal velocity in the aorta ascendens, as we observed in some of our cases and all cerebral vessels, might also reflect a hyperdynamic circulation as described in anemic fetuses. Considering the course of our pregnancies with 'active postponement' in pregnancies with early onset abruptio, subchorionic hematoma and coagulative disorders, the described hemodynamic observations seem to be temporary signs of fetal adaptation which do not necessarily lead to final abruptio and fetal death. In pregnancies with a severe retroplacental clot, however, a dicrotic notch of the umbilical artery waveform was described reflecting the possible tamponade effect or vasoconstriction due to prostaglandin re-

lease[15]. It was postulated that a sudden increase in vascular resistance may be the cause of fetal death. High end diastolic velocities in the umbilical arteries in pregnancies complicated by pre eclampsia and abruptio had up to now already been observed when compared to controls with pre eclampsia alone[8]. This observation has never been further evaluated or incorporated in diagnostic protocols.

Our observations of a rise of end-diastolic blood flow velocity together with a deterioration of the fetal condition have changed our own attitudes and have improved our awareness as regards pregnancies with progressive abruptio and have further helped us to identify patients at risk. A better understanding of the concomitant mechanisms also helps to select and follow pregnancies with early onset abruptio conservatively by active postponement. Our goal is therefore to make further detailed observations in order to specify the etiology and clinical course of abruptio placentae.

SUMMARY

Evaluation protocols for abruptio placentae should take into account independent aspects of the functional changes of environment and fetal organs. Unless we have specific screening tests, as in chronic anemia, or early diagnostic tools, as in chronic placental insufficiency, we have to include tests to detect both eventual and specific risks. Thereby we should be open to new tools and retrospective analysis of our own data.

Laboratory values can indicate disseminated vascular coagulation. At this stage, they can be helpful in differential diagnosis, but not in management decision making when compared to biophysical examination. In contrast to knowledge to date, normal or high end-diastolic velocities in the umbilical arteries or an increase during longitudinal examinations associated with high or increasing end-diastolic velocities in the cerebral vessels may be a warning sign of fetal risk due to abruptio and should not be misinterpreted. Umbilical Doppler measurements alone can be misleading and should always be interpreted in the context of the clinical and multivariate biophysical approach.

Active prolongation of early onset abruptio requires intensive surveillance with frequently performed longitudinal laboratory and biophysical tests interpreted by an experienced obstetrician in a tertiary center. Courage and time-consuming care are prerequisites for good decision making and a successful course in selected cases.

THE FUTURE

Most risk factors of abruptio placentae seem to be compounded by sociodemographic status. At this stage, when there are no defined medical options, sociodemographic prevention programs and counselling of mothers at risk so that they respond to early symptoms should not be neglected. This also holds true for 'environmental fetal diseases', in which an understanding of the etiology, leading to the development of screening programs, is still insufficiently available, except when progressive threats rapidly lead to fetal demise or death.

As described in early onset pre-eclampsia and HELLP syndrome, there might be a variety of underlying immunological, metabolic and mainly vascular disorders. In patients with abruptio of unknown etiology and absence of obstetric risks it therefore seems to be an option to search for other metabolic, coagulative or hemostatic disorders. The prognosis for abruptio placentae, in the discipline of obstetrics, still appears to be poor. In order to rescue fetuses where even the most aware and sporting obstetrician might be too late to rescue fetal life, all efforts should be concentrated on positive attitudes with the goal of a live-born infant with a long-term quality of life.

References

1. Knab, D. R. (1978). Abruptio placentae: an assessment of the time and method of delivery. *Obstet. Gynecol.*, **52**, 625–9
2. Saftlas, A. F., Olson, D. R., Atrash, H. K., Rochat, R. and Rowley, D. (1991). National trends in the incidence of abruptio placentae, 1979–1987. *Obstet. Gynecol.*, **78**, 1081–6
3. Fox, H. (1978). *Pathology of the Placenta.* (London: Saunders)
4. Laurini, R. (1995). Abruptio placentae: from early pregnancy to term. *Ultrasound Obstet. Gynecol.*, **6**. (Suppl. 2) 36
5. Mooney, E. E., Shunnar, A. A., O'Regan, M. and Gillan, J. E. (1994). Chorionic villous haemorrhage is associated with retroplacental haemorrhage. *Br. J. Obstet. Gynaecol.*, **101**, 965–9
6. Page, E. W., King, E. B. and Merril, J. A. (1954). Abruptio placentae: dangers of delayed delivery. *Obstet. Gynecol.*, **3**, 385–93
7. Nolan, T. E., Smith, R. P. and Devoe, L. D. (1993). A rapid test for abruptio placentae: evaluation of a D-dimer latex agglutination slide test. *Am. J. Obstet. Gynecol.*, **169**, 265–9
8. Nyberg, D. A., Cyr, D. R., Mack, L. A., Wilson, D. A. and Shuman, W. P. (1987). Sonographic spectrum of placental abruption. *Am. J. Roentgenol.*, **148**, 161–4
9. Campbell, S., Pearce, J. M. F., Hackett, G. *et al.* (1986). Quantitative assessment of uteroplacental blood flow: early screening test for high risk pregnancies. *Obstet. Gynecol.*, **68**, 649–53
10. Steyn, D. W. and Odendaal, H. J. (1994). Fetal heart rate variability prior to delivery in women with severe hypertension who developed placental abruption. *Br. J. Obstet. Gynaecol.*, **101**, 1005–6
11. Jones, C. T. and Knox-Ritchie, J. W. (1993). The effects of adrenergic blockade on the fetal response to hypoxia. *J. Dev. Phys.*, **5**, 211–22
12. Arabin, B., Bergmann, P. L. and Saling, E. (1987). Simultaneous assessment of blood flow velocity waveforms in uteroplacental vessels, umbilical artery, fetal aorta and common carotid artery. *Fetal Ther.*, **2**, 17–22
13. Bilardo, C. M., Nicolaides, K. H. and Campbell, S. (1990). Doppler measurements of fetal and uteroplacental circulation: relationship with umbilical venous blood gases measured at cordocentesis. *Am. J. Obstet. Gynecol.*, **162**, 115–19
14. Trudinger, B. C., Giles, W. B., Cook, C. M., Bombardieri, J. and Collins, L. (1985). Fetal umbilical artery flow velocity waveforms and placental resistance: clinical significance. *Br. J. Obstet. Gynaecol.*, **92**, 23–30
15. Morrow, R. J. and Knox-Ritchie, J. W. (1988). Uteroplacental and umbilical artery blood velocity waveforms in placental abruption assessed by Doppler ultrasound. Case report. *Br. J. Obstet. Gynaecol.*, **95**, 723–4

What is fetal distress? 35

D. W. Skupski

INTRODUCTION

The term 'fetal distress' has been used for decades to describe a deteriorating status of the fetus when faced with the stress of labor. With the impact of electronic fetal heart rate (FHR) monitoring, many FHR patterns have come to be known as abnormal or pathological, and associated with fetal acidosis; thus the term 'fetal distress'. Electronic fetal monitoring (EFM) has now been in widespread use for the last 20 years or more; a large body of data has been accrued attesting to its use, abuse and ability to detect the fetus in jeopardy. Particularly in the last 10 years, our ability to diagnose the decompensating fetus in labor has improved tremendously. Data are now beginning to accrue that EFM may be beneficial in decreasing perinatal mortality and morbidity. This chapter will review: (1) the history of the development of EFM; (2) the problems of terminology regarding 'fetal distress' and 'asphyxia'; (3) the current thinking regarding the traditional link between intrapartum events and long-term neurological dysfunction; (4) the literature on 'fetal distress' in the form of metabolic acidosis; (5) the intrapartum diagnosis and management of 'fetal distress' as determined by the characteristics of the FHR patterns of EFM, focusing on the latest diagnostic techniques; and (6) data on how physicians actually practise when faced with intrapartum FHR abnormalities.

HISTORY

Almost as soon as the stethoscope was invented by Rene Laennec in 1816, it was adapted to listen to the fetus. The first description of auscultation came from Robert Collins in Dublin in 1832, whose work was expanded on and published by Evory Kennedy[1] in 1833. The first description of alterations of the rate of the auscultated fetal heart came from John Moir in Edinburgh in 1836, who related slowings of the fetal heart rate during the uterine contractions of labor (probably variable decelerations). Subsequent to these reports, significant advancements in the detection of fetal distress awaited the development of EFM. The pioneering work performed in the development of EFM by Hon[2–4] and Hess must be recognized as one of the first steps taken toward the realization that the fetus is a patient. The first attempts at determining the fetal electrocardiogram (ECG) were limited by technical aspects, but ultrasound-based technology soon paved the way for non-invasive EFM. In addition, fetal scalp puncture for the determination of acid-base status was developed through the work of Bretsher and Saling[5]; thus both invasive and non-invasive methods of determining fetal deterioration in labor were available. With the development of fetal vibroacoustic stimulation (VAS)[6–8], the stage is set for a discussion of the current tools available for the diagnosis and management of 'fetal distress' as determined by EFM.

TERMINOLOGY

No consensus can be seen in the terminology used to describe abnormal FHR patterns. The term *fetal distress* is very imprecise, nevertheless, it is commonly used in clinical practice to designate the fetus with metabolic acidosis, or one who has an ominous FHR pattern. Ominous FHR patterns will be described below. *Asphyxia* has been used in the past synonymously with severe metabolic acidosis in the fetus, but more properly consists of severe metabolic or mixed acidosis, Apgar scores < 4 at 5 min or greater, neonatal neurological sequelae such as seizures, coma or hypotonia, and evidence of end organ damage to such organs as the myocardium, kidneys, liver, bowels and central nervous system (CNS)[9]. *Cerebral palsy* refers to long-term permanent neurological damage thought to have occurred either prior to or during labor.

The study of fetal distress has traditionally been approached from four aspects: the infant with a low Apgar score, the fetus or neonate with metabolic acidosis, the interpretation of abnormal FHR patterns, and randomized controlled trials (RCT) of EFM. A fifth approach is the determination of how physicians actually practise when faced with abnormal FHR patterns. These will be reviewed below.

Low Apgar scores

The development of the Apgar score was based on the observation that the 'depressed' neonate often suffered severe morbidity or mortality[10]. The classic and largest study of the risk of perinatal mortality (PNM) and morbidity in the infant with a low Apgar score was published by Nelson and Ellenberg[11] in 1981. This study was based on the 49 000 births in the Collaborative Perinatal Project which was undertaken during the 1960s[12]. These infants were followed and had neurological testing performed up to age 7. Low Apgar scores (0–3) were a risk factor for death and for cerebral palsy, with both these adverse outcomes more likely to occur with a persistently low Apgar score. Among term infants, death in the first year occurred in 34.4, 52.5 and 59.0% of infants with Apgar scores of 0–3 at 10, 15 and 20 min, respectively. Of the survivors ($n = 99$) cerebral palsy developed in 16.7, 36.0 and 57.1% of those with Apgar scores of 0–3 at 10, 15 and 20 min, respectively. Thus it can be seen that persistently low Apgar scores are associated with increasing rates of subsequent long-term major neurological handicap. However, this is not the complete picture. Of infants suffering from persistently low Apgar scores (0–3 at ≥ 10 min) who survived, 80% were free from major handicap at early school age. In addition, 55% of infants later suffering from cerebral palsy had 1-min Apgar scores ≥ 7 and 73% had 5-min Apgar scores ≥ 7. The authors concluded that Apgar scores are poor predictors of long-term neurological outcome.

Although persistently low Apgar scores do indicate a higher risk of long-term neurological disability, they are only a marker and not the cause of this ultimate poor outcome. The large proportion of infants later suffering cerebral palsy who had normal Apgar scores argues against intrapartum causes of cerebral palsy in these patients. The focus of investigations has now shifted to the antepartum period. Apgar scores are important in determining the infant in need of resuscitation, but have a limited role in the study of intrapartum fetal distress.

Fetal acidemia

While EFM was being developed, Bretscher and Saling[5] pursued the establishment of normal values for pH and acid-base status in the fetus in labor, and developed the technique of fetal scalp puncture for the measurement of capillary blood pH[5]. The technique of EFM in determining abnormal FHR patterns followed by the availability of fetal scalp puncture for pH determination was, and remains, a powerful set of tools in the diagnosis of fetal distress caused by developing hypoxia and acidemia. Normal values for intrapartum fetal capillary blood pH have been established[5,13]. The level of pH, as determined by fetal scalp puncture, generally recognized as diagnostic of 'acidemia', is ≤ 7.20[14]. Despite this, it is well known that the level of acidemia at which the fetus is at risk for long-term neurological deficits is ≤ 7.10. In fact, the correlation between fetal acidemia and the subsequent development of cerebral palsy is not great until the fetal cord blood pH is ≤ 7.00[15–18].

Recent studies have evaluated the long-term neurological outcome in infants born with metabolic acidosis. Low and colleagues[16] studied the neurological outcome at 1 year of age of 37 term infants born with metabolic acidosis, defined as an umbilical artery buffer base ≤ 34 mmol/l, and compared these with a control group of 76 term infants born without metabolic acidosis. In addition to a detailed neurological examination, each infant underwent

Bayley scale testing, physical and mental development index scoring and a shortened version of the Uzgiris and Hunt scale. Each infant was classified as normal or as having a major or minor neurological deficit. In infants born with metabolic acidosis, they found no evidence of major or minor deficits (normal) in 22/37 (59%) infants, minor deficits in 10/37 (27%) infants and major deficits in 5/37 (14%) infants. In the control group 70/76 (92%) were normal, 5/76 (7%) had minor deficits and 1/76 (1%) had a major deficit. This elevated rate of both major and minor deficits in the group born with metabolic acidosis, with minor deficits elevated more than major ones, led the authors to conclude that their data support the concept that, beyond a critical threshold of fetal asphyxia, a continuum of casualty exists in the surviving newborn infants. Looking carefully at their data, however, the 7% and 1% rates of minor and major deficits, respectively, in the control group might possibly be evidence that there exist antenatal causes of long-term neurological deficits, which may be worsened by the intrapartum development of metabolic acidosis. Unfortunately, the authors used the term asphyxia synonymously with metabolic acidosis in the fetus, perhaps leading to confusion when attempting to compare their study to others.

Dennis and co-workers[17] studied neurological outcome at 4½ years of 230 infants with measured umbilical artery acid-base status at birth out of a population of 1210 deliveries[17]. Metabolic acidosis was defined as a pH ≤ 7.10 and a base deficit > 12 mmol/l. They divided these into five groups based upon pH, base deficit and Apgar scores. Neurological assessment included Griffiths development scales, the test for reception of grammar, the Rutter behavior screening questionnaire, the Renfrew picture pointing test, the keyhole pegboard test, the tramline square test and a detailed neurological examination. They found no significant associations between acidosis and developmental outcome. The highest proportion of unimpaired children was found among those who were the most severely acidotic at birth (pH < 7.04; base deficit > 12 mmol/l), but this finding was not statistically significant. There were only 10 non-acidotic infants and eight acidotic infants with a 1-min Apgar score 0–3. Although not significant (perhaps due to these very small numbers of patients in each group), they concluded that their findings suggested that metabolic acidosis may be beneficial to long-term neurological outcome.

Fee and colleagues[18] performed a 4-year review of 15 528 neonates, examining the relationship between severe acidosis at birth (defined as a pH ≤ 7.05 and a base deficit ≥ 10 mEq/l) and subsequent neurological dysfunction. Severe metabolic acidosis was found in 142 (0.9%) of these neonates, 110 term and 32 preterm. Neurological assessment at 12–24 months of age included detailed neurological examination, Brazelton neonatal behavioral assessment scale, Bayley scales of infant development and psychomotor and mental development index. They found nine term and 15 preterm neonates with abnormal examinations upon discharge. At long-term follow up, seven of nine term and eight of 15 preterm infants were available for examination. Five of the seven term and eight of the 15 preterm infants demonstrated mild developmental delays or mild tone abnormalities in the first year of life. None showed evidence of a major deficit at 12–24 months of age. They concluded that severe metabolic acidosis was a poor predictor of subsequent neurological dysfunction.

These three studies are illustrative of the problems in evaluating the scientific literature in this area of study. It is probably fair to say that these studies are not comparable because the definition of metabolic acidosis differs, the methods of determining neurological dysfunction differ, and two of the studies are population based and one is a case-control study. However, the conclusions of these studies are conflicting; the data show evidence that:

(1) Beyond a critical threshold, a continuum of casualty exists in terms of an effect of metabolic acidosis on long-term neurological injury;

(2) Metabolic acidosis is protective against long-term neurological injury; and

(3) Metabolic acidosis is a very poor predictor of long-term neurological injury.

These disparate results are the rule rather than the exception in the scientific literature regarding fetal metabolic acidosis and subsequent neurological outcome. These disparate findings have also been taken as evidence that it is not the insult of labor or the development of intrapartum metabolic acidosis that is the cause of cerebral palsy in the majority of cases. The focus is now centering on the antepartum period as the time when long-term neurological damage may occur in the preponderance of cases.

Electronic fetal monitoring

A normal FHR pattern is one where a baseline is discernable at 110–160 beats per minute (bpm), spontaneous accelerations of > 15 bpm amplitude and > 15 s duration are present, and beat-to-beat variability is present (2–5 beats amplitude short-term variation).

Despite the somewhat pessimistic discussion above of the ability to predict long-term neurological dysfunction, EFM has shown utility in detecting the fetus with developing acidemia[19]. Pathological, abnormal, or ominous FHR patterns do occur with reliability when fetal acidemia is progressive[19–21]. Table 1 shows the four pathological FHR patterns most likely to be considered ominous that may be seen during the intrapartum period. These patterns alone may not be ominous. However, when combined with either absent or decreased beat-to-beat variability, or with a lack of FHR accelerations, these are the patterns most likely to indicate that the fetus is either unable to withstand an extrinsic insult (such as uterine tetany) or is developing fetal acidemia due to decreased uteroplacental or umbilical blood flow.

Table 1 *Pathological fetal heart rate patterns most likely to be considered ominous*

Fetal bradycardia (prolonged deceleration)
Recurrent late decelerations
Recurrent severe variable decelerations
Sinusoidal pattern

Ominous FHR patterns

There are three situations where a FHR pattern may be considered ominous, requiring immediate delivery. The first is a severe fetal bradycardia (below 60 bpm) with decreased beat-to-beat variability lasting longer than 15 min. As detailed below (actual physician practice), virtually all authorities would agree that a fetal bradycardia of this severity and duration requires intervention in the form of emergent delivery. Many would act sooner than this admittedly arbitrary limit. The second situation is that of the sinusoidal FHR pattern, when the cause is unknown and when rhesus alloimmunization has been excluded, (particularly when the gestational age is at or near term). The third is when a severely abnormal FHR pattern (Table 1), not qualifying as ominous by the above definition, is persistent and is seen in the presence of some underlying high-risk clinical situation in addition to a cervical examination that indicates that delivery is many hours away (Table 2). Underlying high-risk clinical situations include: severe prematurity (< 32 weeks'), abruptio placentae and intrauterine growth restriction (IUGR).

Fetal bradycardia

Intrapartum fetal bradycardia, also termed prolonged deceleration, is a response of the fetus to an acute event. The causes are listed in Table 3. The usual response of the obstetric team consists of lateral recumbent positioning, intravenous fluid bolus, oxygen administration,

Table 2 *Ominous fetal heart rate (FHR) patterns indicating the need for immediate delivery*

Severe fetal bradycardia (< 60 bpm) with decreased beat-to-beat variability

Unexplained sinusoidal pattern (particularly in the term or near-term gestation), when drug effects and rhesus alloimmunization have been excluded

Severely abnormal FHR patterns, such as in Table 1, in the presence of complicating clinical factors such as:
   severe prematurity (< 32 weeks' gestation)
   abruptio placentae
   intrauterine growth restriction
   anticipation of very long labor

Table 3 *Causes of intrapartum fetal bradycardia*

Uterine tetany
Umbilical cord compression
Epidural anesthesia
Fetal head compression
Rapid descent of the fetal head in the maternal
  pelvis
Maternal valsalva
Maternal aorto-caval compression
Umbilical cord prolapse
Fetal anomaly
Fetal vagal stimulation
Amnioinfusion with cold or room-temperature fluid
Fetal congenital heart block
Maternal hypothermia

vaginal examination to rule out umbilical cord prolapse and rapid descent of the fetal head, and fetal stimulation. If an epidural anesthetic had been placed or reinforced within 20–30 min prior to the bradycardia, ephedrine may also be given in an attempt to increase uterine vascular tone. Uterine tocolytic agents such as terbutaline may also be given. All of these maneuvers are designed to increase uteroplacental or umbilical blood flow, or to detect causes of fetal bradycardia that are amenable to other treatments such as immediate operative vaginal delivery or Cesarean delivery. The overwhelming majority of instances of fetal bradycardia will resolve within 3–10 min of the onset. It should be noted that a transient (5–20 min) period of lack of beat-to-beat variability, tachycardia, and/or late decelerations is often present after recovery from an episode of fetal bradycardia[19]. This probably indicates a respiratory acidemia from which the fetus is able to recover with continued intrauterine oxygen delivery. The appearance of this pattern does not indicate a need for intervention in the form of urgent delivery unless the pattern is persistent.

Late and severe variable decelerations

During uterine contractions, decreased uteroplacental blood flow occurs, and can result in late decelerations, which indicate a transient hypoxia in the fetus. Similarly, umbilical cord compression or stretching may lead to variable decelerations, indicating a decreased umbilical blood flow to the fetus. Variable decelerations are more likely to be associated with fetal acidemia when they are severe; i.e. a decrease of 60 bpm from the baseline FHR, or to < 60 bpm absolute rate, lasting ≥ 60 s. In the case of either late decelerations or severe variable decelerations, three other characteristics of the FHR pattern are particularly important in detecting developing acidemia:

(1) The frequency of the decelerations;

(2) The presence or absence of beat-to-beat variability;

(3) The presence or absence of accelerations of the FHR, either spontaneous or induced.

If late or variable decelerations are recurrent in > 50% of contractions, they can be considered significant, i.e. more likely to be associated with developing fetal acidemia. In addition, if these decelerations are accompanied by a decrease or absence of beat-to-beat variability, or by a lack of spontaneous or induced accelerations, the likelihood of fetal acidemia is increased significantly; perhaps as many as 50% of these fetuses are acidemic[22,23]. In the presence of recurrent late or severe variable decelerations, some maneuvers designed to increase uteroplacental blood flow and fetal oxygenation may be beneficial, including lateral recumbent positioning, intravenous fluid bolus and oxygen administration.

The sinusoidal pattern

The sinusoidal FHR pattern is one associated with chronic, severe fetal anemia. Classically this has been seen in fetuses suffering from hemolytic disease of the fetus due to maternal rhesus alloimmunization. Other causes of fetal anemia can be associated with the sinusoidal pattern, including fetal infection with parvovirus B-19 and chronic fetomaternal hemorrhage. It should be noted, however, that massive, acute fetomaternal hemorrhage may not produce the sinusoidal FHR pattern[19], but will produce the FHR patterns more commonly described for 'fetal distress'. The treatment depends on the cause of fetal anemia, the gestational age, and the availability of the techniques of cordocentesis and intrauterine blood transfusion.

Beat-to-beat variability

It is recognized by most authorities that the presence of beat-to-beat variability (BBV) is a necessary but not sufficient factor in determining the healthy fetus. The presence of BBV indicates an intact fetal CNS-cardiac connection. The most reliable indicator of developing fetal acidemia is in the fetus who begins with normal BBV and shows accelerations of the FHR, then progresses through either severe variable or late decelerations to a lack of accelerations or a decrease in BBV or both. There are many factors that can lead to a decrease in BBV, most commonly changes in fetal behavioral state, i.e. fetal sleep cycles. When BBV has been present in the intrapartum period, and subsequently decreases or becomes absent, a further test of fetal well-being is probably indicated. The single most important factor in predicting a healthy fetus, other than the baseline FHR, is the presence of BBV.

TESTS OF FETAL WELL-BEING

Intrapartum tests of fetal well-being are shown in Table 4. One of these tests is indicated in the presence of persistent intrapartum FHR abnormalities. The type of FHR abnormality, or the suspicion of the clinician that fetal acidemia may be developing, determines which tests of fetal well-being may be the most appropriate. Simply awaiting a change in fetal behavioral state and continuing EFM is often an appropriate choice. Many FHR abnormalities are transient or intermittent. The presence of BBV and/or accelerations can be very reassuring. The tests of scalp stimulation and vibroacoustic

Table 4 *Intrapartum tests of fetal well-being*

Continued electronic fetal monitoring (awaiting a
   change in fetal behavioral state)
Fetal scalp stimulation
Fetal vibroacoustic stimulation
Fetal scalp pH determination

stimulation (VAS) were designed to attempt more rapidly to change the fetal state, inducing fetal movement, and thus a FHR acceleration in response to the stimulation[7,22–24]. It was also noted that accelerations of the FHR during the test of fetal scalp pH is a reliable indicator of fetal well-being[25]. These have been readily accepted in clinical practice as non-invasive alternatives to the option of fetal scalp pH measurement. Fetal scalp puncture for the determination of fetal capillary blood pH in labor has been used in most major centers in the United States as an adjunctive test to detect fetal acidemia when intrapartum FHR abnormalities are present. Previously, it was common practice to perform fetal scalp puncture for determination of pH in many, if not virtually all cases where a fetus developed FHR pattern abnormalities in labor. Currently, many authorities believe that fetal scalp puncture for capillary pH measurement has a much more limited role in the management of intrapartum FHR abnormalities[26,27].

Perhaps the most reliable way to produce an acceleration of the FHR in labor is with VAS[23]. Two studies have shown the reliability of VAS-induced accelerations of the FHR in demonstrating a lack of fetal acidosis[22,23]. Smith and colleagues[22] studied 64 patients with intrapartum FHR abnormalities. First, VAS was performed and within several minutes fetal scalp puncture for capillary blood pH was performed. When an acceleration of the FHR was induced, defined as an increase of ≥ 15 bpm above the baseline lasting ≥ 15 s ($n = 30$), there were no fetuses who demonstrated acidemia by fetal scalp puncture. Conversely, when VAS led to a lack of an acceleration or an inadequate acceleration by their definition ($n = 34$), 53% of fetuses were found to have a fetal scalp pH < 7.25. The authors concluded that VAS may be a reasonable clinical alternative to fetal scalp puncture when a reactive pattern, or the presence of a qualifying acceleration, was observed.

The second study was by Edersheim and co-workers[23], who studied 127 patients with abnormal intrapartum FHR patterns. In 188 instances, VAS was performed followed within several minutes by fetal scalp puncture for determination of capillary blood pH. When a reactive pattern was observed, defined as an increase of the FHR of ≥ 15 bpm above the baseline lasting ≥ 15 s, induced either by VAS ($n = 116$) or by fetal scalp puncture ($n = 10$), there were no instances of scalp pH < 7.20. Conversely, when a reactive response was not observed to either VAS or fetal scalp puncture ($n = 62$), acidosis (pH < 7.20) was demonstrated in 10% of cases, while a pre-acidotic state (pH 7.20–7.25) was seen in 37%. The authors concluded that VAS is less invasive and may be used in some instances in which fetal scalp puncture for pH determination is technically impossible.

In addition to these two studies, Clark and associates[24] showed the utility of fetal scalp stimulation in inducing a reactive response in the non-acidotic fetus in labor. These three studies show the reliability of induced accelerations of the FHR in the intrapartum period in demonstrating a lack of fetal acidemia. Induced accelerations (≥ 15 bpm above baseline lasting for ≥ 15 s) are thus a reliable non-invasive way of ruling out acidemia as a cause of fetal distress. It is important to point out that this only holds for the immediate time at which the test is performed. As demonstrated by Edersheim's study, many patients continue to demonstrate an abnormal FHR pattern, and may require repeat testing to determine whether fetal acidemia may not have subsequently developed during the progression of labor. These studies also demonstrate an important principle of FHR monitoring, which is that it is common to see a healthy fetus with an abnormal or suspicious FHR pattern, but difficult to elicit a normal FHR pattern from the distressed or acidemic fetus. This important observation is what allows us to use intrapartum FHR monitoring to reliably detect the acidotic fetus.

Another important point is that the fetus with CNS damage or a CNS anomaly may demonstrate an abnormal FHR pattern in the absence of fetal acidosis[28]. These types of cases can be very difficult to reliably predict and manage.

THE SECOND STAGE OF LABOR

The second stage of labor has a much higher incidence of abnormal FHR patterns[29]. The causes of this have generally been described as umbilical cord compression or stretching, head compression, a fetal vagal response and a decompensation of the fetus into acidemia[30]. These patterns can also be very difficult to manage. An important component of the FHR pattern that may help in predicting a healthy or non-acidotic fetus in the second stage of labor is the continued presence of BBV. Fetal scalp puncture for determination of scalp pH is used liberally in this situation at our institution.

COMPLICATING CLINICAL SITUATIONS

Several clinical situations may occur during labor and complicate the management of abnormal FHR patterns. These include: abruptio placentae, IUGR, meconium staining of the amniotic fluid, chorioamnionitis and multiple gestations. The principles involved in the interpretation of FHR patterns are not changed in these settings, although abnormalities of the FHR may be more likely to be seen when these clinical entities complicate labor[31-34]. Particularly with abruptio placentae, and perhaps also with both IUGR (seen commonly of course in multiple gestation) and with meconium, the progression of a fetus from a normal acid-base status to a severe metabolic acidosis can be very rapid[35-37].

RANDOMIZED CONTROLLED TRIALS OF ELECTRONIC FETAL MONITORING

Numerous randomized controlled trials have addressed the efficacy of EFM in decreasing perinatal mortality and morbidity. In order to review the large number of these trials which have been performed, it is illustrative to turn to two recent meta-analyses, which have combined many of these trials.

Vintzileos and colleagues[38] evaluated all randomized controlled trials which compared a universally-monitored group with a group undergoing intermittent auscultation. This study approached the topic of perinatal mortality with the assumption that not all perinatal deaths are caused by hypoxia or acidosis. Thus, previous trials of EFM, looking at total perinatal mortality as the end point of analysis, may have incorporated a beta error in their design. The authors combined the results of nine studies, reviewing the papers carefully and contacting the lead authors of the studies, if necessary, to determine which perinatal deaths were due to hypoxia or acidosis. Despite no difference in total perinatal mortality between the EFM and intermittent auscultation groups, they found a significant decrease in perinatal mortality due to hypoxia in the EFM group. This provides the first scientific evidence of a beneficial effect of EFM on perinatal mortality – specifically, perinatal mortality due to hypoxia, the disorder that EFM would be expected to detect. One word of caution should be emphasized, however. If one study[39] is eliminated from the meta-analysis the significant difference evaporates. Thus, the evidence should be viewed as only suggestive, not conclusive.

The second meta-analysis reviewed a larger number of randomized controlled trials of EFM, and looked at a number of outcome measures, including low Apgar scores, neonatal seizures, neonatal intensive care unit admissions and perinatal deaths[40]. Two significant findings were discovered. The first is that there was a decrease in 1-min Apgar scores < 4 in the group undergoing universal EFM. The second is that, neonatal seizures were decreased in the group undergoing universal EFM. These two clinical findings (neonatal seizures and low 1-min Apgar scores) provide for a risk of subsequent long-term neurological dysfunction[37,41,42]. Considering that EFM decreases the occurrence of both the low Apgar score at 1 min and neonatal seizures, this is indirect evidence of a beneficial effect of EFM on subsequent neurological function.

The results of this meta-analysis may be the best scientific data we are able to produce regarding the beneficial effect of EFM for two reasons. The first is that all randomized controlled trials of EFM have shown an increase in the rate of Cesarean delivery in the group undergoing EFM. This is the price we pay for this technology. Presumably this is due to clinicians 'overcalling' abnormal FHR patterns as 'ominous' or indicative of acidosis, i.e. determining that an abnormal FHR pattern requires emergent Cesarean delivery when this is not the case.

The second reason relates to the power of calculations regarding any randomized controlled trial of EFM in evaluating the effect of EFM on the incidence of cerebral palsy. Previously it was assumed that approximately 50% of cerebral palsy was caused by intrapartum events. It is now believed that less than 10% of cerebral palsy is caused by intrapartum events[9,43]. The incidence of cerebral palsy in the general population is very low. Thus, in order to detect any decrease in cerebral palsy obtained by the use of EFM, randomized controlled trials of EFM vs. intermittent auscultation would need a prohibitive number of patients in each arm of the study; this type of study will undoubtedly never be accomplished.

ACTUAL PHYSICIAN PRACTICE

There is conflicting scientific data with regards to the diagnosis of fetal distress by EFM. In addition, there is a dearth of published information on recommended management of intrapartum FHR abnormalities. This prompted our group at the New York Hospital-Cornell University Medical Center to conduct a survey questionnaire on how physicians actually practice when faced with intrapartum FHR abnormalities[44]. To four FHR patterns we felt were most likely to be considered ominous, we added the description of either normal or decreased BBV, providing eight questions on management of these intrapartum FHR patterns. When posing these questions, we asked how long the physician would observe the pattern before making the decision to proceed to Cesarean delivery. Answers were categorical and included a range of observation times from 2–4 min up to > 60 min. Each question also provided a choice that the physician would not decide based on the FHR tracing alone.

This survey was sent to members of the Society of Perinatal Obstetricians, specialists in maternal-fetal medicine (MFM), certified by the American Board of Obstetrics and Gynecology. These physicians are generally considered the most knowledgeable in this area of fetal surveillance.

In addition to other demographic questions, we also queried these physicians on two other areas: the use of tests of intrapartum fetal well-being such as scalp stimulation, VAS and scalp pH, and the impact of other clinical situations such as abruptio placentae, IUGR, meconium, chorioamnionitis and twin gestation on their observation times.

The example of a 'normal' pregnancy was chosen to decrease the variables affecting the physicians' decisions. In other words, a term, cephalic, uncomplicated pregnancy was designated as the case in which the FHR abnormalities developed. Specifically excluded were: fetal anomalies, fetal congenital heart block, maternal complications of pregnancy and imminent vaginal delivery.

The results showed responses from 431/704 (61.2%) physicians surveyed, and the data were analyzed in terms of agreement on each question. Legislative definitions of consensus ($\geq 67\%$ agreement) and strong consensus ($\geq 75\%$ agreement) were adopted[45]. Table 5 shows the results: in five of the eight questions consensus or strong consensus was reached for opting for Cesarean delivery within a certain time. It is important to note that in all four of the FHR patterns in which there was decreased BBV, consensus was able to be reached.

The results of the survey showed that if the clinical situations of abruptio placentae, IUGR and thick meconium were suspected, a consensus of physicians responded that they would decrease their observation times of most of the eight abnormal FHR patterns. For the clinical situations of thin meconium, chorioamnionitis

and twin gestation no consensus was reached. The results of the survey in terms of percentages of physicians answering that they would decrease their observation times in the presence of one of these clinical situations are shown in Table 6.

Although little consensus was reached, many physicians deemed tests of fetal well-being useful in the face of the eight abnormal FHR patterns presented. Table 7 shows the percentages of physicians who answered that they would use one or more of the various tests of fetal well-being when confronted with an abnormal intrapartum FHR pattern.

Implications

This survey shows observation times for abnormal intrapartum FHR patterns for a large number of maternal-fetal medicine physicians prior to deciding upon Cesarean delivery. It was designed not as a prescription for guidelines or 'standards of care' for how long these patterns should be observed, but simply to provide more information to practising physicians in order to fill a very obvious gap in the scientific literature.

MANAGEMENT OF INTRAPARTUM FETAL HEART RATE ABNORMALITIES

A suggested algorithm for the management of intrapartum FHR abnormalities is shown in Figure 1. This algorithm presupposes a lack of factors complicating the pregnancy – either maternal or fetal – which may alter the decision-making process at any time. If other clinical

Table 5 *Abnormal fetal heart rate (FHR) patterns for which consensus was reached for deciding upon Cesarean delivery*

Abnormal FHR pattern	Observation time until decision for Cesarean delivery (min)	Agreement (%)
Late decelerations with decreased BBV	30	78**
Variable decelerations with decreased BBV	30	74*
Bradycardia < 60 bpm with normal BBV	10	68*
Bradycardia < 60 bpm with decreased BBV	10	91**
Bradycardia 60–89 bpm with decreased BBV	10	76**

BBV, beat-to-beat variability; *, consensus; **, strong consensus

Table 6 *Percentages of maternal-fetal medicine specialists who responded that various clinical situations would influence their decision to proceed to Cesarean delivery in the face of intrapartum fetal heart rate (FHR) abnormalities (shorten observation time)*

	Case 1	Case 2	Case 3	Case 4
Normal BBV				
Abruptio placenta	90**	76**	67*	73*
Intrauterine growth restriction	86**	89**	64	68*
Thick meconium	80**	77**	60	66
Chorioamnionitis	59	52	44	48
Twin A	39	38	41	42
Twin B	64	62	49	51
Decreased BBV				
Abruptio placenta	80**	73*	56	68*
Intrauterine growth restriction	80**	77**	58	66
Thick meconium	74*	70*	52	61
Chorioamnionitis	63	55	42	47
Twin A	53	48	40	44
Twin B	65	61	44	51

Case 1, late decelerations in >50% of contractions; case 2, severe variable decelerations; case 3, fetal bradycardia to <60 beats per minute (bpm); case 4, fetal bradycardia between 60–89 bpm; BBV, beat-to-beat variability; *, consensus; **, strong consensus

Table 7 *Percentages of respondents who would employ tests of fetal well-being in the setting of intrapartum fetal heart rate (FHR) abnormalities*[†]

	Tests of fetal well-being (%)		
	FSS	*VAS*	*Scalp pH*
Late decelerations with normal BBV	63	30	77**
Late decelerations with decreased BBV	48	24	56
Variable decelerations with normal BBV	44	21	64
Variable decelerations with decreased BBV	43	22	55
Bradycardia < 60 bpm with normal BBV	32	13	27
Bradycardia < 60 bpm with decreased BBV	24	10	17
Bradycardia 60–89 bpm with normal BBV	46	19	45
Bradycardia 60–89 bpm with decreased BBV	37	15	31

[†], More than one test could be chosen; **, strong consensus; FSS, fetal scalp stimulation; VAS, vibroacoustic stimulation; BBV, beat-to-beat variability

situations are suspected, and the abnormal intrapartum FHR pattern is persistent, consideration should be given to immediate delivery. These clinical situations include, but are not limited to: placenta previa, abruptio placentae, vasa previa, fetal anomalies, fetomaternal hemorrhage, meconium, multiple gestations, IUGR and the anticipation of many hours of labor before delivery (e.g. a long, closed cervix). It should also be emphasized that resuscitative measures should routinely be undertaken when persistent FHR abnormalities appear, including: lateral recumbent positioning, oxygen administration and an intravenous fluid bolus. In addition, if oligohydramnios is known to be present or the abnormal FHR pattern is one of recurrent severe variable decelerations, saline amnioinfusion is strongly recommended[46–48]. It is important that this algorithm is used for decision-making only in the term fetus. The preterm fetus is probably unable to withstand whatever insult may be causing a

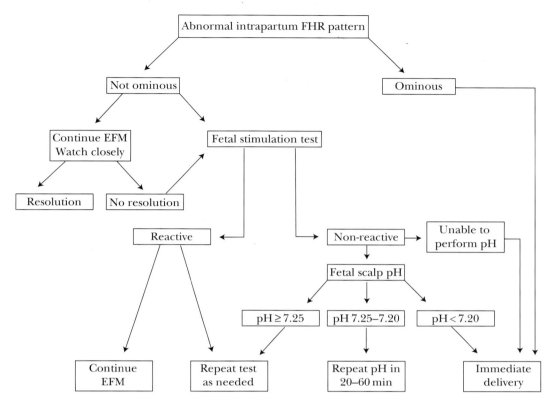

Figure 1 *Algorithm for the management of abnormal intrapartum FHR patterns. FHR, fetal heart rate; EFM, electronic fetal monitoring*

severely abnormal intrapartum FHR pattern for as long as the term fetus, and thus probably deserves intervention in the form of urgent delivery more quickly than the term fetus in the face of these types of FHR abnormalities.

CONCLUSION

Although the initial experience in randomized controlled trials of EFM was disappointing, further expertise has developed in the interpretation of abnormal FHR patterns during the last decade. Our ability to diagnose more accurately the fetus in distress has improved. In addition, we are now better able to determine the causes of observed FHR abnormalities, and thus treat or alleviate these specific problems. The fetus is being treated as a patient, and refinement of diagnostic and therapeutic techniques continues.

References

1. Kennedy, E. (1833). *Observations on Obstetric Auscultation.* (Dublin: Longman)
2. Hon, E. H. (1959). The fetal heart rate patterns preceding death *in utero. Am. J. Obstet. Gynecol.,* **78**, 47–56
3. Hon. E. H. (1958). The electronic evaluation of the fetal heart rate. Preliminary report. *Am. J. Obstet. Gynecol.,* **75**, 1215–30

4. Hon, E. H. and Hess, O. W. (1957). Instrumentation of fetal electrocardiography. *Science*, **125**, 553–55

5. Bretscher, J. and Saling, E. (1967). pH values in the human fetus during labor. *Am. J. Obstet. Gynecol.*, **97**, 906–11

6. Johannson, B., Wedenberg, E. and Westin, B. (1964). Measurement of tone response by the human fetus. A preliminary report. *Acta Otolaryngol.*, **57**, 188–92

7. Read, J. A. and Miller, F. C. (1977). Fetal heart rate acceleration in response to acoustic stimulation as a measure of fetal well-being. *Am. J. Obstet. Gynecol.*, **129**, 512–17

8. Birnholz, J. C. and Benacerraf, B. R. (1983). The development of human fetal hearing. *Science*, **222**, 516–18

9. American College of Obstetricians and Gynecologists (1992). Fetal and neonatal neurologic injury. In *ACOG Technical Bulletin 163*. (Washington, DC: The American College of Obstetricians and Gynecologists)

10. Apgar, V. (1953). A proposal for a new method of evaluation of the newborn infant. *Anesth. Analg.*, **32**, 260

11. Nelson, K. B. and Ellenberg, J. H. (1981). Apgar scores as predictors of chronic neurologic disability. *Pediatrics*, **68**, 36–44

12. Niswander, K. and Gordon, M. (1972). The women and their pregnancies. In *National Institutes of Health Publication*, pp. 73–379. (Bethesda, Maryland: US Department of Health, Education and Welfare)

13. Beard, R. W., Morris, E. D. and Clayton, S. G. (1967). pH of fetal capillary blood as an indicator of the condition of the fetus. *J. Obstet. Gynaecol. Br. Commonw.*, **74**, 812–22

14. American College of Obstetricians and Gynecologists (1995). Umbilical artery blood acid-base analysis. In *ACOG technical bulletin 216*. (Washington, DC: The American College of Obstetricians and Gynecologists)

15. Gilstrap, L. C. III, Leveno, K. J., Burris, J., Williams, M. L. and Little, B. B. (1989). Diagnosis of birth asphyxia on the basis of fetal pH, Apgar score, and newborn cerebral dysfunction. *Am. J. Obstet. Gynecol.*, **161**, 825–30

16. Low, J. A., Galbraith, R. S., Muir, D. W., Killen, H. L., Pater, E. A. and Karchmar, E. J. (1988). Motor and cognitive deficits after intrapartum asphyxia in the mature fetus. *Am. J. Obstet. Gynecol.*, **158**, 356–61

17. Dennis, J., Johnson, A., Mutch, L., Yudkin, P. and Johnson, P. (1989). Acid-base status at birth and neurodevelopmental outcome at four and one-half years. *Am. J. Obstet. Gynecol.*, **161**, 213–20

18. Fee, S. C., Malee, K., Deddish, R., Minogue, J. P. and Socol, M. L. (1990). Severe acidosis and subsequent neurologic status. *Am. J. Obstet. Gynecol.*, **162**, 802–6

19. American College of Obstetricians and Gynecologists (1995). Fetal heart rate patterns: monitoring, interpretation, and management. In *ACOG Technical Bulletin*, 207. (Washington, DC: The American College of Obstetricians and Gynecologists)

20. Myers, R. E., Meuller-Huebach, E. and Adamsons, K. (1973). Predictability of the state of fetal oxygenation from quantitative analysis of the components of late deceleration. *Am. J. Obstet. Gynecol.*, **115**, 1083–94

21. Wakatsuki, A., Murata, Y., Ninomiya, Y., Masaoka, N., Tyner, J. G. and Kutty, K. K. (1992). Autonomic nervous system regulation of baseline heart rate in the fetal lamb. *Am. J. Obstet. Gynecol.*, **167**, 519–23

22. Smith, C. V., Nguyen, H. N., Phelan, J. P. and Paul, R. H. (1986). Intrapartum assessment of fetal well-being: a comparison of fetal acoustic stimulation with acid-base determinations. *Am. J. Obstet. Gynecol.*, **155**, 726–8

23. Edersheim, T. G., Hutson, J. M., Druzin, M. L. and Kogut, E. A. (1987). Fetal heart rate response to vibratory acoustic stimulation predicts fetal pH in labor. *Am. J. Obstet. Gynecol.*, **157**, 1557–60

24. Clark, S. L., Gimovsky, M. L., Miller, F. C. (1984). The scalp stimulation test: a clinical alternative to fetal scalp blood sampling. *Am. J. Obstet. Gynecol.*, **148**, 274–7

25. Clark, S. L., Gimovsky, M. L. and Miller, F. C. (1982). Fetal heart rate response to scalp blood sampling. *Am. J. Obstet. Gynecol.*, **44**, 706–8

26. Clark, S. L. and Paul, R. H. (1985). Intrapartum fetal surveillance: the role of fetal scalp blood sampling. *Am. J. Obstet. Gynecol.*, **153**, 717–20

27. Goodwin, T. M., Milner-Masterson, L. and Paul, R. H. (1994). Elimination of fetal scalp blood sampling on a large clinical service. *Obstet. Gynecol.*, **83**, 971–4

28. Niswander, K. R. (1991). EFM and brain damage in term and post-term infants. *Contemp. Obstet. Gynecol.*, **36**, 39–50

29. Parer, J. T. (1954). Fetal heart rate. In Creasy, R. K. and Resnik, R. (eds.). *Maternal-fetal Medicine: Principles and Practice*, 3rd edn., pp. 298–325. (Philadelphia: W.B. Saunders)

30. Ball, R. H. and Parer, J. T. (1992). The physiological mechanisms of variable decelerations. *Am. J. Obstet. Gynecol.*, **166**, 1683–9

31. Naeye, R. L., Harkness, W. L. and Utts, J. (1977). Abruptio placentae and perinatal death: a prospective study. *Am. J. Obstet. Gynecol.*, **128**, 740–6

32. Low, J. A., Boston, R. W. and Pancham, S. R. (1972). Fetal asphyxia during the antepartum

period in intrauterine growth retarded infants. *Am. J. Obstet. Gynecol.*, **113**, 351

33. Low, J. A., Handley-Derry, M. H., Burke, S. O., *et al.* (1992). Association of intrauterine growth retardation and learning deficits at age 9 to 11 years. *Am. J. Obstet. Gynecol.*, **167**, 1499–1505

34. Yeomans, E., Gilstrap, L. C., Leveno, K. J. and Burris, J. S. (1989). Meconium stained amniotic fluid and neonatal acid-base status. *Obstet. Gynecol.*, **73**, 175–8

35. Westgren, M., Holmqvist, P., Ingemarsson, I., *et al.* (1984). Intrapartum fetal acidosis in preterm infants: fetal monitoring and long-term morbidity. *Obstet. Gynecol.*, **63**, 355

36. Boylan, P. C. and Parisi, V. M. (1994). Fetal acid-base balance. In Creasy, R. K. and Resnik, R. (eds.). *Maternal-fetal Medicine: Principles and Practice*, 3rd edn. (Philadelphia: WB Saunders)

37. Shy, K. K., Luthy, D. A., Bennett, F. C., Whitefield, M., Larson, E. B., van Belle, G., Hughes, J. P., Wilson, J. A. and Stenchever, M. A. (1990). Effects of electronic fetal heart rate monitoring, as compared with periodic auscultation, on the neurologic development of premature infants. *N. Engl. J. Med.*, **322**, 588–93

38. Vintzileos, A. M., Nochimson, D. J., Guzman, E. R., Knuppel, R. A., Lae, M. and Schifrin, B. S. (1995). Intrapartum electronic fetal heart rate monitoring versus intermittent auscultation: a meta-analysis. *Obstet. Gynecol.*, **85**, 149–55

39. Vintzileos, A. M., Antsaklis, A., Varvarigos, I., Papas, C., Sofatzis, I. and Montgomery, J. T. (1993). A randomized trial of intrapartum electronic fetal heart rate monitoring versus intermittent auscultation. *Obstet. Gynecol.*, **81**, 899–907

40. Thacker, S. B., Stroup, D. F. and Peterson, H. B. (1995). Efficacy and safety of intrapartum electronic fetal monitoring: an update. *Obstet. Gynecol.*, **86**, 613–20

41. Nelson, K. B. and Ellenberg, J. H. (1986). Antecedents of cerebral palsy. Multivariate analysis of risk. *N. Engl. J. Med.*, **315**, 81–6

42. Freeman, J. M. and Nelson, K. B. (1988). Intrapartum asphyxia and cerebral palsy. *Pediatrics*, **82**, 240–9

43. Blair, E. and Stanley, F. J. (1988). Intrapartum asphyxia: a rare cause of cerebral palsy. *J. Pediatr.*, **112**, 515–9

44. Skupski, D. W., Chervenak, F. A., McCullough, L. and Horwitz, S. (1996). Cesarean delivery for intrapartum fetal heart rate abnormalities: incorporating survey data into clinical judgement. *Obstet. Gynecol.*, in press

45. Wertz, D. C. and Fletcher, J. C. (eds.) (1989). *Ethics and Human Genetics: a Cross-cultural Perspective.* pp. 11–13. (Berlin: Springer-Verlag)

46. Miyazaki, F. S. and Nevarez, F. (1985). Saline amnioinfusion for relief of repetitive variable decelerations: a prospective randomized study. *Am. J. Obstet. Gynecol.*, **153**, 301–6

47. Strong, T. H. Jr, Hetzler, G., Sarno, A. P. and Paul, R. H. (1990). Prophylactic intrapartum amnioinfusion: a randomized clinical trial. *Am. J. Obstet. Gynecol.*, **162**, 1370–5

48. Sadovsky, Y., Amon, E., Bade, M. E. and Petrie, R. H. (1989). Prophylactic amnioinfusion during labor complicated by meconium: a preliminary report. *Am. J. Obstet. Gynecol.*, **161**, 613–7

Section 5

Clinical perinatology

Calcium supplementation in the prevention of pregnancy-induced hypertensive diseases

36

B. Haddad and S. Uzan

INTRODUCTION

Hypertensive diseases and particularly pre-eclampsia remain a concern for obstetricians as they are still a major cause of maternal and fetal morbidity and mortality. Several authors have hypothesized that because calcium metabolism seems to interfere with vascular sensitivity in non-pregnant subjects it may therefore be involved in the pathogenesis of hypertension. Several trials studying the relationship between calcium supplementation and pregnancy-induced hypertensive diseases, in pregnant women, have been recently published. Results of some of these trials may show a beneficial effect of calcium therapy in reducing the incidence of pregnancy-induced hypertensive diseases. The aim of this chapter is to try to clarify the usefulness of calcium supplementation in the prevention of hypertensive diseases during pregnancy.

PATHOPHYSIOLOGY

Initially, several authors tried to find a relationship between calcium metabolism and hypertensive diseases during pregnancy. In normal pregnancy, urinary calcium excretion is increased when compared to non-pregnant women[1]. It increases during pregnancy reaching a maximum level in the third trimester of pregnancy[2]. Taufield and colleagues[3] studied urinary calcium excretion in 40 women in the third trimester of pregnancy (ten normotensive, five pregnancy-induced hypertension, six chronic hypertension, seven chronic hypertension with pre-eclampsia and 12 pre-eclampsia alone). No dietary or socioeconomic status data

were reported. The authors found a significant decrease of urinary fractional excretion of calcium in pregnancy-induced hypertension. As the Taufield study[3], Hutchesson and colleagues[4] evaluated urinary calcium excretion in pregnant women divided into five groups (84 normotensive women, ten hypertensive women prior to 20 weeks, four hypertensive women prior to 20 weeks with proteinuria, 19 pregnancy-induced hypertension and 21 pregnancy-induced hypertension with proteinuria). Dietary calcium intake, which ranged from 1160 to 1320 mg/day, was not found to be different between the groups. The authors found a reduction in the 24-h urinary calcium excretion in women with hypertensive diseases and particularly in pre-eclamptic women. Sanchez-Ramos and associates[5] reported a study concerning 24-h urinary calcium excretion in 143 pregnant women. Patients were divided in three groups (58 normotensive patients, 52 gestational hypertension and 33 pre-eclampsia). No dietary calcium intake data were available. Patients with pre-eclampsia had significantly lower excretion of total calcium than normotensive women or those with gestational hypertension. Moreover, the authors suggested that a urinary calcium level below 12 mg/dl may help to distinguish pre-eclampsia from other hypertensive diseases of pregnancy. The same author[6] reported a prospective trial studying the relationship between urinary calcium excretion and pre-eclampsia in 103 consecutive nulliparous women. He found that the women who later would develop pre-eclampsia had lower urinary calcium excretion at 10–24 weeks' gestation than that of normotensive women (169 ± 30 vs. 298 ± 15 mg/24 h respectively, $p < 0.05$).

Several authors have tried to explain the mechanism of hypocalciuria observed in pre-eclampsia. Regulation of vitamin D metabolism has given rise to much controversy. In normal pregnancy, Reddy and colleagues[7] found an increase of serum levels of 1,25-dihydroxyvitamin D from the first trimester of the pregnancy until delivery. Serum levels fall acutely to almost normal levels on the third postpartum day. Seely and associates[8] measured serum and urinary calcium and serum calciotropic hormones in the third trimester of pre-eclamptic women ($n = 12$) and of women with normotensive pregnancies ($n = 24$). In agreement with other authors[3-5], they found a decrease of urinary calcium excretion in pre-eclamptic women when compared with normotensive women (2.9 ± 0.7 vs 6.5 ± 0.2 mmol/day, $p < 0.01$). Pre-eclamptic women had lower serum ionized calcium and higher intact serum parathyroid hormone than normotensive women. However, in contrast with the results of Taufield and associates[3] pre-eclamptic women had significantly lower levels of 1,25-dihydroxyvitamin D when compared to normotensive patients, whereas levels of 25-hydroxyvitamin D levels were equivalent in both pre-eclamptic and normotensive women. These findings suggest that in pre-eclampsia, lower serum 1,25-dihydroxyvitamin D levels contribute to suboptimal intestinal absorption of calcium at a time of increased calcium demands, resulting in a decrease of serum ionized calcium, and an increase in parathyroid hormone and hypocalciuria. This hypothesis was not supported by Frenkel and associates[9]. In their study, the authors compared serum parathyroid hormone, 1,25-dihydroxyvitamin D and urinary calcium excretion levels in women with pre-eclampsia ($n = 14$) to women with chronic hypertension ($n = 12$) and women with normal blood pressure ($n = 11$). All patients were in the third trimester of pregnancy. Dietary calcium intake data were not available. As in several other reports[3-5,8], urinary calcium excretion was found to be significantly decreased in pre-eclamptic women (62.1 ± 32.8 mg/24 h)

when compared to chronic hypertensive women (162.6 ± 97.8 mg/24 h) and to normotensive controls (225.6 ± 146.9 mg/24 h) ($p < 0.05$). Serum parathyroid hormone level was found to be significantly the lowest in pre-eclamptic women (9.8 ± 5.5 pg/ml) when compared to that of normotensive (16.4 ± 3.2 pg/ml) or chronic hypertensive women (18.5 ± 2.7 pg/ml) ($p < 0.005$). Moreover, serum levels of 1,25-dihydroxyvitamin D in three groups of patients were not found to be statistically different. More recently, August and associates[10] confirmed the findings of Seely[8] concerning 1,25-dihydroxyvitamin D levels in pre-eclamptic women. In their study, the women included (11 women with pre-eclampsia, nine women with chronic hypertension and 12 normotensive women) were all taking prenatal vitamins that contained 200–600 mg of calcium; dietary calcium intake data were not available. The authors found a significant decrease in serum level of 1,25-dihydroxyvitamin D in women with pre-eclampsia (37.8 ± 15 pg/ml) when compared to that of women with chronic hypertension (75 ± 15 pg/ml, $p < 0.05$), or to that of normal women (65 ± 10 pg/ml, $p < 0.05$). The serum parathyroid hormone level was higher in pre-eclamptic women without being significant.

Hypocalciuria observed in pre-eclampsia could be the consequence of an impaired intestinal absorption combined with a decrease of 1,25-dihydroxyvitamin D levels. Tolaymat and co-workers[11], using calcium isotopes, studied intestinal calcium absorption in 15 pregnant women (eight pre-eclampsia and seven normotensive controls). Although serum levels of 1,25-dihydroxyvitamin D were significantly decreased in pre-eclamptic women, the authors did not find any statistical difference in the fractional intestinal absorption between pre-eclamptic women and normotensive controls. However, they noted that the fraction of dietary calcium appearing in urine was significantly decreased in pre-eclamptic women when compared to that of normotensive controls ($p = 0.008$). The retention site of unexcreted calcium was unidentified by these authors.

To conclude, pregnancy-induced hypertension, and particularly pre-eclampsia, is associated with an alteration of extracellular calcium metabolism, characterized by a decrease of urinary calcium excretion. This phenomenon could be mediated by abnormalities of parathyroid hormone and vitamin D metabolism. However, the etiology of hypocalciuria in pre-eclampsia remains unclear.

CALCIUM SUPPLEMENTATION IN THE PREVENTION OF HYPERTENSIVE DISEASES

Trials concerning the relationship between calcium dietary intake and hypertension have been more consistent in animal models. Meta-analysis of these trials performed by Dumas and colleagues[12] resulted in a lowering of blood pressure in spontaneous hypertensive rats or in other genetic or experimental models of hypertension. In contrast, low-calcium feeding of spontaneous hypertensive rats[13] or normotensive rats[14] resulted in higher blood pressure. However, almost all of these trials concerned young animals and the hypotensive action of calcium diet was not studied in older animals. Moreover, animal studies did not concern calcium diet during pregnancy. Therefore, experimental conditions limit extrapolation of such results to humans.

A decade ago, Belizan and co-workers[15] presented evidence that supports the hypothesis that calcium supplementation reduces blood pressure in pregnant women. In a simple randomized placebo-controlled trial, 36 Guatemalan women, without evidence of previous pathology, were recruited at 15 weeks' gestation and divided into three treatment groups. They were allocated to take elemental calcium 1 g/day ($n = 11$), or 2 g/day ($n = 11$) or a placebo ($n = 14$). Dietary calcium intake before entering the trial was about 700 mg/day, which is similar to that previously reported by the same team. The authors found that women having 2 g/day of calcium had significantly lower blood pressure throughout the second and third trimesters than placebo-treated women.

The review of most important interventional trials showed that study populations could be divided on high-risk and low-risk patients. This separation cannot be established on calcium intake alone for at least two reasons: calcium intake in pregnancy cannot be the sole factor inducing an increase of vascular sensitivity, moreover, in most of these trials, dietary calcium data were not available. Distinguishing populations at high risk can be performed with the roll-over test or angiotensin test. This approach may clarify the effect of calcium supplementation in these populations.

Effect of calcium supplementation in high-risk patients

Lopez-Jaramillo and colleagues[16] reported a prospective randomized double-blind placebo-controlled trial which evaluated the efficacy of calcium in high-risk patients for developing pregnancy-induced hypertension selected by a positive roll-over test at 28–32 weeks' gestation. A total of 56 women were recruited and allocated to take 2 g of calcium ($n = 22$) or a placebo ($n = 34$) from 28–32 weeks' gestation to delivery. The authors found a significant decrease in the incidence of pregnancy-induced hypertension (3/22 vs. 24/34, $p < 0.001$) and proteinuric hypertension (0/22 vs. 8/34, $p < 0.05$) in the calcium-treated group when compared to the placebo group.

Sanchez-Ramos and associates[17] evaluated, in a prospective randomized double-blind clinical trial, the efficacy of calcium supplementation in reducing the incidence of pregnancy-induced hypertension (gestational hypertension and pre-eclampsia) in angiotensin sensitive nulliparas. Angiotensin sensitivity was established between 24 and 28 weeks in women having a positive roll-over test. A total of 67 women were recruited and allocated to take 2 g/day of calcium ($n = 33$) or a placebo ($n = 34$). Four patients (from the calcium group) were excluded from analysis because of lack of information. Calcium supplementation resulted in a significant decrease in the incidence of pre-eclampsia (4/29 vs. 15/34, relative risk 0.37, 95% CI (0.15–0.92)), and pregnancy-induced hypertension (9/29 vs. 22/34, relative risk 0.46, 95% CI (0.25–0.86)) when compared to placebo.

In both trials, calcium supplementation seems to have a beneficial effect in the prevention of pre-eclampsia and pregnancy-induced hypertension in selected high-risk patients.

Effect of calcium supplementation in low-risk women

Villar and associates[18] studied the effect of calcium supplementation on blood pressure in a double-blind placebo-controlled trial. Fifty-two healthy pregnant women, with a negative rollover test performed before 24 weeks of gestation, were enrolled and allocated to take 1.5 g/day of calcium or a placebo from 26 weeks until delivery. The authors found significant decrease of systolic and diastolic blood pressure (4–5 mmHg) in the calcium-treated group when compared to the placebo group ($p < 0.05$), after adjustment for race and initial blood pressure. Although a reduction in the incidence of pregnancy-induced hypertension was found in the calcium-treated group, this decrease was not statistically significant (4% vs. 11.1%); this result can be attributed to the small number of subjects.

Lopez-Jaramillo and colleagues[19] studied, in a prospective double-blind placebo-controlled trial, the efficacy of calcium supplementation in 106 healthy nulliparous women residing in Ecuador. Women were randomly assigned to receive 2 g/day of calcium ($n = 55$) or a placebo ($n = 51$) from 23 weeks' gestation until delivery. Outcome variables were available for 92 women (calcium group, $n = 49$; placebo group, $n = 43$). The authors found a significant decrease in the incidence of pre-eclampsia in the calcium-treated group when compared to the placebo group (2/49 vs. 12/43, odds ratio 0.11, 95% CI (0.02–0.52)). However, the incidence of pre-eclampsia was too high (27.9%) to consider this study population at low-risk.

Villar and Repke[20] studied, in a prospective randomized double-blind placebo-controlled trial, the effect of calcium supplementation on the incidence of preterm delivery. All patients were less than 17 years old, and nearly 80% were nulliparous. These women were allocated to take 2 g of calcium per day ($n = 95$) or a placebo ($n = 95$) from 20 weeks of gestation. In this trial, incidence of pre-eclampsia and pregnancy-induced hypertension were noted. Incidence of these complications was not significantly different in the calcium- or placebo-treated groups (0 vs. 3.4%, respectively, for pre-eclampsia; 3.3% vs. 5.7%, respectively, for pregnancy-induced hypertension).

Belizan and colleagues[21] reported the largest prospective double-blind placebo-controlled trial in women at low-risk from Argentina in order to study the relationship of calcium supplementation and hypertension diseases during pregnancy. A total of 1194 nulliparous were randomly assigned to receive 2 g of calcium per day ($n = 593$) or a placebo ($n = 601$) from 20 weeks until delivery. Before starting calcium or placebo treatment, urinary calcium and creatinine excretions were measured. The overall incidence of hypertensive diseases (pre-eclampsia and gestational hypertension) was significantly decreased in the calcium-treated group when compared to the placebo (9.8 vs. 14.8%, respectively, odds ratio 0.63, 95% CI (0.44–0.7)). The main significant reduction was found in the incidence of gestational hypertension (7.2 vs. 10.7%, respectively, odds ratio 0.64, 95% CI (0.43–0.96)) whereas the incidence of pre-eclampsia was not statistically modified (2.6 vs. 3.9%, respectively, odds ratio 0.65, 95% CI (0.35–1.25)). Moreover, the effectiveness of calcium supplementation was analyzed as a function of urinary excretion of calcium. Among women with low ratio of urinary calcium to creatinine (below 0.62 mmol/mmol) before treatment, the incidence of hypertensive diseases seems to decrease in the calcium supplementation group when compared to the placebo group without reaching statistical significance (7.8 vs. 13.2%, respectively, odds ratio 0.56, 95% CI (0.29–1.09)).

In healthy women calcium supplementation seems to have some beneficial effect in reducing the incidence of pregnancy-induced hypertensive diseases. However, concerning pre-eclampsia, the results of trials, especially the largest one[21], do not support an effective action of calcium intake in reducing the incidence of pre-eclampsia.

Most of the published prospective randomized trials concerned small numbers of subjects. To give a more analytical power to the results of these trials, Carroli and associates[22] undertook a meta-analysis of six randomized trials[16,18–21,23] comparing calcium supplementation to a placebo. This meta-analysis resulted in a significant decrease of hypertension (odds ratio 0.44, 95% CI (0.33–0.59)), of pre-eclampsia (odds ratio 0.34, 95% CI (0.22–0.54)) in calcium-treated groups when compared to placebo groups. Even if these results are encouraging, one could argue about the methodology used in this meta-analysis which combines studies with high-risk and low-risk patients for developing hypertensive disease.

OPTIMAL DOSE AND SIDE-EFFECTS OF CALCIUM SUPPLEMENTATION

Hamet[13] reviewed all trials undertaken since 1987 concerning calcium intake in the prevention of hypertension in non-pregnant subjects. The optimal level of calcium intake has not yet been established. Calcium supplementation levels used in trials ranged from 375 mg/day to 2150 mg/day. In most of these studies, no rationale for the use of calcium doses was given and concurrent calcium intake was not always controlled. However, there is no evidence to support the use of doses higher than 2 g/day in view of the published studies. In trials concerning pregnant women, calcium doses ranged from 500 mg to 2 g per day and as in trials including non-pregnant subjects, daily calcium intake was not always described.

The relationship between calcium intake and urolithiasis in male subjects has been studied in a vary large trial by Curhan and associates[24]. Subjects were stratified into quintiles of calcium intake. The authors demonstrated that dietary calcium intake was inversely correlated with kidney stones when comparing urolithiasis formation in highest (1326 mg/day) and lowest (516 mg/day) group of calcium intake (relative risk 0.56, 95% CI (0.43–0.73), $p < 0.001$). Moreover, no significant association was found between calcium supplementation and risk of kidney stones. The review of interventional trials concerning calcium supplementation during pregnancy did not show any increase of side-effects, and particularly formation of kidney stones.

CONCLUSION

Calcium supplementation seems to have a beneficial effect in reducing the incidence of pregnancy-induced hypertension and pre-eclampsia in women at high risk selected by a positive angiotensin II-test or a roll-over test. However, these methods of selection of high-risk patients are not easily reproducible. This leads to the investigation of other selection modes, such as the one proposed by Belizan and co-workers[21] consisting of using urinary excretion calcium–creatinine ratio below a cut-off, which could be determined in each population. Moreover, it is apparent that calcium supplementation in low-risk patients reduces the rate of pregnancy-induced hypertension, in contrast, this therapy seems not to be effective in reducing the incidence of pre-eclampsia. Therefore, more prospective randomized trials are needed to assure the usefulness of calcium therapy in the prevention of hypertensive diseases in pregnancy.

References

1. Howarth, A. T., Morgan, D. B. and Bayne, R. B. (1977). Urinary excretion of calcium in late pregnancy and its relation to creatinine clearance. *Am. J. Obstet. Gynecol.*, **129**, 499–502

2. Gertner, J. M., Coustan, D. R., Klinger, A. S., Mallette, L. E., Ravin, N. and Broadus, A. E. (1986). Pregnancy as state of physiologic absorptive hypercalciuria. *Am. J. Med.*, **81**, 451–6

3. Taufield, P. A., Ales, K. L., Resnick, L. M., Druzin, M. L., Gertner, J. M. and Laragh, J. H. (1987). Hypocalciuria in pre-eclampsia. *N. Engl. J. Med.*, **316**, 715–18

4. Hutchesson, A. C. J., Macintosh, M. C., Duncan, S. L. B., Forrest, A. R. W. and Macinctosh, M. N. (1990). Hypocalciuria and hypertension in pregnancy: a prospective study. *Clin. Exp. Hypertens. Pregnancy*, **9**, 115–34

5. Sanchez-Ramos, L., Sandroni, S., Andres, F. J. and Kaunitz, A. M. (1991). Calcium excretion in pre-eclampsia. *Obstet. Gynecol.*, **77**, 510–13

6. Sanchez-Romas, L., Jones, D. C. and Cullen, M. T. (1991). Urinary calcium as an early marker for preeclampsia. *Obstet. Gynecol.*, **77**, 685–8

7. Reddy, G. S., Norman, A. W., Willis, D. M., Goltzman, D., Guyda, H., Solomon, S., Philips, D. R., Bishop, J. E. and Mayer, E. (1983). Regulation of vitamin D metabolism in normal human pregnancy. *J. Clin. Endocrinol. Metab.*, **56**, 363–70

8. Seely, E. W., Wood, R. J., Brown, E. M. and Graves, S. W. (1992). Lower serum ionized calcium and abnormal calciotropic hormone level in pre-eclampsia. *J. Clin. Endocrinol. Metab.*, **74**, 1436–40

9. Frenkel, Y., Barkai, G., Maschiach, S., Dolev, E., Zimlichman, R. and Weiss, M. (1991). Hypocalciuria of preeclampsia is independent of parathyroid hormone level. *Obstet. Gynecol.*, **77**, 689–91

10. August, P., Marcaccio, B., Gertner, J. M., Druzin, M. L., Resnick, L. M. and Laragh, J. H. (1992). Abnormal 1,25 dihydroxyvitamin D metabolism in preeclampsia. *Am. J. Obstet. Gynecol.*, **166**, 1295–9

11. Tolaymat, A., Sanchez-Ramos, L., Yergey, A. L., Vierra, N. E., Abrams, S. A. and Edelstein, P. (1994). Pathophysiology of hypocalciuria in preeclampsia. *Obstet. Gynecol.*, **83**, 239–43

12. Dumas, P., Tremblay, J. and Hamet, P. (1994). Stress modulation by electrolytes in salt-sensitive spontaneously hypertensive rats. *Am. J. Med. Sci.*, **307** (Suppl. 1), S130–7

13. Hamet, P. (1995). The evaluation of the scientific evidence for a relationship between calcium and hypertension. *J. Nutr.*, **125**, 311S–400S

14. Belizan, J. M., Pineda, O., Sainz, E., Menendez, L. A. and Villar, J. (1981). Rise of blood pressure in calcium-deprived pregnant rats. *Am. J. Obstet. Gynecol.*, **141**, 163–9

15. Belizan, J. M., Villar, J., Zalazar, A., Rojas, L., Chan, D. and Bryce, G. F. (1983). Preliminary evidence of the effect of calcium supplementation on blood pressure in normal pregnant women. *Am. J. Obstet. Gynecol.*, **146**, 175–80

16. Lopez-Jaramillo, P., Narvaez, M., Felix, C. and Lopez, A. (1990). Dietary calcium supplementation and prevention of pregnancy-induced hypertension. *Lancet*, **335**, 293

17. Sanchez-Ramos, L., Briones, D. K., Kaunitz, A. M., Delvalla, G. O., Gaudier, F. L. and Walker, C. D. (1994). Prevention of pregnancy-induced hypertension by calcium supplementation in angiotensin II-sensitive patients. *Obstet. Gynecol.*, **84**, 349–53

18. Villar, J., Repke, J., Belizan, J. M. and Pareja, G. (1987). Calcium supplementation reduces blood pressure during pregnancy: results of a randomized controlled clinical trial. *Obstet. Gynecol.*, **70**, 317–22

19. Lopez-Jaramillo, P., Narvaez, M., Weigel, R. M. and Yepez, R. (1989). Calcium supplementation reduces the risk of pregnancy-induced hypertension in an Andes population. *Br. J. Obstet. Gynaecol.*, **96**, 648–55

20. Villar, J. and Repke, J. T. (1990). Calcium supplementation during pregnancy may reduce preterm delivery in high-risk populations. *Am. J. Obstet. Gynecol.*, **163**, 1124–31

21. Belizan, J. M., Villar, J., Gonzalez, L., Campodonico, L. and Bergel, E. (1991). Calcium supplementation to prevent hypertensive disorders of pregnancy. *N. Engl. J. Med.*, **325**, 1399–405

22. Carroli, G., Duley, L., Belizan, J. M. and Villar, J. (1994). Calcium supplementation during pregnancy: a systematic review of randomised controlled trials. *Br. J. Obstet. Gynaecol.*, **101**, 753–8

23. Montanaro, D., Boscutti, G., Mioni, G., Driul, P. and Tosolini, G. (1990). Calcium supplementation decreases the incidence of pregnancy-induced hypertension and pre-eclampsia. *Proceedings of 7th World Congress of Hypertension in Pregnancy*, Perugia, Italy

24. Curhan, G. C., Willet, W. C., Rimm, E. B. and Stamfer, M. J. (1993). A prospective study of dietary calcium and other nutrients and the risk of symptomatic kidney stone. *N. Engl. J. Med.*, **328**, 833–8

Preterm prelabor amniorrhexis

N. J. Sebire, S. G. Carroll and K. H. Nicolaides

37

PREVALENCE

Delivery before 37 completed weeks of gestation occurs in less than 10% of pregnancies[1] (Table 1), but accounts for more than 60% of all neonatal deaths and more than 80% of deaths in neonates with birth weight less than 2500 g[2] (Table 2). Approximately one-third of preterm deliveries are associated with preterm prelabor amniorrhexis[3–10] (Table 3).

INFECTION AS A CAUSE OF AMNIORRHEXIS

In a high proportion of pregnancies complicated by preterm labor and preterm prelabor amniorrhexis, the underlying cause may be ascending infection from the lower genital tract. Positive amniotic fluid cultures, with organisms commonly found in the vagina, are present in about 10% of pregnancies in preterm labor with intact membranes and in more than 30% of cases with preterm prelabor amniorrhexis; in those studies that also tested for *Mycoplasma* species the incidence of infection was even higher[11–21] (Table 4). Additionally, *in vitro* studies have demonstrated that although microorganisms can cross intact chorioamniotic membranes, they can also cause damage to membranes by the release of various proteases and this damage is augmented by the host response to infection[22].

Evidence that infection is a cause rather than the consequence of amniorrhexis has been provided by a recent study of 69 pregnancies with prelabor amniorrhexis at 12–36 weeks of gestation in which the diagnosis of intrauterine infection was based on the results of culture of amniotic fluid and fetal blood obtained by amniocentesis and cordocentesis,

Table 1 *Gestation at delivery of 3 891 440 singleton live births during 1989 in the United States of America. From reference 1*

Gestation (weeks)	n	Incidence (%)
< 28	23 766	0.6
28–31	42 788	1.1
32–36	310 927	8.0
37–41	3 038 496	78.1
> 41	475 463	12.2

Table 2 *Causes of neonatal death in England and Wales for all births and those with birth weight less than 2500 g. From reference 2*

Cause of neonatal death	All weights (%)	< 2500 g (%)
Prematurity	62	84
Congenital anomalies	29	22
Non-infectious respiratory disease	24	29
Intrauterine hypoxia	8	4
Infection	6	5
Hemolytic disease of the newborn	< 1	< 1

Table 3 *Studies reporting on preterm prelabor amniorrhexis as a percentage of preterm deliveries. In a total of 30 272 preterm deliveries, 29% were associated with preterm prelabor amniorrhexis*

Authors	n	Preterm delivery (%)
Kaltreider and Kohl (1980)[3]	11 832	34
Naeye and Peters (1980)[4]	6613	32
Johnson *et al.* (1981)[5]	1174	38
Daikoku *et al.* (1982)[6]	477	43
Main *et al.* (1985)[7]	534	40
Meis *et al.* (1987)[8]	206	39
Goldenberg *et al.* (1990)[9]	7991	18
Tucker *et al.* (1991)[10]	1445	28
Total	30 272	29

Table 4 *Incidence of positive amniotic fluid cultures in pregnancies with preterm prelabor amniorrhexis. The mean incidence of positive cultures in those studies that cultured the fluid only for aerobic and anaerobic organisms was 24%, whereas in those that also examined for Mycoplasma species the incidence was 36% (*)*

Authors	Gestation (weeks)	n	Positive cultures (%)
Garite and Freeman (1982)[11]	< 35	86	23
Cotton *et al.* (1984)[12]	< 37	41	14
Broekhuizen *et al.* (1985)[13]	< 37	53	28
Vintzileos *et al.* (1986)[14]	< 35	54	22
Fisk *et al.* (1987)[15]	< 34	20	30
Romero *et al.* (1988)[16]	< 37	221	29*
O'Brien *et al.* (1990)[17]	< 36	27	37
Dudley *et al.* (1991)[18]	< 37	79	37*
Coultrip and Grossman (1992)[19]	< 37	29	41*
Gauthier *et al.* (1992)[20]	< 35	111	48*
Carroll *et al.* (1995)[21]	< 37	82	36*
Total		281/522*	24%/36%*

respectively[23]. In patients with fetal bacteremia there was spontaneous delivery within 5 days of amniorrhexis, whereas in those with negative fetal blood and amniotic fluid cultures the interval between amniorrhexis and delivery was prolonged by up to 5 months, and subsequent cultures of blood obtained from the umbilical cord at delivery or from the neonates were negative. If the amniotic membranes protected against ascending organisms, the incidence of intrauterine infection would be expected to increase with time after amniorrhexis. In contrast, if one of the causes of amniorrhexis was infection, then the incidence of chorioamnionitis would decrease with time after amniorrhexis.

INFECTION AS A CAUSE OF PRETERM DELIVERY

There are essentially three causes of preterm delivery: (1) iatrogenic cause for maternal or fetal indications, such as pre-eclampsia, antepartum hemorrhage or intrauterine growth retardation; (2) preterm prelabor amniorrhexis, where approximately 40% of the cases have evidence of intrauterine infection with organisms found in the lower genital tract; and (3) preterm labor with intact membranes, where about one-tenth of the cases have evidence of intrauterine infection with organisms found in the lower genital tract.

In preterm prelabor amniorrhexis, the evidence that infection may be the cause of subsequent preterm labor and delivery is based on the demonstration that, in the group with intrauterine infection, (1) spontaneous delivery occurs earlier than in those without infection; and (2) there is increased amniotic fluid concentration of prostaglandins, leukotrienes and a variety of inflammatory mediators that can induce uterine contractions.

Interval from amniorrhexis to delivery

Carroll and co-workers[23] reported a study of 69 pregnancies with preterm prelabor amniorrhexis at 12–36 weeks of gestation that were managed expectantly and had spontaneous onset of labor. In all cases cordocentesis and amniocentesis were performed and fetal blood and amniotic fluid were cultured for aerobic and anaerobic bacteria; the amniotic fluid was also cultured for *Mycoplasma* species. In the group with negative fetal blood and amniotic fluid cultures, the median interval from amniorrhexis to delivery was 41 days (range 1–161) and there was an inverse correlation between gestational age at amniorrhexis and the interval between amniorrhexis and delivery (Figure 1). In the group with negative fetal blood but positive amniotic fluid cultures (usually *Mycoplasma* species), the median interval from amniorrhexis to delivery was 9 days (range 1–37),

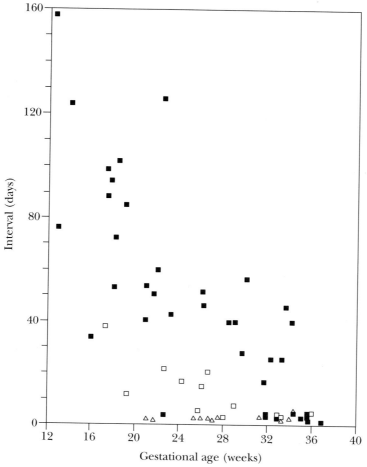

Figure 1 *Median interval (days) between preterm prelabor amniorrhexis and spontaneous onset of labor in patients with negative fetal blood and amniotic fluid cultures (filled squares), negative fetal blood but positive amniotic fluid cultures (open squares) and those with positive fetal blood cultures (triangles). Adapted from reference 23*

and in the group with positive fetal blood cultures the interval was 2 days (range 1–5).

The link between intrauterine infection and labor

The suggested mechanism for the association between intrauterine infection and labor is infection-mediated release of cytokines which stimulate production of prostaglandins that induce uterine contractions. Supportive evidence is provided from a series of studies[24–36] that reported increased amniotic fluid concentrations of prostaglandins, leukotrienes and a

variety of inflammatory mediators in pregnancies with positive amniotic fluid cultures and/or preterm labor; the highest concentrations were observed in cases with both infection and labor (Table 5).

Carroll and associates[32] measured interleukin (IL)-1β concentration in fetal and maternal plasma and amniotic fluid from pregnancies complicated by preterm prelabor amniorrhexis. In patients with positive fetal blood and/or amniotic fluid cultures, plasma and amniotic fluid levels of IL-1β were higher (Figure 2) and the interval between amniorrhexis and onset of labor was shorter than in the non-infected group.

Table 5 *Median amniotic fluid concentration of arachidonic acid metabolites and cytokines in preterm prelabor amniorrhexis or in preterm labor with intact membranes in the presence of positive or negative amniotic fluid cultures (AF)*

Metabolite	Authors	Labor		No labor	
		AF+	AF−	AF+	AF−
PGE$_2$ (pg/ml)	Romero *et al.* (1987)[24]	3143	290	502	278
PGF$_2$ (pg/ml)	Romero *et al.* (1987)[24]	2649	183	340	187
PGF$_2$ (pg/ml)	Romero *et al.* (1989)[25]	720	87	—	—
PGFM (pg/ml)	Romero *et al.* (1989)[25]	1390	510	—	—
PGEM II (pg/ml)	Romero *et al.* (1989)[25]	4143	1485	—	—
12 HETE (μg/ml)	Romero *et al.* (1987)[26]	15	10	10	6
15 HETE (ng/ml)	Romero *et al.* (1987)[27]	1817	386	677	200
5 HETE (ng/ml)	Romero *et al.* (1988)[28]	1876	2052	—	—
LTB$_4$ (pg/ml)	Romero *et al.* (1987)[26]	98	10	16	0
TNF (pg/ml)	Romero *et al.* (1992)[28]	249	< 60	< 60	< 60
TNF (pg/ml)	Hillier *et al.* (1993)[29]	400	0	—	—
TNF (pg/ml)	Romero *et al.* (1989)[30]	750	< 200	—	—
IL-1 (IU/ml)	Romero *et al.* (1989)[31]	100	< 1	< 1	< 1
IL-1α (pg/ml)	Hillier *et al.* (1993)[29]	175	0	—	—
IL-1β (pg/ml)	Hillier *et al.* (1993)[29]	250	0	—	—
IL-1β (IU/ml)	Carroll *et al.* (1995)[32]	—	—	33	19
IL-6 (pg/ml)	Hillier *et al.* (1993)[29]	9500	2000	—	—
IL-6 (pg/ml)	Greig *et al.* (1993)[33]	2592	153		
IL-8 (ng/ml)	Romero *et al.* (1991)[34]	80	< 0.3	—	—
IL-8 (ng/ml)	Cherouny *et al.* (1993)[35]	64	< 1	—	—
Endothelin (fmol/ml)	Romero *et al.* (1992)[36]	150	62	—	—

PG, prostaglandin; HETE, hydroxyeicosatetraenoic acid; LT, leukotriene; TNF, tumor necrosis factor; IL, interleukin

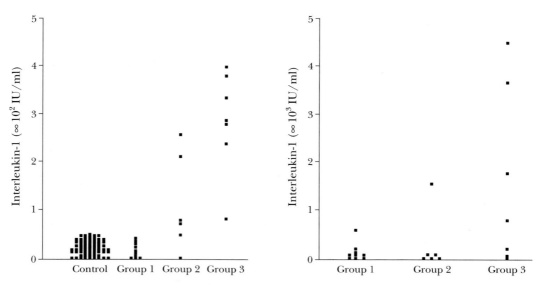

Figure 2 *Fetal plasma (left) and amniotic fluid (right) interleukin-1β concentration in normal pregnancies and in pregnancies complicated by preterm prelabor amniorrhexis. Group 1, no infection; group 2, microbial invasion of the amniotic cavity; group 3, fetal bacteremia. From reference 33*

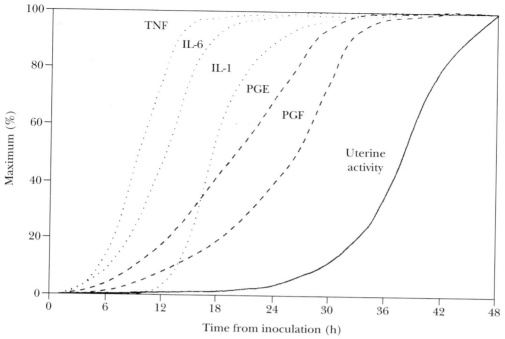

Figure 3 *Temporal relationship between increase in amniotic fluid concentration of cytokines and prostaglandins (PG) and onset of labor following intra-amniotic inoculation of bacteria into rhesus monkeys. TNF, tumor necrosis factor; IL, interleukin. Adapted from reference 38*

Amnion cells, like other epithelial cells, respond to stimulation by one cytokine to produce other cytokines. For example, IL-1β stimulates cultured amnion cells to produce IL-8 mRNA[37]. The temporal relationship between intra-amniotic infection and cytokine production has been demonstrated in a study on chronically instrumented pregnant rhesus monkeys; intra-amniotic inoculation of group B streptococcus was performed on day 130 of gestation[38] (Figure 3). About 10–20 h after inoculation, there was an increase in amniotic fluid concentration of tumor necrosis factor and then interleukins 6 and 1. About 6 h after the initial increase in cytokines, there was a rise in the concentration of prostaglandins E and F. Finally, there was an increase in uterine activity about 30 h after the inoculation. This study also demonstrated that the peak amniotic fluid concentration of prostaglandins in the monkeys with iatrogenic intra-amniotic infection was seven times higher than in those undergoing spontaneous labor at term without infection.

CLINICAL IMPLICATIONS OF PRETERM PRELABOR AMNIORRHEXIS

In pregnancies complicated by preterm prelabor amniorrhexis there are essentially three causes of neonatal death: (1) prematurity; (2) pulmonary hypoplasia; and (3) sepsis.

Prematurity

The survival of preterm infants is mainly dependent on gestation at delivery and birth weight. The survival rate increases from less than 10% before 24 weeks to 90% by 30 weeks (Figure 4). Similarly, survival increases with birth weight from about 10% at 500 g to over 90% at 1500 g (Figure 5).

Pulmonary hypoplasia

In pregnancies with prelabor amniorrhexis that are managed expectantly and result in live births, the risk of neonatal death is related to the gestation at amniorrhexis and decreases from 66% for those with amniorrhexis before 20 weeks to less than 10% when amniorrhexis occurs after 26 weeks[54–59] (Table 6).

Neonatal sepsis

The incidence of neonatal sepsis in the general population is about 0.1–0.8%[60]. In patients with preterm prelabor amniorrhexis the risk of neonatal sepsis is about ten times higher than in the general population, and the risk is increased four-fold in those with positive amniotic fluid cultures compared to those with negative cultures[11–14,19,20,61–72] (Table 7, Figure 6). Additionally, the incidence of neonatal sepsis in pregnancies with preterm prelabor amniorrhexis and in those with preterm labor and intact membranes is inversely related to gestational age (Figure 7).

The reported mortality rate in neonates with congenital systemic bacterial infection varies from 25 to 90%[60,73–76]. However, there is a scarcity of studies comparing mortality in infected neonates to controls matched for gestation at delivery and birth weight. A study that examined 168 infants born at less than 33 weeks of gestation reported that the mortality in the infected group was 33% compared to 17% for those that were not infected[76]. Furthermore, neonatal mortality is higher in those with congenital rather than postnatally acquired sepsis[75].

The long-term prognosis of infants from pregnancies with amniorrhexis is primarily dependent on gestation at delivery. The overall incidence of permanent neurological handicap in infants born prematurely after prelabor amniorrhexis is not higher than in infants born at the same gestation because of other causes. In a

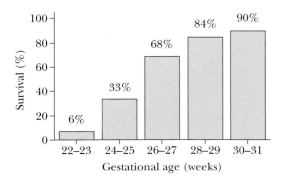

Figure 4 *Postnatal survival of liveborn infants according to gestational age at delivery. The data are derived from nine major recent studies[39–47] on a total of 12 866 liveborn infants delivered at 22–31 weeks*

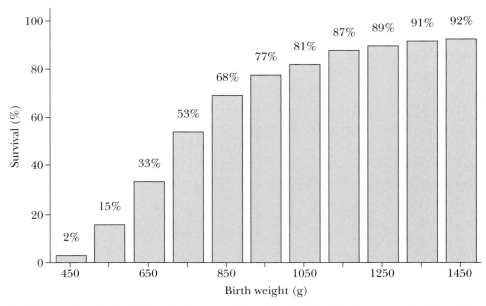

Figure 5 *Postnatal survival of liveborn infants according to birth weight. The data are derived from 12 major recent studies[39,40,42,44–46,48–53] on a total of 26 064 liveborn infants delivered with birth weight of less than 1500 g*

Table 6 *Incidence of postnatal death in live births from pregnancies complicated by preterm prelabor amniorrhexis according to gestational age (weeks) at amniorrhexis. The total results are also illustrated in the figure below*

Authors	n	Incidence of postnatal death (%) by gestation at amniorrhexis			
		< 20	20–24	25–26	27–28
Taylor and Garite (1984)[54]	44	50	75	65	—
Beydoun and Yasin (1986)[55]	54	—	45	24	14
Moretti and Sibai (1988)[56]	107	86	78	37	—
Major and Kitzmiller (1990)[57]	60	—	24	8	—
Morales and Talley (1993)[58]	78	87	46	—	—
Carroll et al (1995)[59]	100	50	37	10	4
Total	443	66	50	33	7

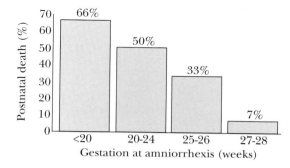

Table 7 *Incidence of neonatal sepsis (positive blood and/or cerebrospinal fluid cultures) in patients with preterm prelabor amniorrhexis. Some of the studies also give the incidence of neonatal sepsis in relation to the results of amniotic fluid culture*

Authors	n	Incidence (%) of neonatal sepsis		
		Total	Amniotic fluid culture	
			Positive	Negative
Seo et al. (1992)[61]	306	8	—	—
Miller et al. (1978)[62]	151	7	—	—
Thibeault and Emmanouilides (1977)[63]	153	3	—	—
Daikoku et al. (1981)[64]	203	1	—	—
Roussis et al. (1991)[65]	99	4	—	—
Wilson et al. (1982)[66]	145	7	—	—
Kappy et al. (1979)[67]	188	1	—	—
Alger et al. (1988)[68]	52	0	—	—
Broekhuizen et al. (1985)[13]	88	4	6	3
Cotton et al. (1984)[12]	61	5	16	3
Bengston et al. (1989)[69]	61	2	—	—
Blott and Greenough (1988)[70]	30	6	—	—
Romero et al. (1993)[71]	110	4	5	3
Gauthier et al. (1992)[20]	111	1	0	2
Garite and Freeman (1982)[11]	86	8	15	3
Coultrip and Grossman (1992)[19]	29	7	17	0
Vintzileos et al. (1986)[14]	54	7	33	0
Fayez et al. (1978)[72]	53	4	—	—
Total	1980	5	8	2

follow-up study of 383 infants born at 26–34 weeks of gestation, the incidence of handicap at 1 year of age in those born after prelabor amniorrhexis was not significantly different from those with idiopathic prematurity[76].

In contrast to the overall outcome of pregnancies with amniorrhexis, infants from pregnancies with clinical chorioamnionitis may have developmental delay. In a follow-up study of 106 infants delivered before 37 weeks of gestation, at 1 year of age the incidence of a low

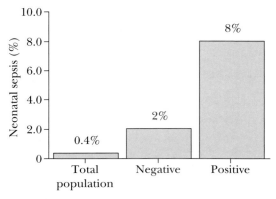

Figure 6 *Incidence of neonatal sepsis in the total population and in pregnancies with preterm prelabor amniorrhexis and positive or negative amniotic fluid cultures*

developmental index score (less than 85/100) was significantly higher in the cases in which preterm delivery was associated with clinical chorioamnionitis[77].

A study of 127 preterm infants who were screened by neonatal cranial ultrasound examinations reported that the incidence of white matter necrosis and periventricular leukomalacia, found in 18% of the cases, was related to both the gestation at delivery and the presence of purulent amniotic fluid[78]. Long-term pulmonary function in infants born after preterm prelabor amniorrhexis may be normal; in a longitudinal study of 22 such infants, serial functional residual capacity measurements were carried out until the age of 2 years, and these were not significantly different from normal controls[79].

CLINICAL MANAGEMENT OF PRETERM PRELABOR AMNIORRHEXIS

Diagnosis of amniorrhexis

The presence of a pool of fluid in the vagina at speculum examination is highly suggestive of amniorrhexis, but a series of tests have been

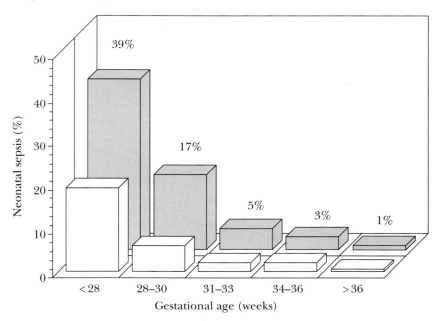

Figure 7 *Incidence of neonatal sepsis in pregnancies with preterm prelabor amniorrhexis (grey columns) and in those with preterm labor and intact membranes (hollow columns) in relation to gestational age. Adapted from reference 61*

used to confirm that this is indeed amniotic fluid. A study evaluating the various tests reported that the best results were obtained with the nitrazine and ferning tests; the sensitivity was around 90%, and the false-positive rate was 17% for the nitrazine test and 6% for the ferning test[80]. A similar sensitivity and false-positive rate was achieved by obtaining a history of 'a gush of fluid from the vagina'.

In patients with suspected amniorrhexis, ultrasound examination may confirm the presence of oligohydramnios. The differential diagnosis would be (1) amniorrhexis; (2) severe uteroplacental insufficiency with fetal growth retardation, and invariably abnormal Doppler results in the umbilical or uterine arteries and fetal vessels; and (3) obstructive uropathy, renal dysplasia or renal agenesis.

Distinction between renal agenesis and amniorrhexis is difficult, because the adrenals may be mistaken for kidneys and vice versa; in both conditions fetal biometry and placental or fetal Doppler results are usually normal. In such cases, further questioning of the patient may reveal a history of intermittent loss of fluid thought to be urine, episodes of vaginal bleeding, or recent increase in vaginal discharge. Additionally, prolonged ultrasound examination may demonstrate fetal bladder filling. Rarely, when there is still uncertainty of the diagnosis, amnioinfusion may be considered; in cases of amniorrhexis, intra-amniotic injection of 100–200 ml of Hartman's solution will invariably cause vaginal loss of fluid within a few minutes. Injection of a water-soluble dye, such as fluorescein, has also been advocated, but this is not necessary.

Non-invasive prediction of intrauterine infection

In the clinical management of pregnancies with amniorrhexis it is aimed to distinguish those without infection, which can be managed expectantly, from those with infection, in which early delivery and/or antibiotic therapy can be undertaken.

Several studies have attempted to predict intrauterine infection non-invasively by assessment of (1) maternal heart rate, temperature, leukocyte count and serum C-reactive protein concentration; (2) cultures of lower genital tract swabs; and (3) fetal assessment by Doppler studies of the placental and fetal circulation, fetal activity, fetal heart rate patterns and amniotic fluid volume. However, a series of recent studies involving culture of amniotic fluid and fetal blood obtained by amniocentesis and cordocentesis have demonstrated that the various methods of maternal assessment do not provide sensitive prediction of infection and have high false-positive rates[21,81] (Tables 8 and 9).

Similarly, in pregnancies with amniorrhexis and intrauterine infection, placental perfusion and fetal oxygenation are normal (Figure 8). Consequently, currently available non-invasive methods for assessment of the fetus will not help distinguish between those with and those without infection, because these tests are designed to detect fetal responses to hypoxia[82] (Table 10).

Invasive diagnosis of intrauterine infection

The diagnosis of intrauterine infection is made by culture of amniotic fluid and fetal blood.

Table 8 *Incidence (%) of maternal pyrexia, tachycardia, leukocytosis and high C-reactive protein in 75 pregnancies with preterm prelabor amniorrhexis. In this study[81] amniocentesis and cordocentesis were performed and the diagnosis of intrauterine infection was made on the basis of positive amniotic fluid and/or fetal blood cultures*

Parameter	Amniotic fluid		Fetal blood	
	Positive	*Negative*	*Positive*	*Negative*
Pyrexia (> 38°C)	7	0	16	0
Tachycardia (> 100 bpm)	14	2	25	3
Leukocytosis (> 15 × 109/l)	14	6	16	8
C-reactive protein	28	15	33	17

Table 9 *True-positive (TP) and false-positive (FP) rates (%) of positive cultures from the lower genital tract in the prediction of positive amniotic fluid and fetal blood cultures in 97 cases of preterm prelabor amniorrhexis. From reference 21*

Organism	Amniotic fluid		Fetal blood	
	TP	FP	TP	FP
Aerobes and/or anaerobes	53	25	40	24
Candida albicans	100	9	100	7
Streptococcus	67	6	50	5
other	45	11	33	13
Mycoplasma species	85	35	—	—
Any organism	76	58	—	—

Table 10 *Incidences (%) of abnormal fetal biophysical profile (BPS) score, fetal tachycardia, reduced fetal heart rate variation and non-reactive non-stress test in patients with preterm prelabor amniorrhexis and positive or negative amniotic fluid or fetal blood cultures. From reference 82*

Parameter	Amniotic fluid		Fetal blood	
	Positive	Negative	Positive	Negative
BPS score (< 7/12)	36	22	50	26
Fetal heart rate (> 95th centile)	14	4	28	3
Fetal heart rate variability (< 5th centile)	28	15	36	15
Non-reactive non-stress test	39	63	50	59

However, the results of culture may not be ready in time for purposeful obstetric intervention, because pregnancies with infection deliver spontaneously within a few days of amniorrhexis. This problem is partly overcome by the use of rapid tests to predict the presence of infection. The most useful test in the amniotic fluid is the Gram stain. This has a high sensitivity (60–80%) and an acceptably low false-positive rate (3–5%) in the prediction of intrauterine infection with aerobic or anaerobic organisms. However, the Gram stain does not identify *Mycoplasma* species, and when these organisms are included the sensitivity of the test is only 40%[21]. In fetal blood a strong suspicion of infection is provided by leukocytosis and neutrophilia[83] (Figure 9).

Need for hospitalization and bedrest?

In the presence of intrauterine infection there is usually spontaneous delivery within 5 days of amniorrhexis. When there is no infection the pregnancy may be prolonged for several months. Traditionally, such patients are hospi-talized for observation and they are often kept in bed with the aim of reducing the loss of amniotic fluid. Such management, despite its major cost, both in economic terms for the health service and family disruption for the individual, is of unproven value. In addition, it has the potential risks of causing thromboembolic complications and leading to infection with resistant organisms. Many patients with preterm prelabor amniorrhexis who fulfil certain criteria (singleton pregnancy, cephalic presentation, more than 72 h from amniorrhexis, no clinical evidence of infection, cervix dilated less than 4 cm), can be managed at home with no increase in adverse maternal or neonatal outcomes[84].

Monitoring uterine activity

The pattern of uterine activity in pregnancies with preterm prelabor amniorrhexis is similar to that of women with intact membranes who later go on to develop preterm labor; within 24 h of the onset of labor there is an increase in the frequency of contractions[85]. Although objective

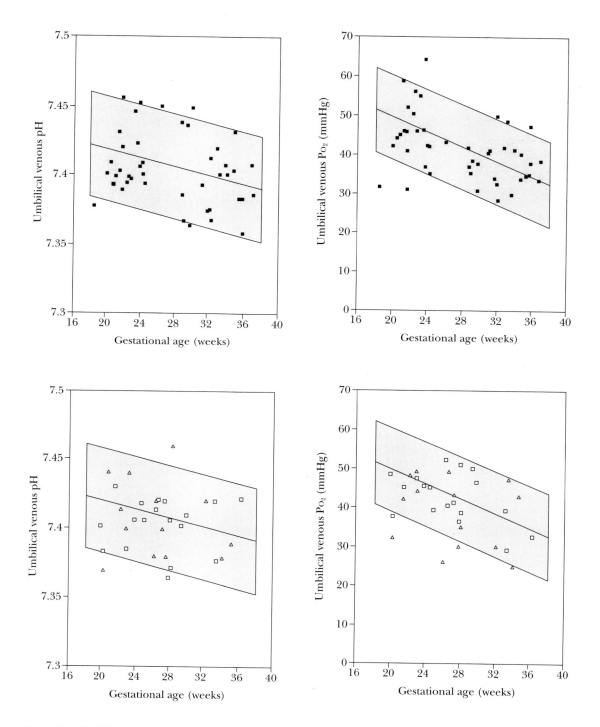

Figure 8 *Umbilical venous blood pH and Po₂ in pregnancies with preterm prelabor amniorrhexis plotted on the appropriate reference range with gestation (mean, 5th and 95th centiles). On the top are those with negative amniotic fluid and fetal blood cultures, on the bottom are those with positive amniotic fluid (open squares) or fetal blood (triangles) cultures. Adapted from reference 83*

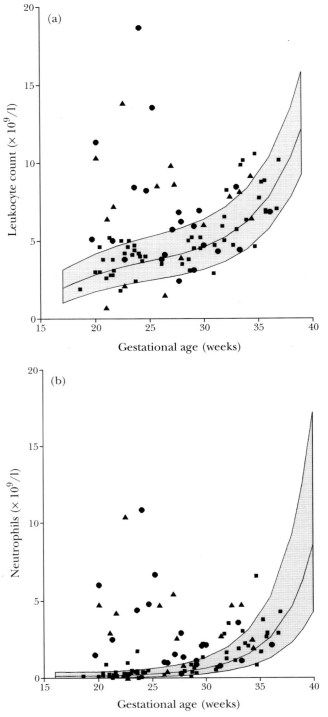

Figure 9 *Fetal leukocyte (a) and neutrophil (b) counts in patients with preterm prelabor amniorrhexis plotted on the appropriate normal range for gestation (shaded area, mean ± 2 SD). Squares, patients with negative fetal blood and amniotic fluid cultures; circles, patients with positive amniotic fluid and negative fetal blood cultures; triangles, patients with positive fetal blood cultures. Adapted from reference 83*

recording of uterine activity may detect increased contraction frequency earlier than maternal subjective assessment, the efficacy of this method of monitoring has not yet been established.

Amnioinfusion

In approximately 2–3% of patients with preterm prelabor amniorrhexis there is apparent 'resealing' of the membranes; they stop leaking fluid from the vagina and fluid reaccumulates in the amniotic cavity. In this group the duration of pregnancy is longer and perinatal mortality is lower than in patients who continue to lose amniotic fluid[86].

For patients who continue to lose amniotic fluid, one suggested option is to insert a cervical suture and then inject a 'fibrin glue' up the cervical canal[87]. However, it is uncertain whether this form of therapy is of any benefit to the mother or fetus. An alternative management is amnioinfusion. In one study an indwelling catheter was introduced through the cervix and held in position by the insertion of a cervical suture[88]. In a study of 84 pregnancies with preterm pre-labor amniorrhexis at less than 33 weeks of gestation, amnioinfusion of antibiotics, together with antiseptic washes of the upper vagina, was associated with a ten-fold reduction in the incidence of positive amniotic fluid cultures at delivery compared to the incidence on admission (from 40% to 4%)[89]. More widespread application of this form of treatment awaits confirmation of the results by other studies.

Antibiotic therapy

The aims of antibiotic therapy are (1) to erradicate occult infection, thereby reducing infectious complications for the mother and fetus; and (2) to interrupt activation of those mechanisms that lead to preterm labor. Although antibiotic therapy is also aimed at reducing the risk of ascending infection, this is probably unnecessary, because in patients with negative amniotic fluid and fetal blood cultures at presentation, subsequent development of intrauterine infec-

tion is unlikely. A potential danger of prophylactic antibiotic use in women with preterm prelabor amniorrhexis is development of resistant organisms. Although there are case reports of neonatal sepsis with resistant organisms following antibiotic therapy for preterm prelabor amniorrhexis, it is not certain whether the use of antibiotics was responsible[90].

Studies assessing the value of antibiotic therapy have not demonstrated a clear benefit on either the incidence of clinical chorioamnionitis or proven neonatal sepsis, but report a small reduction in the incidence of endometritis[91–99] (Table 11). This may be a consequence of the relatively small size of the populations examined and also the 'dilutional' effect of including all patients with amniorrhexis rather than only those with evidence of infection. Nevertheless, the majority of studies have shown a significant prolongation of pregnancy in those receiving antibiotics. This is important, since premature delivery is the major complication of preterm prelabor amniorrhexis. In addition, prolongation of the pregnancy by even 24 h exposes the fetus to the beneficial effect of corticosteroids.

Steroid therapy

There are six randomized studies that have specifically investigated the effect of maternal corticosteroid administration in pregnancies with preterm prelabor amniorrhexis, involving a total of 751 pregnancies[100–105] (Table 12). The data have demonstrated that use of corticosteroids is associated with approximately half as much risk of neonatal death, respiratory distress syndrome and intraventricular hemorrhage, without increased risk of neonatal sepsis or clinical chorioamnionitis.

Tocolytic therapy

In preterm labor after prelabor amniorrhexis there is reluctance to give tocolytics, because amniorrhexis is often associated with infection and there are theoretical worries that tocolytic use may contain a fetus within an infected uterine environment. Additionally, the side effects of the tocolytic agents themselves, such as

Table 11 *Randomized studies on the effect of antibiotic therapy in patients with preterm prelabor amniorrhexis. Comparisons between groups are given as the 95% confidence interval of the odds ratio. This indicates the degree by which an outcome in the treated group differed from that in controls. The definitions of the interval to delivery used in the various studies are shown, and the percentage of patients in each group that had not delivered within the given interval*

Study	n	Chorio-amnionitis	Endometritis	Neonatal sepsis	Definition of interval to delivery	Not delivered (%) Antibiotics	Control
Dunlop et al. (1986)[91]	48	0.67–1.99	—	0.82–24.20			
Amon et al. (1988)[92]	82	0.54–4.80	0.43–5.47	0.02–0.85	> 2 days from randomization	70	44
Johnston et al. (1990)[93]	85	0.07–0.60	0.15–0.89	0.22–17.90	> 6 days from randomization	45	18
McGregor et al. (1991)[94]	55	0.45–2.90	—	—	median (days) from randomization	8	2
Christmas et al. (1992)[95]	94	0.62–4.57	0.05–2.33	0.23–19.20	> 6 days from admission	42	15
Mercer et al. (1992)[96]	220	0.42–1.69	0.36–3.17	0.45–2.18	> 6 days from randomization	27	18
Lockwood et al. (1993)[97]	72	—	—	0.13–3.00	mean (days) from amniorrhexis	11	6
Owen et al. (1993)[98]	117	0.29–0.82	0.11–1.21	0.08–1.35	mean (days) from amniorrhexis	12	7
Ernest and Givner (1994)[99]	144	0.07–0.75	0.05–3.26	—	mean (days) from amniorrhexis	4	3
Total	917	0.54–1.06	0.38–0.96	0.42–1.11			

Table 12 *Randomized studies on the effect of maternal corticosteroids on maternal and fetal outcome in women with preterm prelabor amniorrhexis at less than 34 weeks. The outcome measures examined in each study are shown with their pooled odds ratios (OR) and 95% CI*

Author	n	Steroid	Outcome
Garite et al. (1981)[100]	159	betamethasone	1, 2, 5
Schmidt et al. (1984)[101]	41	hydrocortisone	5
Iams et al. (1985)[102]	73	betamethasone	1, 2, 4, 5, 6
Nelson et al. (1985)[103]	68	betamethasone	1, 4, 5, 6
Morales et al. (1986)[104]	245	dexamethasone	1, 3, 4, 5, 6
Morales et al. (1989)[105]	165	betamethasone	1, 3, 4, 5, 6

1, Clinical chorioamnionitis, OR 0.73 (0.48–1.10)
2, Maternal endometritis, OR 2.97 (1.43–6.18)
3, Intraventricular hemorrhage, OR 0.51 (0.26–0.99)
4, Perinatal mortality, OR 0.65 (0.36–1.17)
5, Respiratory distress syndrome, OR 0.45 (0.33–0.62)
6, Neonatal sepsis, OR 1.22 (0.56–2.62)

tachycardia, may mask signs of maternal infection.

Two randomized studies examining the value of prophylactic tocolytic therapy in a total of 90 patients with preterm prelabor amniorrhexis and no evidence of clinical infection at 25–36 weeks of gestation reported that the proportion of women remaining undelivered 10 days after amniorrhexis was not significantly higher in those receiving oral prophylactic tocolysis (24%), compared to those receiving placebo (18%)[91,106].

Table 13 *Studies investigating the use of tocolytic agents in preterm labor after prelabor amniorrhexis*

Authors	n	Delivery within 7 days (%)	
		Tocolysis	*Controls*
Christensen *et al.* (1980)[107]	30	79	94
Garite *et al.* (1987)[108]	79	69	68

Randomized studies on women with preterm labor after prelabor amniorrhexis reported that the use of intravenous tocolysis was not associated with a significant prlongation of pregnancy[107,108] (Table 13).

RECOMMENDED MANAGEMENT

In patients with suspected amniorrhexis the diagnosis may be confirmed by performing a sterile speculum examination and testing the fluid with a nitrazine indicator. Digital cervicovaginal examination should be avoided. The value of cervicovaginal swabs for culture is uncertain. Ultrasound examination should be performed, to exclude fetal defects, to estimate fetal weight and to determine the presentation. Amniocentesis and also cordocentesis, in centers with the appropriate experience, are essential for the diagnosis/exclusion of subclinical infection. The Gram stain and leukocyte count will provide an early (within 1 h) indication of possible infection, but this requires confirmation by culture, which provides results within 2 days.

Management of patients with negative cultures

In this group, subsequent development of infection is unlikely and there is no need for hospitalization or bedrest. Patients with amniorrhexis at > 34 weeks are best managed expectantly, awaiting spontaneous vaginal delivery; there is no need for antibiotics, steroids or tocolytics. In the group with amniorrhexis at 24–34 weeks, the main risk is that of prematurity and therefore, the aim is to prolong the pregnancy. Corticosteroids are of proven value and should be given. There is no evidence that the use of prophylactic antibiotics is beneficial. If labor starts, tocolytics should be administered and for breech presentation, if the gestation is less than 32 weeks, delivery by Cesarean section may be preferable to vaginal delivery. If amniorrhexis occurs at < 24 weeks, the main risks are those of miscarriage/preterm delivery and pulmonary hypoplasia. Termination of the pregnancy is one of the options to be discussed with the parents. In those who continue with the pregnancy, the value of chronic amnioinfusion in reducing the incidence of pulmonary hypoplasia requires further investigation.

Management of patients with positive cultures

This group will go into spontaneous labor within a few days of amniorrhexis. The main risks to the baby are those of prematurity and sepsis. Additionally, the mother is at risk of infectious complications. These patients should be hospitalized and receive appropriate antibiotic therapy. Patients with amniorrhexis at > 34 weeks are best managed by induction of labor and intrapartum administration of antibiotics. Those with amniorrhexis at 24–34 weeks are best managed expectantly. The use of corticosteroids is beneficial and there is no associated increase in risk of clinical chorioamnionitis or neonatal sepsis. Antibiotics should be administered, but the optimal regime and effectiveness need to be assessed by further studies. If labor starts, tocolytics should not be given and if the presentation is breech, Cesarean section may be preferable to vaginal delivery. If amniorrhexis occurs at < 24 weeks, the main risk is progression to miscarriage or preterm delivery of a septic infant. Management options to be discussed with the parents include termination of the pregnancy or aggressive attempts to prevent early delivery, including maternal antibiotic therapy, and in addition, possible amnioinfusion with antimicrobial agents.

References

1. Department of Health Statistics and Research (SR28) (1993). Annual summaries of LHS 27/1 returns. *United States Annual Vital Statistics Reports*, Vol. I, *Natality. 1989.* (Washington: Department of Health)
2. Department of Health Statistical Office (1993). *Mortality Statistics. Perinatal and infant: Social and Biological Factors. England and Wales.* (London: Office of Population Censuses and Surveys)
3. Kaltreider, D. F. and Kohl, S. (1980). Epidemiology of preterm delivery. *Clin. Obstet. Gynecol.*, **23**, 17–32
4. Naeye, R. L. and Peters, E. C. (1980). Causes and consequences of premature rupture of fetal membranes. *Lancet*, **1**, 192–4
5. Johnson, J. W. C., Daikoku, N. H., Niebyl, J. R., Johnson, T. R. B., Khouzami, V. A. and Witter, F. R. (1981). Premature rupture of the membranes and prolonged latency. *Obstet. Gynecol.*, **57**, 547–55
6. Daikoku, N. H., Kaltreider, D. F., Khouzami, V. A., Spence, M. and Johnson, J. W. C. (1982). Premature rupture of membranes and spontaneous preterm labor: maternal endometritis risks. *Obstet. Gynecol.*, **59**, 13–19
7. Main, D. M., Gabbe, S. G., Richardson, D. and Strong, S. (1985). Can preterm deliveries be prevented? *Am. J. Obstet. Gynecol.*, **151**, 892–8
8. Meis, P. J., Ernest, J. M. and Moore, M. L. (1987). Causes of low birth weight births in public and private patients. *Am. J. Obstet. Gynecol.*, **156**, 1165–8
9. Goldenberg, R. L., Davis, R. O., Copper, R. L., Corliss, D. K., Andrews, J. B. and Carpenter, A. H. (1990). The Alabama Preterm Birth Prevention Project. *Obstet. Gynecol.*, **75**, 933–9
10. Tucker, J. M., Goldenberg, R. L., Davis, R. O., Copper, R. L., Winkler, C. L. and Hauth, J. C. (1991). Etiologies of preterm birth in an indigent population: is prevention a logical expectation? *Obstet. Gynecol.*, **77**, 343–7
11. Garite, T. J. and Freeman, R. K. (1982). Chorioamnionitis in the preterm gestation. *Obstet. Gynecol.*, **54**, 539–45
12. Cotton, D. B., Hill, L. M., Strassner, H. T., Platt, L. D. and Ledger, W. J. (1984). Use of amniocentesis in preterm gestation with ruptured membranes. *Obstet. Gynecol.*, **63**, 38–48
13. Broekhuizen, F. F., Gilman, M. and Hamilton, P. R. (1985). Amniocentesis for Gram stain and culture in preterm premature rupture of the membranes. *Obstet. Gynecol.*, **66**, 316–21
14. Vintzileos, A. M., Campbell, W. A., Nochimson, D. J., Weinbaum, P. J., Escoto, D. T. and Mirochnick, M. H. (1986). Qualitative amniotic fluid volume versus amniocentesis in predicting infection in preterm premature rupture of the membranes. *Obstet. Gynecol.*, **67**, 579–83
15. Fisk, N. M., Fysh, J., Child, A. G., Gatenby, P. A., Jeffery, H. and Bradfield, A. H. (1987). Is C-reactive protein really useful in preterm premature rupture of the membranes. *Br. J. Obstet. Gynaecol.*, **94**, 1159–64
16. Romero, R., Quintero, R., Oyarzun, E., King Wu, Y., Sabo, V., Mazor, M. and Hobbins, J. C. (1985). Intraamniotic infection and the onset of labor in preterm premature rupture of the membranes. *Am. J. Obstet. Gynecol.*, **159**, 661–6
17. O'Brien, W. F., Knuppel, R. A., Morales, W. J., Angel, J. L. and Torres, C. T. (1990). Amniotic fluid alpha 1-antitrypsin concentration in premature rupture of the membranes. *Am. J. Obstet. Gynecol.*, **162**, 756–9
18. Dudley, J., Malcolm, G. and Ellwood, D. (1991). Amniocentesis in the management of preterm premature rupture of the membranes. *Aust. NZ J. Obstet. Gynaecol.*, **31**, 331–6
19. Coultrip, L. L. and Grossman, J. H. (1992). Evaluation of rapid diagnostic tests in the detection of microbial invasion of the amniotic cavity. *Am. J. Obstet. Gynecol.*, **167**, 1231–42
20. Gauthier, D. W., Meyer, W. J. and Bieniarz, A. (1992). Biophysical profile as a predictor of amniotic fluid culture results. *Obstet. Gynecol.*, **80**, 102–5
21. Carroll, S. G., Papaioannou, S., Ntumazah, I. L., Philpott-Howard, J. and Nicolaides, K. H. (1996). Lower genital tract swabs in the prediction of intrauterine infection in preterm prelabour amniorrhexis. *Br. J. Obstet. Gynaecol.*, in press
22. Schoonmaker, J. N., Lawellin, D. W., Lunt, B. and McGregor, J. A. (1989). Bacteria and inflammatory cells reduce chorioamniotic membrane integrity and tensile strength. *Obstet. Gynecol.*, **74**, 590–5
23. Carroll, S. G., Ville, Y., Greenough, A., Gamsu, H., Patel, B., Philpott-Howard, J. and Nicolaides, K. H. (1995). Preterm prelabour amniorrhexis: intrauterine infection and interval between membrane rupture and delivery. *Arch. Dis. Child.*, **72**, F43–6
24. Romero, R., Emamian, M., Wan, M., Quintero, R., Hobbins, J. C. and Mitchell, M. D. (1987). Prostaglandin concentrations in amniotic fluid of women with intra-amniotic infection and preterm labor. *Am. J. Obstet. Gynecol.*, **157**, 1461–7
25. Romero, R., Wu, Y. K., Sirtori, M., Oyarzun, E., Mazor, M., Hobbins, J. C. and Mitchell, M. D.

(1989). Amniotic fluid concentrations of prostaglandin F2a, 13, 14-dihydro-15-keto-prostaglandin F2a (PGFM) and 11-deoxy-13, 14-dihydro-15-keto-11, 16-cyclo-prostaglandin E2 (PGEM-II) in preterm labor. *Prostaglandins*, **37**, 149–61

26. Romero, R., Quintero, R., Emamian, M., Wan, M., Grzyboski, C., Hobbins, J. C. and Mitchell, M. D. (1987). Arachidonate lipoxygenase metabolites in amniotic fluid of women with intraamniotic infection and preterm labor. *Am. J. Obstet. Gynecol.*, **157**, 1454–60

27. Romero, R., Wu, Y. K., Mazor, M., Hobbins, J. C. and Mitchell, M. D. (1988). Amniotic fluid 5-hydroxyeicosatetraenoic acid in preterm labor. *Prostaglandins*, **36**, 180–9

28. Romero, R., Mazor, M., Sepulveda, W., Avila, C., Copeland, D. and Williams, J. (1992). Tumor necrosis factor in preterm and term labor. *Am. J. Obstet. Gynecol.*, **166**, 1576–87

29. Hillier, S. L., Witkin, S. S., Krohn, M. A., Watts, D. H., Kiviat, N. B. and Eschenbach, D. A. (1993). The relationship of amniotic fluid cytokines and preterm delivery, amniotic fluid infection, histologic chorioamnionitis and chorioamnion infection. *Obstet. Gynecol.*, **81**, 941–8

30. Romero, R., Manogue, K. R., Mitchell, M. D., Wu, Y. K., Oyarzun, E., Hobbins, J. C. and Cerami, A. (1989). Cachectin–tumor necrosis factor in the amniotic fluid of women with intraamniotic infection and preterm labor. *Am. J. Obstet. Gynecol.*, **161**, 336–41

31. Romero, R., Brody, D. T., Oyarzun, E., Mazor, M., King Wu, Y., Hobbins, J. C. and Durum, S. K (1989). Interleukin-1: a signal for the onset of parturition. *Am. J. Obstet. Gynecol.*, **160**, 1117–23

32. Carroll, S. G., Abbas, A., Ville, Y., Meher-Homjii, H. and Nicolaides, K. H. (1995). Fetal plasma and amniotic fluid interleukin-1 concentration in pregnancies complicated by preterm prelabour amniorrhexis. *J. Clin. Pathol.*, **48**, 368–71

33. Greig, P. C., Ernest, J. M., Teot, L., Erikson, M. and Talley, R. (1993). Amniotic fluid interleukin-6 levels correlate with histological chorioamnionitis and amniotic fluid cultures in patients in premature labor with intact membranes. *Am. J. Obstet. Gynecol.*, **169**, 1035–44

34. Romero, R., Ceska, M., Avila, C., Mazor, M., Behnke, E. and Lindley, I. (1991). Neutrophil attractant/activating peptide-1/interleukin-8 in term and preterm parturition. *Am. J. Obstet. Gynecol.*, **165**, 813–20

35. Cherouny, P. H., Pankuch, G. A., Romero, R., Botti, J. J., Kuhn, D. C., Demers, L. M. and Appelbaum, P. C. (1993). Neutrophil attractant/activating peptide-1/interleukin-8: association with histologic chorioamnionitis, preterm delivery and bioactive fluid leukoattractants. *Am. J. Obstet. Gynecol.*, **169**, 1299–303

36. Romero, R., Avila, C., Edwin, S S. and Mitchell, M. D. (1992). Endothelin-1,2 levels are increased in the amniotic fluid of women with preterm labor and microbial invasion of the amniotic cavity. *Am. J. Obstet. Gynecol.*, **166**, 95–9

37. Trautman, M. S., Dudley, D. J., Edwin, S. S., Collmer, D. and Mitchell, M. D. (1992). Amnion cell biosynthesis of interleukin-8: regulation by inflammatory cytokines. *J. Cell Physiol.*, **153**, 38–43

38. Gravett, M. G., Witkin, S. S., Haluska, G. J., Edwards, J. L., Cook, M. J. and Novy, M. J. (1994). An experimental model for intraamniotic infection and preterm labor in rhesus monkeys. *Am. J. Obstet. Gynecol.*, **171**, 1660–7

39. Hack, M. and Fanaroff, A. A. (1989). Outcomes of extremely low birth weight infants between 1982 and 1988. *N. Eng. J. Med.*, **321**, 1642–7

40. Wood, B., Katz, V., Bose, C., Goolsby, R. and Kraybill, E. (1989). Survival and morbidity of extremely premature infants based on obstetric assessment of gestational age. *Obstet. Gynecol.*, **74**, 889–92

41. Ferrara, T. B., Hoekstra, R. E., Gaziano, E., Knox, G. E., Couser, R. J. and Fangman, J. J. (1989). Changing outcome of extremely premature infants (< 26 weeks gestation and < 750 g): survival and follow up at a tertiary center. *Am. J. Obstet. Gynecol.*, **161**, 1114–18

42. Kilbride, H. W., Daily, D. K., Clafin, K., Hall, R. T., Maulik, D. and Grundy, H. O. (1990). Improved survival and neurodevelopmental outcome for infants less than 801 g birthweight. *Am. J. Perinatol.*, **7**, 160–5

43. Working Group on the Very Low Birthweight Infant (1990) European community collaborative study of outcome of pregnancy between 22 and 28 weeks gestation. *Lancet*, **336**, 782–4

44. Hack, M., Horbar, J. D., Malloy, M. H., Tyson, J. E., Wright, E. and Wright, L. (1991). Very low birth weight outcomes of the national institute of child health and human development neonatal network. *Pediatrics*, **87**, 587–96

45. Phelps, D. L., Brown, D. R., Tung, B., Cassady, G., McClead, R. E., Purohit, D. M. and Palmer, E. A. (1991). 28 day survival rates of 6676 neonates with birth weights of 1250 grams or less. *Pediatrics*, **87**, 7–17

46. Copper, R. L., Goldenberg, R. L., Creasy, R. K., DuBard, M. B., Davis, R. O., Enthan, S. S., Iams, J. D. and Cliver, S. P. (1993). A multicenter study of preterm birth weight and gestational age specific neonatal mortality. *Am. J. Obstet. Gynecol.*, **168**, 78–84

47. Whyte, H. E., Fitzhardinge, P. M., Shennan, A. T., Lennox, K., Smith, L. and Lacy, J. (1993). Extreme immaturity: outcome of 568 pregnancies of 23–26 weeks gestation. *Obstet. Gynecol.*, **82**, 1–7

48. Powers, W. and Hegwood, P. D. (1989). Survival and ventilatory course of a regional cohort of very low birthweight (501–1500 g) infants. *Am. J. Perinatol.*, **6**, 427–31

49. Resnick, M. B., Carter, R. L., Ariet, M., Bucciarelli, R. L., Evans, J. H., Furlough, R. R., Ausbon, W. W. and Curran, J. S. (1989). Effect of birth weight, race, and sex on survival of low birth weight infants in neonatal intensive care. *Am. J. Obstet. Gynecol.*, **161**, 184–7

50. Vermont–Oxford Trials Network Database Project (1993). The Vermont–Oxford trials Network: very low birth weight outcomes for 1990. *Pediatrics*, **91**, 540–5

51. Victorian Infant Collaborative Study Group (1991). Improvement of outcome for infants for birth weight under 1000 g. *Arch. Dis. Child.*, **66**, 765–9

52. Alberman, E. and Botting, B. (1991). Trends in prevalence and survival of very low birth weight infants, England and Wales; 1983–7. *Arch. Dis. Child.*, **66**, 1304–9

53. Howell, E. M. and Vert, P. (1993). Neonatal intensive care and birth weight specific perinatal mortality in Michigan and Lorraine. *Pediatrics*, **91**, 464–9

54. Taylor, J. and Garite, T. J. (1984). Premature rupture of membranes before fetal viability. *Obstet. Gynecol.*, **64**, 615–20

55. Beydoun, S. N. and Yasin, S. Y. (1986). Premature rupture of the membranes before 28 weeks: conservative management. *Am. J. Obstet. Gynecol.*, **155**, 471–9

56. Moretti, M. and Sibai, B. M. (1988). Maternal and perinatal outcome of expectant management of premature rupture of membranes in the midtrimester. *Am. J. Obstet. Gynecol.*, **159**, 390–6

57. Major, C. A. and Kitzmiller, J. L. (1990). Perinatal survival with expectant management of midtrimester rupture of membranes. *Am. J. Obstet. Gynecol.*, **163**, 838–44

58. Morales, W. J. and Talley, T. (1993). Premature rupture of membranes at < 25 weeks: a management dilemma. *Am. J. Obstet. Gynecol.*, **168**, 503–7

59. Carroll, S. G., Blott, M. and Nicolaides, K. H. (1995). Preterm prelabor amniorrhexis: outcome of livebirths. *Obstet. Gynecol.*, **86**, 18–25

60. Gerdes, J. S. (1991). Clinicopathologic approach to the diagnosis of neonatal sepsis. *Clin. Perinat.*, **18**, 361–81

61. Seo, K., McGregor, J. A. and French, J. I. (1992). Preterm birth is associated with increased risk of maternal and neonatal infection. *Obstet. Gynecol.*, **79**, 75–80

62. Miller, J. M., Pupkin, M. J. and Crenshaw, C. (1978). Premature labor and preterm rupture of the membranes. *Am. J. Obstet. Gynecol.*, **132**, 1–6

63. Thibeault, D. W. and Emmanouilides, G. C. (1977). Prolonged rupture of fetal membranes and decreased frequency of respiratory distress syndrome and patent ductus arteriosus in preterm infants. *Am. J. Obstet. Gynecol.*, **129**, 43–6

64. Daikoku, N. H., Kaltreider, F., Johnson, T. R. B., Johnson, J. W. C. and Simmons, M. A. (1981). Premature rupture of membranes and preterm labor: neonatal infection and perinatal mortality risks. *Obstet. Gynecol.*, **58**, 417–25

65. Roussis, P., Rosemond, R. L., Glass, C. and Boehm, F. H. (1991). Preterm premature rupture of membranes: detection of infection. *Am. J. Obstet. Gynecol.*, **165**, 1099–104

66. Wilson, J. C., Levy, D. L. and Preston, L. W. (1982). Premature rupture of membranes prior to term: consequences of nonintervention. *Obstet. Gynecol.*, **60**, 601–6

67. Kappy, K. A., Cetrulo, C. L., Knuppel, R. A., Ingardia, C. J., Sbarra, A. J., Scerbo, J. C. and Mitchell, G. W. (1979). Premature rupture of the membranes: a conservative approach. *Am. J. Obstet. Gynecol.*, **134**, 655–61

68. Alger, L. S., Lovchik, J. C., Hebel, J. R., Blackmon, L. R. and Crenshaw, M. C. (1988). The association of *Chlamydia trachomatis*, *Neisseria gonorrhoeae* and group B streptococci with preterm PROM and pregnancy outcome. *Am. J. Obstet. Gynecol.*, **159**, 397–404

69. Bengston, J. M., Van Marter, L. J., Barss, V. A., Greene, M. F., Tuomala, R. E. and Epstein, M. F. (1989). Pregnancy outcome after premature rupture of the membranes at or before 26 weeks gestation. *Obstet. Gynecol.*, **73**, 921–6

70. Blott, M. and Greenough, A. (1988). Neonatal outcome after prolonged rupture of the membranes starting in the second trimester. *Arch. Dis. Child.*, **63**, 1146–50

71. Romero, R., Yoon, B. H., Mazor, M., Gomez, R., Gonzalez, R., Diamond, M. P., Baumann, P., Araneda, H., Kenney, J. S., Cotton, D. B. and Sehgal, P. (1993). A comparative study of the diagnostic performance of amniotic fluid glucose, white blood cell count, interleukin-6, and Gram stain in the detection of microbial invasion in patients with premature rupture of membranes. *Am. J. Obstet. Gynecol.*, **169**, 839–51

72. Fayez, J. A., Hasan, A. A., Jona, H. S. and Miller, G. L. (1978). Management of premature

rupture of the membranes. *Obstet. Gynecol.*, **52**, 17–21

73. Placzek, M. M. and Whitelaw, A. (1983). Early and late neonatal septicemia. *Arch. Dis. Child.*, **58**, 728–31

74. Boyer, K. M., Gadzala, C. A., Burd, L. I., Fisher, D. E., Paton, J. B. and Gotoff, S. P. (1983). Selective intrapartum chemoprophylaxis of neonatal group B streptococcal early onset disease. I. Epidemiologic rationale. *J. Infect. Dis.*, **148**, 795–801

75. Ohlsson, A. and Vearncombe, M. (1987). Congenital and nosocomial sepsis in infants born in a regional perinatal unit: cause, outcome, and white blood cell response. *Am. J. Obstet. Gynecol.*, **156**, 407–13

76. Shennan, A. T. Milligan, J. E. and Hoskins, E. M. (1985). Perinatal factors associated with death or handicap in very preterm infants. *Am. J. Obstet. Gynecol.*, **151**, 231–8

77. Hardt, N. S., Kostenbauder, M., Ogburn, M., Behnke, M., Resnick, M. and Cruz, A. (1985). Influence of chorioamnionitis on long term prognosis in low birth weight infants. *Obstet. Gynecol.*, **65**, 5–9

78. Bejar, R., Wozniak, P., Allard, M., Benirschke, K., Vaucher, Y., Coen, R., Berry, C., Schragg, P., Villegas, I. and Resnick, R. (1988). Antenatal origin of neurologic damage in newborn infants. *Am. J. Obstet. Gynecol.*, **159**, 357–63

79. Thompson, P., Greenough, A., Nicolaides, K. H. and Blott, M. (1990). Chronic respiratory morbidity following prolonged and preterm rupture of membranes. *Arch. Dis. Child.*, **65**, 878–80

80. Friedman, M. L. and McElin, T. W. (1969). Diagnosis of ruptured fetal membranes. Clinical study and review of the literature. *Am. J. Obstet. Gynecol.*, **104**, 544–50

81. Carroll, S. G., Papaioannou, S., Davies, E. T. and Nicolaides, K. H. (1995). Maternal assessment in the prediction of intrauterine infection in preterm prelabour amniorrhexis. *Fetal Diagn. Ther.*, **10**, 290–6

82. Carroll, S. G., Papaioannou, S. and Nicolaides, K. H. (1995). Assessment of fetal activity and amniotic fluid volume in pregnancies complicated by preterm prelabor amniorrhexis. *Am. J. Obstet. Gynecol.*, **172**, 1427–35

83. Carroll, S. G. and Nicolaides, K. H. (1995). Fetal hematological response to intrauterine infection in preterm prelabor amniorrhexis. *Fetal Diagn. Ther.*, **10**, 279–85

84. Carlan, S. J., O'Brien, W. F., Parsons, M. T. and Lense, J. J. (1993). Preterm premature rupture of membranes: a randomised study of home versus hospital management. *Obstet. Gynecol.*, **81**, 61–4

85. Campbell, B. A., Newman, R. B. and Stramm, S. L. (1991). Uterine activity after premature rupture of the membranes. *Am. J. Obstet. Gynecol.*, **165**, 422–5

86. Johnson, J. W. C., Egerman, R. S. and Moorhead, J. (1990). Cases with ruptured membranes that reseal. *Am. J. Obstet. Gynecol.*, **163**, 1024–32

87. Baumgarten, K. and Moser, S. (1986). The technique of fibrin adhesion for premature rupture of the membranes during pregnancy. *J. Perinat. Med.*, **14**, 43–7

88. Ogita, S., Imanaka, M., Matsumoto, M., Oka, T. and Sugawa, T. (1988). Transcervical amnioinfusion of antibiotics: a basic study for managing premature rupture of membranes. *Am. J. Obstet. Gynecol.*, **158**, 23–7

89. Ogita, S., Mizuno, M., Takeda, Y., Arai, M., Sugawa, T., Kuwabara, Y., Hashimoto, T., Nishijima, M. and Imanaka, M. (1988). Clinical effectiveness of a new cervical indwelling catheter in the management of premature rupture of the membranes: a Japanese collaborative study. *Am. J. Obstet. Gynecol.*, **159**, 336–41

90. McDuffie, R. S., McGregor, J. A. and Gibbs, R. S. (1993). Adverse perinatal outcome and resistant Enterobacteriaceae after antibiotic usage for premature rupture of the membranes and group B streptococcus carriage. *Obstet. Gynecol.*, **82**, 487–9

91. Dunlop, P. D. M., Crowley, P. A., Lamont, R. F. and Hawkins, D. F. (1986). Preterm ruptured membranes, no contractions. *J. Obstet. Gynecol.*, **7**, 92–6

92. Amon, E., Lewis, S. V., Sibai, B. M., Villar, M. A. and Arheart, K. L. (1988). Ampicillin prophylaxis in preterm premature rupture of the membranes: a prospective randomised study. *Am. J. Obstet. Gynecol.*, **159**, 539–43

93. Johnston, M. M., Sanchez-Ramos, L., Vaughn, A. J., Todd, M. W. and Benrubi, G. I. (1990). Antibiotic therapy in preterm premature rupture of the membranes: a randomised, prospective, double blind trial. *Am. J. Obstet. Gynecol.*, **163**, 743–7

94. McGregor, J. A., French, J. I. and Seo, K. (1991). Antimicrobial therapy in preterm premature rupture of membranes: results of a prospective, double-blind, placebo-controlled trial of erythromycin. *Am. J. Obstet. Gynecol.*, **165**, 632–40

95. Christmas, J. T., Cox, S. M., Andrews, W., Dax, J., Leveno, K. J. and Gilstrap, L. C. (1992). Expectant management of preterm ruptured membranes: effects of antimicrobial therapy. *Obstet. Gynecol.*, **80**, 759–62

96. Mercer, B. M., Moretti, M. L., Prevost, R. R. and Sibai, B. M. (1992). Erythromycin therapy in

preterm premature rupture of the membranes: a prospective, randomised trial of 220 patients. *Am. J. Obstet. Gynecol.*, **166**, 794–802

97. Lockwood, C. J., Costigan, K., Ghidini, A., Wein, R., Chien, D., Brown, B. L., Alvarez, M. and Cetrulo, C. L. (1993). Double blind, placebo controlled trial of piperacillin prophylaxis in preterm membrane rupture. *Am. J. Obstet. Gynecol.*, **169**, 970–6

98. Owen, J., Groome, L. J. and Hauth, J. C. (1993). Randomised trial of prophylactic antibiotic therapy after preterm amnion rupture. *Am. J. Obstet. Gynecol.*, **169**, 976–81

99. Ernest, J. M. and Givner, L. B. (1994). A prospective, randomised, placebo-controlled trial of penicillin in preterm premature rupture of membranes. *Am. J. Obstet. Gynecol.*, **17**, 516–21

100. Garite, T. J., Freeman, R. K., Linzey, E. M., Braly, P. S. and Dorchester, W. L. (1981). Prospective randomised study of corticosteroids in the management of premature rupture of the membranes and the premature gestation. *Am. J. Obstet. Gynecol.*, **141**, 508–14

101. Schmidt, P. L., Simms, M. E., Strassner, H. T., Paul, R. H., Mueller, E. and McCart, D. (1984). Effect of antepartum glucocorticoid administration upon neonatal respiratory distress syndrome and perinatal infection. *Am. J. Obstet. Gynecol.*, **148**, 178–86

102. Iams, J. D., Talbert, M. L., Barrows, H. and Sachs, L. (1985). Management of preterm prematurely ruptured membranes: a prospective randomised comparison of observation versus steroids and timed delivery. *Am. J. Obstet. Gynecol.*, **151**, 32–8

103. Nelson, L. H., Meis, P. J., Hatjis, C. G., Ernest, J. M., Dillard, R. and Schey, H. M. (1985). Premature rupture of membranes: a prospective, randomised evaluation of steroids, latent phase, and expectant management. *Obstet. Gynecol.*, **66**, 55–8

104. Morales, W. J., Diebel, N. D., Lazar, A. J. and Zadrozny, D. (1986). The effect of antenatal dexamethasone administration on the prevention of respiratory distress syndrome in preterm gestations with premature rupture of membranes. *Am. J. Obstet. Gynecol.*, **154**, 591–5

105. Morales, W. J., Angel, J. L., O'Brien, W. F. and Knuppel, R. A. (1989). Use of ampicillin and corticosteroids in premature rupture of membranes: a randomised study. *Obstet. Gynecol.*, **73**, 721–6

106. Levy, D. and Warsof, S. L. (1985). Oral ritodrine and preterm premature rupture of membranes. *Obstet. Gynecol.*, **66**, 621–33

107. Christensen, K. K., Ingemarsson, I., Leideman, T., Solum, H. and Svenningsen, N. (1980). Effect of ritodrine on labour after premature rupture of the membranes. *Obstet. Gynecol.*, **55**, 187–90

108. Garite, T. J., Keegan, K. A., Freeman, R. K. and Nageotte, M. P. (1987). A randomised trial of ritodrine tocolysis versus expectant management in patients with premature rupture of membranes at 25 to 30 weeks gestation. *Am. J. Obstet. Gynecol.*, **157**, 388–93

Clinical implications of automated blood pressure monitoring in pregnancy

38

J. Rigó Jr and Z. Papp

INTRODUCTION

In past years, numerous studies have been published which have emphasized the significance of blood pressure monitoring in the definitive diagnosis of hypertension and the care of hypertensive patients. Several important facts have been discovered, due to the application of blood pressure monitoring. Recently it has been found that the false-positive 'hypertension' diagnosis rate, according to office blood pressure measurements, is 20–25%[1,2]. It is well known that the data obtained by ambulatory blood pressure monitoring show a closer relationship with left ventricular hypertrophy and muscle mass than blood pressure values measured in the outpatient department[3,4]. An attenuated circadian rhythm of blood pressure has occurred in all renal and most endocrine forms of secondary hypertension[5,6].

Blood pressure monitoring creates new approaches in the diagnosis and treatment of hypertension in pregnancy. The applications of blood pressure monitoring during pregnancy have been studied by many, and have led to some controversy, indicating the necessity to survey the experiences and knowledge obtained to date.

REVIEW OF METHODOLOGY AND TECHNICAL PROBLEMS OF BLOOD PRESSURE MONITORING

Blood pressure monitoring techniques enable blood pressure to be measured with reliable accuracy at optional intervals. There are at least 20 types of non-invasive, automatic devices that can measure, record and store the systolic and diastolic blood pressure and pulse frequency values. All of the devices are computer-controlled.

At the present time, there are no international standards for the frequency of measurement in pregnancy. Commonly, daytime 4–6, night-time at least 2 measurements/h are recommended. Although, at least 50 blood pressure values/day are necessary for the evaluation of the blood pressure profile[7].

The analysis of recordings is carried out by computer. Universally accepted parameters, characterizing the blood pressure profile, have not yet been defined. Generally, 24-h, daily and nightly average values, their standard deviations, and minimum–maximum values are analyzed. The diurnal index is also a useful parameter for characterization of the diurnal rhythm. Diurnal variability of blood pressure can also be evaluated by a chronobiological method (cosinor analysis). The reproducibility of the 24-h, daily and nightly average values has been confirmed[8].

According to our observations, performed by ABPM 02 monitor, there are strong, significant correlations between the systolic and diastolic blood pressure average values obtained during the first 24-h of monitoring, and subsequent, repeated 24-h monitoring applications in normotensive pregnant women[9] (Figures 1 and 2; Table 1).

Devices can be assigned to two groups, according to the blood pressure measuring methods employed. In the first group, oscillometric devices sense the oscillations in the brachialis artery. These oscillations are

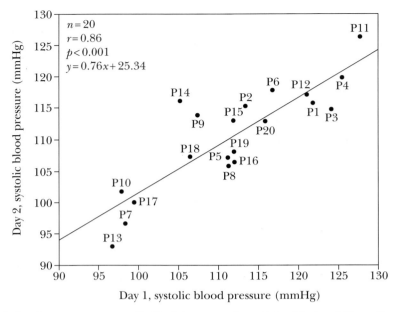

Figure 1 *Correlation between average systolic blood pressure values obtained by two 24-h continuous blood pressure monitoring applications in normotensive pregnancies*

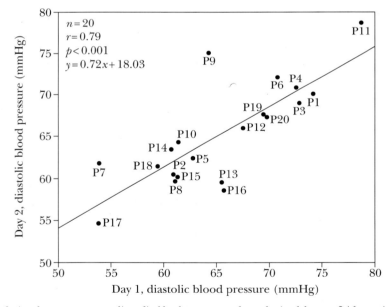

Figure 2 *Correlation between average diastolic blood pressure values obtained by two 24-h continuous blood pressure monitoring applications in normotensive pregnancies*

conducted by tube to the monitor, where the signals are analyzed. In the second group, the auscultatory ambulatory technique uses the Korotkoff method to measure blood pressure. Korotkoff sounds are sensed by a microphone built into the cuff. The accuracy of this measurement is influenced by the position of the microphone, its sensitivity and environmental noise.

Table 1 *Average values of 24-h blood pressure monitoring measurements in normotensive pregnant women*

| | Blood pressure (mmHg) | | | |
| | Systolic | | Diastolic | |
Patient	Day 1	Day 2	Day 1	Day 2
P 1	122	116	74	70
P 2	113	115	61	61
P 3	124	115	73	69
P 4	125	120	73	71
P 5	111	107	63	62
P 6	117	118	71	72
P 7	98	97	54	62
P 8	111	106	61	60
P 9	107	114	64	75
P10	98	102	61	64
P11	128	126	79	79
P12	121	117	68	66
P13	97	93	66	60
P14	105	116	61	64
P15	112	113	61	60
P16	112	107	66	59
P17	99	100	54	55
P18	107	107	59	61
P19	112	108	70	67
P20	116	113	70	68

The oscillometric technique has several advantages. Patient compliance during the 24-h period when the monitor is connected to the patient is better, because there is no microphone that has to be positioned above the brachialis artery. The ambient noise has no effect on measurements, either. The disadvantage of this method is that muscle contraction or movement of the arm can, and usually does, disturb the accuracy of measured data[10,11].

In clinical practice, 'bedside' or 'ambulatory' blood pressure monitoring is employed. Strict bedrest provides a more standardized condition for continuous blood pressure monitoring. Portable blood pressure monitors fastened to the waist of the patient do not disturb the patient's daily activities. Therefore, portable blood pressure monitors are suitable for outpatient monitoring, giving valuable information about the variability of blood pressure at home or at work, etc.

In pregnancy, the measurement of diastolic blood pressure, according to Korotkoff phases IV or V, involves a persistent controversy. Blood pressure monitors define the diastolic value closer to Korotkoff phase V than to Korotkoff phase IV[12–15]. However, Korotkoff phase IV is recommended as the accepted diastolic blood pressure in pregnancy by several organizations and societies[16,17], because Korotkoff phase V cannot be determined in a population segment of pregnant women, due to hyperkinetic circulation. Johenning and Baron[18] reviewed those studies which reported the frequency of undetectable Korotkoff phase V in pregnancy. They found that Korotkoff phase V could not be determined in only < 10% of gravid women. In addition, determination of Korotkoff phase IV includes more significant observer variability. To establish the quality of a sound (muffling) is more difficult to sense the disappearance of the sound. Therefore, determination of Korotkoff phase IV involves significant risk of observer bias.

Another controversial issue is the difference between Korotkoff phases IV and V. The mean value of the difference probably has no clinical significance, because the reported mean differences were only 4.5 mmHg[19], 6.2 mmHg[20], and 12.5 mmHg[21]. Our observation confirms this hypothesis. In our study, diastolic blood pressure was determined by the Korotkoff method in 100 normotensive and 20 hypertensive pregnant women in a sitting position. The mean difference between Korotkoff phases IV and V was 6.45 ± 3.01 mmHg[22].

Finally, Korotkoff phase V is closer to the true diastolic blood pressure measured directly than Korotkoff phase IV[19]. Therefore, it is doubtful that by measuring Korotkoff phase V, rather than Korotkoff phase IV, automatic devices present a minor methodological disadvantage, if any.

Recently, a new concern has arisen, as a comparison of oscillometric and auscultatory techniques in the determination of blood pressure in pre-eclamptic women has shown that oscillometric devices under-recorded both systolic and diastolic blood pressures. The mean differences between auscultatory and oscillometric observations were 5.4 mmHg and 14.8 mmHg for systolic and diastolic observations, respectively, and in normotensive pregnancies these mean differences were 2.4 mmHg and 7.5 mmHg, respectively[23]. A conflicting observation was made by Shennan and co-workers[24], who also employed an oscillometric device (SpaceLabs) and did not find a systematic error associated with the degree of hypertension in severe pre-eclampsia. Nevertheless, the inaccuracy of the oscillometric method in severe pre-eclampsia has not been found by other authors. Therefore, further studies are necessary to examine the validity of this concern.

All of the blood pressure monitoring devices can be used only after a complex validation procedure, according to the recommendations of the American Association for the Advancement of Medical Instrumentation[25] or the British Hypertension Society[26]. It is suggested that blood pressure monitors should be validated separately in non-pregnant and pregnant patients, because of the special characteristics of circulation in pregnancy. According to the recommendations of the British Hypertension Society, the grading criteria are based on a cumulative percentage of test readings that differ from the standard. These grades vary from 'A' to 'D'. 'A' is the best, based on the percentage of measurements differing by < 5, < 10, and < 15 mmHg from the actual blood pressure[26].

Lately, patient compliance has also been investigated during blood pressure monitoring. At present, the weight of the monitoring equipment is significantly less, due to technical development. However, other factors may cause several inconveniences leading to decreased patient compliance. According to Halligan and associates[27] arm restriction was not a significant complaint, while arm discomfort was the subject of complaint in up to 50% of the patients. It is remarkable that 40% of the patients have experienced sleep disturbance[27]. Davies and co-workers[28] have shown by continuous electroencephalography that blood pressure monitors cause appreciable arousal from sleep together with simultaneous blood pressure increases. According to this finding, this effect should be taken into account when blood pressure readings are evaluated.

Patient compliance can be influenced by the occurrence of edema and petechiae distal to the cuff. Paresis of the ulnar nerve due to blood pressure monitoring has also been described[29].

CLINICAL DATA OBTAINED BY BLOOD PRESSURE MONITORING DURING PREGNANCY

Although numerous studies have been published which provide systolic and diastolic blood pressure values obtained by monitoring in normal uncomplicated pregnancies, there is no international consensus concerning reference values. Basic data on systolic and diastolic blood pressure values have been published by Cornélissen and colleagues[30]. The authors computed 90% prediction limits of systolic and diastolic blood pressures values, to be used as a reference set, based on measurements at 1-h intervals during three trimesters in 223 pregnant women. Cugini and associates[31] also defined mean systolic and diastolic blood pressure values and 90% tolerance intervals for 24-h measurements in a smaller normotensive pregnant population. Valuable baseline data were published by Halligan and co-workers[27], who performed ambulatory blood pressure monitoring in 100 Caucasian primigravidas during the three trimesters. A total of 496 ambulatory 24-h recordings were analyzed. There were no differences in daytime or night-time systolic blood pressures between the 9th and 33rd gestational weeks, but significant increases were observed in both daytime and night-time values from the 33rd to the 40th weeks. In daytime and night-time measurements, the diastolic blood pressure decreased between the 18th and 24th weeks; however, it increased from the 30th to the 40th weeks[27]. In addition, further exact studies must be carried out for the determination of reference blood pressure values in normal pregnancies.

Blood pressure monitoring can be very useful in the process of ruling out 'white coat hypertension'. The significance of 'white coat hypertension' in pregnancy has not been adequately explored. The etiology of this phenomenon is not entirely elucidated; however, psychic influences (anxiety and conditioned responses) have been implicated[32]. Based on our own observations, patients exhibiting 'white coat hypertension' require more vigilant prenatal care. In those patients who, in an outpatient setting, were hypertensive, but who, during inpatient stay, with 24-h blood pressure monitoring, were normotensive, we observed complications of hypoxia (e.g. intrauterine growth retardation, meconium-stained amniotic fluid, pathological cardiotocogram, etc.) which are usually associated with pregnant patients who are continuously hypertensive during their entire pregnancy[33,34].

It might be supposed that short-time blood pressure monitoring (of 1 h duration) could help in distinguishing 'white coat hypertension' from more established, chronic hypertension. Mooney and Dalton[35] measured at 5-min intervals for 1 h the blood pressures of 51 third-trimester pregnant women who were diagnosed as hypertensive (by using conventional blood pressure measurements), but who were normotensive before the third trimester of pregnancy. Of these women, 37% showed average systolic values of > 140 mmHg, and of this group, 68% developed severe hypertension later in the third trimester; 63% of the women were found to have blood pressure averages of < 140 mmHg during the 1-h monitoring, and thus were classified as normotensive; 3% of this group became seriously hypertensive at a later stage of their third trimester. Therefore, according to Mooney and Dalton[35], the 1-h blood pressure monitoring profile has more predictive value and provides more information than conventional blood pressure measurements taken during prenatal outpatient visits.

Diurnal variation of blood pressure was already described in non-pregnant subjects in the last century[36]. This characteristic feature of blood pressure can also be observed in normotensive pregnant women[37–40]. This circadian rhythm of blood pressure can be followed during the entire pregnancy[41], but, according to Halligan and associates[27], there is blunting of the day/night difference in the third trimester.

Generally, blood pressure rises in the early morning, reaches the first peak in midmorning, and has a second peak in early evening. After that it falls progressively. The lowest blood pressure values occur between 0.00 and 4.00[39,42]. The second peak (in the early evening) was not found in studies conducted by Mooney and associates[43] who could not identify significant daytime variation between 10.00 and 22.00.

It is interesting that circadian rhythm is not influenced by antihypertensive drug therapy in chronic hypertensive pregnant women[38,39]. From antihypertensive therapy studies, an important finding has emerged which indicates that mean nocturnal decrease of blood pressure is significantly greater in normotensive and chronically hypertensive pregnancies than in pre-eclampsia. In pre-eclamptic women, the circadian rhythm of the blood pressure may be completely deranged[38,40] – even peak values can occur around midnight[44]. It is also interesting that the circadian rhythm of pre-eclampsia does not depend on the severity of pre-eclampsia; both mild and severe pre-eclampsia have similar circadian rhythms[45]. In addition, according to Cugini and colleagues[46], systolic and diastolic blood pressures lose circadian rhythmicity in pre-eclamptic pregnancies complicated by fetal distress. They found higher 'hyperbaric impact' (the integral of the excess of blood pressure in relation to time) values in this group of pre-eclamptic pregnant women, which can indicate a more severe atrial load.

Miyamoto and co-workers[47] documented a clear circadian rhythm of plasma concentration of atrial natriuretic peptide in severe pre-eclampsia. The maximum values were observed at midnight. This finding can support the theory that atrial wall distension might be associated with a significant rise in blood pressure. The circadian rhythm of atrial natriuretic peptide may reflect the changes in atrial load caused by changes in either the peripheral vascular tone or the circulation blood volume[47].

Several theories have been put forward to explain the physiological mechanism of absent or reversed nocturnal blood pressure fall in pre-eclamptic pregnancies. Miyamoto and colleagues[48] described abnormal thermal conductivity of the skin in pre-eclamptic patients. This conductivity was higher at night than during the day, similar to the changes in mean arterial pressure. These observations may indicate that nocturnal hypertension in pre-eclampsia could be caused by an increased plasma volume, which is due to shift of extracellular fluid from the extravascular to the intravascular compartments[48]. This hypothesis of mobilizing fluid from the interstitial space into the intravascular compartment has also been suggested by others[38,42]. Beilin and associates[49] proposed that failure of angiotensin II, epinephrine (adrenaline) or norepinephrine (noradrenaline) to fall adequately at night could have a significant influence on blood pressure in pre-eclampsia. Nevertheless, these theories must be confirmed by further studies.

There are some studies that have focused on the possibility of predicting pre-eclampsia by using results obtained through blood pressure monitoring. Kyle and colleagues[50] employed blood pressure monitoring in the 18th and 28th weeks of gestation in 162 normotensive nulliparous pregnant women. There were no circadian rhythm disturbances observed in women who later developed pre-eclampsia. If 85 mmHg in mean arterial pressure was designated as the cut-off point, then higher pressures in the 28th week of pregnancy had 65% sensitivity and 31% positive predictive value for development of future pre-eclampsia. It is noteworthy that, in those women who later developed pre-eclampsia, significantly higher pulse rates were found, both during the day and while sleeping during the night, in the 18th and 28th weeks of pregnancy. When results from tests using heart frequency and mean arterial pressure parameters were combined, then the sensitivity and positive predictive values were 53% and 45%, respectively[50].

Halligan and associates[51] conducted 24-h blood pressure monitoring in 100 pregnant patients. In four cases, pre-eclampsia developed. Three of the four had elevated mean nocturnal systolic blood pressure measurements greater than the 95th centile at 18–24 weeks of gestation. These measurements preceded the clinical detection of pre-eclampsia by 13–21 weeks[51].

Benedetto and co-workers[52] used chronobiological parameters for the evaluation of the predictive value of blood pressure monitoring in pregnancy-induced hypertension. In those patients who later developed overt hypertension, systolic and diastolic blood pressure MESORs (midline estimated statistic of rhythm) and systolic blood pressure amplitudes were significantly higher in the second trimester. Moreover, in these patients systolic and diastolic 'hyperbaric impacts' and 'percentage time excesses' (the percentage of time with blood pressure excess during a 24-h period) were also elevated between the 20th and 24th weeks of pregnancy.

Tranquilli and colleagues[53] also observed a significant increase of diastolic blood pressure MESOR values during the 20th week of pregnancy in those patients who developed pregnancy-induced hypertension of IUGR during the second half of pregnancy.

Currently, an ongoing study in Dublin, Ireland is tabulating data from blood pressure monitoring in 1000 normotensive women between the 18th and 24th weeks of pregnancy. Data thus obtained may provide additional information about predicting the development of pre-eclampsia[10].

In summary, it is evident that blood pressure monitoring can provide important information for the diagnosis and treatment of hypertension in pregnancy. One of the advantages of blood pressure monitoring is that by employing simple methodology, a large quantity of accurate, dependable data can be obtained about blood pressure changes in pregnant women – especially pressure variations in the home setting. The disadvantages are the lack of uniform standard parameters for the definition of hypertension in pregnancy and the high cost of equipment. It is also true, however, that, by using blood pressure monitoring, savings can be achieved by eliminating excessive clinic visits and unnecessary pharmacological antihypertensive therapy.

It is quite conceivable that, in the future, the classification of hypertension in pregnancy will be influenced by blood pressure monitoring, provided that there is a consensus regarding the normal limits of blood pressure in pregnancy. It is expected that blood pressure monitoring will help in determining the significance of 'white coat' and 'borderline' blood pressure elevations in pregnancy.

Furthermore, in the future, it is to be expected that the therapeutic effects and results of antihypertensive interventions in pregnant patients can be more accurately assessed.

ACKNOWLEDGEMENTS

We would like to thank Peter Csepes, MD (New York, USA) for his insights and advice during the writing of this chapter.

References

1. Pickering, T. G., James, G. D., Boddie, C., Harshfield, G. A., Blank, S. and Laragh, J. H. (1988). How common is white coat hypertension? *J. Am. Med. Assoc.*, **259**, 225–8

2. Hoegholm, A., Kristensen, K. S., Madsen, N. H. and Svendsen, T. L. (1992). White coat hypertension diagnosed by 24-h ambulatory monitoring: examination of 159 newly diagnosed hypertensive patients. *Am. J. Hypertens.*, **5**, 64–70

3. Drayer, J. I., Weber, M. A. and DeYoung, J. L. (1983). BP as a determinant of cardiac left ventricular muscle mass. *Arch. Intern. Med.*, **143**, 90–2

4. Prisant, L. M. and Carr, A. A. (1990). Ambulatory blood pressure monitoring and echocardiographic left ventricular wall thickness and mass. *Am. J. Hypertens.*, **3**, 81–9

5. Middeke, M. and Schrader, J. (1994). Nocturnal blood pressure in normotensive subjects and those with white coat, primary, and secondary hypertension. *Br. Med. J.*, **308**, 630–2

6. Schrader, J., Schoel, G., Kandt, M., Warneke, G., Ruschitzka, F., Rath, W. and Scheler, F. (1991). Bedeutung der 24-Stunden-Blutdruckmessung bei sekundarer Hypertonie. *Z. Kardiol.*, **80** (Suppl. 1), 21–7

7. Thibonnier, M. (1992). Ambulatory blood pressure monitoring. When is it warranted? *Postgrad. Med.*, **91**, 263–74

8. James, G. D., Pickering, T. G., Yee, L. S., Harshfield, G. A., Riva, S. and Laragh, J. H. (1988). The reproducibility of average ambulatory, home, and clinic pressures. *Hypertension*, **11**, 545–9

9. Rigó, J. Jr, Paulin, F. and Varga, I. (1996). Reproducibility of the results obtained by 24-hour blood pressure monitoring in normotensive pregnancy (in Hungarian). *Magy. Nöorv. L.*, **59**, 13–16

10. Halligan, A., Shennan, A., Thurston, H., de Swiet, M. and Taylor, D. (1995). Ambulatory blood pressure measurement in pregnancy: the current state of the art. *Hypertens. Pregn.*, **14**, 1–16

11. Rigó, J. Jr and Papp, Z. (1995). Significance of automatic blood pressure monitoring in pregnancy. In Kurjak, A., Latin, V. and Rippmann, E. (eds.) *Advances on the Pathophysiology of Pregnancy*, pp. 189–96. (Rome: CIC Edizioni Internazionali)

12. Brown, M. A. and Adsett, D. (1991). Automated blood pressure recording in pregnancy. *J. Clin. Exp. Hypertens. Pregn.*, **B10**, 7–19

13. Greer, I. A. (1993). Ambulatory blood pressure in pregnancy: measurement and machines. *Br. J. Obstet. Gynaecol.*, **100**, 887–9

14. Shennan, A. H., Kissane, J. and de Swiet, M. (1993). Validation of the SpaceLabs 90207 ambulatory blood pressure monitor for use in pregnancy. *Br. J. Obstet. Gynaecol.*, **100**, 904–8

15. Franx, A. van der Post, J. A. M., Elfering, I. M., Veerman, D. P., Merkus, H. M. W. M., Boer, K. and van Montfrans, G. A. (1994). Validation of automated blood pressure recording in pregnancy. *Br. J. Obstet. Gynaecol.*, **101**, 66–9

16. Petrie, J. C., O'Brien, E. T., Littler, W. A. and de Swiet, M. (1986). Recommendations on blood pressure measurement. *Br. Med. J.*, **293**, 611–15

17. World Health Organization Study Group (1987). *The Hypertensive Disorders of Pregnancy*, Technical Report, series no. 758. (Geneva: World Health Organization)

18. Johenning, A. R. and Barron, W. M. (1992). Indirect blood pressure measurement in pregnancy: Korotkoff phase IV versus phase V. *Am. J. Obstet. Gynecol.*, **167**, 577–80

19. Raftery, E. B. and Ward, A. P. (1968). The indirect method of recording blood pressure. *Cardiovasc. Res.*, **2**, 210–18

20. Clark, S., Hofmeyr, G. J., Gaots, A. J. S. and Redman, C. W. G. (1991). Ambulatory blood pressure monitoring during pregnancy: validation of the TM-2420 monitor. *Obstet. Gynecol.*, **77**, 152–5

21. Villar, J., Repke, J., Markush, L., Calvert, W. and Rhoads, G. (1989). The measuring of blood pressure during pregnancy. *Am. J. Obstet. Gynecol.*, **161**, 1019–24

22. Rigó, J. Jr, Paulin, F. and Toth, M. (1996). Blood pressure measurement in pregnancy. Comparison of ABPM 02 blood pressure monitor and Korotkoff method (in Hungarian). *Magy. Nöorv. L.*, in press

23. Quinn, M. (1994). Automated blood pressure measurement devices: a potential source of morbidity in preeclampsia? *Obstet. Gynecol.*, **170**, 1303–7

24. Shennan, A., de Swiet, M. and Halligan, A. (1995). Accuracy of oscillometric blood pressure measurements in preeclampsia. *Am. J. Obstet. Gynecol.*, **172**, 1325–6

25. Association for the Advancement of Medical Instrumentation (1987). *American National Standard for Electronic or Automated Sphygmomanometers.* (Washington, DC: AAMI)

26. O'Brien, E., Petrie, J., Littler, W., de Swiet, M., Padfield, P. L., O'Malley, K., Jamieson, M. Altman, D., Bland, M. and Atkins, N. (1990). The British Hypertension Society protocol for the evaluation of automated and semi-automated blood pressure measuring devices with special reference to ambulatory systems. *J. Hypertens.*, **8**, 607–19

27. Halligan, A., O'Brien, E., O'Malley, K., Mee, F., Atkins, N., Conroy, R., Walshe, J. J. and Darling, M. (1993). Twenty-four-hour ambulatory blood pressure measurement in a primigravid population. *J. Hypertens.*, **11**, 869–73

28. Davies, R. J. O., Jenkins, N. E. and Stradling, J. R. (1994). Effect of measuring ambulatory blood pressure on sleep and on blood pressure during sleep. *Br. Med. J.*, **308**, 820–3

29. Burris, J. F., Brinkley, R. R., Riggs, M. C. and Mroczek, W. J. (1988). Adverse events associated with 24-hour ambulatory sphygmomanometry. *J. Am. Med. Assoc.*, **260**, 2508–9

30. Cornélissen, G., Halberg, F., Kopher, R., Kato, J., Maggioni, C., Tamura, K., Otsuka, K., Miyake, Y., Ohnishi, M., Satoh, K., Rigó, J. Jr, Paulin, F., Adam, Z., Zaslavskaya, R. M., Work, B. and Carandente, F. (1991). Halting steps in Minnesota toward international blood pressure (BP) rhythm-specified norms (chronodesms) during pregnancy. *Chronobiologia*, **18**, 72–3

31. Cugini, P., Di Palma, L., Battisti, P., Leone, G., Pachi, A., Paesano, R., Masella, C., Stirati, G., Pierucci, A., Rocca, A. R. and Morabito, S. (1992). Describing and interpreting 24-hour blood pressure patterns in physiologic pregnancy. *Am. J. Obstet. Gynecol.*, **166**, 54–60

32. Rayburn, W. F., Scnoor, T. A., Brown, D. L. and Smith, C. V. (1993). 'White coat' hypertension during pregnancy. *Hypertens. Pregn.*, **12**, 191–7

33. Rigó, J. Jr, Paulin, F. and Ádám, Zs. (1990). Results of non-invasive 24 hour blood pressure measurement in hypertensive and normotensive pregnant women. In Kovács, L., Herczeg, J., Resh, B. and Rippman, E. T. (eds.) *Perinatal Perspectives Caring for High-risk Fetus and Mother*, pp. 509–13. (Szeged: Albert Szent-Györgyi Medical University)

34. Rigó, J. Jr, Paulin, F. and Ádám, Zs. (1990). Continuous blood pressure and pulse rate recording in pregnant women hospitalized due to hypertension (in Hungarian). *Magy. Nöorv. L.*, **53**, 327–30

35. Mooney, P. and Dalton, K. J. (1990). An 'admission challenge test' to predict severe hypertension in pregnancy? *Eur. J. Obstet. Gynecol. Reprod. Biol.*, **35**, 41–9

36. Zadek, M. (1881). Die Messung des Blutdrucks am Menschen mittels des Bauschen Apparates. *Z. Klin. Med.*, **2**, 509–51

37. Seligman, S. A. (1971). Diurnal blood pressure variation in pregnancy. *J. Obstet. Gynaecol. Br. Commonw.*, **78**, 417–22

38. Redman, C. W. G., Beilin, L. J. and Bonnar, J. (1976). Variability of blood pressure in normal and abnormal pregnancy. In Lindheimer, M. D., Katz, A. I. and Zuspan, F. P. (eds.) *Hypertension in Pregnancy*, pp. 53–60. (New York: Wiley)

39. Murnaghan, G. A., Mitchell, R. and Ruff, S. (1980). Circadian variation of blood-pressure in pregnancy. In Bonnar, J., MacGilivray, I. and Symonds, M. (eds.) *Pregnancy Hypertension*, pp. 107–12. (Lancaster: MTP Press)

40. Ruff, S. C., Mitchell, R. H. and Murnaghan, G. A. (1982). Long-term variations of blood pressure rhythms in normotensive pregnancy and pre-eclampsia. In Sammour, M. B., Symonds, E. M. and Zuspan, F. P. (eds.) *Pregnancy Hypertension*, p. 129. (Cairo: Ain Shams University Press)

41. Papadopoulous, L., Papanikolaou, S. Y., Elisaf, M., Ziakka, S. T., Kalaitzidis, R., Theodoru, J., Pappas, H., Mantzios, G., Papanikolaou, N. and Siamopoulos, K. C. (1993). Ambulatory blood pressure monitoring in normotensive pregnant women. In *Proceedings of International Symposium Hypertension in Pregnancy*, pp. 71–3. (Kallithea: Aristotle University of Thessaloniki; New York: Winthrop University Hospital State University)

42. Sawyer, M. D., Lipshitz, J., Anderson, G. D., Dilts, P. V. Jr and Halperin, L. (1981). Diurnal and short-term variation of blood pressure: comparison of preeclamptic, chronic hypertensive, and normotensive patients. *Obstet. Gynecol.*, **58**, 291–6

43. Mooney, P., Dalton, K. J., Swindells, H. E., Rushant, S., Cartwright, W. and Juett, D. (1990).

Blood pressure measured telemetrically from home throughout pregnancy. *Am. J. Obstet. Gynecol.*, **163**, 30–6

44. Redman, C. W., Beilin, L. J. and Bonnar, J. (1976). Reversed diurnal blood pressure rhythm in hypertensive pregnancies. *Clin. Sci. Mol. Med.*, (Suppl. 3), 687s–689s

45. Sumioki, H., Shimokawa, H., Miyamoto, S., Uezono, K., Utsunomiya, T. and Nakano, H. (1989). Circadian variations of plasma natriuretic peptide in four types of hypertensive disorder during pregnancy. *Br. J. Obstet. Gynaecol.*, **96**, 922–7

46. Cugini, P., Leone, G., Antonicoli, S., Lucia, P., Letizia, C., Di Palma, J., Cogliati, A., Moscarini, M. and Caserta, D. (1988). Blood pressure monitoring from a biostatistical and clinical viewpoint for predicting fetal distress in preeclamptic pregnancy. *Gynecol. Obstet. Invest.*, **25**, 239–48

47. Miyamoto, S., Shimokawa, H., Sumioki, H., Touno, A. and Nakano, H. (1988). Circadian rhythm of plasma atrial natriuretic peptide, aldosterone, and blood pressure during the third trimester in normal and preeclamptic pregnancies. *Am. J. Obstet. Gynecol.*, **158**, 393–9

48. Miyamoto, S., Shimokawa, H., Sakai, K., Matsumoto, N. and Nakano, H. (1989). A possible explanation for nocturnal hypertension in preeclamptics. *J. Clin. Exp. Hypertens. Preg.*, **B8**, 495–506

49. Beilin, L. J., Deacon, J., Michael, C. A., Vandongen, R., Layor, C. M., Barden, A. E. and Davidson (1982). Circadian rhythms of blood pressure and pressor hormones in normal and hypertensive pregnancy. *Clin. Exp. Pharmacol. Physiol.*, **9**, 321–6

50. Kyle, P. M., Clark, S. J., Buckley, D., Kissane, J., Coats, A. J. S., de Swiet, M. and Redman, C. W. G. (1993). Second trimester ambulatory blood pressure in nulliparous pregnancy: a useful screening test for pre-eclampsia? *Br. J. Obstet. Gynaecol.*, **100**, 914–19

51. Halligan, A. J., O'Brien, E., O'Malley, R., Walshe, J. J. and Darling, M. R. N. (1993). 24-hour ambulatory blood pressure measurement in pregnancy. *Br. J. Obstet. Gynaecol.*, **100**, 290

52. Benedetto, G., Narducci, P. L., Rondoni, F., Betti, R. and Angeli, G. (1993). Non invasive 24-hour monitoring of blood pressure. In Cosmi, E. V. and Di Renzo, G. C. (eds.) *Abstract Book of 2nd World Congress of Perinatal Medicine*, pp. 8–9, Rome and Florence

53. Tranquilli, A. L., Harfouche, I., Rezai, B., Conti, C., Garzetti, G. G. and Romanini, C. (1993). Midtrimester diastolic mesor predicts subsequent PIH and IUGR. In Cosmi, E. V. and Di Renzo, G. C. (eds.) *Abstract Book of 2nd World Congress of Perinatal Medicine*, p. 147. (Rome and Florence)

Twinning and twins

39

I. Blickstein and M. Smith-Levitin

INTRODUCTION

There is no doubt that twin gestations pose special challenges for the healthcare provider, for the mother, and for the fetuses themselves. The impact of the risks on overall perinatal morbidity and mortality is changing as the frequency of twin gestations is steadily increasing and reaching, according to several authorities, epidemic proportions[1]. At the same time, our understanding of the twinning process, and our ability to diagnose, treat and even prevent some of the complications is improving.

Twins were once thought of as monsters and divine punishment for maternal misbehavior[2]. In the present era of perinatal medicine, where the fetus is considered to be a patient from an early gestational age, twins are thought of as two distinct patients. Multiple gestations, however, are a unique situation in fetal medicine as what is in the best interest of one fetus may be detrimental to its co-fetus or fetuses. This chapter, in keeping with the philosophy of the fetus as a patient, focuses on the fetal aspects of twin pregnancies from conception through their intrauterine development to their delivery.

EPIDEMIOLOGY OF TWINS

The incidence of multifetal pregnancies, including twins, has increased significantly over the last 20 years. Luke[3] found that twin births have increased at twice the rate of singletons since 1973 in a population-based analysis of all live births in the United States between 1960 and 1990. The frequency of twins was 1 in 43 births (2–3%) in 1990 which is two times higher than the usually quoted rate of 1–1.2%.

There are primarily two reasons for this increase. The first is the more widespread use of assisted reproductive technologies (ART)[4].

Ovulation induction, alone, leads to twins 7–50% of the time depending on which agent is used[5]. The second reason is the recent trend toward delayed childbirth. The proportion of births to women over age 30 doubled from 1973 to 1990, and there is a greater natural incidence of twins among older women (Figure 1)[4,6,7]. Older women also have decreased natural fecundity necessitating the use of ART more frequently.

The use of ART will probably change the naturally different epidemiologies of monozygotic (MZ) and dizygotic (DZ) twins. It has been generally accepted that the rate of MZ twinning is a biological constant (4/1000 deliveries), comprising about one-third of the twin population (DZ : MZ = 2 : 1)[8]. Some observations have cast doubt on this paradigm. Yoshida[9] has shown that a 1 : 1 ratio better represents the relative zygosity in the naturally occurring Japanese twin population, which suggests that racial differences in MZ twinning rates cannot be excluded.

Unlike with MZ twinning, several factors have been firmly associated with an increased rate of spontaneous DZ twins. Most importantly, higher twinning rates in specific races and in families with twins suggest a genetic predisposition. The best example comes from the Yorubas in western Nigeria. The rate of liveborn twins in this tribe is 4–5%, of which 92% are DZ. Nylander[10] found that mothers who have had twins previously have a much greater tendency toward twinning than mothers who have not, that fathers do not contribute to the twinning tendency, and that mothers who are themselves twins do not have a higher tendency toward twinning. These observations are consistent with either a tendency toward twinning that is acquired or one that is determined by multiple

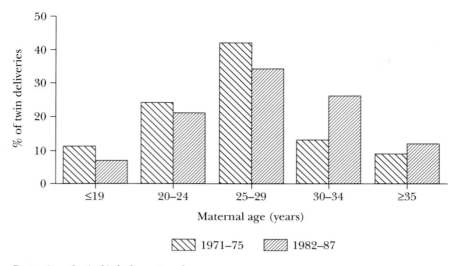

Figure 1 *Proportion of twin births by maternal age*

genes. Recently, Meulemans and associates[11] investigated three-generational pedigrees of mothers of spontaneous DZ proband twins. Complex segregation analysis showed that the trait of 'having DZ twins' was inherited as an autosomal monogenic dominant with a gene frequency of 0.035 and a female-specific penetrance of 0.1.

Women with a familial tendency toward twins may have some selective advantage for having a successful twin pregnancy. Eriksson[12] has provided evidence that mothers who are siblings of triplets have a high rate of having twins and may have better physical capacity than other women for carrying a multiple gestation. This concept is further supported by the observation that the perinatal outcome of a second pair of twins is significantly better than the outcome of a previous set delivered to the same woman[13].

The pathogenesis of the twinning process

Theories relating to the twinning process have changed drastically over the centuries, particularly for monozygotic twins. Monozygotic twins result from the fertilization of one ovum by one sperm leading to two fetuses with the same genetic make-up. Dizygotic twins result from the fertilization of two separate ova by two separate sperm leading to two fetuses that are genetically dissimilar. The advent of reproductive endocrinology has rendered these definitions inadequate.

Dizygotic twins should be classified as a reproductive *disorder*, since they usually result from the production of more than one egg in a single cycle, whether naturally or artificially. Cases of superfecundation and interval ovulation are also referred to as twins. Although superfetation has not been documented in humans, pregnancies resulting from the simultaneous transfer of two cryopreserved embryos achieved in different cycles may be regarded as iatrogenic superfetation. Similarly, two *in-vitro* fertilization (IVF) embryos from one cycle, even if transferred at different times to produce two successive singleton pregnancies, are 'twins' according to the definition above. Furthermore, the combinations of a fetus and hydatidiform mole and an intra- and extrauterine (heterotopic) pregnancy are twins. A special subset of DZ twins, who will be discussed later, are those who remain after reduction of higher-order multiples.

Monozygotic twins, on the other hand, should be classified as a reproductive *anomaly* since they result from a pathogenic splitting of a single zygote and are associated with a unique set of abnormalities. For example, the incidence of congenital malformations in monozygotic twins is 2–4-fold higher than in dizygotic twins, the syndrome of twin–twin transfusion affects only MZ twins[14], and the relative risk of fetal mortality after 28 weeks' gestation for a MZ pair is 2–3-fold higher than for a DZ pair[15].

Surprisingly, the rate of MZ twinning is increased with ART as has been demonstrated by the East Flanders Prospective Twin Study[16]. Zygotic splitting is significantly higher in pregnancies following ovulation induction[17] and possibly after IVF-embryo transfer (ET)[18]. Increased MZ twinning seems to be unrelated to the mode of conception, whether with induction of ovulation only, IVF-ET, gamete intrafallopian tube transfer, zygote intrafallopian tube transfer, or to the use of fertility enhancing drugs, whether with clomiphene citrate or gonadotropins.

It is not as yet known why MZ twins are more frequent after ART procedures. The most compelling speculation is that the exposure of the zona pellucida surrounding the early embryo, to biochemical or mechanical trauma, which creates a *locus minoris resistentiae* in the zona, leads to herniation of the blastocyst and eventually to monozygotic splitting. Recent observations from pregnancies following zona manipulation support this speculation. Cohen[19] has pointed to the increased risk of MZ twinning following application of assisted hatching[20]. Further support for this theory comes from a case report of a healthy MZ twin pair that was the result of transfer of a frozen-thawed blastocyst in which the thickness of the zona pellucida was reduced by gentle rubbing with a microneedle[21]. Alikani and colleagues[22] observed six MZ twin pregnancies resulting from replacement of embryos, with either naturally thin zonae pellucidae or with zonae that had been breached during micromanipulation, for subzonal sperm insertion or assisted hatching.

The latter set of observations is of particular interest since the literature seems to take for granted Corner's[23] 'critical stages' theory which explains the distinct morphogenetic changes in MZ twinning and placentation. According to this theory, the ultimate chorionicity depends on the developmental stage at the time of blastocyst splitting. It follows that only dichorionic, MZ twins will result if ART manipulates the embryo at Corner's critical stage I (circa day 2, postovulation). To date, all the reported cases with documented placentation have had a monochorial placenta[21,22]. Admittedly, series of zona manipulation are not large enough to support or refute Corner's postulations. It must be recalled, however, that none of these critical stages has been experimentally proven. Corner described these stages only as a model for understanding the morphogenesis of MZ twinning. Our current concept of MZ placentation, which is the key to understanding the unique pathology of twinning, will probably continue to change with additional evidence from iatrogenic MZ twins.

THE FIRST-TRIMESTER TWIN GESTATION

Diagnosis of twins

It is of utmost importance to diagnose a twin gestation as early as possible. Twins that are diagnosed well before labor have a better outcome than twins that are diagnosed intrapartum[24]. Biochemical testing in early pregnancy can suggest a multiple gestation. Higher than normal values of pregnancy markers such as β-human chorionic gonadotropin (β-hCG) and human placental lactogen have been associated with twinning, but they have not been specific enough nor have they been cost effective to be used as a screen for a multiple gestation.

Ultrasonography has become indispensable for the first-trimester diagnosis, and later management, of twins (Table 1). In the United States, however, where controversy exists regarding routine sonography, pregnant women do not necessarily receive an ultrasound examination, particularly not in the first trimester. At least women who are at high risk of having twins such as women who have used ART, who have uterine size greater than expected for dates, or who present with early hyperemesis gravidarum should have an early sonogram.

The first indication of twins is the finding of two gestational sacs which can be seen as early as 4–5 weeks' gestation with a transvaginal probe[25]. This finding also excludes a diagnosis

Table 1 *Benefits of sonography in twin gestations*

First trimester
Documentation of twins
Determination of chorionicity and amnionicity
Crown–rump length determination for early
   dating and early normal growth
Screening for some anomalies
Guidance for chorionic villus sampling

Second trimester
Screening and diagnosis of anomalies
Guidance for amniocentesis
Biometry for early growth patterns and
   determination of early discordance
Diagnosis of twin–twin transfusion syndrome

Third trimester
Biometry for growth patterns, evidence of
   intrauterine growth retardation and discordance
Fetal status assessment
   amniotic fluid index
   biophysical profile
   Doppler flow studies
Fetal presentation

Intrapartum
Fetal presentation
Guidance for external cephalic version of the
   second twin

of monoamniotic twins even before embryonic structures can be identified. The sonographic findings can also significantly aid in the diagnosis of chorionicity. The presence of two separate placental discs, often located on opposite uterine surfaces, is absolute evidence of a DZ twin gestation. If the placentas are close to one another or appear as one, the gestation can be DZ or MZ. Attention must then be turned to the dividing membrane. A monochorionic membrane may be too illusive for sonography giving the false impression of a monoamniotic gestation. The definite diagnosis of monoamniotic twins should thus be deferred to a more advanced gestational age. A thick membrane with four layers, which can occasionally be counted, is consistent with a dichorionic gestation. Unfortunately, the data relating the sonographic measurements of intertwin membrane thickness to chorionicity are, at best, conflicting. For example, Brass and co-workers[26] were able to correctly assign the chorionicity of 33 out of 34 twin pregnancies. In contrast, Stagiannis and

associates[27] found that measurement of the dividing membrane thickness had high intra- and interobserver variation, but this was in the second and third trimester. The 'twin peak' sign is reliable proof of dichorionicity[28]. It is a triangular projection of tissue from the chorionic plate into a cleft between the membranes.

Although a determination of the chorionicity does not necessarily establish the zygosity since an MZ twin pair can result in a monochorionic or dichorionic placenta, the early diagnosis of a monochorionic gestation is important for many reasons that will be discussed below. It may be necessary, in certain cases, to resort to more sophisticated methods of zygosity determination such as DNA fingerprinting[29]. It is currently unknown how many twins will benefit, and to what extent, from early diagnosis of chorionicity since it is unknown how many spontaneous twins, who have a much greater chance of having a monochorionic placenta, are diagnosed and evaluated in the first trimester[18].

Early fetal demise

Since the implementation of sonography, it has become evident that the number of twins observed at delivery is markedly less than the number of twin pregnancies identified by first-trimester sonography. This 'vanishing twin' syndrome was initially accepted with some scepticism. However, studies combining serial sonograms with histological confirmation of the vanished twin have proven that early embryonic or fetal disappearance in multiple pregnancies does occur. As seen in Figure 2, the first-trimester appearance of two live embryos rather than just two gestational sacs improves the chances of a live birth of two, or even of one, baby[30]. For this reason, the obstetrician should be cautious in counselling couples regarding the diagnosis of a twin gestation too early.

Before a diagnosis of two gestational sacs could be made sonographically, most of these pregnancies would not have been classified as a twin gestation. This presents a problem in the epidemiology of twins in that the true denominator for outcome calculations is not really known[1]. Ideally, this number should include all

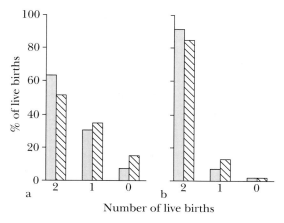

Figure 2 *The percentage of live births after an initial finding of two gestational sacs (a) vs. two live embryos (b). Graph represents data collected by Dickey and colleagues[30] from 227 twin pregnancies following infertility treatment. Maternal age < 30 years (stippled bars) and > 30 years (hatched bars)*

postconception twins. Including only cases in which two fetal heart beats are initially documented and subsequent scans reveal one viable fetus results in a quoted incidence of twins (3.3%) that is low[31]. If all suspected twin gestations are included, the incidence increases to 5–5.4%[31].

Looking at these numbers from another perspective reveals a 21.2% disappearance rate, which is comparable to the background rate of spontaneous abortion in the first trimester. This figure indicates that a twin has only a slightly higher risk of embryonal demise compared to a singleton. The observed difference between the incidence of postconception and delivered twins may, therefore, be attributed to events in the second and third trimesters.

Although the prognosis for the remaining twin appears to be good, the 'vanishing twin' syndrome is not always just a sonographic phenomenon. There is some speculation that the 'vanishing twin' syndrome may be the result of a twin–twin transfusion syndrome (TTTS) of very early onset. Evidence for this comes from the frequent association of the vanishing twin syndrome with marginal or velamentous insertions of the umbilical cord in the surviving twin[32,33], which have also been found more commonly in cases of twin–twin transfusion syn-

drome[34,35]. Since TTTS affects only MZ twins, it is possible that MZ twins are more frequent than we realize, but their spontaneous reduction (by the 'vanishing twin' phenomenon) leads to the artificially greater occurrence of DZ twinning.

Early fetal growth

Anatomical and sonographic studies have indicated that growth rates of twins in the first 20 weeks of pregnancy are similar to those of singletons. The average fetal size in relation to menstrual age is equivalent for twins and singletons within about 6–7 days in early pregnancy[36]. The use of crown–rump length to establish good gestational dating is accurate and important in twins since they have such a high incidence of growth problems later. Iffy and colleagues[36] found that twin fetuses have the same linear growth and weight gain prior to mid-gestation, that most twins tend to begin their development within a time span of about 24 h, that there is a close intrapair relation between length and weight during the first 18 weeks of gestation, and that growth disparity probably begins at mid-gestation[36].

While intertwin discordant growth is more pronounced in the second half of gestation, there is evidence suggesting that intertwin size disparity can begin in the first trimester. For example, discordant twin growth following IVF-ET that ultimately resulted in an apparently healthy pair with a 26.6% weight discordance was diagnosed in the first trimester by different crown–rump lengths.[37] Early growth discordance, however, can be indicative of a more serious problem[38]. Weissman and co-workers[39] described five twin pregnancies with crown–rump length differences of more than 5 days in which the smaller twin was affected by a major congenital anomaly. Thus, a finding of first-trimester intertwin growth discordance warrants a meticulous sonographic search for congenital anomalies[16].

Congenital anomalies in twins

It is generally accepted that there is an increased incidence of fetal anomalies in twin gestations.

However, there are opposing views regarding whether twins do have more anomalies than singletons[40,41]. Some of the placental, membrane and cord abnormalities as well as some of the structural abnormalities are unique to twins and may be related to the twinning process itself. Others are the same as those seen in singletons.

Congenital anomalies that are more frequent among twins may be grouped into four categories (Table 2). These groups are different from those proposed by Schinzel and associates[42] who categorized structural defects in twins according to three presumed etiologies: limited uterine space, disruption of blood flow and early defects in morphogenesis.

Anomalies in MZ twins, which are unequivocally increased 2–4 fold, is particularly interesting. Sir Francis Galton[43], in 1875, even pointed out that the genetic identity of MZ twins makes them uniquely suited for evaluation of the 'relative powers of nature and nurture'. This observation probably initiated and stimulated scientific efforts that use twins as a model for the interaction between genotype and the environment[44]. The high rate of concordance of the anomalies in MZ twins is probably due to the genetic homogeneity of the pair. Another theory purports that the hypothetical teratogen which causes MZ twinning also causes malformations, and, therefore, leads to anomaly concordance.

Table 2 *Categories of congenital anomalies that are more frequent among twins*

Structural malformations
Neural tube defects
Congenital heart disease
Hydrocephalus
Urogenital sinus malformations

Malformations that are unique to MZ twins
Amniotic band syndrome
Acardiac twin
Conjoined twins
Twin embolization syndrome (microcephaly, hydranencephaly, porencephalic cysts, intestinal atresia, aplasia cutis)

Placental abnormalities
Deformations due to intrauterine crowding

The risk of chromosomal abnormalities is also increased in twin gestations. Consider, for example, the risk of trisomy 21. Assuming that the probability of non-disjunction is the same for each twin, a patient carrying twins will have a risk of having at least one affected fetus at a younger maternal age than she would for having an affected singleton. Rodis and colleagues[45] provided convincing data demonstrating that a 33-year-old patient with a twin gestation has a risk of Down syndrome in at least one of her twins equivalent to that of a 35-year-old with a singleton gestation. Since twins are more frequent among older patients who have a priori greater risk of aneuploidy, a greater proportion of twin pregnancies will be at increased risk.

Hunter and Cox[46] quantified the theoretical increased genetic risk of a twin pregnancy. Based on the 2 : 1 ratio between DZ and MZ twins, they calculated the risk to be 5/3 times the empirical age risk. However, this risk must always be compared to the risk of complications following invasive prenatal diagnostic procedures, which will be discussed later, and to the abortion rate for twin gestations without invasive diagnostic procedures.

First trimester prenatal diagnosis

Ideally, congenital anomalies should be diagnosed as early as possible. Unfortunately, the modalities for prenatal diagnosis in the first trimester are limited. Some anomalies, such as anencephaly, should be carefully sought during transvaginal sonography. In addition, sonographic markers for chromosomal abnormalities such as nuchal translucency thickness, can be used as a screening tool. In twins, this sonographic method has three obvious advantages: it is harmless, it provides a detectable marker to ensure correct identification of the affected twin, and it is discernible early enough for the option of selective reduction in the first trimester. Pandya and co-workers[47] described a series of eight twin pregnancies karyotyped at 10–14 weeks' gestation in which a nuchal translucency thickness of more than 2.5 mm was found in nine of the ten trisomic fetuses. Larger samples are clearly needed to confirm the predictivity of nuchal translucency measurements in twin pregnancies.

First-trimester chorionic villus sampling (CVS) is an invasive method that may be superior to second-trimester amniocentesis. Wapner and associates[48] prospectively evaluated the relative risks and accuracy of the two methods in twin gestations. They did not find a significant difference in the procedure-related loss of the entire pregnancy (3% for CVS vs. 3–5% for amniocentesis) or in the total fetal loss rate (4–5% for CVS vs. 9–10% for amniocentesis) up to 28 weeks' gestation. However, if only normal cases were considered, the total fetal loss rate was significantly lower in the CVS group. These data demonstrate that CVS is at least as safe as amniocentesis in twin gestations.

Multifetal pregnancy reduction

The issue of numerical reduction in twin pregnancies is rarely raised. However, as twins are more and more the result of reduction from higher-order multiples, the topic deserves some in-depth attention here. The procedure most commonly involves injection of potassium chloride into the fetal thorax transcervically or transabdominally under direct ultrasound guidance late in the first trimester[49]. The overall pregnancy loss rate (8–13%), gestational age at delivery, birthweight, incidence of pregnancy complications, and neonatal morbidity and mortality are all improved when triplets or greater are reduced to twins[49,50]. However, the clear improvement in outcome of triplets recently[51] as well as some questions which are often not addressed raise some ethical issues regarding the reduction of triplets to twins.

The way that the perinatal mortality rate is calculated, for one, affects the quoted statistics. Almost all studies compare the mortalities between twins that were reduced from triplets and non-reduced triplets or non-reduced twins[49,52]. If we take into account the total number of embryos at the beginning of a multifetal pregnancy, the apparent outcomes will be different. First, a comparison between triplets that are reduced and non-reduced triplets will show an advantage for the reduced ones, since some of the reduced fetuses would have spontaneously reduced. Therefore, a substantial rate of spontaneous reductions among triplets will improve the apparent outcome of the twins that were reduced from triplets[53]. In addition, one-third of the fetuses who are presently excluded from the vital statistics would then be included as losses, thereby reducing the favorable outcome rates for reduced triplets[54].

A second question arises when one considers which embryo or embryos to reduce. One can never be certain that the non-reduced fetuses are better off than those who were reduced. It is a strange concept in fetal medicine that a given embryo be subjected to selective continuance or selective birth[55]. This unique situation may represent one of the ultimate paradoxes of modern reproductive techniques in that it may be seen from one view as 'wrongfully and cynically manipulating and expending potential lives in the interest of selfish expediency' and from another view as 'acting in the patient's best interest to achieve a successful pregnancy'[56]. It is a tragedy when a serious anomaly is diagnosed in one twin in the second trimester when embryos that may have been normal fetuses were eliminated earlier.

In order to avoid such undesirable circumstances, each embryo would have to be tested for anomalies prior to selection of the ones to be reduced. This logical approach has been proposed, as an alternative use of embryo reduction, by Brambati and associates[57]. They have suggested that high-order multiples be induced in couples who are at high risk for genetic disorders followed by early prenatal testing of each embryo and selective termination of the affected ones. In other words, they suggest using fetal reduction as an alternative to preimplantation diagnosis. This is in contrast to the original intention of the procedure which was basically to mend what ovulation induction caused.

The final question that must be entertained is whether the remaining twins should be considered as normal twins. This question is the most pertinent to our discussion. The collaborative study did find an inverse relationship between the starting and finishing number of fetuses to loss rates and gestational age at delivery suggesting that the remaining fetuses do retain a 'feature' of the original number[49]. Yovel and colleagues[58] attempted to answer the question by comparing twins resulting from reduction of IVF triplets to IVF twins. They found significantly lower birth weight among the twins that had started as triplets despite similar gestational ages at delivery. The invasive reduction procedure or the effect of the remaining tissue from the reduced sac were suggested explanations for this observation. Smith-Levitin and Kowalik's[58,59] comparison of a large series of twins resulting from reduction of high-order multiples to expectantly managed triplets and twins, on the other hand indicates that twins resulting from embryo reduction behave, in all ways, almost the same as twins. Although multifetal embryo reduction clearly improves outcomes in high-order multiple gestations, the ultimate ramifications have yet to be fully elucidated.

THE SECOND TRIMESTER

Prenatal diagnosis

The modalities available for prenatal diagnosis, except for CVS which is discussed above, are largely in the second trimester. Although prenatal diagnosis in twins is associated with unique problems and needs a special approach, twin pregnancies often have more indications for prenatal diagnosis than other pregnancies.

Maternal serum markers are now routinely offered to women with singleton pregnancies, regardless of their risk factors, as a screen for structural (neural tube and abdominal wall, primarily) and chromosomal abnormalities. It is difficult to assess maternal serum α-fetoprotein levels in twins, however, as they will normally be much higher than in singletons. For example, levels up to four multiples of the mean are associated with normal anatomy in twins[61]. Even higher levels are expected after multifetal embryo reduction in the first trimester rendering the test useless for assessing the risk of neural tube defects in this setting[62]. Regrettably, there are similar problems with the use of α-fetoprotein, estriol and hCG as a screen for triso-

mies in twins. Presently, there is no standard, non-invasive screening test for anomalies in multiple gestations that has reasonable sensitivity and specificity.

The clinician has at least two invasive methods with well-documented predictive value to choose from. The largest experience has been with standard amniocentesis at 14–19 weeks. In a single-center study involving 336 multiples, Anderson and co-workers[63] found a 3.6% abortion rate up to 28 weeks' gestation, which was comparable to the 3.7% rate found by Pruggmayer and colleagues[64] in a multicenter study of 529 cases. The former study also found an increase in abortion rate in mothers over 40 years of age that was not confirmed in the latter, possibly because it did not include data from chromosomally and sonographically abnormal pregnancies. The results demonstrate that although abortion rates following amniocentesis in twin gestations are markedly higher than in singletons, they do not greatly exceed the normal biological loss rate in twin pregnancies.

All prenatal diagnostic procedures in twins should be performed under continuous real-time ultrasound guidance, and there must be certainty that each gestational sac is sampled separately. This can be accomplished by injecting the first sac with a small amount of dye such as indigo carmine after the aliquot of amniotic fluid is removed. The absence of blue fluid upon sampling the second sac ensures that the second fetus was, indeed, sampled. If the dye is shaken to create tiny air bubbles prior to injection, the bubbles will outline the boundaries of the sac which can be of additional help, especially for confirmation of a monoamniotic gestation. Dye injection is not risk free. Methylene blue, in particular, has been implicated in the cause of hemolytic anemia, fetal liver damage and fetal intestinal obstruction[64]. Sonographic identification, alone, can be adequate and will be safer when the accessible fluid pockets are clearly on opposite sides of the dividing membrane.

Funipuncture for rapid karyotyping of fetal lymphocytes can be performed in multiple pregnancies as well, and it should be done for the same indications as in singletons. An accurate risk assignment, however, is not available due to the paucity of data on cordocentesis in twins. One potential complication is that the dividing membrane may be punctured, whether inadvertently or deliberately (i.e. when the cord of one fetus is only accessible by traversing the sac of the other), thereby iatrogenically creating a monoamniotic cavity[65]. Incidentally, this can also happen during amniocentesis.

Selective termination

When a discordant chromosomal or structural anomaly is found in a twin gestation, a dilemma is encountered by both patients and practitioners. They must decide between termination of the entire pregnancy despite the presence of an otherwise normal co-twin, continuation of the entire pregnancy on behalf of the normal twin despite bringing the other, possibly severely handicapped, child to life, or selective termination of the affected fetus[66].

Selective termination is associated with a higher pregnancy-loss rate than multifetal embryo reduction. This has been attributed to the later gestational age at which the procedure is performed, often because the diagnosis of the anomaly cannot be made until well into the second trimester. The risk of losing the entire pregnancy is 14.4% for procedures performed after 16 weeks[67]. Given this significant risk, the benefit of a selective termination in cases where the anomaly is lethal is questionable.

The dilemma is even harder when the discordant anomaly is found in a monochorionic twin pregnancy with suspected vascular communication. In such cases, the twin embolization syndrome may lead to death or severe impairment of the healthy co-twin[66]. One way to potentially prevent this from occurring is to selectively reduce the affected twin by occluding its umbilical cord or by removing it via hysterotomy. The risks from these highly invasive procedures are self evident. There are not unequivocal solutions to these unique and distressing problems so the recommendations must be individualized depending on the circumstances and the parents' wishes.

Twin–twin transfusion syndrome

Twin–twin transfusion syndrome (TTTS), stuck-twin syndrome and polyhydramnios-oligohydramnios syndrome (POS) are all terms applied to a unique complication of monochorial gestations that is often recognized in the second trimester. The syndrome has recently been a major focus of twin research[14]. The diagnosis of TTTS was traditionally based on a postnatal finding of discordant hemoglobin and hematocrit values as well as discordant birth weight. In the late 1980s, investigators found that such discordant values occurred, at a similar rate, in twins from dichorionic and monochorionic gestations, and therefore concluded that a definitive diagnosis of TTTS cannot be made based on such findings[68]. Now, sonographic criteria for the diagnosis of TTTS enable a reasonably accurate antepartum diagnosis to be made. These include a monochorionic pregnancy with a growth discrepancy of > 20% in estimated fetal weight, severe oligohydramnios in the smaller twin's sac, and polyhydramnios in the larger twin's sac.

Although a substantial number of the studies published since 1990 have merely confirmed the previously reported observations, some recent advances have truly added to our understanding and ability to treat the syndrome. The central role of the monochorionic placenta in TTTS is well recognized. The twins are perfectly normal until they react to the hemodynamic changes caused by the 'opening' of intertwin transplacental anastomoses. Evaluation of the angioarchitecture of monochorionic placentas has demonstrated that the anastomoses involved in TTTS are significantly fewer, more likely to be solitary and of deep arteriovenous type than those of monochorionic placentas without the syndrome[69]. It has been maintained that the superficial anastomoses compensate for the hemodynamic imbalance set up by the deep anastomoses and that TTTS may result when there is an imbalance caused by a lack of superficial anastomoses.

The frequently documented association of velamentous cord insertion with TTTS has led to some theories regarding the pathogenesis of the syndrome and some treatment sugges-tions[34,35]. Fries and colleagues[34], for example, suggested that the cord may be compressed at its membraneous insertion which would lead to reduced blood flow, decreased renal perfusion and decreased urine production in that twin; while, at the same time, leading to increased shunting and polyhydramnios in the other twin causing further compression of the cord. Am-niocentesis with removal of significant amounts of fluid may, therefore, be successful in the treatment of TTTS because it reduces this com-pressive force.

Our understanding of the progression of TTTS in both twins has become clearer as our surveillance techniques have become more sophisticated. In the recipient twin, for ex-ample, there is often an absence of atrioventric-ular valve regurgitation during the early stages of TTTS, followed by the appearance of partial systolic regurgitation which progresses to holosystolic insufficiency, and finally to fetal hydrops[70]. This and other echocardiographic observations have been supported by Doppler studies. A recent study of the fetal circulatory events in TTTS describes characteristics of con-gestive heart failure due to hypervolemia in the recipient's circulation and decreased venous re-turn due to hypovolemia and increased after-load due to increased placental resistance in the donor's circulation[71]. Together, these findings suggest that cardiac decompensation and hemodynamic changes play a central role in the pathogenesis of TTTS.

Autopsy findings from fetuses that have suc-cumbed to TTTS have also contributed to our understanding of the syndrome. In the past, it was theorized that death of one fetus resulted in embolization of some undetermined thrombo-plastin-like material via the vascular com-munications to the surviving twin causing brain lesions[68]. The occurrence of such embolic phe-nomena has been challenged by several studies which suggest, instead, that acute hypotensive ischemia of the brain is the main cause of mor-bidity in the surviving twin[73–75]. Either way, it would seem that the surviving twin may be in immediate danger of death or severe damage following the death of its co-twin. Fortunately,

and for unclear reasons, this does not com-monly occur, and thus death of one twin does not necessarily indicate prompt delivery before term of the surviving twin[14].

Several treatment options have emerged for TTTS. Simple feticide of the donor, which was popular for a brief period, has fallen out of favor because of the risk of damage to the recipient. Methods such as occlusion of the umbilical cord by fetoscopic ligation, vascular embolization[76], or insertion of thrombogenic coils[77], which eliminate the connections between the two fetuses, are currently preferred. Still, they sacri-fice one twin leading to a minimum mortality rate of 50%.

There are also treatment modalities that at-tempt to save both twins. Laser ablation of the placental vascular communications is perhaps the most logical method as it treats the cause of TTTS. Since the first anecdotal reports in humans in the late 1980s, results of two relatively large preliminary series are available that both report a 53% survival[78,79]. The cases with sur-vivors were delivered at mean gestational ages of greater than 32 weeks. The interval between the laser procedure and delivery was 6–17 weeks in one study[78] and 0–21 weeks in the other[79]. Both groups have reached the conclusion that TTTS can be treated effectively by fetoscopic laser occlusion of the communicating placental ves-sels, albeit the total survival rates are only some-what higher than the minimum survival rates after feticide.

Decompression amniocentesis, which was proposed more than half a century ago, is cur-rently the only alternative treatment to placen-tal laser surgery which does not employ feticide. Until 1989, the calculated overall perinatal mor-tality was about 55%[14]. Several series in the last 5 years have provided confusing results. For example, there have been four articles, exclud-ing series of less than five cases, that have rec-ommended amniocentesis, three of which were from the same Arizona center[80–83]. Four articles from different centers, however, have ques-tioned the utility of the procedure[84–87]. Prospec-tive comparisons between amniocentesis, laser surgery and feticide are needed in order to establish accurate survival figures before absolute recommendations can be made regarding treatment for TTTS.

THE THIRD TRIMESTER

Growth

It has long been recognized that twins do not behave merely as two singletons who happen to share the same uterine cavity for a given period of time[88]. This view is based on numerous observations which show a mean lower birth weight for twins than for singletons. Leroy and colleagues[89] confirmed the results of four previous large-scale studies of intrauterine growth as estimated from live births at gestational ages ranging from 28 to 42 weeks[89]. Birth weights of twins were quite similar to those of singletons until the first weeks of the third trimester when some ill-defined conditions began to restrict twin growth. Yet, large numbers of twins are born who are appropriate for gestational age (AGA), even by singleton standards, indicating that the conditions which predispose to restricted growth in twins do not affect all twin pregnancies. Some twins, often born to multiparous mothers, are even 'macrosomic'[90,91].

If twins do have different growth patterns from singletons, then specific growth curves generated for twins should be used. Attempts at establishing normograms of fetal weight gain throughout twin pregnancies, which are dependent on actual birth weights, have been made[92], but there are some major concerns about their accuracy. Because twins have a high rate of premature birth which is, itself, abnormal, growth curves based on a high proportion of preterm deliveries will be biased. To date, accurate growth charts for twins are not available, and clinicians must, therefore, compare individual twin growth to the more well-established singleton curves[93].

The accuracy of sonographic biometry for assessment of twin growth has also been evaluated[92–95]. Although all sonographic parameters are generally smaller in twins than in singletons, the anthropometric values obtained from the neonates only reveal delays in birth weight and abdominal circumference[94]. This observation was the first, of many, to suggest that sonographic head measurements in twins might be inaccurate, possibly secondary to intrauterine crowding[93–95]. A more reliable estimate of fetal weight will likely be obtained if formulas, which incorporate femur length and abdominal circumference, are applied.

Although both fetuses of a twin pair share the same uterine cavity, they do not necessarily share the same environment and they may exhibit discordant growth. Discordant pairs who are full term and appropriately grown for gestational age have good perinatal outcomes suggesting their growth discordance is not always the result of a pathological process[96,97]. It may be physiological. For example, the second, or non-presenting, twin will deliver less traumatically if smaller and is more often smaller as shown in Figure 3[98]. A study of unlike sex twins in which the expected birth weight difference between female and male twins was only apparent in male-first, female-second pairs further suggests that growth discordance may be a birth order dependent event[99].

In contrast, there are some discordantly grown twins who have increased morbidity and mortality, albeit they often have severe growth discordance (> 25%) and evidence of intrauterine growth retardation[98,100]. Other risk factors are implied by the results of a study that found mortalities only in second twins who were discordant by more than 20% and delivered preterm[101]. Since it is frequently difficult to predict, antenatally, which pairs are truly at risk, it is important accurately to diagnose and closely follow most discordant pairs[102]. Similarly, discordance, per se, is not an indication for early delivery or Cesarean section[102]. The benefit of early intervention may outweigh the risks of prematurity, however, in a twin pregnancy with progressive growth divergence and signs suggestive of fetal jeopardy, just as with cases of fetal growth retardation in singletons.

Some investigators have demonstrated that estimated fetal weight (EFW) differences, alone, are not accurate for estimating actual birth weight differences[95,103–107]. An intertwin difference in abdominal circumference > 20 mm, however, has repeatedly been found to be a

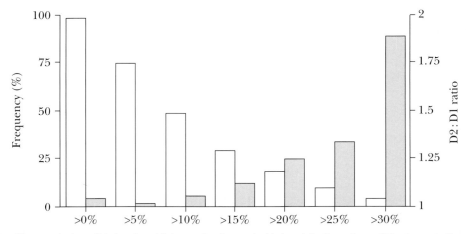

Figure 3 *The association of birth order with increasing intertwin birth weight discordance. D1 represents discordant pairs in which the smaller twin is the presenting fetus; D2 represents discordant pairs in which the smaller twin is the non-presenting fetus; frequency, hollow bars; D2 : D1 ratio, gray bars. Data are based on 400 consecutive pairs*

relatively good predictor of discordance[107–109]. A difference of > 15% in the systolic to diastolic Doppler velocimetry ratio of the umbilical arteries has also been shown to be predictive[110], especially when it complements differences in the biometric indices (biparietal diameter > 6 mm, abdominal circumference > 20 mm, femur length > 5 mm, transverse cerebellar diameter > 4 mm).

Preterm delivery

Premature twins account for a large share of perinatal mortality and morbidity even though they make up only 2% of live births[3,111]. Preterm premature rupture of the membranes, occurring in 7.4% of twins compared to 3.7% of singletons, is a cause of many of these preterm births[112]. The high rate of premature delivery (48%), due to many causes, results in high rates of low and very low birth weight infants (VLBW)[3]. Some twins may have adapted techniques for reducing preterm labor in their mothers. There is some evidence, for example, that a pair will position itself so as to occupy the least space, thereby minimizing uterine distension and subsequent contractions[113,114]. Neither the advances made in prenatal diagnosis and treatment nor the institution of prophylactic measures such as bed rest, hospitalization, tocolytics, or cervical cerclage have been effective in reducing prematurity rates or improving the perinatal outcome of twins.

The development of specialized antenatal care programs for multiple gestations, however, may have some impact. Ellings and co-workers[115] found that women with twins who attended a specialized, multidisciplinary clinic had lower rates of VLBW infants with fewer neonatal intensive care unit admissions and lower perinatal mortality compared to women who were not followed as closely[115]. The improvement in outcome was attributed to intensive preterm birth prevention, education, individualization of prenatal care and frequent maternal assessment by a consistent care provider.

In addition, birth weight has been shown to be the most important factor for predicting morbidity and mortality in twins, with the risk decreasing by 40% for every 250-g increase in weight[95]. As poor maternal weight gain is associated with all measures of intrauterine growth, weight gains of at least 35 lbs should be recommended in twin gestations to maximize birth weight[114,115]. Dietary counselling, which will help a patient meet the extra nutritional requirements, can be provided in specialty clinics.

Antepartum testing with non-stress tests and biophysical profiles has proven validity in multiple gestations, and they are indicated, especially

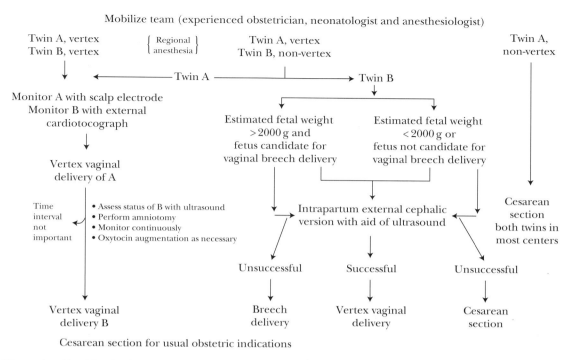

Figure 4 *Algorithm for the intrapartum management of twin gestation. Adapted from Chervenak and colleagues[127]*

in higher-risk twins (monochorionic pairs, discordantly-grown pairs, intrauterine growth retardation of one, or both twins, maternal medical complications or postdates). The availability of monitors that can test twins simultaneously allows observations of *in utero* interactions between twins which may add to our knowledge of this interesting phenomenon[118]. One of the few new suggestions for fetal surveillance in multiple pregnancies is magnetocardiography, but larger series are needed to confirm the promising preliminary results[119].

Timing of delivery

Since twins are delivered at an earlier gestational age than singletons, it is possible that twins mature earlier and become post-term earlier. There is currently no accepted gestational age which denotes term in twins. It has been shown that neonatal morbidity, even in twins, improves significantly with increasing gestational age until 38 weeks and that mortality nadirs at 38–39 weeks[120]. For this reason, un-

complicated twins, in our opinion, should not be electively delivered prior to 38 weeks. The possible risk attributed to 'post-term' twins was recently evaluated by Chien and Loy[120] who did not find a rise in mortality after 38–39 weeks.

Intrapartum management

The question of whether malpresentation of twins is an, a priori, indication for Cesarean section was apparently settled by the end of the 1980s. It is now generally accepted that a trial of labor may be permitted for all vertex first twins when no contraindication exists for the vaginal birth of the non-vertex twin[121,122]. An algorithm for the intrapartum management of these pairs is suggested in Figure 4. Abdominal delivery has been recommended for breech first twins, however, mainly on the grounds that the safety of vaginal delivery for these pairs has not been established. Opponents of this view argue that if the criteria are met for vaginal delivery of a breech singleton, then vaginal delivery of the breech first twin should be no different. Indeed, recent retrospective studies have suggested that vaginal delivery may be as safe as abdominal delivery for breech-vertex pairs[123,124].

The increased frequency of Cesarean sections in the general population will certainly increase the frequency of patients with twins who have had a Cesarean in a previous pregnancy. Until recently, there were only sporadic documentations of successful twin vaginal births after Cesarean section (VBAC). Strong and colleagues[125] reported a successful VBAC rate of 72% in their series of 56 twin pregnancies and concluded that a trial of labor appears to be a safe option in such situations.

CONCLUSION

In conclusion, there are still significant emotional, physical and financial risks to twin gestations despite recent improvements in our understanding of the twinning process and in our ability to manage some of the complications. As successful reproductive technologies become more widely available, the number of twin gestations will continue to increase. So too, must the current trend toward research in all aspects of multiple gestations with the most important goal being to improve overall perinatal outcome. Although this goal is more easily defined than achieved, the fetuses, our patients, deserve the best, possible chance.

References

1. Hecht, B. R. (1993). Iatrogenic multifetal pregnancy. *Assist. Reprod. Rev.*, **3**, 75–87
2. Thijssen, J. M. (1987). Twins as monsters: Albertus Magnus's theory of the generation of twins and its philosophical context. *Bull. Hist. Med.*, **61** 237–46
3. Luke, B. (1994). The changing pattern of multiple births in the United States: maternal and infant characteristics, 1973 and 1990. *Obstet. Gynecol.*, **84**, 101–6
4. Jewell, S. E. and Yip, R. (1995). Increasing trends in plural births in the United States. *Obstet. Gynecol.*, **85**, 229–32
5. Schenker, J. G., Yarkoni, S. and Granat, M. (1981). Multiple pregnancies following induction of ovulation. *Fertil. Steril.*, **35**, 105
6. Keith, L., Ellis, R., Berger, G. S. and Depp, R. (1980). The Northwestern University multi-hospital twin study: a description of 588 twin pregnancies and associated pregnancy loss, 1971 to 1975. *Am. J. Obstet. Gynecol.*, **138**, 781–9
7. Spellacy, W. N., Handler, A. and Ferre, C. D. (1990). A case-control study of 1253 twin pregnancies from a 1982–1987 perinatal data base. *Obstet. Gynecol.*, **75**, 168–71
8. Bulmer, M. G. (1960). The familial incidence of twinning. *Ann. Hum. Genet.*, **24**, 1
9. Yoshida, K. (1993). Physiopathology in multiple pregnancy with special reference to twin placentation. *Perinat. Symp.* (Jpn.), **11**, 81–6
10. Nylander, P. P. S. (1970). The inheritance of DZ twinning: a study of 18 737 maternities in Ibadan, Western Nigeria. *Acta Genet. Med. Gemellol.*, **19**, 36–9
11. Meulemans, W. J., Lewis, C. M., Boomsma, D. I., Derom, C. A., Yan den Berghe, H., Orlebeke, J. F., Ylietnick, R. F. and Derom, R. (1994). Genetic modelling of dizygotic twinning among relatives of spontaneous dizygotic twins. The 9th International Workshop on Multiple Pregnancy, Herzliya, Israel, (abstr.) *Isr. J. Obstet. Gynecol.*, **5** (Suppl.), 11
12. Eriksson, A. W. (1990). Twinning in families of triplets. *Acta Genet. Med. Gemellol.*, **39**, 279–93
13. Blickstein, I. and Borenstein, R. (1989). Recurrent spontaneous twinning. *Acta Genet. Med. Gemellol.*, **38**, 279–83
14. Blickstein, I. (1990). The twin–twin transfusion syndrome. *Obstet. Gynecol.*, **76**, 714–22
15. Rydhstrom, H. (1993). The dividing membrane and late fetal death in twin pregnancy. Abstracts of 8th International Workshop on Multiple Pregnancy, Helsingborg, Sweden, May, p. 23
16. Derom, C., Derom, R., Ylietnick, R., Maes, H. and Yan den Berghe, H. (1993). Iatrogenic multiple pregnancies in East Flanders, Belgium. *Fertil. Steril.*, **60**, 493–6
17. Derom, C., Ylietnick, R., Derom, R., Yan den Berghe, H. and Thiery, M. (1987). Increased monozygotic twinning rate after ovulation induction. *Lancet*, **1**, 1236–8
18. Edwards, R. G., Mettler, L. and Walters, D. E. (1986). Identical twins and *in vitro* fertilization. *J. In-Vitro Fert. Embryo Transfer*, **3**, 114–7

19. Cohen, J. (1991). Assisted hatching of human embryos. *J. In-Vitro Fertil. Embryo. Transfer*, **8**, 179–90

20. Skupski, D. W., Streltzoff, J., Hutson, J. M., Rosenwaks, Z., Cohen, J. and Chervenak, F. A. (1995). Early diagnosis of conjoined twins in a triplet pregnancy following *in-vitro* fertilization and assisted hatching. *J. Ultrasound Med.*, **14**, 611–7

21. Nijs, M., Yanderzwalmen, P., Segal-Bertin, G., Geerts, L., Roosendaal, E., Segal, L., Schoysman-Deboeck, A. and Schoysman, R. (1993). A monozygotic twin pregnancy after application of zona rubbing on a frozen-thawed blastocyst. *Hum. Reprod.*, **8**, 127–9

22. Alikani, M., Noyes, N., Cohen, J. and Rosenwaks, Z. (1994). Monozygotic twinning in the human is associated with the zona pellucida architecture. *Hum. Reprod.*, **9**, 1318–21

23. Corner, G. W. (1955). The observed embryology of human single-ovum twins and other multiple births. *Am. J. Obstet. Gynecol.*, **70**, 933–51

24. Chervenak, F. A., Youcha, S. and Johnson, R. E. (1984). Antenatal diagnosis and perinatal outcomes in a series of 385 consecutive twin pregnancies. *J. Rep. Med.*, **29**, 727–30

25. Blumenfeld, Z., Rottem, S. and Elgali, S. (1988). Transvaginal sonographic assessment of early embryological development. In Timor-Tritsch, I. E. and Rottem, S. (eds.) *Transvaginal Sonography*, pp. 95–7. (New York: Elsevier Science)

26. Brass, Y. A., Benacerraf, B. R. and Frigoletto, F. D. (1985). Ultrasonographic determination of chorion type in twin gestation. *Obstet. Gynecol.*, **66**, 779–83

27. Stagiannis, K. D., Sepulveda, W., Southwell, D., Price, D. A. and Fisk, N. M. (1995). Are ultrasonographic measurements of intertwin membrane thickness reliable in determining chorionicity? A reproducibility study. The 15th Annual Meeting of the Society of Perinatal Obstetricians, Atlanta, GA, (abstr.) *Am. J. Obstet. Gynecol.*, **172**, 352

28. Finberg, H. J. (1992). The 'twin peak' sign: reliable evidence of dichorionic twinning. *J. Ultrasound Med.*, **11**, 571–7

29. Appelman, Z., Manor, M., Magal, N., Caspi, B., Shohat, M., and Blickstein, I. (1994). Prenatal diagnosis of twin zygosity by DNA 'fingerprint' analysis. *Prenat. Diag.*, **14**, 307–9

30. Dickey, R. P., Olar, T. T., Curole, D. N., Taylor, S. N., Rye, P. H. and Matulich, E. M. (1990). The probability of multiple births when multiple gestational sacs or viable embryos are diagnosed at first trimester ultrasound. *Hum. Reprod.*, **5**, 880–2

31. Landy, H. J., Weiner, S., Corson, S. L., Batzer, F. R. and Bolognese, R. J. (1986). The 'vanishing twin': ultrasonographic assessment of fetal disappearance in the first trimester. *Am. J. Obstet. Gynecol.*, **155**, 14–19

32. Jauniaux, E., Elkazen, N., Leroy, F., Wilkin, P., Rodesch, F. and Hustin, J. (1988). Clinical and morphologic aspects of the vanishing twin phenomenon. *Obstet. Gynecol.*, **72**, 577–81

33. Yoshida, K. (1993). Confirmation of the vanishing twin. *Presented at the 8th International Workshop on Multiple Pregnancy*, Helsingborg, Sweden, May, abstr. p. 27

34. Fries, M. H., Goldstein, R. B., Kilpatrick, S. J., Golbus, M. S., Callen, P. W. and Filly, R. A. (1993). The role of velamentous cord insertion in the etiology of twin–twin transfusion syndrome. *Obstet. Gynecol.*, **81**, 569–74

35. Mari, G., Uerpairojkit, B., Abuhamad, A., Martinez, E. and Copel, J. (1995). Velamentous insertion of the cord in polyhydramnios-oligohydramnios twins. Abstracts of the 15th Annual Meeting of the Society of Perinatal Obstetricians Atlanta, Georgia (abstr.) *Am. J. Obstet. Gynecol.*, **172**, 291

36. Iffy, L., Jakobovits, A., Lavenhar, M. A., Najem, R., Hopp, L. and Jakobovits, A. A. (1993). A study of early fetal growth patterns in twin pairs. *Acta Anat.*, **148**, 176–80

37. Ahiron, R. and Blickstein, I. (1993). Persistent discordant twin growth following IVF-ET. *Acta Genet. Med. Gemellol.*, **42**, 41–4

38. Blickstein, I. and Lancet, M. (1988). The growth discordant twin. *Obstet. Gynecol. Surv.*, **43**, 509–15

39. Weissman, A., Achiron, R., Lipitz, S., Blickstein, I. and Mashiach, S. (1994). The first trimester growth-discordant twin: an ominous prenatal finding. *Obstet. Gynecol.*, **84**, 110–14

40. Ghai, Y. and Yidyasagar, D. (1988). Morbidity and mortality factors in twins. *Clin. Perinatol.*, **15**, 123–40

41. Little, J. and Bryan, E. (1986). Congenital anomalies in twins. *Semin. Perinatol.*, **10**, 54–64

42. Schinzel, A. A., Smith, D. W. and Miller, J. R. (1979). Monozygotic twinning and structural defects. *J. Pediatr.*, **95**, 921–30

43. Galton, F. (1875). The history of twins as a criterion of the relative powers of nature and nurture. *Fraser's Magazine*, **12**, 566–76

44. Hrubec, Z. and Robinette, C. D. (1984). The study of twins in medical research. *N. Engl. J. Med.*, **310**, 435–41

45. Rodis, J F., Egan, J. F., Craffey, A., Ciarleglio, L., Greenstein, R. M. and Scorza, W. E. (1990). Calculated risk of chromosomal abnormalities in twin gestations. *Obstet. Gynecol.*, **76**, 1037–41

46. Hunter, A. and Cox, D. (1979). Counseling problems when twins are discovered at genetic amniocentesis. *Clin. Genet.*, **16**, 34–42
47. Pandya, P. P., Hilbert, F., Snijders, R. J. M. and Nicolaides, K. H. (1995). Nuchal translucency thickness and crown–rump length in twin pregnancies with chromosomally abnormal fetuses. *J. Ultrasound Med.*, **14**, 565–8
48. Wapner, R., Johnson, A., Davis, G., Urban, A., Morgan, P. and Jackson, L. (1993). Prenatal diagnosis in twin gestations: a comparison between second-trimester amniocentesis and first-trimester chorionic villus sampling. *Obstet. Gynecol.*, **82**, 49–56
49. Evans, M. I., Dommergues, M., Timor-Tritsch, I., Zador, I. E., Wapner, R. J., Lynch, L., Dumez, Y., Goldberg, J. D., Nicolaides, K. H., Johnson, M. P., Golbus, M. S., Boulot, P., Aknin, A. J., Monteagudo, A. and Berkowitz, R. L. (1994). Transabdominal versus transcervical and transvaginal multifetal pregnancy reduction: international collaborative experience of more than one thousand cases. *Am. J. Obstet. Gynecol.*, **170**, 902–9
50. Lipitz, S., Reichman, B., Uval, J., Shalev, J., Achiron, R., Barkai, G., Lusky, A. and Mashiach, S. (1994). A prospective comparison of the outcome of triplet pregnancies managed expectantly or by multifetal reduction to twins. *Am. J. Obstet. Gynecol.*, **170**, 874–9
51. Lipitz, S., Reichman, B., Paret, G., Modan, M., Shalev, J., Serr, D. M., Mashiach, S. and Frenkel, Y. (1989). The improving outcome of triplet pregnancies. *Am. J. Obstet. Gynecol.*, **161**, 1279–84
52. Macones, G. A., Schemmer, G., Pritts, E., Weinblatt, Y. and Wapner, R. J. (1993). Multifetal reduction of triplets to twins improves perinatal outcome. *Am. J. Obstet. Gynecol.*, **169**, 982–6
53. Blumenfeld, Z., Dirnfeld, M., Abramovici, H., Amit, A., Bronshtein, M. and Brandes, J. M. (1992). Spontaneous fetal reduction in multiple gestations assessed by transvaginal ultrasound. *Br. J. Obstet. Gynaecol.*, **99**, 333–7
54. Blickstein, I. (1994). Should the reduced embryos be considered in outcome calculations of multifetal pregnancy reduction? *Am. J. Obstet. Gynecol.*, **171**, 866–7
55. Baldwin, V. J. and Wittmann, B. K. (1990). Pathology of intragestational intervention in twin-to-twin transfusion syndrome. *Pediatr. Pathol.*, **10**, 79–93
56. Brahams, D. (1987). Assisted reproduction and selective reduction of pregnancy. *Lancet*, **2**, 1409–10
57. Brambati, B., Formigli, L., Mori, M. and Tului, L. (1994). Multiple pregnancy induction and selective fetal reduction in high genetic risk couples. *Hum. Reprod.*, **168**, 799–804
58. Yovel, I., Yaron, Y., Lessing, J. B., David, M. P., Peyser, M. R. and Amit, A. (1994). Outcome of multiple pregnancy reduction of triplets to twins: a comparison to IVF twin pregnancies. The 9th International Workshop on Multiple Pregnancy, Herzeliya, Israel, (abstr.) *Isr. J. Obstet. Gynecol.*, **5** (Suppl.), 8
59. Smith-Levitin, M., Kowalik, A., Birnholz, J., Hutson, J. M., Skupski, D., Rosenwaks, Z. and Chervenak, F. A. (1996). Comparison of birthweights of twin and triplet gestations resulting from embryo reduction of higher order gestations to birthweights of twin and triplet gestations using a novel way to correct for gestational age at delivery. Sixteenth Annual Meeting of The Society of Perinatal Obstetricians, Kamuela, Hawaii. *Am. J. Obstet. Gynecol.*, **174**, 346
60. Kowalik, A. Smith-Levitin, M., Moy, F., Hutson, J. M., Skupski, D., Rosenwaks, Z. and Chervenak, F. A. (1996). Pregnancy related complications in twin gestations resulting from multifetal embryo reduction as compared to non-reduced twin and triplet pregnancies. Sixteen Annual meeting of The Society of Perinatal Obstetricians, Kamuela, Hawaii. *Am. J. Obstet. Gynecol.*, **174**, 346
61. Johnson, J. M., Harman, C. R., Evans, J. A., MacDonald, K. and Manning, F. A. (1990). Maternal Serum α-fetoprotein in twin pregnancy. *Am. J. Obstet. Gynecol.*, **162**, 1020–5
62. Lynch, L. and Berkowitz, R. L. (1993). Maternal serum α-fetoprotein and coagulation profiles after multifetal pregnancy reduction. *Am. J. Obstet. Gynecol.*, **169**, 987–90
63. Anderson, R. L., Goldberg, J. D. and Golbus, M. S. (1991). Prenatal diagnosis in multiple gestation: 20 years experience with amniocentesis. *Prenat. Diagn.*, **11**, 263–70
64. Pruggmayer, M. R. K., Jahoda, M. G. J., Yan der Pol, J. G., Baumann, P., Holzgreve, W. and Karkut, G. (1992). Genetic amniocentesis in twin pregnancies: results of a multicenter study of 529 cases. *Ultrasound Obstet. Gynecol.*, **2**, 6–10
65. Megory, E., Weiner, E., Shalev, E. and Ohel, G. (1991). Pseudomonoamniotic twins with cord entanglement following genetic funipuncture. *Obstet. Gynecol.*, **78**, 915–7
66. Golbus, M. S., Cunningham, N., Goldberg, J. D., Anderson, R., Filly, R. and Callen, P. (1988). Selective termination of multiple gestation. *Am. J. Med. Genet.*, **31**, 339–48
67. Evans, M. I., Goldberg, J. D., Dommergues, M., Wapner, R. J., Lynch, L., Dock, B. S., Horenstein, J., Golbus, M. S., Rodeck, C. H., Dumez, Y., Holzgreve, W., Timor-Tritsch, I., Johnson,

M. P., Isada, N. B., Monteagudo, A. and Berkowitz, R. L. (1994). Efficacy of second-trimester selective termination for fetal abnormalities: international collaborative experience among the worlds largest centers. *Am. J. Obstet. Gynecol.*, **171**, 90–4

68. Danskin, F. H. and Neilson, J. P. (1989). Twin-to-twin transfusion syndrome: what are appropriate diagnostic criteria? *Am. J. Obstet. Gynecol.*, **161**, 365–9

69. Bajoria, R., Wigglesworth, J. and Fisk, N. M. (1995). Angioarchitecture of monochorionic placentas in relation to the twin–twin transfusion syndrome. *Am. J. Obstet. Gynecol.*, **172**, 856–63

70. Gembruch, U., Bald, R., Fahnenstich, H., Arabin, B. and Hansmann, M. (1994). Echocardiographic function in cases of twin–twin transfusion syndrome (TTTS). The 4th World Congress of Ultrasound in Obstetrics and Gynecology, Budapest, Hungary, (abstr.) *Ultrasound Obstet. Gynecol.*, **4**, 183

71. Hecher, K., Ville, Y., Snijders, R. and Nicolaides, K. (1995). Doppler studies of the fetal circulation in twin–twin transfusion syndrome. *Ultrasound Obstet. Gynecol.*, **5**, 318–24

72. Sherer, D. M., Abramowicz, J. S., Jaffe, R., Smith, S. A., Metlay, L. A. and Woods, J. R. (1993). Twin–twin transfusion with abrupt onset of microcephaly in the surviving recipient following spontaneous death of the donor twin. *Am. J. Obstet. Gynecol.*, **169**, 85–8

73. Grafe, M. R. (1993). Antenatal cerebral necrosis in monochorionic twins. *Pediatr. Pathol.*, **13**, 15–19

74. Okamura, K., Murotsuki, J., Tanigawara, S., Uehara, S. and Yajima, A. (1994). Funipuncture for evaluation of hematologic and coagulation indices in the surviving twin following co-twin's death. *Obstet. Gynecol.*, **83**, 975–8

75. Larroche, J. C., Girard, N., Narcy, F. and Fallet, C. (1994). Abnormal cortical plate (polymicrogyria), heterotopias and brain damage in monozygous twins. *Biol. Neonate.*, **65**, 343–52

76. Dommergues, M., Mandlbrot, L., Delezoide, A. L., Aubry, M. C., Fermont, L., Caputo-Mahieu, D. and Dumez, Y. (1995). Twin–twin transfusion syndrome: selective feticide by embolization of the hydropic fetus. *Fetal. Diagn. Ther.*, **10**, 26–31

77. Bebbington, M. W., Wilson, R. D., Machan, L. and Wittmann, B. K. (1995). Selective feticide in twin transfusion syndrome using ultrasound-guided insertion of thrombogenic coils. *Fetal. Diagn. Ther.*, **10**, 32–6

78. De Lia, J. E., Kuhimann, R. S., Harstad, T. W. and Cruikshank, D. P. (1995). Fetoscopic laser ablation of placental vessels in severe previable twin–twin transfusion syndrome. *Am. J. Obstet. Gynecol.*, **172**, 1202–8

79. Ville, Y., Hyett, J., Hecher, K. and Nicolaides, K. (1995). Preliminary experience with endoscopic laser surgery for severe twin–twin transfusion syndrome. *N. Engl. J. Med.*, **332**, 224–7

80. Urig, M. A., Clewell, W. H. and Elliott, J. P. (1990). Twin–twin transfusion syndrome. *Am. J. Obstet. Gynecol.*, **163**, 1522–6

81. Elliott, J. P., Urig, M. A. and Clewell, W. H. (1991). Aggressive therapeutic amniocentesis for treatment of twin–twin transfusion syndrome. *Obstet. Gynecol.*, **77**, 537–40

82. Pinette, M. G., Pan, Y., Pinette, S. G. and Stubblefield, P. G. (1993). Treatment of twin–twin transfusion syndrome. *Obstet. Gynecol.*, **82**, 841–6

83. Elliott, J. P., Sawyer, A. T., Radin, T. G. and Strong, R. E. (1994). Large volume therapeutic amniocentesis in the treatment of hydramnios. *Obstet. Gynecol.*, **84**, 1025–7

84. Gonsoulin, W., Moise, K. J. Jr, Kirshon, B., Cotton, D. B., Wheeler, J. M. and Carpenter, R. J. Jr (1990). Outcome of twin–twin transfusion diagnosed before 28 weeks of gestation. *Obstet. Gynecol.*, **75**, 214–6

85. Grischke, E. M., Boos, R., Schmidt, W. and Bastert, G. (1990). Twin pregnancies with fetofetal transfusion syndrome. *Z. Geburtshilfe. Perinatol.*, **194**, 17–21

86. Saunders, N. J., Snijders, R. J. and Nicolaides, K. H. (1992). Therapeutic amniocentesis in twin–twin transfusion syndrome appearing in the second trimester of pregnancy. *Am. J. Obstet. Gynecol.*, **166**, 820–4

87. Weiner, C. P. and Ludomirski, A. (1994). Diagnosis, pathophysiology, and treatment of chronic twin-to-twin transfusion syndrome. *Fetal Diagn. Ther.*, **9**, 283–90

88. Gedda, L., Brenci, G. and Gatti, I. (1981). Low birthweight in twins versus singletons: separate entities and different implications for child growth and survival. *Acta Genet. Med. Gemellol.*, **39**, 1–8

89. Leroy, B., Lefort, F., Neveu, P., Risse, R. J., Trevise, P. and Jeny, R. (1982). Intrauterine growth charts for twin fetuses. *Acta Genet. Med. Gemellol.*, **31**, 199–206

90. Blickstein, I. and Weissman, A. 'Macrosomic' twinning: a study of growth promoted twins. *Obstet. Gynecol.*, **76**, 822–4

91. Blickstein, I., Zalel, Y. and Weissman, A. (1995). Pregnancy order: a factor influencing birth weight in twin gestations. *J. Reprod. Med.*, **40**, 443–6

92. Yarkoni, S., Reece, E. A., Holford, T., O'Connor, T. Z. and Hobbins, J. C. (1987). Estimated

fetal weight in the evaluation of growth in twin gestations: a prospective longitudinal study. *Obstet. Gynecol.*, **69**, 636–9

93. Rodis, J. F., Vintzileos, A. M., Campbell, W. A. and Nochimson, D. J. (1990). Intrauterine fetal growth in discordant twin gestations. *J. Ultrasound Med.*, **9**, 443–8

94. Sokol, M. L., Tamura, R. K., Sabbagha, R. E., Thomas, C. and Yaisrub, N. (1984). Diminished biparietal diameter and abdominal circumference growth in twins. *Obstet. Gynecol.*, **64**, 235–8

95. Leyon, J. (1993). Fetal weight prediction by ultrasound in twin pregnancy: clinical usefulness. *Abstracts of the 8th International Workshop on Multiple Pregnancy*, Helsingborg, Sweden, May, abstr. p. 24

96. Blickstein, I., Shoham-Schwartz, Z. and Lancet, M. (1988). Growth discordancy in appropriate-for-gestational-age term twins. *Obstet. Gynecol.*, **72**, 582–4

97. Fraser, D., Pickard, R., Picard, E. and Leiberman, J. R. (1994). Birth weight discordance, intrauterine growth retardation and perinatal outcomes in twins. *J. Reprod. Med.*, **39**, 504–8

98. Blickstein, I., Shoham-Schwartz, Z., Lancet, M. and Borenstein, R. (1987). Characterization of the growth discordant twin. *Obstet. Gynecol.*, **70**, 11–15

99. Blickstein, I. and Weissman, A. (1990). Birth weight discordancy in male-first and female-first pairs of unlike-sexed twins. *Am. J. Obstet. Gynecol.*, **162**, 661–3

100. Blickstein, I. and Lancet, M. (1988). The growth discordant twin. *Obstet. Gynecol. Survey*, **43**, 509–15

101. Blickstein, I., Ben-Hur, H. and Borenstein, R. (1992). The perinatal outcome of twin pregnancies complicated with pre-eclampsia. *Am. J. Perinatol.*, **9**, 256–8

102. Blickstein, I. (1991). The definition, diagnosis, and management of growth discordant twins: an international census survey. *Acta Genet. Med. Gemellol.*, **40**, 345–51

103. Watson, W. J., Yalea, F. A. and Seeds, J. W. (1991). Sonographic evaluation of growth discordance and chorionicity in twin gestation. *Am. J. Perinatol.*, **8**, 342–4

104. MacLean, M., Mathers, A., Walker, J. J., Cameron, A. D. and Howat, R. (1992). The ultrasonic assessment of discordant growth in twin pregnancies. *Ultrasound Obstet. Gynecol.*, **2**, 30–4

105. Schwartz, D., Goyert, G., Daoud, Y., Wright, E., Zazula, P., Copes, J., Seabolt, L. and Boyce, M. (1993). Evaluation of twin discordance by second and third trimester ultrasound. The 13th Annual Meeting of the Society of Perinatal Ob-

stetricians, San Francisco, CA, (abstr.) *Am. J. Obstet. Gynecol.*, **168**, 351

106. Shah, Y. G., Sherer, D. M., Gragg, L. A., Casaceli, C. J. and Woods, J. R. (1994). Diagnostic accuracy of different ultrasonographic growth parameters in predicting discordancy in twin gestation: a different approach. *Am. J. Perinatol.*, **11**, 199–204

107. Hill, L. M., Guzick, D., Chenevey, P., Boyles, D. and Nedzesky, P. (1994). The sonographic assessment of twin growth discordancy. *Obstet. Gynecol.*, **84**, 501–4

108. Storlazzi, E., Vintzileos, A. M., Campbell, W. A., Nochimson, D. J. and Weinbaum, P. J. (1987). Ultrasonic diagnosis of discordant fetal growth in twin gestations. *Obstet. Gynecol.*, **69**, 363–7

109. Blickstein, I., Friedman, A., Caspi, B. and Lancet, M. (1989). Ultrasonic prediction of growth discordancy by intertwin difference in abdominal circumference. *Int. J. Gynecol. Obstet.*, **29**, 121–4

110. Kurmanavicius, J., Hebisch, G., Huch, R. and Huch, A. (1992). Umbilical artery blood flow velocity waveforms in twin pregnancies. *J. Perinat. Med.*, **20**, 307–12

111. Gardner, M. O., Goldenberg, R. L., Cliver, S. P., Tucker, J. M., Nelson, K. G. and Copper, R. L. (1995). The origin and outcome of preterm twin pregnancies. *Obstet. Gynecol.*, **85**, 553–7

112. Mercer, B. M., Crocker, L. G., Pierce, W. F. and Sibai, B. M. (1993). Clinical characteristics and outcome of twin gestation complicated by preterm premature rupture of the membranes. *Am. J. Obstet. Gynecol.*, **168**, 1467–73

113. Blickstein, I. and Lancet, M. (1989). Second-breech presentation in twins – a possible adaptive measure to promote fetal growth? *Obstet. Gynecol.*, **73**, 700–3

114. Blickstein, I., Namir, R., Weissman, A. and Diamant, Y. (1993). The influence of birth order and presentation on intrauterine growth of twins. *Acta Genet. Med. Gemellol.*, **42**, 151–8

115. Ellings, J. M., Newman, R. B., Hulsey, T. C., Bivins, H. A. Jr and Keenan, A. (1993). Reduction of very low birth weight deliveries and perinatal mortality in a specialized, multidisciplinary twin clinic. *Obstet. Gynecol.*, **81**, 387–91

116. Luke, B., Minogue, J., Witter, F. R., Keith, L. G. and Johnson, T. R. (1993). The ideal twin pregnancy: patterns of weight gain, discordancy, and length of gestation. *Am. J. Obstet. Gynecol.*, **169**, 588–97

117. Luke, B., Keith, L., Johnson, T. R. and Keith, D. (1991). Pregravid weight, gestational weight gain and current weight of women delivered of twins. *J. Perinat. Med.*, **19**, 333–40

118. Sherer, D. M., D'Amico, M. L., Cox, C., Metlay, L. A. and Woods, J. R. (1994). Association of *in-utero* behavioral patterns of twins with each other as indicated by fetal heart rate reactivity and nonreactivity. *Am. J. Perintol.*, **11**, 208–12

119. Schuessler, M., Van Leeuwen, P., Bettermann, H. and Hatzmann, W. (1994). Magnetocardiography for analysis of fetal heart rate parameters in multiple pregnancy. The 9th International Workshop on Multiple Pregnancy, Herzliya, Israel, (abstr.) *Isr. J. Obstet. Gynecol.*, **5** (Suppl), 2

120. Chien, E. and Loy, G. (1995). Timing of delivery in twin gestation. The 15th Annual Meeting of the Society of Perinatal Obstetricians, Atlanta, GA (abstr.) *Am. J. Obstet. Gynecol.*, **172**, 292

121. Blickstein, I., Schwartz, Z., Lancet, M. and Borenstein, R. (1987). Vaginal delivery of the second twin in breech presentation. *Obstet. Gynecol.*, **69**, 774–6

122. Fishman, A., Grubb, D. K. and Kovacs, B. W. (1993). Vaginal delivery of nonvertex second twin. *Am. J. Obstet. Gynecol.*, **168**, 861–4

123. Blickstein, I., Weissmann, A., Ben-Hur, H., Borenstein, R. and Insler, V. (1993). Vaginal delivery for breech-vertex twins. *J. Reprod. Med.*, **38**, 879–82

124. Ophir, E., Markovitz, J., Odeh, M., Stolro, E. and Oettinger, M. (1994). Is it necessary to perform Cesarean section in management of delivery of breech-first twin? The 9th International Workshop of Multiple Pregnancy, Herzliya, Israel, (abstr.) *Isr. J. Obstet. Gynecol.*, **5** (Suppl.), 1

125. Strong, T. H. Jr, Phelan, J. P., Ahn, M. O. and Sarno, A. P. (1989). Vaginal birth after Cesarean delivery in the twin gestation. *Am. J. Obstet. Gynecol.*, **161**, 29–32

126. Contantine, G. and Redman, C. W. (1987). Cesarean delivery of the second twin. *Lancet*, **1**, 618–9

127. Chervenak, F. A., Johnson, R. E., Youcha, S., Hobbins, J. C. and Berkowitz, R. L. (1985). Intrapartum management of twin gestation. *Obstet. Gynecol.*, **65**, 119–24

Management of intrauterine growth retardation

40

G. C. Di Renzo and G. Luzi

INTRODUCTION

Fetal birth weight is considered to be one of the most important indices in the prediction of fetal outcome. The incidence of neonatal birth weight of less than 2500 g is near 7% of all births, but half of this figure reflects neonatal deaths[1]. Fetuses with intrauterine growth retardation (IUGR) have a high risk for perinatal morbidity and mortality. Furthermore, the causes of the IUGR can exert their effects after birth. This is demonstrated by a reduction of the ability to learn in the children who suffered from IUGR[2]. Moreover, there is no agreement on the assessment of the damage caused by altered fetal growth, and this might be due to an inaccurate nosologic approach to the problem.

Fetal IUGR is a symptom that has several causes. The approach to IUGR includes three steps: the diagnosis of the symptom, the identification of the cause or causes and the monitoring of fetal health[3].

DIAGNOSIS OF THE SYMPTOM

For correct identification of a symptom, a correct definition is required. The definition of IUGR is unclear and unsatisfactory. The definition of IUGR most used in clinical practice is that which results in a birth weight equal to or below the 10th centile for that gestational age[4]. This definition is unsatisfactory, because: (1) it is a neonatological definition, which is based on the birth weight and only presumes the presence of fetal IUGR; (2) there are some fetuses that have a birth weight below the 10th centile but are normally developed; (3) there are fetuses that have a birth weight higher than the 10th centile and have suffered IUGR with respect to their potential growth[5]; and (4) there are great differences between the various standard curves of birth weight – the difference between several 10th centile values can be greater than 300 g[6]. All definitions based on the birth weight have these limits. The neonatal ponderal index (BW × 100/CHL[3], where BW is the birth weight in grams and CHL is the crown–heel length in centimeters) below the 10th centile seems to be able to identify subjects with poor neonatal outcome[7], but it is a neonatological definition. It may be better to define a fetus with IUGR as a neonate which has a birth weight below its own genetic potential for growth[8]. This definition involves the identification of the standard of growth for every fetus. The definition does not consider the delay of growth. This is a dynamic phenomenon and requires an evaluation during the period of gestation. The most common mistake is the confusion between fetal 'size' and fetal 'growth'[9]. Fetal growth determination requires at least two evaluations during pregnancy. The evaluation of the measurements for monitoring the growth of the fetus needs the exact date of the pregnancy.

Indirect detection of the symptom of IUGR is possible in several ways: evaluation of the weight of the pregnant woman, or evaluation of the fundal height of the uterus. Today, however, fetal growth is evaluated by echographic examination. A sequence of measurements of the anthropometric parameters is required during the course of pregnancy. The biparietal diameter of the fetal head was the first anthropometric parameter utilized to monitor fetal growth[10]. Later, several others parameters were used in order to assess fetal growth, but the sensitivity of the majority of these is too low to utilize them for growth retardation screening (Table 1). The

Table 1 *Ability of some fetal anthropometric measurements to detect intrauterine growth retardation*

	Sensitivity (%)	Specificity (%)	PPV	NPV
Biparietal diameter < 10th centile	75	70	21	96
Femur length < 10th centile	45	97	64	94
Mean abdominal diameter < 10th centile	70	96	49	98
Abdominal circumference < 10th centile	95	60	21	99
Estimated fetal weight	65	96	65	96
Fetal ponderal index < 30th centile	77	82	35	96

PPV, positive predictive value; NPV, negative predictive value

most useful parameters for the detection of IUGR appear to be those that have the indirect capacity to evaluate the quantity of fat tissues. The evaluation of the total intrauterine volume and the fetal ponderal index is subject to many miscalculations, related to the complexity of the formulae for their calculation[11,12]. The best parameter to detect IUGR is evidence of irregular growth in the measurement of the fetal abdominal circumference between two echographic evaluations[13]. Considering that IUGR is a dynamic phenomenon and that the best parameter to evaluate this is the abdominal circumference, in our opinion a useful perinatological definition of fetal IUGR must include the evaluation of fetal abdominal circumference. We therefore define IUGR as a delay of the growth of the fetus estimated as a decrease of 25 centiles in the measure of the abdominal circumference, according to the standard curve at that gestational age, and in subsequent echographic evaluations performed at least 2 weeks subsequently.

IDENTIFICATION OF THE CAUSES

There are several causes that can induce IUGR and these act through various pathogenic mechanisms (Tables 2 and 3). A correct diagnosis of the causes is required for correct monitoring of fetal conditions and the best treatment of the disease. There is a great difference in the various problems which can cause fetal growth disturbances and affect fetal prognosis. The clinical and obstetric history of the pregnant woman may be useful to identify the maternal diseases that could affect fetal growth. It is also important to have information on the socioeconomic status of the mother and an evaluation of

Table 2 *Maternal causes of fetal intrauterine growth retardation*

Environmental
Low socioeconomic status
Pollution: air and water contaminants

Nutritional
Poor caloric intake
Unbalanced nutrients intake
Malnutrition

Gastroenteric diseases
Chronic enteritis
Enteric resections
Malabsorption diseases

Pulmonary diseases
Asthma
Cystic fibrosis
Respiratory failure

Cardiovascular diseases
Cardiac diseases
Hypertension
Pre-eclampsia

Renal diseases
Renal failure

Hematological diseases
Anemia
Hematological neoplasia
Malaria

Drug addiction
Alcohol abuse
Drug abuse
Smoking

Uterine anomalies
Fibroids
Uterine malformations

the structural characteristics of the parents of the fetus affected by suspected IUGR[14]. It is necessary to carry out a physical examination, a blood test and an electrocardiogram. Drug and

Table 3 *Placental and fetal causes of intrauterine growth retardation*

Placentation anomalies
Placenta previa

Placental anomalies
Chorioangioma

Umbilical cord anomalies
Single umbilical artery
Anomalies of cord insertion

Multiple pregnancies
Twin pregnancies
High-grade multiple pregnancies

Chromosomal anomalies
Deletions (4p-, 5p-, 13q-, 21q-)
Trisomies (21, 13, 18)
Turner's syndrome

Genetic anomalies
Metabolic diseases

Isolated fetal malformations
Micro-anencephaly
Cardiovascular defects
Gastroenteric malformations
Genitourinary malformations
Skeletal dysplasia

Viral infections
Human immunodeficiency virus
Cytomegalovirus
Herpes simplex virus
Rubella virus/parvovirus B19

Bacterial infections
Syphilis
Listeriosis

Protozoal infections
Toxoplasmosis
Chagas' disease

alcohol abuse should be investigated. Echographic examinations may be useful to identify fetal malformations or markers of chromosomal alterations, even though the ability of these examinations to identify such conditions have a sensitivity of about 50%[15]. Apart from this, the echographic examination will also allow the determination of the placental site, uterine malformations and cord anomalies. When a severe alteration of fetal growth is present in early gestation, it may be due to a chromosomal or genetic defect of the fetus; in this case, or in the presence of signs of high maternal risk for chromosomal diseases, amniocentesis or cordocentesis may be performed to identify the defect.

It is essential to perform tests to identify feto-maternal infections (TORCH, syphilis, HIV) and, in presence of characteristic fetal signs, to investigate the possibility of parvovirus B19 in fetal blood[16–18], even though the incidence of these as a cause of fetal IUGR is as low as 10%[1].

The greater part of fetal IUGR is due to alterations in the balance of the fetomaternal unit, with subsequent alteration of uteroplacental exchanges and fetal hypoxia. The only direct test is the determination of the PO_2 in a sample of fetal blood, but this procedure is extremely invasive and potentially dangerous for the fetus and its use is not recommended in clinical routine. However, it is possible to detect some fetomaternal signs induced by the metabolic and homeostatic alterations which cause IUGR.

In the presence of IUGR, a reduction of the expansion of the maternal plasma volume[19] and an increase in the maternal blood viscosity at low shear rate have been demonstrated and this last fact seems to be related to the grade of fetal IUGR[20]. The increase of resistance to blood flow in the uteroplacental circulation seems to be present in a majority of cases of fetal growth disturbances.

Doppler evaluations of the uterine artery flow velocity waveforms between 16 and 22 weeks of gestation may give information on these maternal modifications. Recently, it has been reported that the presence of a bilateral notch in one or both uterine arteries has a sensitivity of near 75% to predict severe fetal complications[21]. The specificity of the test may be improved by the evaluation of the maternal blood viscosity at low shear rate. The decrease of uterine blood flow and/or placental exchange capability leads to a reduced supply to the fetus of oxygen, glucose and other essential nutrients[22,23]. In the presence of hypoxia, the fetus shows growth reduction, typical of hemodynamic modifications known as the 'brain-sparing effect'; these modifications are protective against hypoxic insult and consist of an increase of blood flow to the brain, liver and the heart and the decrease of flow to the periphery[24,25]. The identification of these fetal hemodynamic modifications by Doppler velocimetry performed on the peripheral vessels (e.g. umbilical artery, aorta, renal artery) and cerebral vessels (e.g. middle cerebral artery, internal carotid artery) is strongly related to the existence of a fetal hypoxic state[26]. The ratio between the flow indices of the fetal middle cerebral artery and the umbilical artery (cerebro–placental ratio) below two standard deviations seems to be a good indirect index to predict fetal hypoxemic status[27] (Figure 1). Recently it has been reported that the fetal vessel which is more sensitive to the initial hypoxia is the middle cerebral artery[28,29]. The middle cerebral artery is the principal branch of the circle of Willis and the direct continuation of the internal carotid artery. It also supplies a great part of the brain. We observed that the subcortical part of the middle cerebral artery (or M2 segment) reacted earlier than the first part of the vessel (or M1 segment) and the ratio between the flow indices of the two parts of the vessels (M1/M2) became higher than two standard deviations in the presence of an initial fetal

hypoxic state[30]. The evidence of these Doppler flow signs in fetal hemodynamics is related to an alteration of the fetal growth due to the hypoxic conditions.

MONITORING OF FETAL HEALTH

The greater part of fetal growth retardation is due to causes that are able to produce fetal hypoxia. The fetal adaptation to the hypoxic state is progressive and 'protective' for the fetus against the possible damage (fetal compensation phase); if the hypoxia is severe and prolonged, a failure of the fetal adaptation mechanisms (fetal decompensation phase) is then apparent. In the presence of hypoxia, the fetal hemodynamics undergo modifications, with a prevalence of the blood flow to the brain, liver, adrenals and heart. Other mechanisms of adaptation are the decrease of the fetal growth rate until growth stops, a reduction of fetal movements and some metabolic modifications, such as the increase of erythropoietin plasma concentrations with a concomitant increase in the number of the red blood cells[31]. The aim of fetal monitoring in the presence of a hypoxic state is to prevent the decompensation phase, characterized by a deficiency in the hemodynamic situation and by fetal cardiac failure. Figure 2 shows the sequence of events which most probably follow the progressive hypoxic state. In the case of IUGR, the tests proposed for fetal surveillance are: echographic evaluation of the fetal growth rate, Doppler velocimetry, amniotic fluid volume assessment, non-stress test (NST), fetal biophysical profile, behavioral state analysis and the contraction stress test (CST)[32–35]. Doppler velocimetry seems to be the most sensitive method for monitoring the fetus affected by growth retardation, from the early stage of the hypoxic state. As indicated previously, the first fetal vessel that responds to hypoxia is the middle cerebral artery. We observed that, in the presence of the small variations in the oxygen requirement of the brain, it is possible for a regional vasodilation to take place in the cerebral circulation. In the presence of a decrease of the pulsatility index (PI) in only the subcortical

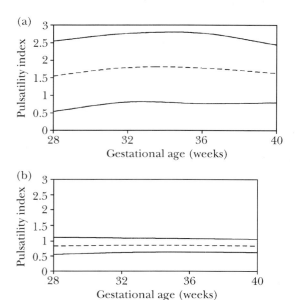

Figure 1 *Standard curves (mean ± 2SD) of the cerebro-placental ratio (a) and the M1/M2 ratio of the segments of the middle cerebral artery (b)*

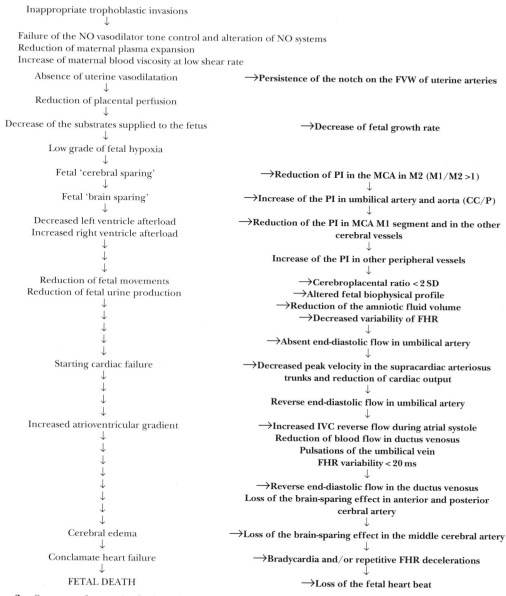

Inappropriate trophoblastic invasions
↓
Failure of the NO vasodilator tone control and alteration of NO systems
Reduction of maternal plasma expansion
Increase of maternal blood viscosity at low shear rate

Absence of uterine vasodilatation   →**Persistence of the notch on the FVW of uterine arteries**
↓
Reduction of placental perfusion
↓
Decrease of the substrates supplied to the fetus   →**Decrease of fetal growth rate**
↓
Low grade of fetal hypoxia
↓
Fetal 'cerebral sparing'   →**Reduction of PI in the MCA in M2 (M1/M2 >1)**
↓   ↓
Fetal 'brain sparing'   →**Increase of the PI in umbilical artery and aorta (CC/P)**
↓   ↓
Decreased left ventricle afterload   →**Reduction of the PI in MCA M1 segment and in the other**
Increased right ventricle afterload   **cerebral vessels**
↓   ↓
↓   **Increase of the PI in other peripheral vessels**
↓   ↓
Reduction of fetal movements   →**Cerebroplacental ratio < 2 SD**
Reduction of fetal urine production   →**Altered fetal biophysical profile**
↓   →**Reduction of the amniotic fluid volume**
↓   →**Decreased variability of FHR**
↓   ↓
↓   →**Absent end-diastolic flow in umbilical artery**
↓   ↓
Starting cardiac failure   →**Decreased peak velocity in the supracardiac arteriosus**
↓   **trunks and reduction of cardiac output**
↓   ↓
↓   **Reverse end-diastolic flow in umbilical artery**
↓   ↓
Increased atrioventricular gradient   →**Increased IVC reverse flow during atrial systole**
↓   **Reduction of blood flow in ductus venosus**
↓   **Pulsations of the umbilical vein**
↓   **FHR variability < 20 ms**
↓   ↓
↓   →**Reverse end-diastolic flow in the ductus venosus**
↓   **Loss of the brain-sparing effect in anterior and posterior**
↓   **cerebral artery**
↓   ↓
Cerebral edema   →**Loss of the brain-sparing effect in the middle cerebral artery**
↓   ↓
Conclamate heart failure   →**Bradycardia and/or repetitive FHR decelerations**
↓   ↓
FETAL DEATH   →**Loss of the fetal heart beat**

Figure 2 *Sequence of events in the fetus during hypoxia. NO, nitric oxide; FVW, flow velocity waveform; PI, pulsatility index; M1/M2, ratio of the segments of the middle cerebral artery (MCA); C/P, cerebroplacental ratio; FHR, fetal heart rate*

segment (M2) of the middle cerebral artery, the birth weight of the fetus was significantly reduced. The initial sign of fetal hypoxia may be the appearance of the 'cerebral sparing effect' characterized by the increase in the ratio of the PI between the M1 and M2 segments (M1/M2 more than 1)[30]. The reduction of the PI in the initial segment of the middle cerebral artery or M1 segment and in the other cerebral vessels normally follows the increase of the resistance in the umbilical artery and it is possible to observe an increase of the resistance in other peripheral vessels; in the presence of the brain-sparing effect there is a re-distribution of the cardiac output to allow the increase of cerebral blood flow[33]. The cerebroplacental ratio can be considered as the Doppler flow expression of the brain-sparing effect[34]; the decrease of this ratio below two standard deviations is a sign of incipient severe hypoxia and in its presence we may observe anomalies of the fetal biophysical profile, reduction of the fetal heart rate variability and reduction of amniotic fluid volume. The abilities of prenatal tests to detect fetal distress are shown in Table 4.

The introduction 15 years ago of the biophysical profile in the fetal surveillance of high-risk pregnancies was based on the observation of five fetal 'activities': fetal breathing movements, fetal tone, active fetal movements, the amount of amniotic fluid and the characteristics of the fetal heart rate; a profile is considered to be pathological when the score is below 6[35]. In the case of a score between 10 and 8, the perinatal mortality is 1–0.03%, and when the score is 0–4[36,37], the mortality may be as high as 60%. Over the last few years, several modifications have been made to the original version of the biophysical profile[38–40]; recently the adaptation of the biophysical profile to a computer-assisted environment seems to have improved the ability of the test to detect fetal distress[41]. The fetal biophysical profile may be used in the monitoring of fetal conditions when the cerebroplacental ratio is below two standard deviations. The antepartum monitoring of fetal heart rate is probably the most used test for fetal surveillance, but the modification of the tracing, which is indicative of severe fetal distress (such as bradycardia and late decelerations), is late in the fetal hypoxic sequence; it appears in the last stage of the fetal hemodynamic decompensation phase, often when there is already fetal damage caused by hypoxia[33–44]. The objective evaluation of the variability of the fetal heart rate does not show great sensitivity in identifying the fetus before any hemodynamic decompensation occurs. The objective analysis of the fetal heart rate variability by a computerized fetal heart rate monitor seems to provide better prediction. A variability in the fetal heart rate of less than 20 mv is considered in a fetus affected by growth retardation as a probable sign of incipient hemodynamic decompensation. Absent end-diastolic flow on the flow velocity waveform of the umbilical artery can be considered as a sign of a strong increase of the placental and peripheral resistance to blood flow. Absent

Table 4 *Ability of the prenatal tests to detect fetal distress. Data collected from reference 27, 35, 41, 43, 45*

	Sensitivity (%)	Specificity (%)	PPV (%)	NPV (%)
Amniotic fluid index	13	95	47	77
Amniotic pocket < 2 cm	7	96	36	77
Cardiotocography				
Fisher's score < 8	36	88	58	75
Reactivity	17	97	69	72
Computerized analysis of FHR (fetal acidosis)	70	93	—	—
Biophysical profile				
Biophysical profile < 6	30	91	61	74
Computerized biophysical profile	86	89	77	93
Doppler velocimetry				
FVW of umbilical artery	65.1	78.6	51.5	—
Cerebroplacental ratio < 1	75	95	83	88
ARED flow in umbilical artery	87	95	83	97
Behavioral state analysis (S2F)	78	95	90	92

PPV, positive predictive value; NPV, negative predictive value; FHR, fetal heart rate; FVW, flow velocity waveform; ARED, absent or reversed end-diastolic flow

end-diastolic flow may also be found in fetuses with various congenital anomalies, such as heart disease, kidney disease and fetal infection[44]; in the fetus with absent end-diastolic flow, the incidence of chromosomal anomalies is reported to be 8–14%[46]. However, the appearance in the umbilical arteries of absent end-diastolic flow in the sequence of fetal hemodynamic compensation may indicate the beginning of the decompensation phase; in cases of reverse end-diastolic flow in the umbilical artery the fetal prognosis is more severe than with absent end-diastolic flow[47]. Obviously, with absent end-diastolic flow in the umbilical artery, the obstetrician should be aware of the increased fetal risk involved and should, therefore, apply appropriate and strict surveillance measures; however, the benefits of an emergency delivery as a consequence of this observation are uncertain. With the progression of the deteriorating fetal condition, it has been observed that the peak velocity on the supracardiac arteriosus trunks and cardiac output decreased progressively rather than showing the expected rise with gestation[48]. Concomitantly in the fetal venous circulation signs of increasing pressure have been observed as the increase of the percentage of reverse flow in the inferior vena cava[49], reduction of peak velocity during atrial contraction and absent or reverse diastolic flow in the ductus venosus[50,51]. In the cerebral circulation, a loss of vasodilation of the cerebral vessel has been described[52]; the disappearance of the cerebral vasodilation is reported to occur earlier in the anterior and the posterior cerebral arteries and later in the middle cerebral artery[53]. This fact may be due to the autoregulation capability of the cerebral circulation and to the particular anatomic situation of the circle of Willis, which favors the blood flow in the middle cerebral artery. In the presence of an incipient cardiovascular disaster, the last attempt to protect the most important cerebral district is the concentration of the cerebral blood flow in the middle cerebral artery. Damage to the cerebral tissue in the occipital and frontal part of the brain produces an edema that increases the loss of vasodilation in the middle cerebral artery. The cardiac insufficency causes a fall in the cerebral blood flow, indicated by the increase of umbilical vein pulsation[54], which appears in the last period of fetal life as a dicrotic pulsation (Color plates 36–39). Late decelerations and severe bradycardia occur in this terminal stage[55]. A flow chart of fetal surveillance in the presence of growth retardation is shown in Figure 3.

THERAPEUTIC APPROACHES TO FETAL GROWTH RETARDATION

Clinical trials of the therapy for fetal growth retardation are usually related to the noxae which cause the symptom. The early onset of severe IUGR may be caused by a genetic or chromosomal anomaly. This accounts for up to 40% of cases in which chromosomal anomalies are linked to severe fetal growth retardation; on the other hand, approximately 10% of the fetuses that have malformations are small for gestational age[56]. In these cases it may be suggested to the mother that she consider a termination of the pregnancy; if the decision is to continue the pregnancy, the parents should be informed of the life expectancy of their baby.

In case of congenital infections, therapy should act against the etiological agents of the disease. When maternal pathologies capable of altering fetal growth are present, these should be treated as well. There are several fetal–maternal and placental causes which may produce fetal intrauterine growth alteration due to inadequate support of substrates through the placenta; the majority affect the uteroplacental blood flow (with the sequence previously mentioned) while others may act on the quality of the substrates present in the maternal blood. It is very important to be able to differentiate between the two groups. The NO (nitric oxide) test, which we recently proposed, is able to detect the lack of an appropriate nitric oxide system in pregnancy and to identify a group of fetuses with IUGR caused by a failure in maternal adaptation to pregnancy[57]. The test consists in the sublingual administration to the mother of 0.3 mg of glyceryl trinitrate and the evaluation by Doppler velocimetry of the flow

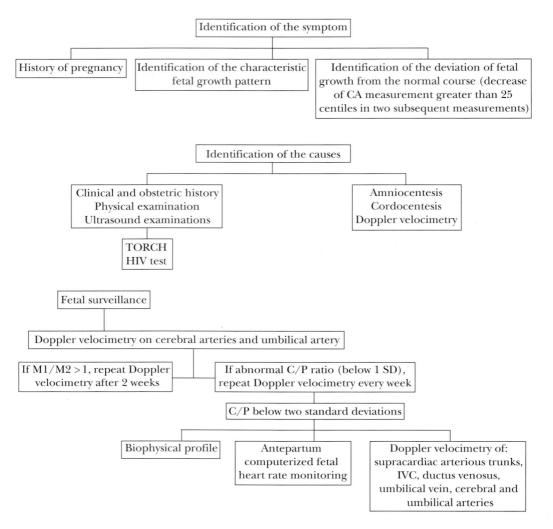

Figure 3 *Fetal surveillance in the presence of growth retardation. CA, cerebral artery; M1/M2, ratio of segments of the middle cerebral artery; C/P, cerebroplacental ratio; IVC, inferior vena cava*

velocity waveform of the placental uterine artery; a decrease in the uterine artery resistance index (RI) of over 20% and/or the disappearance of the protodiastolic notch is considered as 'positive' for the test and may select cases which can benefit from treatment with nitric oxide donor agents[58]. In these cases the administration (intravenous, sublingual, oral or transdermic) of nitric oxide donor agents may be considered an etiologic therapy for IUGR; this treatment is reported to improve the uteroplacental blood flow and correct the alteration

of several maternal cell types (such as platelet anomalies)[59] present in this type of fetal growth alteration.

Other methods which may modify uteroplacental blood flow are bedrest[60], administration of tocolytic agents[61] and/or antiaggregant agents[62]. Bedrest did not show any particular benefit in pregnancies complicated by fetal IUGR[63], but obviously it is not contraindicated. Tocolytic agents proposed for the treatment of IUGR are mainly β-mimetic agents; in this case, also, there is no evidence of benefit of the use

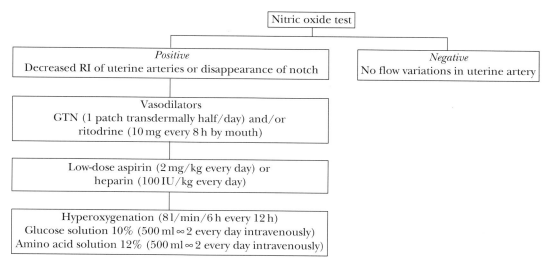

Figure 4 *Clinical management of fetuses with intrauterine growth retardation due to placental insufficiency. RI, resistance index; GTN, glycerol trinitrate*

of these agents[64]. The treatment with low-dose aspirin or dipyridamole has been proposed by some authors, but this modality has not yet shown consistent results[65,66]. Heparin may be used to reduce maternal blood viscosity in severe IUGR[67]. Maternal hyperoxygenation seems to improve the perinatal outcome of fetuses with growth retardation[68]; however, it should not be used continuously, since oxygen therapy has been shown also to have noxious effects on the fetus[69]. The intra-amniotic or maternal administration of glucose or amino acids has been reported to improve birth weight in fetuses with IUGR[70]. Other trials are needed to confirm early reports. It is to be kept in mind that if premature delivery is indicated, fetal lung maturation should be induced in case of pregnancy before the 34th week of gestation. In Figure 4, our clinical management of fetal IUGR is shown.

References

1. Pollack, R. N. and Divon, M. Y. (1992). Intrauterine growth retardation: definition, classification and etiology. *Clin. Obstet. Gynecol.*, **35**, 99–113
2. Low, J. A., Handely-Derry, M. G. and Burke, S. O. (1992). Association of intrauterine growth retardation and learning deficits at age 9 to 11 years. *Am. J. Obstet. Gynecol.*, **167**, 1499–506
3. Cosmi, E. V., Luzi, G., Anceschi, M. M., Coata, G. and Di Renzo, G. C. (1994). Fetal intrauterine growth retardation: pathophysiologic and diagnostic aspects. In Genazzani, A. R., D'Ambrosio, G. and Genezzani, A. D. (eds.) *Growth and Differentiation in Reproductive Organs*, pp. 111–18. (Rome: CIC International Edition)
4. Lubchenco, L. O., Hamsman, C. and Dressler, C. (1963). Intrauterine growth as estimated from liveborn birth weight data at 24 to 42 weeks of gestation. *Pediatrics*, **32**, 793–801
5. Chard, T., Costeloe, K. and Leaf, A. (1992). Evidence of growth retardation in neonates of apparently normal weight. *Eur. J. Obstet. Gynecol. Rep. Biol.*, **45**, 59–64
6. Goldenberg, R. L., Cutter, G. R., Hoffman, H. J., Foster, J. M., Nelson, K. G. and Haunt, J. C. (1989). Intrauterine growth retardation: standard for diagnosis. *Am. J. Obstet. Gynecol.*, **161**, 271–8
7. Patterson, R. M. and Pouliot, M. R. (1987). Neonatal morphometric and perinatal

outcome: who is growth retarded? *Am. J. Obstet. Gynecol.*, **157**, 691–9

8. Chard, T., Yoong, A. and Macintosh, M. (1993). The myth of fetal growth retardation at term. *Br. J. Obstet. Gynaecol.*, **100**, 1076–8

9. Altman, D. G. and Hytten, F. E. (1989). Intrauterine growth retardation: let's be clear about it. *Br. J. Obstet. Gynaecol.*, **96**, 1127–32

10. Thompson, H. E., Holmes, J. H. and Gottesheld, J. (1965). Fetal development as determined by ultrasonic pulse echo techniques. *Am. J. Obstet. Gynecol.*, **92**, 44–52

11. Gomari, P., Berkowitz, R. L. and Hobbins, J. C. (1977). Prediction of intrauterine volume. *Am. J. Obstet. Gynecol.*, **127**, 255–60

12. Vintzileos, A. M., Lodeiro, J. G., Feinstein, S. J., Campbell, W. A., Weinbaum, P. J. and Nochimson, D. J. (1986). Value of fetal ponderal index in predicting growth retardation. *Obstet. Gynecol.*, **67**, 584–9

13. Chang, T. C., Robson, S. C., Boys, M. J. and Spencer, J. A. D. (1992). Prediction of small gestational age infant: which ultrasound measurement is best? *Obstet. Gynecol.*, **80**, 44–8

14. Sciscione, A., Longman, R., Lantz, H. and Callan, N. (1994). Adjustment of birth weight for maternal characteristics improves prediction of morbidity and mortality in the growth retarded infant. *Am. J. Obstet. Gynecol.*, **170** (Suppl.), 346

15. Levi, S., Schaaps, J. P., De Havay, P., Coulon, R. and Defoort, P. (1995). End-result of routine ultrasound screening for congenital anomalies: the Belgian Multicentric Study 1984–92. *Ultrasound Obstet. Gynecol.*, **5**, 366–71

16. Amstei, M. S. (1985). Specific viral infections: rubella, herpes simplex, varicella zoster. In Sciarra, J. J. (ed.) *Gynecology and Obstetrics*, vol. 3, pp. 46–62. (Philadelphia: Harper & Row)

17. Knox, G. E. (1985). Specific viral infection: cytomegalovirus. In Sciarra, J. J. (ed.) *Gynecology and Obstetrics*, vol. 3, pp. 36–45. (Philadelphia: Harper & Row)

18. Carrera, J. M. and Di Renzo, G. C. (1993). *Recommendations and Protocols for Prenatal Diagnosis. Report of the European Study Group on Prenatal Diagnosis.* (Barcellona: Salvat)

19. Salas, S. P., Rosso, P., Espinoza, R., Robert, J., Valdez, G. and Donoso, E. (1993). Maternal volume expansion and hormonal changes in women with idiopathic fetal growth retardation. *Obstet. Gynecol.*, **81**, 1029–35

20. Luzi, G., Coata, G., Chiaradia, E., Caserta, G., Anceschi, M. M., Cosmi, E. V. and Di Renzo, G. C. (1994). Maternal haemodynamic and haemorrheologic considerations in fetal IUGR. *J. Perinat. Med.*, **22** (Suppl. 1), 193–8

21. Campbell, S., Kurdi, W. and Harrington, K. (1995). Doppler ultrasound of the uteroplacental circulation in early prediction of pre-eclampsia and intrauterine growth retardation. *Ultrasound Obstet. Gynecol.*, **6** (Suppl. 2), 29

22. Economides, D. L. and Nicolaides, K. H. (1989). Blood glucose and oxygen tension in small for gestational age fetuses. *Am. J. Obstet. Gynecol.*, **160**, 385–9

23. Cetin, I., Corbetta, G., Sereni, L. P., Marconi, A. M., Bozzetti, P. and Pardi, G. (1990). Umbilical amino acid concentration in normal and growth retarded fetuses sampled *in utero* by cordocentesis. *Am. J. Obstet. Gynecol.*, **162**, 253–61

24. Rudolph, A. M. and Heymann, M. A. (1970). Circulatory changes during growth in the fetal lamb. *Circ. Res.*, **26**, 289–99

25. Jones, M. D., Sheldon, R. E., Peeters, L. L., Makowski, E. L. and Meschia, G. (1978). Regulation of cerebral blood flow in ovine fetus. *Am. J. Physiol.*, **235**, 162–6

26. Bilardo, C. M., Nicolaides, K. H. and Campbell, S. (1988). Doppler measurements of fetal and uteroplacental circulation: relationship with umbilical venous blood gas measured at cordocentesis. *Early Hum. Dev.*, **8**, 213–23

27. Di Renzo, G. C., Luzi, G., Cucchia, G. C., Caserta, G., Fusaro, P., Perdikaris, A. and Cosmi, E. V. (1992). The role of Doppler technology in the evaluation of fetal hypoxia. *Early Hum. Dev.*, **29**, 259–63

28. Mori, A., Iwashita, M. and Takeda, Y. (1993). Haemodynamic changes in IUGR fetuses with chronic hypoxia evaluated by fetal heart rate monitoring and Doppler measurement of blood flow. *Med. Biol. Eng. Comput.*, **3**, 49–58

29. Veille, J. C. and Penry, M. (1993). Effect of maternal administration of 3% carbon dioxide on umbilical artery and fetal renal and middle cerebral artery Doppler waveforms. *Am. J. Obstet. Gynecol.*, **167**, 1668–71

30. Luzi, G., Coata, G., Caserta, G., Cosmi, E. V. and Di Renzo, G. C. (1996). Doppler velocimetry of different sections of the fetal middle cerebral artery in relation to perinatal outcome. *J. Perinat. Med.*, in press

31. Snijders, R. J. M., Abbas, A., Melby, O., Ireland, R. M. and Nicolaides, K. H. (1993). Fetal plasma erythropoietin concentration in severe growth retardation. *Am. J. Obstet. Gynecol.*, **168**, 615–19

32. Vintzileos, A. M. (1995). Antepartum fetal surveillance. *Clin. Obstet. Gynecol.*, **38**, 1–2

33. Arduini, D., Rizzo, G. and Romanini, C. (1995). Fetal cardiac function in growth retardation. In Arduini, D., Rizzo, G. and Romanini, C. (eds.) *Fetal Cardiac Function*, pp. 91–101 (Carnforth UK: Parthenon Publishing)

34. Arbeille, P., Body, G. and Saliba, E. (1988). Fetal cerebral circulation assessment by Doppler

ultrasound in normal and pathologic pregnancies. *Eur. J. Obstet. Gynecol. Reprod. Biol.*, **29**, 261–6

35. Manning, F. A., Platt, L. D. and Sipos, L. (1980). Antepartum fetal evaluation: development of a fetal biophysical profile. *Am. J. Obstet. Gynecol.*, **136**, 787–97

36. Manning, F. A., Harman, C. R., Menticoglou, S. and Morrison, I. (1991). Assessment of fetal well being with ultrasound. *Obstet. Gynecol. Clin. North Am.*, **18**, 891–905

37. Baskett, T. F., Gray, J. H., Prewett, S. J., Young, L. M. and Allen, A. C. (1984). Antepartum fetal assessment using fetal biophysical profile score. *Am. J. Obstet. Gynecol.*, **148**, 630–9

38. Shah, D. M., Brown, J. E., Sayer, S. I., Fleischer, A. C. and Boehm, F. H. (1989). A modified scheme for biophysical profile scoring. *Am. J. Obstet. Gynecol.*, **160**, 586–95

39. Carrera, J. M., Mallafré, J. and Torrents, M. (1994). The fetal biophysical profile. In Kurjak, A. (ed.) *The Fetus as a Patient*, pp. 231–44. (Carnforth, UK: Parthenon Publishing)

40. Vintzileos, A. M., Campbell, W. A., Ingradia, C. J. and Nochimson, D. J. (1993). The fetal biophysical profile and its predictive value. *Obstet. Gynecol.*, **62**, 271–83

41. Devoe, L. D. (1995). Computerized fetal biophysical assessment. *Clin. Obstet. Gynecol.*, **38**, 121–31

42. Weiner, Z., Farmakides, G., Schneider, E., Schulman, H., Kellner, L., Plancher, S. and Maulik, D. (1994). Computerized analysis of fetal heart rate variation in post-term pregnancy: prediction of fetal distress and acidosis. *Am. J. Obstet. Gynecol.*, **171**, 1132–8

43. Maulik, D. (1995). Doppler ultrasound velocimetry for fetal surveillance. *Clin. Obstet. Gynecol.*, **38**, 91–111

44. Weiner, Z., Farmakides, G., Shulman, H. and Penny, B. (1994). Central and peripheral hemodynamic changes in fetuses with absent end dyastolic velocity in umbilical artery; correlation with computerized fetal heart rate. *Am. J. Obstet. Gynecol.*, **170**, 509–15

45. Schneider, E., Shulman, H., Farmakides, G. and Chan, L. (1992). Clinical experience with antepartum computerized fetal heart rate monitoring. *J. Matern. Fetal Invest.*, **2**, 41–4

46. Rizzo, G., Pietropoli, A., Capponi, A. and Romanini, C. (1994). Chromosomal abnormalities in fetuses with absent end-diastolic velocity in umbilical artery: analysis of risk factors for an abnormal karyotype. *Am. J. Obstet. Gynecol.*, **171**, 827–31

47. Rochelson, B., Shulman, H., Fermakides, J., Bracero, L., Ducey, J., Fleisher, A., Penny, B. and Winter, D. (1987). The significance of absent end diastolic velocity in umbilical artery velocity waveform. *Am. J. Obstet. Gynecol.*, **156**, 1213–17

48. Rizzo, G., Arduini, D. and Romanini, C. (1992). Fetal cardiac function in intrauterine growth retardation. *Am. J. Obstet. Gynecol.*, **165**, 876–82

49. Rizzo, G., Arduini, D. and Romanini, C. (1992). Inferior vena cava flow velocity waveforms in appropriate and small for gestational age fetuses. *Am. J. Obstet. Gynecol.*, **166**, 1271–80

50. Rizzo, G., Pietropolli, A., Bufalino, L. M., Soldano, S., Arduini, D. and Romanini, C. (1993). Ductus venosus systolic to peak velocities ratio in appropriate and small for gestational age fetuses. *J. Matern. Fetal Invest.*, **3**, 198

51. Goncalves, L. F., Romero, R., Silva, M., Ghezzi, F., Soto, A., Munoz, H. and Ghidini, A. (1995). Reverse flow in the ductus venosus: an ominous sign. *Am. J. Obstet. Gynecol.*, **172** (Suppl. 1), 266

52. Chandran, R., Serra-Serra, V., Sellers, S. M. and Redman, C. W. G. (1991). Fetal middle cerebral artery flow velocity waveforms; a terminal pattern. Case report. *Br. J. Obstet. Gynaecol.*, **98**, 937–9

53. Luzi, G., Clerici, G., Taddei, F. and Di Renzo, G. C. (1995). Cerebral circulation in normal and growth retarded fetuses. *Ultrasound Obstet. Gynecol.*, **6** (Suppl. 2), 71

54. Indick, J. H., Chen, V. and Reed, K. L. (1991). Association of umbilical venous with inferior vena cava blood flow velocities. *Obstet. Gynecol.*, **77**, 551–7

55. Bekedam, D. J., Visser, G. H. A., van der Zee, A. G. J., Snijder, R. A. and Poeleman-Weesjes, G. (1990). Abnormal umbilical artery waveform patterns in growth retarded fetuses: relationship to antepartum late heart rate decelerations and outcome. *Early Hum. Dev.*, **24**, 79–90

56. Khoury, M. J., Erickson, J. D., Cordero, J. F. and McCarthy, B. J. (1988). Congenital malformation and intrauterine growth retardation: a population study. *Pediatrics*, **82**, 83–90

57. Luzi, G., Abubakari, M. N., Clerici, G., Caserta, G. and Di Renzo, G. C. (1995). Feto-maternal haemodynamics during maternal glyceryl trinitrate sublingual administration. *J. Soc. Gynecol. Invest.*, **2**, 177

58. Di Renzo, G. C., Caserta, G., Iammarino, G., Clerici, G. and Luzi, G. (1995). The NO test in the management of hypertensive pregnancies and IUGR. *Ultrasound Obstet. Gynecol.*, **6** (Suppl. 2), 29

59. Ramsay, B., De Bleder, A., Campbell, S., Moncada, S. and Martin, J. F. (1994). A nitric oxide donor improves uterine artery diastolic blood flow in normal early pregnancy and in women at high risk of pre-eclampsia. *Eur. J. Clin. Invest.*, **24**, 76–85

60. Cunningham, F. C., McDonald, P. C., Gant, N., Leveno, K. and Gilstrap, L. C. (1993). *Williams Obstetrics*, 19th edn, p. 881. (Newark: Appleton & Lange)

61. Lippert, T. H., DeGrandi, P. B., Romer, V. M. and Fridirich, R. (1980). Hemodynamic changes in placenta, myometrium and heart after administration of the uterine relaxant ritodrine. *Int. J. Clin. Pharmacol. Ther. Toxicol.*, **18**, 15–19

62. Wallenburg, H. S. C. and Rotmans, N. (1987). Prevention of recurrent idiopathic fetal growth retardation by low-dose aspirin and dipyridamole. *Am. J. Obstet. Gynecol.*, **157**, 1230–9

63. Laurin, J. and Perrson, P. H. (1987). The effect of bed-rest in hospital on fetal outcome in pregnancies complicated by intrauterine growth retardation. *Acta Obstet. Gynecol. Scand.*, **66**, 407–12

64. Cabero, L., Cerquiera, M. J., Del Solar, L., Bellart, J. and Esteban-Altirriba, J. (1988). Long term hospitalization and beta-mimetic therapy in the treatment of intrauterine growth retardation of unknown etiology. *J. Perinat. Med.*, **16**, 453–61

65. Uzan, S., Beaufils, M., Breart, G., Bazin, B., Capirant, C. and Paris, J. (1991). Prevention of fetal growth retardation with low-dose aspirin: findings of the EPREDA trial. *Lancet*, **337**, 1427

66. Italian Study of Aspirin in Pregnancy (1993). Low-dose aspirin in the prevention and treatment of intrauterine growth retardation and pregnancy induced hypertension. *Lancet*, **341**, 396

67. Takeda, Y. (1993). Intrauterine treatment of the growth retarded fetus. In Di Renzo, G. C., Cosmi, E. V. and Hawkins, D. P. (eds.) *Recent Advances in Perinatal Medicine*, pp. 67–78. (London: Harwood)

68. Battaglia, C., Artini, P. G., D'Ambrogio, G., Galli, P. A., Segre, A. and Genazzani, A. R. (1993). Maternal hyperoxygenation in the treatment of intrauterine growth retardation. *Am. J. Obstet. Gynecol.*, **167**, 430

69. Arding, J. E., Owens, J. A. and Robinson, J. S. (1993). Should we try to supplement the growth retarded fetus? A cautionary tale. *Br. J. Obstet. Gynaecol.*, **99**, 707–12

70. Mesaki, N., Kubo, T. and Iwasaki, H. (1980). A study of the treatment for intrauterine growth retardation. *Acta Obstet. Gynecol. Jpn.*, **32**, 879–88

The diabetic fetus

41

Y. Ezra and J. G. Schenker

INTRODUCTION

The incidence of diabetes (all types) in pregnancy is between 1.5 and 11.3%, this variation is mainly due to age and ethnic differences[1-6]. The fetus of a mother with gestational diabetes mellitus (GDM) is prone to complications starting in the first trimester of pregnancy until after birth and into adult life. Fetal and neonatal complications consist of major and minor malformations, spontaneous abortions or stillbirth, macrosomia or growth restriction (IUGR), prematurity, birth trauma and asphyxia, and postpartum respiratory distress syndrome (RDS), hypoglycemia, hypocalcemia, polycythemia, and hyperbilirubinemia. The offspring of a diabetic mother has an increased risk of glucose handling disorders, obesity, and psychomotor and intellectual disorders in adult life. Appropriate counselling should be given to the mother during and after pregnancy.

Prevention of fetal complications depends on appropriate control of maternal blood glucose levels, and early recognition and treatment of maternal complicating conditions, such as threatened preterm labor, diabetic ketoacidosis, infections and pre-eclampsia, as well as fetal complications, such as congenital malformations, macrosomia, IUGR, birth trauma and asphyxia. In the postpartum period, attention should be drawn to the potential metabolic disorder, polycythemia and RDS of the newborn infant.

In pregnancy, there are two main types of disorders of the carbohydrate metabolism, the gestational and the pregestational diabetes mellitus (PGDM). Gestational diabetes mellitus and PGDM differ in their rate of complications and in their obstetric management.

THE DIFFERENCES BETWEEN GESTATIONAL DIABETES MELLITUS AND PREGESTATIONAL DIABETES MELLITUS

Pure GDM is considered to be a disorder of glucose handling limited to pregnancy, but it is not a maternal disease. This disorder is usually resolved after birth, and may or may not arise in future pregnancies.

On the other hand, PGDM is a maternal disease that may affect the pregnancy starting in the periconceptional period. If maternal glycemic control is not optimal, major and minor fetal malformations may result. Pregestational diabetes mellitus complicated with vasculopathy is more hazardous to the fetus, and is associated with higher risk of spontaneous abortions, preterm labor, IUGR, and stillbirth.

Glycemic control can be achieved in GDM patients by diet or insulin treatment, but PGDM can be controlled only by insulin injections. Oral hypoglycemic drugs are not the treatment of choice during pregnancy.

Diabetic ketoacidosis is a relatively rare complication resulting from failure of glycemic control and is more frequent in PGDM than in GDM pregnancies. This condition will also be discussed later.

CONGENITAL MALFORMATIONS

Congenital anomalies occur in PGDM and not in GDM pregnancies[7]. The incidence of major anomalies in infants born to uncontrolled PGDM mothers is estimated to be between 5 and 12.9%[8-18], and this rate is 2–5 times more frequent than in the normal population. The contribution of diabetes-associated congenital malformations to the perinatal mortality rate may be up to 50%[19–21].

Congenital anomalies seen among infants of diabetic mothers involve almost all the body systems[20,22,23].

The risk of central nervous system malformations in the diabetic infant is increased by 2–19-fold, and anencephaly is the most frequent, followed by open spina bifida, and holoprosencephaly[22,24,25]. There is a 4–7-fold increase in the risk of cardiac anomalies, mainly ventricular septal defects, but also coarctation of the aorta, situs inversus, and transposition of the great arteries[22,26–28]. A fetal echocardiogram is required in every PGDM pregnancy at 20–22 weeks' gestation in order to detect cardiac anomalies. Accelerated cardiac growth and septal hypertrophy are also a frequent finding in fetuses of diabetic mothers, regardless of their glycemic control[29,30]. The most frequent anomalies of the skeletal system are those of the vertebrae and limbs[31,32]. Of the defects of the vertebrae, hemivertebra is the most frequent[33]. The most typical, but not pathognomonic anomaly of the diabetic fetus is the sacral agenesis or caudal regression syndrome, which is 200–400 times more common in infants of diabetics than in non-diabetic mothers[22,34,35]. This syndrome is characterized by a combination of osseous deficiencies of the sacrum, coccyx, and the lower limbs, in addition to cleft lips and palate, congenital cardiac anomalies, microcephaly, and renal anomalies[36,37]. The ultrasonographic findings of the caudal regression syndrome are distinct from that of sirenomelia by marked oligohydramnios, and suspected renal agenesis. The latter syndrome is not common in diabetic pregnancies. The rate of renal anomalies and genitourinary malformations is also increased in diabetic infants[20,22,24,38,39]. Most of the renal anomalies consist of renal agenesis, hydronephrosis and duplication of the collecting system. Gastrointestinal malformations are increased up to five times in diabetics and the common lesions are imperforate anus, small bowel atresia and small left colon syndrome. Identification of small bowel atresia may be made by the findings of oligohydramnios and the double-bubble sign.

Many etiological factors have been mentioned in association with congenital anomalies in the infants of diabetic women, including metabolic abnormalities, such as hyperglycemia and hyperinsulinemia, hypoglycemia, ketoacidosis, glutathione depletion, decreased intracellular myoinositol, inhibition of somatomedin, arachidonic acid deficiency, maternal vasculopathy and genetic susceptibility.

Hyperglycemia has been demonstrated in humans and animals to act as a teratogen during critical periods of organogenesis[40–43]. Insulin treatment early in pregnancy has been shown to reduce malformations in infants of diabetic mothers[9]. Many clinical studies used glycosilated hemoglobin (HgbA1c) levels during the first trimester of human pregnancy as evidence for glycemic control; normal values were considered to be 8.5% or less[9,10,12,44]. Higher levels of HgbA1c were found to be associated with a malformation rate of up to 22%[8,10]. Not all studies agreed that an association exists between glycemic control and fetal malformation rate, because diabetic embryopathy may occur in the presence of normal HgbA1c levels[12].

The role of hyperglycemia in the pathogenesis of dysmorphogenesis is still unclear. One possible suggested mechanism was a functional failure of the yolk-sac which would result in skeletal and neural defects in the embryo due to nutritional deficiency and hypoxia[45,46]. Glutathione depletion and oxidative stress associated with the hyperglycemic state in rat embryo culture was also suggested as a possible mechanism for embryopathy[47]. Functional deficiency of arachidonic acid was another mechanism suggested by Goldman and colleagues[48] and others[49] to affect adversely fetal growth and development. Supplementation with arachidonic acid was associated with decreased incidence of congenital malformations compared to a hyperglycemic non-treated group[48], and with *in vitro* reversal of ultrastructural abnormalities in rat embryos[50]. Sorbitol increase due to hyperglycemia may result in a proportional decrease in myoinositol in rats[51,52]. The competition between glucose and myoinositol may lead to intracellular depletion that can be associated with a teratogenic effect, such as a diabetic cataract[49].

The role of hypoglycemia as a teratogen is questionable. Some *in vitro* studies in rodents demonstrated dysmorphogenesis when short periods of hypoglycemia were induced early in embryogenesis[53–56]. In humans, there is no evidence for a teratogenic effect of hypoglycemia. Some of the earlier studies showed a lower rate of malformations in women who had more hypoglycemic episodes[15], but recent studies failed to find any association between hypoglycemia and congenital malformations[12,57,58]. Insulin was suspected, by some authors, to have a teratogenic effect in animals but today there is no evidence to support this effect in humans[14]. It is unclear if there is any exposure of the fetus to insulin during organogenesis, since insulin is produced only after embryogenesis is completed, and maternal insulin transport through the placenta was only demonstrated in earlier animal studies[59,60].

The inhibition of glycolysis has been proposed by Freinkel and associates[61] to be associated with congenital malformations. When they added D-mannose to the culture medium of rat embryos, inhibition of glycolysis occurred and resulted in IUGR and neural tube closure defects.

Somatomedin inhibitors produced structural defects and growth impairment in animals, and it was speculated that this effect may be an adjunct to hyperglycemia and hyperketonemia[62,63]. To date, no human data are available to support this mechanism.

Maternal vasculopathy was considered to be associated with increased incidence of congenital anomalies based on an earlier report from 1964[64]. Later studies showed no association at all[13,65], or only a slight and non-significant increase in diabetic women with vasculopathy[66].

In conclusion, it seems that there is no single factor which is responsible for the pathogenesis of fetal congenital malformations, and a multifactorial etiology is more reasonable to consider.

MACROSOMIA

The most significant fetal complication in pregnancies with GDM or PGDM is macrosomia that might lead to birth trauma and asphyxia in labor. Entrapment of the shoulders in labor is a life-threatening condition, and the surviving newborn may suffer from traumatic injuries, such as brachial plexus palsy of the Erb's type, and clavicular fractures. The macrosomic fetus may also suffer from birth asphyxia as a result of prolonged labor and difficulties in body extraction.

Twenty to twenty-five per cent of the fetuses of diabetic mothers may suffer from macrosomia and its related complications[67]. Macrosomia is defined by some authors according to the absolute birth weight of 4000–4500 g. Others attribute to 'large for a gestational age' when birth weight is more than 90th percentile (dependent on specific population growth curves). The incidence of infants weighing more than 4500 g is ten-fold higher in diabetic than in non-diabetic women[68,69]. Fetuses of PGDM mothers with no vasculopathy suffer more frequently from macrosomia than fetuses of mothers with end-organ involvement, such as the nephropathies[15]. The macrosomic fetus has disproportional growth of the trunk and shoulders when compared to the head, and this makes it prone to difficulties during vaginal delivery[70,71]. Head and neck trauma may be associated with severe intrapartum asphyxia. Although shoulder dystocia is also common in non-diabetic fetuses weighing more than 4000 g, the diabetic fetus will have a two-fold increase in occurrence. The incidence of shoulder dystocia is 10% in non-diabetic fetuses of more than 4000 g, and 22% in fetuses of more than 4500 g, but in diabetic fetuses, the incidence is 23% and 50%, respectively[80]. In a very large retrospective study, Langer and colleagues[72] found that the incidence of shoulder dystocia in diabetics with macrosomic fetuses weighing more than 4250 g, was 8%. The principal contributors to the increased risk of shoulder dystocia were birth weight, diabetes and labor abnormalities.

Ultrasonic fetal weight estimation has limited accuracy in predicting macrosomia prior to planned delivery, especially with fetuses of more than 4000 g[73,74]. It was also speculated that increased body fat in fetuses of diabetic mothers is associated with sonographic overestimation of fetal weight[75]. Most formulae which were developed for the calculation of fetal weight *in utero*, were based on the measurement of abdominal circumference with a combination of other parameters such as the biparietal diameter, head circumference, or femur length[73,76–78]. Formulae based on abdominal circumference alone were suggested to be as effective as other more complex and more simple ones[79].

The ability to predict shoulder dystocia of the macrosomic fetuses in diabetics is still very limited. Many studies have been conducted in order to select the high-risk fetus for birth trauma, especially for shoulder dystocia. Parameters of labor such as prolonged second stage and delay or arrest of descent have a low prediction rate[80–82]. More accurate but less feasible techniques are the measurement of humeral soft tissue thickness[83], individualized birth weight ratio[84] and maternal body mass index[85]. According to several studies[80,82,86–88], only a few cases could be predicted on the basis of abnormal labor course or other prelabor parameters. There is also a debate as to the mode of delivery of macrosomic fetuses of diabetic mothers. Some authors have recommended an elective Cesarean section whenever the estimated fetal weight is equal or more than 4000 g[80], 4250 g[72], or 4500 g[81], and if the decision is made to allow vaginal delivery, mid-pelvic instrumental procedures should be avoided.

The effectiveness of tight glycemic control in the prevention of macrosomia is still controversial[89–91]. Fasting plasma glucose levels of < 105 mg/dl and/or 2-h postprandial values of < 120 mg/dl achieved by diet only, are considered to be satisfactory by most authorities, and only higher glucose levels necessitate insulin therapy. Langer and Mazze[92] considered fasting glucose levels of 95 mg/dl or more to justify insulin therapy in GDMs, in order to reduce the incidence of macrosomia. In insulin treated women, the target of treatment is daily mean glucose levels of 95 mg/dl[93]. Coustan and Imarah[94] suggested that prophylactic insulin therapy of patients who otherwise could be controlled by diet only, also reduces the frequency of macrosomia, but others have failed to confirm these findings[95].

Macrosomia is believed to be the result of the increase in fetal insulin secretion, which occurs in response to maternal hyperglycemia that leads to fetal hyperglycemia. An increase in fetal pancreatic β-cell mass has been found starting from the second trimester of the pregnancy[96]. Insulin and C-peptide levels in amniotic fluid and cord blood were increased[97,98] and correlated well with newborn subcutaneous skin-fold measurements[99,100]. Fetal insulin in Rhesus monkeys was found to act as a growth factor enhancing glycogen and protein synthesis, and lypogenesis[101].

SPONTANEOUS ABORTIONS

Uncontrolled PGDM women are considered to be at higher risk for spontaneous abortions[102–106]. The exact rate of abortions in this group is unknown, and according to different studies it varies between 6 and 29%[102,103]. A few authors used abnormal HgbA1c levels as evidence of the association of poor diabetic control and increased abortion rate[12,105,107]. The incidence of abortions could be minimized by tight glycemic control during the periconceptional period, and with modern management of diabetic women with insulin-dependent diabetes, the abortion rate should not be increased above that of the non-diabetic population[104,108,109]. Patients with vasculopathies also had low incidence of abortions when treated appropriately[110,111].

FETAL MORTALITY

In the past, fetal mortality was known to be an unexpected event occurring in 10–30% of PGDM pregnancies[112], but today, the incidence is decreasing and is associated frequently with maternal complications, such as diabetic vasculopathy, poor glycemic control, diabetic ketoacidosis, polyhydramnios, fetal macrosomia and severe pre-eclampsia[110]. Fetal death is more frequent during the third trimester of pregnancy[113], and the cause of fetal death is unclear. Animal studies have suggested that the cause of fetal death in diabetic vasculopathy may be related to reduced uterine blood flow leading to chronic asphyxia and IUGR; when severe growth restriction will result in intra-uterine death. Poor glycemic control and diabetic ketoacidosis may be associated with fetal death by causing severe metabolic changes of the fetal compartment, with resulted hypoxia, hypokalemia and dehydration. Hyperglycemia and the resulting fetal hyperinsulinemia may be associated with increased oxygen consumption and an elevated basal metabolic rate, which, in conjunction with reduced placental blood flow due to maternal dehydration, may also cause fetal death.

PRETERM LABOR

Preterm labor is reported to be three-fold higher in uncontrolled diabetes[114,115]. Although polyhydramnios is expected to be the most frequent factor associated with preterm labor, this was not demonstrated in any of the controlled studies. Miodovnik and associates[115] found that premature rupture of the membranes and previous preterm labor were associated more significantly with preterm labor. The use of β-sympathomimetics, such as terbutaline, for the prevention or treatment of preterm labor, should be discouraged as they may aggravate glucose intolerance and ketoacidosis by increasing hepatic glucogenolysis[116–118]. Magnesium sulfate has no adverse effect on glycemic control, thus it may be considered as the drug of choice for diabetic patients with threatened preterm labor.

MATERNAL DIABETIC KETOACIDOSIS

Maternal diabetic ketoacidosis (DKA) is a rare condition, affecting mainly PGDM pregnancies but may also occur in GDM pregnancies. The incidence is decreasing and has been reported

to be between 1.73 and 9.3%[119,120]. The risk for both the mother and the fetus is due to the resultant metabolic acidosis and intracellular dehydration that may lead to tissue damage. The fetus may suffer from hypoxemia resulting from decreased uterine blood flow and reduced red cell oxygen delivery. Fetal cardiac arrest may be the consequence of potassium deficiency[121]. With appropriate treatment, maternal death is rare but fetal mortality has been reported to be as high as 35–90%[121–123]. Kilvert and colleagues[119], in a recent retrospective study of 635 insulin-treated diabetic pregnancies between 1971 and 1990, found only one fetal death out of seven DKA episodes occurring during the second and third trimesters of pregnancy. They concluded that DKA has an infrequent occurrence and is not associated with high fetal loss.

Management of pregnant women suffering from DKA includes aggressive fluid resuscitation, correction of hypokalemia, hyperglycemia and ketoacidosis. In the case of fetal distress, saving the fetus should be weighed against the risks associated with emergency Cesarean section and anesthesia of the mother with severe DKA. Prompt correction of maternal DKA by itself has been reported to be associated with reversal of the adverse fetal metabolic condition, with improvement of fetal heart rate tracing and delivery of a healthy newborn[124,125].

FETAL SURVEILLANCE

Fetal surveillance in the third trimester is aimed at identifying, as early as possible, any change in fetal well-being, in order to anticipate preterm labor, IUGR, or intrauterine death. An outpatient clinic which has the ability to perform all the tests needed for the evaluation of the specific maternal and fetal parameters, is the common practice in most centers today.

When to start fetal surveillance? Most authors divide diabetic pregnancies into two groups according to the need for insulin and the level of glycemic control. Pregnant women with well-controlled GDM who require insulin and those with uncomplicated PGDM, are followed similarly, since their risk for fetal death is low. They may start weekly fetal assessment at 28–30 weeks' gestation, and increase to twice weekly thereafter until 40 weeks. The high-risk group includes those with complicated PGDM with vasculopathy or hypertension, and a significant risk for IUGR and shoulder dystocia. These patients should start fetal assessment at 26 weeks' gestation and early delivery may be needed. In a recent study, Lagrew and co-workers[126] examined, during a 10-year period, the histories of 614 patients according to the time when fetal compromise became evident. The very high-risk pregnancies were those of diabetic women with any vasculopathy who had early occurrence of hypertension in pregnancy and IUGR. They concluded that in high-risk patients, fetal assessment should be started as early as 26 weeks' gestation, and in other diabetics fetal assessment may be delayed to 32 weeks' gestation.

Maternal assessment of fetal movements was suggested by Sadovsky[127] as a simple and inexpensive tool. The method of fetal movement count has a very low false negative rate, and in diabetics, it was found that the interval between the decrease in fetal activity and fetal demise was shorter than in other high-risk conditions, therefore, maternal self-assessment of fetal movements should be performed at least every 8 h, and if a decrease in fetal activity is noticed, the woman should contact the delivery room for further evaluation. Women with GDM may start to count daily fetal movements from the 26th–27th weeks of gestation.

Electronic fetal heart rate tracing known as the non-stress test (NST), is a simple and relatively reliable test of fetal well-being used in many centers for the follow-up of diabetic patients[128–130]. It is performed weekly until the 32nd week of gestation, and twice weekly thereafter.

The contraction stress test (CST) was suggested as a better predictor for fetal well-being[131]. When performed in well-controlled diabetic patients, negative CST predicted fetal survival for 1 week[132]. The false positive rate of CST is up to 69%, and this may cause unnecessary interventions.

The fetal biophysical profile (BPP) is used more commonly today for the detection of intrauterine compromise in high-risk fetuses[129,130,133]. This test is a non-invasive test but its superiority over the NST or CST was never proven, yet it may be used as a complementary test in the antenatal assessment. Landon and associates[130] used the BPP when a non-reactive NST occurred in a group of 114 patients with and without diabetic vasculopathy. Salvesen and co-workers[133] studied the correlation between BPP and fetal heart rate (FHR) testing, and measurement of umbilical venous blood glucose concentration and blood gases, up to 24 h before delivery at 27–39 weeks' gestation. They found that in the group of women with diabetic nephropathy, the predictive value of BPP and FHR was limited as compared to fetal pH in cord blood. Girz and colleagues[134] described a group of well-controlled diabetic women with satisfactory antepartum assessment that included a weekly NST from the 28th week of gestation until the 34th week, and twice weekly thereafter. In spite of reassuring glycemic control and fetal testing, there was a two-fold increase in stillbirth rate when compared to a non-diabetic group of patients.

Ultrasound examinations may contribute some useful information during pregnancy, but their limitations should not be overlooked. A detailed ultrasound examination should be performed at mid-trimester when, together with maternal α-fetoprotein performed at 16–17 weeks' gestation, it may detect fetal malformations, especially the open neural tube defects[135]. Fetal echocardiogram should also be performed at 20–22 weeks' gestation in every diabetic patient to exclude most of the cardiac anomalies. Ultrasonographic assessment of fetal growth should be performed every 4–6 weeks because early detection of macrosomia or IUGR will assist the caregivers to optimize glycemic control, and to plan the timing and mode of delivery. In spite of the common use of ultrasonic estimation of fetal weight, there are large discrepancies in the ability of ultrasound to identify accurately the macrosomic fetus, and differences of more than 10% may be found between the sonographic estimation and the actual infant weight in labor even when using different calculation methods[73,74,76]. Therefore many attempts have been made to improve the ability of ultrasound to estimate fetal weight. Serial measurements of the abdominal circumference were suggested to be very useful in identifying the macrosomic fetus[79,136,137], and humeral soft tissue thickness assessment was found to be more sensitive in predicting macrosomia than was the usual ultrasound estimated fetal weight, but it was less specific[138].

In recent years, Doppler umbilical artery velocimetry has been used concurrently with the sonographic estimation of fetal growth in cases of suspected IUGR[137]. Since the incidence of complicating pre-eclampsia and reduced placental blood flow is higher in insulin-dependent diabetic patients with or without vasculopathy, earlier detection of reduced blood flow would be helpful in preventing IUGR becoming more severe. Dicker and associates[139] found no association between maternal glucose levels and the systolic/diastolic ratio in diabetic pregnancies, and Doppler flow studies of the uterine arteries in patients with diabetic vasculopathy failed to identify the women at risk for the development of placental insufficiency[140,141]. Thus normal Doppler investigations should not be relied on as reassuring[142], but impaired flow may suggest fetal compromise, and then attention could be drawn to the fetus at risk[142]. Doppler flow study should be reversed for high-risk cases when placental insufficiency is suspected[143].

NEONATAL COMPLICATIONS

The management of GDM and PGDM has an important influence on the incidence of morbidity and mortality of the newborn infant during the immediate postpartum period. Neonatal hypoglycemia is presumably caused by reactive hyperinsulinemia resulting in maternal hyperglycemia before and during labor. The control of maternal hyperglycemia in labor by infusion of glucose and insulin, to maintain plasma glucose levels between 100 and 130 mg/dl, may reduce the incidence of neonatal hypoglycemic episodes[144]. Severe neonatal hypoglycemia may be associated with neurological sequelae, and awareness of the neonatologist and early supportive treatment is mandatory.

The incidence of neonatal hypocalcemia and hypomagnesemia is increased in infants born to diabetic mothers[145]. The pathogenesis of this phenomenon is not clear, but it was speculated to be associated with relative neonatal hypoparathyroidism. Diabetic control was suggested to be one of the affecting factors on the incidence of hypocalcemia and a predictive scoring system was suggested by Mimouni and co-workers[146] who used cord blood calcium and magnesium levels.

Polycythemia was found in one-third of the infants born to diabetic mothers in the first few hours of life[147]. Increased hematopoiesis and erythropoietin levels found in the cord blood of PGDM fetuses and neonates, may be the result of chronic intrauterine hypoxia in less optimally-controlled PGDM[148,149]. Polycythemia is associated with hyperviscosity of the blood, leading to multiple organ involvement because of microthrombi formation. Reducing the infant's hematocrit to less than 55% may decrease the risk of this complication.

Hyperbilirubinemia is frequent in the newborn infants of diabetics, and is associated with prematurity and polycythemia.

The incidence of transient cardiomyopathy was found to be increased in infants born to diabetic mothers. In a recent study Veille and colleagues[30] studied 64 fetuses of diabetic women by M-mode echocardiogram between 20 and 41 weeks' gestation. Ventricular septal hypertrophy was found in 75% of the fetuses of diabetics, and cardiomegaly was also frequently found in this group. They concluded that larger septum and cardiac dimensions in fetuses of diabetic women may represent a specific diabetic cardiomyopathy. The mechanism of this complication is unknown but it may be associated with hypertrophy resulting from hyperinsulinemia in poorly-controlled patients[150,151].

Respiratory distress syndrome (RDS) in a newborn infant is associated with significant morbidity and mortality. Clinically it appears as tachypnea, grunting, nasal flaring and intercostal retractions. The cause of RDS is attributed to surfactant deficiency or dysfunction, that leads to decreased lung compliance and hypoxia. Infants born to diabetic mothers have an increased risk of RDS, especially when associated with preterm deliveries and Cesarean sections[152,153]. In the last decade, due to better glycemic control, there has been a decrease in elective preterm delivery rate and less Cesarean sections have been performed in diabetic women.

Several earlier studies suggested that a delay in biochemical lung maturity may occur even in uncomplicated diabetic pregnancies. Hyperinsulinemia and hyperglycemia were found in animal studies to be associated with inhibition of surfactant production by the fetal type-II pneumocytes[154,155]. High glucose levels have recently been shown to inhibit fetal lung maturation *in vitro*[156]. When looking at the relevant literature, there is some contradictory evidence regarding the contribution of diabetes *per se* to the risk of neonatal RDS. In a large Italian multicenter study of 1624 newborn infants, the risk for RDS was associated with low birth weight and gestational age of less than 31 weeks at delivery, but not with GDM or PGDM[157]. In a historical cohort analysis, Hunter and co-workers[158] found, in a group of 230 infants of insulin-dependent diabetic mothers, that neonatal morbidity (including RDS) was determined more by the gestational age at delivery than by maternal diabetes of the degree of glycemic control. Mimouni and colleagues[152] found that an increased rate of RDS in 127 newborn infants of insulin-dependent diabetics was not a direct result of diabetes, but was associated with the higher rate of elective Cesarean sections and gestational age at delivery.

In clinical practice, there is a debate as to which is the best test to perform before delivering a diabetic mother, in order to predict fetal lung maturity. The lecithin/sphingomyelin (L/S) ratio was found to have false positive results in almost 15% of uncontrolled cases when values of more than 2 were used, and many authors suggested values of 3.5 or more to be consistent with true pulmonary maturity in diabetics[159]. The presence of phosphatidylglycerol in the amniotic fluid is considered to be supe-

rior over the L/S ratio test in predicting the fetus at low-risk for the development of RDS, because it is a marker of completed pulmonary maturation[160,161]. Optical density of the amniotic fluid at 650 nm was recently suggested as a more reliable test for the prediction of RDS in the infant of the diabetic mother[162]. Other tests are the TDxFLx assay[163] and the NBD-PC fluorescence polarization assay[164], that were suggested as highly reliable predictors of fetal lung maturity in clinical practice.

The prevalence of RDS can be reduced by proper glycemic control of diabetic pregnant women. Controlling the diabetes will prevent the need for early delivery of an immature infant in order to avoid fetal death *in utero*. Successful prevention of macrosomia will reduce the need for elective Cesarean sections, and this will have a further effect on RDS rate.

WHEN TO DELIVER THE FETUS OF THE DIABETIC MOTHER AND HOW?

It is agreed by most authorities that GDM patients controlled by diet only can be delivered at term or when spontaneous labor starts, but never beyond 42 weeks' gestation. For more than a decade, it has been agreed that delivery in well-controlled insulin-dependent GDM and PGDM can also be delayed until 40 weeks' gestation, or until the onset of spontaneous labor[165,166]. With more frequent spontaneous deliveries, the Cesarean section rate is expected to decrease and so is the incidence of RDS. The Cesarean section rate in diabetic pregnancies was lowered to 19% and 22% in 1986[167] and 1992[168], respectively, compared to earlier reports of up to 72%[169,170].

The decision about the timing of delivery is based on the quality of glycemic control, the occurrence of maternal complications such as pre-eclampsia, deteriorating renal functions and retinopathy, and the fetal condition. When complications occur, delivery should not be delayed beyond 38 weeks' gestation, preferably after fetal lung maturity is tested.

When considering the mode of delivery, fetal weight estimation is an important factor. In a very large study, Langer and associates[72] found that the risk of shoulder dystocia is significantly increased in deliveries of diabetic infants weighting 4250 g or more. They recommended elective Cesarean section in these cases to avoid this complication. With the new techniques and knowledge of labor induction, it is advisable to consider elective induction if fetal weight estimation becomes close to 4000 g, even in well-controlled diabetics, in order to avoid further fetal growth and higher risk of birth trauma and asphyxia.

WHAT SHOULD THE INFANT BORN TO A DIABETIC MOTHER EXPECT FROM ADULT LIFE?

Beyond the early neonatal hypoglycemia and polycythemia, that may result in neurological damage and renal vein thrombosis, the newborn infant may be expected to carry into adult life some sequelae associated with the pregnancy. Non-lethal congenital malformations are the result of periconceptional poor glycemic control. Macrosomia is associated with higher risk of birth trauma, and further neurological damage to the brachial plexus. Obesity is expected to be more frequent in adults who were macrosomic *in utero*[171–175]. Jahrig and co-workers[174] studied 160 infants of diabetic mothers and found that purely macrosomic infants showed a tendency towards obesity and length acceleration in their fourth year of life. Pettitt and colleagues[175] reviewed the long-term effects of the diabetic pregnancy on the offspring among the Pima Indians of Arizona, and found that they were more obese and had more diabetes than the offspring of women who became diabetic after the index pregnancy, or remained non-diabetic.

Glycemic control during pregnancy may affect the development of brain cells leading to behavioral and cognitive dysfunction later in life[172]. Maternal ketonemia was reported by some authors[176,177] to be associated with poor intellectual performance in later life. Others found that there was no association between maternal acetonuria and IQ until the age of 11 years[178]. Rizzo and associates[179] performed a neonatal behavioral assessment on 73 well-controlled PGDM patients, 112 GDM patients and 24 non-diabetic patients. They found significant correlation between second- and third-trimester glycemic and neurobehavioral deficits. Early IUGR in poorly-controlled diabetics was reported to be associated with psychomotor deficits at the age of 4 years[180].

There is a debate as to whether the offspring of diabetic women have an increased risk of diabetes later in adult life. Some authors[181,182] found that the risk of diabetes mellitus is more significant when related to diabetes in the fathers and not to diabetes in pregnancy. Others[183,184] found that offspring of diabetic mothers have a 3% incidence, or a 20-fold increased risk for diabetes in adult life[183,184]. When they studied 89 women with GDM, Knowler and colleagues[185] found that 35% of them were offspring of diabetic mothers and only 7% of diabetic fathers.

References

1. Green, J. R., Pawson, I. G., Schumacher, L. B., Perry, J. and Kretchmer, N. (1990). Glucose tolerance in pregnancy: ethnic variation and influence of body habitus. *Am. J. Obstet. Gynecol.*, **163**, 86

2. Kirshon, B. and Wait, R. B. (1990). Incidence of gestational diabetes: effects of race. *Tex. Med.*, **86**, 88

3. Mazze, R. S. and Krogh, C. L. (1992). Gestational diabetes mellitus: now is the time for detection and treatment. *Mayo Clin. Proc.*, **67**, 995

4. Magee, M. S., Walden, C. E., Benedetti, T. J. and Knopp, R. H. (1993). Influence of diagnostic criteria on the incidence of gestational diabetes and perinatal morbidity. *J. Am. Med. Assoc.*, **269**, 609

5. Shelley-Jones, D. C., Wein, P., Nolan, C. and Beischer, N. A. (1993). Why do Asian-born women have a higher incidence of gestational

diabetes? An analysis of racial differences in body habitus, lipid metabolism and the serum insulin response to an oral glucose load. *Aust. NZ J. Obstet. Gynaecol.*, **33**, 114

6. Moses, R. G., Griffiths, R. D. and McPherson, S. (1994). The incidence of gestational diabetes mellitus in the Illawarra area of New South Wales. Illawarra Area Health Service, New South Wales, Australia. *Aust. NZ J. Obstet. Gynaecol.*, **34**, 425

7. Langer, O., Huff, R., Xanakis, E. and Berkus, M. (1994). Is there an increased incidence of congenital anomalies in women with gestational diabetes? (Abstr.) *Am. J. Obstet. Gynecol.*, **170**, 273

8. Miller, E., Hare, J. W., Cloherty, J. P. *et al.* (1981). Elevated maternal hemoglobin A1c in early pregnancy and major congenital anomalies in infants of diabetic mothers. *N. Engl. J. Med.*, **304**, 1331

9. Fuhrmann, K., Reiher, H., Semmler, K., Fischer, F., Fischer, M. and Glockner, E. (1983). Prevention of congenital malformations in infants of insulin-dependent diabetic mothers. *Diabetes Care*, **6**, 219

10. Ylinen, K., Aula, P., Stenman, U. H., Kesaniemi-Kuokkanen, T. and Teramo, K. (1984). Risk of minor and major fetal malformations in diabetics with high haemoglobin A1c values in early pregnancy. *Br. Med. J.*, **289**, 345

11. Steel, J. M. (1985). Prepregnancy counselling and contraception in the insulin-dependent diabetic patient. *Clin. Obstet. Gynecol.*, **28**, 553

12. Mills, J. L., Knopp, R. H., Simpson, J. L. *et al.* (1988). The NICHD-Diabetes in Early Pregnancy Study: lack of relation of increased malformation rates in infants of diabetic mothers to glycemic control during organogenesis. *N. Engl. J. Med.*, **318**, 671

13. Greene, M. F., Hare, J. W., Cloherty, J. P., Benacerraf, B. R. and Soeldner, J. S. (1989). First trimester hemoglobin A1c and risk for major congenital malformations and spontaneous abortion in diabetic pregnancy. *Teratology*, **39**, 225

14. Reece, E. A., Gabrielli, S. and Abdalla, M. (1988). The prevention of diabetes-associated birth defects. *Semin. Perinatol.*, **12**, 292

15. Pedersen, J. F. (ed.) (1977). Congenital malformations. In *The Pregnant Diabetic and her Newborn*, 2nd edn. p. 191. (Copenhagen: Munksgaard)

16. Omori, Y., Minei, S., Testuo, T., Nemoto, K., Shimizu, M. and Sanaka, M. (1994). Current status of pregnancy in diabetic women. A comparison of pregnancy in IDDM and NIDDM mothers. *Diabetes Res. Clin. Pract.*, **24** (Suppl.), 273

17. Aucott, S. W., Williams, T. G., Hertz, R. H. and Kalhan, S. C. (1994). Rigorous management of insulin-dependent diabetes mellitus during pregnancy. *Acta Diabetol.*, **31**, 126

18. Goto, M. P. and Goldman, A. S. (1994). Diabetic embryopathy. *Curr. Opin. Pediatr.*, **6**, 486

19. Karlsson, K. and Kjellmer, I. (1972). The outcome of diabetic pregnancies in relation to the mother's blood sugar level. *Am. J. Obstet. Gynecol.*, **112**, 213

20. Mills, J. L. (1982). Malformations in infants of diabetic mothers. *Teratology*, **25**, 385

21. Simpson, J. L., Elias, S., Martin, A. O. *et al.* (1983). Diabetes in pregnancy, Northwestern University Series (1977–1981). I. Prospective study of anomalies in offspring of mothers with diabetes mellitus. *Am. J. Obstet. Gynecol.*, **146**, 263

22. Kucera, J. (1971). Rate and type of congenital anomalies among offspring of diabetic women. *J. Reprod. Med.*, **7**, 61

23. Cousins, L. (1983). Congenital anomalies among infants of diabetic mothers: etiology, prevention, prenatal diagnosis. *Am. J. Obstet. Gynecol.*, **147**, 333

24. Reece, E. A. and Hobbins, J. C. (1986). Diabetic embryopathy: pathogenesis, prenatal diagnosis, and prevention. *Obstet. Gynecol. Surv.*, **41**, 325

25. Milunsky, A. (1982). Prenatal diagnosis of neural tube defects. The importance of serum alpha-fetoprotein screening in diabetic pregnant women. *Am. J. Obstet. Gynecol.*, **142**, 1030

26. Rowland, T. W., Hubbell, J. P. and Nadas, A. S. (1973). Congenital heart disease in infants of diabetic mothers. *J. Pediatr.*, **83**, 815

27. Shields, L. E., Gan, E. A., Murphy, H. F., Sahn, D. J. and Moore, T. R. (1993). The prognostic value of hemoglobin A1c in predicting fetal heart disease in diabetic pregnancies. *Obstet. Gynecol.*, **81**, 954

28. Ferencz, C., Rubin, J. S., McCarter, R. J. and Clark, E. B. (1990). Maternal diabetes and cardiovascular malformations: predominance of double outlet right ventricle and truncus arteriosus. *Teratology*, **41**, 319

29. Rizzo, G., Arduini, D. and Romanini, C. (1992). Accelerated cardiac growth and abnormal cardiac flow in fetuses of type I diabetic mothers. *Obstet. Gynecol.*, **80**, 369

30. Veille, J. C., Sivakoff, M., Hanson, R. and Fanaroff, A. A. (1992). Interventricular septal thickness in fetuses of diabetic mothers. *Obstet. Gynecol.*, **79**, 51

31. Farquhar, J. W. (1969). Prognosis for babies born to diabetic mothers in Edinburgh. *Arch. Dis. Child.*, **44**, 36

32. Leveno, K. J., Hauth, J. C., Gilstrap, L. C. *et al.* (1979). Appraisal of 'rigid' blood glucose control during pregnancy of the overtly diabetic woman. *Am. J. Obstet. Gynecol.*, **135**, 853

33. Grix, A. (1982). Malformations in infants of diabetic mothers. *Am. J. Med. Genet.*, **13**, 131

34. Mills, J. L., Baker, L. and Goldman, A. S. (1979). Malformations in infants of diabetic mothers occur before the seventh gestational week: implications for treatment. *Diabetes*, **28**, 292

35. Twickler, D., Budorick, N., Pretorius, D., Grafe, M. and Currarino, G. (1993). Caudal regression versus sirenomelia: sonographic clues. *J. Ultrasound Med.*, **12**, 323

36. Dignan, P. J. (1981). Teratogenic risk and counselling in diabetes. *Clin. Obstet. Gynecol.*, **24**, 149

37. Baxi, L., Warren, W., Collins, M. H. and Timor-Tritsch, I. E. (1990). Early detection of caudal regression syndrome with transvaginal scanning. *Obstet. Gynecol.*, **75**, 486

38. Mackenzie, F. M., Kingston, G. O. and Oppenheimer, L. (1994). The early prenatal diagnosis of bilateral renal agenesis using transvaginal sonography and color Doppler ultrasonography. *J. Ultrasound Med.*, **13**, 49

39. Gabbe, S. G. (1977). Congenital malformations in infants of diabetic mothers. *Gynecol. Surv.*, **32**, 125

40. Baker, L., Egler, J. M., Klein, S. H. and Goldman, A. S. (1981). Meticulous control of diabetes during organogenesis prevents congenital lumbosacral defects in rats. *Diabetes*, **30**, 955

41. Sadler, T. W. and Horton, W. E. Jr (1983). Effects of maternal diabetes on early embryogenesis: the role of insulin and insulin therapy. *Diabetes*, **32**, 1070

42. Freinkel, N. (1988). Diabetic embryopathy and fuel mediated organ teratogenesis: lessons from animal models. *Horm. Metab. Res.*, **20**, 473

43. Eriksson, R. S. M., Thundberg, L. and Eriksson, U. J. (1989). Effects of interrupted insulin treatment on fetal outcome of pregnant diabetic rats. *Diabetes*, **38**, 764

44. Leslie, R. D. G., Pyke, D. A., John, P. N. and White, J. M. (1978). Haemoglobin A1 in diabetic pregnancy. *Lancet*, **2**, 958

45. Pinter, E., Reece, E. A., Leranth, C. Z. *et al.* (1986). Yolk sac failure in embryopathy due to hyperglycemia: ultrastructural analysis of yolk sac differentiation associated with embryopathy in rat conceptuses under hyperglycemic conditions. *Teratology*, **33**, 73

46. Reece, E. A., Pinter, E., Leranth, C. Z. *et al.* (1985). Ultrastructural analysis of malformations of the embryonic neural axis induced by in vitro hyperglycemic conditions. *Teratology*, **32**, 263

47. Trocino, R. A., Akazawa, S., Ishibashi, M. *et al.* (1995). Significance of glutathione depletion and oxidative stress in early embryogenesis in glucose-induced rat embryo culture. *Diabetes*, **44**, 992

48. Goldman, A. S., Baker, L., Piddington, R., Marx, B., Herold, R. and Egler, J. (1985). Hyperglycemia-induced teratogenesis is mediated by a functional deficiency of arachidonic acid. *Proc. Natl. Acad. Sci. USA*, **82**, 8227

49. Kuhn, D. C., Crawford, M. A., Stuart, M. J., Botti, J. J. and Demers, L. M. (1990). Alterations in transfer and lipid distribution of arachidonic acid in placentas of diabetic pregnancies. *Diabetes*, **39**, 914

50. Pinter, E., Reece, E. A., Leranth, C. Z. *et al.* (1986). Arachidonic acid prevents hyperglycemia-associated yolk sac damage and embryopathy. *Am. J. Obstet. Gynecol.*, **155**, 691

51. Hod, M., Star, S., Passonneau, J. V., Unterman, T. G. and Freinkel, N. (1986). Effect of hyperglycemia on sorbitol and myo-inositol content of cultured rat conceptus: failure of aldose reductase inhibitors to modify myo-inositol depletion and dysmorphogenesis. *Biochem. Biophys. Res. Commun.*, **140**, 974

52. Weigensberg, M., Garcia-Palmer, F. and Freinkel, N. (1987). Competition between glucose and myo-inositol for transport in the embryo: a possible contributor to the embryopathy of hyperglycemia? *Clin. Res.*, **35**, 863

53. Buchanan, T. A., Schemmer, J. K. and Freinkel, N. (1986). Embryotoxic effects of brief maternal insulin-induced hypoglycemia during organogenesis in the rat. *J. Clin. Invest.*, **78**, 643

54. Sadler, T. W. and Hunter, E. S. III (1987). Hypoglycemia: how little is too much for the embryo? *Am. J. Obstet. Gynecol.*, **157**, 190

55. Ellington, S. K. L. (1987). Development of rat embryos cultured in glucose-deficient media. *Diabetes*, **36**, 1372

56. Akazawa, M., Akazawa, S., Hashimoto, M. *et al.* (1989). Effects of brief exposure to insulin-induced hypoglycemic serum organogenesis in rat embryo culture. *Diabetes*, **38**, 1573

57. Kitzmiller, J. L., Gavin, L. A., Gin, G. D. *et al.* (1991). Preconception management of diabetes continued through early pregnancy prevents the excess frequency of major congenital anomalies in infants of diabetic mothers. *J. Am. Med. Assoc.*, **265**, 731

58. Buchanan, T. A. and Sipos, G. F. (1989). Lack of teratogenic effect of brief maternal

insulin-induced hypoglycemia in rats during late neurolation. *Diabetes*, **38**, 1063

59. Pitkin, R. M. and Reynolds, W. A. (1969). Insulin transfer across the hemochorial placenta. *Obstet. Gynecol.*, **33**, 626

60. Gitlin, D., Kumate, J. and Morales, C. (1965). On the transport of insulin across the human placenta. *Pediatrics*, **35**, 65

61. Freinkel, N., Lewis, N. J., Akazama, S. *et al.* (1984). The honeybee syndrome: implication of the teratogenicity of mannose in rat-embryo culture. *N. Engl. J. Med.*, **310**, 223

62. Sadler, T. W., Phillips, L. S., Balkan, W. and Goldstein, S. (1986). Somatomedin inhibitors from diabetic rat serum after growth and development of mouse embryos in culture. *Diabetes*, **35**, 861

63. Sadler, T. W., Hunter, E. S. III, Wynn, R. E. and Phillips, L. S. (1989). Evidence for a multifactorial origin of diabetes-induced embryopathies. *Diabetes*, **38**, 70

64. Molsted-Pedersen, L., Tygstrup, I. and Pedersen, J. (1964). Congenital malformations in newborn infants of diabetic women. *Lancet*, **1**, 1123

65. Damm, P. and Molsted-Pedersen, L. (1989). Significant decrease in congenital malformations in newborn infants of an unselected population of diabetic women. *Am. J. Obstet. Gynecol.*, **161**, 1163

66. Miodovnik, M., Mimouni, F., St John Dignan, P. *et al.* (1988). Major malformations in infants of IDDM women: vasculopathy and early first-trimester poor glycemic control. *Diabetes Care*, **11**, 713

67. Gabbe, S. G., Mestman, J. H., Freeman, R. K. *et al.* (1977). Management and outcome of class A diabetes mellitus. *Am. J. Obstet. Gynecol.*, **127**, 465

68. Spellacy, W. N., Miller, S., Winegar, A. *et al.* (1985). Macrosomia – maternal characteristics and infant complications. *Obstet. Gynecol.*, **66**, 158

69. Elliot, J. P., Garite, T. J., Freeman, R. K. *et al.* (1982). Ultrasonic prediction of fetal macrosomia in diabetic patients. *Obstet. Gynecol.*, **60**, 159

70. Modanlou, H. D., Komatsu, G., Freeman, R. K. *et al.* (1982). Large-for-gestational age neonates: anthropometric reasons for should dystocia. *Obstet. Gynecol.*, **60**, 417

71. Brans, Y. W., Shannon, D. L., Hunter, M. A. *et al.* (1983). Maternal diabetes and neonatal macrosomia. II. Neonatal anthropometric measurements. *Early. Hum. Dev.*, **8**, 297

72. Langer, O., Berkus, M. D., Huff, R. W. and Samueloff, A. (1991). Shoulder dystocia: should the fetus weighing greater than or equal

to 4000 grams be delivered by Cesarean section? *Am. J. Obstet. Gynecol.*, **165**, 831

73. McLaren, R. A., Puckett, J. L. and Chauhan, S. P. (1995). Estimators of birth weight in pregnant women requiring insulin: a comparison of seven sonographic models. *Obstet. Gynecol.*, **85**, 565

74. Benson, C. B., Doubilet, P. M. and Sallzman, D. H. (1987). Sonographic determination of fetal weights in diabetic pregnancies. *Am. J. Obstet. Gynecol.*, **156**, 441

75. Bernstein, I. M. and Catalano, P. M. (1992). Influence of fetal fat on the ultrasound estimation of fetal weight in diabetic mothers. *Obstet. Gynecol.*, **79**, 561

76. Hadlock, F. P., Harrist, R. B., Carpenter, R. J. *et al.* (1984). Sonographic estimation of fetal weight. *Radiology*, **150**, 535

77. Campbell, S. and Wilkin, D. (1975). Ultasonic measurement of fetal abdomen circumference in the estimation of fetal weight. *Br. J. Obstet. Gynaecol.*, **82**, 689

78. Ferrero, A., Maggi, E., Giancotti, A., Torcia, F. and Pachi, A. (1994). Regression formula for estimation of fetal weight with use of abdominal circumference and femur length: a prospective study. *J. Ultrasound Med.*, **13**, 823

79. Pedersen, J. F. and Molsted-Pedersen, L. (1992). Sonographic estimation of fetal weight in diabetic pregnancy. *Br. J. Obstet. Gynaecol.*, **99**, 475

80. Acker, D., Sachs, B. P. and Friedman, E. A. (1985). Risk factors for shoulder dystocia. *Obstet. Gynecol.*, **66**, 762

81. el-Madany, A. A., Jallad, K. B., Radi, F. A., el-Hamdan, H. and O'deh, H. M. (1991). Shoulder dystocia: anticipation and outcome. *Int. J. Gynaecol. Obstet.*, **34**, 7

82. Keller, J. D., Lopez-Zeno, J. A., Dooley, S. L. and Socol, M. L. (1991). Shoulder dystocia and birth trauma in gestational diabetes: a five-year experience. *Am. J. Obstet. Gynecol.*, **165**, 928

83. Sood, A. K., Yancey, M. and Richards, D. (1995). Prediction of fetal macrosomia using humeral soft tissue thickness. *Obstet. Gynecol.*, **85**, 937

84. Sanderson, D. A., Wilcox, M. A. and Johnson, I. R. (1994). Relative macrosomia identified by the individualized birthweight ratio (IBR). A better method of identifying the at risk fetus. *Acta Obstet. Gynecol. Scand.*, **73**, 246

85. Wolfe, H. M., Zador, I. E., Gross, T. L., Martier, S. S. and Sokol, R. J. (1991). The clinical utility of maternal body mass index in pregnancy. *Am. J. Obstet. Gynecol.*, **164**, 1306

86. O'Leary, J. A. and Leonetti, H. B. (1990). Shoulder dystocia: prevention and treatment. *Am. J. Obstet. Gynecol.*, **162**, 5

87. Bassaw, B., Roopnarinesingh, S., Mohammed, N., Ali, A. and Persad, H. (1992). Shoulder dystocia: an obstetrical nightmare. *West Indian Med. J.*, **41**, 158

88. Nocon, J. J., McKenzie, D. K., Thomas, L. J. and Hansell, R. S. (1993). Shoulder dystocia: an analysis of risks and obstetric maneuvers. *Am. J. Obstet. Gynecol.*, **168**, 1732

89. Coustan, D. R., Berkowitz, R. L. and Hobbins, J. C. (1980). Tight metabolic control of overt diabetes in pregnancy. *Am. J. Med.*, **68**, 845

90. Willman, S. P., Lereno, K. J., Guzick, D. S. *et al.* (1986). Glucose threshold for macrosomia in pregnancy complicated by diabetes. *Am. J. Obstet. Gynecol.*, **154**, 470

91. Langer, O., Rodriguez, D. A., Xenakis, E. M., McFarland, M. B., Berkus, M. D. and Arrendondo, F. (1994). Intensified versus conventional management of gestational diabetes. *Am. J. Obstet. Gynecol.*, **170**, 1036

92. Langer, O. and Mazze, R. M. (1988). The relationship between large for gestational age infants and glycemic control in women with gestational diabetes. *Am. J. Obstet. Gynecol.*, **159**, 1478

93. Langer, O. (1993). Management of gestational diabetes. *Clin. Perinatol.*, **20**, 603

94. Coustan, D. R. and Imarah, J. (1984). Prophylactic insulin treatment of gestational diabetes reduces the incidence of macrosomia, operative delivery, and birth trauma. *Am. J. Obstet. Gynecol.*, **150**, 836

95. Persson, B., Stangenberg, M. and Hasson, U. *et al.* (1985). Gestational diabetes mellitus: comparative evaluation of two treatment regimens, diet versus insulin and diet. *Diabetes*, **34** (Suppl. 2), 101

96. Reiher, H., Fuhrmann, K., Noack, S. *et al.* (1983). Age-dependent insulin secretion of the endocrine pancreas *in vitro* from fetuses of diabetic and nondiabetic patients. *Diabetes Care*, **6**, 446

97. Falluca, F., Garguilo, P., Troili, F. *et al.* (1985). Amniotic fluid insulin, C-peptide concentrations and fetal morbidity in infants of diabetic mothers. *Am. J. Obstet. Gynecol.*, **153**, 534

98. Milner, R. D. and Hill, D. H. (1984). Fetal growth control: the role of insulin and related peptides. *Clin. Endocrinol.*, **21**, 415

99. Enzi, G., Inelman, E. M., Caretta, F. *et al.* (1980). Development of adipose tissue in newborns of gestational diabetic and insulin-dependent diabetic mothers. *Diabetes*, **29**, 100

100. Whitelow, A. (1977). Subcutaneous fat in newborn infants of diabetic mothers: an indication of quality of diabetic control. *Lancet*, **1**, 15

101. Susa, J. B., McCormick, K. L., Widness, J. A. *et al.* (1979). Chronic hyperinsulinemia in the fetal Rhesus monkey. Effects on fetal growth and composition. *Diabetes*, **28**, 1058

102. Miodovnik, M., Lavin, J. O., Knowles, H. C. *et al.* (1984). Spontaneous abortion among insulin-dependent diabetic women. *Am. J. Obstet. Gynecol.*, **150**, 372

103. Miodovnik, M., Minouni, F., Siddiqi, T. A. *et al.* (1988). Periconceptional metabolic status and risk for spontaneous abortion in insulin-dependent diabetic pregnancies. *Am. J. Perinatol.*, **5**, 368

104. Rosenn, B., Miodovnik, M., Combs, C. A., Khoury, J. and Siddiqi, T. A. (1994). Glycemic thresholds for spontaneous abortion and congenital malformations in insulin-dependent diabetes mellitus. *Obstet. Gynecol.*, **84**, 515

105. Hanson, U., Persson, B. and Thunell, S. (1990). Relationship between haemoglobin A1C in early type 1 (insulin-dependent) diabetic pregnancy and the occurrence of spontaneous abortion and fetal malformation in Sweden. *Diabetologia*, **33**, 100

106. Katz, V. L. and Kuller, J. A. (1994). Recurrent miscarriage. *Am. J. Perinatol.*, **11**, 386

107. Miodovnik, M., Skillman, C., Holroyde, J. C. *et al.* (1985). Elevated maternal hemoglobin A1 in early pregnancy and spontaneous abortion among insulin-dependent diabetic women. *Am. J. Obstet. Gynecol.*, **153**, 439

108. Healy, K., Jovanovic-Peterson, L. and Peterson, C. M. (1995). Pancreatic disorders of pregnancy. Pregestational diabetes. *Endocrinol. Metab. Clin. North Am.*, **24**, 73

109. Coulam, C. B. and Stern, J. J. (1994). Endocrine factors associated with recurrent spontaneous abortion. *Clin. Obstet. Gynecol.*, **37**, 730

110. Reece, E. A., Lockwood, C. J., Tuck, S., Coulehan, J., Homko, C., Wiznitzer, A. and Puklin, J. (1994). Retinal and pregnancy outcomes in the presence of diabetic proliferative retinopathy. *J. Reprod. Med.*, **39**, 799

111. Nielsen, G. L. and Nielsen, P. H. (1994). Results of 312 pregnancies among white class B-F mothers in northern Jutland from 1976 to 1992. *Dan. Med. Bull.*, **41**, 115

112. Gabbe, S. G. (1980). Management of diabetes in pregnancy: six decades of experience. In Pitkin, R. M. and Zlatnik, F. (eds.) *The Yearbook of Obstetrics and Gynecology*, p. 37. (Chicago: Year Book Medical Publishers)

113. North, A. F., Mazumdar, S. and Logrillo, V. M. (1977). Birth weight, gestational age, and perinatal death in 5471 infants of diabetic mothers. *J. Pediatr.*, **90**, 444

114. Molested-Pedersen, L. (1979). Preterm labor and perinatal mortality in diabetic pregnancy: obstetric consideration. In Sutherland, H. W. and Stowers, J. M. (eds.) *Carbohydrate Metabolism*

in Pregnancy and the Newborn, p. 392. (Berlin: Springer-Verlag)

115. Miodovnik, M., Minouni, F., Siddiqi, T. A. *et al.* (1988). High spontaneous premature labor rate in insulin-dependent diabetes (IDD) pregnant women: an association with poor glycemic control. *Obstet. Gynecol.*, **72**, 175

116. Diamond, M., Vaughn, W. and Sayler, S. (1985). Efficacy of outpatient management of insulin-dependent diabetic pregnancies. *J. Perinatol.*, **5**, 2

117. Regenstein, A. C., Belluomini, J. and Katz, M. (1993). Terbutaline tocolysis and glucose intolerance. *Obstet. Gynecol.*, **81**, 739

118. Peterson, A., Peterson, K., Tongen, S., Guzman, M., Corbett, V., Langer, O. and Mazze, R. (1993). Glucose intolerance as a consequence of oral terbutaline treatment for preterm labor. *J. Fam. Pract.*, **36**, 25

119. Kilvert, J. A., Nicholson, H. O. and Wright, A. D. (1993). Ketoacidosis in diabetic pregnancy. *Diabet. Med.*, **10**, 278

120. Cousins, L. (1987). Pregnancy complications among diabetic women: review 1965–1985. *Obstet. Gynecol. Surv.*, **42**, 140

121. Kitzmiller, J. L. (1982). Diabetic ketoacidosis and pregnancy. *Contemp. Obstet. Gynecol.*, **20**, 141

122. Bhagwanjee, S., Muckart, D. J., Hodgson, R. E. and Naidoo, J. (1995). Fatal foetal outcome from diabetic ketoacidosis in pregnancy. *Anaesth. Intensive Care*, **23**, 234

123. Montoro, M. N., Myers, V. P., Mestman, J. H., Xu, Y., Anderson, B. G. and Golde, S. H. (1993). Outcome of pregnancy in diabetic ketoacidosis. *Am. J. Perinatol.*, **10**, 17

124. Hagay, Z. J., Weissman, A., Lurie, S. and Insler, V. (1994). Reversal of fetal distress following intensive treatment of maternal diabetic ketoacidosis. *Am. J. Perinatol.*, **11**, 430

125. LeBue, C. and Goodlin, R. C. (1978). Treatment of fetal distress during diabetic ketoacidosis. *J. Reprod. Med.*, **20**, 201

126. Lagrew, D. C., Pircon, R. A., Towers, C. V., Dorchester, W. and Freeman, R. K. (1993). Antepartum fetal surveillance in patients with diabetes: when to start? *Am. J. Obstet. Gynecol.*, **168**, 1820

127. Sadovsky, E. (1981). Fetal movements and fetal health. *Semin. Perinatol.*, **5**, 131

128. Phelan, J. P. (1981). The nonstress test: a review of 3000 tests. *Am. J. Obstet. Gynecol.*, **139**, 7

129. Landon, M. B., Langer, O., Gabbe, S. G., Schick, C. and Brustman, L. (1992). Fetal surveillance in pregnancies complicated by insulin-dependent diabetes mellitus. *Am. J. Obstet. Gynecol.*, **167**, 617

130. Landon, M. B. and Gabbe, S. G. (1993). Fetal surveillance in the pregnancy complicated by diabetes mellitus. *Clin. Perinatol.*, **20**, 549

131. Freeman, R. K. (1982). Contraction stress testing for primary fetal surveillance in patients at high risk for uteroplacental insufficiency. *Clin. Perinatol.*, **9**, 265

132. Evertson, L. R., Gauthier, R. J. and Collea, J. V. (1978). Fetal demise following negative contraction stress tests. *Obstet. Gynecol.*, **130**, 424

133. Salvesen, D. R., Freeman, J., Brudenell, J. M. and Nicolaides, K. H. (1993). Prediction of fetal acidaemia in pregnancies complicated by maternal diabetes mellitus by biophysical profile scoring and fetal heart rate monitoring. *Br. J. Obstet. Gynaecol.*, **100**, 227

134. Girz, B. A., Divon, M. Y. and Merkatz, I. R. (1992). Sudden fetal death in women with well-controlled, intensively monitored gestational diabetes. *J. Perinatol.*, **12**, 229

135. Greene, M. F. and Benacerraf, B. (1991). Prenatal diagnosis in diabetic gravidas: utility of ultrasound and MSAFP screening. *Obstet. Gynecol.*, **77**, 420

136. Landon, M. B., Mintz, M. G. and Gabbe, S. G. (1989). Sonographic evaluation of fetal abdominal growth: predictor of the large-for-gestational age infants in pregnancies complicated by diabetes mellitus. *Am. J. Obstet. Gynecol.*, **160**, 115

137. Landon, M. B., Gabbe, S. G., Bruner, J. P. *et al.* (1989). Doppler umbilical artery velocimetry in pregnancy complicated by insulin dependent diabetes mellitus. *Obstet. Gynecol.*, **73**, 961

138. Sood, A. K., Yancey, M. and Richards, D. (1995). Prediction of fetal macrosomia using humeral soft tissue thickness. *Obstet. Gynecol.*, **85**, 937

139. Dicker, D., Goldman, J. A., Yeshaya, A. and Peleg, D. (1990). Umbilical artery velocimetry in insulin dependent diabetes mellitus (IDDM) pregnancies. *J. Perinat. Med.*, **18**, 391

140. Zimmermann, P., Kujansuu, E. and Tuimala, R. (1992). Doppler velocimetry of the umbilical artery in pregnancies complicated by insulin-dependent diabetes mellitus. *Eur. J. Obstet. Gynecol. Reprod. Biol.*, **47**, 85

141. Salvesen, D. R., Higueras, M. T., Brudenell, J. M., Drury, P. L. and Nicolaides, K. H. (1992). Doppler velocimetry and fetal heart rate studies in nephropathic diabetes. *Am. J. Obstet. Gynecol.*, **167**, 1297

142. Johnstone, F. D., Steel, J. M., Haddad, N. G., Hoskins, P. R., Greer, I. A. and Chambers, S. (1992). Doppler umbilical artery flow velocity waveforms in diabetic pregnancy. *Br. J. Obstet. Gynaecol.*, **99**, 135

143. Brown, M. A., North, L. and Hargood, J. (1990). Uteroplacental Doppler ultrasound in routine antenatal care. *Aust. NZ J. Obstet. Gynaecol.*, **30**, 303

144. Anderson, O., Hertel, J., Schmolker, L. *et al.* (1985). Impact of maternal plasma glucose at delivery on the risk of hypoglycemia of infants of insulin-treated diabetic mothers. *Acta Pediatr. Scand.*, **74**, 268

145. Tsang, R. C., Kleinman, L., Sutherland, J. M. *et al.* (1972). Hypoclacemia in infants of diabetic mothers: studies in Ca, P and Mg metabolism and in parathormone responsiveness. *J. Pediatr.*, **80**, 384

146. Mimouni, F., Loughead, J., Miodovnik, M., Khoury, J. and Tsang, R. C. (1990). Early neonatal predictors of neonatal hypocalcemia in infants of diabetic mothers: an epidemiologic study. *Am. J. Perinatol.*, **7**, 203

147. Gamsu, H. R. (1978). Neonatal morbidity in infants of diabetic women. *J. R. Soc. Med.*, **71**, 211

148. Mamopoulous, M., Bili, H., Tsantali, C., Assimakopoulos, E., Mantalenakis, S. and Farmakides, G. (1994). Erythropoietin umbilical serum levels during labor in women with preeclampsia, diabetes, and preterm labor. *Am. J. Perinatol.*, **11**, 427

149. Salvesen, D. R., Brudenell, J. M., Snijders, R. J., Ireland, R. M. and Nicolaides, K. H. (1993). Fetal plasma erythropoietin in pregnancies complicated by maternal diabetes mellitus. *Am. J. Obstet. Gynecol.*, **168**, 88

150. Weber, H. S., Botti, J. J. and Baylen, B. G. (1994). Sequential longitudinal evaluation of cardiac growth and ventricular diastolic filling in fetuses of well controlled diabetic mothers. *Pediatr. Cardiol.*, **15**, 184

151. Reller, M. D., Tsang, R. C., Meyer, R. A. *et al.* (1985). Relationship of prospective diabetes control in pregnancy to neonatal cardiorespiratory function. *J. Pediatr.*, **106**, 86

152. Mimouni, F., Miodovnik, M., Whitsett, J. A. *et al.* (1987). Respiratory distress syndrome in infants of diabetic mothers in the 1980s: no direct adverse effect of maternal diabetes with modern management. *Obstet. Gynecol.*, **69**, 191

153. Robert, M. F., Neff, R. K., Hubble, J. P. *et al.* (1976). Association between maternal diabetes and the respiratory-distress syndrome in the newborn. *N. Engl. J. Med.*, **294**, 357

154. Hallman, M. and Wermer, D. (1982). Effects of maternal insulin or glucose infusion on the fetus: study on lung surfactant phospholipids, plasma myoinositol, and fetal growth in the rabbit. *Am. J. Obstet. Gynecol.*, **142**, 817

155. Smith, B. T., Giroud, C. J. P., Robert, M. *et al.* (1975). Insulin antagonism of cortisol action on lecithin synthesis by cultures of fetal lung cells. *J. Pediatr.*, **7**, 953

156. Gewolb, I. H., and Torday, J. S. (1995). High glucose inhibits maturation of the fetal lung *in vitro*. Morphometric analysis of lamellar bodies and fibroblast lipid inclusion. *Lab. Invest.*, **73**, 59

157. Luerti, M., Parazzini, F., Agarossi, A., Bianchi, C., Rocchetti, M. and Bevilacqua, G. (1993). Risk factors for respiratory distress syndrome in the newborn. A multicenter Italian survey. Study Grouup for Lung Maturity of the Italian Society of Perinatal Medicine. *Acta Obstet. Gynecol. Scand.*, **72**, 359

158. Hunter, D. J., Burrows, R. F., Mohide, P. T. and Whyte, R. K. (1993). Influence of maternal insulin-dependent diabetes mellitus on neonatal morbidity. *Can. Med. Assoc. J.*, **149**, 47

159. Whittle, M., Wilson, A., Whitfield, C. *et al.* (1982). Amniotic fluid phosphatidylglycerol and lecitin/sphingomyelin ratio in the assessment of fetal lung maturity. *Br. J. Obstet. Gynaecol.*, **89**, 727

160. Landon, M. B., Gabbe, S. G., Piana, R. *et al.* (1987). Neonatal morbidity in pregnancy complicated by diabetes mellitus: predictive value of maternal glycemic profiles. *Am. J. Obstet. Gynecol.*, **156**, 1089

161. Cunningham, M. D., Desai, N. S., Thompson, S. A. *et al.* (1978). Amniotic fluid phosphatidylglycerol in diabetic pregnancies. *Am. J. Obstet. Gynecol.*, **131**, 719

162. Kjos, S. L., Walther, F. J., Montoro, M., Paul, R. H., Diaz, F. and Stabler, M. (1990). Prevalence and etiology of respiratory distress in infants of diabetic mothers: predictive value of fetal lung maturation tests. *Am. J. Obstet. Gynecol.*, **163**, 898

163. Apple, F. S., Bilodeau, L., Preese, L. M. and Benson, P. (1994). Clinical implementation of a rapid, automated assay for assessing fetal lung maturity. *J. Reprod. Med.*, **39**, 883

164. Chen, C., Roby, P. V., Weiss, N. S., Wilson, J. A., Benedetti, T. J. and Tait, J. F. (1992). Clinical evaluation of the NBD-PC assay for prediction of fetal lung maturity. *Obstet. Gynecol.*, **80**, 688

165. Gabbe, S. G. (1985). Management of diabetes mellitus in pregnancy. *Am. J. Obstet. Gynecol.*, **153**, 824

166. Drury, M. I., Stronge, J. M., Foley, M. E. *et al.* (1983). Pregnancy in the diabetic patient: timing and mode of delivery. *Obstet. Gynecol.*, **62**, 279

167. Stronge, J. M., Foley, M. E. and Drury, M. I. (1986). Diabetes mellitus and pregnancy. *N. Engl. J. Med.*, **58**, 314

168. Lurie, S., Matzkel, A., Weissman, A., Gotlibe, Z. and Friedman, A. (1992). Outcome of pregnancy in class A1 and A2 gestational diabetic patients delivered beyond 40 weeks' gestation. *Am. J. Perinatol.*, **9**, 484

169. Kitzmiller, J. L., Cloherty, J. P., Younger, M. D. *et al.* (1978). Diabetic pregnancy and perinatal morbidity. *Am. J. Obstet. Gynecol.*, **131**, 560

170. Roversi, G. D., Gargiulo, M., Nicolini, U. *et al.* (1979). A new approach to the treatment of diabetic pregnant women. *Am. J. Obstet. Gynecol.*, **135**, 567

171. Pettit, D. J., Bennett, P. H., Knowler, W. C. *et al.* (1985). Gestational diabetes mellitus and impaired glucose intolerance during pregnancy: long term effects on obesity and glucose tolerance in the offspring. *Diabetes*, **34** (Suppl.), 119

172. Freinkel, N. (1980). The Banting lecture: of pregnancy and progeny. *Diabetes*, **29**, 1023

173. Silverman, B. L., Landsberg, L. and Metzger, B. E. (1993). Fetal hyperinsulinism in offspring of diabetic mothers. Association with the subsequent development of childhood obsity. *Ann. NY Acad. Sci.*, **699**, 36

174. Jahrig, D., Stiete, S. and Jonas, C. (1993). Offspring of diabetic mothers. Problems of morbidity. *Diabetes Metab.*, **19**, 207

175. Pettitt, D. J., Nelson, R. G., Saad, M. F., Bennett, P. H. and Knowler, W. C. (1993). Diabetes and obesity in the offspring of Pima Indian women with diabetes during pregnancy. *Diabetes Care*, **16**, 310

176. Churchill, J. A., Berendes, H. W. and Nemore, J. (1969). Neuropsychological defects in children of diabetic mothers. *Am. J. Obstet. Gynecol.*, **105**, 257

177. Stenhens, J. A., Baker, G. L. and Kitchell, M. (1977). Outcome at ages 1, 3, and 5 of children born to diabetic women. *Am. J. Obstet. Gynecol.*, **127**, 408

178. Persson, B. and Gentz, J. (1984). Follow up of children of insulin dependent and GDM mothers. Neuropsychological outcome. *Acta Pediatr. Scand.*, **73**, 349

179. Rizzo, T., Freinkel, N., Metzger, B. E., Hatcher, R., Burns, W. J. and Barglow, P. (1990). Correlation between antepartum maternal metabolism and newborn behavior. *Am. J. Obstet. Gynecol.*, **163**, 1458

180. Petersen, M. N., Pedersen, S. A., Greisen, G. *et al.* (1988). Early growth delay in diabetic pregnancy: relationship to psychomotor development at age 4. *Br. Med. J.*, **296**, 598

181. Warram, J. H., Krolewski, A. S., Gottliev, M. S. *et al.* (1984). Differences in risk of insulin-dependent diabetes in offspring of diabetic mothers and diabetic fathers. *N. Engl. J. Med.*, **311**, 149

182. McFarland, K. F., Edwards, J. G., Strickland, A. L. *et al.* (1988). Incidence of diabetes mellitus in parents and grandparents of diabetic children. *Clev. Clin. J. Med.*, **55**, 217

183. Farquhar, J. W. (1969). Prognosis of babies born to diabetic mothers in Edinburgh. *Arch. Dis. Child.*, **44**, 36

184. Persson, B., Gentz, J. and Miller, E. (1984). Follow-up of children of insulin dependent (Type I) and gestational diabetic mothers. Growth pattern, glucose tolerance, insulin response, and HLA types. *Acta Pediatr. Scand.*, **73**, 778

185. Knowler, W. C., Pettit, D. J., Kunzelman, C. L. *et al.* (1985). Genetic and environmental determinants of non-insulin diabetes mellitus. *Diabetes Res. Clin. Pract.*, **1** (Suppl.), 309

Biochemical markers of preterm delivery

42

S. R. Inglis

INTRODUCTION

Preterm delivery is the leading cause of perinatal morbidity and mortality worldwide. Gestational age at birth and birth weight are primary determinants of an infant's chance of achieving his biological potential. Six to 10% of infants in the US are born weighing less than 2500 g (low birth weight) or before completing 37 weeks' gestation (preterm)[1,2]. Significantly, rates of preterm birth in the US have been increasing since 1985[1]. Despite advances in obstetric and perinatal care during the past several decades, the rate of preterm births has remained unchanged or has risen[3,4]. Specifically, the extensive use of tocolytic agents has done little to reduce perinatal morbidity and mortality[5,6]. Despite its pivotal role in management, rapid identification of patients at risk for preterm delivery is difficult. Strategies designed to prevent prematurity have focused on identification of epidemiological risk factors associated with preterm birth and placement of women considered 'at risk' into special antenatal care programs[7]. History of preterm birth in a prior pregnancy is the strongest indicator of risk for preterm birth identified by epidemiological studies[8]. Women with a single prior preterm birth, which followed preterm labor or premature rupture of membranes, have a 3-fold increased risk for preterm birth in the current pregnancy[8]. This risk increases further with the number of prior preterm births experienced by the woman. The reasons for experiencing recurrent premature birth are unclear. Continued presence of psychological stressors, behavioral patterns and genetic factors have all been proposed. Recent data suggest that prior reproductive tract infection may persist as a subclinical infection in these women. Alternatively, the mother's local immune system may be sensitized by past infection in ways that perturb subsequent pregnancies. The biological processes resulting in cervical softening and shortening (ripening) are intimately involved in the development of preterm labor. Premature cervical dilatation and effacement (shortening) detected by digital examination is well established as an important predictor of preterm birth[9]. However, measurement by digital examination is subject to considerable variability between examiners, and concern has been raised about increased risk of infection and preterm rupture of membranes from repeated digital cervical examinations which can displace cervical mucus and increase the risk of infection and preterm birth[9–11]. Transvaginal ultrasonographic imaging of the cervix provides a more precise and reproducible measure of cervical change than can be detected by digital examination and does not impair cervical host defenses[9,10,12].

Prospective evaluation of both low- and high-risk women has shown that the presence of ultrasound-detected short cervical length is associated with a 2–5 times increased risk for preterm birth[9,10,12]. Importantly, up to 75% of women with a history of prior preterm birth or second-trimester loss had evidence of shortened cervical length and/or presence of cervical funnelling (dilatation of the internal cervical os). Whether or not these cervical changes represent preclinical evidence that the events leading to parturition have begun, or if these changes represent women more susceptible to subsequent insults remains to be determined.

The cervix is composed primarily of collagen, which is vulnerable to the effects of bacterial and/or host mediated proteolytic enzymes. The action of exogenous proteases and collagenase on an already shortened cervix could accelerate the processes towards preterm birth. Identification of potential joint effects of preclinical cervical change and other independent risk factors will lead to effective risk-reduction strategies. Intervention programs have provided intensive antenatal surveillance for preterm labor symptoms and early intervention with bed rest or tocolytics[7]. None of these programs have focused on etiologically based treatments. Well-controlled evaluations of these programs show no statistically or clinically important benefits[13]. Lack of effect may result from poor selection of women to study, i.e. poor identification of risk status, and/or ineffective treatment strategies. Current methods of detecting patients at risk for preterm delivery rely on obstetric history, demographic factors, or premonitory symptoms that are neither sensitive nor specific[14]. Identification of biologically-based causally-associated factors and targeting specific treatments for these factors may lead to more effective preventive strategies. Recently, several biological conditions or changes during pregnancy have been recognized as risk markers for preterm birth. Biochemical markers may represent factors which can be used to detect evidence of preclinical disease, or impending preterm labor or rupture of membranes prior to clinical recognition of symptoms. Earlier and more accurate detection of disease should provide greater opportunities for preventive intervention. Accurate identification of women and babies at risk for preterm birth can allow the identification and treatment of reproductive tract infections early in pregnancy, cerclage and/or molecular biology based treatments.

INFLAMMATORY BIOCHEMICAL MARKERS

Biochemical markers may be grouped by the presumptive mechanism or source of the marker. The interleukins and tumor necrosis factor are inflammatory mediators produced in response to intrauterine infection. Although the pathophysiological processes by which preterm labor is initiated are not completely under-

stood, increasing information supports a role for inflammatory processes initiated within the uterine decidua and fetal membrane weakening via prostaglandin mediated mechanisms. It is estimated that at least 20% of premature neonates are born to mothers with intra-amniotic infection[15–17]. Intra-amniotic infection has been associated with markedly elevated levels of inflammatory mediators or cytokines, such as interleukin-1, interleukin-6 and tumor necrosis factor-α, in the amniotic fluid[18–21]. The inflammatory mediators stimulate prostaglandin synthesis by a variety of uterine tissues. The prostaglandins lead to parturition[22–26]. Elevated cytokine levels in the amniotic fluid are associated with preterm labor refractory to tocolysis, resulting in preterm delivery[26,27]. Elevated levels of tumor necrosis factor-α measured non-invasively from the lower genital tract can predict preterm delivery[28].

It is possible that inflammatory biochemical changes seen during preterm delivery are secondary to labor rather than infectious processes. The three principal arguments that may be used to support this are:

(1) The widely differing results in patients who have preterm deliveries;

(2) The presence of the biochemical markers may be explained on the basis of the amount of time the patient has been in labor; and

(3) Prostaglandin levels are not elevated until 18 h after the onset of preterm labor.

In our study as well as many others, control for labor is performed through the cervical status. In our patients undergoing evaluation for threatened preterm labor that resulted in preterm delivery, 37% had a long and closed cervix. In those patients both tumor necrosis factor-α and fetal fibronectin still predicted preterm delivery. Using the amount time in labor as an argument is fraught with error unless one controls for the different patient responses to the labor process. Specifically, patients are instructed to immediately bring to medical attention any symptoms of preterm labor but to wait as long as possible before arriving at the hospital with symptoms of term labor. The apparent absence of prostaglandins in the amniotic fluid for a period of time certainly does not rule out their presence or action at the fetal membrane, decidual and myometrial level. The absence of inflammatory changes in some patients having a preterm delivery may be explained by another process, e.g. a space-confining lesion in the uterus or abruption causing the delivery. It is not our contention that all preterm deliveries are secondary to infection and inflammation.

Interleukin-6 is a major mediator of the host response to infection and tissue injury. It has been studied in pregnancy. It is produced by endometrial stromal cells, decidual and macrophages in response to interleukin-1 and tumor necrosis factor-α[24]. Interleukin-6 is normally present at low levels in human amniotic fluid in the second and third trimester[24]. Spontaneous labor at term is associated with a modest elevation of interleukin-6 levels in the amniotic fluid[24]. However, intra-amniotic infections are associated with a dramatic increase of amniotic fluid interleukin-6 levels[24,26].

Tumor necrosis factor-α is a cytokine produced by activated macrophages in response to a variety of stimuli, including bacterial products, viruses and parasites. Endotoxin (lipopolysaccharide), a component of the cell wall of Gram-negative bacteria, can also stimulate decidual cells to produce tumor necrosis factor[29]. Tumor necrosis factor-α triggers the release of prostaglandin E_2 by amnion cells[29]. No detectable tumor necrosis factor-α was found in the amniotic fluids of women in the mid-trimester, third trimester, or during normal spontaneous labor[20,21,25]. However, parturition in the setting of microbial invasion of the amniotic cavity is associated with high levels of tumor necrosis factor-α in the amniotic fluid[25,26].

In our center we were interested to see whether these inflammatory changes could be detected in the lower genital tract and whether their presence predicted preterm delivery. Among the 38 patients admitted to the hospital with threatened preterm labor, 16 (42.1%) delivered prior to 37 weeks' gestation. The presence of tumor necrosis factor-α was associated with preterm delivery. Women positive for tumor necrosis factor-α had a greater than 6-fold increased risk of preterm birth. Tumor necrosis factor-α (51–180 pg/ml) was detected in nine (56.3%) women who delivered prior to 37 weeks and (70–95 pg/ml) in two (9.1%) women delivering at 37 weeks or later ($p < 0.005$). The prevalence of interleukin-6 (50–770 pg/ml) was also high in women who delivered prior to 37 weeks (nine of 16, 56.3%), but due to the frequent occurrence of this cytokine (51–320 pg/ml) in women who delivered at 37 weeks or later (six of 22, 27.3%), the difference did not reach significance. However, when the data for the two cytokines, tumor necrosis factor-α and interleukin-6, were combined 88% of the women who delivered preterm, as opposed to 27% of women who delivered at term, were positive and the presence of cervico-vaginal cytokines was associated with greater than a 3-fold increased risk of preterm delivery ($p < 0.001$)[28].

FETAL FIBRONECTIN

Fibronectins are large glycoproteins that bind cells to the extracellular matrix[30]. They are a family of ubiquitous proteins found in the plasma and extracellular matrix. Although similar in structure to two other isoforms of this protein, fetal fibronectin is distinguished immunochemically by a unique epitope resulting from alternate splicing of the primary messenger RNA transcript. Fetal fibronectin is specific to the fetus and trophoblast. High concentrations are found in the amniotic fluid. Immunohistochemical studies demonstrated fetal fibronectin throughout the chorion layer of the fetal membranes, and between the uterine decidua and intervillous space and the cytotrophoblastic cell columns[30].

Elevated levels of fetal fibronectin in cervical and vaginal secretions during the second and third trimester have ben associated with an increased risk of preterm delivery[31,32]. Since fetal fibronectin is normally present in amniotic fluid and placental tissue, its appearance in the cervix and vagina is suggestive of mechanical or inflammatory-mediated damage to the integrity of the membranes[31]. Cross-sectional studies which examined women with symptoms of preterm labor or rupture of membranes, and longitudinal prospective cohort studies of low-risk women, report that the presence of vaginal or cervical fetal fibronectin is associated with 4–9-fold increased risk of preterm delivery[30,33]. Preliminary information shows that fetal fibronectin can be recovered from cervical fluid approximately 3 weeks prior to the onset of preterm labor or preterm rupture of membranes[30].

Mechanical or inflammatory processes resulting from preterm contractions or ascending infection may disrupt the uteroplacental or chorion-decidua tissues causing the release of fetal fibronectin. To date, no studies have reported results of testing for coexisting reproductive tract infections in association with the detection of fetal fibronectin. In our study an independent association between an inflammatory response identified by the presence of cytokines and the presence of elevated levels of fetal fibronectin was found[28]. This indicates that cytokines may induce the production or release of fetal fibronectin in the fetal membranes or decidua. Interestingly, fetal fibronectin may be degraded by proteolytic enzyme activity from both bacteria and inflammatory cells[34]. Further release of proteolytic enzymes by bacteria or an inflammatory process could lead to the destruction of fetal fibronectin and disruption of the chorion-decidua interface. Documentation of associations between specific reproductive tract infections, virulence factors or placental villitis and the presence of fetal fibronectin would provide support for the idea that infection contributes to the release of fetal fibronectin. Identification of a specific marker for infection-mediated preterm birth may facilitate the treatment of specific infections and the prolongation of pregnancy.

In our study we found that women who were positive for fetal fibronectin during threatened preterm labor had almost a 5-fold increased risk for preterm birth. Fetal fibronectin (0.11–1.87 µg/ml) was detected in seven (43.8%) patients who delivered preterm and (0.11–1.0 µg/ml) in two (9.1%) who delivered at term ($p < 0.05$)[28].

ELASTASE, PROTEASE AND PHOSPHOLIPASE A$_2$

The infections most commonly implicated as risk factors for preterm birth include: *Chlamydia trachomatis*, *Trichomonas vaginalis*, bacterial vaginosis and possibly *Mycoplasma hominis*[35]. These microorganisms produce a variety of so-called virulence factors which may serve to perturb the integrity and natural functioning of reproductive tract tissues[36]. Many of the microorganisms directly produce the enzymes phosphokinase A$_2$ and C[36,37]. These enzymes may lead to the release of arachidonic acid from the maternal cell membrane fatty acid tissue stores[36]. Alternatively, microorganisms may stimulate an inflammatory response and the release of inflammatory mediators (cytokines), such as interleukin-1-β, tumor necrosis factor and platelet activating factor, which lead to the release of maternal phospholipase and/or arachidonic acid[34]. Increased availability of the substrate, arachidonic acid, would facilitate synthesis of prostaglandins by maternal decidual or fetal amnion cells. Increasing laboratory and clinical research supports these potential pathways for preterm birth.

Microorganisms also produce a variety of proteolytic enzymes, including collagenase, elastases, IgA protease, sialidase and mucinases, which may degrade the maternal mucous membrane and endocervical host defenses. They may also directly weaken the fetal membranes[35–40]. The presence of enzymes such as sialidase, which breaks down mucin and facilitates bacterial attachment (the first step in establishing bacterial infection), may represent an early sign, or potential for disease progression, i.e. spread of the infection into the uterus and above.

Similarly, proteases may act as immunogenic agents and activate the host inflammatory response. Release of these inflammatory mediators may then be responsible for prostaglandin activation. Alternatively, the proteolytic enzymes may act directly on cervical collagen and the amniochorion leading to premature cervical ripening and weakening of the fetal membranes and subsequent premature rupture of the membranes[39]. Phospholipase A$_2$ may also directly contribute to the disruption of collagen biosynthesis, cervical ripening and membrane weakening[36]. Phospholipase A_2 action may involve direct release of arachidonic acid and subsequent prostaglandin synthesis by maternal tissues[36].

Vaginal fluid levels of sialidase, phospholipase A_2, prostaglandin E_2 and interleukin-1-β are greatly increased among women with bacterial vaginosis[36–40]. The role of these putative virulence factors during pregnancy has not been studied in women. However, such microbe-produced substances (e.g. collagenase) along with similar enzyme-produced substances of such virulence factors within the vagina may predispose to premature cervical ripening, preterm labor or preterm premature rupture of membranes. An association between virulence factor presence and shortened cervical length or funnelling would support these processes.

PROLACTIN

Prolactin is produced by the decidua, maternal adenohypophysis and fetal pituitary. Decidual production of prolactin is induced by the α-subunit of human chorionic gonadotropin. Prolactin then diffuses across the membranes to the amniotic cavity. The role of the prolactin is not clear, but it may suppress the synthesis of prostaglandins and augment fetal lung maturity. High levels of prolactin are found in the amniotic fluid from the second trimester onwards. Prolactin measured in the washings of the ectocervix and vaginal fornices predicted those patients likely to deliver at ≤ 34 weeks' gestation, a shorter latency to delivery, and lower birth weight[41]. The question of whether prolactin is actively produced and shed through the cervix or is instead leaked subclinically through the membranes is unclear.

ESTRIOL

Considerable information suggests that fetal and maternal endocrine mechanisms are involved in the biology of both term and preterm parturition. Unlike testing hormone levels in serum or urine, salivary fluid levels reflect only

unbound unconjugated (biologically active) estrogen and progesterone[42]. More than 90% of estriol is derived from fetal sources and rises approximately 3 weeks prior to the onset of term labor[43]. In fact, one study found that labor does not occur spontaneously post-term (after 42 weeks' gestation) without this rise in estriol[44]. Increases of maternal estriol have been associated with the induction of uterine changes important in parturition.

METALLOPROTEINASE

Metalloproteinases are a family of enzymes, including collagenase, gelatinase and stromelysins, that break down tissues. There are naturally occurring inhibitors of these enzymes called tissue inhibitors of metalloproteinases. During pregnancy, large amounts of these inhibitors are found in the amniotic fluid but the serum levels are lower than in the non-pregnant state. Furthermore, it has been found that the serum levels significantly increase in both term and preterm labor states vs. no labor[45].

MATERNAL SERUM α-FETOPROTEIN

Screening for maternal serum levels of α-fetoprotein is recommended for all pregnant women because of well-established associations between high maternal serum α-fetoprotein levels (greater than 2.5 times the median level) and the presence of neural tube defects and low levels with aneuploidy[46]. Approximately 2–3% of all women screened have elevated maternal serum α-fetoprotein levels which cannot be explained by correction of gestational age assessment, presence of multiple gestations, fetal death, or presence of an anomalous fetus[46]. Increasing information suggests that high levels of maternal serum α-fetoprotein in the presence of a structurally normal fetus is associated with increased risk for multiple adverse pregnancy outcomes. Among these studies, a 2–10-fold increase in risk for preterm birth associated with unexplained elevated maternal serum α-fetoprotein has been noted[46–48]. Preterm rupture of membranes, intrauterine growth retardation, stillbirth, pregnancy-induced hypertension and placental abruption are also increased significantly[46–48]. Whether or not the increase in preterm births associated with elevated maternal serum α-fetoprotein is related to medially indicated preterm births, such as those following pregnancy-induced hypertension and abruption, from those following preterm rupture of membranes or from idiopathic preterm labor, has not been examined. Different preventive strategies may be required to impact on each of these subtypes of preterm births.

α-fetoprotein is produced by the fetal liver and enters the maternal serum by crossing the placenta or through diffusion across the amniochorion[47]. Presence of an abnormally high maternal serum level is thought to reflect early gestational placental dysfunction or damage to the maternoplacental barrier[49]. Evidence at delivery of either placental inflammation (villitis) or old thrombosis has been demonstrated among up to 70% of women who had an elevated second-trimester maternal serum α-fetoprotein level[50]. Pathophysiological processes which could lead to such early placental damage remain unclear; however, chronic infection and inflammation of the uterine lining (decidua) or acute ascending infection may play important roles in disruption of placental development and function

SUMMARY

It is clear that the cause of spontaneous preterm delivery is poorly understood. No biochemical marker is perfect in its prediction of preterm delivery. It is likely that still undefined host factors influence cytokine release which then triggers the cascade leading to expulsion of the fetus. Cytokines and fetal fibronectin are occasionally present in the lower genital tracts of women during uneventful pregnancies and only at the time of the initiation of contractions is the appearance of these compounds indicative of ensuing pregnancy complications. Localized immune system activation undoubtedly takes place in the vicinity of the cervix to prevent vaginal microorganisms from ascending to the uterus. The initiation and extent of cytokine production in response to various stimuli is under genetic control[51] and would be expected to vary between individuals. The association between the presence of tumor necrosis factor-α, interleukin-6 and fetal fibronectin in the lower genital tract suggests that a localized inflammatory event and subsequent membrane damage may be responsible for fibronectin leakage from the amniotic cavity into the cervix. Alternatively, cytokines may be capable of inducing fetal fibronectin production in the fetal membranes, decidual tissues, or cervix.

Thus, under circumstances where amniocentesis is not available or is not performed for a variety of reasons analysis of lower genital tract secretions of women with threatened preterm labor for tumor necrosis factor-α plus interleukin-6 and/or fetal fibronectin could be of value in planning subsequent monitoring and treatment of these women. Numerous studies have reported fetal fibronectin in the cervical mucus identifying women at high risk for preterm delivery[20,31]. Further refinements of these and other analyses to identify patients at risk for preterm birth will lead to development of prospective randomized controlled trials of preventive therapy. Perhaps then we will be more effective in reducing the prevalence of preterm labor and delivery.

References

1. Center for Disease Control (1990). Low birthweight – United States. *Pediatr. Ann.*, **15**, 191–201
2. Paneth, N. (1986). Etiologic factors in cerebral palsy. *Ped. Ann.*, **15**, 191–201
3. Committee to Study the Prevention of Low Birth Weight. Division of Health Promotion and Disease, Institute of Medicine (1985). Preventing low birth weight. (Washington, DC: National Academy Press)

4. Creasy, R. K. (1993). Preterm birth prevention: where are we? *Am. J. Obstet. Gynecol.*, **145**, 1223–30

5. Boylan, P. and O'Driscoll, K. (1983). Improvement in the perinatal mortality rate attributed to spontaneous preterm labor without use of tocolytic agents. *Am. J. Obstet. Gynecol.*, **145**, 781–3

6. The Canadian Preterm Labor Investigators Group (1992). Treatment of preterm labor with the beta-adrenergic agonist ritodrine. *N. Engl. J. Med.*, **327**, 308–12

7. Iams, J., Johnson, F. and Creasy, R. (1988). Prevention of preterm birth. *Clin. Obstet. Gynecol.*, **31**, 599–613

8. Bakketeig, L., Hoffman, H. and Harley, E. (1979). The tendency to repeat gestational age and birth weight in successive births. *Am. J. Obstet. Gynecol.*, **135**, 1086–103

9. Gomex, R., Galasso, M. and Romero, R. (1994). Ultrasonographic examination of the uterine cervix is better than cervical digital examination as a predictor of the likelihood of premature delivery in patients with preterm labor and intact membranes. *Am. J. Obstet. Gynecol.*, **171**, 956–64

10. Andersen, H., Nugent, C., Wanty, S. and Hayashi, R. (1996). Prediction of risk for preterm delivery by ultrasonographic measurement of cervical length. *Am. J. Obstet. Gynecol.*, **163**, 859–67

11. Lenihan, J. (1996). Relationship of antepartum pelvic examination to premature rupture of the membranes. *Obstet. Gynecol.*, **63**, 33–7

12. Ayers, J., DeGrood, R., Compton, A., Barclay, M. and Ansbacher, R. (1987). Sonographic evaluation of cervical length in pregnancy: diagnosis and management of preterm cervical effacement in patients at risk for premature delivery. *Obstet. Gynecol.*, **71**, 939–44

13. Main, D., Richardson, D., Hadley, C. and Gabbe, S. (1989). Controlled trial of preterm labor detection program: efficacy and costs. *Obstet. Gynecol.*, **74**, 873–7

14. Main, D. M., Gabbe, S. G., Richardson, D. and Strong, S. (1985). Can preterm deliveries be prevented? *Am. J. Obstet. Gynecol.*, **151**, 892–8

15. Romero, R., Mazor, M., Wheyey, Y. K. *et al.* (1988). Infection in the pathogenesis of preterm labor. *Semin. Perinatol.*, **12**, 262–79

16. Romero, R., Quintero, M., Oyarzun, E. *et al.* (1988). Intraamniotic infection and the onset of labor in preterm rupture of membranes. *Am. J. Obstet. Gynecol.*, **159**, 661–6

17. Romero, R., Sirtori, M., Oyarzun, E. *et al.* (1989). Prevalence, microbiology, and clinical significance of intraamniotic infection in women with preterm labor and intact membranes. *Am. J. Obstet. Gynecol.*, **161**, 817–24

18. Romero, R., Mazor, M., Brandt, F. *et al.* (1992). Interleukin-1α and interleukin-1β in preterm and term human parturition. *Am. J. Reprod. Immunol.*, **27**, 117–23

19. Romero, R., Avila, C., Samthanam, U. and Sehgal, P. (1990). Amniotic fluid interleukin-6 in preterm labor. Association with infection. *J. Clin. Invest.*, **85**, 1392–400

20. Romero, R., Mazor, M., Supulveda, W., Avila, C., Copeland, D. and Williams, J. (1992). Tumor necrosis factor in preterm labor and term labor. *Am. J. Obstet. Gynecol.*, **166**, 1576–87

21. Hillier, S. L., Witkins, S. S., Krohn, M. A., Watts, D. H., Kiviat, N. D. and Eschenbach, D. A. (1993). The relationship of amniotic fluid cytokines and preterm delivery, amniotic fluid infection, histologic chorioamnionitis, and chorioamnion infection. *Obstet. Gynecol.*, **81**, 941–8

22. Novy, M. J. and Liggins, G. C. (1980). Role of prostaglandins, prostacyclin and thromboxanes in the physiologic control of the uterus and in parturition. *Semin. Perinatol.*, **4**, 45–66

23. Romero, R., Brody, D. T., Oyarzun, E. *et al.* (1989). Infection and labor. III. Interleukin-1: a signal for the onset of parturition. *Am. J. Obstet. Gynecol.*, **160**, 117–23

24. Romero, R., Durum, S., Dinarello, C. A., Ovarazun, E., Hobbins, J. C. and Mitchell, M. D. (1989). Interleukin-1 stimulates prostaglandin biosynthesis by human amnion. *Prostaglandins*, **37**, 13–22

25. Romero, R., Manogue, K. R., Mitchell, M. D. *et al.* (1989). Infection and labor. IV. Cachectin-tumor necrosis factor in the amniotic fluid of women with intraamniotic infection and preterm labor. *Am. J. Obstet. Gynecol.*, **161**, 336–41

26. Romero, R., Wu, Y. K., Avila, C., Oyarzun, E. and Mitchell, M. D. (1989). Bacterial endotoxin and tumor necrosis factor stimulate prostaglandin production by human decidua. *Prostagl. Leuk. Essential Fatty Acids*, **37**, 183–6

27. Romero, R., Supulveda, W., Kenney, J. S., Archer, L. E., Allison, A. C. and Sehgal, P. (1992). Interleukin 6 determination in the detection of microbial invasion of the amniotic cavity. *Ciba Found. Symp.*, **167**, 205–20

28. Inglis, S. R., Jeremias, J., Kuno, K., Lescale, K., Peeper, O., Chervenak, F. and Witkin, S. (1994). Detection of tumor necrosis factor-α, interleukin-6, and fetal fibronectin in the lower genital tract during pregnancy: relation to outcome. *Am. J. Obstet. Gynecol.*, **171**, 5–10

29. Casey, M. L., Cox, S. M., Beutler, B., Milewich, L. and MacDonald, P. C. (1989). Cachectin/tumor necrosis factor-α formation in human decidua. Potential role of cytokines in infection-induced preterm labor. *J. Clin. Invest.*, **83**, 430–6

30. Lockwood, C. J., Senyei, A. E., Desche, M. R. *et al.* (1991). Fetal fibronectin in cervical and

vaginal secretions as a predictor of preterm delivery. *N. Engl. J. Med.*, **325**, 669–74

31. Nageotte, M. P., Casal, D. and Senyei, A. E. (1994). Fetal fibronectin in patients at increased risk for premature birth. *Am. J. Obstet. Gynecol.*, **170**, 20–5

32. Eriksen, N. L., Parisi, V. M., Daoust, S., Flamm, B., Garite, T. J. and Cox, S. M. (1992). Fetal fibronectin: a method of detecting the presence of amniotic fluid. *Obstet. Gynecol.*, **80**, 451–4

33. Lockwood, C. J., Wein, R., Lapinski, R. *et al.* (1993). The presence of cervical and vaginal fetal fibronectin predicts preterm delivery in an inner-city obstetric population. *Am. J. Obstet. Gynecol.*, **169**, 798–804

34. Jackson, G. M., Edwin, S. S., Varner, M. W., Casal, D. and Mitchell, M. D. (1993). Regulation of fetal fibronectin production in human chorion cells. *Am. J. Obstet. Gynecol.*, **169**, 1431–5

35. McGregor, J. A. (1988). Prevention of preterm birth: new initiatives based on microbial-host interactions. *Obstet. Gynecol. Surv.*, **43**, 1–14

36. McGregor, J. A., French, J. I., Jones, W. *et al.* (1992). Associations of cervico/vaginal infections with increased vaginal fluid phospholipase A_2 activity. *Am. J. Obstet. Gynecol.*, **167**, 1588–94

37. McGregor, J. A., Lawellin, D., Franco-Buff, A., Todd, J. K. and Makowski, E. L. (1986). Protease production by microorganisms associated with reproductive tract infection. *Am. J. Obstet. Gynecol.*, **154**, 109–14

38. McGregor, J. A., French, J. I., Jones, W. *et al.* (1994). Bacterial vaginosis is associated with prematurity and vaginal fluid mucinase and sialidase: results of a controlled trial of topical clindamycin cream. *Am. J. Obstet. Gynecol.*, **170**, 1048–60

39. Schoonmaker, J. N., Lawellin, D., Lunt, B. and McGregor, J. A. (1989). Bacteria and inflammatory cells reduce chorioamniotic membrane integrity and tensile strength. *Obstet. Gynecol.*, **74**, 590–6

40. Platz-Christensen, J. J., Brandberg, A. and Wiqvist, N. (1992). Increased prostaglandin concentrations in the cervical mucus of pregnant women with bacterial vaginosis. *Prostaglandins*, **2**, 133–41

41. O'Brien, J. M., Peeler, G. H., Pitts, D. W., Salama, M. M., Sibai, B. M. and Mercer, B. M. (1994). Cervicovaginal prolactin: a marker for spontaneous preterm delivery. *Am. J. Obstet. Gynecol.*, **171**, 1107–11

42. Darne, J., McGarrigle, H. H. G. and Lachelin, G. (1987). Increased saliva estriol to progesterone ratio before idiopathic preterm delivery: a possible predictor of preterm labor? *Br. Med. J.*, **294**, 270–2

43. Darne, J., McGarrigle, H. H. G. and Lachelin, G. (1987). Saliva oestriol, oestradiol, oestrone and progesterone levels in pregnancy: spontaneous labour at term is preceded by a rise in the saliva oestriol: progesterone ratio. *Br. J. Obstet. Gynaecol.*, **87**, 227–35

44. Maron, D. J., McGarrigle, H. H. G. and Lachelin, G. (1992). Lack of normal increase in saliva estriol/progesterone ratio in women with labor induced at 42 weeks gestation. *Am. J. Obstet. Gynecol.*, **167**, 1563–4

45. Clark, I., Morrison, J., Hackett, G., Powell, E., Cawston, T. and Smith, S. (1994). Tissue inhibitor of metalloproteinases: serum levels during pregnancy and labor, term and preterm. *Obstet. Gynecol.*, **83**, 532–7

46. Brazerol, W. F., Grover, S. and Donnenfeld, A. E. (1994). Unexplained elevated maternal serum alphafetoprotein levels and perinatal outcome in an urban clinic population. *Am. J. Obstet. Gynecol.*, **171**, 1030–5

47. Williams, M. A., Hickok, D. E., Zingheim, R. W. *et al.* (1992). Elevated maternal serum alpha-fetoprotein levels and midtrimester placental abnormalities in relation to subsequent adverse pregnancy outcomes. *Am. J. Obstet. Gynecol.*, **167**, 1032–7

48. Milunshy, A., Jicks, S. S., Bruell, C. L. *et al.* (1989). Predictive values, relative risks, and overall benefits of high and low maternal serum alpha-fetoprotein screening in singleton pregnancies: new epidemiologic data. *Am. J. Obstet. Gynecol.*, **161**, 291–7

49. Berkeley, A. S., Killackey, M. A. and Cederquist, L. L. (1983). Elevated maternal serum alpha-fetoprotein levels associated with breakdown in fetal-maternal placental barrier. *Am. J. Obstet. Gynecol.*, **146**, 859–61

50. Salafia, C. M., Silberman, L., Herrera, N. E. and Mahoney, M. J. (1988). Placental pathology at term associated with elevated midtrimester maternal serum alpha-fetoprotein concentration. *Am. J. Obstet. Gynecol.*, **158**, 1064–6

51. Jeremias, J., Kalo-Klein, A. and Witkins, S. S. (1991). Individual differences in tumor necrosis factor-α and interleukin-1 production by viable and heat-killed *Candida albicans. J. Med. Vet. Mycol.*, **29**, 157–63

Early onset pre-eclampsia and HELLP syndrome

43

J. van Eyck, W. P. F. Fetter and B. Arabin

INTRODUCTION

At present, pre-eclampsia and hemolysis, elevated liver enzymes and low platelet count (HELLP) syndrome can be considered as one of the main causes of maternal mortality in Western countries. About 10–15% of all pregnant women will develop hypertensive disorders with 3–5% developing pre-eclampsia. Pre-eclampsia is defined, according to the International Society for the Study of Hypertension in Pregnancy (ISSHP), as diastolic blood pressure > 90 mmHg (Korotkoff IV) in combination with proteinuria of at least 0.3 g/24 h. HELLP syndrome is defined as the combination of hemolysis (haptoglobin < 1.0 g/l), elevated liver enzymes (ASAT and ALAT > 30 U/l) and low platelet count (< 100×10^9/l)[1].

In pre-eclampsia and HELLP syndrome trophoblast invasion is inadequate. Among other possible factors, disturbed immune response towards trophoblast invasion seems to play a major role[2]. Trophoblast hypoxia activates several toxic substances, such as free oxygen radicals, cytokines[3] and proteolytic enzymes, resulting in endothelium damage[4,5]. The injured endothelium produces less vasodilatatory substances, such as prostacyclin (prostaglandin I_2) and nitric oxide, and more endothelin, which is a potent vasoconstrictor[5]. Increased vessel wall permeability leads to edema (capillary leak syndrome) and further reduction of the maternal plasma volume (hemoconcentration). When combined with vasoconstriction this leads to increased platelet aggregation, resulting in raised production of thromboxane and serotonin, inducing further vasoconstriction. Thrombi are formed in the systemic microcirculation, including the uteroplacental vascular bed. Microangiopathic thrombocytopenia and hemolysis may also develop.

As a result of all these mechanisms maternal hemodynamics become disturbed, characterized by decreased plasma volume, low cardiac output and low intravasal filling pressure. The subsequent increased peripheral vascular resistance and high blood pressure can be interpreted as compensatory mechanisms[6]. All these processes may lead to reduced organ perfusion, resulting in dysfunction of kidneys, liver, brain and placenta. In this way the disturbed maternal hemodynamics induce a hostile environment for the fetus. The risks for the fetus are growth retardation, hypoxia and possibly abruptio placentae, increasing perinatal and neonatal morbidity and mortality and possibly reducing long-life quality of the infant.

The only causal therapy is removal of the trophoblast. Therefore, delivery has been recommended as soon as the diagnosis is made[7,8]. However, before 32 weeks' gestation, this type of management is significantly associated with all the neonatal problems of prematurity. With respect to pathophysiology it is known, that maternal hemodynamics are disturbed. Evaluation and symptomatic correction of maladapted maternal hemodynamics may improve the maternal condition and placental perfusion, thereby providing the fetus with a less hostile environment. Prolongation of pregnancy in this way offers the opportunity to stabilize maternal hemodynamics prior to intervention and allows administration of corticosteroids to stimulate fetal lung maturation[6].

At present, an increasing number of research projects focus on the development of preventive

563

measures[9]. Especially for primigravidas early recognition of the possible risks, as well as the number of validated preventive measures, are still limited. This situation is not so surprising, taking into account that the etiology of pre-eclampsia and HELLP syndrome is still obscure.

CLINICAL EXPERIENCE

We present a systematic functional evaluation of combined maternal and fetal hemodynamics in pregnancies complicated by early onset pre-eclampsia and HELLP syndrome. During recent years our hospital has developed into a referral center for high-risk perinatal care for the north east part of the Netherlands. In 1993 and 1994, a total of 46 out of 295 transferred pregnancies presented with early onset severe pre-eclampsia and HELLP syndrome. The population presented in this chapter consists of the 39 pregnancies for which 1-year neonatal follow-up is available.

Gestational age of these 39 pregnancies at admission varied between 24 and 32 weeks. All women were treated at our intensive care unit using a stepwise protocol according to the systematic antenatal functional evaluation (SAFE)-concept[10].

Admission

Routine obstetric examination was performed including actocardiotocography, real-time ultrasound of fetal size, morphology, neuromotor appearance and color Doppler examination of the uteroplacental, umbilical, cerebral and, nowadays also, venous circulation. Laboratory tests were undertaken including hemoglobin count, clotting status, liver and kidney function tests and haptoglobin level. Unless there were signs of severe fetal distress requiring immediate delivery, women were transferred to the intensive care unit. Corticosteroids were administered to stimulate lung maturation.

Evaluation of maternal hemodynamics

A Swan–Ganz catheter, for central monitoring of maternal hemodynamics, and a peripheral intra-arterial catheter, for continuous monitor-ing of blood pressure, were inserted. A strict fluid balance was maintained and proteinuria quantified. Maternal hemodynamics were documented by measurements of blood pressure, pulmonary capillary wedge pressure (PCWP), cardiac output and systemic vascular resistance (SVR) (Table 1). Almost all patients initially had low intravasal filling pressure and low cardiac output in combination with high blood pressure and high systemic vascular resistance.

Correction of maternal hemodynamics

Initially we corrected the decreased intravascular filling status by plasma volume expansion in an attempt to reach normal values (Table 1).

Volume expansion leads to an increase in cardiac output and filling pressure reflected by PCWP. As a result SVR and blood pressure usually decrease. If SVR did not drop sufficiently, vasodilatatory drugs were added intravenously, while constantly maintaining the filling pressure at the corrected levels. In our department we use dihydralazin and ketanserin. Correction of maternal hemodynamics was usually achieved within 24 h. The aim of this procedures was to restore optimal organ and placental perfusion.

Vasodilatation to reduce blood pressure without prior plasma volume expansion may lead to a further decrease in the intravasal filling pressure which can be disastrous for the already compromised fetus.

Maternal and fetal monitoring during prolongation of pregnancy

At regular intervals maternal hemodynamics were checked and optimized, using the information obtained by the Swan–Ganz catheter. Laboratory tests which were performed at admission were repeated on a daily basis. During and after optimizing maternal hemodynamics the fetal condition was evaluated.

Fetal monitoring was performed by continuous actocardiotocography and frequent Doppler measurements. After having optimized and stabilized the maternal condition the Swan–Ganz catheter was removed, after which the patient was transferred to the perinatal high

Table 1 *Evaluation of pregnancies (n = 39) complicated by pre-eclampsia and hemolysis, elevated liver enzymes and low platelet count (HELLP) syndrome before and after correction*

	Mean values at admission	Mean values after correction	Mean values before delivery	Normal values
Hemodynamic parameter				
RRsystole (mmHg)	168	150	160	100–150
RRdiastole (mmHg)	101	88	96	60–90
PCWP (mmHg)	8	11	12	10–14
Cardiac output (l/min)	6.4	8.3	7.8	7–10
SVR (ds/cm^5)	1604	1035	1170	1000–1400
Laboratory findings				
Platelets ($n \times 10^9$/l)	138	114	110	> 100
ASAT (U/l)	102	45	46	< 30
ALAT (U/l)	109	60	61	< 30
LDH (U/l)	585	446	477	< 320
Haptoglobin (g/l)	0.5	0.5	0.6	1.0–3.0
Blood flow actocardiogram				
Umbilical artery PI	1.89	1.54	1.93	< 1.7
Internal cerebral artery PI	1.25	1.21	1.13	> 1.4
Biophysical profile (FAS)	5.5	6.8	4.9	> 6

PCWP, pulmonary capillary wedge pressure; SVR, systemic vascular resistance; ASAT and ALAT, liver transaminases; LDH, lactic dehydrogenase; PI, pulsatility index; FAS, Fetal Assessment Score

care unit. Cesarean section was performed when there were signs of fetal distress or aggravation of the maternal condition, due to the progression of pre-eclampsia and HELLP syndrome despite therapy being given.

Maternal and fetal outcome and 1-year neonatal follow-up

From the total group of 46 pregnancies with pre-eclampsia and HELLP syndrome who were admitted to our hospital in 1993 and 1994, three babies died *in utero*, one after abruptio placentae at 26 weeks' gestation and two after decisions not to intervene by Cesarean section, in the case of fetal distress because of extreme prematurity and estimated fetal weight of < 500 g. Four neonates died in the first week after birth because of one each of the following: intracranial hemorrhage, candida sepsis, respiratory distress syndrome IV and trisomy 13. Gestational age at birth of these four babies varied between 27 and 29 weeks. Our study population consisted of the remaining 39 women and their babies. On average, pregnant women remained in the intensive care unit for 5 days. In all women hemodynamics were corrected within 24 h (Table 1). Aver-

age SVR and blood pressure fell, whereas PCWP and cardiac output increased. Simultaneously normal liver function was restored and a further abrupt fall in platelet count was prevented (Table 1). Concomitantly with the correction of maternal hemodynamics and condition, Doppler flow measurements obtained from the umbilical artery also showed rapid improvement, whereas pulsatility index (PI) values obtained from the internal carotid artery remained reduced (Table 1). The actocardiotocogram improved in 15/39 pregnancies. In 20 pregnancies the actocardiotocogram was normal at admission and remained normal, whereas in three pregnancies it was and remained pathological despite correction of maternal hemodynamics. Only one fetus demonstrated deterioration of fetal heart rate (FHR)-pattern associated with increasing contractions directly after optimizing maternal hemodynamics. Mean prolongation of pregnancy, after admission to the intensive care unit, was 6 days, allowing sufficient time to give corticosteroids to stimulate fetal lung maturity and stabilize the maternal condition prior to intervention. Thirty-eight women were delivered by Cesarean section, indications included fetal distress (*n* = 25), deterioration of maternal

Table 2 *Neonatal morbidity of survivors (n = 39)*

	Gestational age at delivery (completed weeks)				
Neonatal complications	27	28	29	30	31
Bronchopulmonary dysplasia	3/8	3/7	1/5	1/9	—
Intraventricular hemorrhage	1/8	—	1/5	—	—
Periventricular leukomalacia	1/8	—	—	—	—
Sepsis	3/8	2/7	—	2/9	3/10
Retinopathy	1/8	—	—	—	—

symptoms ($n = 10$) or a combination of both ($n = 3$). One mother delivered vaginally uneventfully. One day after Cesarean section one woman developed liver rupture, which was successfully managed. Mean gestational age at delivery was 29 weeks (range 27–31) and mean birth weight was 1040 g (range 640–1450). Mean Apgar score after 5 min was 8 (range 5–10) and mean umbilical cord pH was 7.22 (range 7.0–7.4).

Immediately after birth, all 39 babies were admitted to the neonatal intensive care unit. Mean neonatal Therapeutic Intervention Scoring System (TISS) score at admission was 21 (range 8–40). Thirty-three neonates needed temporary artificial ventilation. In all neonates ultrasonic examinations of the brain were performed to detect intraventricular hemorrhage (IVH) and periventricular leukomalacia (PVL). All neonates were examined for retinopathy.

Twenty-seven babies had an uneventful neonatal course, and in the group of babies born after 30 weeks there was no major morbidity. Results of neonatal morbidity are shown in Table 2.

One-year follow-up was performed using standard protocols for evaluation of psychomotor development. A total of 33 babies developed normally and in five babies psychomotor development was suspect. Only one baby had an abnormal test result. This baby was born at 29 weeks and had an intraventricular hemorrhage grade III during the neonatal period.

Postpartum screening and implications for prevention

The incidence of pre-eclampsia and HELLP syndrome is increased in women suffering from

Table 3 *Disorders associated with early onset pre-eclampsia (n = 16)*

Underlying disorder	Positive tests (n)
Protein S deficiency	2
Protein C deficiency	0
Antithrombin III deficiency	0
Activated protein C resistance	3
IgM anticardiolipin	1
Lupus anticoagulant	0
Hyperhomocysteinemia	4
Diabetes	1
Renal dysfunction	5

diseases which are associated with pre-existing endothelial dysfunction, including diabetes, renal dysfunction and chronic hypertension, and vascular thrombosis, including hypercoagulability due to deficiency of protein S, protein C, antithrombin III and activated protein C (APC)-resistance, metabolic diseases like hyperhomocysteinemia and the presence of circulating antibodies, such as lupus anticoagulant and anticardiolipin antibodies[9]. Sixteen women in our study population were examined for possible underlying disorders. In only five women were all tests negative. In the remaining 11 women a total of 16 positive test results were found (Table 3). Three women had a combination of several underlying disorders.

DISCUSSION

In order to interpret the data properly it should be emphasized that our hospital has a regional function for tertiary perinatal care. Adequate intensive care facilities are present, as well as expertise and experience with respect to invasive hemodynamic monitoring of women with severe early onset pre-eclampsia and HELLP syndrome. Almost all mothers were transferred to our hospital in a late stage of the disease.

At admission, it seems from our results that, filling pressure was slightly lowered (mean PCWP 8 mmHg). It should be emphasized, however, that this slightly reduced PCWP is the result of a raised SVR, subsequently leading to hypertension. In this way hypertension is a compensatory mechanism, to maintain filling pressure and blood flow to the organs. In absolute terms, blood flow is reduced and obviously not capable of guaranteeing adequate perfusion of several organs including the placenta. The combination of reduced SVR and increased PCWP after correction reflects raised perfusion and blood flow which are beneficial in temporizing hemolysis and reducing platelet aggregation.

Blood pressure and organ function are restored, the latter documented in our data by improved liver function. Correction of maternal hemodynamics does not immediately result in normalization of the platelet count. Restoration to normal values takes more time, since platelet production in the bone marrow is limited. However, as soon as production exceeds destruction the platelet count will increase. In summary, optimizing maternal hemodynamics improves maternal condition, which is beneficial when operative intervention is required.

With respect to the fetus, PI values obtained from the umbilical artery temporarily improved after correction of maternal hemodynamics. This phenomenon has already been reported by Karsdorp and colleagues[11]. Actocardiotocograms also temporarily improved in 15/39 pregnancies, whereas in 20/39 cases actocardiotocograms remained normal after optimizing. Both phenomena indicate that the fetal condition is also, at least temporarily, improved, which is beneficial with respect to our efforts to prolong gestation. The neonatal morbidity rate was relatively low. For a proper interpretation and evaluation of our perinatal management, it is very important to evaluate not only maternal, fetal and neonatal results, but also long-term follow-up of the babies. Evaluation of psychomotor development is continuing and is promising to date.

Screening procedures in women with a history of severe early onset pre-eclampsia and HELLP syndrome appear to be worthwhile since the chance of a positive test result is high. Furthermore, it should be realized that in almost all disorders (Table 3), preventive measures are relatively simple. In addition to low dose aspirin therapy[12], subcutaneous heparin is administered in protein S, protein C and AT3 deficiency and APC-resistance, whereas hyperhomocysteinemia is corrected by folic acid and pyridoxin.

Screening for underlying disorders can even be beneficial if no further pregnancies are desired, since it may be helpful in the choice of contraception. Oral contraception is contraindicated in hypercoagulability. Furthermore, sisters and offspring may benefit from revealed disorders which are hereditary.

SUMMARY

Temporizing management of pregnancies, complicated by severe early onset pre-eclampsia and HELLP syndrome may improve fetal and neonatal, as well as maternal, outcome. This management should, however, be restricted to tertiary centers for perinatal care with adequate intensive care facilities, expertise and experience. The stepwise protocol for monitoring fetomaternal hemodynamics, according to the SAFE concept may be helpful.

Taking into account neonatal mortality and morbidity, as well as the compromised maternal condition we do not recommend prolonging pregnancies with severe pre-eclampsia and HELLP syndrome, beyond 31 weeks, when maternal hemodynamics are optimized and corticosteroids are given.

Not only short-term fetomaternal evaluation but also long-term follow-up of babies from this group is very important for a critical appraisal of applied management. It should be emphasized that women with severe early onset pre-eclampsia and HELLP syndrome form a select group at high risk for underlying disorders[9]. Screening programs may provide tools for preventive measures and advice even beyond the scope of only the next pregnancy. People practising first- and second-line obstetrics should be aware of early signs and risk factors, such as specific complaints and hemoconcentration. General, obstetric and family history may also provide useful information for estimating the chance of developing this disease.

THE FUTURE

In recent years management options with respect to pre-eclampsia and HELLP syndrome have remained limited and can frequently only be applied in a late stage of the disease. In no small part, this is caused by the fact, that the etiology is still obscure. Tests for early diagnosis and prediction have been presented in the past, such as the roll-over test[13], increased vascular reactivity to angiotensin II infusion[14], plasma cellular fibronectin concentration[15], Doppler velocimetry of the uterine arteries[16,17], etc. Sensitivity and specificity, however, still have to be improved.

A more complete understanding of the pathophysiology and underlying disorders, using medical epidemiology, molecular biology and human genetics should contribute to the search for the mysterious 'factor X'. Focusing on these aspects may produce solutions for the problems related to early diagnosis, therapy and even for preventive measures, with the goal of a live-born infant with life-long life quality.

Moreover, it should be our goal to prevent both, mother and child becoming long-term patients.

ACKNOWLEDGEMENTS

Dr G. A. Dekker and Dr. L. L. H. Peeters for the analysis of underlying disorders and Dr F. Bodewes for the analysis of neonatal follow-up.

References

1. Weinstein, L. (1982). Syndrome of hemolysis, elevated liver enzymes and low platelet count: a severe consequence of hypertension in pregnancy. *Am. J. Obstet. Gynecol.*, **142**, 159–67
2. Redman, C. W. G. (1990). The fetal allograft. *Fetal Med. Rev.*, **2**, 21–43
3. Hill, J. A. (1992). Cytokines considered critical in pregnancy. *Am. J. Reprod. Immunol.*, **28**, 123–6
4. Roberts, J. M., Tayler, R. N., Muscy, T. J., Rodgers, G. M., Hubel, C. A. and McLaughlin, M. K. (1989). Pre-eclampsia: an endothelial cell disorder. *Am. J. Obstet. Gynecol.*, **161**, 1200–4
5. Morris, N. H., Eaton, B. M. and Dekker, G. A. (1996). Nitric oxide, the endothelium, pregnancy and preeclampsia. *Br. J. Obstet. Gynaecol.*, **103**, 4–15
6. Visser, W. and Wallenburg, H. C. S. (1995). Temporizing management of severe preeclampsia with and without the HELLP syndrome. *Br. J. Obstet. Gynaecol.*, **102**, 111–17
7. Weinstein, L. (1985). Preeclampsia-eclampsia with hemolysis, elevated liver enzymes and thrombocytopenia. *Obstet. Gynecol.*, **66**, 657–60
8. Sibai, B. M., Taslimi, M. M., El Nazer, A., Amon, E., Mabie, B. C. and Ryan, G. M. (1986). Maternal-perinatal outcome associated with the syndrome of hemolysis, elevated liver enzymes and low platelets in severe preeclampsia. *Am. J. Obstet. Gynecol.*, **155**, 501–9
9. Dekker, G. A., de Vries, J. I. P., Doelitzsch, P. M., Huijgens, P. C. M., von Blomberg, B. M. E., Jakobs, C. and van Geijn, H. P. (1995). Underlying disorders associated with severe early-onset preeclampsia. *Am. J. Obstet. Gynecol.*, **173**, 1042–8
10. Arabin, B., Snyders, R., Mohnhaupt, A., Ragosch, V. and Nicolaides, K. H. (1993). Evaluation of the fetal assessment score in pregnancies at risk for intrauterine hypoxia. *Am. J. Obstet. Gynecol.*, **169**, 549–54
11. Karsdorp, V. H. M., van Vugt, J. M. G., Dekker, G. A. and van Geijn, H. P. (1992). Reappearance of end-diastolic velocities in the umbilical artery following maternal volume expansion: a preliminary study. *Obstet. Gynecol.*, **80**, 679–83
12. CLASP Collaborative Group (1994). A randomized trial of low-dose aspirin for the prevention and treatment of preeclampsia among 9346 pregnant women. *Lancet*, **343**, 619–29
13. Gant, N. F., Chand, S., Worley, R. J. *et al.* (1971). A clinical test useful for predicting the development of acute hypertension of pregnancy. *Am. J. Obstet. Gynecol.*, **120**, 1–7
14. Gant, N. F., Daley, G. L., Chand, S. *et al.* (1973). A study of angiotensin II pressure response

throughout primigravid pregnancy. *J. Clin. Invest.*, **52**, 2682–9

15. Lazarchick, J., Stubbs, J. M., Romein, L. *et al.* (1986). Predictive value of fibronectin levels in normotensive gravid women destined to become preeclamptic. *Am. J. Obstet. Gynecol.*, **154**, 1050–2

16. Campbell, S., Pearce, J. M. F., Hackett, G. *et al.* (1986). Quantitative assessment of utero-placental blood flow: early screening test for high risk pregnancies. *Obstet. Gynecol.*, **68**, 649–53

17. Bower, S., Bewley, S. and Campbell, S. (1993). Improved prediction of preeclampsia by two stage screening of uterine arteries using the early diastolic notch and color Doppler imaging. *Obstet. Gynecol.*, **82**, 78–83

Post-term pregnancy: fetal considerations

44

H. N. Winn

INTRODUCTION

Post-term pregnancy is defined as a gestation of more than 42 weeks or 294 days from the onset of the last normal menstrual cycle which was followed by conception 2 weeks later. Postmaturity syndrome or dysmaturity refers to a constellation of neonatal physical findings reflecting the wasting of subcutaneous fat as initially described by Clifford[1]. At birth, infants with dysmaturity have one or a combination of the following features: wrinkled, dry, cracked and desquamated skin, thin extremities, meconium-stained nails and skin, and a very alert look. Although dysmaturity occurs more frequently in post-term pregnancies, it is evident in pregnancies complicated by severe intrauterine growth retardation (IUGR) at other gestational ages as well.

The etiology of post-term gestation remains unknown. The placenta and fetal pituitary and adrenal glands appear to play a role in the onset of spontaneous labor. Gestation has been prolonged in pregnancies complicated by placental sulfatase insufficiency, fetal anencephaly, or fetal adrenal hypoplasia or aplasia[2]. Whether the underproduction of estrogens (estradiol and estriol) in these clinical situations is the culprit remains to be answered. Interestingly, labor has been initiated in post-term pregnancies with intra-amniotic injection of cortisol[3]. It appears that there is a delicate inter-relationship between fetal steroid production, placental metabolism and prostaglandin production which brings about the onset of labor in the normal gestation. More work is needed to shed light on this important issue.

Post-term gestation occurs in about 10% of pregnancies and is associated with a significant perinatal morbidity[4,5] mainly from an increased incidence of macrosomia, dysmaturity and intrapartum fetal distress. In addition, compared to normal term pregnancy, the fetal mortality rate doubles and quadruples at 43 and 44 completed weeks of gestation, respectively[6]. Although the high-risk nature of post-term pregnancy has been recognized since the beginning of the century, the best management approach remains to be determined.

DETERMINATION OF GESTATIONAL AGE

Determination of gestational age is the most important initial step in the post-term pregnancy management. Interestingly, one study demonstrated that all of the pregnancies which had been diagnosed as post-term based on the certain last menstrual periods actually were term pregnancies when basal body temperature was used to ascertain ovulation[7]. Mislabelling term as post-term pregnancies will result in escalated medical costs from unnecessary testing, wasting the physician's and patient's time, and creating an emotional strain on the patient.

The traditional methods of gestational dating, such as uterine size, the timing of the audible fetal heart sounds by either the fetoscope or the doptone, and the onset of the fetal movement perceived by the mother, are not accurate enough in most instances to be clinically useful. Ultrasound examinations, obtained at the appropriate time, can be used to predict gestational age with a high degree of accuracy. The crown–rump length (CRL) can predict the gestational age within 2.7 days from the 7th to the 14th weeks of gestation when the average of three independent measurements is used[8]. The biparietal diameter (BPD) and femur length (FL) are the two useful parameters in estimating gestational age during the second trimester. The accuracy of BPD or FL in gestational dating is about 1 week with 95% confidence limits until about 26 weeks[9–11]. It should be noted that to use the BPD for gestational dating, the cephalic index, which is the ratio of the BPD to the occipitofrontal diameter, has to be in the normal range of 74–83%[12]. The cerebellum is located in the posterior fossa of the cranium and its transverse diameter (TD) can be easily measured. During the second trimester, the linear relationship of the TD with the gestational age permits the convenient estimation of gestational age in weeks by measurement of the TD in millimeters with a high degree of accuracy[13]. Since the TD is not affected by the head shape, the TD can replace the BPD in dating the pregnancy when the cephalic indices fall outside the normal range. The above ultrasonographic parameters are not reliable for gestational dating, with an error of up to 3 weeks, during the third trimester. The extremity ossification centers, which appear as echodense structures, can be useful for gestational dating during this stage of gestation. The presence of distal femoral epiphysis, proximal tibial epiphysis and proximal humeral epiphysis generally indicates gestational ages of at least 32 weeks, 34 weeks and 36 weeks of gestation, respectively[14–17]. It should be noted that the timing of the appearance of the epiphyses is affected by the fetal gender with earlier occurrence in female fetuses[18,19]. If routine ultrasound examination ever becomes a reality, one ultrasound examination at 18–19 weeks of gestation should be sufficient to accomplish both the screening of fetal anomalies and the determination of gestational age.

PRENATAL ASSESSMENT OF FETAL WELL-BEING

The controversy in the management of post-term pregnancies arises when the cervix is non-inducible. In this clinical setting, the increased risk of perinatal mortality and mor-bidity associated with expectant management has to balance against the increased maternal morbidity and mortality associated with a higher incidence of Cesarean section due to failed induction. It becomes apparent that expectant management of post-term pregnancies is possible only if fetal well-being can be assured. Although many methods of fetal surveillance, either biochemically or biophysically, have been proposed and clinically utilized over the years, only the commonly used modalities of fetal assessment such as non-stress test (NST), biophysical profile (BPP) evaluation of amniotic fluid, and Doppler blood flow will be addressed.

The non-stress test

This test has been extensively used for the evaluation of fetal well-being in postdate pregnancies since its introduction. Its popularity rests on its ease of use and interpretation. The current protocol for NST as developed by Evertson and Paul[20] includes observing the fetal heart rate (FHR) pattern for a period of 10–40 min. A reactive NST is defined as having two accelerations of FHR, with at least 15 beats per minute (bpm) above the baseline FHR and lasting at least 15 s for each acceleration, during a 20-min observational window. The NST is non-reactive if there are no such FHR accelerations during the 40-min observational period. Although the NST does not directly address the placental insufficiency problem, it monitors the essential endpoint of the pregnancy itself, the fetus. Generally, a reactive NST is reassuring and indicates a non-hypoxic fetus. The incidence of stillbirth within a week of reactive NST among postterm pregnancies ranges from 2.8/1000 to 24/1000[21–23]. Since stillbirth can occur within 2–5 days after a reactive NST[22–24], NST should be done at least twice weekly, if it is the only test used to assess fetal well-being in post-term pregnancies. A non-reactive NST does not necessarily mean fetal distress and requires further evaluation with either a contraction stress test (CST) or an ultrasound examination.

The biophysical profile

The biophysical profile, as introduced by Manning and colleagues[25], consists of an ultrasound evaluation of the amniotic fluid, fetal biophysical characteristics such as breathing movement (FBM), body movement (FM) and tone (FT), in addition to a standard NST. Each of the five variables is assigned a score of 0 or 2 depending on whether it is abnormal or normal. The BPP was developed based on the assumption that the presence of normal FBM, FM and FT reflects a non-depressed fetal central nervous system. In the original study of 216 high-risk patients with 40% of patients being post-term, no perinatal mortality was noted within a week of a normal fetal biophysical profile (normal amniotic fluid, FBM, FM and FT) regardless of the result of the NST. On the other hand, a poor BPP (a total score of 4/10 or less), which presumably reflected fetal hypoxemia, was associated with a significantly increased perinatal mortality and morbidity. In this study the NST rather than the BPP was used for fetal assessment[25]. Subsequently, the BPP was used in the clinical management of 12 620 high-risk pregnancies complicated by post-term, suspected intrauterine growth retardation, hypertension, diabetes and others with a patient distribution of 11.6%, 20.8%, 17.5%, 9.2% and 40.9%, respectively. The false negative rate of the BPP, i.e. stillbirth occurring within a week of a normal BPP with a total score of at least 8/10, was 0.634/1000. One stillbirth occurred in a post-term pregnancy within 5 days of a normal BPP[25]. Similarly to the NST and CST, a poor BPP does not necessarily mean impending fetal distress because of the inherent cyclicity of the fetal biophysical characteristics during a 24-h period. In fact, one study showed that the accuracy of an abnormal BPP in predicting poor neonatal outcomes in post-term gestation is only 14%[26].

The biophysical profile appears to be an excellent modality of assessing fetal well-being in post-term pregnancies. First of all, being non-invasive and easily applied, the BPP can be performed in an outpatient setting. Second, the BPP has a very low false negative rate that is comparable to that of the CST. In fact, no peri-natal mortality was observed when twice-weekly BPP alone was used for fetal assessment in the management of post-term pregnancies. Furthermore, excellent perinatal outcomes with a reduction of the Cesarean section rate were observed when expectant management was carried out in the presence of normal BPP[27]. Third, compared to NST or CST, the BPP is associated with a much lower percentage of equivocal or abnormal tests[28]. Thus, the expense of time, labor and patients' anxiety associated with false testing is reduced. Fourth, until routine ultrasound examination of the fetus in early pregnancy becomes a reality, the BPP provides the opportunity to evaluate fetal anatomy. Finally, it permits the detection of oligohydramnios which has an ominous prognosis in post-term pregnancy.

Even though oligohydramnios is an important clinical finding, its definition remains unsettled. Proposed definitions include:

(1) The average of the two diameters measured in two perpendicular planes of the largest cord-free pocket of amniotic fluid is < 1 cm[28]; and

(2) Amniotic fluid index is < 5 cm.

The latter is obtained by adding the vertical diameters of the largest cord-free pocket of amniotic fluid, one from each quadrant[29,30]. When the average of the two diameters is 1–2 cm, the amniotic fluid index is considered marginal[31]. The pathogenesis of oligohydramnios probably includes placental insufficiency and reduced fetal urine production[32]. It should be noted that although the reduction in amniotic volume is usually a gradual process, oligohydramnios can occasionally develop acutely over a 24-h period[33].

Cord compression secondary to oligohydramnios rather than uteroplacental insufficiency is a major cause of intrapartum fetal distress as revealed by FHR monitoring in post-term gestation[34,35]. In addition, one fetal death occurred 2 days after a BPP score of 8/10 with the only abnormal variable being oligohydramnios[36]. It appears that the BPP should be done twice weekly if it is the only prenatal testing used for fetal assessment and that termination of the expectant management may be considered when oligohydramnios is detected.

The Doppler blood flow study

Doppler ultrasound has been used to measure the relative blood flow velocity in various parts of the human body for quite some time, and its utility in obstetrics is currently being investigated. Its major potential application involves predicting fetal distress and elucidating one of the mechanisms of intrauterine growth retardation: fetoplacental blood flow insufficiency. The relative blood flow is measured by different indices obtained from the Doppler flow velocity waveform such as:

(1) The S/D ratio of the peak systolic frequency shift (S) to peak end-diastolic frequency shift (D);

(2) The pulsatility index (PI) (PI = (S − D)/M where M represents the mean frequency shift); and

(3) The resistance index (RI) (RI = (S − D)/S).

These indices are related to the vascular resistance beyond the point of measurement. Another Doppler velocimetry parameter, the time-averaged mean velocity, has also been studied in post-term pregnancies[37,38]. In uncomplicated pregnancies, blood flow in the uterine, umbilical, fetal middle cerebral, fetal descending thoracic or renal arteries as reflected by these indices does not significantly change as gestational age advances beyond 40 weeks of gestation[37–41]. Thus, it does not appear that there is a significant increase in placental resistance to blood flow in post-term pregnancy as once thought. In a comparison of post-term pregnancies with and without perinatal complications, such as oligohydramnios, intrapartum fetal distress or low 5-min Apgar score, the change in the S/D ratios of uterine arteries has not been found to be significantly different, while that of the umbilical artery has not been consistently reported[38,41–43]. Among these Doppler blood flow indices, the absence of the end-diastolic frequency shift (D) from the umbilical

artery waveform appears to be a useful marker in predicting fetal distress. In a study of 534 patients[40], absent end-diastolic frequency shift had a positive predictive value of 91% for fetal distress during the first stage of labor. Another promising direct parameter of fetal blood flow, the time-averaged mean velocity in the fetal descending thoracic aorta, has been found to be significantly decreased in post-term pregnancies complicated by oligohydramnios, meconium-stained amniotic fluid, abnormal NST or fetal distress. The latter may necessitate Cesarean section delivery[38]. Similarly, the S/D ratio of the fetal internal carotid artery has been found to be elevated in complicated post-term pregnancies[43]. At present, there are insufficient data to determine whether Doppler blood flow offers a better method of identifying fetuses at risk for poor perinatal outcomes in the expectant management of post-term gestation. Doppler blood flow velocimetry could play a role in identifying a subset of post-term patients with abnormal prenatal testings, such as reduced amniotic fluid volume or nonreactive NST, who have an increased risk of fetal compromise during the peripartum period.

PRENATAL MANAGEMENT

Once the diagnosis of post-term pregnancy is made, a plan of management with the goal of optimal maternal and perinatal outcomes should be discussed with the patient and carried out in a timely manner. Unfortunately, the best approach to the management of post-term pregnancy remains to be determined. The main concern with elective induction of labor of all pregnancies at 42 weeks of gestation regardless of cervical status is increased maternal morbidity from a higher rate of Cesarean section due to failed induction[44]. However, this concern has not been supported by many randomized clinical trials[45–48]. A recent large randomized clinical trial revealed that there was no significant difference in the perinatal mortality and morbidity and the Cesarean section rates between expectant management and induction of labor at 41.0 weeks of gestation. Furthermore, intracervical administration of 0.5 mg of prostaglandin E_2

was not more effective than placebo in cervical ripening[48]. If active management of patients with post-term pregnancies and unripe cervices (Bishop score of 5 or less) is to be pursued, a 2.5-mg prostaglandin E_2 suppository could be placed in the posterior vaginal fornix, with close monitoring of uterine contractions and FHRs for the next 2 h as an outpatient. Induction of labor with intravenous oxytocin can be initiated 12 h later[48]. Cervical ripening has also been tried with intravaginal insertion of 100 µg tablets of misoprostol (prostaglandin E_1)[49]. It remains to be determined if intravaginal administration of prostaglandin E_1 or prostaglandin E_2 is more effective than placebo in cervical ripening.

The incidences of fetal macrosomia and perinatal morbidity and mortality rise significantly as early as 41.0 weeks[50–53], thus fetal evaluation should be started no later than this gestational age. The initial step involves assessing fetal weight and amniotic fluid volume by an ultrasound examination. Evaluation of fetal well-being with a combination of twice-weekly NST and weekly evaluation of amniotic volume is adequate and can be conveniently carried out as an outpatient. If both tests are normal, the patient can be allowed to await spontaneous labor or ripening of her cervix. Weekly cervical examination should be done. The presence of abnormal fetal testing, such as variable decelerations, oligohydramnios, non-reactive NST, positive CST, or BPP of less than 6/10, indicates that termination of the pregnancy should be considered. In addition, induction of labor is advisable whenever the cervix is inducible. The question of how long expectant management should continue remains debatable. It is not unreasonable to electively terminate the pregnancy at 44 completed weeks of gestation in view of a very high risk of perinatal mortality beyond this gestational age.

INTRAPARTUM MANAGEMENT

The perinatal morbidity of post-term pregnancies does not stop once the decision of induction of labor is made. The post-term fetuses are at an increased risk of perinatal hypoxia, severe birth injury from shoulder dystocia and meconium aspiration.

Meconium aspiration

The frequency of meconium-stained amniotic fluid in post-term pregnancies ranges from 22% at 42 weeks to 44% at a later gestation[54] compared to 11.3% in term high-risk pregnancies[55]. Advanced gastrointestinal maturation may play a major role since passage of meconium is infrequently observed before 32 weeks. Although meconium may pass in response to fetal distress, the presence of meconium-stained amniotic fluid *per se* without concomitant biochemical or biophysical abnormalities does not necessarily mean impending fetal distress[54,56]. Thus, post-term pregnancies with meconium-stained amniotic fluid and negative CST can be expectantly managed without increased perinatal morbidity and mortality[54]. Meconium tends to be thick in the case of post-term gestation because of the frequent concomitant oligohydramnios. The merit of peripartum detection of thick meconium lies in the timely initiation of preventive measures to reduce the morbidity associated with meconium aspiration syndrome. Suction of the meconium from the infant's nasopharynx and posterior oropharynx before delivery of the chest and endotracheal suction of the meconium below the infant's vocal cords immediately after delivery have been shown to be effective in reducing the morbidity of the meconium aspiration syndrome. Recently, amnioinfusion has been advocated to reduce the neonatal morbidity associated with meconium aspiration syndrome, probably by diluting the meconium in the amniotic fluid. Intrapartum amnioinfusion has been shown to significantly reduce the incidence of meconium below the vocal cords, neonatal acidemia, and the need for positive pressure ventilation resuscitation during the neonatal period[57].

Perinatal hypoxia

Post-term fetuses are at risk of distress during labor from either cord compression due to oligohydramnios or placental insufficiency.

Abnormal FHR patterns during labor or neonatal hypoxia have been observed in 12–30% of post-term pregnancies with normal antenatal testings[23,58,59]. As a result, these fetuses should be closely monitored during labor so that timely and appropriate intervention can be carried out. Amnioinfusion has also been used to relieve repetitive variable decelerations and prolonged decelerations commonly caused by cord compression presumably by restoring the cushioning effect of the amniotic fluid[60–62]. One prospective study has shown that, in the presence of oligohydramnios secondary to premature rupture of membranes, patients who have received prophylactic amnioinfusion have significantly higher umbilical arterial and venous pH values than those who have not. Fortunately, the mean umbilical arterial and venous pH values for both groups are within normal limits[63]. The value of prophylactic intrapartum amnioinfusion in parturients with oligohydramnios from either post-term or premature rupture of membranes in improving perinatal outcomes remains to be determined.

Shoulder dystocia

Since the fetus may continue to grow during the post-term period, macrosomia may ensue[64]. The incidence of fetal macrosomia in post-term pregnancies is about 25% compared with 10.2% in term pregnancies[50,51,58,65,66]. Since the risk of shoulder dystocia increases with higher birth weight, should dystocia is a potential problem. An estimate of fetal weight by ultrasound examination should be obtained if a large fetus is clinically suspected, recognizing that the error in predicting fetal weight by ultrasound is about 10–15%. It is not unreasonable to perform elective Cesarean section if the fetal weight is estimated to be about 5000 g because dysfunctional labor and/or shoulder dystocia are the likely outcomes in this clinical setting. Besides macrosomia, other risk factors for shoulder dystocia, such as prolonged second stage of labor, operative vaginal delivery and diabetes[67], should also

be recognized. Ultrasonography has also been utilized to predict shoulder dystocia in addition to estimating fetal weight. For example, a difference between the fetal chest circumference and the biparietal diameter of > 14 mm has been associated with a 3–13% risk of shoulder dystocia in pregnant diabetic patients[68]. Unfortunately, the accuracy of predicting shoulder dystocia with ultrasonography has so far remained limited.

To minimize the perinatal morbidity and mortality associated with shoulder dystocia, those who manage post-term pregnancies should have a high index of suspicion for this condition and be prepared to perform skillfully those maneuvers affecting the delivery before permanent damage has occurred.

In summary, the post-term gestation represents a high-risk clinical situation with a potentially significant obstetric mortality and morbidity. Although the ideal management of this clinical entity remains to be determined, any expectant management plan should include the following:

(1) Determine the date of confinement early in the gestation, and obtain the ultrasound examination for dating if necessary;

(2) Monitor the fetus closely and consider delivery when fetal well-being cannot be assured; and

(3) Be well prepared for the potential perinatal complications such as perinatal asphyxia, meconium aspiration and shoulder dystocia.

Hopefully, with a well-designed plan of management and the patient's cooperation, excellent perinatal outcomes can be obtained without unnecessarily increased maternal morbidity and mortality. It is somewhat reassuring to know that post-term gestation *per se* without perinatal hypoxia does not appear to adversely affect the offsprings' mental and physical development as measured by intelligence quotient and physical milestones, respectively[69].

References

1. Clifford, S. H. (1954). Postmaturity with placental dysfunction. *Pediatrics*, **44**, 1
2. Naeye, R. L. (1978). Causes of perinatal mortality: excess of prolonged gestations. *Am. J. Epidemiol.*, **108**, 429
3. Nwosu, V. C., Wallach, E. E. and Bolognese, R. J. (1966). Initiation of labor by intraamniotic cortisol instillation in prolonged human pregnancy. *Am. J. Obstet. Gynecol.*, **96**, 901
4. Fleischer, A., Schulman, H., Farmakides, G., *et al.* (1985). Antepartum nonstress test and the postmature pregnancy. *Am. J. Obstet. Gynecol.*, **66**, 80
5. Vorherr, H. (1975). Placental insufficiency in relation to postterm pregnancy and fetal postmaturity. *Am. J. Obstet. Gynecol.*, **125**, 1
6. McClure-Browne, J. C. (1963). Postmaturity. *Am. J. Obstet. Gynecol.*, **85**, 573
7. Saito, M., Yazawa, K., Hashiguchi, A. *et al.* (1972). Time of ovulation and prolonged pregnancy. *Am. J. Obstet. Gynecol.*, **112**, 31
8. Robinson, H. P. and Fleming, J. E. (1975). A critical evaluation of sonar 'crown–rump length' measurements. *Br. J. Obstet. Gynaecol.*, **82**, 702
9. Campbell, S. (1969). The prediction of fetal maturity by ultrasonic measurement of the biparietal diameter. *J. Obstet. Gynaecol. Br. Commonw.*, **76**, 603
10. O'Brien, G. D., Queenan, J. T. and Campbell, S. (1985). Assessment of gestational age in the second trimester by real-time ultrasound measurement of the femur length. *Am. J. Obstet. Gynecol.*, **151**, 304
11. Sabbagha, R. E., Barton, B. A., Barton, F. B., *et al.* (1976). Sonar biparietal diameter. I. Analysis of percentile growth differences in two normal populations using same methodology. *Obstet. Gynecol.*, **126**, 479
12. Hadlock, F. P., Deter, R. L., Carpenter, R. J. *et al.* (1981). Estimating fetal age: effect of head shape of BPD. *Am. J. Roentgenol.*, **137**, 83
13. Goldstein, I., Reece, E. A., Pilu, G. *et al.* (1987). Cerebellar measurements with ultrasonography in the evaluation of fetal growth and development. *Am. J. Obstet. Gynecol.*, **156**, 1065
14. Chinn, D. H., Bolding, D. B., Callen, P. W. *et al.* (1983). The lateral cerebral ventricle in early second trimester. *Radiology*, **148**, 529
15. Goldstein, I., Lockwood, C., Belanger, K. *et al.* (1988). Ultrasonographic assessment of gestational age with the distal femoral and proximal tibial ossification center in the third trimester. *Am. J. Obstet. Gynecol.*, **158**, 127
16. Mahony, B. S., Barei, J. D., Killan, A. P. *et al.* (1986). Epiphyseal ossification centers in the assessment of fetal maturity. Sonographic correlation with amniocentesis lung profile. *Radiology*, **159**, 521
17. Tabsh, R. M. A. (1984). Correlation of ultrasonic epiphyseal centers and the lecithin/sphingomyelin ratio. *Obstet. Gynecol.*, **64**, 92
18. Kuhns, L. R. and Finnstrom, O. (1976). New standards of ossification of the newborn. *Radiology*, **119**, 655
19. Mahony, B. S., Callen, P. W. and Filly, R. A. (1985). Distal femoral epiphyseal ossification center in the assessment of third trimester menstrual age. Sonographic identification and measurement. *Radiology*, **155**, 201
20. Evertson, L. R. and Paul, R. H. (1978). Antepartum fetal heart rate testing: the nonstress test. *Am. J. Obstet. Gynecol.*, **132**, 895
21. Khouzami, V. A., Johnson, J. W. C., Daikoku, N. H. *et al.* (1983). Comparison of urinary estrogens, contraction stress tests and nonstress tests in the management of postterm pregnancy. *J. Reprod. Med.*, **28**, 23
22. Barss, V. A., Frigoletto, F. D. and Diamond, F. (1985). Stillbirth after nonstress testing. *Obstet. Gynecol.*, **65**, 541
23. Miyazaki, F. S. and Miyazaki, B. A. (1981). False reactive nonstress tests in postterm pregnancies. *Am. J. Obstet. Gynecol.*, **140**, 269
24. Eden, R. D., Gergely, R. Z., Schifrin, B. S. *et al.* (1982). Comparison of antepartum testing schemes for the management of the postdate pregnancy. *Am. J. Obstet. Gynecol.*, **144**, 683
25. Manning, F. A., Platt, L. D. and Sipos, L. (1980). Antepartum fetal evaluation: development of a fetal biophysical profile. *Am. J. Obstet. Gynecol.*, **136**, 6
26. Hann, L., McArdle, C. and Sachs, B. (1987). Sonographic biophysical profile in the postdate pregnancy. *J. Ultrasound Med.*, **6**, 191
27. Johnson, J. M., Harman, C. R., Lange, I. R. and Manning, A. (1986). Biophysical profile scoring in the management of the postterm pregnancy: an analysis of 307 patients. *Am. J. Obstet. Gynecol.*, **154**, 2
28. Manning, F. A., Morrison, I., Lang, I. R. *et al.* (1985). Fetal assessment based on fetal biophysical profile scoring: experience in 12 620 referred high-risk pregnancies. *Am. J. Obstet. Gynecol.*, **151**, 3
29. Phelan, J. P., Platt, L. D., Yeh, S. *et al.* (1985). The role of ultrasound assessment of amniotic fluid volume in the management of the post-date pregnancy. *Am. J. Obstet. Gynecol.*, **151**, 304
30. Phelan, J. P., Smith, C. V., Broussard, P. *et al.* (1987). Amniotic fluid volume assessment with

the four-quadrant technique at 36–42 weeks' gestation. *J. Reprod. Med.*, **32**, 540

31. Chamberlain, P. F., Manning, F. A., Morrison, I., Harman, C. R. and Lange, I. R. (1984). Ultrasound evaluation of amniotic fluid volume. *Am. J. Obstet. Gynecol.*, **150**, 245

32. Trimmer, K. J., Leveno, K. J., Peters, M. T. and Kelly, M. A. (1990). Observations on the cause of oligohydramnios in prolonged pregnancy. *Am. J. Obstet. Gynecol.*, **163**, 1900

33. Clement, D., Schifrin, B. S. and Kates, R. B. (1987). Acute oligohydramnios in postdate pregnancy. *Am. J. Obstet. Gynecol.*, **157**, 884

34. Bochner, C. J., Medearis, A. L., Davis, J. *et al.* (1987). Antepartum predictors of fetal distress in postterm pregnancy. *Am. J. Obstet. Gynecol.*, **157**, 353

35. Leveno, K. J., Quirk, J. G., Cunningham, F. G. *et al.* (1984). Prolonged pregnancy – observations concerning the cause of fetal distress. *Am. J. Obstet. Gynecol.*, **150**, 465

36. Phelan, J. P., Platt, L. D., Leh, S. Y. *et al.* (1985). The role of ultrasound assessment of amniotic fluid volume in the management of the postdate pregnancy. *Am. J. Obstet. Gynecol.*, **151**, 304

37. Rightmire, D. A. and Campbell, S. (1987). Fetal and maternal Doppler blood flow parameters in postterm pregnancies. *Obstet. Gynecol.*, **69**, 6

38. Battaglia, C., Larocca, E., Lanzani, A., Coukos, G. and Genazzani, A. R. (1991). Doppler velocimetry in prolonged pregnancy. *Obstet. Gynecol.*, **77**, 213

39. Arduini, D. and Rizzo, G. (1991). Fetal renal artery velocity waveforms and amniotic fluid volume in growth-retarded and post-term fetuses. *Obstet. Gynecol.*, **77**, 370

40. Pearce, J. M. and McParland, P. J. (1991). A comparison of Doppler flow velocity waveforms, amniotic fluid columns, and the nonstress test as a means of monitoring post-dates pregnancies. *Obstet. Gynecol.*, **77**, 204

41. Guidetti, D. A., Divon, M. Y., Cavalieri, R. L., Langer, O. and Merkatz, I. R. (1987). Fetal umbilical artery flow velocimetry in postdate pregnancies. *Am. J. Obstet. Gynecol.*, **157**, 1521

42. Fischer, R. L., Kuhlman, K. A., Depp, R. and Wapner, R. J. (1991). Doppler evaluation of umbilical and uterine-arcuate arteries in the postdates pregnancy. *Obstet. Gynecol.*, **78**, 363

43. Brar, H. S., Horenstein, J., Medearis, A. L., Platt, L. D., Phelan, J. P. and Paul, R. H. (1989). Cerebral, umbilical, and uterine resistance using Doppler velocimetry in postterm pregnancy. *J. Ultrasound Med.*, **8**, 187

44. Gibb, D. M. F., Cardozo, L. D., Studd, J. W. W. and Cooper, P. (1982). Prolonged pregnancy: is induction of labor indicated? a prospective study. *Br. J. Obstet. Gynaecol.*, **89**, 292

45. Witter, F. R. and Weitz, C. M. (1987). A randomized trial of induction at 42 weeks gestation versus expectant management for postdates pregnancies. *Am. J. Perinatol.*, **4**, 3

46. Rayburn, W., Gosen, R., Ramadei, C., Woods, R. and Scott, J. (1988). Outpatient cervical ripening with prostaglandin E2 gel in uncomplicated postdate pregnancies. *Am. J. Obstet. Gynecol.*, **158**, 1417

47. Dyson, D. C., Miller, P. D. and Armstrong, M. A. (1987). Management of prolonged pregnancy: induction of labor versus antepartum fetal testing. *Am. J. Obstet. Gynecol.*, **156**, 928

48. The National Institute of Child Health and Human Development; Network of Maternal-Fetal Medicine Units (1994). A clinical trial of induction of labor versus expectant management in postterm pregnancy. *Am. J. Obstet. Gynecol.*, **170**, 716

49. Fletcher, H., Mitchell, S., Frederick, J., Simeon, D. and Brown, D. (1994). Intravaginal misoprostol versus dinoprostone as cervical ripening and labor-inducing agents. *Obstet. Gynecol.*, **83**, 244

50. Arias, F. (1987). Predictability of complications associated with prolongation of pregnancy. *Obstet. Gynecol.*, **70**, 101

51. Chervenak, J. L., Divon, M. Y., Hirsch, J., Girz, B. A. and Langer, O. (1989). Macrosomia in the postdate pregnancy: is routine ultrasonographic screening indicated? *Am. J. Obstet. Gynecol.*, **161**, 753

52. Guidetti, D. A., Divon, M. Y. and Langer, O. (1989). Postdate fetal surveillance: is 41 weeks too early? *Am. J. Obstet. Gynecol.*, **161**, 91

53. Bochner, C. J., Williams, J., Castro, L., Medearis, A., Hobel, C. J. and Wade, M. (1988). The efficacy of starting postterm antenatal testing at 41 weeks as compared with 42 weeks of gestational age. *Am. J. Obstet. Gynecol.*, **159**, 550

54. Knox, E. G., Huddleston, J. R., Flowers, C. E. *et al.* (1979). Management of prolonged pregnancy: results of a prospective randomized trial. *Am. J. Obstet. Gynecol.*, **134**, 4

55. Mandelbaum, B. (1973). Gestational meconium in the high-risk pregnancy. *Obstet. Gynecol.*, **42**, 87

56. Miller, F. C., Sacks, D. A., Yeh, S. Y. *et al.* (1973). Significance of meconium during labor. *Am. J. Obstet. Gynecol.*, **115**, 3

57. Sadovsky, Y., Amon, E., Bade, M. E. and Petrie, R. H. (1989). Prophylactic amnioinfusion during labor complicated by meconium: a preliminary report. *Am. J. Obstet. Gynecol.*, **161**, 613

58. Freeman, R. K., Garite, T. J., Modanlou, H. *et al.* (1981). Postdate pregnancy: utilization of contraction stress testing for primary fetal surveillance. *Am. J. Obstet. Gynecol.*, **140**, 128

59. Rochard, F., Schifrin, B. S., Goupil, F. *et al.* (1976). Nonstressed fetal heart rate monitoring

in the antepartum period. *Am. J. Obstet. Gynecol.*, **126**, 699

60. Miyazaki, F. S. and Taylor, N. A. (1983). Saline amnioinfusion for relief of variable or prolonged decelerations. *Am. J. Obstet. Gynecol.*, **146**, 670

61. Owen, J., Henson, B. V. and Hauth, J. C. (1990). A prospective randomized study of saline solution amnioinfusion. *Am. J. Obstet. Gynecol.*, **162**, 1146

62. Schrimmer, D. B., Macri, C. J. and Paul, R. H. (1991). Prophylactic amnioinfusion as a treatment for oligohydramnios in laboring patients: a prospective, randomized trial. *Am. J. Obstet. Gynecol.*, **165**, 972

63. Nageotte, M. P., Freeman, R. K., Garite, T. J. and Dorchester, W. (1985). Prophylactic intrapartum amnioinfusion in patients with preterm premature rupture of membranes. *Am. J. Obstet. Gynecol.*, **153**, 557

64. McLean, F. H., Boyd, M. E., Usher, R. H. and Kramer, M. S. (1991). Postterm infants: too big or too small? *Am. J. Obstet. Gynecol.*, **164**, 619

65. Boyd, M. E., Usher, R. H. and McLean, F. H. (1983). Fetal macrosomia: prediction, risks, proposed management. *Obstet. Gynecol.*, **61**, 715

66. Golditch, I. M. and Kirkman, K. (1978). The large fetus: management and outcome. *Obstet. Gynecol.*, **52**, 26

67. Benedetti, T. J. and Gabbe, S. G. (1978). Shoulder dystocia: a complication of fetal macrosomia and prolonged second stage of labor with mid-pelvic delivery. *Obstet. Gynecol.*, **52**, 526

68. Elliott, J. P., Garite, T. J., Freeman, R. K. *et al.* (1982). Ultrasonic prediction of fetal macrosomia in diabetic patients. *Obstet. Gynecol.*, **60**, 159

69. Shime, J., Librach, C. L., Gare, D. J. and Cook, C. J. (1986). The influence of prolonged pregnancy on infant development at one and two years of age: a prospective controlled study. *Am. J. Obstet. Gynecol.*, **154**, 341

Congenital toxoplasmosis: old and new perspectives

45

E. Schiff and S. Mashiach

PARASITOLOGY

Toxoplasmosis is an infection caused by the parasite *Toxoplasma gondii*. This organism belongs to the phylum Protozoa and the subphylum of apical complex organisms that includes the plasmodium, coccidea, sarcocystis, isospora and toxoplasmia. Several members of this subclass exist, but *Toxoplasma gondii* is the most common and best known.

Toxoplasma gondii is an intracellular parasite. It is a crescent-shaped unicellular organism, approximately 12 μm long and 6 μm wide. One end is pointed, with a conoid projection thought to be the 'cell mouth' organelle. Under the electron microscope one can distinguish a system of 15 longitudinal fibrils, the toxonemes, extending to the pointed end. These are thought to account for the active motility of the organism and its ability to penetrate cells.

Toxoplasma is able to parasitize a variety of hosts including humans, other mammals and birds. The only known host, however, in which the parasite undergoes gametogenesis is the cat family. The parasite is secreted as an oocyst in the feces of the infected cat and becomes infective within 4–5 days. When ingested by its host, the infective oocyst penetrates the intestinal tissue and is carried by the blood in leukocytes to various areas of the body; especially the reticuloendothelial system, the central nervous system (CNS), the skeletal muscles and the eyes, probably because of their lower ability to resist the infection. When cells of these organs are infected, pseudocysts are formed. If the cyst ruptures, the tachysoites can eventually circulate and infect other cells.

HUMAN INFECTION

Human beings can be infected either by ingested oocysts originating from the feces of infected cats or by ingested cysts originating from improperly cooked meat, such as pork, beef or poultry, containing cysts or pseudocysts. The parasite invades the lymphatic system and bloodstream and gives rise to cyst formation in various organs. A lesion caused by acquired toxoplasmosis (which is also typical of congenital toxoplasmosis) is seen in the fundus of the human eye in the form of a heavily pigmented central choroidal cystic lesion.

VERTICAL TRANSMISSION AND FETAL INFECTION

Pregnant women infected by oocysts or cysts may experience a parasitemia. In most cases of acute maternal toxoplasmosis the disease is subclinical. According to different reports, 60–90% of pregnant patients had no symptoms while seroconverted due to acute disease. When apparent clinically, the disease may manifest as a flu-like syndrome with fever, fatigue, sore throat, maculopapular rash and non-tender lymphadenopathy, which is most commonly cervical. Some women may have hepatosplenomegaly, and a certain percentage may have ocular symptoms such as haziness of vision, photophobia, etc. Blood smears may show lymphocytosis and abnormal-looking lymphocytes, and fundoscopy may show yellow clusters indicative of focal necrotizing chorioretinitis. In healthy immunocompetent pregnant women, however, the disease, even when clinically evident, is usually mild and always self-limiting.

While the organism is circulating in the blood, it may reach the placenta as well as any other organ. There is little information on the toxoplasmatic infection process in the human placenta. Nevertheless, a recent report[1] of infected placentae showed interesting findings of hydropic changes, local infarctions, areas of calcification and, most consistently, low-grade chronic villitis with mononuclear inflammatory infiltrates. From the placental villi the organism may invade the fetal circulation and cause acute fetal infection. It is important to note that the placental infection may continue long after the parasitemia, and therefore vertical transmission to the fetus may occur at a later stage and not only around the time of parasitemia. This means that secondary prevention by chemotherapy for women with acute toxoplasmosis in pregnancy should be continued throughout pregnancy to reduce the risk of placental–fetal transmission.

According to several studies in the 1970s, the overall average chance of vertical transmission to the fetus from untreated primary maternal toxoplasmosis during pregnancy is approximately one in three. The incidence of vertical transmission is strongly dependent on gestational age. The average transmission rate in the first trimester, without exposure to chemotherapy, is around 15%, rising to 70% in the late third trimester. The well known series of Daffos and co-workers[2], reported in 1988 in the *New England Journal of Medicine* included 748 parturients with acute toxoplasmosis in pregnancy. In this series, among untreated patients the rate of fetal infection during the first trimester was 12%.

In general, approximately 70% of infected fetuses have undetectable subclinical illness at delivery and should be kept under observation. It is important to realize that in contrast to transmission that depends on trophoblast thickness, the risk of clinically apparent disease and of increased severity in the congenitally infected fetus rises significantly at the time of organ development during the early weeks of gestation. Based on information by Stray-Pedersen and Jenum[3], the risk of severe clinical congenital disease is 25% before the 20th gestational week and 0% thereafter. Those with severe disease either die *in utero* or at a young age, or have severe sequelae necessitating institutional care. Among those infected after 20 weeks, 90% have subclinical illness while the rest have mild disease and no more than 15% need institutional care.

EPIDEMIOLOGY

Information has accumulated over several years in connection with the rates of maternal immunity and of acquired toxoplasmosis during pregnancy. As Table 1 shows, an immunity rate of 21–78% against toxoplasma was observed among different populations of pregnant women, depending on geographical location and probably influenced by general hygiene status as well as by cultural factors such as diet, cooking practices, etc. Large-scale studies from Belgium and Austria have demonstrated that immunity at the beginning of pregnancy has significantly decreased over the past 20 years from 50–70% down to 37–47%, even though the average maternal age rose significantly during that period.

As for acquiring acute infection during pregnancy, the rates vary from 1.6/1000 in Australia up to 12/1000 in recent years in certain parts of Belgium and France. It should be noted that these numbers are based on 1000 seronegative pregnant women. The ratio would be totally different if it were based on the total number of deliveries, especially in a country like France, where only 20% are seronegative at the beginning of pregnancy. It should also be noted that

Table 1 *Maternal immune status to toxoplasma in different countries*

Country	Year published	Number studied	Immune (%)
Belgium	1992	20 901	47
Finland	1992	16 733	21
Austria	1992	167 041	37
Nigeria	1992	352	78
India	1991	200	77
Australia	1991	10 207	35
Sweden	1991	1086	21

the various rates are based on different laboratory diagnostic techniques.

PRIMARY PREVENTION

An interesting issue is the impact of primary prevention on the incidence of acquired toxoplasma infection in pregnancy. Traditionally, primary prevention includes education about avoiding undercooked meat, and detailed instructions for handling cats during pregnancy. At least two recent studies have addressed this issue. The first[4] reported a 63% reduction in seroconversion rates during pregnancy, attributed to primary prevention among 11 286 consecutive parturients receiving education over 12 years. In the second, Stray-Pedersen and Jenum[3], who developed a mathematical model for calculating cost vs. benefit in programs for prevention of congenital toxoplasmosis, indicated that, depending on general cost variables, a health education program can result in reduction of 30–60% in the rate of congenital toxoplasmosis. Thus, the primary prevention is clearly effective and is well accepted, irrespective of the debate over strategies for secondary prevention. Health education on avoiding toxoplasmosis during pregnancy should therefore become part of the standard obstetric care in every country and by every physician. Presumably, this would also significantly reduce the total cost of secondary prevention.

In addition to education, research aimed at the development of a vaccine strategy has been concentrating for several years on the identification and molecular characterization of surface antigens of the organism's proliferative stage, the tachyzoite. Capron and associates[5] recently described four major immunogens that were shown by various techniques to be common to different stages of the parasite. Molecular cloning of these proteins is now under way. Some progress can therefore be expected in this field in the coming years. Obviously, many of the queries and controversies associated with the prevention of congenital toxoplasmosis would become irrelevant once an efficient vaccine were developed.

SECONDARY PREVENTION

The principle of secondary prevention is based on the serodiagnosis and timing of acute maternal toxoplasmosis during pregnancy. There are several tests in current use for detection of antitoxoplasma antibodies. For Immunoglobulin G (IgG) detection, most laboratories still use the cheap and simple indirect immunofluorization test. Other laboratories use direct or indirect hemagglutination tests and in Europe the complement fixation test is also commonly used for IgG detection. Enzyme-linked immunosorbent assay (ELISA), though probably even more sensitive and specific, is not widely used for IgG, because of its relatively higher cost. Many laboratories, however, still consider the dye test named after Sabin and Feldman as the 'gold standard' for specific and sensitive IgG measurement, in spite of its major disadvantage of using live organisms for the test. It should be emphasized that in all of these tests for detection of IgG, positive results take 2–3 weeks to develop, and reach peak levels only after 8–12 weeks. All, including the Sabin Feldman test, are difficult to interpret in terms of a diagnosis of acute infection, unless regular tests are performed at short intervals. Other tests aimed at identification of acute disease, such as indirect immunofluorescence specific for IgM and hemagglutination tests, have been used during the last decade for IgM determination. In line with this approach, many laboratories have switched to ELISAs for IgM detection.

Interestingly, several recent studies[6,7] have obtained inconsistent results when comparing different commercial automated enzyme immunoassays for IgG and IgM, a finding that calls into question their reliability. Some of the kits had unacceptable rates of false-positive or false-negative findings. These discrepancies between the results of laboratories using different kits are a source of confusion for physicians in many countries. In recent years some of the larger laboratories have started using the immunosorbent agglutination assay, at least for IgM detection, since it has been shown that this method, in addition to being cheaper, has greater sensitivity and can improve the serodiagnosis of congenital toxoplasmosis when compared to the commercial ELISA kits[8].

Some interesting data on techniques for differentiating between acute and late onset infection have been reported in recent years. At least two well-designed studies[9,10] have demonstrated that the IgA type of anti-toxoplasma antibodies may be even more sensitive and useful than IgM for the diagnosis of recently acquired infection and for follow-up of illness in the fetus and neonate. Indeed, several of the French groups reported their last series using the IgA ELISA kit as a main factor in fetal diagnosis. Others[11] have presented convincing evidence that detection of IgE anti-toxoplasma antibodies using ELISA or immunosorbent agglutination assays is at least as useful as IgM or IgA in the diagnosis of recently acquired acute disease. Similarly, it has been suggested that measurement of IgG avidity, i.e. the proportion of antibodies with relatively high affinity, may be helpful, because acute infection is characterized by low avidity, and so a special ELISA for avidity determination has been developed. Other authors have proposed a specific type of IgM anti-4–5 kDa antigen, measurements of IgG subtypes, or *in vitro* assessment of IgG secretion by lymphoid cells as alternative indicators of recently acquired infection. A major advance in serodiagnosis occurred with the development of ELISA and immunosorbent agglutination assays, as well as immunoblotting techniques for the specific detection of IgA and IgM targeted towards the surface antigen of the organism known as P30 antigen. Over the past years, a number of reports have confirmed the marked sensitivity mainly of the anti-P30 of the IgA type for diagnosis of acute infection, in comparison to the traditional non-specific IgM antibodies[12,13].

An important study by Roos and colleagues[14] represents a new approach using the latest and most specific available techniques of serodiagnosis for decision analysis in large-scale pregnant populations. These authors screened 2104 parturients at 8, 17 and 28 weeks of gestation, using the IgG direct agglutination assay and the IgM immunosorbent agglutination assay. The patients who were IgM positive at some stage underwent differential serology by two steps. The first included the dye test, the immunofluorescence test and the complement fixation test. If one or more of these were positive, the patient then underwent the second step, involving anti-P30 IgM and IgA by ELISA or immunoblotting. The authors successfully identified all 12 women with acute infection in pregnancy (6 per 1000 pregnancies or 10 per 1000 nonimmune women) while at the same time avoiding unnecessary invasive procedures that might have been recommended if no second-stage differential serodiagnosis was performed.

FETAL DIAGNOSIS

The next controversial, although exciting and challenging, issue is fetal diagnosis in cases of established maternal acute toxoplasmosis in pregnancy. During the last 10 years most of the information on this subject has come from the group of Daffos. In their large New England study published in 1988[2], they reported proven congenital infection in 42 out of 746 women with acute toxoplasmosis in pregnancy. Of the 42 infected fetuses, 39 (93%) were diagnosed by a combination of ultrasound findings, cordocentesis and amniocentesis with inoculation of mice. It should be noted that the sensitivity of the ultrasound findings for congenital infection in this large series was 45%, that of the total fetal IgM test was 52%, and that of indirect infection indicators, such as platelet or white blood cell counts, lactate dehydrogenase or aspartate aminotransferase concentrations, was between 19 and 57%. Therefore, based on Daffos' data, even though the specificity of the fetal blood tests is as high as 97–100%, when the tests are all negative there is still a 40–50% chance of congenital disease that may be diagnosed later by the bioassay.

In addition, a French group recently presented their experience with fetal diagnosis in relatively large numbers of infected mothers[15]. A successful prenatal diagnosis rate of 83% among 192 infected mothers was found. The cumulative sensitivity of specific fetal IgM or IgA was 65%. Ultrasound identified only four out of 20 congenitally infected babies. These authors also found that first-trimester maternal infection was associated with a fetal disease rate of only 4%. Among mothers infected after 28 weeks there was a 53% chance of vertical transmission, but only one of these babies had clinical mild disease. Hence, the main conclusions from these French studies are that although ultrasonography and fetal blood sampling are seriously limited in sensitivity, applying them routinely in women with well established infection during pregnancy may dramatically reduce the rate of unnecessary pregnancy terminations and may provide important information as to the mode of chemotherapy needed.

A dramatic improvement in the sensitivity and promptness of the diagnosis of fetal toxoplasma infection can be expected in the near future, once the polymerase chain reaction (PCR) technique becomes more easily available. Perhaps, because of the intensive research associated with AIDS patients, the ability to identify components of the parasite using PCR in human sera or body fluids was achieved earlier than anticipated. The experimental data published during the past 4 years indicate that this technique is highly promising. At least five groups have reported their experience with maternal and fetal samples. Some used the sequence related to the P30 surface antigen, whereas others used other sequences. Regardless of the sequence used, all groups reported a sensitivity of 80–100% in detecting the parasite antigen in infected amniotic fluid or serum samples. The results were usually available within 24 h and the technique was sensitive enough for a signal to be observed with only one parasite in the sample. The most promising study[16], in 1994, described the results of PCR targeted to the B1 antigen in 339 amniotic fluid samples of infected pregnant women. PCR was positive in all 34 cases with traditional laboratory evidence of fetal infection, as well as in three infected offspring in whom the usual tests were negative. Therefore, the PCR performed better than conventional parasitological methods, with a sensitivity of 97.4% and a negative predictive value of 99.7%, and of course within a very much shorter time. We estimate that within 2 or 3 years amniocentesis and PCR will become the standard method of fetal diagnosis in cases of maternal toxoplasma infection.

CHEMOTHERAPY

Acute acquired toxoplasmosis is not treated in immunocompetent children or adults unless there is significant organ involvement, such as encephalitis or myocarditis. It is well accepted today, however, that primary infected pregnant women should be treated once the infection is recognized, in order to reduce the risk of vertical transmission. As was mentioned earlier, the placenta acts as a reservoir, supplying viable organisms to the fetus throughout pregnancy. In other words, transmission may occur long after the parasitemia clears up. For this reason, the rationale is that therapy suggested to the infected mother can prevent fetal infection and perhaps even modify the severity of infection in the fetus that actually was infected.

The efficacy of treatment in pregnancy is difficult to evaluate, because it is dependent on several factors: the screening procedure, gestational age at the time of infection, how soon the infection was detected, whether parasites had already reached the fetus by the time therapy began, etc. Furthermore, the drugs available today can be expected only to slow down the multiplication of parasites but not to eliminate the tissue cysts. Other complicating factors are related to the ability of the drugs to cross the placental barrier and the possibility that they may cause teratogenic or adverse effects.

Which drugs are available and what do we know about them? Pyrimethamine, an antimalarial drug given in combination with sulfonamides, has been accepted since the 1970s as the best therapy for toxoplasmosis in humans. Both components are inhibitors of folate metabolism and thus prevent proliferation of the parasite in its acute stages. The drug without sulfonamide is eight times less effective. The dosage is 0.5–1 mg/kg/day. The drug enters the CNS and thus may be of value in fetal CNS involvement. A possible side effect is bone marrow suppression and pancytopenia. For this reason, folinic acid should be added (0.05–0.1 mg/kg/day or every 48 h). Although theoretically there is a risk of teratogenic side effects, according to numerous studies this risk is negligible, and thus use of the drug in pregnancy is approved (for patients with malaria even in the first trimester). The most commonly used combinations are pyrimethamine plus 1–2 g/day of sulfadiazine or two tablets per week of Fansidar®, containing 25 mg of pyrimethamine and 500 mg sulfadoxine. The sulfonamides are uncommonly associated with the Stevens–Johonson hypersensitivity reaction as well as with crystalluria and possible neonatal hyperbilirubinemia.

Spiramycin, a macrolide antibiotic, has been used extensively in Europe as an alternative or additional drug. It has intracellular antiparasitic activity and its uniqueness lies in the fact that its concentration in placental tissue is up to five times higher than in serum. The recommended daily dosage is approximately 3 g, which contains 9 mIU. This drug penetrates the fetal circulation to a much lower degree than does pyrimethamine, and also does not penetrate the CNS. Spiramycin has no teratogenic effects whatsoever and can be used in every pregnant woman. Also, side effects occur only very rarely.

For nearly 30 years now, two chemotherapeutic regimes have been employed, mostly in central Europe, in the treatment of primary toxoplasmosis in pregnant women. The original studies from Austria and France on several hundreds of infected pregnant women reported a 50–70% reduction in the incidence of congenital infection and a corresponding reduction in the isolation of the organism from the placenta. The incidence of placental infection was reduced from 25 to 8% in the first trimester, 54 to 19% in the second trimester and 65 to 44% in the third. However, since the reduction in clinically apparent infection was no more than 10–15% it was concluded that the drug reduces the risk of maternofetal infection by up to 60% but does not significantly modify the pattern of infection in an already infected fetus. Several studies published in the French literature in the 1980s claimed that the combination of pyrimethamine and sulfadiazine is more effective than spiramycin, and, furthermore, leads to a significant reduction in the number of severely

congenitally infected babies and a shift from less severe to subclinical forms. More recently, pyrimethamine in combination with a longer acting sulfonamide, sulfadoxine, which has a half-life of 8 days, has been tried in pregnancies with evidence of infected offspring. The suggested schedule was pyrimethamine 50 mg and sulfadoxine 1000 mg, that is two tablets of Fansidar, each week, alternating with daily administration of spiramycin until delivery.

THE SCREENING DILEMMA

Congenital toxoplasmosis: to screen or not to screen? This is an old public health controversy. The American College of Obstetricians and Gynecologists does not recommend routine screening in the United States for maternal infection in pregnancy. Several authors have provided calculations in an attempt to resolve the dilemma. Joss and co-workers[17] calculated the cost to society of congenital toxoplasmosis estimated to occur annually in Scotland and compared it to the cost of preventing the disease by screening and treatment. For a three-stage screening program they found that the screening cost was 0.7–1.2 times the society cost and concluded that a screening program should be adopted in their population. Of course, a major issue in this decision is the infection rate of non-immune mothers in the specific population. Stray-Pedersen and Jenum, in their 1992 publication[3] of the mathematical model for cost vs. benefit, concluded that screening programs are of economic benefit to society if the incidence of maternal toxoplasmosis in pregnancy is at least 1–1.5 per 1000 deliveries. There are, of course, medicolegal issues in addition to economic cost vs. benefit considerations, which will not be discussed in this chapter.

CONCLUSIONS

(1) Primary prevention is highly important in preventing congenital toxoplasmosis and should be part of the management protocol of every obstetrician.

(2) Serodiagnosis is complicated and should be performed only by competent laboratories with the knowledge and facilities for differential tests. Otherwise, the results will be a large number of unnecessary invasive procedures and pregnancy terminations.

(3) A combination of ultrasound, parasitology methods, serology and indirect signs can identify approximately 80% of infected fetuses. However, the polymerase chain reaction is expected to become the method of choice, with even higher sensitivity and negative predictive values than are obtainable at present.

(4) Continuous chemotherapy is recommended. Following maternal and fetal diagnosis, it should be given according to the suggested European protocols. Physicians should be aware of the possible side effects.

(5) The use of screening programs is still a debatable issue. However, it seems that in populations with seroconversion of more than 1.5 per 1000 deliveries, screening might be of cost benefit to society.

References

1. Abdel-Salam, A. M., Eissa, M. H., Mangoud, A. M., Eissa, T. M. and Morsy, T. A. (1990). Pathological examination of the placenta in human cases of toxoplasmosis. *J. Egypt. Soc. Parasitol.*, **20**, 549–54
2. Daffos, F., Forestier, F., Capella-Pavlovsky, M. *et al.* (1988). Prenatal management of 746 pregnancies at risk for congenital toxoplasmosis. *N. Engl. J. Med.*, **318**, 271–8
3. Stray-Pedersen, B. and Jenum, P. (1992). Economic evaluation of preventive programs against congenital toxoplasmosis. *Scand. J. Infect. Dis.* (Suppl.), **84**, 86–96
4. Foulon, W., Naessens, A. and Derde, M. P. (1994). Evaluation of the possibilities for preventing congenital toxoplasmosis. *Am. J. Perinatol.*, **11**, 57–62
5. Capron, A., Cesbron-Delauw, M. F. and Darcy, F. (1990). New molecular approaches to the diagnosis and prevention of toxoplasmosis (French). *Bull. Acad. Natl. Med.*, **174**, 387–92
6. Naessens, A., Houninolx, W., Foulon, W. and Lauwera, S. (1993). Evaluation of seven commercially available enzyme immunoassays for immunoglobulin G and M antibody detection of *Toxoplasma gondii. Immunol. Infect. Dis.*, **3**, 258–62
7. Cubitt, W. D., Ades, A. E. and Peckham, C. S. (1992). Evaluation of five commercial assays for screening antenatal sera for antibodies to *Toxoplasma gondii. J. Clin. Pathol.*, **45**, 435–8
8. Skinner, L. J., Chatterton, J. M., Joss, A. W., Moir, I. L. and Ho-Yen, D. O. (1989). The use of an IgM immunosorbent agglutination assay to diagnose congenital toxoplasmosis. *J. Med. Microbiol.*, **28**, 125–8
9. Stepick-Biek, P., Thulliez, P., Araujo, F. G. and Remington, J. S. (1990). IgA antibodies for diagnosis of acute congenital and acquired toxoplasmosis. *J. Infect. Dis.*, **162**, 270–3
10. Bessieres, M. H., Roques, C., Berrebi, A., Barre, V., Cazaux, M. and Seguela, J. P. (1992). IgA antibody response during acquired and congenital toxoplasmosis. *J. Clin. Pathol.*, **45**, 605–8
11. Wong, S. Y., Hajdu, M. P., Ramirez, R., Thulliez, P., McLeod, R. and Remington, J. S. (1993). Role of specific immunoglobulin E in diagnosis of acute toxoplasma infection and toxoplasmosis. *J. Clin. Microbiol.*, **31**, 2952–9
12. Gross, U., Roos, T., Appoldt, D. and Heesemann, J. (1992). Improved serological diagnosis of *Toxoplasma gondii* infection by detection of immunoglobulin A (IgA) and IgM antibodies against P30 by using the immunoblot technique. *J. Clin. Microbiol.*, **30**, 1436–41
13. Decoster, A., Darcy, F., Caron, A. *et al.* (1992). Anti-P30 IgA antibodies as prenatal markers of congenital toxoplasma infection. *Clin. Exp. Immunol.*, **87**, 310–15
14. Roos, T., Martius, J., Gross, U. and Schrod, L. (1993). Systematic serologic screening for toxoplasmosis in pregnancy. *Obstet. Gynecol.*, **81**, 243–50
15. Partlong, F., Boulot, P., Issert, E. *et al.* (1994). Fetal diagnosis of toxoplasmosis in 190 women infected during pregnancy. *Prenat. Diagn.*, **14**, 191–8

16. Hohlfeld, P., Daffos, F., Costa, J. M., Thulliez, P., Forestier, F. and Vidaud, M. (1994). Prenatal diagnosis of congenital toxoplasmosis with a polymerase-chain-reaction test on amniotic fluids. *N. Engl. J. Med.*, **331**, 695–9

17. Joss, A. W., Chatterton, J. M. and Ho-Yen, D. O. (1990). Congenital toxoplasmosis: to screen or not to screen? *Public Health*, **104**, 9–20

Fetal and neonatal aspects of myasthenia gravis

46

V. Váradi

INTRODUCTION

Myasthenia gravis is a relatively serious disease which can influence the condition of the fetus and neonate. The importance of this impact is confirmed by numerous publications and Fennell and Ringel[1] and Plauché[2] have written excellent reviews on this subject.

HISTORY

In the first three decades of the 20th century the clinical features of myasthenia gravis were completely defined. Excess fatiguability results in diplopia, ptosis and weakness of facial, neck and extremity muscles. Chewing and swallowing can be difficult, so that the threat of aspiration is always present. Occasionally, respiratory distress predominates over all other symptoms.

As early as 1895 the treatment with physostigmine was suggested by Jolly[3] and in the 1930s it was successfully administered. At the same time acetylcholine was defined as a transmitter at the motor endplate. Physostigmine was followed by pyridostigmine with a longer duration of action and fewer side-effects[4].

Although thymectomy was used, as early as 1913, for the treatment of patients with myasthenia gravis and Graves disease, in 1936 the first successful thymectomy was performed for myasthenia gravis in a young woman with thymoma. With the development of surgery, anesthesia and respiratory care thymectomy became the second, but rather controversial, mode of therapy, because only slightly more than half of patients improve and the improvement may not be noted until years after the operation[5–8].

In the last two decades the role of autoimmunity in the pathogenesis of myasthenia gravis has been established. The discovery of diminished acetylcholine receptors in myasthenic postjunctional folds, circulating antibodies to acetylcholine receptors and the localization of antibody to acetylcholine receptors on the postsynaptic membrane suggests that the immunological abnormality in myasthenia gravis is humorally mediated[9–12]. This information led to the successful use of corticosteroids[13]. Other immunosuppressive drugs (azathioprine, cyclosporine) are also used in refractory cases[14,15]. Recently, the use of intravenous immunoglobulins has provided a substantial therapeutic advance in the treatment of myasthenia gravis along with other autoimmune diseases[16]. Plasmapheresis leads to a temporary fall of anti-acetylcholine receptor antibody titer and the improvement of myasthenic symptoms so it has become widely accepted in the treatment of myasthenic crisis. Improvement is usually short-lived without concomitant immunosuppressive therapy[17–19].

CLINICAL FEATURES AND DIAGNOSIS

The clinical diagnosis of myasthenia gravis is suspected with a history of skeletal muscle weakness. Repetitive exercise demonstrates rapid loss of muscle strength. Muscle strength is restored with anticholinesterase drugs.

Skeletal muscle weakness can be identified by the patient repeatedly squeezing your hand or flexing her arm against resistance. Sophisticated confirmatory studies including bulb reography, single-fiber electromyography, nerve-conduction studies, repetitive nerve stimulation and vital capacity determination accurately document the degree of loss of strength and establish a baseline against which to measure response to treatment.

Edrophonium chloride (Tensilon®) is the favored short-acting anticholinesterase medication to test the restoration of muscle strength. Injection of 2–10 mg of edrophonium (Tensilon test) results in prompt restoration of strength to the involved skeletal muscle. The drooping lids of ophthalmoplegia regress, and the slurred speech of dysarthria disappears.

In the neonatal period the diagnosis of transient myasthenia gravis is usually apparent in the presence of the clinical syndrome in the infant of a myasthenic mother. The onset of this disorder in approximately two-thirds of cases is within the first hours after birth, although this often occurs after an apparently normal period immediately following delivery. In 80% of patients onset is apparent within 24 h and the latest onset is 3 days. The characteristic neurological features are usually dramatic and evolve rapidly (Table 1).

The disturbance of cranial nerve musculature is a prominent feature. Nearly all patients exhibit feeding difficulties with weakness of sucking and swallowing. Tube feeding is required in approximately one-third of patients. Respiratory difficulties occur in two-thirds and are due to the inability to handle pharyngeal secretions and to weakness of the respiratory muscles. The cry is weak and facial diplegia is obvious in approximately 60% of affected infants. Generalized muscle weakness is recognized in 69% of the cases and hypotonia is marked in about 48%. Hypotonia in some degree is an almost constant feature. However,

Table 1 *Characteristic neurological features of myasthenia gravis in the neonate*

	Incidence (%)
Feeding disturbance	87
Generalized muscle weakness	69
Respiratory disturbance	65
Weak cry	60
Facial weakness	54
Marked hypotonia	48
Tube feeding required	31
Ptosis	15
Oculomotor disturbance	8

tendon reflexes are normally active and no fasciculation can be seen. In contrast to the most common congenital syndrome eye signs are uncommon, ptosis is apparent in only 15% of patients and oculomotor disturbance is seen in less than 10%[20].

Plauché[2], in his overviewing report, summarizes laboratories now able to determine titers of antibodies to various components of the myoneural junction. Anti-acetylcholine receptor protein precipitating antibodies were the first to be identified and are the most commonly used markers. The acetylcholine receptor-blocking antibodies may more accurately identify the myasthenic process[2].

Precipitating antibodies are detected using acetylcholine receptor complexed to iodinated α-bungarotoxin prepared from venom of the krait (*Bungarus caerulens*) by the method described by Lindstrom[21]. Approximately 80% of affected myasthenia gravis patients have significant titers of acetylcholine receptor-precipitating antibodies. Some authors caution against relating antibody levels to the severity, course, or prognosis of myasthenia gravis[22–25].

CLASSIFICATION

The categorization of myasthenic disorders was standardized in a classic article by Osserman and Genkins[26] in 1961 and expanded by Genkins and colleagues[27] in 1987 (Table 2).

EPIDEMIOLOGY

The prevalence of myasthenia gravis is between two and ten cases per 100 000 people. It can affect both sexes at all ages but most large studies contain twice as many female as male patients. It is markedly more common in young women. The onset of the disease before or during the childbearing years occurs in a significant proportion of women, so it is important to know the effect of this disease on pregnancy, the neonate and the puerperium.

Familial clustering of myasthenia cases exceeds that expected based on incidence figures, but no consistent HLA type or Mendelian inheritance pattern has been recognized[28,29].

Table 2 *Categories of myasthenic disorders*

Neonatal myasthenia
Adult myasthenia
  Stage I: Pure ocular myasthenia
  Stage I/A: Ocular symptoms with only electrophysiological evidence of generalization
  Stage II/A: Mild generalized myasthenia, predominantly skeletal (arms and legs)
  Stage II/B: Mild generalized myasthenia with bulbar symptoms (dysphagia, dysarthria and respiratory
    difficulties)
  Stage III: Acute fulminating myasthenia with progression from ocular symptoms to severe disability
    within 6 months
  Stage IV: Late severe generalized myasthenia
  Remission stage: Relief of all myasthenic symptoms, no further improvement with anticholinesterase
    medication. There may be residual fixed muscle function deficits

Engle[30] hypothesizes that the myasthenia gravis manifestations include several distinct genetic forms: an infantile autosomal recessive form, a hereditary X-linked form principally in non-white females at puberty and an acquired form that affects older men of all races.

Mediastinal thymic tumors, either lymphoblastic or epithelial, were found in 10% of fatal myasthenia gravis cases. Thymic lymph follicle hyperplasia was found in 75% of cases without thymomas.

Myasthenia gravis is associated with a number of other autoimmune diseases/systemic lupus, rheumatoid arthritis, Hashimoto's thyroiditis, autoimmune hemolytic anemia, polymyositis, sarcoidosis, ulcerative colitis, scleroderma, celiac disease, immune-complex nephritis and pernicious anemia[28].

PREGNANCY AND MYASTHENIA GRAVIS

Myasthenia gravis, when associated with pregnancy, has several features that make it a high-risk disease. According to the literature about one-third of the affected pregnant women improve during their pregnancy, one-third remain stable and one-third have an exacerbation of symptoms[1]. Exacerbations can occur in all three trimesters and therapeutic termination of pregnancy does not demonstrate consistent benefit in cases of first-trimester exacerbation[28]. Several other authors have had the same experience[31–33]. In addition, exacerbation has been described after termination probably due to surgery and/or anesthesia.

The exacerbation of symptoms during pregnancy is thought to correlate with a rise in progesterone and its influence on mineralocorticoids[34]. The role of previous thymectomy in exacerbation is controversial. Plauché[35] noted that equal proportions of thymectomized and non-thymectomized patients exhibit exacerbations. Others found lower maternal morbidity and mortality in the thymectomy rather than in the non-thymectomy group[18].

Cohen and co-workers[36] in 1976 first proposed an association between myasthenia gravis and pre-eclampsia. Duff[8] also found such cases and speculated that altered immune status might be an etiological factor in pre-eclampsia. Benshushan and associates[37] describe the serious therapeutic dilemmas which may arise when pre-eclampsia complicates pregnancy in a myasthenic patient. No pre-eclampsia was found by Plauché[35] in 10 myasthenic pregnancies reported in 1979. Similarly we did not find increased incidence of pre-eclampsia among 16 myasthenic mothers either[38].

FETAL MYASTHENIA GRAVIS

Severe cases of neonatal myasthenia gravis may be expressed prenatally as arthrogryposis or polyhydramnios[39–42].

Fetal myasthenia gravis could cause polyhydramnios and weak movement *in utero*. Polyhydramnios is associated with abnormalities of fetal swallowing[43]. In our series of 16 pregnancies of myasthenic mothers we found that polyhydramnios accompanies pregnancy of a myasthenic mother if the fetus is severely affected[38]. Verspyck and colleagues[44] describe an infant whose mother had no signs of neuromuscular disease. The case presented with severe polyhydramnios at 31 weeks. Sonographic and invasive work-up showed only an absence of fetal swallowing. At birth the infant had severe muscle weakness and respiratory distress. He also had high titers of antiacetylcholinesterase receptor antibodies of maternal origin. Antiacetylcholine receptor antibodies were also found in stored samples of fetal serum and amniotic fluid. Antiacetylcholine receptor antibody testing should be considered in cases of unexplained polyhydramnios[44].

In utero paralysis might also result in arthrogryposis as reported in three offspring of two mothers with myasthenia gravis[45,46]. Dinger and Prager[47] reported 11 newborn infants born to myasthenic mothers with distal arthrogryposis, severe hypotonia and respiratory distress who were unresponsive to the administration of pyridostigmine bromide. Of the 11, five were stillborn or died within the first day of life. The surviving children had profound weakness and needed ventilatory assistance for a long period. The severity of these few cases contrasts with the numerous reports of benign and transitory signs of neonatal myasthenia[47]. Barnes and co-workers[48] reported a sibship in which the syndrome of congenital arthrogryposis occurred in two male and two female neonates, three of whom died. Others have also reported the risk of recurrence of fetal arthrogryposis[49,50]. In subsequent pregnancies the extremely high risk of this association is indicated. In cases of arthrogryposis the lack of fetal movement is responsible for joint contractures. Fetuses without breathing movements, due mostly to paralysis of the diaphragm, may, in addition, develop pulmonary hypoplasia. Using serial plasmapheresis in an affected mother, who had given birth to a newborn infant with arthrogryposis in her previous pregnancy, the prevention of the same disease in the next pregnancy was possible[51]. Real-time ultrasonographic evaluations of the fetuses of myasthenic mothers can be used to monitor fetal movements and to detect the development of joint contractures *in utero*[50,52]. Early detection of reduced fetal limb motion is a challenge because of the wide variability of normal limb motion as the fetus goes in and out of sleep phases.

Another promising possibility for the intrauterine screening for affected fetuses is the use of intrapartum vibroacoustic stimulation. In as much as fetal acoustic stimulation results in a fetal reaction resembling the startle response of the newborn infant, Orvieto and associates[53] think it will be worthwhile performing this test antenatally in the next encountered fetuses of myasthenic mothers in order to assess its role in the prediction of neonatal myasthenia gravis.

The heterogeneity of prenatal presentations is poorly understood. Verspyck and colleagues[44] suggest antiacetylcholine receptor antibody testing in cases of unexplained polyhydramnios, even in the absence of past or present maternal symptoms of myasthenia gravis. Antiacetylcholine receptor antibodies can be found in affected cases not only in the serum of the mother and umbilical cord serum, but also in the amniotic fluid[40].

Attempts may be made to decrease the amount of circulating antibody crossing to the fetus. Interventions may include starting or increasing corticosteroid therapy, therapy with azathioprine, or serial plasmapheresis. Thymectomy is not usually performed during pregnancy[54].

LABOR AND DELIVERY

In the intrapartum period, fatigue in the mother increases, and may precipitate a myasthenic crisis[54]. During labor and delivery all myasthenia medications should be administered parenterally because of unpredictable gastrointestinal absorption of oral medication and prolonged gastric emptying. Administration of magnesium sulfate in the case of preeclampsia is contraindicated. Paralysis after magnesium has been described in patients with known myasthenia gravis, and there is a report to describe this paralysis as the initial or only manifestation of the disease[55]. The physical stress of labor and delivery increases myasthenic weakness. It is necessary to observe the patient in labor for signs of respiratory impairment[2].

Symptoms of respiratory distress can be non-specific and include irritability and restlessness. Arterial blood gases should be monitored and supplemental oxygen administered. In case of respiratory failure (hypoxia and hypercarbia) mechanical ventilation has to be instituted. Special attention should be paid to excessive tracheobronchial secretions in ventilator dependent cases.

The incidence of Cesarean section is not higher during the delivery of myasthenic patients. Vacuum extractor is recommended to shorten the second stage of labor[49]. In our series of 16 myasthenic pregnant women the frequency of Cesarean section was the same as in the normal pregnant population[38]. In mild and moderate myasthenia cases regional anesthesia is preferred for vaginal delivery by most authorities[56–59]. Rolbin and colleagues[57] and Burke[54] recommended epidural anesthesia to prevent fatigue. Esterase local anesthetics are contraindicated because of the decreased cholinesterase enzyme activity in myasthenic patients[60]. A mid-type local anesthetic (lidocaine) can be used for epidural anesthesia, and episiotomy as well, because it is metabolized normally.

For the patient with bulbar and respiratory involvement who requires Cesarean section general endotracheal anesthesia with halothane is recommended[28,57]. One should be aware of the fact, that myasthenic patients are very sensitive to stress, anesthetics and non-depolarizing muscle relaxants and that exacerbations are frequent in the postpartum period. That is why, apart from the bulbar involvement, only for obstetric indications should a Cesarean section be carried out.

PUERPERIUM AND BREAST FEEDING

In one-third of myasthenic pregnancy cases exacerbation occurs in the postpartum period, but there can also be improvement[61]. In a few cases remission occurred during pregnancy, which was followed by exacerbation after delivery. Postpartum deterioration can be sudden and devastating due to respiratory failure. Maternal death in myasthenic mother can be related either to worsening of myasthenic symptoms or treatment complications[2].

There are no predictive factors that identify the mother at risk for peripartum exacerbation of myasthenia gravis, or the newborn infant at risk for neonatal myasthenia. Optimal care for the parturient is achieved through a team approach involving the obstetrician, neurologist and pediatrician[62].

The issue of breast feeding has not been completely resolved for mothers with myasthenia gravis. Maternal antiacetylcholine receptor antibodies may pass to the newborn infant through breast milk and accentuate neonatal myasthenia. Muscarine symptoms (nausea, emesis, abdominal cramping, profuse diarrhea, etc.) have been described in the infants of women taking anticholinesterase agents. It seems appropriate to avoid breast feeding in the presence of postpartum myasthenic exacerbation, high titers of antiacetylcholine receptor antibodies, or in newborn infants with proven sensitivity to maternal anticholinesterase ingestion[28,63].

NEONATAL MYASTHENIA GRAVIS

Newborn and childhood myasthenia gravis has three forms. Neonatal myasthenia is a transitory disorder of the newborn of myasthenic mothers caused by the passive transfer of antibodies from mother to infant.

The congenital form of myasthenia gravis is a non-immunological disease resulting from a presynaptic and/or postsynaptic structural defect[64]. Only a few cases with congenital myasthenia have been reported in the literature, the most common symptoms being bilateral eyelid ptosis, ophthalmoparesis, easy fatiguability, respiratory and feeding difficulties. This form of myasthenia gravis will usually present as an emergency, primarily as respiratory failure associated with inhalation of gastric or oral secretions and/or lower respiratory tract infection. The child will usually have a history of having been floppy from birth (no progression of weakness except daily fluctuations) with classical fatigue of both bulbar and generalized musculature. There may be a positive history of siblings, cousins, or parents being involved[64]. Calderon-Gonzalez and co-workers[65] reported a congenital myasthenia case with dysphagia as the only clinical manifestation seen since the first days of the child's life confirming the diagnosis using a repetitive supramaximal stimulation test and obtaining excellent results with pyridostigmine. They concluded that although this is a rare form of the disease, congenital neonatal myasthenia should be considered in the differential diagnosis of newborn infants with difficulties in swallowing. The repetitive supramaximal stimulation test is the first choice of diagnostic procedure to be used in the neonatal period.

Another manifestation of congenital myasthenia is reported by Beydon and colleagues[66] in the form of esophageal dysfunction. Gastroesophageal reflux was diagnosed during the first weeks of life in a girl. Later the infant developed weakness of the eyelids and extraocular muscles; subcutaneous neostigmine completely removed the symptoms in a few minutes. Neuromuscular transmission tests showed a progressive decrease in eyelid muscle response on repetitive stimulation of the nerve, with a pattern of postsynaptic defects that was corrected by edrophonium chloride injection. Neither the girl nor her mother had acetylcholine receptor antibodies[66].

The chronic juvenile form of myasthenia gravis may occur at any time from birth to puberty. It is distinguished from the transient neonatal disorder by the self generation of acetylcholine receptor antibodies. Ophthalmoplegia is the predominant sign in most cases of juvenile myasthenia.

The occurrence of transitory neonatal myasthenia cannot be predicted by the course or severity of the maternal disease, by the presence or absence of thymectomy, or by the level of maternal acetylcholine receptor antibodies[18,67,68]. In fact a mother in complete remission may have a child with neonatal myasthenia gravis[69]. There is some evidence that mothers who have one child with myasthenia gravis are at increased risk for the second child developing the same syndrome[38,70]. Delmis and associates[71] observed an inverse relationship between

neonatal myasthenia and duration of disease in mothers. Incidence of neonatal myasthenia was higher in newborn infants born by mothers with a short duration of myasthenia gravis.

The exact mechanism for the development of neonatal myasthenia gravis is unclear. Passive transfer of acetylcholine receptor antibodies occurs to some degree in all children born to myasthenic mothers and not just in those who develop the syndrome. A longer half-life of acetylcholine receptor antibody was also noted in infants who developed neonatal myasthenia gravis. Anti-idiotypic antibodies identified differences in antibody specificity between the affected and unaffected children[72,73]. It is thought that children who develop neonatal myasthenia gravis may transiently synthesize antiacetylcholine receptor antibodies.

ACETYLCHOLINE RECEPTOR ANTIBODIES IN NEWBORN INFANTS OF MOTHERS WITH MYASTHENIA GRAVIS

Lefvert and Osterman[72] emphasize that antibodies to acetylcholine receptor are found in most patients with myasthenia gravis and the defect in neuromuscular transmission is attributed to these antibodies. A circulating factor had been suspected, because 8–18% of infants born to myasthenic mothers are affected by transient muscular weakness that is electrophysiologically and pharmacologically similar to the adult disease. The causative factor was presumed to be transferred from mother to neonate through the placenta. Keesey and colleagues[74] reported that the incidence of neonatal myasthenia was highly related to maternal antiacetylcholine antibody titer. However, there are other explanations:

(1) Only one of several subtypes of antibodies detected by the immunoprecipitation method might interact with acetylcholine receptors in neonatal postsynaptic membrane to cause the syndrome.

(2) Different infants might have different susceptibilities to the development of a

neuromuscular block because of local neuromuscular junction factors.

(3) Some humoral substances might inhibit the biological effects of antibody *in vivo* by blocking antibody binding to acetylcholine receptors in the infants.

Monnier and Fulpius[75] and Brenner and associates[76] suggest that α-fetoprotein inhibits the binding of antibody to acetylcholine receptor *in vitro*. This may be one explanation for the occurrence of unaffected infants of mothers with high titers[33]. Others did not find any significant effect of α-fetoprotein on the binding of acetylcholine receptor antibodies to receptor-toxin complex. In a study of 15 pregnancies the mothers showed no consistent pattern of exacerbations and remissions in parallel with the changing levels of α-fetoprotein that occur in pregnancy. Some children have symptoms at birth, which also seems to contradict the importance of α-fetoprotein as the main protective factor[72].

The binding of antibodies to endplate determinants other than acetylcholine receptors has been postulated by Melber[77]. In his case he demonstrates the placental transfer of acetylcholine-receptor negative serum produced myasthenia.

Neonatal myasthenia provided early evidence of a circulating factor, thought to be maternal IgG receptor antibody. The presence of acetylcholine receptor antibodies in the serum of both healthy and affected children born to myasthenic mothers has been demonstrated repeatedly[12]. Since the maternal antibodies are found in all infants, some additional factors must trigger the neonatal disease. It does not seem to depend on high maternal titer alone[72].

Although there are several reports on the birth of an affected child after normal siblings, the birth of an infant with neonatal myasthenia gravis increases the chance that the subsequent children will be similarly affected[33,38]. Neonatal myasthenia cannot be related to duration or severity of maternal disease, to any alteration in the maternal symptoms during pregnancy, or to thymectomy[78]. A mother in complete remission may give birth to an affected child.

Others found a significant difference between the half-life of the acetylcholine receptor antibody in newborn infants with the features of neonatal myasthenia gravis and unaffected infants, although the antibody concentration in the cord blood was equally high. The rapid disappearance of the antibody from the circulation of healthy children and the persistence of antibody in affected ones may be due to a transient synthesis of antibody in the child[72]. Moreover, it is known that the fetuses are capable of synthesizing IgG as early as the 20th week of pregnancy[79] and synthesis at birth has also been noted[80]. According to Tzartos and colleagues[81] although in a few cases significant differences in antibody specificities were observed between mothers and infants, whether myasthenic or not, generally the antigen specificities of the antibodies in sera from infants were similar to those of their mothers. Furthermore, no characteristic differences were detected between the antibody repertoires of mothers who transferred the disease and those who did not.

In the case of an affected child, different idiotypes should be found in mother and child. Lefvert and Osterman[72] evaluated this theory by subgrouping the antibodies according to IgG class, isoelectric spectra, binding properties and reaction with anti-idiotypic antibody. They found different amounts of cross-reacting acetylcholine receptor antibody idiotype in mother and child at birth in two patients with neonatal myasthenia. These differences increased after a few weeks. One patient seemed to synthesize receptor antibodies that reacted very well with the anti-idiotypic antibody. In the other patient the infant produced antibodies that did not react with anti-idiotypic antibody. In normal children and their mothers no such differences in acetylcholine receptor antibody reactivity with the anti-idiotypic antibody were found. Nakao and associates[73] also found that the binding properties of the maternal antibodies did not correspond to those found in a child with neonatal myasthenia. These findings support the theory that the receptor antibodies found at birth in neonatal myasthenia are not all transferred from the mother and that the affected children synthesize receptor antibodies even before birth. Failure of exchange transfusions to produce sustained lowering of the antibody titer also supports the theory of ongoing synthesis in the child. Antibody production in the child may be due to transfer of a cell clone from the mother. Another theory is that the passively transferred maternal antibodies may bind to and damage the endplate in the child, triggering occasional antibody synthesis. Although antibody levels do not seem to correlate well with the severity of generalized muscle weakness in adult myasthenia gravis, Keesey and co-workers[82] found that in neonatal myasthenia there appears to be at least a qualitative correlation between the falling antibody level and increasing strength. Although the antibodies to acetylcholine receptors accelerate the degradation of acetylcholine receptors, their titer level does not predict the magnitude of generalized symptoms.

Vernet der Garabedian and colleagues[83] investigated the specificities of autoantibodies directed against the acetylcholine receptor for embryonic and adult muscle. Acetylcholine receptors were studied in 22 mothers with myasthenia gravis and their newborn infants using human fetus and normal adult muscle preparations. In all 22 mothers had transmitted myasthenia gravis to their neonates with, in three cases, antenatal injury. A clear correlation was found between the occurrence of neonatal myasthenia gravis and the high overall level of antiacetylcholine receptor antibodies (embryonic or adult muscle acetylcholine receptors). However, a strong correlation was also found between the occurrence of neonatal myasthenia gravis and the ratio of antiembryonic acetylcholine receptor to antiadult muscle (Te/Ta) acetylcholine receptor antibodies ($p < 0.0002$). Taken together, these data suggest that autoantibodies directed against the embryonic form of the acetylcholine receptor could play a predominant role in the pathogenesis of neonatal myasthenia gravis. Paradoxically, the three cases with antenatal injury, presumably the most severe form of neonatal myasthenia gravis, were not associated with high Te/Ta. At the clinical level these observations could prove helpful in the prediction of transmission of neonatal myasthenia gravis[83].

MANAGEMENT OF NEONATAL MYASTHENIA GRAVIS

It is necessary to observe the newborn infants of every myasthenic mother carefully for signs of weakness of skeletal muscles, particularly those that control breathing and swallowing. The infant may require support with anticholinesterase drugs until such weakness subsides, usually for about 3 weeks.

In the early postnatal period an obscure respiratory inadequacy and hypoventilation might be the signs of transient myasthenia gravis even in the absence of known maternal disease. In these cases an edrophonium chloride challenge test should be performed to rule out myasthenia gravis. In the myasthenic newborn infant the need for ventilatory support declines immediately after the edrophonium administration[38,84,85].

MONITORING

In a crisis situation (acute worsening of symptoms) the myasthenia gravis patient must be monitored primarily for respiratory and pharyngeal function, other muscle weakness is of secondary importance[64]. The cardinal rule must be preservation of respiratory and pharyngeal function. Myasthenia gravis is a disease not only of weakness but also of fatigue, therefore strength assessment must be made in reference to time: time of last medication and time of last examination.

Monitoring of the respiratory system should include:

(1) Clinical observations for signs of gasping, inability to handle secretions, cyanosis, increasing respiratory rate initially, followed by a decrease, and increasing cardiac rate initially, followed by a decrease.

(2) Laboratory investigation – chest roentgenogram, arterial blood-gas tensions and pH.

(3) Assessment of recovery of respiratory function.

   (a) Clinical observation for signs of return of diaphragmatic movement, and maintenance of color, heart rate and state of well-being whilst the patient is disconnected from the ventilator.

   (b) Laboratory investigation – repetitive measurement of arterial blood-gas tensions and pH; careful attention should be paid to the quality and character of tracheal secretion; cultures should be obtained.

Monitoring of the neurological system should include:

(1) Assessment of oculomotor function (ptosis, dysconjugate gaze);

(2) Assessment of motor function or other cranial nerve function and proximal and distal somatic muscle groups. Fasciculations indicate overmedication;

(3) Assessment of responsiveness to anticholinesterase medication.

Monitoring of the autonomic system should include:

(1) Observation of patient for signs of anticholinesterase excess (cholinergic stimulation, profuse sweating, lacrimation, salivation, bradycardia, small pupils, diarrhea);

(2) Checking for signs of atropine-like agent excess: dry skin, dilated pupils, altered mental status, tachycardia, hypertension.

Pharyngeal assessment for dysphagia should be performed hourly to prevent inhalation pneumonia.

Monitoring of the renal-metabolic system should include:

(1) Ensuring adequate nutrition;

(2) Assessment of serum Ca for hypercalcemia, as at every patient immobilized for a long period of time;

(3) Assessment of character and frequency of stools and prevention of constipation.

TREATMENT

The symptoms usually reach their zenith in 24–72 h and then slowly improve over the next few weeks or months. The severity of symptoms dictates the extent of therapy. If the child is only mildly affected, anticholinesterase medication is probably the best choice. Neostigmine methylsulfate may be used since it can be given both orally and parenterally, however, it has more cholinergic side-effects. The usual starting dose is 0.02 mg/kg parenterally or orally. Pyridostigmine bromide (Mestinone®) is probably the drug of choice, since it has fewer side-effects, but it is available only for oral administration. The usual starting dose is 0.3 mg/kg every 3–8 h, given half an hour before feedings. The dose should be adjusted to optimize strength and minimize side-effects. Occasionally, a parasympatholytic drug (atropine) is given to reduce excessive secretion. Medication can usually be tapered and then discontinued by age 4–10 weeks.

Alternatively, if the child is in respiratory or pharyngeal failure, preservation of respiratory or pharyngeal function by mechanical ventilation in addition to nasogastric feeding is obviously appropriate. Blood exchange

Table 3 *Drugs which are hazardous in cases of neonatal myasthenia gravis*[64]

Drugs to be avoided
Membrane stabilizers
procainamide
quinine
quinidine
Muscle relaxants
diazepam (Valium)
baclofen (Lioresal)
chlordiazepoxide (Librium)
Drugs to be used with caution
Antibiotics
aminoglycosides
tetracycline
Endocrine or steroidal compounds
corticosteroids
corticotropin (ACTH)
Membrane stabilizers
phenytoin (Dilantin)
carbamazepine (Tegretol)
valproic acid (Depakene)

transfusions (two blood volumes) have been found to be quite effective. The passive transmitted antineuromuscular junction antibodies are thought to be removed. With blood volume exchange, mechanical ventilation and nasogastric feeding can be discontinued much earlier and the difficult problem of determining the proper dose of anticholinesterase is avoided. Early exchange transfusion has been suggested for the newborn infant who is severely affected[34]. The idea came from a case, where an infant with transient neonatal myasthenia gravis had a double volume exchange transfusion because of maternal-fetal blood group incompatibility. This seemed to accelerate both the decline in antiacetylcholine antibody titer and clinical improvement[86]. We had five neonatal myasthenic cases who responded readily to blood exchange transfusions[38]. Plasmapheresis with a special technique also has the same effect[87].

At least one child whose mother was on anticholinesterase medication during her pregnancy has been reported to have severe cholinergic symptoms which persisted for the first 10 weeks of life. Because of the profuse salivation and lacrimation, atropine (0.01 mg/kg every 6 h) was necessary to control these symptoms. A list of drugs which are hazardous in cases of myasthenia gravis is shown in Table 3.

References

1. Fennell, D F. and Ringel, S. P. (1987). Myasthenia gravis and pregnancy. *Obstet. Gynecol. Surv.*, **41**, 414–21
2. Plauché, W. C. (1991). Myasthenia gravis in mothers and their newborns. *Clin. Obstet. Gynecol.*, **34**, 82–99
3. Jolly (1895). Cited by Harvey, A. M. (1970). Myasthenia gavis. The first 100 years in perspective. *Trans. Am. Clin. Climatol. Assoc.*, **82**, 149
4. Osserman, K. E. (1958). *Myasthenia Gravis.* (New York: Gruna and Stratton)
5. Buckingham, J. M., Howard, F. M., Bernatz, P. E., Payne, W. S. and Harrison, E. G. (1976). The value of thymectomy in myasthenia gravis. A computer-assisted matched study. *Ann. Surg.*, **184**, 453–8
6. Papatestas, A. E., Genkins, G. and Jaretzki, A. (1978). Symposium on therapeutic controversies: myasthenia gravis. Cervical thymectomy. *Trans. Am. Neurol. Assoc.*, **103**, 286–91
7. Plauché, W. C. (1964). Myasthenia gravis in pregnancy. *Am. J. Obstet. Gynecol.*, **88**, 404–9
8. Duff, G. B. (1979). Preeclampsia and the patient with myasthenia gravis. *Obstet. Gynecol.*, **54**, 355–8
9. Drachman, D. B. (1978). Myasthenia gravis. *N. Engl. J. Med.*, **298**, 136–42, 186–93
10. Lindstrom, J. M., Seybold, M. E., Lennon, V. A., Whittingham, S. and Duane, D. D. (1976). Antibody to acetylcholine receptors in myasthenia gravis: prevalence, clinical correlates and diagnostic value. *Neurology*, **26**, 1054–9
11. Bender, A. N., Ringel, S. P., Engel, W K., Daniels, M. P. and Vogel, Z. (1975). Myasthenia gravis: a serum factor binding acetylcholine receptors of the human neuromuscular junction. *Lancet*, **1**, 607–9
12. Engel, A G. (1979). Myasthenia gravis. In Vinken, P. J., Bruyn, G. W. and Ringel, S. P. (eds.) *Handbook of Clinical Neurology*, Vol. 41, pp. 95–145. (Amsterdam: North-Holland Publishing Co)
13. Johns, T. R. (1977). Treatment of myasthenia gravis: long-term administration of corticosteroids with remarks on thymectomy. In Griggs, R. C. and Moxley, R. T. (eds.), *Treatment of Neuromuscular Diseases*, 3rd edn., pp. 99–122. (New York: Raven Press)
14. Mertens, H. G., Balzereit, F. and Leipert, M. (1969). The treatment of severe myasthenia gravis with immunosuppressive agents. *Neurology*, **2**, 321–39
15. Frey, F. J. (1990). Cyclosporin in autoimmune diseases. *Schweiz. Med. Wochenschr.*, **120**, 772–86
16. Bardare, M. and Dellepiane, R. M. (1991). Current developments in the use of intravenous immunoglobulins. *Minerva Pediatr.*, **43**, 665–74
17. Lisak, R. P. and Schotland, D. L. (1978). Plasmapheresis in the treatment of myasthenia gravis. In Symposium on therapeutic controversies: myasthenia gravis. *Trans. Am. Neurol. Assoc.*, **103**, 292–302
18. Eden, R. D. and Gall, S. A. (1983). Myasthenia gravis and pregnancy: a reappraisal of thymectomy. *Obstet. Gynecol.*, **62**, 328–33
19. Havard, C. W. and Fonseca, V. (1990). New treatment approaches to myasthenia gravis. *Drugs*, **39**, 66–73

20. Volpe, J. J. *Neurology of the Newborn*, 3rd edn., pp. 621–6. (Philadelphia, London, Toronto, Montreal, Sydney, Tokyo: W.B. Saunders Company)

21. Lindstrom, J. (1977). An assay for antibodies to human AChR in serum from patients with myasthenia gravis. *Clin. Immunol. Immunopathol.*, **7**, 36–43

22. Vernet der Garbedian, B., Eymard, B., Bach, J. F. and Morel, E. (1989). Alpha-bungarotoxin blocking antibodies in neonatal myasthenia gravis: frequency and selectivity. *J. Neuroimmunol.*, **21**, 41–7

23. Elias, S. B., Butler, I. and Appel, S. H. (1979). Neonatal myasthenia gravis in an infant of a myasthenic mother in remission. *Ann. Neurol.*, **6**, 72–5

24. Heilbronn, E. (1979). Short review of progress in experimental myasthenia gravis bearing on the pathogenesis of myasthenia gravis. *Prog. Brain Res.*, **49**, 459–63

25. Roses, A. D., Olanow, C. W., McAdams, M. W. and Lane, R. J. M. (1981). No direct correlation between serum AChRab levels and clinical state of individual patients with myasthenia gravis. *Neurology (New York)*, **31**, 220–4

26. Osserman, K. E. and Genkins, G. (1961). Studies in myasthenia gravis: review of a twenty year experience in over 1200 patients. *Mt. Sinai J. Med. (New York)*, **38**, 497–537

27. Genkins, G., Kornfeld, P., Papatestas, A. E., Bender, A. N. and Motta, R. J. (1987). Clinical experience in more than 2000 patients with myasthenia gravis. *Ann. NY Acad. Sci.*, **505**, 500–13

28. Mitchell, P. J. and Bebbington, M. (1992). Myasthenia gravis in pregnancy. *Obstet. Gynecol.*, **80**, 178–81

29. Ahlsten, G., Lefvert, A. K., Osterman, P. O., Stalberg, E. and Safwenberg, J. (1992). Follow-up study of muscle function in children of mothers with myasthenia gravis during pregnancy. *J. Child. Neurol.*, **7**, 264–9

30. Engel, A. G. (1980). Morphologic and immunologic findings in myasthenia gravis and EMG syndromes. *J. Neurol. Neurosurg. Psychiatry*, **43**, 577–89

31. Hay, D. M. (1969). Myasthenia gravis in pregnancy. *Br. J. Obstet. Gynaecol.*, **76**, 323–9

32. Viets, H. R., Schwab, R. S. and Brazier, M. A. B. (1942). The effects of pregnancy on the course of myasthenia gravis. *J. Am. Med. Assoc.*, **119**, 236–42

33. Namba, T., Brown, S. B. and Grob, D. (1970). Neonatal myasthenia gravis: report of two cases and review of the literature. *Pediatrics*, **45**, 488–504

34. Frenkel, M. and Ehrlich, E. N. (1964). Influence of progesterone and mineralocorticoids upon myasthenia gravis. *Ann. Intern. Med.*, **60**, 971–81

35. Plauché, W. C. (1979). Myasthenia gravis in pregnancy: an update. *Am. J. Obstet. Gynecol.*, **135**, 691–7

36. Cohen, B. A., London, R. S. and Goldstein, P. J. (1976). Myasthenia gravis and pre-eclampsia. *Obstet. Gynecol.*, **45**, (Suppl. 1), 35s

37. Benshushan, A., Rojansky, N. and Weinstein, D. (1994). Myasthenia gravis and pre-eclampsia. *Isr. J. Med. Sci.*, **30**, 229–33

38. Váradi, V., Nagy, A., György, I., Machay, T. and Papp, Z. (1995). Transitorikus újszülöttkori myasthenia gravis. *Orv. Hetil.*, **136**, 401–5

39. Stoll, C., Ehret-Mentre, M. C., Treisser, A. and Tranchant, C. (1991). Prenatal diagnosis of congenital myasthenia with arthrogryposis in a myasthenic mother. *Prenat. Diagn.*, **11**, 17–22

40. Morel, E., Bach, J. F., Briard, M. L. and Aubry, J. P. (1984). Neonatal myasthenia gravis. Anti-acetylcholine receptor antibodies in the amniotic fluid. *J. Neuroimmunol.*, **6**, 313–17

41. Moutard-Codou, M. L., Delleur, M. M., Dulac, O., Morel, E., Voyer, M. and de Gamara, E. (1987). Myasthénie néo-natale sévère avec arthrogrypose. *Nouv. Presse Méd.*, **16**, 615–18

42. Vincent, A., Newland, C., Brueton, L., Beeson, D., Riemersma, S., Huson, S. M. and Newsom-Davies, J. (1995). Arthrogryposis multiplex congenita with maternal autoantibodies specific for a fetal antigen. *Lancet*, **346**, 24–5

43. Lloyd, J. R. and Clatworthy, H. W. (1958). Hydramnios as an aid to the early diagnosis of congenital obstruction of the alimentary tract: a study of the maternal and fetal factors. *Pediatrics*, **21**, 903–9

44. Verspyck, E., Mandelbrot, L., Dommergues, M., Huon, C., Woimant, F., Baumann, C. and Garabedian, B. V. (1993). Myasthenia gravis with polyhydramnios in the fetus of an asymptomatic mother. *Prenat. Diagn.*, **13**, 539–42

45. Shepard, M. K. (1971). Arthrogryposis multiplex congenita in sibs. *Birth Defects*, **7**, 127

46. Holmes, L. B., Driscoll, S. G. and Bradley, W. G. (1979). Multiple contractures in newborn of mother with myasthenia gravis. *Pediatr. Res.*, **13**, 486

47. Dinger, J. and Prager, B. (1993). Arthrogryposis multiplex in a newborn of a myasthenic mother. Case report and literature. *Neuromuscul. Disord.*, **3**, 335–9

48. Barnes, P. R., Kanabar, D. J., Brueton, L., Newsom-Davies, J., Huson, S. M., Mann, N. P. and Hilton-Jones, D. (1995). Recurrent congenital arthrogryposis leading to a diagnosis of myasthenia gravis in an initially asymptomatic mother. *Neuromuscul. Disord.*, **5**, 59–65

49. Tranchant, C., Ehret, C., Labouret, P., Gasser, B. and Warter, J. M. (1991). Arthrogryposis and

maternal myasthenia gravis. Risk of recurrence. *Rev. Neurol. Paris*, **147**, 62–4

50. Flagg, C. (1991). Myasthenia gravis. When the patient is pregnant. *Registered Nurse (USA)*, **54**, 57

51. Carr, S. R., Gilchrist, J. M., Abuelo, D. N. and Clark, D. (1991). Treatment of antenatal myasthenia gravis. *Obstet. Gynecol.*, **78**, 485–9

52. Vajsar, J., Sloane, A., MacGregor, D. L., Ronen, G. M., Becker, L. E. and Jay, V. (1995). Arthrogryposis multiplex congenita due to congenital myasthenic syndrome. *Pediatr. Neurol.*, **12**, 237–41

53. Orvieto, R., Levy, T., Peleg, D. and Ben-Rafael, Z. (1994). The role of intrapartum vibroacoustic stimulation in the prediction of neonatal myasthenia gravis. *Med. Hypotheses*, **42**, 129–30

54. Burke, M. E. (1993). Myasthenia gravis and pregnancy. *J. Perinat. Neonatal Nurs.*, **7**, 11–21

55. Bashuk, R. G. and Krendel, D. A. (1990). Myasthenia gravis presenting as weakness after magnesium administration. *Muscle Nerve*, **13**, 708–12

56. McNall, P. G. and Jafarnia, M. R. (1965). Management of myasthenia gravis in obstetrical patients. *Am. J. Obstet. Gynecol.*, **92**, 518–25

57. Rolbin, S. H., Levinson, G., Shnider, S. M. and Wright, R. G. (1978). Anesthetic consideration for myasthenia gravis and pregnancy. *Anesth. Analg.*, **57**, 441–7

58. Perry, C. P., Hilliard, G. D., Gilstrap, L. C. and Harris, R. E. (1975). Myasthenia gravis in pregnancy. *Ala. J. Med. Sci.*, **12**, 219–21

59. Foldes, F. F. and McNall, P. G. (1962). Myasthenia gravis. A guide for anaesthesiologist. *Anaesthesiology*, **23**, 837

60. Foldes, F. F. (1959). Factors which alter the effects of muscle relaxants. *Anaesthesiology*, **20**, 464–504

61. Giwa-Osagie, O. F., Newton, J. R. and Larcher, V. (1981). Obstetrical performance of patients with myasthenia gravis. *Int. J. Gynecol. Obstet.*, **19**, 267–70

62. Ohta, M., Matsubara, F., Hayashi, K., Nakao, K. and Nishitani, H. (1981). Acetylcholine receptor antibodies in infants of mothers with myasthenia gravis. *Neurology (New York)*, **31**, 1019–22

63. Brenner, T., Shahin, R., Steiner, I. and Abramsky, O. (1992). Presence of anti-acetylcholine receptor antibodies in human milk: possible correlation with neonatal myasthenia gravis. *Autoimmunity*, **12**, 315–16

64. Cook, J. D. (1984). Myasthenia gravis. In Levin, D. L., Morriss, F. C. and Moore, G. C. (eds.) *A Practical Guide to Pediatric Intensive Care*, 2nd edn., pp. 155–66. (St Louis, Toronto, Princeton: C.V. Mosby Company)

65. Calderon-Gonzalez, R., Alonso-Rivera, C. G., Elizondo-Vazquez, J. and Calderon-Sepulveda, R. (1990). Congenital myasthenia gravis. Presentation of a case with dysphagia as the only clinical manifestation. *Bol. Med. Hosp. Infant Mex.*, **47**, 851–5

66. Beydon, N. Faure, C., Mayer, M. and Bourrillon, A. (1993). Congenital myasthenia gravis with esophageal involvement. *Arch. Fr. Pediatr.*, **50**, 219–22

67. Plauché, W. C. (1983). Myasthenia gravis. *Clin. Obstet. Gynecol.*, **26**, 592–604

68. Gutmann, L. and Seybold, M. E. (1980). Acetylcholine receptor antibodies in absence of neonatal myasthenia gravis. *Arch. Neurol.*, **37**, 738

69. Elias, S. B., Butler, I. and Appel, S. (1979). Neonatal myasthenia gravis in an infant of a myasthenic mother in remission. *Ann. Neurol.*, **6**, 72–5

70. Yerushalmy, J., van der Berg, B., Erhardt, C. L. and Jacobziner, H. (1965). Birth weight and gestation as indices of immaturity. *Am. J. Dis. Child.*, **109**, 43–57

71. Delmis, J., Drazancic, A., Jusic, A. and Petric, M. (1990). Myasthenia gravis in pregnancy. *Lijec. Vjesn.*, **112**, 301–4

72. Lefvert, A. K. and Osterman, P. O. (1983). Newborn infants to myasthenic mothers: a clinical study and an investigation of acetylcholine receptor antibodies in 17 children. *Neurology*, **33**, 133–8

73. Nakao, K., Nishitani, H., Suzuki, M., Ohta, M. and Hayashi, K. (1977). Anti-acetylcholine receptor IgG in neonatal myasthenia gravis. *N. Engl. J. Med.*, **297**, 169

74. Keesey, J., Lindstrom, J., Cokely, H. and Hermann, C. (1977). Anti-acetylcholine receptor antibody in neonatal myasthenia gravis. *N. Engl. J. Med.*, **296**, 55

75. Monnier, V. L. and Fulpius, B. W. (1977). A radio-immunoassay for the quantitative evaluation of anti-human acetylcholine receptor antibodies in myasthenia gravis. *Clin. Exp. Immunol.*, **29**, 16–22

76. Brenner, T., Beyth, Y. and Abramsky, O. (1980). Inhibitory effect of alpha-fetoprotein on the binding of myasthenia gravis antibody to acetylcholine receptors. *Proc. Natl. Acad. Sci. USA*, **77**, 3635–9

77. Melber, D. (1988). Maternal-fetal transmission of myasthenia gravis with acetylcholine-receptor antibody. *N. Engl. J. Med.*, **318**, 996–7

78. Levinson, A. I., Zweiman, N. and Lisak, R. P. (1987). Immunopathogenesis and treatment of myasthenia gravis. *J. Clin. Immunol.*, **7**, 187–97

79. van Furth, R., Schuit, H. R. E. and Hijmans, W. (1965). The immunological development of the human fetus. *J. Exp. Med.*, **122**, 1173–88

80. Ropartz, C., Rivat, L. and Rousseau, P. U. (1965). La transmission des facteurs Gm et Inv de la

mère a l'enfant nouveau-né. *Ann. Genet. (Paris)*, **8**, 39–43

81. Tzartos, S. J., Efthimiadis, A., Morel, E., Eymard, B. and Bach, J. F. (1990). Neonatal myasthenia gravis: antigenic specificities of antibodies in sera from mothers and their infants. *Clin. Exp. Immunol.*, **80**, 376–80

82. Keesey, J., Lindstrom, J., Cokely, H. and Herrmann, C. (1977). Anti-acetylcholine receptor antibody in neonatal myasthenia gravis. *N. Engl. J. Med.*, **296**, 55

83. Vernet der Garabedian, R., Lacokova, M., Eymard, B., Morel, E., Faltin, M., Zajac, J., Sadovsky, O., Dommergues, M., Tripon, P. and Bach, J. F. (1994). Association of neonatal myasthenia gravis with antibodies against the fetal acetylcholine receptor. *J. Clin. Invest.*, **94**, 555–9

84. Jones, W. R. (1994). Autoimmune disease and pregnancy. *Aust. NZ J. Obstet. Gynaecol.*, **34**, 251–8

85. Bianchi, D. W. and Van Marter, L. J. (1994). An approach to ventilator-dependent neonates with arthrogryposis. *Pediatrics*, **94**, 682–6

86. Donat, J. F., Donat, J. R. and Lennon, V. A. (1981). Exchange transfusion in neonatal myasthenia gravis. *Neurology*, **31**, 911–12

87. Seggia, J. C. and Abreu, P. (1992). Plasmapheresis in neurology. Critical analysis of indications and protocols. *Arq. Neuropsiquiatr.*, **50**, 324–8

Surfactant therapy for neonatal respiratory distress syndrome

47

T. Fujiwara

INTRODUCTION

Soon after the discovery of lung surfactant[1], Avery and Mead[2] proposed the role of surfactant deficiency as a major pathophysiological factor in the neonatal respiratory distress syndrome (RDS). In 1980, we reported the first successful administration of a reconstituted bovine surfactant given in a liquid form, instilled into the airways of preterm infants with RDS[3]. Since then, several thousand infants with RDS have received exogenous surfactants in controlled trials. The efficacy of this treatment has been confirmed, and surfactant therapy is now part of the routine management of infants with immature lungs all over the world. Surfactant therapy represents a major breakthrough in the treatment and survival of preterm infants. The results of clinical trials have been extensively discussed in recent reviews[4,5] and books[6-8].

In this chapter, some of the controversial issues regarding current clinical trials evaluating the efficacy of prophylaxis and treatment of RDS with different surfactants and also the issues regarding the optimization of surfactant ther-apy, based on our own experience of 15 years of work in this field, will be discussed.

TYPES OF SURFACTANT FOR CLINICAL USE

The surfactants available for clinical use can be classified into three categories: an organic solvent extract of animal lung lavage or of minced lung saline solution extract with or without additives, natural surfactant isolated from human amniotic fluid, and synthetic surfactants. Four bovine-based and one porcine-based surfactants have been prepared by different techniques (Table 1). All of these surfactants contain hydrophobic proteins SP-B and SP-C, but no SP-A. Synthetic surfactants based on synthetic lipids and proteins produced by recombinant DNA technology or direct synthesis are still at the developmental stage.

The 'best' surfactant for treating infants with RDS has not yet been clearly identified. One of the criteria for an optimal surfactant is that it

Table 1 *Surfactant preparations, dosage and volume for clinical use*

Preparation	Source	Dose (phospholipids, mg/kg)	Volume (ml/kg)
Surfactant TA	bovine	100	3
Survanta®	bovine	100	4
CLSE	bovine	90–100	3
Infasurf®	bovine	90–100	3
Alveofact®*	bovine	50	1.2
Curosurf®	porcine	100–200	1–2.5
Amniotic-fluid surfactant	human	60	3
ALEC	DPPC/PG/7 : 3	100	1
Exosurf®	DPPC/hexadecanol tyloxapol/NaCl	67.5	5

CLSE, calf lung surfactant extract (Rochester, USA); DPPC, dipalmitoyl phosphatidylcholine; PG, phosphatidylglycerol; ALEC, artificial lung expanding compound; *, SF-RI 1, Thomae GmbH, Germany

should convert the pulmonary mechanics (pressure-volume curves and compliance) and the degree of alveolar expansion of the lungs of surfactant-deficient animals to levels equal to those of mature term animals[6]. Inasmuch as there is little information available concerning the *in vivo* dose–response relationships between different surfactants, Maeta and colleagues[9,10] performed a randomized blind study comparing the dose-response of different surfactant preparations in prematurely delivered rabbit fetuses (gestation, 27 days) with mature controls (gestation, 30 days). This study showed that Surfactant TA (Surfacten®, Tokyo Tanabe, Japan) satisfied this criterion for an optimal surfactant with a dose of only 30 mg/kg, while other surfactants including Survanta® (Abbott Laboratories, Chicago, USA), a modification of Surfactant TA, required a dose of more than 100 mg/kg to show similar improvement. Synthetic surfactants (Exosurf® (Burroughs Wellcome, USA) and artificial lung expanding compound (ALEC, Pumactant, Britannia Pharmaceuticals, UK)) failed to improve both pulmonary mechanics and alveolar expansion of these animals even with a dose of 200 mg/kg.

CLINICAL RESPONSE TO SURFACTANTS

Rescue treatment

Rescue trials have used surfactants to treat infants with established RDS in order to modify the course of RDS. There have been 13 randomized trials of different surfactants in a rescue mode, 11 of which reported sequential changes in the fraction of inspired oxygen (FiO$_2$) after surfactant administration[11-21]. This author feels that, where possible, a combination of similar trials using the same surfactant would be of use to the neonatologist in assessing the benefit of surfactant treatment. A single-dose rescue treatment with Surfactant TA has been evaluated in three controlled randomized clinical trials[11-13]. Thus, the data from three rescue trials using a single dose of Surfactant TA, and those from two rescue trials using a single dose

of Survanta[14,15] were combined, and the combined data were used for comparison with the combined or single data from other trials. The severity of RDS is reflected in the level of the FiO$_2$ required to maintain normal arterial oxygenation.

Figure 1 shows a comparison of the effect of different surfactant preparations on oxygenation over the first 96 h after treatment. The trials that reported the FiO$_2$ values at 0, 6, 12, 24, 48, 72 or 96 h after treatment have been selected for this comparison. All the trials showed significant improvements in respiratory status. The larger the difference in the FiO$_2$ level between the treated and control infants the better the effect. It is clear from Figure 1 that the magnitude and speed of action of naturally-derived surfactants exceed those reported for synthetic surfactants. However, none of the trials reported the reduction of the mean FiO$_2$ value to less than 0.3 at 6 h post-treatment, which is equivalent to that required for ventilated infants without lung disease, indicating that rescue treatment does not cure RDS completely, leaving some infants with some degree of lung injury. Although all the studies demonstrated that surfactant therapy can reverse the pulmonary surfactant deficiency, there are some differences in response among the different surfactants.

The suboptimal response seen in these trials may be related to several factors, such as some degree of early lung injury due to surfactant deficiency occurring before surfactant therapy, some degree of structural immaturity, pathological conditions of RDS other than surfactant deficiency, or the quality of surfactant. The major concern about the use of naturally-derived surfactant is quality control. Treatment with 'suboptimal' surfactant may require larger and multiple doses to show the magnitude of response equivalent to that seen with a single dose of 'optimal' surfactant.

Head-to-head clinical trials comparing the efficacy of different surfactants have recently been reported. In a multicenter randomized trial, Horbar and colleagues[22] compared the efficacy of Exosurf with Survanta for the rescue treatment of RDS. Infants treated with Survanta required significantly less oxygen and lower

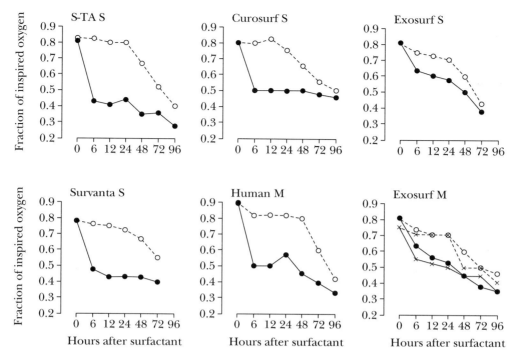

Figure 1 *Sequential changes in oxygen requirements in rescue trials of different surfactants. S-TA S, data combined from the three trials of surfactant TA[11–13]; Survanta S, data combined from the two trials of Survanta[14,15]; Curosurf S, data from the single trial of Curosurf[16]; Human M, data combined from the two trials of human amniotic fluid surfactant[17,18]; Exosurf S, data combined from the single trial of Exosurf[19]; Exosurf M; data combined from the two trials of Exosurf[20,21]; S, single dose; M, multiple dose; ○- - -○, placebo; ●——●, surfactant treated; x——x, surfactant-treated; x- - -x, placebo*

ventilatory pressure than those treated with Exosurf, but there were no significant differences between the two surfactants in the incidence of death or bronchopulmonary dysplasia. Also in a recent randomized blinded trial, Alvarado and co-workers[23] showed a clear difference in efficacy between Survanta and Exosurf for the treatment of established RDS. The majority of the Exosurf group (33/39) required all four doses of surfactant compared to less than half of the Survanta group (16/33, 48%; $p < 0.01$). The reductions pre- and 12 h post-treatment were significantly greater for the Survanta group compared to the Exosurf group for ventilator rate and FiO_2. The Survanta group also had shorter durations of mechanical ventilation, supplemental oxygen and hospitalization. However, the acute effects of these surfactants are again clearly suboptimal.

Prophylactic treatment

The goal of delivery-room treatment, referred to as prophylactic treatment, is to prevent both RDS and any injury to the preterm surfactant-deficient lung that might result from mechanical ventilation. Eleven randomized trials using different surfactants have been reported. Eight of these trials reported sequential changes in FiO_2 values at 6–72 h of age[24–30]. These values are shown in Figure 2. If prophylactic treatment prevents RDS completely, the treated infants should have FiO_2 of less than 0.3 shortly after birth. However, all prophylactic trials except that of Merritt and associates[27] included 40–60% normal infants in both surfactant-treated and control groups. Consequently, the FiO_2 values reported in the majority of trials must have been greater than indicated by the data for all infants with or without RDS. Only the trial of Merritt and colleagues[27] showed the FiO_2

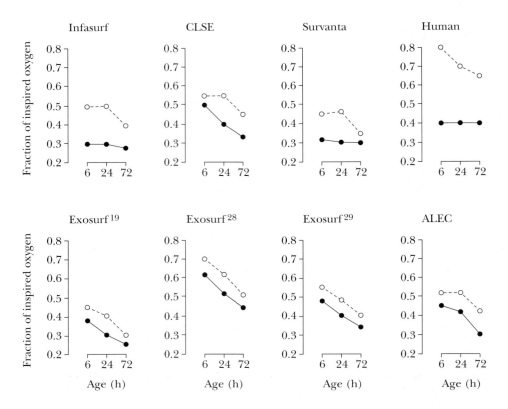

Figure 2 *Sequential changes in oxygen requirements in prophylactic trials of different surfactants. Infasurf[24]; calf surfactant extract, CLSE[25]; Survanta[26]; Human[27]; three trials of Exosurf[19,28,29]; artificial lung expanding compound, ALEC[30]; o- - -o, placebo; ●——●, surfactant-treated*

of 0.8 for the control group at 6 h of age, indicating that only the infants who were destined to severe RDS received surfactant. Unfortunately, a multiple-dose human surfactant used in this trial did not prevent RDS completely. Other trials using different surfactants showed significant reductions in the severity of RDS, but did not achieve the goal of prevention of RDS.

Outcome data from trials

The meta-analysis of the outcome data derived from all the trials of different surfactants reported by Soll[8] showed that the absolute decrease in overall neonatal mortality was 41% by rescue treatment and 40% by prophylactic treatment. Surfactant treatment resulted in a striking decrease in pneumothorax and other air leaks[8].

Once a neonate has been born prematurely, the prevention of bronchopulmonary dysplasia rests on preventing RDS. However, as noted in the previous section, the individual results of prophylactic trials have not provided conclusive evidence that surfactant therapy, either a single- or multiple-dose strategy at birth, offers all premature neonates protection against RDS. The incidence of bronchopulmonary dysplasia was not consistently lower, although it was reduced in individual studies.

Prophylaxis vs. rescue treatment

There is considerable controversy about the timing of surfactant therapy. The relative effectiveness of administering surfactant prophylactically compared with waiting until RDS develops was assessed in six controlled trials

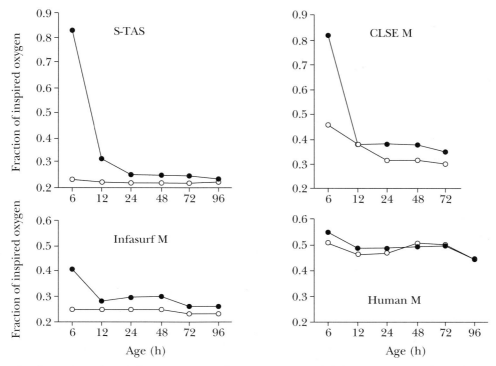

Figure 3 *Comparison of prophylaxis vs. rescue surfactant treatment with different surfactants. S-TA, Surfactant TA[31]; CLSE, calf lung surfactant extract M[32]; Infasurf M[33]; Human M[34];* ●——●, *rescue treatment;* ○——○, *prophylaxis; S, single dose; M, multiple dose*

using different surfactants[31–36]. Of these trials, four trials reported sequential changes in FiO_2 requirements at 6, 12, 24, 48, 72 or 96 postnatal hours, which are shown in Figure 3.

In the trial using a single dose of Surfactant TA[31], the mean FiO_2 of the rescue group at 6 h of age was 0.8, indicating that moderate to severe RDS developed by 6 h of age before surfactant treatment, whereas the mean FiO_2 in the prophylactic-treatment group at age 6 h was below 0.3, which is equivalent to that required for intubated infants without lung disease, and this beneficial effect was sustained over the first 96 h. A similar improvement in oxygenation was seen in the trial with multiple dose Infasurf® (ONY Inc., Buffalo, USA) reported by Dunn and associates[33]. However, inasmuch as the rescue-treatment group of the latter trial, as in most other trials, included a substantial number of infants without surfactant deficiency, by their study design, the FiO_2 value must have been greater than indicated by the data for infants in

the prophylactic- and rescue-treatment groups. The same criticism can be applied to other trials except the trial using human surfactant reported by Merritt and co-workers[34]. As shown in Table 2, most studies allowed for inclusion of normal infants in the range of 20–60% in both treatment strategies. In contrast, only the trial of Surfactant TA did not include normal infants in the rescue group[31]. An important feature of this trial design was the identification of infants with surfactant deficiency by the stable micro-bubble test[37,38] in gastric aspirates obtained at birth. This is of paramount importance to evaluate the true effect of surfactant therapy and also to avoid unnecessary exposure of surfactant to otherwise normal infants.

The incidence of bronchopulmonary dysplasia was reduced only in the trial of a single dose of Surfactant TA, regardless of which bronchopulmonary dysplasia criterion was used and despite a relatively small sample size. This finding was confirmed by a subsequent multicenter

Table 2 *Documentation of surfactant deficiency in randomized clinical trials of prophylaxis vs. rescue treatment*

Trial	Surfactant deficiency	RDS in rescue group (%)	Estimate of normal infants in prophylaxis group (%)
Konishi *et al.*, 1994[31]	SM test in GA	100	0
Merritt *et al.*, 1991[34]	L/S < 2.0 absence of PG	80	20
Kendig *et al.*, 1991[32]	not determined	58	42
Dunn *et al.*, 1991[33]	L/S ≥ 2.0*	48	52
Kattwinkel *et al.*, 1993[36]	not determined	43	57
Egberts *et al.*, 1993[35]	not determined	52	48

RDS, respiratory distress syndrome; SM, stable microbubble stability; GA, gastric aspirates; L/S, lecithin/sphingomyelin ratio; PG, phosphatidylglycerol; *infants with amniotic fluid L/S ratio ≥ 2.0 were not enrolled in the trial

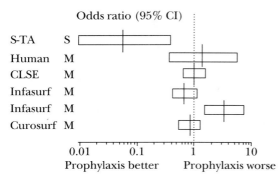

Figure 4 *Effects of prophylaxis and rescue surfactant treatment on bronchopulmonary dysplasia. The odds ratios and 95% confidence intervals (CI) were estimated for the difference in incidence of bronchopulmonary dysplasia reported by Konishi and colleagues[31] using Surfactant TA (S-TA), Merritt and associates[34] using human amniotic fluid surfactant (Human), Kendig and co-workers[32] using calf lung surfactant extract (CLSE), Kattwinkel and colleagues[32] using Infasurf, Dunn and associates[33] using Infasurf, and Egberts and co-workers[35] using Curosurf. S, single dose; M, multiple dose. A value of less than 1 suggests prophylaxis advantages over rescue treatment*

controlled study[39]. In contrast, the trial of multiple-dose Infasurf[33] showed a significant increase in the incidence of bronchopulmonary dysplasia (Figure 4).

Both Kendig and associates[32] and Kattwinkel and co-workers[36] demonstrated a decrease in mortality in infants receiving prophylactic treatment. The trial of a single dose of Surfactant TA was not designed to evaluate mortality, and neonatal mortality rate was 6% in the prophylactic-treatment group and 12% in the rescue-treatment group, despite inclusion of only infants with moderate to severe RDS.

In the largest randomized trial, the OSIRIS (open study of infants at high risk of or with respiratory insufficiency) collaborative group[40] studied early treatment (< 2 h of age) compared with delayed selective treatment in 2690 preterm infants at high risk of RDS. Earlier treatment led to a small but significant reduction in the death or oxygen dependence at term-adjusted age (relative risk 0.84, 95% confidence interval 0.76–0.93).

Single- vs. multiple-dose treatment

Dunn and colleagues[41] compared single vs. multiple doses of Infasurf. They studied 75 infants of 30–36 weeks' gestation randomized to receive a single dose vs. up to four doses if required by clinical status. Both groups showed a marked improvement in oxygenation, and multiple doses sustained the improvement in oxygenation, but there was no difference in ventilatory requirements or time to extubation. Speer and associates[42] also compared single with multiple doses of Curosurf® (Chiesi Farmaceutici, Parma, Italy) in a multicenter randomized controlled trial. Infants weighing 700–2000 g less than 15 h of age with severe RDS were randomized into a single- ($n = 176$) or multiple-dose ($n = 167$) treatment. Both groups received an initial dose of 200 mg/kg, while the multiple-dose group received additional doses (100 mg/kg each) of Curosurf at 12 and 24 h if they still required mechanical ventilation with $FiO_2 > 0.21$. In both groups there was a rapid improvement in oxygenation as reflected by a three-fold increase in arterial–alveolar oxygen tension ratio (a/A pO_2) within 15 min after surfactant administration, and peak inspiratory pressure and mean airway pressure (MAP) could be reduced significantly during the first 6 h after surfactant treatment. This study showed that the multiple-dose treatment was associated with a significant reduction in overall neonatal mortality (21 vs. 13%, $p < 0.05$ by logistic regression). The incidence of pneumothorax was also reduced from 18 to 9% ($p < 0.01$). There was no difference in the incidence of bronchopulmonary dysplasia.

A multicenter prospective randomized trial comparing single- vs. multiple-dose strategies in infants with moderate to severe RDS (birth weight 700–1299 g) was recently conducted in Japan[43]. This study showed that infants in the multiple-dose group (the second dose, 40% at < 6 h; the third, 12% at 12–24 h; the fourth, 4% at 24–36 h of age, when infants required $FiO_2 \geq$ 0.3 and/or MAP $\geq$ 6 cmH$_2$O) had significantly higher a/A pO_2 levels (near normal) and significantly fewer bronchopulmonary dysplasias than those in the single-dose group (5 vs. 22%, $p = 0.006$). This specific effect of multiple-dose therapy on bronchopulmonary dysplasia (odds ratio, 0.06 or 94% reduction, $p = 0.001$) was confirmed by logistic regression analysis.

COHORT STUDY

During the past 13 years (1982–1994), ventilated infants with RDS were consecutively treated with Surfactant TA at our NICU. Clinical response and outcome in preterm infants with only moderate to severe RDS receiving Surfactant TA were compared for the three periods (period 1, 1982–86; period 2, 1987–91; period 3, 1992–94)[10]. The results of the first decade (periods 1 and 2) have been reported previously[44].

Neonatal characteristics

The characteristics of the patient population are given in Table 3. The percentage of RDS patients born in our unit significantly increased from 53% in period 1 to 64% in period 2 ($p < 0.01$) and to 86% in period 3 ($p < 0.01$).

Every measure was taken to avoid intrapartum asphyxia. Consequently, the incidence of Cesarean section significantly increased over the three periods.

The percentage of infants receiving antenatal corticosteroids was 3% and 4% in periods 1 and 2, respectively, but it significantly increased to 61% in period 3 ($p < 0.01$). According to the standard protocol recommended by Liggins[45], we administered four doses each of betamethasone, 5 mg intravenously, at 12-h intervals. Amniocentesis, for the prediction of lung maturity, was rarely performed. Instead, we performed the stable microbubble test, originally described by Pattle and colleagues[37], on gastric aspirate obtained at birth. The clinical value of this test for the prediction of RDS was reported by Chida and associates[38]. This test can supply results within 10 min. The positive predictive value (the prediction of RDS) is 96%. This test was used in two controlled trials of rescue surfactant therapy[13,46] and in three controlled trials comparing prophylaxis with rescue surfactant treatment[31,43,47] in Japan, to define a population of infants with surfactant therapy. In these studies all of the infants included in the rescue arm of the prophylactic trials developed moderate to severe RDS.

Surfactant administration

Infants who had surfactant sufficiency and required intubation and mechanical ventilation were usually observed without receiving surfactant, and if they developed RDS requiring FiO_2 > 0.4 and MAP > 7 cmH$_2$O with abnormal chest radiographs compatible with RDS, they were treated with surfactant.

During the period 1, we dispersed one vial (100 mg phospholipid) of surfactant in 4 ml of saline by sonication to give a phospholipid concentration of 25 mg/ml. During the periods 2 and 3, the following changes occurred in the dispersion technique and dosing:

(1) The surfactant was dispersed in saline by gentle swirling instead of sonication;

(2) The volume of saline was 3 ml instead of 4 ml;

Table 3 *Patient characteristics in cohort study of preterm infants with moderate to severe respiratory distress syndrome (RDS)*

	Period 1 (n = 78)	Period 2 (n = 132)	Period 3 (n = 76)
Birth weight (g)	1285	1336	1197
Gestational age (weeks)	29	29	28
Male (%)	69	64	57
Born with RDS (%)	53*	76	86***
5 min Apgar score	6.1*	7	6.9***
Maternal tocolysis (%)	32*	77	84***
Maternal steroids (%)	3	4**	61***
PROM (> 24 h) (%)	10	15	17
Cesarean section (%)	31	41	72***
Dosage of surfactant (mg/kg)	114*	120	127***
Age at treatment (h)	6*	4.2**	1.7***
Retreatment (%)	5*	4**	33***

Period 1, 1982–1986; period 2, 1987–1991; period 3, 1992–1994;
PROM, premature rupture of membranes. Statistical significance
*period 1 vs.2; **period 2 vs. 3; ***period 1 vs. 3

(3) The dosing schedule was one vial for an infant weighing less than 1000 g, 1.5 vials for an infant weighing 1000–1500 g, and two vials for an infant weighing more than 1500 g.

Surfactant suspension was administered as five aliquots given over a period of approximately 5 min with the infant in different positions. After surfactant administration, initial adjustments were made for FiO_2 and then for peak inspiratory pressure and rate to maintain normal blood gas values.

Inborn infants (infants born in this unit but not infants transferred from elsewhere) born with RDS with proven surfactant deficiency requiring ventilatory support were treated with surfactant at the earliest possible time after birth. The timing of treatment became significantly earlier in period 3 than in periods 1 and 2 (Table 3).

Each infant was evaluated for the presence of a patent ductus arteriosus (PDA) with left-to-right shunting using standard clinical, radiographic and echocardiographic criteria. A large shunt PDA was diagnosed by two-dimensional echocardiography and a color Doppler echocardiographic technique. If a significant PDA was demonstrated, mefenamic acid was used for its closure.

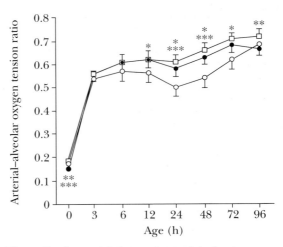

Figure 5 *Sequential changes in arterial–alveolar oxygen tension (a/A pO₂) ratios during the first 96 h after administration of Surfactant TA in infants with moderate to severe RDS for the three periods. Period 1, 1982–86 (○——○); period 2, 1987–91 (●——●); period 3, 1992–94 (□——□). Results are mean and 95% confidence intervals; *period 1 vs. 2; **period 2 vs. 3; ***period 1 vs. 3; are all significant*

Response to surfactant therapy

Sequential changes in arterial–alveolar oxygen tension ratio (a/A pO_2 ratio) following surfactant therapy for the three periods are shown in Figure 5. Rapid and sustained improvement was observed in a/A pO_2 ratios following surfactant therapy, but the improvement was better in periods 2 and 3 than in period 1. Note that the a/A pO_2 value at 3 h post surfactant treatment was above 0.5, which is equivalent to that of the intubated infants without lung disease, indicating that surfactant therapy nearly normalizes the respiratory status of preterm infants with moderate to severe RDS.

We defined response types by the changes in ventilatory index ($FiO_2 \times MAP \times paO_2^{-1}$), which considers both FiO_2 and MAP to normalize paO_2. Excluded for this assessment of response type were infants with mild RDS before surfactant therapy. Based on ventilatory index, the severity of RDS was categorized as 'near normal' (ventilatory index < 0.03, FiO_2 < 0.3 and MAP < 6 cmH_2O), mild (ventilatory index ≥ 0.03, $FiO_2 \geq 0.3$ and MAP ≥ 6 cmH_2O), mod-

erate (ventilatory index ≥ 0.047, $FiO_2 \geq 0.4$ and MAP ≥ 7 cmH_2O), or severe (ventilatory index ≥ 0.133, $FiO_2 \geq 0.8$ and MAP ≥ 10 cm H_2O) to maintain paO_2 at 60–80 mmHg and $paCO_2$ < 50 mmHg[45]. The results of this analysis are shown in Table 4. When evaluated at 6 h post-treatment, the overall surfactant treatment response was better in periods 2 and 3 than in period 1 (Cochran–Mantel–Haenszel χ^2 test, $p = 0.001$ for periods 1 vs. 3). In period 3, the proportion of good responders was 92%, relapsers 1% and poor responders 7%. Within 12 h of surfactant therapy, 95% of the infants with moderate to severe RDS treated in period 3 required minimal ventilatory support equivalent to that of most ventilated infants without lung disease (Figure 6), and required significantly fewer days on the

Table 4 *Response types in infants with moderate to severe respiratory distress syndrome receiving Surfactant TA by period*

	Period 1, 1982–86 (n = 78)	Period 2, 1987–91 (n = 132)	Period 3, 1992–94 (n = 76)	Study, 1982–94 (n = 286)
Good response	56 (72%)	118 (89%)	70 (92%)	244 (85%)
Relapse	14 (18%)	8 (6%)	1 (1%)	23 (8%)
Poor response	8 (10%)	6 (5%)	5 (7%)	19 (7%)

Period 1 vs. 2, Cochran–Mantel–Haenszel (CMH) $\chi^2 = 10.32$, $p < 0.001$; period 1 vs. 3, CHM $\chi^2 = 9.446$, $p < 0.001$; period 2 vs. 3, not significant

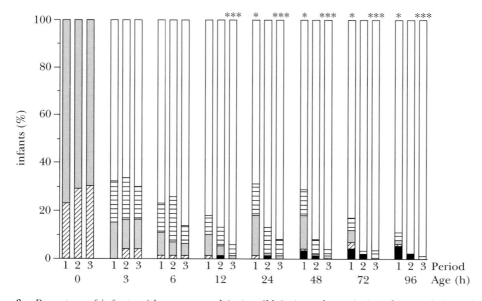

Figure 6 *Percentage of infants with near normal (□), mild (▬), moderate (▩) and severe (▨) respiratory distress syndrome at various time intervals after the administration of Surfactant TA for the three time periods. *Period 1 vs. 2 significant; ***period 1 vs. 3 significant*

Table 5 *Outcomes of infants with moderate to severe respiratory distress syndrome treated with Surfactant TA by period*

	Period 1 (n = 78)	Period 2 (n = 132)	Period 3 (n = 76)
Hospital death	10 (13%)	6 (5%)	1 (1%)***
Sepsis/pneumonia	2 (3%)	6 (5%)	4 (5%)
Hypotension	22 (28%)	27 (20%)	15 (20%)
Pulmonary interstitial emphysema	9 (12%)	5 (4%)	1 (1%)***
Pneumothorax/pneumomediastinum	7 (9%)	9 (7%)	0 (0%)***
Patent ductus arteriosus	57 (73%)	66 (50%)	36 (47%)***
Hemorrhagic lung edema	5 (6%)	7 (5%)	3 (4%)
Intraventricular hemorrhage (grade ≥ 2)	12 (15%)	14 (11%)	2 (3%)***
Necrotizing enterocolitis	2 (3%)	1 (0.8%)	1 (1%)
Retinopathy of prematurity	18/68 (26%)	19/126 (15%)	9/75 (12%)***
O_2 at 36 conceptional weeks	15/68 (22%)*	11/126 (9%)	7/75 (9%)***
O_2 at 40 conceptional weeks	7/68 (10%)*	3/126 (2%)	2/75 (3%)

Period 1, 1982–86; period 2, 1987–91; period 3, 1992–94.
*period 1 vs.2; **period 2 vs. 3; ***period 1 vs. 3; statistically significant (by the two-tailed Fisher exact test)

respirator. Logistic regression analysis showed that the good response was associated with the absence of intractable hypotension, sepsis/pneumonia, and air leaks and the use of tocolytic agents and lower pretreatment ventilatory index. Poor response was associated with intractable hypotension, increased pretreatment ventilatory index, vaginal delivery, RDS-mimicking sepsis/pneumonia and premature rupture of membranes (PROM) of > 24 h.

Outcome

The outcome of infants with moderate to severe RDS treated with Surfactant TA is shown in Table 5. The hospital death rate was significantly lower in period 3 than in period 1 (1 vs. 13%, p < 0.01). The incidence of intracranial hemorrhage (≥ Papille's grade 2) was 3% in period 3 and 15% in period 1 (p < 0.01). The incidence of bronchopulmonary dysplasia beyond 36 weeks' gestational age was also significantly lower in period 3 than in period 1 (9 vs. 22%, p < 0.05). Thus, it is important to point out that the increased survival rate in infants with moderate to severe RDS during the past 13 years has not been followed by parallel increases in intracranial hemorrhage and bronchopulmonary dysplasia.

Factors affecting outcome

There have been changing patterns in the management of premature infants during the last 13 years. The proportion of infants born with RDS increased from 53% in period 1 to 86% in period 3, that of Cesarean section increased from 31% in period 1 to 72% in period 3, and that of maternal use of corticosteroids increased from 3 to 61%; the differences between period 1 and period 3 are all significant. Timing of surfactant administration also became earlier in period 3 than in period 1 (mean age 1.7 vs. 6.0 h, p < 0.01).

Logistic regression analysis revealed that the significant factors reducing mortality and incidence of intracranial hemorrhage are the increased proportions of inborn infants with RDS and Cesarean section delivery, and the earlier administration of surfactant, but not the maternal use of corticosteroids.

The hospital death rate was associated with intracranial hemorrhage, increasing age at treatment, relapse response, birth weight and lowest pretreatment base excess. Bronchopulmonary dysplasia was associated with no use of tocolytic agents, increasing age at treatment, air leaks, large shunt PDA and relapse response. Although the frequency of antenatal steroid use has changed in the three periods, 3% for period 1, 4% for period 2 and 61% for period 3

($p < 0.01$), the adjustment for exposure to antenatal steroids did not affect the odds ratios for bronchopulmonary dysplasia or intracranial hemorrhage, and antenatal steroid use was not significantly associated with either, as assessed by logistic regression analysis. One explanation for the lack of effect of the antenatal steroids may be the relatively lower prevalence of RDS (30–40%) and lower percentage receiving steroids in our unit during the first decade (periods 1 and 2). Also, it may be that the true effect of antenatal steroid therapy[48,49], is masked by the improvement in outcome resulting from surfactant therapy. Further studies are needed to address this issue.

Clinical tolerance

Surfactant TA administration has been well tolerated in our single- and multicenter randomized trials, in which it did not increase the incidence of complications of RDS in premature infants (500–1750 g birth weight), including retinopathy of prematurity, patent ductus arteriosus (PDA), pulmonary hemorrhage, pneumonia/septicemia and necrotizing enterocolitis.

The RDS mortality rate in infants weighing 500–1500 g at birth from the 114 NICUs (about 50%) was compared in the presurfactant period of 1984–1987 ($n = 3641$) and the postsurfactant period of 1988–1990 ($n = 3085$)[50]. This population study suggested that the introduction of Surfactant TA has led to decreased mortality in this RDS population (odds ratio, 0.61; 95% confidence interval (CI), 0.55–0.68; $p < 0.001$). When the first year (1988), in which surfactant was widely introduced, was compared with the year preceding surfactant release (1987), the RDS mortality rate was also significantly decreased (odds ratio, 0.78; 95% CI, 0.64–0.96; $p = 0.019$).

CONCLUSIONS AND PERSPECTIVES

The goal of surfactant therapy is to improve the respiratory status of infants with RDS and prevent injury of the immature lung. Respiratory improvements reported in clinical trials of prophylactic and rescue treatment using either single or multiple doses of a synthetic surfactant or various natural surfactants, appear to be less optimal than those we observed in a similar population of infants treated with Surfactant TA during the period of 1987–1992[44]. During the subsequent 3 years (1992–94), we observed that within 12 h after treatment with Surfactant TA 95% of the infants with moderate to severe RDS required minimal ventilatory support equivalent to that of ventilated infants without lung disease and that the proportion of such infants increased to 98% during the subsequent hours. In this group of good responders there were fewer intracranial hemorrhage and bronchopulmonary dysplasia and no hospital deaths occurred. The optimization of surfactant therapy achieved by us may have been attributed to several factors.

(1) Employment of a more active perinatal approach which minimized the factors affecting surfactant response and outcome;

(2) Use of antenatal corticosteroid;

(3) Identification of infants with surfactant deficiency by means of a rapid test on gastric aspirate obtained at birth, which allowed the earlier administration of surfactant to the selected preterm infants;

(4) Retreatment for relapsers;

(5) Earlier pharmacological intervention for a large left-to-right shunting through the patent ductus arteriosus.

Whilst natural surfactants seem to have an advantage over synthetic ones, there is also evidence that natural surfactants differ in their effects. Most surfactants available for clinical use have not undergone *in-vivo* dose-response studies using the standard animal model. Any new generation of surfactants should undergo rigorous *in-vivo* quality control to exert optimal response, such as we observed with our surfactant in an animal model as well as preterm infants with RDS. Data presented in this article will provide guidelines for the optimization of surfactant therapy.

ACKNOWLEDGEMENTS

This work was supported by a grant from The Japanese Ministry of Education, Science and Culture (project 02454274).

References

1. Pattle, R. E. (1955). Properties, function and origin of the alveolar lining layer. *Nature (London)*, **15**, 1125–6

2. Avery, M. E. and Mead, J. (1959). Surface properties in relation to atelectasis and hyaline membrane disease. *Am. J. Dis. Child.*, **97**, 517–23

3. Fujiwara, T., Maeta, H., Chida, S., Watabe, Y. and Abe, T. (1980). Artificial surfactant therapy in hyaline-membrane disease. *Lancet*, **1**, 55–9

4. Jobe, A. (1993). Pulmonary surfactant therapy. *N. Engl. J. Med.*, **328**, 861–8

5. Halliday, H. L. (1995). Overview of clinical trials comparing natural and synthetic surfactants. *Biol. Neonate*, **67** (Suppl.), 32–47

6. Fujiwara, T. and Robertson, B. (1992). Pharmacology of exogenous surfactant. In Robertson, B., Van Golde, L. M. G. and Batenburg, J. J. (eds.) *Pulmonary Surfactant from Molecular Biology to Clinical Practice*, pp.561–92. (Amsterdam, London, New York, Tokyo: Elsevier Science Publishers)

7. Smith, B. T. (1992). Clinical experience with modified natural surfactant. In Robertson, B., Van Golde, L. M. G. and Batenburg, J. J. (eds.) *Pulmonary Surfactant from Molecular Biology to Clinical Practice*, pp.593–604. (Amsterdam, London, New York, Tokyo: Elsevier Science Publishers)

8. Soll, R. F. (1995). Clinical trials of surfactant therapy in the newborn. In Robertson, B. and Taeusch, W. H. (eds.) *Surfactant Therapy for Lung Disease*, pp.407–41. (New York, Basel, Hong Kong: Marcel Dekker, Inc.)

9. Maeta, H. (1995). Dose-effects of exogenous surfactants on neonatal pulmonary mechanics and morphology: comparison of different surfactants. *J. Iwate Med. Ass.*, **47**, 37–49

10. Fujiwara, T., Konishi, M., Chida, S., Shimada, S. and Maeta, H. (1995). Summary of 15 years experience with exogenous surfactant therapy. *Appl. Cardiopulmonary Pathophysiol.*, **5**, 34–6

11. Gitlin, J. D., Soll, R. F., Parad, R. B., Feldman, H. A., Lucey, J. F. and Taeusch, H. W. (1987). A randomized controlled trial of exogenous surfactant for the treatment of hyaline membrane disease. *Pediatrics*, **79**, 31–7

12. Raju, T. N. K., Bhat, R., McCulloch, K. M., Maeta, H., Vidyasagar, D. *et al.* (1987). Double-blind controlled trial of single-dose treatment with bovine surfactant in severe hyaline membrane disease. *Lancet*, **1**, 651–5

13. Fujiwara, T., Konishi, M., Chida, S., Okuyama, K., Ogawa, Y., Takeuchi, Y., Nishida, H., Kito, H., Fufimura, M., Nakamura, H. and Hashimoto, T. (1990). Surfactant replacement therapy with a single dose postventilatory dose of a reconstituted bovine surfactant in preterm neonates with respiratory distress syndrome: final analysis of a multicenter, double-blind, randomized trial and comparison with similar trials. *Pediatrics*, **86**, 753–64

14. Horbar, J. D., Soll, R. F., Sutherland, J. M., Philip, A. G. S., Kotagal, U., Little, G. A., Edwards, W. H., Vidyasagar, D., Raju, T. N K., Jobe, A. H., Ikegami, M., Mullet, M. D., Mullett, M. D., Myerberg, D. Z., McAuliff, T. L. and Lucey, J. F. (1989). A multicenter randomized placebo-controlled trial of surfactant therapy for respiratory distress syndrome. *N. Engl. J. Med.*, **320**, 959–65

15. Horbar, J. D., Soll, R. F., Schachinger, H., Kewitz, G., Versmold, H. T., Linder, W., Duc, G., Mieth, D., Linderkamp, O., Zilow, E. P., Lemburg, P., von Loewenich, V., Brand, M., Minoli, I., More, G., Riegel, K. P., Roos, R., Weiss, L. and Lucey, J. F. (1990). A European multicenter randomized controlled trial of single dose surfactant therapy for idiopathic respiratory distress syndrome. *Eur. J. Pediatr.*, **149**, 416–23

16. Collaborative European Multicenter Study Group (1988). Surfactant replacement therapy for severe neonatal respiratory distress syndrome: an international randomized clinical trial. *Pediatrics*, **82**, 683–91

17. Hallman, M., Merritt, T. A., Jarvenpaa A. L., Boynton. B., Mannino, F., Gluck, L., Moore, T. and Edwards, D. (1985). Exogenous human surfactant for treatment of severe respiratory distress syndrome: a randomized prospective clinical trial. *J. Pediatr.*, **106**, 963–9

18. Lang, M. J., Rhodes, P. G., Reddy, O., Kurth, C. G., Merritt, T. A. and Hall, R. T. (1990). A

controlled trial of human surfactant therapy for severe respiratory distress syndrome in very low birth weight infants. *J. Pediatr.*, **116**, 295–30

19. Phibbs, R. H., Ballard, R. A., Clements, J. A., Heilbron, D. C., Phibbs, C. S., Schlueter, M. A., Sniderman, S. H., Tooley, W. H. and Wakley, A. (1991). Initial clinical trial of Exosurf, a protein-free synthetic surfactant, for the prophylaxis and early treatment of hyaline membrane disease. *Pediatrics*, **88**, 1–9

20. Long, W., Thompson, T., Sundell, H., Schumacher, R., Volbeg, F., Guthrie, R. and the American Exosurf Neonatal Study Group (1991). Effects of two rescue doses of a synthetic surfactant on morality rate and survival without bronchopulmonary dysplasia in 700- to 1350-gram infants with respiratory distress syndrome. *J. Pediatr.*, **118**, 595–605

21. Long, W., Corbet, A., Cotton, R. *et al.* (1991). A controlled trial of synthetic surfactant in infants weighing 1250 g or more with respiratory distress syndrome. *N. Engl. J. Med.*, **325**, 1696–1703

22. Horbar, J. D., Wright, L. L., Sol, R. F., Wright, E. C., Fanaroff, A. A., Korones, S. B., Shankaran, S., Oh, W., Fletcher, B. D., Bauer, C. R., Tyson, J. E., Lemons, J. A., Donovan, E. F., Stoll, B. J., Stevenson, D. D., Papile, L. A. and Philips, J. III (1994). A multicenter randomized trial comparing two surfactants for the treatment of neonatal respiratory distress syndrome. *J. Pediatr.*, **123**, 757–66

23. Alvarado, M., Hinoce, R., Hakanson, D. and Gross, S. (1993). Clinical trial of Survanta vs. Exosurf therapy in infants < 1500 g with respiratory distress syndrome (RDS). *Pediatr. Res.*, **33**, 1865 A

24. Enhorning, G., Shennan, A., Possmayer, F., Dunn, M., Chen, C. P. and Milligan, J. (1985). Prevention of neonatal respiratory distress syndrome by tracheal instillation of surfactant: a randomized clinical trial. *Pediatrics*, **76**, 145–53

25. Kendig, J. W., Notter, R. H., Cox, C., Aschner, I. L., Bernstein, R. M., Hendricks-Munoz, K., Maniscalco, W. M., Metlay, L. A., Phelps, D. L., Sinkin, R. A., Wood, B. P. and Shapiro, D. L. (1988). Surfactant replacement therapy at birth: final analysis of a clinical trial and comparisons with similar trials. *Pediatrics*, **82**, 756–62

26. Soll, R. F., Hoekstra, R. E., Fangman, J. J., Corbet, A. J., Adams, J. M., James. L. S., Schulze, K., Oh, W., Roberts, J. D., Dorst, J. P., Kramer, S. S., Gold, A. J., Zola, E. M., Horbar, J. D., McAuliffe, T. L. and Lucey, J. F. (1990). Multicenter trial of single-dose modified bovine surfactant extract (Survanta) for prevention of respiratory distress syndrome. *Pediatrics*, **85**, 1092–102

27. Merritt, T. A., Hallman, M., Bloom, B. T., Berry, C., Benrischke, K., Sahn, D., Key, T., Edwards, D., Jarvenppa, A. L., Pohjavuori, M., Kankaanpa, K., Kunnas, M., Paatero, H., Rapola, J. and Jaaskelainen, J. (1986). Prophylactic treatment of very premature infants with human surfactant. *N. Engl. J. Med.*, **315**, 785–90

28. Stevenson, D., Walther, F., Long, W., Sell, M., Pauly, T., Gong, A., Easa, D., Pramanik, A., Le-Blanc, M., Anday, E., Dhanireddy, R., Burchfield, D., Corbet, A. and the American Exosurf Neonatal Study Group I (1992). Controlled trial of a single dose of synthetic surfactant at birth in premature infants weighing 500 to 699 grams. *J. Pediatr.*, **120**, S3–S12

29. Corbet, A. J., Goldman, S. A., Lombardy, L., Mammel, M. A. and Long, W. A. (1991). Decreased mortality in small premature infants treated at birth with a single dose of synthetic surfactant: a multicenter trial. *J. Pediatr.*, **118**, 277–84

30. Morley, C. J., Greenough, A., Miller, N. G., Bangham, A. D., Pool, J., Wood, S., South, M., Davis, J. A. and Vyas, H. (1988). Randomized trial of artificial surfactant (ALEC) given at birth to babies from 23 to 24 weeks gestation. *Early Hum. Dev.*, **17**, 41–54

31. Konishi, M., Chida, S., Cho, K. and Fujiwara, T. (1994). A prospective, randomized study of preventive versus rescue surfactant treatment in premature babies with surfactant deficiency. *J. Jpn. Pediatr. Soc.*, **98**, 1057–66

32. Kendig, J. W., Notter, R. H., Cox, C., Reubens, L. J., Davis, J. M., Manisgalco, W. M., Sinkin, R. A., Bartoletti, A., Dweck, H. S., Horgan, M. J., Rismberg, H., Phelps, Đ. L. and Shapiro, D. L. (1991). A comparison of surfactant as immediate prophylaxis and as rescue therapy in newborns of less than 30 weeks' gestation. *N. Engl. J. Med.*, **324**, 865–71

33. Dunn, M. S., Shennan, A. T., Zayack, D. and Possmayer, F. (1991). Bovine surfactant replacement therapy in neonates of less than 30 weeks' gestation – a randomized controlled trial of prophylaxis versus treatment. *Pediatrics*, **87**, 377–86

34. Merritt, T. A., Hallman, M., Berry, C., Pohjavuori, M., Edwards, D. K., Jaaskelainen, J., Grafe, M., Vaucher, Y., Wozniak, P., Heldt, G. and Rapola, J. (1991). Randomized, placebo-controlled trial of human surfactant given at birth versus rescue administration in very low birth weight infants with lung immaturity. *J. Pediatr.*, **118**, 581–94

35. Egberts, J., de Winter, J. P., Sedin, G., de Kleine, M. J. K., Broberger, U., van Bel, F., Curstedt, T. and Robertson, B. (1993). Comparison of prophylaxis and rescue treatment with Curosurf in

babies less than 30 weeks gestation: a randomized trial. *Pediatrics*, **92**, 768–74

36. Kattwinkel, J., Bloom, B. T., Delmore, P., Davis, C. L., Farrell, E., Friss, H., Lung, A. L., King, K. and Mueller, D. (1993). Prophylactic administration of calf lung surfactant extract is more effective than early treatment of respiratory distress syndrome in neonates of 29 to 32 weeks gestation. *Pediatrics*, **92**, 90–8

37. Pattle, R. E., Kratzing, C. C., Parkinson, C. E., Graves, L., Robertson, R. D., Robards, G. J., Currie, J. O., Parsons, J. H. and Sutherland, P. D. (1979). Maturity of fetal lungs tested by production of stable microbubbles in amniotic fluid. *Br. J. Obstet. Gynaecol.*, **86**, 615–22

38. Chida, S., Fujiwara, T., Konishi, M., Takahashi, H. and Sasaki, M. (1993). Stable microbubble test for predicting the risk of respiratory distress syndrome. II. Prospective evaluation of the test on amniotic fluid and gastric aspirate. *Eur. J. Pediatr.*, **152**, 152–6

39. Japanese Surfactant TA study group (1994). A multicenter, randomized comparison of prophylaxis and rescue surfactant treatment in premature infants with RDS weighing 700–1299 gm at birth. (Abstr. 75) *Acta Neonat. Jpn.*, **30**, 597

40. The OSIRIS Collaborative Group (1992). Early versus delayed neonatal administration of a synthetic surfactant – the judgements of OSIRIS. *Lancet*, **340**, 1363–69

41. Dunn, M. S., Shennan, A. T. and Possmayer, F. (1991). Single versus multiple-dose surfactant replacement therapy in neonates of 30 to 36 weeks' gestation with respiratory distress syndrome. *Pediatrics*, **87**, 377–86

42. Speer, C. P., Robertson, B., Curstedt, T., Halliday, H. L., Compagnone, D., Gefeller, O., Harms, K., Herting, E., McClure, G., Reid, M., Tubman, R., Herin, P., Noack, G., Kokm, J., Koppe, J., van Sonderen, L., Laufkotter, E., Kohler, W., Boenisch, H., Albrecht, K., Hanssler, L., Haim, M., Otetomo, S. B., Okken, A., Altfeld, P. C., Groneck, P., Rachel, W., Relier, J. P. and Walti, H. (1992). Randomized European multicenter trial of surfactant replacement therapy for severe neonatal respiratory distress syndrome: single versus multiple doses of Curosurf. *Pediatrics*, **89**, 13–20

43. Japanese Surfactant TA study group (1994). A multicenter randomized comparison of the single-dose versus multiple-dose surfactant treatment in premature infants with respiratory distress syndrome (RDS). (Abstr. 78) *Acta Neonat. Jpn.*, **30**, 599

44. Konishi, M., Chida, S., Shimada, S., Kasai, T., Murakami, Y., Cho, K., Fujii, Y., Maeta, H. and Fujiwara, T. (1992). Surfactant replacement therapy in premature babies with respiratory distress syndrome: factors affecting the response to surfactant and comparison of outcome from 1982–86 and 1987–91. *Acta Pediatr. Jpn.*, **34**, 617–30

45. Liggins, G. C. (1990). Antenatal corticosteroids. In Nelson, N. M. (ed.) *Current Therapy in Neonatal-Perinatal Medicine-2*, pp.1–3. (Toronto, Philadelphia: B. C. Deckker Inc.)

46. Konishi, M., Fujiwara, T., Naito, T., Takeuchi, Y., Ogawa, Y., Inukai, K., Fujimura, M., Nakamura, H. and Hashimoto, T. (1988). Surfactant replacement therapy in neonatal respiratory distress syndrome. A multi-centre, randomized clinical trial: comparison of high vs low-dose of Surfactant TA. *Eur. J. Pediatr.*, **147**, 20–5

47. Konishi, M., Fujiwara, T., Chida, S., Maeta, H., Shimada, S., Kasai, T., Fuji, Y. and Murakami, Y. (1992). A prospective, randomized trial of early versus late administration of a single dose of Surfactant-TA. *Early Hum. Dev.*, **29**, 275–82

48. Farrell, E. E., Silver, R. K., Kimberlin, C. V., Wolf, E. S., and Dusik, J. M. (1989). Impact of antenatal dexamethasone administration on respiratory distress syndrome in surfactant treated infants. *Am. J. Obstet. Gynecol.*, **161**, 623–33

49. Jobe, A. H., Mitchell, B. R. and Gunkel, J. H. (1993). Beneficial effects of the combined use of prenatal corticosteroids and postnatal surfactant on preterm infants. *Am. J. Obstet. Gynecol.*, **168**, 508–13

50. Itabashi, K., Masano, H., Tsukosi, T., Takeuchi, T., Hayashi, T., Imai, Y., Endo, T., Kure, A., Mizuno, K. and Okuyama, K. (1991). National neonatal mortality rate before and after introduction of surfactant therapy. *The 9th Surfactant-TA Study Meeting*, pp.17–23 (Tokyo Tanabe Company)

Index

abdominal circumference to femur length ratios, 62
abdominal cysts, color Doppler in diagnosis of, 40
abdominal tumors,
    adrenal, 290
    hepatic, 289
    ovarian cysts, 291
    renal, 290
    spleen, 292
    varieties of, 288
abdominal wall malformations, and abnormal
    karyotype, 221
abortion (spontaneous),
    anembryonic pregnancy, 346
    biology of, 345
    classification of and pathological examination of
        yolk sac, 23
    in pregestational diabetes, 542
    macroscopic presentation in first trimester, 434
    prediction of by ultrasound, 345
    responses to, 345
    subchorionic hematoma as a risk factor for, 34
    use of color Doppler in cases of subchorionic
        hematoma to predict risk of, 36
abortion (missed),
    amniotic fluid excess in, 352
    body length and, 349
abruptio placentae,
    classification, 445
    clinical experience of, 446
    clinical significance, 441
    Doppler velocimetry in, 452
    Doppler velocity waveforms of umbilical artery in,
        448
    early onset, 450
    end-diastolic blood flow increase in umbilical
        artery, 449
    etiology, 433
    fetal hypoxia and anemia in, 387
    histological examination of, 435, 440
    importance, 445
    in first and second trimesters, 433–9
    in third trimester, 439–41
    incidence, 433, 445
    infection-induced or decidual vasculopathy, 442
    morphology of, 439
    outcome in grade 2–3, 446
    physiopathology of, 441
    prostaglandin E and, 437
acetylcholine receptor antibodies in offspring of
    myasthenia gravis mothers, 594
achondroplasia, molecular diagnosis of, 121
acid–base levels,
    in normal fetus cf. distressed, 456
    metabolic acidosis, 457
acidemia (fetal), acid–base levels in normal fetus cf.
    distressed, 456

acidosis, metabolic, 457
acrania, contrast medium radiographic study of, 113
actocardiography,
    augmented,
        fetal breathing, 421
        fetal hiccupping, 420
    fetal distress measurement by, 417
    fetal distress prediction by, 418
    fetal hiccupping movements, 416
    fetal response to light, 420
    fetal response to sound, 419
    principles of, 415
    pseudosinusoidal fetal heart rate pattern, 417
adenovirus type II, congenital cerebral infection with,
    198
amniocentesis,
    color Doppler and, 39
    detection rates of cf. color Doppler, 45
    in twin pregnancies, 514
    justification of in cases of isolated fetal structural
        malformations, 244
    serial drainage for twin–twin transfusion syndrome,
        276
amnioinfusion after amniorrhexis, 489
amniorrhexis,
    age at and pulmonary hypoplasia risk, 481
    amnioinfusion for, 489
    antibiotic therapy after, 489
    arachidonic acid metabolite levels after, 480
    clinical implications of, 481
    clinical management of, 484
    cytokine levels after, 480, 481
    diagnosis, 484
    fetal leukocyte counts in, 488
    fetal neutrophil counts in, 488
    infection as a cause of, 477
    interval to preterm delivery after, 478
    invasive prediction of intrauterine infections after,
        485
    need for hospitalization, 486
    neonatal sepsis and, 482
    non-invasive prediction of intrauterine infections
        after, 485
    prevalence, 477
    recommended management,
        patients with negative cultures, 491
        patients with positive cultures, 491
    steroid therapy after, 489
    tocolytic therapy after, 489
    umbilical venous blood measures in, 487
    uterine activity monitoring after, 486
anembryonic pregnancy, ultrasound diagnosis of, 346
anemia (fetal),
    clinical experience with, 424
    evaluation of, 423
    in progressive abruptio placentae, 387

in red blood cell alloimmunization, 386
    liver length in, 425
    management, 426
    spleen perimeter, 426
anencephaly,
    detection by neuroscanning, 170
    links with abnormal karyotype, 21
aneuploidy,
    color Doppler in diagnosis of, 43
    femur length and, 246
    fetal biometry and, 245
    links with fetal structural anomalies, 243
aneurysm of vein of Galen,
    color Doppler in diagnosis of, 40
    differential diagnosis from arachnoid cyst, 285
antibiotic therapy after amniorrhexis, 489
aortic circulation, role in fetal hypoxia, 366
Apert syndrome, molecular diagnosis of, 122
Apgar scores, low and neonatal morbidity and mortality, 456
arachidonic acid, levels of metabolites in preterm labor with and without amniorrhexis, 480
arachnoid cyst,
    color Doppler in diagnosis of, 40
    differential diagnosis from intracranial teratoma, 285
Arnold–Chiari malformation, detection by neuroscanning, 174
arthrogryposis multiplex congenita, three-dimensional ultrasound of, 81
aspirin, low-dose in pregnancy for hypertension, 409
assisted reproductive technologies, increased incidence of twins with, 507

B-mode imaging,
    thermal effects of, 13, 18
'banana sign' in spinal dysraphism, 172
beat-to-beat variability, 460
biochemical markers for preterm delivery, 555
biparietal diameter to femur length ratio, 62
    trisomy 21 prediction from, 247
bladder, imaging of for malformations, 39
blood transfusions, use in red blood cell alloimmunization, 427
blood pressure monitoring,
    1-hour monitoring, 500, 501
    24-hour monitoring, 498, 499
    clinical data obtained by, 500
    diurnal variations in pressure, 501
    methodology of, 497
    technical problems of, 497
    use in prediction of pre-eclampsia, 502
    'white-coat' hypertension, 500
blood vessels of fetal brain, neuroscanning of, 168
bradycardia, 458

calcium metabolism and pregnancy-induced hypertension, 471
calcium supplementation,
    effect of in high-risk patients, 473
    effect of in low-risk patients, 474
    in pregnancy-induced hypertension, 473

    optimal dose, 475
    side-effects, 475
cardiac arrhythmia, in embryo, 351
cardiac bypass, in fetal lamb, 307
cardiac malformations,
    color Doppler in diagnosis of, 40
    diagnosis in first trimester, 140
cardiotocography (antepartum computerized),
    baseline fetal heart rate, 394
    characteristics of, 393
    clinical considerations for, 395
    development of, 393
    fetal heart rate variations with gestational age, 395
    interpretation of, 394
    intrauterine growth retardation and, 397
    pregnancy-induced hypertension and, 397
    use in red blood cell alloimmunization, 429
caudal regression syndrome, 540
cavitation, bioeffects of in ultrasound, 17
central nervous system malformations, in pregestational diabetes, 540
cephalocele,
    associated with chromosomal syndromes, 172
    detection by neuroscanning, 171
    links with abnormal karyotype, 217
cerebellar diameter, 64
cerebral circulation,
    cerebrovascular reactivity, 365
    changes in hypoxia, 373
    regional, 365
    role in fetal hypoxia, 364
cerebral palsy,
    rate with and without fetal monitoring, 379
    rate with term and preterm delivery, 381
cerebral resistance indices, in fetal hypoxia, 360–2
cervical lymphangioma, 284
cervical teratoma, 283–4
Chediak–Higashi disease, molecular diagnosis of compatible stem cells for transplantation in, 130
chest tumors,
    cardiac, 288
    lung,
        cystic adenomatoid malformation, 286, 287
        differential diagnosis of, 287
choledochal cyst, 290
chorioamnionitis, in abruptio placentae, 439
chorionic villus sampling, color Doppler and, 39
chorionicity of twins, 510
choroid plexus cysts, 286
    detection by neuroscanning, 169
    predictive value of, 44
choroid plexus papilloma, 285
choroidal artery, persistence of and chromosomal defects, 43
chromosomal anomalies,
    and fetal malformation, 213
    association with intrauterine growth retardation, 50
    cardiovascular malformations, 217
    central nervous system malformations, 215
    color Doppler in diagnosis of, 42
    cystic hygroma, 221

gastrointestinal and abdominal wall defects, 220
methods of screening for, 213, 214, 229
predictive value of color Doppler in, 43, 44
respiratory malformations, 223
single umbilical artery as a sign of, 42
skeletal malformations, 223
tissue echogenicity and, 96
urinary tract malformations, 219
cleft lip and palate, three-dimensional ultrasound of, 80
clubfoot, three-dimensional ultrasound of, 82
congenital adrenal hyperplasia, molecular diagnosis of, 123
congenital anomalies,
association with intrauterine growth retardation, 50
increased incidence of in twins, 511
congenital cardiopathies,
cf. normal fetus with color Doppler, 42
color Doppler in diagnosis of,
advantages, 41
limitations, 41
fetal surgery for, 267
congenital cerebral infections,
adenovirus, 198
congenital syphilis, 193
cytomegalovirus, 185
enteroviruses, 197
equine encephalitis virus, 198
herpes simplex viruses, 191
human immunodeficiency virus, 194
Lyme disease, 198
lymphocytic choriomeningitis virus, 198
parvovirus, 198
rubella, 190
toxoplasmosis, 188
Trypanosoma cruzi, 198
varicella, 196
congenital complete heart block,
fetal cardiac pacing, 304
medical therapy, 304
pathophysiology, 303
prevention, 304
treatment rationale, 303
congenital cystic adenomatoid malformation, 286, 287
algorithm for management of, 263
fetal surgery for, 262
congenital diaphragmatic hernia,
algorithm for management of, 261
fetal surgery for, 260–2
congenital heart defects,
associated with other disorders, 154
epidemiology, 147
fetal heart examination, 149
incidence, 147
second trimester fetal examination, 148
team approach to suspicion of, 154
ultrasound in first trimester, 140
congenital heart disease, fetal cardiac intervention in, 297
congenital heart malformations, links with abnormal karyotype, 218

congenital malformations in pregestational diabetes mellitus, 539
congenital thrombocytopenic purpura, molecular diagnosis of, 130
cordocentesis for red blood cell alloimmunization, 428
corpus callosum, neuroscanning of, 163
corpus callosum agenesis, links with abnormal karyotype, 217
counselling,
directive vs. non-directive, 4
strength of and severity of fetal anomaly, 4
craniofacial anomalies, fetal surgery for, 266
craniosynostosis syndromes, molecular diagnosis of, 122
cystic fibrosis, molecular diagnosis of, 125
cystic hygroma,
and abnormal karyotypes, 221
differential diagnosis from cervical teratoma, 283
cystic hygromas, nuchal, 229
cytokines,
levels after amniorrhexis, 480, 481
cytomegalovirus,
clinical manifestations, 186
detection of fetal infection by neuroscanning, 177
epidemiology, 185
microbiology, 185
pathogenesis, 186
prenatal diagnosis, 186
prevention, 187
prognosis, 187
therapy, 188

Dandy–Walker anomaly, 216, 244
decelerations, late and severe, 459
densitometry,
gain-assisted densitometric evaluation of sonograms, 97
in assessment of tissue echogenicity, 95
diabetes,
fetal surveillance in, 543
gestational cf. pregestational, 539
macrosomia in, 541
maternal ketoacidosis, 543
neonatal complications in,
hyperbilirubinemia, 545
hypoglycemia, 545
polycythemia, 545
respiratory distress syndrome, 545
transient cardiomyopathy, 545
pregestational, congenital malformations in, 539
risks in adult life of offspring, 547
spontaneous abortion in, 542
when to deliver, 546
Doppler,
cardiac malformations, 140
cardiovascular hemodynamics in first trimester, 139
cerebral and umbilical resistance indices in fetal hypoxia, 360–2
cerebroplacental ratio, hypoxia and outcome, 362
color,
aneuploidy diagnosis by, 43

as an adjunct to invasive techniques, 39
diagnosis of twin–twin transfusion syndrome by, 272
distinction of subchorionic fluid from subchorionic blood by, 438
future role in prenatal diagnosis, 47
malformation diagnosis with, 39
    abdominal, 40
    cardiopathies, 41
    central nervous system, 40
    thoracic, 40
predictive value of in chromosomal defects, 43, 44
subchorionic hematoma studies with, 35
trisomy 21 detection by, 45, 46
yolk sac studies, 27
fetal well-being assessment, 574
flowmetry,
    characteristics of, 399
    hypoxemia prediction by, 402
    interpretation of readings, 400
    intrauterine growth retardation prediction by, 401
    patterns in fetal hypoxemia, 400
    patterns in normal pregnancy, 399
hypertension prediction by, 405
thermal effects of, 13, 18
trials of in hypertension prediction, 407
use in fetal hypoxia, 359
use in red blood cell alloimmunization, 429
use in selecting patients for aspirin treatment, 410
velocimetry in abruptio placentae, 452
velocity waveforms of umbilical artery in abruptio placentae, 448
Down syndrome, see under trisomy 21
ductus arteriosus, premature closure of, 306
duodenal atresia, 220
dysanthropometry, 61, 65

early pregnancy loss, see abortion (spontaneous)
echocardiography,
    fetal transesophageal, 309
    in late first trimester, 137
elastase, biochemical marker for preterm delivery, 558
embryo,
    anomaly recognition with more detailed resolution, 353
    body length and missed abortion, 349
    cardiac arrhythmia in, 351
    cardiac motion in, 348, 350
    heart rate, 350
    normal growth patterns, 353
    ultrasound visualization of, 347
encephalocele, color Doppler in diagnosis of, 40
endoscopic laser coagulation, of communicating placental vessels in twin–twin transfusion syndrome, 273
enteroviruses, congenital cerebral infection with, 197
equine encephalitis viruses, congenital cerebral infection with, 198
esophageal atresia, 220
estriol, biochemical marker for preterm delivery, 559
ethics,

and fetus viability, 3
concept of fetus as a patient, 2
criteria for rigorous analysis of,
    clarity, 5
    clinical adequacy, 6
    clinical applicability, 6
    coherence, 6
    completeness, 7
    consistency, 6
definition of, 1
implications for counselling, 4
independent moral status of fetus, 3
limitations of consensus, 7
limitations of law and, 7
limitations of philosophy of, 7
limitations of religion and, 7
of molecular diagnosis of diseases with manifestation after birth or in adulthood, 129
of routine ultrasound examinations, 208–10
pitfalls, 7
principles of in medicine, 1
exencephaly, 354
color Doppler in diagnosis of, 40

femur length, and aneuploidy, 246
fetal anomalies, detection by routine ultrasound examinations, 203
fetal balloon valvuloplasty, 300
fetal behavioral states, classification by actocardiography, 415
fetal breathing movements, augmented actocardiography of, 421
fetal cardiac catheterization by fetoscopy, 308
fetal cardiac intervention,
    cardiac lesions suitable for, 298
    fetal balloon valvuloplasty, 300
    selection criteria for, 297
    selection for in valvar obstructions, 301
fetal cardiac surgery, animal studies, 306–8
fetal distress,
    ability of tests to detect, 532
    actocardiographic prediction of, 418
    Apgar scores, 456
    cf. well-being, 460
    definition of, 455
    fetal acidemia, 456
    history of, 455
    in abruptio placentae, 449
    in second stage of labor, 461
    measurement of, 417
    terminology used in, 455
fetal dysanthropometry, 61, 65
fetal growth,
    abdominal circumference to femur length ratios, 62
    biparietal diameter to femur length ratios, 62, 247
    cerebellar diameter, 64
    fetal weight to femur length cubed ratios, 63
    head circumference to abdominal circumference ratios, 63
    placental weight, 66
    subcutaneous adipose tissue, 66

fetal growth curves, 61
fetal heart examination, detailed description of, 149
fetal heart rate,
    antepartum computerized cardiotocography for
        investigation of, 393–9
    beat-to-beat variability, 460
    bradycardia, 458
    cerebral palsy incidence and, 379, 381
    consensus on patterns indicating need for
        Cesarean delivery, 463
    correlation with fetal movement, 419
    in diabetic patients, 544
    in trisomies 13, 18, 19 and 21, 235
    late and severe variable decelerations, 459
    management of intrapartum abnormalities, 463
        algorithm for, 465
    nuchal translucency and, 235
    patterns considered ominous, 458
    patterns of and fetal distress, 455
    reduction of perinatal mortality by, 379
    sinusoidal pattern, 459
    variations with gestational age, 395
fetal hiccupping, augmented actocardiography of, 420
fetal hydrops, in red blood cell alloimmunization, 428
fetal malformations, suitable for prenatal surgical
    correction, 258
fetal monitoring,
    cerebral palsy incidence and, 379, 381
    consensus on heart rate patterns indicating need
        for Cesarean delivery, 463
    electronic, 455, 458–60
    in prolongation of pregnancy, 564
    increased Cesarean rate with, 462
    Laennec and, 455
    long-term experience with, 379–83
    method of, 380
    randomized controlled trials, 461
    reduction of perinatal mortality by, 379
fetal mortality in pregestational diabetes, 542
fetal movement,
    actocardiographic measurement of, 415
    correlation with fetal heart rate, 419
    hiccupping, 416
fetal scalp pH determination, 460
fetal scalp stimulation, 461
fetal stem cell transplantation, 265
fetal structural anomalies, links to aneuploidy, 243
fetal surgery, see under surgery
fetal surveillance in diabetic mothers, 543
fetal weight estimation formulas, 60
fetal weight for gestational age data, 52
fetal weight to femur length cubed ratios, 63
fetal well-being,
    assessments for,
        biophysical profile, 573
        Doppler blood flow study, 574
        non-stress test, 572
    fetal scalp pH determination, 460
    fetal scalp stimulation, 461
    intrapartum tests of, 460
    measures of in diabetic mothers, 544

vibroacoustic stimulation, 460
fetoscopy,
    cf. open fetal surgery, 262
    fetal cardiac catheterization by, 308
fetus,
    environmental risk factors, 388
    recognition of risks to, 385
fibronectin (fetal), biochemical markers for preterm
    delivery, 557
fissures, neuroscanning of, 165
foramen ovale, premature closure of, 305
four-chamber view of fetal heart, 138
    role in prenatal diagnosis, 149
    sensitivity in detecting defects, 153
funiculocentesis, color Doppler and, 39
funipuncture, 514

gain-assisted densitometric evaluation of sonograms, 97
gastrointestinal malformations, and abnormal
    karyotype, 220
gastroschisis,
    and abnormal karyotype, 221
    color Doppler in diagnosis of, 40
gestational age, determination of, 571
gyri, neuroscanning of, 165

head circumference to abdominal circumference
    ratios, 63
HELLP (hemolysis, elevated liver enzymes and low
    platelet count) syndrome,
    clinical experience with, 564
    definition, 563
    fetal hypoxia in, 387
    future management of, 568
    maternal and fetal outcome after, 565
    maternal hemodynamics in, 564
    screening after and prevention, 566
hemangioma,
    color Doppler in diagnosis of, 40
    hepatic, 289
hematoma,
    marginal, 437, 438
    retroplacental, 434
    subchorionic,
        clinical outcome of pregnancies with, 34
        color Doppler studies of, 35
        first ultrasound studies of, 33
        mistaken for blighted twin, 36
        recognition by ultrasound 434
        use of color Doppler to predict abortion risk of,
            36
hemodynamics in HELLP syndrome, 564
hemoglobinopathies, molecular diagnosis of, 123
hemolysis, after red blood cell alloimmunization, 424
hemorrhage,
    intraventricular, 382
    ultrasound-induced, 14
herpes simplex viruses,
    clinical manifestations, 191
    diagnosis, 192
    epidemiology, 191

microbiology, 191
pathogenesis, 191
prevention, 192
prognosis, 192
therapy, 192
hexadactyly, three-dimensional ultrasound of, 82
holoprosencephaly,
    alobar, 354
        detection by neuroscanning, 176
    detection by neuroscanning, 174
    link with trisomy 13, 215
    semilobar, detection by neuroscanning, 176
horseshoe kidney in trisomy 18, 219
human immunodeficiency virus,
    clinical manifestations, 195
    diagnosis, 196
    epidemiology, 194
    microbiology, 194
    pathogenesis, 194
    prevention, 196
    prognosis, 196
    therapy, 196
hydrocephalus, detection by neuroscanning, 173
hydrocephaly,
    color Doppler in diagnosis of, 40
    links with abnormal karyotype, 215
hydronephrosis,
    and abnormal karyotype, 219
    bilateral,
        algorithm for management of, 265
        fetal surgery for, 265
hyperbilirubinemia, 545
hyperechogenic lung lesions, 287
hyperechogenicity, intestinal, predictive value of, 44
hyperglycemia,
    as a teratogen, 540
    role in dysmorphogenesis, 540
hypocalciuria, 472
hypochondroplasia, molecular diagnosis of, 121
hypoglycemia, 545
hypoxemia,
    Doppler flowmetry patterns in, 400
    prediction from Doppler flowmetry, 402
hypoxia,
    perinatal, 55
    sequence of events in fetus during, 531
hypoxia (fetal),
    aortic circulation and, 366
    case report, 371
    cerebral circulation and, 364
    cerebral circulation changes in, 373
    definition of, 359
    Doppler indices and, 359
    in early onset pre-eclampsia, 387
    in HELLP (hemolysis, elevated liver enzymes and low
        platelet count) syndrome, 387
    in progressive abruptio placentae, 387
    induction in lambs, 367–70
    renal circulation and, 366
    resistance indices in, 360–2
    umbilical circulation changes and, 363

venous circulation and, 367

indomethacin,
    •in twin–twin transfusion syndrome, 276
    use in fetal valvar obstruction, 300
infections,
    as a cause of amniorrhexis, 477
    as a cause of preterm delivery, 478
    congenital cerebral,
        adenovirus, 198
        congenital syphilis, 193
        cytomegalovirus, 185
        enteroviruses, 197
        equine encephalitis viruses, 198
        herpes simplex viruses, 191
        human immunodeficiency virus, 194
        Lyme disease, 198
        lymphocytic choriomeningitis virus, 198
        parvovirus, 198
        rubella, 190
        toxoplasmosis, 188
        Trypanosoma cruzi, 198
        varicella, 196
    cytomegalovirus, detection of fetal infection by
        neuroscanning, 177
    in placental abruptions, 438
    invasive prediction of intrauterine, 485
    link between intrauterine infection and labor, 479
    non-invasive prediction of intrauterine, 485
    role in intrauterine growth retardation, 529
    toxoplasmosis,
        chemotherapy for, 585
        detection of fetal infection by neuroscanning, 178
        epidemiology, 582
        fetal diagnosis, 584
        fetal infection, 581
        parasitology, 581
        primary prevention, 583
        screening dilemma, 586
        secondary prevention, 583
        vertical transmission, 581
insulin, treatment in early pregnancy of diabetic
    mothers, 540
interleukins, biochemical markers for preterm delivery,
    556
intracranial tumors,
    choroid plexus cysts, 286
    choroid plexus papilloma, 285
    teratoma diagnosis cf. arachnoid cyst, 285
    teratomas, 284
intrauterine growth retardation,
    cardiotocographic studies of, 397
    case report with fetal hypoxia, 371
    catch-up growth and, 50
    causes of, 49
    cf. small-for-gestational-age infants, 51
    clinical management when due to placental
        insufficiency, 535
    clinical screening for, 58
    congenital abnormality incidence in association with,
        50

definition, 49, 67, 527
diagnosis, 527
division into categories, 49
Doppler flow velocity waveform prediction trials, 407
early management of, 409
fetal causes, 529
fetal distress in, 532
fetal health monitoring, 530
fetal surveillance during, 534
follow-up evaluation of infants with, 50
identification of the causes, 528
incidence, 405, 527
infections and, 529
maternal causes of, 528
maternal risk factors for, 58
measurement of, 528
neonatal morbidity associated with, 52
neonatal outcome parameters, 53
placental causes, 529
prediction from Doppler flowmetry, 401
preterm delivery and, 55
therapy for, 533
ultrasonic diagnosis of, 59

ketoacidosis, 543
kidney,
    agenesis, color Doppler in diagnosis of, 40
    ectopic, color Doppler in diagnosis of, 40
Klippel–Trenaunay–Weber syndrome, 292

labor, link with intrauterine infection, 479
laparoscopy (fetal),
    development of, 327
    difficulty levels of, 327–9
    equipment, 331
    instrumentation, 333
    principles of, 329
    techniques,
        extracorporeal knotting, 340
        intracorporeal knotting, 337
        suturing, 335
    training approach, 334
large-for-gestational-age infants,
    labor and delivery complications of, 58
    perinatal problems of, 57
law,
    limitations of and ethics, 7
    malpractice, 7
'lemon sign' in spinal dysraphism, 172
light, fetal response to, 420
liver tumors, hemangiomas (small and large), 289
Lyme disease, congenital cerebral infection with, 198
lymphocytic choriomeningitis virus, congenital
    cerebral infection with, 198

macrosomia, 541
malpractice laws, 7
maternal diabetic ketoacidosis, 543
maternal serum α-fetoprotein, biochemical marker for
    preterm delivery, 559

maternal serum biochemistry, nuchal translucency
    and, 236
meconium aspiration, 575
megacystis, contrast medium radiographic study of, 111
meningomyelocele, detection by neuroscanning, 173
mesoblastic nephroma, cf. neuroblastoma, 290
metabolic acidosis, 457
metalloproteinase, biochemical marker for preterm
    delivery, 559
Miller–Dieker syndrome, 215
miscarriage, see abortion (spontaneous)
molecular diagnosis,
    acquired disease, 129
    conditions that can be tested, 134
    congenital adrenal hyperplasia, 123
    congenital thrombocytopenic purpura, 130
    consequences of, 131
    craniosynostosis syndromes, 122
    cystic fibrosis, 125
    hemoglobinopathies, 123
    Huntington disease, 128
    in cases with abnormal signs on standard
        investigation, 121
    in cases with affected family member, 121
    in cases with ethnic links, 121
    muscular dystrophies, 126
    of compatible stem cells for transplantation, 130
    of diseases with manifestation after birth or in
        adulthood, 128
    paternity, 130
    rhesus isoimmune disease, 130
    risks of, 133
    skeletal dysplasias, 121
    sources of error in, 132
molecular genetics,
    advances in, 119
    fetal molecular medicine, 119
    see also molecular diagnosis
mosaicism, prediction of by color Doppler, 44
multifetal pregnancy reduction, 513
multiple pregnancy,
    multifetal pregnancy reduction in, 513
    nuchal translucency in, 238
    see also twins
muscular dystrophy,
    Becker, molecular diagnosis of, 126
    Duchenne, molecular diagnosis of, 126
myasthenia gravis,
    acetylcholine receptor antibodies in offspring, 594
    breast feeding in, 593
    classification, 590
    clinical features, 589
    diagnosis, 589
    epidemiology, 590
    fetal, 591
    history of, 589
    labor and delivery in, 592
    monitoring of, 596
    neonatal, 593
        management of, 596
    pregnancy and, 591

puerperium, 593
treatment, 597
myelomeningocele,
    fetal surgery for, 266
    three-dimensional ultrasound of, 81

neonatal sepsis, and amniorrhexis, 482
neural tube defects,
    detection by neuroscanning, 170
    links with abnormal karyotype, 216
neuroblastoma, 288
    cf. mesoblastic nephroma, 290
    differential diagnosis from intracranial teratoma, 285
    differential diagnosis from sacrococcygeal teratoma,
        282
neuroscanning,
    anomalies of fetal brain,
        choroid plexus cysts, 169
        cytomegalovirus, 177
        holoprosencephaly, 175
        hydrocephalus, 173
        neural tube defects,
            anencephaly, 170
            cephalocele, 171
            spinal dysraphism, 172
        toxoplasmosis, 177
        ventriculomegaly, 173
    blood vessels of fetal brain, 168
    corpus callosum, 163
    gyri, sulci and fissures, 165
    normal prenatal brain anatomy,
        first trimester, 160
        second trimester, 161
    posterior fossa, 165
    scanning technique, 160
        in second trimester, 162
    subarachnoid spaces and cisterns, 164
    ultrasound equipment for, 159
    ventricular system, 163
nitroglycerin, use after open fetal surgery, 258
non-stress test, 572
nuchal cystic hygromas, 229
nuchal edema, 230
nuchal fluid, abnormal, 229
nuchal fold thickness, trisomy 21 detection from, 248
nuchal translucency,
    assessment of thickness of, 230
        increase with maternal age, 231
        measurement, 230
        repeatability, 231
    fetal heart rate and, 235
    in multiple pregnancies, 238
    increased and lethality of trisomy 21, 237
    increased in chromosomally normal fetuses, 239
    links with chromosomal defects, 231
    maternal serum biochemistry and, 236
    pathological findings in trisomic fetuses with, 236
    predictive value of, 44
    screening in high-risk populations, 232
    screening in unselected populations, 233–5
    use in screening for chromosomal defects, 229

oligohydramnios, color Doppler use in, 40
omphalocele,
    and abnormal karyotype, 221
    three-dimensional ultrasound of, 82
ossification centers,
    radiographic analysis of, 106, 107
osteochondrodysplasia, three-dimensional ultrasound
    of, 83
ovarian cysts, 290, 291

palate fissure, color Doppler in diagnosis of, 40
parvovirus B19, congenital cerebral infection with, 198
periventricular leukomalacia, 382
phospholipase A$_2$, biochemical marker for preterm
    delivery, 558
placenta,
    abruption of, 433–43
    abruption of and fetal hypoxia and anemia, 387
    contrast medium radiographic study of, 114
    see also abruptio placentae
placental insufficiency, intrauterine growth retardation
    management, 535
placental weight, 66
pleural effusions,
    chromosomal anomalies and, 317
    conservative management, 318
        intrapartum thoracocentesis, 318
    effect on lung development, 317
    incidence of, 317
    pleuroamniotic shunting, 319
pleuroamniotic shunting, 319
    infant follow-up after, 324
    maternal morbidity after, 324
    pregnancy outcome after, 320
    technique of, 319
    value in diagnosis, 325
polycythemia, 545
ponderal index, 51
post-term pregnancy,
    definition, 571
    etiology, 571
    fetal well-being assessment,
        biophysical profile, 573
        Doppler blood flow study, 574
        non-stress test, 572
    gestational age determination in, 571
    intrapartum management,
        meconium aspiration, 575
        perinatal hypoxia, 575
        shoulder dystocia, 576
    prenatal management, 574
posterior fossa, neuroscanning of, 165
pre-eclampsia,
    clinical experience, 564
    definition, 563
    Doppler flow velocity waveform prediction trials, 407
    early management of, 409
    early onset, associated disorders, 566
    fetal hypoxia in, 387
    future management of, 568
    incidence, 405

low-dose aspirin treatment for, 409
maternal hemodynamics in, 564
outcomes, 565
pathophysiology of, 471
postpartum screening and prevention, 566
prediction by Doppler, 405
prediction using blood pressure monitoring, 502
pregnancy reduction, 513
pregnancy-induced hypertension,
blood pressure monitoring in, 497
calcium metabolism and, 471
calcium supplementation,
in high-risk patients, 473
in low-risk patients, 474
optimal dose, 475
side-effects, 475
cardiotocographic studies of, 397
pathophysiology of, 471
premature closure,
of ductus arteriosus, 306
of foramen ovale, 305
prenatal diagnosis,
amniocentesis, 514
in first trimester, 512
in second trimester, 514
molecular genetics in, 119
see also molecular diagnosis
preterm delivery,
biochemical markers for, 555
elastase, 558
estriol, 559
fetal fibronectin, 557
interleukins, 556
maternal serum α-fetoprotein, 559
metalloproteinase, 559
phospholipase A$_2$, 558
prolactin, 559
protease, 558
tumor necrosis factors, 556
in twins, 518
infection as a cause of, 478
interval from amniorrhexis to, 478
intrauterine growth retardation and, 55
preterm labor, in pregestational diabetes, 543
prolactin, biochemical marker for preterm delivery,
559
prostaglandin E, placental abruption and, 437
protease, biochemical marker for preterm delivery, 558
pseudosinusoidal fetal heart rate pattern,
actocardiographic detection of, 417
pulmonary development, effect of pleural effusions
on, 317
pulmonary hypoplasia, risk of and gestational age at
amniorrhexis, 481
pulmonary sequestration, color Doppler in diagnosis
of, 40
pyelectasis, predictive value of, 44

radiography,
contrast medium studies,
acrania, 113
arterio- and venograms, 112
cavities and cysts, 112
central nervous system, 109
gastrointestinal tract, 110
megacystis by obstructed urethra, 111
placenta, 114
subarachnoid cysts, 110
trisomy 18, 110, 111
urogenital tract, 111
diagnosis of fetal disease in, 103
methods used, 104
skeletal analysis by,
anthropometric analysis, 106
general characteristics, 105
ossification centers, 106
thanatophoric dysplasia, 105
soft tissue analysis by,
constriction rings, 104
gas accumulation in infection, 104
maceration, 104, 105
subdermic edema, 104, 113
RADIUS (Routine Antenatal Diagnostic Imaging with
Ultrasound) study, 206
red blood cell alloimmunization,
clinical experience with, 424
fetal adaptation to, 423
fetal anemia and, 386
future management of, 430
hemolysis after, 424
incidence, 423
liver length, 425
management, 426
non-invasive diagnostic tests for, 424
spleen perimeter, 426
renal agenesis, color Doppler in diagnosis of, 40
renal anomalies in pregestational diabetes, 540
renal circulation, role in fetal hypoxia, 366
renal cortical cysts (microscopic) and trisomy 13, 219
renal hypoplasia in triploidy, 219
renal tumors, mesoblastic nephroma, 290
respiratory distress syndrome, surfactant therapy for,
603–14
respiratory system malformations, and abnormal
karyotypes, 223
respiratory distress syndrome in diabetes, 545
rhabdomyoma of heart, 288
rhesus isoimmune disease, molecular diagnosis of, 130
rubella,
diagnosis, 190
epidemiology, 190
microbiology, 190
pathogenesis, 190
prevention, 191
prognosis, 190
therapy, 191

sacral agenesis, 540
sacrococcygeal teratoma,
algorithm for management of, 264
associated anomalies, 282
delivery techniques, 283

differential diagnosis of, 282
fetal surgery for, 262, 283
prognosis, 283
staging of, 281
ultrasonic diagnosis of, 282
safety of routine ultrasound examination, 13, 203
scoliosis, three-dimensional ultrasound of, 83
selective fetocide, in twin–twin transfusion syndrome, 276
selective termination, 515
semilunar valvar obstruction,
fetal balloon valvuloplasty, 300
fetal cardiac intervention, treatment rationale, 298
history of, 299
medical therapy, 300
pathophysiology, 299
sex chromosome abnormalities, prediction of by color Doppler, 44
shoulder dystocia, 576
sinusoidal pattern of fetal heart rate, 459
skeletal dysplasias, molecular diagnosis of, 121
skeletal malformations and abnormal karyotypes, 223
skin tumors, 292
small-for-gestational-age infants,
cf. intrauterine growth retardation, 51
preterm delivery and, 55, 56
ultrasonic diagnosis of, 59
sound, fetal response to, 419
spina bifida,
detection by neuroscanning, 173
links with abnormal karyotype, 216
three-dimensional ultrasound of, 81
spinal dysraphism, detection by neuroscanning, 172
steroid therapy, after amniorrhexis, 489
Sturge–Weber syndrome, 292
subarachnoid cysts, contrast medium radiographic study of, 110
subarachnoid spaces and cisterns, neuroscanning of, 164
sulci, neuroscanning of, 165
surfactants,
administration, 609
clinical response to, 604
cohort study, 609–13
outcome, 612
prophylactic treatment, 605
rescue cf. prophylaxis, 606
rescue treatment, 604
response to, 610
single-dose cf. multiple dose, 608
tolerance, 613
types in clinical use, 603
use in respiratory distress syndrome, 603–14
surgery,
bilateral hydronephrosis, 265
cardiac anomalies, 267
congenital diaphragmatic hernia, 260
craniofacial anomalies, 266
effect on future pregnancies, 258
fetal malformations that could be treated in this way, 258
fetal stem cell transplantation, 265

future of, 267
healing after in fetus, 266
laparoscopic,
development of, 327
difficulty levels of, 327–9
instrumentation, 331
knotting, 337–41
principles of, 329
suturing, 335–41
technique, 335
training approaches, 334
management of mother and fetus, 258
maternal complications after, 257
myelomeningocele, 266
open surgery cf. fetoscopy, 262
pleuroamniotic shunting, 319–25
risks and benefits of, 257
sacrococcygeal teratoma, 262, 283
see also cardiac intervention
twin–twin transfusion syndrome, 266
urethral obstruction, 264
syphilis (congenital),
clinical manifestations, 193
diagnosis, 193
epidemiology, 193
microbiology, 193
pathogenesis, 193
prevention, 194
prognosis, 194
therapy, 194

temperature,
bioeffects, 16
indices for safe ultrasound, 15
raised by ultrasound,
negative effects on fetus,
animal studies, 14
human studies, 13
safe changes, 13
teratoma, sacrococcygeal, color Doppler in diagnosis of, 41
terbutaline, use after open fetal surgery, 258
tetralogy of Fallot, 306
thanatophoric dysplasia,
molecular diagnosis of, 121
radiographic analysis of, 105
three-dimensional ultrasound of, 80
thoracocentesis, intrapartum, 318
three-dimensional ultrasound,
advantages of in prenatal diagnosis, 83
arthrogryposis multiplex congenita, 81
cleft lip and palate, 80
clubfoot, 82
examination technique, 76
future of, 86
hexadactyly, 82
methods of, 75
myelomeningocele, 81
normal fetal face, 79
normal left ear, 79
normal left upper arm, 80

normal male genitalia, 80
omphalocele, 82
orthogonal image display, 76
osteochondrodysplasia, 83
problems with, 85
scoliosis, 83
spina bifida, 81
surface view, 77
thanatophoric dysplasia, 80
transparent and X-ray views, 79
trisomy 13, 80
trisomy 18, 78, 80, 81
volume data acquisition, 76
volume data storage, 81
tissue echogenicity,
   densitometry in assessment of, 95
   impediments to assessment of, 89, 89–95
   qualitative assessment of, 95
   quantitative assessment of, 95
tocolytic therapy, after amniorrhexis, 489
toxoplasmosis,
   chemotherapy for, 585
   clinical manifestations, 189
   detection of fetal infection by neuroscanning, 178
   diagnosis, 189
   epidemiology, 188, 582
   fetal diagnosis, 584
   fetal infection, 581
   microbiology, 188
   parasitology, 581
   pathogenesis, 188
   prevention, 189
      primary, 583
      secondary, 583
   prognosis, 189
   screening for, 586
   therapy, 189
   vertical transmission, 581
transducer, role in tissue echogenicity, 91
transient cardiomyopathy, 545
triploidy,
   prediction of by color Doppler, 44
   renal hypoplasia in, 219
trisomy 13,
   and holoprosencephaly, 215
   congenital heart malformations in, 217
   fetal heart rate in, 235
   prediction of by color Doppler, 44
   renal cortical cysts (microscopic) in, 219
   skeletal malformations in, 223
   three-dimensional ultrasound of, 80
trisomy 18,
   congenital heart malformations in, 217
   contrast medium radiographic study of, 110, 111
   fetal heart rate in, 235
   horseshoe kidney in, 219
   prediction of by color Doppler, 44
   skeletal malformations in, 223
   three-dimensional ultrasound of, 78, 80, 81
trisomy 19, fetal heart rate in, 235
trisomy 21,

congenital heart malformations in, 217
fetal heart rate in, 235
lethality and nuchal translucency increase, 237
pleural effusions in, 317
prediction of by color Doppler, 44
prenatal diagnosis in the past, 243
risk adjustment using ultrasound examination, 248
risk evaluation with color Doppler, 45, 46
skeletal malformations in, 223
three-dimensional ultrasound of, 78
ultrasound markers for, 248
Trypanosoma cruzi, congenital cerebral infection with, 198
tumor necrosis factors, biochemical markers for preterm delivery, 556
tumors, *see under* specific tumor
tumors of the neck, 283–4
twin–twin transfusion syndrome, 515–17
   diagnosis, 272
   fetal surgery for, 266
   management,
      endoscopic laser coagulation of communicating placental vessels, 273
      expectant, 275
      laser coagulation cf. amniodrainage, 277
      medical therapy with indomethacin, 276
      selective fetocide, 276
      serial amniodrainage, 276
   pathophysiology of, 271
   treatment options, 516
twins,
   acardiac, color Doppler in diagnosis of, 41
   algorithm for intrapartum management, 519
   benefits of use of ultrasound in, 510
   blighted, 349
   blighted cf. subchorionic hematoma, 36
   chorionicity, 510
   congenital anomalies in, 511
   diagnosis of, 509
   early fetal demise, 510
   early fetal growth, 511
   epidemiology, 507
   growth discordance, 511
   growth in third trimester, 517
   incidence of live births after diagnosis of, 511
   increased incidence with use of assisted reproductive technologies, 507
   maternal age and incidence, 508
   pathogenesis of twinning process, 508
   prenatal diagnosis, in second trimester, 514
   prenatal diagnosis of congenital anomalies in first trimester, 512
   preterm delivery in, 518
   radiographic view of growth retarded, 108
   selective termination in, 515
   timing of delivery, 519

ultrasound,
   B-mode imaging, thermal effects of, 13
   benefits of its use in twin gestations, 510
   bioeffects induced by, 18

cardiac malformations, 140
cavitation-induced bioeffects and, 17
clinical trials of, 204
color Doppler,
 in prenatal diagnosis,
  for chromosomal defects, 42
  for congenital cardiopathies, 41
  for malformations, 39
  with invasive techniques, 39
diagnosis of twin–twin transfusion syndrome by, 272
Doppler,
 cerebroplacental ratio, hypoxia and outcome, 362
 thermal effects of, 13
  spectral vs. color, 18
Doppler flowmetry, 399
early pregnancy visualization, 347
evaluation of fetal anatomy and malformations with, 75
fetal growth estimation by, 61–7
fetal transesophageal echocardiography, 309
fetal weight curves by, 57
four-chamber view of fetal heart, 138
hemorrhage induced by, 14
in late first trimester, 137
indications for use, 52
intrauterine growth retardation diagnosis by, 59
markers for trisomy 21, 248
maximum allowable intensities, 16
mechanical indices for, 15
neuroscanning, 159
normal cardiac anatomy, 138
normal fetal heart examination, 149
of subchorionic hematomas, 33
prediction of early pregnancy loss by, 345
risk adjustment for trisomy 21 using, 248
routine examination with,
 clinical trials of, 204
 cost of, 210
 detection of anomalies by, 203
 ethics of, 208
 RADIUS study, 206
 safety, 203
safety of, 13–18
see also neuroscanning
small-for-gestational-age infant diagnosis by, 59
thermal effects of, 13
 animal studies, 14
 human studies, 13
thermal indices for, 15
three-dimensional, 75–86
tissue echogenicity, 89–100
transducer heating, 13
use in early pregnancy, 355
use in gestational age estimation, 571
yolk sac studies with,
 abnormal pregnancy, 25
 normal pregnancy, 25
umbilical arteries, single, as a sign of chromosomal defects, 42
umbilical artery,

Doppler velocity waveforms of in abruptio placentae, 448
end-diastolic blood flow increases in abruptio placentae, 449
umbilical circulation, increased resistance in, 43
umbilical circulation changes in fetal hypoxia, 363
umbilical cord,
 pseudocysts of, 43
 shortening of, 43
umbilical resistance indices, in fetal hypoxia, 360–2
umbilical vein, anomalous position of and hepatic malformations, 40
urethral obstruction,
 consequences of, 264
 radiograph of megacystis caused by, 111
urinary tract malformations,
 and abnormal karyotype, 220
 horseshoe kidney and trisomy 18, 219
 hydronephrosis, and abnormal karyotype, 219
 microscopic renal cortical cysts and trisomy 13, 219
 renal hypoplasia, and triploidy, 219
urinary tract obstruction, fetal surgery for, 263
uterine activity, monitoring of after amniorrhexis, 486
uterine artery,
 flow velocity waveform in hypertensive pregnancies, 406
 flow velocity waveform in normal pregnancies, 406

valvar obstruction, 299
varicella,
 congenital, 196
 diagnosis, 197
 perinatal, 196
 prevention, 197
 prognosis, 197
 therapy, 197
venous circulation, role in fetal hypoxia, 367
ventricular system, neuroscanning of, 163
ventriculomegaly,
 borderline, 224
 detection by neuroscanning, 173
 links with abnormal karyotype, 215
viability, definition of, 3
vibroacoustic stimulation, 460
vitelline stalk, color Doppler studies of, 27
von Hippel–Lindau syndrome, 292

Wilms' tumor, 290
World Federation for Ultrasound in Medicine and Biology (WFUMB), 13

X-rays, see radiography
xeroradiography, description of, 103

yolk sac,
 calcification of, 25, 26
 color Doppler studies of, 27
 development of human, 21
 double, 26
 fibrosis of, 25
 function of human, 21

hypoplastic, 24
mean gestational sac diameter, 26
morphological classification of secondary, 24
necrosis of, 25
pathological examination and abortion
    classification, 23

ultrasound of in abnormal pregnancy, 25
ultrasound of in normal pregnancy, 25
ultrasound studies of, 25
ultrasound visualization of, 347
vascularization of in abnormal pregnancy, 28